To my twin sons, Leonard and Patrick, and singletons, Andrew and Michael.

Contents

Section IV. Diseases and Disorders

Contributors

Irfan Ahmad, MD
Clinical Assistant Professor of Pediatrics
School of Medicine
University of California, Irvine
and
Pediatric Subspecialty Faculty
Children's Hospital of Orange County
Orange, California
Necrotizing Enterocolitis and Spontaneous Intestinal Perforation

Marilee C. Allen, MD
Professor of Pediatrics
The Johns Hopkins University School of Medicine
Co-Director of the NICU Developmental Clinic, Kennedy-Kreiger Institute
Baltimore, Maryland
Follow-up of High-Risk Infants, Counseling Parents Before High-Risk Delivery

Gad Alpan, MD, MBA
Professor of Clinical Pediatrics
New York Medical College
Maria Fareri Children's Hospital
Westchester Medical Center
Valhalla, New York
Patent Ductus Arteriosus, Persistent Pulmonary Hypertension of the Newborn, Infant of a Drug-Abusing Mother

April L. Anderson, PharmD
Neonatal Clinical Pharmacist
Winnie Palmer Hospital for Women and Babies
Orlando, Florida
Commonly Used Medications

Hubert O. Ballard, MD
Assistant Professor of Pediatrics
Division of Neonatology
Department of Pediatrics
University of Kentucky College of Medicine
Lexington, Kentucky
Apnea and Periodic Breathing

Fayez M. Bany-Mohammed, MD, FAAP
Associate Clinical Professor
Division of Neonatology
Department of Pediatrics
University of California at Irvine
UCI Medical Center
Orange, California
Chlamydial Infection, Gonorrhea, Hepatitis, Human Immunodeficiency Virus (HIV), Meningitis, Methicillin-Resistant Staphylococcal Aureus (MRSA) Infections, Parvovirus B19 Infection, Respiratory Syncytial Virus (RSV), Sepsis, Syphilis, TORCH Infections, Ureaplasma Urealyticum Infection, Varicella-Zoster Infections

Julia S. Barthold, MD
Associate Chief, Division of Urology
A.I. duPont Hospital for Children
Wilmington, Delaware
and
Associate Professor, Urology and Pediatrics
Jefferson Medical College of Thomas Jefferson University
Philadelphia, Pennsylvania
Surgical Diseases of the Newborn: Urologic Disorders

Jason K. Baxter, MD, MSCP
Assistant Professor
Director, Division of Research
Department of Obstetrics and Gynecology
Thomas Jefferson University
Philadelphia, Pennsylvania
Antepartum and Intrapartum Fetal Assessment

Daniel Beals, MD
Associate Clinical Professor
University of Cincinnati
Department of General and Thoracic Surgery
Cincinnati Children's Hospital Medical Center
Cincinnati, Ohio
Neonatal Bioethics

Dhilip R. Bhatt, MD
Neonatologist
Kaiser Permanente
Claremont, California
Isolation Guidelines

Michael B. Bober, MD, PhD
Assistant Professor
Department of Pediatrics
Thomas Jefferson University
Philadelphia, Pennsylvania
and
Co-Director, Skeletal Dysplasia Program
Nemours Children's Clinic
Division of Medical Genetics
Wilmington, Delaware
Common Multiple Congenital Anomaly
  Syndromes

Maria Teresa Canola, RN,
  MSN/MPH, CIC
Infection Control Practitioner
Department Administrator Infection Control
Kaiser Permanente Hospital
Fontana, California
Isolation Guidelines

Daniel Canter, MD
Instructor, Urology
University of Pennsylvania
Philadelphia, Pennsylvania
Hematuria, Renal Failure (Acute), Urinary
  Tract Infection

Gary E. Carnahan, MD, PhD
Director of Transfusion Medicine
Assistant Professor
Department of Pathology
College of Medicine
University of South Alabama
University of South Alabama Children's and
  Women's Hospital
Mobile, Alabama
Blood Component Therapy

Pasquale Casale, MD
Assistant Professor
Department of Urology
University of Pennsylvania
Children's Hospital of Pennsylvania
Philadelphia, Pennsylvania
Hematuria, Renal Failure (Acute), Urinary
  Tract Infection

Kara Cole, PA-C
Physician Assistant
Division of Pediatric Surgery
University of Kentucky Children's Hospital
Lexington, Kentucky
Surgical Diseases of the Newborn: Abdominal
  Masses, Abdominal Wall Defects,
  Alimentary Tract Obstruction, Diseases of
  the Airway, Tracheobronchial Tree and
  Lungs, Retroperitoneal Tumors

Carol M. Cottrill, MD, FAAP, FACC
Professor of Pediatrics
Department of Pediatrics
University of Kentucky
Lexington, Kentucky
Defibrillation and Cardioversion, Arrhythmia,
  Congenital Heart Disease

M. Douglas Cunningham, MD
Clinical Professor of Pediatrics
School of Medicine
University of California, Irvine
and
Consulting Neonatologist
University of California Medical Center
Orange, California
Body Water, Fluid, and Electrolytes, Exchange
  Transfusion, Calcium Disorders
  (Hypocalcemia, Hypercalcemia),
  Enteroviruses and Parechoviruses,
  Hydrocephalus and Ventriculomegaly,
  Intracranial Hemorrhages, Lyme Disease
  and Pregnancy, Magnesium Disorders
  (Hypomagnesemia, Hypermagnesemia),
  Aerosol Therapy in Neonates, Emergency
  Medications and Therapy for Neonates

Lauren Davey, PA-C, MMS, MSPH
Physician Assistant
Department of Pediatric Genetics
Alfred I. duPont Hospital for Children
Wilmington, Delaware
Common Multiple Congenital Anomaly
  Syndromes

Nirmala S. Desai, MBBS
Professor of Pediatrics
Division of Neonatology
Department of Pediatrics
University of Kentucky Medical Center
Lexington, Kentucky
*Newborn Screening, Nutritional Management,
Management of the Extremely Low
Birthweight Infant During the First Week
of Life, Intrauterine Growth Restriction
(Small for Gestational Age), Osteopenia
of Prematurity*

Kevin Dysart, MD
Assistant Professor of Pediatrics
Thomas Jefferson University
Philadelphia, Pennsylvania
Nemours Children's Clinics
Philadelphia, Pennsylvania, and Wilmington,
Delaware
Infant of a Diabetic Mother

Fabien G. Eyal, MD
Professor of Pediatrics
Chief and Louise Lenoir Locke Professor of
Neonatology
Medical Director, Intensive Care Nurseries
University of South Alabama Children's and
Women's Hospital
Mobile, Alabama
*Blood Component Therapy, Temperature
Regulation, Sedation and Analgesia in a
Neonate, ABO Incompatibility, Anemia,
Bronchopulmonary Dysplasia, Meconium
Aspiration, Rh Incompatibility,
Thrombocytopenia and Platelet Dysfunction*

Catherine A Finnegan, MS, CRNP
Neonatal Nurse Practitioner
Department of Neonatology
Johns Hopkins Bayview Medical Center
Baltimore, Maryland
*Venous Access: Percutaneous Central Venous
Catheterization*

Tricia Lacy Gomella, MD
Part-Time Assistant Professor of Pediatrics
Department of Pediatrics
The Johns Hopkins University School of
Medicine
Baltimore, Maryland
*Assessment of Gestational Age, Newborn
Physical Examination, Section II: Procedures,
Section III: On-Call Problems, Transient
Tachypnea of the Newborn*

Janet E. Graeber, MD
Associate Professor of Pediatrics
Chief, Section of Neonatology
Department of Pediatrics
West Virginia University School of Medicine
Robert C. Byrd Health Science Center
Morgantown, West Virginia
*Eye Disorders of the Newborn and
Retinopathy of Prematurity*

Deborah L. Grider, RNC
Neonatal Intensive Care Unit Research Nurse
Coordinator
Division of Neonatology
Department of Pediatrics
University of Kentucky
Lexington, Kentucky
*Management of the Extremely Low Birth-
weight Infant During the First Week of Life*

George W. Gross, MD
Professor of Radiology
Director, Division of Pediatric Radiology
Department of Diagnostic Radiology
University of Maryland Medical System
Baltimore, Maryland
Neonatal Radiology

Wayne E. Hachey, DO, MPH
Director, Preventive Medicine
Office of the Assistant Secretary of Defense
(Health Affairs)
Department of Defense
Pentagon, Virginia
Meconium Aspiration

Charles R. Hamm Jr., MD
Professor and Vice Chair of Pediatrics
University of South Alabama College of Medicine
Mobile, Alabama
Respiratory Management

Pui Man (Julia) Ho, PharmD
Pharmacy Clinical Specialist
Department of Pharmacy
Children's Hospital of The King's Daughters
Norfolk, Virginia
Commonly Used Medications

Pip M. Huang-Hidestrand, MD
Resident Physician, Pediatrics
Children's Hospital of Wisconsin
Milwaukee, Wisconsin
Defibrillation and Cardioversion

H. Jane Huffnagle, DO, FAOCA
Associate Professor of Anesthesiology
Thomas Jefferson University
Philadelphia, Pennsylvania
and
Director of Obstetric Anesthesia
Thomas Jefferson University Hospital
Philadelphia, Pennsylvania
Obstetric Anesthesia and the Neonate

Virginia Hustead, MD
Medical Director of ECMO Services
Department of Neonatology
Children's Hospital of Minnesota
Minneapolis, Minnesota
*Extracorporeal Membrane Oxygenation of
the Newborn*

Joseph A. Iocono, MD
Assistant Professor of Surgery and Pediatrics
University of Kentucky
Lexington, Kentucky
and
Director, Pediatric Trauma Program
Associate Director, Minimally Invasive
Surgery Center
Kentucky Children's Hospital
Lexington, Kentucky
*Surgical Diseases of the Newborn: Abdominal
Masses, Abdominal Wall Defects,
Alimentary Tract Obstruction, Diseases of
the Airway, Tracheobronchial Tree and
Lungs, Retroperitoneal Tumors*

Jamieson E. Jones, MD
Attending Neonatologist
Palomar-Pomorado Health Systems and Rady
Children's Hospital of San Diego
and
Clinical Instructor, Pediatrics
University of California
San Diego, California
*Complementary and Alternative Medical
Therapies in Neonatology*

Robert J. Kuhn, PharmD
Professor
Department of Pharmacy Practice and Science
University of Kentucky College of Pharmacy
Lexington, Kentucky
Commonly Used Medications

Christoph U. Lehmann, MD
Associate Professor
Department of Pediatrics
Johns Hopkins University
Baltimore, Maryland
Studies for Neurologic Evaluation

William G. MacKenzie, MD, FRCS(C)
Chairman, Department of Orthopedic Surgery
A.I. duPont Hospital for Children
Wilmington, Delaware
and
Assistant Professor
Department of Orthopaedic Surgery
Jefferson Medical College
Thomas Jefferson University
Philadelphia, Pennsylvania
Orthopedic and Musculoskeletal Problems

Barbara McKinney, PharmD
Neonatal Clinical Pharmacist
Department of Pharmacy
Christiana Hospital
Newark, Delaware
*Aerosol Therapy in Neonates, Emergency
Medications and Therapy for Neonates,
Commonly Used Medications*

Ambadas Pathak, MD
Assistant Professor Emeritus
Department of Pediatrics
The Johns Hopkins University School
of Medicine
Baltimore, Maryland
and
Clinical Associate Professor of Pediatrics
University of Maryland School of Medicine
Baltimore, Maryland
Seizures in the Neonate

David A. Paul, MD
Attending Neonatologist
Christiana Care Health System
Newark, Delaware
and
duPont Hospital for Children
Wilmington, Delaware
and
Associate Professor of Pediatrics
Thomas Jefferson University
Philadelphia, Pennsylvania
Multiple Gestation

Kurlen S. E. Payton, MD
Postdoctoral Fellow
Department of Neonatology
The Johns Hopkins University Hospital
Baltimore, Maryland
Rash and Dermatologic Problems

Stephen A. Pearlman, MD
Clinical Professor of Pediatrics
Thomas Jefferson University
Fellowship Director, Neonatology
Jefferson Medical College and Christiana
    Care Health System
Director of Medical Education, Pediatrics
Christiana Care Health System/duPont
    Hospital for Children
Associate Director, Neonatology, Christiana
    Care Health System
Philadelphia, Pennsylvania
Management of the Late Preterm Infant

Keith J. Peevy, JD, MD
Professor of Pediatrics and Neonatal Medicine
Department of Pediatrics
University of South Alabama
Mobile, Alabama
Polycythemia and Hyperviscosity

Judith D. Polak, MSN, NNP-BC
Clinical Instructor
Department of Pediatrics
West Virginia University
Morgantown, West Virginia
*Eye Disorders of the Newborn and
    Retinopathy Prematurity*

Andrew R. Pulito, MD
Professor of Surgery and Pediatrics
University of Kentucky
Surgeon-in-Chief, Kentucky Children's Hospital
Lexington, Kentucky
*Surgical Diseases of the Newborn: Abdominal
    Masses, Abdominal Wall Defects,
    Alimentary Tract Obstruction, Diseases of
    the Airway, Tracheobronchial Tree and
    Lungs, Retroperitoneal Tumors*

Rakesh Rao, MD
Assistant Professor
Division of Newborn Medicine
Department of Pediatrics
Washington University in St. Louis
St. Louis, Missouri
*Nutritional Management, Intrauterine Growth
    Restriction (Small for Gestational Age),
    Osteopenia of Prematurity*

Tracey L. Robinson, RN
Research Nurse Coordinator
Department of Neonatology
Kentucky Children's Hospital
Lexington, Kentucky
*Management of the Extremely Low
    Birthweight Infant During the First
    Week of Life*

Sarah J. Rosen, MD
Clinical Instructor
Department of Obstetrics and Gynecology
Thomas Jefferson University
Philadelphia, Pennsylvania
Antepartum and Intrapartum Fetal Assessment

Jack Sills, MD
Medical Director, NICU
University of California, Irvine Medical Center
Clinical Professor
Department of Pediatrics
University of California, Irvine
Orange, California
Perinatal Asphyxia

Lizette C. Sistoza, MD, FAAP
Staff Neonatologist
Division of Neonatology
Department of Pediatrics
Arrowhead Regional Medical Center
Colton, California
Air Leak Syndromes

Kendra Smith, MD
Associate Professor
Division of Neonatology
Department of Pediatrics
University of Washington
Seattle, Washington
*Extracorporeal Membrane Oxygenation of
    the Newborn*

Ganesh Srinivasan, MD, DM
Assistant Professor
Department of Pediatrics and Child Health
    (Neonatology)
University of Manitoba
Winnipeg, Manitoba
Canada
Thyroid Disorders

Thomas P. Strandjord, MD
Associate Professor of Pediatrics
Department of Pediatrics
University of Washington
Seattle, Washington
Resuscitation of the Newborn

Theodora A. Stavroudis, MD
Assistant Professor of Pediatrics
USC Division of Neonatal Medicine
Children's Hospital Los Angeles and
    LAC+USC Medical Center
Keck School of Medicine
University of Southern California
Los Angeles, California
Studies for Neurologic Evaluation

Wendy J. Sturtz, MD
Attending Neonatologist
Department of Neonatology
Christiana Care Health System
Newark, Delaware
Infant Transport

Outi K. T. Tammela, MD
Docent in Neonatology
Head of Division of Neonatology
Department of Pediatrics
Pediatric Research Center
Tampere University Hospital
Tampere, Finland
*Hyaline Membrane Disease (Respiratory
    Distress Syndrome)*

Ahmed M. Thabet, MD
Pediatric Orthopedic Fellow
Department of Orthopedics
A.I. duPont Hospital for Children
Nemours Children Clinics
Wilmington, Delaware
and
Lecturer of Orthopedic Surgery
Orthopedic Surgery Department
Benha Medical School
Benha, Egypt
Orthopedic and Musculoskeletal Problems

Christiane Theda, MD, PhD, MBA
Assistant Professor
Johns Hopkins University
Baltimore, Maryland
and
Visiting Geneticist
Victoria Clinical Genetics Services
Neonatologist, Newborn Emergency Transfer
    Service
Melbourne, Victoria, Australia
*Disorders of Sex Development, Inborn Errors
    of Metabolism with Acute Neonatal Onset,
    Neural Tube Defects*

Deborah J. Tuttle, MD
Assistant Professor of Pediatrics
Jefferson Medical College of Thomas
    Jefferson University Hospital
Philadelphia, Pennsylvania
and
Attending Neonatologist
Christiana Care Health System
Wilmington, Delaware
Consulting Editor

Cherry Uy, MD, FAAP
Associate Clinical Professor
Division of Neonatology
Department of Pediatrics
University of California, Irvine
Orange, California
*Section IV: Diseases and Disorders:
    Hyperbilirubinemia, Direct (Conjugated
    Hyperbilirubinemia); Hyperbilirubinemia,
    Indirect (Unconjugated Hyperbilirubinemia)*

Louis Weinstein, MD
Paul A. and Eloise B. Bowers Professor and
    Chair
Department of Obstetrics and Gynecology
Thomas Jefferson University
Philadelphia, Pennsylvania
Antepartum and Intrapartum Fetal Assessment

Richard M. Whitehurst, Jr., MD
Associate Professor
Division of Neonatology
Department of Pediatrics
University of South Alabama
Mobile, Alabama
ABO Incompatibility, Rh Incompatibility

Regina Winner, ARNP, MSN
Director, NICU
Central Baptist Hospital
Lexington, Kentucky
Newborn Screening

Michael Zayek, MD
Associate Professor
Division of Neonatology
Department of Pediatrics
University of South Alabama
Mobile, Alabama
*Bronchopulmonary Dysplasia,
    Thrombocytopenia and Platelet Dysfunction*

Preface

I am pleased to present the sixth edition of *Neonatology*. Since the first edition was published in 1988, *Neonatology: Management, Procedures, On-Call Problems, Diseases, and Drugs* continues to be widely accepted both in the United States and internationally. To date, various editions of this book have been translated into eight languages: Polish, Portuguese, Russian, Spanish, Yugoslavian, Turkish, Greek, and Chinese (short form). This worldwide acceptance is only made possible because of the contributions of our outstanding group of associate editors and contributors.

The specialty of neonatology continues to advance and the sixth edition has been completely updated to reflect the changes in our dynamic field. We have kept our basic format in this edition but changed most sections to alphabetical listings to make it easier to locate a chapter quickly. Section I, "Basic Management," is not alphabetical but is organized in a logical way with "Antepartum and Intrapartum Fetal Assessment" and "Obstetric Anesthesia" in the beginning and "Follow-up of High-Risk Infants" and "Neonatal Bioethics" at the end.

Some very interesting chapters are new to this edition. Section I now includes "Newborn Screening," which includes a discussion of some of the 29 screening tests recommended by the American College of Medical Genetics. Other additions include "Blood Component Therapy," "Management of the Late Preterm Infant," a relatively new area that focuses on the unique problems of late preterm infants, and "Complementary and Alternative Medical Therapies in Neonatology." Many families and practitioners are now interested in the complementary and alternative topic, another relatively new area in neonatology. The chapter includes a discussion of topics such as aromatherapy and sound and music therapy. "Defibrillation and Cardioversion" was added to the Procedure section and reviews indications and techniques.

The very popular and practical Section III, "On-Call Problems," was thoroughly updated and has the new chapter "Rash and Dermatologic Problems." The "On-Call Problems" continue to be the most popular and most commonly used section in the book. In Section IV, "Diseases and Disorders," the following sections are new: "Enteroviruses and Parechoviruses," "Eye Disorders of the Newborn and Retinopathy of Prematurity," "Methicillin-Resistant *Staphylococcal Aureus* (MRSA) Infections," "Orthopedic and Musculoskeletal Problems," "Parvovirus B19," "*Ureaplasma Urealyticum* Infections," and the new "Urologic Disorders".

Experienced users of the book will take note of the extensive revision and additions to Section V, "Neonatal Pharmacology." The sixth edition now contains one of the most comprehensive lists of neonatal medications available in a manual. We have combined the two tables on effects of drugs and substances taken during pregnancy and the effects of drugs and substances on breast-feeding to one table to make it more user friendly. The appendix has many new abbreviations, an updated blood pressure table to include very low birthweight infants, new growth charts, and a very useful isolation guideline table.

We are fortunate to have contributors from all over the United States with a good representation of all geographic regions. Contributors from Egypt, Finland, Australia and Canada help further internationalize the book. It is important to have many different centers represented because there are many different methods of caring for infants. Where appropriate, we have tried to include several different approaches to the management of the neonate. We recognize that some areas of neonatology are generally accepted as standard of care, whereas others are more controversial. The areas of controversy are noted as such in the text. For areas that are more controversial, it is always best to follow your local institutional guidelines.

I would like to thank Drs. Doug Cunningham and Fabien Eyal, my valued associate editors; Dr. Deborah Tuttle, consulting editor; Dr. Barbara McKinney; and all contributors to this and previous editions of the book. I also express my appreciation to Dr. Anne Sydor, Alyssa Fried, Harriet Lebowitz and the entire editorial and production staff at McGraw-Hill and their colleagues abroad for their extensive assistance during the two year journey to complete this edition. A special thanks to my husband, Lenny, who helped me extensively concerning matters of editorial content, and my children, Leonard, Patrick, Andrew, and Michael, who helped troubleshoot computer issues and tolerated many sacrifices while I worked on the book.

Lastly, I would like to acknowledge the origins of this book. The idea of the manual was developed during my neonatal fellowship at the University of Kentucky. I had the unique opportunity to finish my fellowship at Johns Hopkins University where I completed the project and added a new group of authors and ideas.

Please visit our new web site www.neonatologybook.com for additional information on this book and for links to enhanced online content for images in this edition, indicated by the symbol [✪].

Any suggestions and comments about this manual are always welcome. Correspondence should be addressed to:

Tricia Lacy Gomella, MD
c/o McGraw-Hill Medical Publishers
Two Penn Plaza, 23th Floor
New York, NY 10121-2298
Or
editor@neonatologybook.com

Tricia Lacy Gomella, MD
June, 2009

1 Antepartum and Intrapartum Fetal Assessment

PRENATAL DIAGNOSIS

I. **First-trimester screening.** Maternal serum can be analyzed for certain biochemical markers that, in combination with ultrasound measurement of the fetal nuchal translucency (NT), can be used to calculate a risk assessment for trisomies 18 and 21. In the first trimester, these serum markers are the free β-human chorionic gonadotropin (hCG) and pregnancy-associated plasma protein A (PAPP-A). Free β-hCG is elevated and PAPP-A is decreased in a pregnancy affected by Down syndrome. First-trimester screening is an effective screening tool, with a detection rate of 82–87% for trisomy 21 with a 5% false-positive screen rate. First-trimester screening is performed between 10 4/7 and 13 6/7 weeks' gestation and requires confirmation of a chromosomal abnormality by an invasive genetic test. The results are available to the patient early enough that chorionic villus sampling (CVS) is an option for diagnostic testing.

II. **Second-trimester screening.** For patients who present after 13 6/7 weeks or choose not to undergo first-trimester screening, the quadruple screen test (Quad screen) is an option. The Quad screen yields a risk assessment for trisomies 18 and 21; unlike first-trimester screening, though, it also provides a risk assessment for open neural tube defects. It involves analyzing levels of maternal serum alpha fetoprotein (MSAFP), total hCG, unconjugated estriol, and inhibin A between 15 and 21 weeks' gestation. In a pregnancy affected by Down syndrome, both MSAFP and unconjugated estriol are low; hCG and inhibin A are elevated. The Quad screen has a detection rate of 81% for Down syndrome at a 5% false-positive screen rate. Like first-trimester screening, the Quad screen requires an invasive test to confirm the diagnosis of a chromosomal abnormality (ie, amniocentesis).

For those patients who chose to undergo first-trimester screening and/or a CVS, neural tube defect screening in the form of a second-trimester MSAFP level should be offered. This maternal serum analyte is elevated in the presence of an open neural tube defect. Evidence exists that focused ultrasound during the second trimester is an effective tool for detecting an open neural tube defect.

III. **Sequential, contingent sequential, and integrated screening.** These options involve a combination of first- and second-trimester screening. Specifically with the integrated screen, an ultrasound measurement of the fetal NT is performed between 10 4/7 and 13 6/7 weeks. In addition, maternal serum levels of PAPP-A are obtained in the first trimester and the Quad screen obtained in the second trimester. The results are reported when all the tests are complete. In sequential screening, NT, PAPP-A, and free β-hCG are measured in the first trimester followed by a Quad screen in the second trimester. The results are reported to the patient after completion of the first-trimester portion of the test and then again after the second-trimester portion. Although this test has a high sensitivity, it has a high false-positive rate because it involves two independent tests. The contingent sequential screen does the first-trimester portion of the sequential testing and follows with the Quad screen when an elevated risk is noted. The contingent sequential screening has an excellent detection rate and a low false-positive rate, and it is the most cost-effective screening tool for trisomy 21. It is for these reasons that it is becoming the most recommended.

IV. **Ultrasound testing.** Ultrasound examination is used in the following circumstances:

A. **Determination of pregnancy viability.** This is important in the first trimester when fetal heart motion can be detected at 6 weeks' gestation by an abdominal scan and a few days earlier by transvaginal ultrasound. Once the crown rump length is ≥5 mm, fetal heart motion should be seen. Ultrasound is also used in the case of a suspected fetal demise later in pregnancy.

B. **Calculation of gestational age.** Measurement of the crown-rump length between 6 and 14 weeks' gestation allows for the most accurate assessment of gestational age, to within 5 days. After the first trimester, a combination of biparietal diameter, head circumference, abdominal circumference, and femur length is used to estimate gestational age and fetal weight. Measurements in the second trimester are accurate to within ~10–14 days and in the third trimester to within 14–21 days.

C. **Diagnosis of multiple pregnancy and determination of chorionicity and amnionicity.** The determination of chorionicity and amnionicity is made by ultrasound examination of the fetal membranes and is best done as early as possible in the first trimester but after 6 weeks and prior to 14 weeks' gestation.

D. **Measurement of nuchal translucency.** An increased NT, best measured between 10 4/7 and 13 6/7 weeks, correlates with an elevated risk for chromosomal abnormalities such as trisomy 21 or 18. In addition, even those gestations with normal chromosomes but an increased NT have an elevated risk of adverse pregnancy outcomes, including fetal cardiac defects and intrauterine fetal demise. Measurement of NT alone has a detection rate for trisomy 18 and trisomy 21 that is less than the Quad screen. Therefore, it is not recommended as a sole screening test for aneuploidy without serum analysis.

E. **Anatomic survey.** A large number of congenital anomalies can be diagnosed reliably by ultrasonography, including anencephaly, hydrocephalus, congenital heart defects, gastroschisis, omphalocele, spina bifida, renal anomalies, diaphragmatic hernia, cleft lip and palate, and skeletal dysplasia. Identification of these anomalies before birth can help determine the safest method of delivery and the support personnel needed at delivery.

Ultrasonography can also aid in determining fetal gender for patients in whom this determination impacts the likelihood of a known X-linked genetic disorder.

F. **Visual guidance.** Ultrasound is used for guidance during procedures such as amniocentesis, CVS, percutaneous umbilical blood sampling (PUBS), and some fetal surgeries (placement of bladder or chest shunts).

G. **Assessment of growth and fetal weight.** Ultrasonography is useful to detect and monitor both intrauterine growth restriction (IUGR) (estimated fetal weight <10%) and fetal macrosomia (estimated fetal weight >90%). Evidence is accumulating that maternal size and race should be considered in customizing the fetal weight for determination of IUGR. Estimation of fetal weight is also important in counseling patients regarding expectations after delivering a premature infant. Ultrasound assessment for fetal weight by an experienced sonographer is accurate within 10–20% of actual weight.

H. **Assessment of amniotic fluid volume.** Amniotic fluid volume may be assessed objectively with ultrasound by measuring the maximum vertical pocket (MVP) or amniotic fluid index (AFI; total of cord-free deepest vertical pockets in four quadrants) in cm.

1. **Oligohydramnios (decreased amniotic fluid).** This condition is defined as an AFI of <5 cm or an MVP <2 cm or <10% on a gestational age–dependent scale. Oligohydramnios is associated with an increase in fetal morbidity and mortality. Spontaneous rupture of membranes is the most common cause. Other maternal causes include placental insufficiency, chronic hypertension, and postdates gestation. Multiple fetal anomalies such as renal agenesis, bladder outlet obstruction, karyotypic abnormalities, and severe cardiac disease can also result in oligohydramnios. The kidneys and the bladder can be seen with ultrasonography by ~14–15 weeks' gestation.

2. **Polyhydramnios (excess of amniotic fluid).** This is defined as an AFI >25 cm or an MVP >8 cm. It has been associated with fetal anomalies, including anencephaly and other neural tube defects, gastrointestinal obstruction such as duodenal atresia, multiple gestation with twin-twin transfusion syndrome, and nonimmune

hydrops fetalis. Maternal causes include diabetes mellitus. Most cases of third-trimester polyhydramnios are idiopathic; however, the risk for fetal anomalies increases with the severity of the polyhydramnios.

I. **Assessment of placental location and presence of retroplacental hemorrhage.** This is useful in suspected cases of placenta previa or placenta accreta. Most cases of abruptio placentae are not diagnosed by ultrasonography because abruption is a clinical diagnosis.

J. **Assessment of fetal well-being**

   1. **Biophysical profile.** Ultrasonography is used to assess fetal movements, fetal breathing, fetal tone, and amniotic fluid volume.

   2. **Doppler studies.** Doppler ultrasonography of fetal vessels, particularly the umbilical artery, is a useful adjunct in the management of high-risk pregnancies, especially those complicated by IUGR. Changes in the vascular Doppler pattern (ie, increased systolic/diastolic ratios and absent or reversed end-diastolic flow in the umbilical artery) signal elevations in placental vascular resistance. These abnormalities correlate with an increased risk for perinatal morbidity and mortality. In high-risk pregnancies, assessment of the middle cerebral artery is useful for evaluating for the presence of fetal anemia, and uterine artery Doppler may be useful in the prediction and evaluation of preeclampsia. The overall use of Doppler ultrasonography has been associated with a 15–55% decrease in perinatal mortality in high-risk pregnancies; however, no benefit in using this technique has been demonstrated in screening a low-risk population.

V. **Amniocentesis.** Amniotic fluid can be analyzed for prenatal diagnosis of karyotypic abnormalities, genetic disorders (for which testing is available), fetal blood type and hemoglobinopathies, fetal lung maturity, monitoring the degree of isoimmunization by measurement of the content of bilirubin in the fluid, and for the diagnosis of chorioamnionitis. Testing for karyotypic abnormalities is usually done at 16–20 weeks' gestation. A sample of amniotic fluid is removed under ultrasound guidance. Fetal cells in the fluid can be grown in tissue culture for genetic study. With visual guidance from the ultrasound, the pregnancy loss rate related to amniocentesis is usually quoted at between 1/200 and 1/1600. Early amniocentesis (before 14 weeks) is associated with a significantly higher rate of fetal loss and limb deformities, and consequently it is not generally recommended. Indications for amniocentesis include the following:

   A. **Any woman at an increased risk of aneuploidy** (ie, trisomies 13, 18, and 21) either by history or abnormal first- or second-trimester screening tests.

   B. **Any woman who has had a child with a chromosomal abnormality.**

   C. **Those in whom X-linked disorders are suspected,** as well as for autosomal recessive disorders when both parents are carriers of the trait in question.

   D. **Ruling out inborn errors of metabolism.**

VI. **Chorionic villus sampling.** CVS is a technique used for first-trimester genetic studies, and it is usually performed between 10 4/7 and 12 6/7 weeks' gestation. Chorionic villi are withdrawn from the placenta, either through a needle inserted through the abdomen or through a transcervical catheter. The cells obtained are identical to those of the fetus and are grown and analyzed. Results can be obtained quickly via fluorescence in situ hybridization (FISH) rapid chromosome analysis, thus enabling the patient to have a diagnosis before the end of the first trimester. Indications are the same as for amniocentesis. Reported complications after CVS are pregnancy loss and limb abnormalities; however, if CVS is performed after 10 weeks' gestation, there appears to be no increased incidence of limb reduction defects. Pregnancy loss rates after CVS are similar to amniocentesis but are highly operator dependent.

VII. **Percutaneous umbilical blood sampling.** Under ultrasound guidance, a needle is placed transabdominally into the fetal umbilical artery or vein. Samples of fetal blood can be obtained for karyotype, viral studies, fetal blood type, hematocrit, or platelet count. This also provides a route for in utero transfusion of red blood cells or platelets. PUBS is most often used in cases of severe hemolytic disease of the fetus with or without hydrops, such as that due to Rh or atypical antibody isoimmunization.

ANTEPARTUM TESTS OF FETAL WELL-BEING

I. **Nonstress test.** The nonstress test (NST) is used to detect intact fetal central nervous system function and the lack of acidosis. Fetal well-being is confirmed if the baseline heart rate is normal and there are periodic accelerations in the fetal heart rate. These accelerations are often associated with fetal movement. The following guidelines can be used, although there may be variations between institutions.

A. **Reactive NST.** In a 20-min monitoring period, there are at least two accelerations of the fetal heart rate peaking 15 beats/min above the baseline fetal heart rate, each acceleration lasting at least 15 s. In a fetus <32 weeks' gestation, the accelerations must reach 10 beats/min above the baseline and last at least 10 s. The perinatal mortality within 1 week after a reactive NST is ~ 1.9/1000.

B. **Nonreactive NST.** Fetal heart rate does not meet the established criteria during a prolonged period of monitoring (usually at least 1 h). *Note:* There are many causes of a nonreactive NST besides fetal compromise, including fetal sleep cycle, chronic maternal smoking, and exposure to medications such as central nervous system depressants and propranolol. Because of this low specificity (the false-positive rate is ~75–90%), a nonreactive NST should be followed by more definitive testing such as a biophysical profile or a contraction stress test.

II. **Biophysical profile.** The biophysical profile (BPP) (Table 1–1) is another test used to assess fetal well-being, often when the NST is nonreactive. An NST is performed along with an ultrasound examination to evaluate fetal breathing movements, gross body movements, tone, and amniotic fluid volume. The BPP is useful after 26–28 weeks. A score of 8–10 is considered normal, 4–6 indicates possible chronic asphyxia, and 0–2 predicts high perinatal mortality. The lower the BPP score, the higher the likelihood of fetal acidemia. The biophysical variables appear as gestational age increases in the order of fluid, tone, movement, breathing, and reactive NST, and the variables disappear in reverse order as fetal acidemia progresses.

The BPP scoring system has since been modified to include an NST and AFI, the modified BPP. In many centers, this has become the primary mode of antepartum fetal surveillance. The stillbirth rate within 1 week of a normal BPP or a modified BPP is the same at 0.8/1000.

III. **Contraction stress test.** The contraction stress test (CST) is used to assess a fetus at risk for uteroplacental insufficiency. Monitors are placed on the mother's abdomen to record the fetal heart rate and uterine contractions continuously. An adequate test consists of three contractions, each lasting 40–60 s within a period of 10 min. If sufficient contractions do not occur spontaneously, the mother is instructed to perform nipple

Table 1–1. BIOPHYSICAL PROFILE SCORING SYSTEM USED TO ASSESS FETAL WELL-BEING

Variable	Normal (2)	Abnormal (0)
Fetal breathing	One episode >30 s in 30 min	None or episode <30 s in 30 min
Body movement	Three or more movements in 30 min	Two or less movements in 30 min
Fetal tone	One episode of active limb or trunk extension with flexion in 30 min	No movement in 30 min
Nonstress test	Reactive	Nonreactive
Amniotic fluid	One pocket of amniotic fluid >2 cm or more in two perpendicular planes	No fluid pockets or pocket <2 cm in two perpendicular planes

Modified from Manning FA et al: Fetal biophysical profile scoring: a prospective study in 1184 high-risk patients. *Am J Obstet Gynecol* 1981;140(3):289–294. Reprinted with permission from Elsevier Science.

stimulation or oxytocin is administered by intravenous pump. If oxytocin is needed to produce contractions for the CST, it is called an oxytocin challenge test (OCT). Normally, the fetal heart rate increases in response to a contraction and no decelerations occur during or after the contraction. If late decelerations occur during or after contractions, uteroplacental insufficiency may be present. The CST may be contraindicated in patients with placenta previa, those who have had a previous cesarean section with a vertical incision, and those with high-risk factors for preterm delivery (ie, premature rupture of membranes or cervical insufficiency). Test results are interpreted as follows:

A. **Negative (normal) test.** No late decelerations occur during adequate uterine contractions (three in 10 min). The baseline fetal heart rate is normal. This result is associated with a very low perinatal mortality rate of 0.3/1000 in the week following the test.

B. **Positive (abnormal) test.** Late decelerations occur with at least two of three contractions over a 10-min interval. A positive CST is associated with an increased risk of perinatal morbidity or mortality and indicates that delivery is usually warranted.

C. **Equivocal (suspicious) test.** A late deceleration occurs with one of three contractions over a 10-min interval. Prolonged fetal monitoring is usually recommended, and the CST should be repeated in 24 h.

INTRAPARTUM TESTS OF FETAL WELL-BEING

I. **Fetal heart rate monitoring.** Continuous fetal heart rate monitoring has become the standard clinical practice for a patient in labor. However, it does not improve perinatal mortality or morbidity compared with intermittent auscultation of the fetal heart rate. To date, no studies have been performed comparing intrapartum monitoring with no monitoring during labor, and it is unlikely that this will ever be done. What continuous fetal monitoring does allow is to have a labor unit with less nursing staff. The only clear medical benefit to continuous fetal monitoring in labor is a decrease in neonatal seizures, although it is unclear if this has had any impact on long-term neurologic outcomes. Continuous fetal monitoring in labor is associated with an increase in the rates of both cesarean sections and operative vaginal deliveries. Fetal heart rate monitoring may be internal, with an electrode attached to the fetal scalp, or external, with a monitor attached to the maternal abdomen.

A. **Baseline fetal heart rate.** The baseline fetal heart rate is the rate maintained apart from periodic variations, rounded to the nearest 5 beats/min over a 10-min period. The normal fetal heart rate is 110–160 beats/min. Fetal tachycardia is present at >160 beats/min. Causes of fetal tachycardia include maternal or fetal infection, fetal hypoxia, thyrotoxicosis, and maternal use of drugs such as parasympathetic blockers or β-mimetic agents. Fetal bradycardia is defined as a heart rate of <110 beats/min. Common causes of bradycardia include hypoxia, complete heart block, and maternal use of drugs such as β-blockers.

B. **Variability.** In the normal mature fetus, there are rapid fluctuations in the baseline fetal heart rate. This variability indicates a functioning sympathetic–parasympathetic nervous system interaction and is the most sensitive indicator of fetal well-being. An amplitude range from peak to trough of 6–25 beats/min indicates moderate variability and suggests the absence of fetal hypoxia. Marked variability occurs when >25 beats/min is noted. Minimal variability is quantified as <5 beats/min; absent variability refers to an amplitude range that is undetectable. Decreased variability may be caused by severe hypoxia, anencephaly and other fetal neurologic abnormalities, complete heart block, and maternal use of drugs such as narcotics or magnesium sulfate. In addition, variability is decreased during normal fetal sleep cycles. The terms *beat-to-beat* versus *long-term variability* have no clinical significance and are no longer used in practice.

C. **Accelerations.** Accelerations are often associated with fetal movement and are an indication of fetal well-being. The presence of accelerations suggests the absence of any acidosis.

D. **Decelerations.** There are three types of decelerations (Figure 1–1).

1. **Early decelerations.** Early decelerations result from physiologic head compression and occur secondary to an intact vagal reflex tone, which follows minor, transient fetal hypoxic episodes. These are benign and not associated with fetal compromise. They appear as mirror images of the contraction pattern.

2. **Late decelerations.** Late decelerations are a result of uteroplacental insufficiency (UPI) and indicate the presence of fetal hypoxia. Potential causes include maternal hypotension, sometimes as a result of supine positioning or regional anesthesia, as well as uterine hypertonicity. More chronic causes of UPI, such as hypertension, postdates gestation, and preeclampsia may predispose a fetus to the development of late decelerations. Although by themselves they reflect only a decreased oxygen tension for the fetus, their persistence may lead to the development of fetal acidemia and eventual compromise. The nadir occurs after the contraction peaks, with the shape demonstrating a gradual decrease and slow return to baseline.

3. **Variable decelerations.** Variable decelerations result from abrupt compression of the umbilical cord. They can also be seen as a consequence of cord stretch, as in

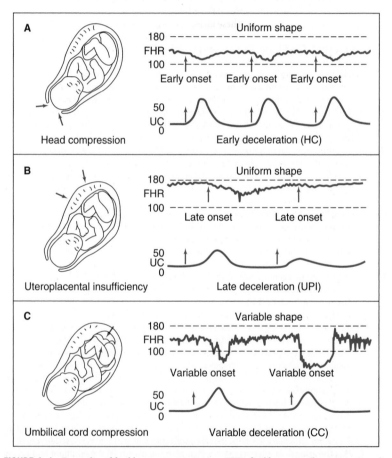

FIGURE 1–1. Examples of fetal heart rate monitoring. FHR, fetal heart rate (beats per minute); UC, uterine contraction (mm Hg); HC, head compression; UPI, uteroplacental insufficiency; CC, cord compression. (*Modified and reproduced, from McCrann JR, Schifrin BS: Fetal monitoring in high-risk pregnancy.* Clin Perinatol *1974;1:149 with permission from Elsevier Science.*)

phases of rapid fetal descent, and with a cord prolapse. Variable decelerations tend to increase in the setting of oligohydramnios. The majority of these decelerations are benign and not predictive of an acidemic fetus. However, severe variable decelerations (those lasting >60 s), especially in the setting of decreased variability and/or tachycardia, may portend a compromised fetus. They have a V or W nonuniform shape with a rapid descent and return to baseline. If the time from baseline to the nadir of the deceleration is 30 s or longer, the deceleration cannot be considered variable; it must be either an early or a late deceleration.

E. **Interpretation of electronic fetal monitoring (EFM).** According to the 2008 National Institute of Child Health and Human Development (NICHD) workshop report on electronic fetal monitoring (EFM), fetal heart rate (FHR) patterns can be classified in one of three categories: I (Normal), II (Indeterminate), or III (Abnormal). A Category I FHR pattern has four characteristics: normal baseline rate (110–160 bpm), moderate variability (6–25 bpm), absence of late or variable decelerations, and absence or presence of early decelerations or accelerations. In the setting of these findings, there is a high likelihood of a normally oxygenated fetus. Conversely, the new NICHD guidelines label four FHR patterns as abnormal, predictive of abnormal fetal acid-base status. These include a sinusoidal heart rate, defined as a pattern of regular variability resembling a sine wave, with fixed periodicity of 3–5 cycles/ min and amplitude of 5–40 bpm. A sinusoidal pattern may indicate fetal anemia caused by fetomaternal hemorrhage or alloimmunization. The other three abnormal FHR patterns in Category III are diagnosed when **baseline FHR variability is absent** and any one of the following is present: recurrent late decelerations, recurrent variable decelerations, or bradycardia. Category II comprises all FHR patterns not in Category I or III. Category II tracings are not predictive of abnormal fetal acid–base status. When a Category II tracing is identified, a fetal scalp stimulation test may help identify fetuses in which acid–base status is normal.

II. **Fetal scalp blood sampling.** Fetal scalp blood sampling had been used during labor to determine the fetal acid-base status when the fetal heart rate tracing was nonreassuring or equivocal. Its reliability and reproducibility for clinical decision making is questionable. Many practitioners have little experience in obtaining the sample, and therefore it is not commonly used in clinical care.

III. **Scalp stimulation/vibroacoustic stimulation.** An acceleration in fetal heart rate in response to either manual stimulation of the fetal presenting part or vibroacoustic stimulation through the maternal abdomen has been associated with a fetal pH of >7.20. These tests are often used in labor to determine fetal well-being; however, a lack of fetal response to stimulation is not predictive of acidemia.

IV. **Fetal pulse oximetry.** This technique was designed as an adjunct to fetal heart rate monitoring in labor and involves the placement of a fetal pulse oximeter transcervically next to the fetal cheek. Its goal is to reduce the number of unnecessary interventions for nonreassuring fetal heart rate tracings. Normal fetal oxygen saturation as measured by pulse oximetry (**Spo_2**) is 30–70%. A prolonged oxygen saturation of <30% for >10 min correlates to an increased risk of fetal metabolic acidosis. The American College of Obstetricians and Gynecologists (ACOG) does not endorse the use of this type of monitor, and it currently is no longer clinically available.

TESTS OF FETAL LUNG MATURITY

I. **Testing strategies.** A mature result from any fetal lung maturity test indicates a very low likelihood of neonatal respiratory distress syndrome (RDS). The positive predictive value of all of the tests is poor, ranging from 30 to 60%, implying that an immature result does not correlate well to the presence of RDS. ACOG therefore recommends that if the first test result is immature, a subsequent test be performed in a sequential fashion to confirm fetal lung immaturity. The choice and availability of tests for fetal lung maturity are institution dependent.

II. **Lecithin-sphingomyelin (L-S) ratio.** Lecithin, or phosphatidylcholine, is a phospholipid that can be measured specifically in amniotic fluid. It is a principal active component of surfactant and is manufactured by type II alveolar cells. Sphingomyelin is a phospholipid found predominantly in body tissues other than the lungs. The L-S ratio compares levels of lecithin, which gradually increase after 28 weeks to levels of sphingomyelin, which remain constant. The L-S ratio is usually 1:1 by 31–32 weeks' gestation and 2:1 by 35 weeks' gestation. The following are guidelines to L-S ratios:

A. **L-S ≥2:0: Mature.**

B. **L-S <2:0: Immature.**

Some disorders are associated with delayed lung maturation, and higher than normal L-S ratios may be needed before fetal lung maturity is ensured. The two most common disorders are diabetes mellitus and Rh isoimmunization complicated by fetal hydrops. Acceleration of fetal lung maturity is seen in sickle cell disease, maternal narcotic addiction, prolonged rupture of membranes, chronic maternal hypertension, IUGR, and smoking. Differences may also occur in various racial groups. The L-S ratio measurement can be affected by the presence of blood or meconium. In addition, the L-S ratio is costly, difficult to perform, and time consuming compared with other tests available.

III. **Phosphatidylglycerol.** Phosphatidylglycerol (PG) appears in amniotic fluid at ~35 weeks, and levels increase at 37–40 weeks. This substance is a useful marker for lung maturation late in pregnancy because it is the last surfactant to appear in the fetal lung. It is reported as either present or absent, and its presence is a strong marker that RDS will not occur. PG levels are not affected by blood or meconium contamination and can also be performed on vaginal pool specimens from patients who have ruptured membranes.

IV. **Surfactant/Albumin ratio by TDx fetal lung maturity (TDx FLM II).** This test (Abbott Laboratories, Abbott Park, IL) measures the relative concentrations of surfactant and albumin (milligrams of surfactant per gram of albumin) in amniotic fluid, which increases with increasing lung maturity. TDx FLM II has several advantages over the L-S ratio: less technical expertise is required, it is performed more easily and results are available quicker. Like the L-S ratio, blood and meconium can interfere with the results. Results are interpreted in the following ways:

A. **≤39 mg/g: Immature.**

B. **40-54 mg/g: Indeterminate.**

C. **≥55 mg/g: Mature.**

V. **Lamellar body count (LBC).** After its secretion by type II pneumocytes, surfactant is packaged into storage granules called lamellar bodies. This test uses a standard hematologic cell counter to count these lamellar bodies. Like the TDx FLM II, this test provides quicker results and is easier to perform than the L-S ratio at an equal or better sensitivity. Both blood and meconium can affect the interpretation of this test.

Selected References

Alfirevic Z, Neilson JP: Doppler ultrasonography in high-risk pregnancies: systematic review with meta-analysis. *Am J Obstet Gynecol* 1995;172:1379-1387.

American College of Obstetricians and Gynecologists. ACOG Practice Bulletin, No. 70: Intrapartum fetal heart rate monitoring. *Obstet Gynecol* 2005;106:1453-1460.

American College of Obstetricians and Gynecologists. ACOG Practice Bulletin, No. 9: Antepartum fetal surveillance. *Obstet Gynecol* 1999;93(2):285-291.

American College of Obstetricians and Gynecologists. ACOG Practice Bulletin, No. 97: Fetal lung maturity. *Obstet Gynecol* 2008;112(3):717-726.

Ball RH et al: First- and second-trimester evaluation of risk for Down syndrome. *Obstet Gynecol* 2007;110:10-17.

Dildy GA: Fetal pulse oximetry: current issues. *J Perinat Med* 2001;29:5-13.

American College of Obstetricians and Gynecologists. ACOG Practice Bulletin, No. 258: Fetal pulse oximetry. *Obstet Gynecol* 2001;98:523-524.

Freeman RK et al: Basic pattern recognition. In *Fetal Heart Rate Monitoring*, 3rd ed. Philadelphia: Lippincott Williams & Wilkins, 2003:63-85.

Macones GA, et al: The 2008 National Institute of Child Health and Human Development workshop report on electronic fetal monitoring: update on definitions, interpretation, and research guidelines. *Obstet Gynecol* 2008;112:661-666.

Malone FD et al: First-trimester or second-trimester screening, or both, for Down's syndrome. *N Engl J Med* 2005;353:2001-2011.

Manning FA: Fetal biophysical profile: a critical appraisal. *Clin Obstet Gynecol* 2002;45: 975-985.

Manning FA et al: Fetal biophysical profile scoring: a prospective study in 1184 high-risk patients. *Am J Obstet Gynecol* 1981;140:289-294.

National Institute of Child Health and Human Development Research Planning Workshop: Electronic fetal heart rate monitoring: research guidelines for interpretation. *Am J Obstet Gynecol* 1997;177:1385-90.

Nicolaides KH: Nuchal translucency and other first-trimester sonographic markers of chromosomal abnormalities. *Am J Obstet Gynecol* 2004;191:45-67.

Porter TF, Clark SL: Vibroacoustic and scalp stimulation. *Obstet Gynecol Clin North Am* 1999; 26(4):657-669.

Wilson RD: Amniocentesis and chorionic villus sampling. *Curr Opin Obstet Gynecol* 2000; 12:81-86.

2 Obstetric Anesthesia and the Neonate

During birth, the status of the fetus can be influenced by obstetric analgesia and anesthesia. Care in choosing analgesic and anesthetic agents can often prevent respiratory depression in the newborn, especially in high-risk deliveries.

I. **Placental transfer of drugs.** Drugs administered to the mother may affect the fetus via placental transfer or, less commonly, may cause a maternal disorder that affects the fetus (eg, maternal drug-induced hypotension may cause fetal hypoxia). All anesthetic and analgesic drugs cross the placenta to some degree. Flow-dependent passive diffusion is the usual mechanism.

Most anesthetic and analgesic drugs have a high degree of lipid solubility, a low molecular weight (<500), and variable protein-binding and ionization capabilities. These characteristics lead to a rapid transfer across the placenta. Local anesthetics and narcotics (lipid-soluble, un-ionized) cross the placenta easily, whereas neuromuscular blocking agents (highly ionized) are transferred slowly.

II. **Analgesia in labor**
   A. **Inhalation analgesia.** Inhalation analgesia is rarely used in the United States due to the availability of regional anesthesia and because several problems limit its routine use:
      1. **The need for specialized vaporizers.**
      2. **The concern regarding pollution of the labor and delivery environment** with waste anesthetic gases.
      3. **Incomplete analgesia.**
      4. **The potential for maternal amnesia.**
      5. **The potential for the loss of protective airway reflexes** and pulmonary aspiration of gastric contents.

Note: Entonox (a mixture of 50% oxygen and 50% nitrous oxide) is widely used outside the United States.

B. Pudendal block and paracervical block. Paracervical block may be associated with severe fetal bradycardia caused by decreased uteroplacental/fetoplacental perfusion from increased uterine activity or a direct vasoconstrictive effect of the local anesthetic, and it is now rarely used. If a paracervical block is performed, the fetal heart rate (FHR) must be monitored. Pudendal blocks have little direct effect on the fetus. However, seizures have been reported after both pudendal and paracervical blocks. Paracervical blocks are used in the first stage of labor, and pudendal blocks during the second stage.

C. Opioids. All intravenously administered opioids are rapidly transferred to the fetus and cause dose-related respiratory depression and alterations in the Apgar and neurobehavioral scores.

1. **Meperidine (Demerol)** can cause severe neonatal depression (measured by Apgar scoring) if the drug is administered 2–3 h before delivery. Depression is manifested as respiratory acidosis, decreased oxygen saturation, decreased minute ventilation, and increased time to sustained respiration. Fetal normeperidine (a meperidine metabolite that may cause significant respiratory depression) increases with longer intervals between drug administration and delivery. Levels are highest 4 h after intravenous administration of the drug to the mother. The half-life of meperidine is 13 h in neonates, whereas that of normeperidine is 62 h.

2. **Morphine** has a delayed onset of action and may cause greater neonatal respiratory depression than meperidine.

3. **Butorphanol (Stadol) and nalbuphine (Nubain)** are agonist-antagonist narcotic agents that cause less respiratory depression than morphine because they demonstrate a ceiling effect for respiratory depression with increasing doses. Decreases in FHR variability, sinusoidal FHR patterns, fetal tachycardia, and fetal bradycardia have all been reported following maternal administration of nalbuphine, unlike butorphanol.

D. Opioid antagonist (naloxone [Narcan]). Naloxone should never be administered to neonates of women who have received chronic opioid therapy because it may precipitate acute withdrawal symptoms. Naloxone may be used to reverse respiratory depression caused by acute maternal opioid administration during labor.

E. Sedatives and tranquilizers

1. **Barbiturates.** Barbiturates cross the placenta rapidly and can have pronounced neonatal effects (eg, somnolence, flaccidity, hypoventilation, and failure to feed) that may last for days. Effects are intensified if opioids are used simultaneously. This is usually not an issue when barbiturates are used as an induction to general anesthesia for an emergent cesarean delivery. Barbiturates are rapidly redistributed into the maternal tissues prior to placental transfer, and when they cross the placenta, are preferentially uptaken by the fetal liver.

2. **Benzodiazepines (diazepam [Valium], lorazepam [Ativan], and midazolam [Versed]).** These agents cross the placenta rapidly and equilibrate within minutes after intravenous administration. Fetal levels are often higher than maternal levels. Diazepam given in low doses (<10 mg) may cause decreased beat-to-beat variability and tone but has little effect on Apgar scores and blood gas levels. Larger doses of diazepam may persist for days and can cause hypotonia, lethargy, decreased feeding, and impaired thermoregulation, with resulting hypothermia. All benzodiazepines share these features; however, diazepam is the most thoroughly studied of the benzodiazepine series. In addition, benzodiazepines are less frequently used because they induce childbirth amnesia in the mother. Midazolam may be used to induce general anesthesia. Anesthetic induction with midazolam is safe for the mother, although low 1-min Apgar scores and transient neonatal hypotonia may be seen.

3. **Phenothiazines.** Phenothiazines are rarely used today because they may induce hypotension via central α-blockade. Phenothiazines are sometimes combined with

a narcotic (neuroleptanalgesia). Innovar, a combination drug containing the narcotics fentanyl and droperidol, may be safe because of the relatively short half-life of the agents.

4. **Ketamine (Ketaject, others).** Ketamine may be used for dissociative analgesia. Doses >1 mg/kg may cause uterine hypertonia, neonatal depression (low Apgar scores), and abnormal neonatal muscle tone. Doses normally used in labor (0.1–0.2 mg/kg) are relatively safe, producing minimal effects in the mother and the neonate.

F. **Lumbar epidural analgesia.** Lumbar epidural analgesia is the most frequently used invasive anesthetic technique for childbirth. Maternal pain and catecholamine levels are reduced (catecholamines cause prolonged incoordinate labor and decreased uterine blood flow), which may lead to diminished maternal hyperventilation and improved fetal oxygen delivery. Vasospasm of uterine arteries in pregnancy-induced hypertension may be corrected. Labor epidural analgesia lasting >4 h is associated with maternal temperature increases of up to 1°C. This may lead to neonatal sepsis evaluation and antibiotic treatment if these treatments are done on the basis of intrapartum maternal temperature.

Local anesthetic (eg, bupivacaine, lidocaine) is usually continuously infused through an epidural catheter placed in a lumbar [L2-3, L3-4, L4-5]) interspace. Alternatively, repeated injections through the catheter may be used. Small doses of an opioid may be added; these have little effect on the neonate. Maternal hypotension caused by sympathetic blockade is easily treated with fluid administration or intravenous ephedrine.

G. **Intrathecal opioid analgesia.** Intrathecal opioids (sufentanil or fentanyl with or without morphine) provide first-stage labor analgesia with minimal motor and sympathetic nerve block. Intrathecal opioids are frequently administered when the fetal head is still high in the pelvis. Transient FHR changes occur in 10–15% of cases, usually without adverse neonatal outcome, although cesarean delivery has been necessary in some cases.

H. **Caudal epidural analgesia.** Caudal epidural analgesia blocks the sacral nerve roots and provides excellent pain relief in the second stage of labor. Caudal analgesia is not used during the first stage of labor because the large doses needed to block the T11-T12 nerve roots increase pelvic muscle relaxation and impair fetal head rotation. Because fetal intracranial local anesthetic injection can occur, this technique is now rarely used.

I. **Local anesthetics.** All of the regional anesthetic/analgesic techniques (eg, epidural or spinal) and local blocks (eg, pudendal) depend on the use of local anesthetic agents. Bupivacaine is the most commonly used agent because of its longer half-life, and when dilute solutions are used, it produces excellent sensory analgesia with minimal motor blockade.

1. **Lidocaine (Xylocaine).** Placental transfer of lidocaine is significant, but Apgar scores are not affected in healthy neonates. Acidotic fetuses accumulate larger amounts of lidocaine through pH-induced ion trapping.

2. **Bupivacaine (Marcaine).** Bupivacaine is theoretically less harmful than lidocaine for the fetus because it has a higher degree of ionization and protein binding than lidocaine. Maternal toxicity leading to convulsions and cardiac arrest has been reported after inadvertent intravascular injection. Bupivacaine, in very low concentrations, is the most commonly used local anesthetic agent for continuous labor analgesia.

3. **Chloroprocaine (Nesacaine).** After systemic absorption, chloroprocaine is rapidly broken down by pseudocholinesterase; thus very little reaches the placenta or fetus. Neurobehavioral studies indicate no difference between controls and neonates whose mothers were given chloroprocaine. However, because of its short duration and significant motor blockade, chloroprocaine is not useful for continuous labor analgesia.

4. **Ropivacaine (Naropin).** Ropivacaine is similar to bupivacaine but produces less motor block and maternal cardiotoxicity. Neurologic and adaptive capacity scores are somewhat better in infants whose mothers received epidural ropivacaine rather than bupivacaine for labor analgesia.

5. **Levobupivacaine (Chirocaine).** Levobupivacaine is the purified levorotary enantiomer of racemic bupivacaine. Like ropivacaine, it has less potential for cardiotoxicity than bupivacaine.

J. **Psychoprophylaxis.** The **Lamaze technique** of prepared childbirth involves class instruction for prospective parents. The process of childbirth is explained, and exercises, breathing techniques, and relaxation techniques are taught to relieve labor pain. However, the popular assumption that the neonate benefits if the mother receives no drugs during childbirth may not be true. Pain and discomfort may cause psychological stress and hyperventilation in the mother, which can negatively impact the neonate; supplemental anesthesia may be needed. Approximately 50–70% of women who have learned the Lamaze method request drugs or an anesthetic block during labor. Other analgesic techniques include transcutaneous electric nerve stimulation (TENS), hypnosis, and acupuncture.

III. **Anesthesia for cesarean delivery.** Aortocaval compression may decrease placental perfusion; the mother should be positioned supine with the bed tilted left side down or a wedge placed under the right hip. Regional anesthesia is the technique of choice for most cesarean deliveries because it is generally safer for both mother and baby. If immediate delivery is indicated, general anesthesia is often used because it has the shortest induction time, although neonates do as well with regional anesthesia.

A. **Spinal anesthesia.** Spinal anesthesia (injection of local anesthetic directly into the cerebrospinal fluid) requires a tenth of the drug needed for epidural anesthesia (drug injection into the epidural space). Maternal and fetal drug levels are low. Hypotension may occur rapidly but can be attenuated by administering 1.5–2.0 L of a balanced salt solution intravenously. Intravenous ephedrine or small doses of phenylephrine can also be used to manage the hypotension. Anesthesia is induced more rapidly with spinal than with epidural anesthesia. Abnormalities in Early Neonatal Neurobehavioral Scores (ENNSs) are more common after general anesthesia than spinal anesthesia for cesarean delivery. ENNS evaluates the effects of maternal medications on newborn neurobehavior. It includes 15 observations of muscle tone and power, reflexes, and response to stimuli; 11 observations of infant wakefulness; assessment of habituation, and overall general neurobehavioral status.

B. **Lumbar epidural anesthesia.** Placental transfer of local anesthetics occurs, but drug effects can be detected only by neurobehavioral testing. Maternal hypotension may occur but to a lesser extent than with spinal anesthesia.

C. **General anesthesia.** General anesthesia is used in the following circumstances: strong patient preference, emergency delivery (eg, in cases of hemorrhage or fetal bradycardia), and contraindications to regional anesthesia (eg, maternal coagulopathy, maternal neurologic problems, sepsis, or infection). After induction of anesthesia, the mother is maintained on a combination of nitrous oxide and oxygen with low doses of inhaled halogenated agents or intravenous drugs. Opioids or benzodiazepines are rarely given until the cord is clamped.

1. **Agents used in general obstetric anesthesia**

a. **Premedication.** Cimetidine (Tagamet) or ranitidine (Zantac) (H_2 receptor antagonists) may be used to decrease gastric volume and increase gastric pH to help prevent aspiration pneumonitis. Metoclopramide (Reglan) may be given to speed gastric emptying. The neonate is not affected by these agents. Premedications traditionally used in surgery (eg, atropinics, opioids, and benzodiazepines) are rarely given.

b. **Thiopental (Pentothal).** Thiopental (4 mg/kg) may be used to induce general anesthesia. Peak fetal concentrations occur within 2–3 min. Apgar scores are not affected by thiopental at the 4 mg/kg dose. Metabolites may affect the neonatal electroencephalogram (EEG) for several days and depress the sucking response.

  c. **Ketamine (Ketalar).** Ketamine (1 mg/kg) is used to induce anesthesia, although it is usually reserved for severe asthmatics (because of its bronchodilator properties) and patients with mild to moderate hypovolemia when cesarean delivery is emergent. Neonatal neurobehavioral test scores after ketamine administration are slightly better than those after thiopental administration.

  d. **Muscle relaxants.** Muscle relaxants, which are highly ionized, cross the placenta only in small amounts and have little effect on the neonate.

    i. **Succinylcholine (Anectine, others)** crosses the placenta in minimal amounts. In twice-normal doses, it is detectable in the fetus, but no respiratory effects are seen until the dose is 5 times normal or both mother and fetus have abnormal pseudo-cholinesterase levels or activity.

    ii. **Atracurium (Tracrium), cisatracurium (Nimbex), vecuronium (Norcuron), and rocuronium (Zemuron)** are medium-duration nondepolarizing muscle relaxants. In clinical doses, an insufficient amount of drug crosses the placenta to affect the neonate.

    iii. **Pancuronium (Pavulon) and tubocurarine (Tubarine)** are long-duration muscle relaxants that do not affect the neonate when administered in clinical doses.

  e. **Nitrous oxide** has rapid placental transfer. Prolonged administration of high (>50%) concentrations of nitrous oxide can result in low Apgar scores because of neonatal anesthesia and diffusion hypoxia. Concentrations up to 50% are safe, but neonates may need supplemental oxygen after delivery, especially if the interval between anesthetic induction and delivery is long.

  f. **Halogenated anesthetic agents** (isoflurane [Forane], enflurane [Ethrane], sevoflurane [Ultane], desflurane [Suprane], and halothane [Fluothane]) are used to maintain general anesthesia. Beneficial effects include decreased maternal catecholamines, increased uterine blood flow, and improved maternal anesthesia compared with nitrous oxide alone. Low concentrations of these agents rarely cause neonatal anesthesia. If anesthesia occurs, it is transient because these volatile agents are readily exhaled. High concentrations may decrease uterine contractility. The lowest effective concentration is chosen, and the agent is promptly discontinued after delivery to decrease uterine atony and prevent excessive blood loss.

2. **Neonatal effects of general anesthesia.** Maternal hypoxia resulting from aspiration or failed endotracheal intubation can cause fetal hypoxia. Maternal hyperventilation ($PaCO_2$ <20 mm Hg) decreases placental blood flow and shifts the maternal oxyhemoglobin curve to the left, which can lead to fetal hypoxia and acidosis. Fetal oxygen saturation increases with increases in maternal oxygen partial pressure up to a maternal PaO_2 of 300 mm Hg.

3. **Interval between incision of the uterus and delivery.** Incision and manipulation of the uterus causes reflex uterine vasoconstriction, resulting in fetal asphyxia. Long intervals between uterine incision and delivery (>90 s) are associated with significant lowering of Apgar scores. If the interval is >180 s, low Apgar scores and fetal acidosis may result. Regional anesthesia decreases reflex vasoconstriction; therefore, the incision-to-delivery interval is less important. The interval may be prolonged with breech, multiple, or preterm delivery; if there is uterine scarring; or if the fetus is large.

4. **Regional versus general anesthesia**

  a. **Apgar scores.** Early studies showed that neonates were less depressed on 1- and 5-min Apgar scores with regional compared with general anesthesia. New general anesthetic techniques lower Apgar scores at 1 min only. This represents transient sedation (ie, temporary neonatal general anesthesia) rather than asphyxia. If the interval between induction and delivery is short, there is less difference between the effects of regional and general anesthesia. If a prolonged delivery time is anticipated, regional anesthesia is preferred because the neonate is less sedated. It is important to note that low Apgar scores secondary to sedation do not have the negative prognostic value of low Apgar scores secondary to asphyxia, provided that the neonate is adequately resuscitated.

b. **Acid-base status.** The differences in acid-base status are minimal and probably not significant. Infants of diabetic mothers may be less acidotic with general than with regional anesthesia because regional anesthesia-induced hypotension may exacerbate any existing uteroplacental insufficiency.

c. **Neurobehavioral examinations** are used to detect subtle changes in the neonate in the first few hours after birth. After delivery, there is a 1-h period of alertness, followed by a 3- to 4-h period of deep sleep and decreased responsiveness. The **ENNS** (defined previously) was initially developed to detect neurobehavioral changes 2–8 h after birth (the half-life of most local anesthetics). These changes are usually manifested as decreased tone in an otherwise alert infant. The **Neonatal Neurologic and Adaptive Capacity Score (NNACS)** uses portions of the **ENNS, Brazelton Neonatal Behavioral Assessment Scale,** and **Amiel-Tison Neurologic Examination.** This score is more weighted toward assessment of neonatal tone and is helpful in differentiating abnormalities caused by birth trauma versus drug effects. Early neurobehavioral examinations show clear-cut advantages of regional compared with general anesthesia. Although infants of mothers receiving spinal and epidural anesthesia had similar results at 15 min, by 2 h the epidural group had lower scores. This probably reflects higher local anesthetic uptake.

Selected References

Abboud TK et al: Maternal, fetal, and neonatal responses after epidural anesthesia with bupivacaine, 2-chloroprocaine, or lidocaine. *Anesth Analg* 1982;61:638-644.

Akamatsu TH et al: Experiences with the use of ketamine for parturition: I. Primary anesthesia for vaginal delivery. *Anesth Analg* 1974;53:284-287.

Amiel-Tison C et al: A new neurologic and adaptive capacity scoring system for evaluating obstetric medications in full-term newborns. *Anesthesiology* 1982;56:340-350.

Bland BAR et al: Comparison of midazolam and thiopental for rapid sequence anesthetic induction for elective cesarean section. *Anesth Analg* 1987;66:1165-1168.

Clark RB, Seifen AB: Systemic medication during labor and delivery. *Obstet Gynecol Annu* 1983;12:165-197.

Cohen SE et al: Intrathecal sufentanil for labor analgesia—sensory changes, side effects, and fetal heart rate changes. *Anesth Analg* 1993;77:1155-1160.

Datta S, Brown WU: Acid-base status in diabetic mothers and their infants following general or spinal anesthesia for cesarean section. *Anesthesiology* 1977;47:272-276.

Datta S et al: Neonatal effect of prolonged anesthetic induction for cesarean section. *Obstet Gynecol* 1981;58:331-335.

Eisenach JC: The pain of childbirth and its effect on the mother and the fetus. In Chestnut DH (ed): *Obstetric Anesthesia Principles and Practice,* 3rd ed. Philadelphia: Elsevier Mosby, 2004:292.

Gambling DA et al: A randomized study of combined spinal-epidural analgesia versus intravenous meperidine during labor. *Anesthesiology* 1998;89:1336-1344.

Gerhard T et al: Use of naloxone to reverse narcotic respiratory depression in the newborn infant. *J Pediatr* 1977;90:1009-1012.

Jouppila P et al: Lumbar epidural analgesia to improve intervillous blood flow during labor in severe preeclampsia. *Obstet Gynecol* 1982;59:158-161.

Kuhnert BR et al: Meperidine and normeperidine levels following meperidine administration during labor: II. Fetus and neonate. *Am J Obstet Gynecol* 1979;133:909-914.

Kuhnert BR et al: Effects of low doses of meperidine on neonatal behavior. *Anesth Analg* 1985;64:335-342.

Lee A et al: A quantitative systematic review of randomized controlled trials of ephedrine versus phenylephrine for the management of hypotension during spinal anesthesia for cesarean delivery. *Anesth Analg* 2002;94:920-926.

Lieberman E et al: Epidural analgesia, intrapartum fever and neonatal sepsis evaluation. *Pediatrics* 1997;99:415-419.

Marx GF et al: Fetal-neonatal status following cesarean section for fetal distress. *Br J Anaesth* 1984;56:1009-1013.

Ravlo O et al: A randomized comparison between midazolam and thiopental for elective cesarean section anesthesia. II. Neonates. *Anesth Analg* 1989;68:234-237.

Scanlon JW et al: Neurobehavioral responses of newborn infants after maternal epidural anesthesia. *Anesthesiology* 1974;40:121-128.

Shnider SM et al: Uterine blood flow and plasma norepinephrine changes during maternal stress in the pregnant ewe. *Anesthesiology* 1979;50:524-527.

Stienstra R et al: Ropivacaine 0.25% vs. bupivacaine 0.25% for continuous epidural analgesia in labor: a double-blind comparison. *Anesth Analg* 1995;80:285-289.

Wakefield ML: Systemic analgesia: parenteral and inhalational agents. In Chestnut DH (ed): *Obstetric Anesthesia Principles and Practice,* 3rd ed. Philadelphia: Elsevier Mosby, 2004:311.

Way WL et al: Respiratory sensitivity of the newborn infant to meperidine and morphine. *Clin Pharm Ther* 1965;6:454-461.

3 Resuscitation of the Newborn

About 10% of all newborns require some assistance to begin breathing after birth, and ~1% require extensive resuscitation efforts. Newborn resuscitation cannot always be anticipated in time to transfer the mother before delivery to a facility with specialized neonatal support. Therefore, every hospital with a delivery suite should have an organized, skilled resuscitation team and appropriate equipment available (Table 3–1).

I. **Normal physiologic events at birth.** Normal transitional events at birth begin with initial lung expansion, generally requiring large negative intrathoracic pressures, followed by a cry (expiration against a partially closed glottis). Umbilical cord clamping is accompanied by a rise in systemic blood pressure and massive stimulation of the sympathetic nervous system. With onset of respiration and lung expansion, pulmonary vascular resistance decreases, followed by a gradual transition (over minutes to hours) from fetal to adult circulation, with closure of the foramen ovale and ductus arteriosus.

II. **Abnormal physiologic events at birth.** The asphyxiated newborn undergoes an abnormal transition. Acutely with asphyxiation the fetus develops **primary apnea,** during which spontaneous respirations can be induced by appropriate sensory stimuli. If the asphyxial insult persists about another minute, the fetus develops deep gasping for 4–5 minutes, followed by a period of **secondary apnea,** during which spontaneous respirations cannot be induced by sensory stimulation. Death occurs if secondary apnea is not reversed by vigorous ventilatory support within several minutes. Because one can never be certain whether an apneic newborn has primary or secondary apnea, resuscitative efforts should proceed as though secondary apnea is present.

Table 3-1. EQUIPMENT FOR NEONATAL RESUSCITATION

Standard Equipment Setup

Radiant warmer

Stethoscope

Oxygen source with warmer and humidifier

Suction source, suction catheter, and meconium "aspirators"

Nasogastric tubes

Apparatus for bag-and-mask ventilation

Ventilation masks

Laryngoscope (handles, No. 00, 0, and 1 blades; batteries)

Endotracheal tubes (2.5, 3.0, 3.5, and 4.0 mm)

Drugs

Epinephrine (1:10,000 solution)

Volume expanders (normal saline, Ringer's lactate, 5% albumin, O-negative whole blood [cross-matched against the mother's blood])

Clock (Apgar timer)

Syringes, hypodermic needles, and tubes for collection of blood samples

Equipment for umbilical vessel catheterization

Warm blankets

Additional Equipment Setup

All of the above plus the following:

Pressure manometer for use during ventilation

Oxygen blender

Heart rate and blood gas monitoring equipment

Micro–blood gas analysis availability

Umbilical vessel catheter setup (ready to insert)

Transcutaneous oxygen tension or saturation monitor

Camera

Plastic bags for "micro-preemies"

Humidified gas

III. **Preparation for high-risk delivery.** Preparation for a high-risk delivery is often the key to a successful outcome. Cooperation between the obstetric and pediatric staff is important. Knowledge of potential high-risk situations and appropriate interventions is essential (Table 3–2). It is useful to have an estimation of weight and gestational age (Table 3–3), so that drug dosages can be calculated and the appropriate endotracheal tube (see Table 28–1) and umbilical catheter size can be chosen. While waiting for the infant to arrive, it is useful

Table 3-2. SOME HIGH-RISK SITUATIONS FOR WHICH RESUSCITATION MAY BE ANTICIPATED

High-Risk Situation	Primary Intervention
Preterm delivery	Intubation, lung expansion
Thick meconium	Endotracheal suction
Acute fetal or placental hemorrhage	Volume expansion
Hydrops fetalis	Intubation, paracentesis, or thoracentesis
Polyhydramnios: gastrointestinal obstruction	Nasogastric suction
Oligohydramnios: pulmonary hypoplasia	Intubation, lung expansion
Maternal infection	Administration of antibiotics
Maternal diabetes	Early glucose administration

Table 3–3. **EXPECTED BIRTHWEIGHT (50TH PERCENTILE) AT 24–38 WEEKS' GESTATION**

Gestational Age (wk)	Birthweight (g)
24	700
26	900
28	1100
30	1350
32	1650
34	2100
36	2600
38	3000

Based on data published in Battaglia FC, Lubchenco LO: A practical classification of newborn infants by weight and gestational age. *J Pediatr* 1967;71:159.

to think through potential problems, steps that may be undertaken to correct them, and which member of the team will handle each step. Provided there is both time and opportunity, resuscitative measures should be discussed with the parents. This is particularly important when the fetus is at the limit of viability or when life-threatening anomalies are anticipated.

IV. **Assessment of the need for resuscitation.** The Apgar score (Appendix B) is assigned at 1, 5, and, occasionally, 10–20 min after delivery. It gives a fairly objective retrospective idea of how much resuscitation a term infant required at birth and the infant's response to resuscitative efforts. It is, however, not particularly useful during resuscitation. During resuscitation, simultaneous assessment of respiratory activity, heart rate, and skin color provides the quickest and most accurate evaluation of the need for continuing resuscitation. For preterm infants, Apgar scores may be particularly misleading (even in assessment of the response to resuscitation) because of developmental differences in tone and response to stimulation.

A. **Respiratory activity.** Respiratory activity is assessed by observing chest movement or listening for breath sounds. If there is no respiratory effort or the effort is poor, the infant needs respiratory assistance by either manual stimulation or positive-pressure ventilation.

B. **Heart rate.** The heart rate is typically evaluated by listening to the apical beat or feeling the pulse by lightly grasping the base of the umbilical cord. The evaluator should tap out each beat so that all team members can hear it. If no heart rate can be heard or felt, ventilatory efforts should be halted for a few seconds so that this finding can be verified by another team member. Pulse oximetry is also useful for monitoring heart rate during resuscitation.

C. **Skin color.** Assessment of skin color may be difficult when there is severe bruising, especially in preterm infants. Marked acrocyanosis may also complicate the picture. Looking at the mucous membranes of the mouth may be helpful under these circumstances. Bluish coloring indicates central cyanosis, and oxygen supplementation or assisted ventilation is needed. Pinkish membranes indicate normal oxygen levels, and resuscitation may not be needed. Pulse oximetry can yield a more accurate assessment of oxygen saturations than visualization of the newborn infant's color.

V. **Technique of resuscitation.** The American Heart Association (AHA) and American Academy of Pediatrics' (AAP) *Textbook of Neonatal Resuscitation* (5th ed., 2006) provides the standard of care used in most delivery services for the resuscitation of newborns.

A. **Ventilatory resuscitation**

1. **General measures**

a. **Suctioning.** First, nasal and oropharyngeal secretions should be partially removed with a brief period of suctioning using either a bulb syringe or a suction catheter. More prolonged suctioning delays resuscitation and may cause a profound vagal response in the infant.

b. **Positive-pressure ventilation.** Most infants can be adequately ventilated with a bag and mask provided that the mask is the correct size with a close seal around the mouth and nose and there is an appropriate flow of gas to the bag (Figure 3–1). Respiratory rate should be 40–60 breaths/min, or 30 breaths/min if accompanying chest compressions. Peak pressures of 20–25 cm H_2O are usually sufficient, but initial pressures as high as 30–40 cm H_2O may be required. The stomach should be emptied during and after prolonged bag-and-mask ventilation by orogastric suctioning. The AAP and AHA recommend that 100% oxygen be used when positive-pressure ventilation is used in resuscitation of term infants, but there is **controversial** evidence supporting the use of 21% oxygen in positive-pressure ventilation. The AAP and AHA recommend that when oxygen concentrations <100% are used and the infant is not improving by 90 s following birth, the concentration should be increased to 100%.

c. **Endotracheal intubation.** Endotracheal intubation should be performed when indicated. However, multiple unsuccessful attempts at intubation by inexperienced persons may make a difficult situation worse. In these cases, it may be best to continue mask ventilation until experienced help arrives. An alternative to endotracheal intubation when intubation attempts are unsuccessful and mask ventilation is not effective is placement of a laryngeal mask airway.

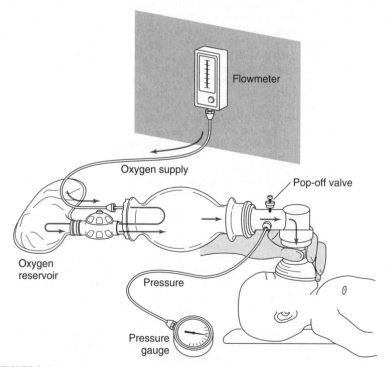

FIGURE 3–1. Bag-and-mask ventilation of the neonate.

Absolute indications for aggressive ventilatory support with endotracheal intubation are difficult to list here because institutional guidelines and clinical situations vary widely. The procedure for endotracheal intubation and some general guidelines are discussed in Chapter 28.

2. **Specific measures**

   a. **Term infant with meconium staining.** Infants born through thick meconium may aspirate this inflammatory material in utero (gasping), during delivery, or immediately after birth. The sickest of these infants have usually aspirated in utero and generally also have reactive pulmonary vasoconstriction. Gregory and associates were among the first to show that endotracheal suctioning at birth was beneficial. More recently, the AAP and the AHA recommended endotracheal suctioning when meconium is present in the amniotic fluid and the infant is not vigorous (e.g., without good muscle tone, good respirations, and heart rate >100 beats/min). **Clinical judgment** is always important in deciding whether or not aggressive endotracheal suctioning is necessary. Meconium aspiration is discussed in detail in Chapter 100. A randomized multicenter trial of intrapartum suctioning (ie, suctioning before delivery of the chest) of the hypopharynx has not shown any reduction in the risk of meconium aspiration syndrome, and this procedure is no longer recommended.

      i. **In nonvigorous infants (heart rate <100, poor tone, or poor respiratory effort), perform endotracheal suctioning. Do not stimulate the infant but proceed directly to intubate the trachea and apply suction directly to the endotracheal tube.** Suctioning with a negative pressure of 80–100 mm Hg can be done directly from the wall unit via a connector (meconium aspirator) to the endotracheal tube. Suction is applied as the endotracheal tube is slowly withdrawn.

      ii. **If meconium has been suctioned "below the cords," suctioning should be repeated after reintubation.** Prolonged or repeated suctioning is not recommended because it will exacerbate the preexisting asphyxial insult.

      iii. **The procedures just described may be continued for up to 2 min after delivery,** but then other resuscitative measures (particularly ventilation) must be started.

      iv. **If meconium-stained fluid is reported at <34 weeks' gestation,** one of the following situations should be suspected:
         (a) The fetus is a growth-restricted term infant.
         (b) The fluid may actually be purulent (consider *Listeria* or *Pseudomonas*).
         (c) The fluid may actually be bile stained (consider proximal intestinal obstruction).

   b. **Term infant with perinatal asphyxia**

      i. **Initially all infants without meconium-stained amniotic fluid should be dried and have their oropharynx suctioned.** If the infant is not vigorous (strong cry, good tone) a brief period of tactile stimulation, by rubbing the back and/or tapping the soles of the feet, can be used. Follow immediately by evaluating respirations, heart rate, and color.

      ii. **A term infant with a heart rate of <100 beats/min and no spontaneous respiratory activity requires positive-pressure ventilation.** If brief tactile stimulation fails to stimulate adequate respirations, positive-pressure ventilation should be initiated at 40–60 breaths/min. If this is not successful in stimulating spontaneous respiratory effort or an improved heart rate, airway patency and positioning of the mask should be confirmed, then peak inflating pressures should be adjusted as necessary to expand the lungs. If bag-and-mask ventilation is ineffective or prolonged positive-pressure ventilation is necessary, endotracheal intubation is indicated.

      iii. **A term infant with a heart rate of >100 beats/min but with poor skin color and weak respiratory activity requires stimulation (rubbing the** back or tapping the soles of the feet are often effective), supplemental oxygen blown across the face, and occasionally bag-and-mask ventilation to expand the lungs. Most of these infants respond with improved skin color and good spontaneous respiratory effort by 5 min of age.

   c. Preterm infant. Preterm infants weighing <1200 g most often require immediate lung expansion in the delivery room.

      i. **If intubation is required,** a smaller (2.5- or 3-mm internal diameter) endotracheal tube is selected.

      ii. **Although high-peak inflating pressures may initially be needed to expand the lungs,** as soon as the lungs "open up" the pressure should be quickly decreased to as low as 20–25 cm H_2O by the end of the resuscitation if the clinical course permits.

      iii. **If available, one of several forms of liquid surfactant may be administered intratracheally as prophylaxis for respiratory distress syndrome** (see Chapters 7 and 89). However, surfactant is not a resuscitative medication and should be administered only to a stable neonate with a correctly placed endotracheal tube.

B. Cardiac resuscitation. During delivery room resuscitation, efforts should be directed first to assisting ventilation and providing supplemental oxygen. A sluggish heart rate usually responds to these efforts.

   1. If the heart rate continues to be <60 beats/min in spite of 30 s of positive-pressure ventilation, chest compression should be initiated. The thumbs are placed on the lower third of the sternum, between the xiphoid and the line drawn between the nipples (Figure 3–2). Alternatively, the middle and ring

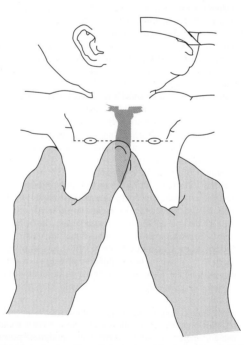

FIGURE 3–2. Technique of external cardiac massage (chest compression) in the neonate. Note the position of the thumbs on the lower third of the sternum, between the xiphoid and the line drawn between the nipples.

finger of one hand can be placed on the sternum while the other hand supports the back. The sternum is compressed a third of the anteroposterior diameter of the chest at a regular rate of 90 compressions/min while ventilating the infant at 30 breaths/min, synchronized so every three compressions are followed by one breath. The heart rate should be checked periodically and chest compression discontinued when the heart rate is >60 beats/min.

2. **An infant with no heart rate (a true Apgar of 0) who does not respond to ventilation and oxygenation may be considered stillborn.** Prolonged resuscitative efforts are a matter for ethical consideration. The AAP and AHA state that if there is no heart rate after 10 min of adequate resuscitation efforts, discontinuation of resuscitation efforts may be appropriate.

C. **Drugs used in resuscitation.** (See also Emergency Medications and Therapy for Neonates, inside the front and back covers.) The *Textbook of Neonatal Resuscitation* recommends giving medications if the heart rate remains <60 beats/min despite adequate ventilation and chest compressions for a minimum of 30 s.

1. **Route of administration**

   a. **The umbilical vein** is the preferred route for rapid drug administration in the delivery room. A no. 3.5 or 5F umbilical catheter should be inserted just until blood is easily withdrawn (usually 2–4 cm); this should avoid inadvertent placement in the hepatic or portal vein. Formal umbilical vein catheterization is discussed in Chapter 38.

   b. **The endotracheal tube** is the fastest route for administration of epinephrine in the delivery room, but absorption is variable. This route may be used while vascular access is being obtained. See Chapter 28 for medications that can be administered by this route.

   c. **Alternate routes** of administration include peripheral venous (Chapter 37) and interosseous routes (Chapter 35).

2. **Drugs**

   a. **Epinephrine** may be necessary during resuscitation when adequate ventilation, oxygenation, and chest compression have failed and the heart rate is still <60 beats/min. This drug causes peripheral vasoconstriction, enhances cardiac contractility, and increases heart rate. **The dose is 0.1–0.3 mL/kg of 1:10,000 solution given intravenously or 0.3–1 mL/kg of 1:10,000 if given by the endotracheal tube.** This may be repeated every 3–5 min.

   b. **Volume expanders.** Hypovolemia should be suspected in any infant requiring resuscitation, particularly when there is evidence of acute blood loss with extreme pallor despite adequate oxygenation, poor peripheral pulse volume despite a normal heart rate, long capillary refill times, or poor response to resuscitative efforts. **Appropriate volume expanders include O-negative whole blood (cross-matched against the mother's blood), 10 mL/kg; Ringer's lactate, 10 mL/kg; and normal saline, 10 mL/kg. All are given intravenously over 5–10 min.**

   c. **Naloxone hydrochloride.** Naloxone (Narcan) is a narcotic antagonist and can be administered to an infant with respiratory depression unresponsive to ventilatory assistance whose mother has received narcotics within 4 h before delivery. The initial corrective action is positive-pressure ventilation. One major contraindication to the use of naloxone is the newborn infant of a mother chronically exposed to narcotics. These infants should never receive Narcan because acute withdrawal symptoms may develop. **The intravenous or intramuscular dosage for Narcan is 0.1 mg/kg.** Two concentrations of naloxone are available: 0.4 mg/mL and 1.0 mg/mL. The dose may be repeated every 5 min as necessary. It should be emphasized that the half-life of Narcan is shorter than that of narcotics.

   d. **Dextrose.** The blood glucose concentration should be checked within 30 min after delivery in asphyxiated term infants, infants of diabetic mothers, and preterm infants, especially those whose mothers received tocolysis with ritodrine. Large boluses of dextrose should be avoided, even when the blood sugar is <25 mg/dL. To avoid wide swings in blood glucose, give a small bolus of **10% dextrose in water (2 mL/kg intravenously), and then begin an intravenous infusion of 10% dextrose at a rate of 4–6 mg/kg/min (80–100 mL/kg/day).**

e. **Sodium bicarbonate** is usually not useful during the acute phase of neonatal resuscitation. Without adequate ventilation and oxygenation, it will not improve the blood pH and may worsen cerebral acidosis. After prolonged resuscitation, however, sodium bicarbonate may be useful in correcting documented metabolic acidosis. **Give 1–2 mEq/kg intravenously at a rate of 1 mEq/kg/min or slower.**

f. **Atropine and calcium.** Although previously used during resuscitation of the asphyxiated newborn, **atropine and calcium are no longer recommended** by the AAP or the AHA.

D. Other supportive measures

1. **Temperature regulation.** Although some degree of cooling in a newborn infant is desirable because it provides a normal stimulus to respiratory effort, excessive cooling increases oxygen consumption and exacerbates acidosis. This is a problem especially for preterm infants, who have thin skin, decreased stores of body fat, and increased body surface area. Heat loss may be prevented by the following measures.

   a. **Dry the infant thoroughly immediately after delivery.**

   b. **Maintain a warm delivery room.**

   c. **Place the infant under a prewarmed radiant warmer** (Chapter 6). Cover extremely preterm infants (<28 weeks' gestation or <1000 g) with plastic wrap or a plastic bag up to the neck.

2. **Preparation of the parents for resuscitation.** Initial resuscitation usually occurs in the delivery room with one or both parents present. It is helpful to prepare the parents in advance, if possible. Describe what will be done, who will be present, who will explain what is happening, where the resuscitation will take place, where the father should stand, why crying may not be heard, and where the infant will be taken after stabilization.

Selected References

Battaglia FC, Lubchenco LO: A practical classification of newborn infants by weight and gestational age. *J Pediatr* 1967;71(2):159-163.

Dawes GS: *Foetal & Neonatal Physiology.* Year Book, 1968.

Gregory GA et al: Meconium aspiration in infants—a prospective study. *J Pediatr* 1974; 85(6):848-852.

Kattwinkel J: *Textbook of Neonatal Resuscitation,* 5th ed. American Academy of Pediatrics and American Heart Association, 2006.

Merril JD, Ballard RA: Resuscitation in the delivery room. In: Taeusch HW et al (eds): *Avery's Diseases of the Newborn,* 8th ed. Philadephia: Elsevier Saunders, 2005;349-363.

O'Donnell CP et al: Clinical assessment of infant colour at delivery. *Arch Dis Child Fetal Neonatal Ed* 2007; 92(6):F465-F467.

Richmond S, Goldsmith JP: Air or 100% oxygen in neonatal resuscitation? *Clin Perinatol* 2006;33:11-27.

Vain NE et al: Oropharyngeal and nasopharyngeal suctioning of meconium-stained neonates before delivery of their shoulders: multicentre, randomised controlled trial. *Lancet* 2004;364(9434):597-602.

Watkinson M: Temperature control of premature infants in the delivery room. *Clin Perinatol* 2006;33(1):43-53.

Wiswell TE et al: Delivery room management of the apparently vigorous meconium-stained neonate: results of the multicenter, international collaborative trial. *Pediatrics* 2000;105(1 Pt 1):1-7.

4 Assessment of Gestational Age

Gestational age can be determined prenatally by the following techniques: date of last menstrual period, date of first reported fetal activity (quickening usually occurs at 16–18 weeks), first reported heart sounds (10–12 weeks by Doppler ultrasound examination), and ultrasound examination (very accurate if obtained before 20 weeks' gestation). The most reliable measure of gestational age is done prenatally during the first trimester. Postnatal gestational age assessment is unreliable in infants that are extremely premature and postterm. The American Academy of Pediatrics recommends that all newborns be classified by birthweight and gestational age. The most common techniques for determining gestational age in the immediate postnatal period are discussed in this chapter.

I. **Classification.** Infants are classified as **preterm** (<37 weeks), **term** (37–41 6/7 weeks), or **postterm** (≥42 weeks). Refinements developed in neonatal assessment have provided additional classifications based on a combination of features.

  A. **Small for gestational age (SGA)** is defined as 2 standard deviations below the mean weight for gestational age or below the 10th percentile (see Appendix E). (For a full discussion, see Chapter 97.) SGA is commonly seen in infants of mothers who have hypertension or preeclampsia or who smoke. This condition is associated with maternal factors (chronic disease, malnutrition, conditions affecting the blood flow and oxygenation in the placenta), placental factors (infarction, previa, abruption, anatomic malformations, etc.) and fetal factors (congenital infections [TORCH; see Chapter 127], chromosomal abnormalities, dysmorphic syndromes, and other congenital anomalies).

  B. **Appropriate for gestational age (AGA).** See Appendix E.

  C. **Large for gestational age (LGA)** is defined as 2 standard deviations above the mean weight for gestational age or above the 90th percentile (see Appendix E). LGA can be seen in infants of diabetic mothers (see Chapter 94), infants with Beckwith-Wiedemann syndrome and other syndromes, constitutionally large infants with large parents, or infants with hydrops fetalis.

II. **Methods of determining postnatal gestational age**

  A. **Rapid delivery room assessment.** The most useful clinical signs in differentiating among premature, borderline mature, and full-term infants are (in order of usefulness): creases in the sole of the foot, size of the breast nodule, nature of the scalp hair, cartilaginous development of the earlobe, and scrotal rugae and testicular descent in males. These signs and findings are listed in Table 4–1, which enables one to make a rapid assessment at delivery.

  B. **New Ballard Score.** The Ballard maturational score has been expanded and updated to include extremely premature infants. It has been renamed the New Ballard Score (NBS). The score now spans from 10 (correlating with 20 weeks' gestation) to 50 (correlating with 44 weeks' gestation). It is best performed at <12 h of age if the infant is <26 weeks' gestation. If the infant is >26 weeks' gestation, there is no optimal age of examination up to 96 h.

    1. **Accuracy.** The examination is accurate whether the infant is sick or well to within 2 weeks of gestational age. It overestimates gestational age by 2–4 days in infants between 32 and 37 weeks' gestation.

    2. **Criteria.** The examination consists of six neuromuscular criteria and six physical criteria. The neuromuscular criteria are based on the understanding that passive tone is more useful than active tone in indicating gestational age.

    3. **Procedure.** The examination is administered twice by two different examiners to ensure objectivity, and the data are entered on the chart (Figure 4–1). This form is available in most nurseries. The examination consists of two parts: neuromuscular

Table 4–1. **CRITERIA FOR RAPID GESTATIONAL ASSESSMENT AT DELIVERY**

Feature	36 Wk and Earlier	37–38 Wk	39 Wk and Beyond
Creases in soles of feet	One or two transverse creases; posterior three fourths of sole smooth	Multiple creases; anterior two thirds of heel smooth	Entire sole, including heel, covered with creases
Breast nodule[a]	2 mm	4 mm	7 mm
Scalp hair	Fine and woolly; fuzzy	Fine and woolly; fuzzy	Coarse and silky; each hair single-stranded
Earlobe	No cartilage	Moderate amount of cartilage	Stiff earlobe with thick cartilage
Testes and scrotum	Testes partially descended; scrotum small, with few rugae	?	Testes fully descended; scrotum normal size, with prominent rugae

[a]The breast nodule is not palpable before 33 weeks. Underweight full-term infants may have retarded breast development.

Usher R et al: Judgment of fetal age: II. Clinical significance of gestational age and objective measurement. *Pediatr Clin North Am* 1966;13:835. Modified and reproduced with permission from Elsevier Science.

maturity and physical maturity. The 12 scores are totaled, and maturity rating is expressed in weeks of gestation, estimated by using the chart provided on the form. Part 2 of the form (Figure 4–2) is then used to plot gestational assessment against weight, length, and head circumference to determine whether the infant is SGA, AGA, or LGA. These are the so-called **Lubchenco charts.**

a. **Neuromuscular maturity**

   i. **Posture.** Score 0 if the arms and legs are extended, and score 1 if the infant has beginning flexion of the knees and hips, with arms extended; determine other scores based on the diagram.

   ii. **Square window.** Flex the hand on the forearm between the thumb and index finger of the examiner. Apply sufficient pressure to achieve as much flexion as possible. Visually measure the angle between the hypothenar eminence and the ventral aspect of the forearm. Determine the score based on the diagram.

   iii. **Arm recoil.** Flex the forearms for 5 s; then grasp the hand and fully extend the arm and release. If the arm returns to full flexion, give a score of 4. For lesser degrees of flexion, score as noted on the diagram.

   iv. **Popliteal angle.** Hold the thigh in the knee-chest position with the left index finger and the thumb supporting the knee. Then extend the leg by gentle pressure from the right index finger behind the ankle. Measure the angle at the popliteal space and score accordingly.

   v. **Scarf sign.** Take the infant's hand and try to put it around the neck posteriorly as far as possible over the opposite shoulder and score according to the diagram.

   vi. **Heel to ear.** Keeping the pelvis flat on the table, take the infant's foot and try to put it as close to the head as possible without forcing it. Grade according to the diagram.

b. **Physical maturity.** These characteristics are scored as shown in Figure 4–1.

   i. **Skin.** Carefully look at the skin and grade according to the diagram. Extremely premature infants have sticky, transparent skin and receive a score of −1.

   ii. **Lanugo hair** is examined on the infant's back and between and over the scapulae.

Name _____ Date/Time of birth _____ Sex _____

Hospital No. _____ Date/Time of exam _____ Birth weight _____

Race _____ Age when examined _____ Length _____

Apgar score: 1 minute _____ 5 minutes _____ 10 minutes _____ Head circ. _____

Examiner _____

SCORE

Neuromuscular _____

Physical _____

Total _____

Maturity rating

Score	Weeks
−10	20
−5	22
0	24
5	26
10	28
15	30
20	32
25	34
30	36
35	38
40	40
45	42
50	44

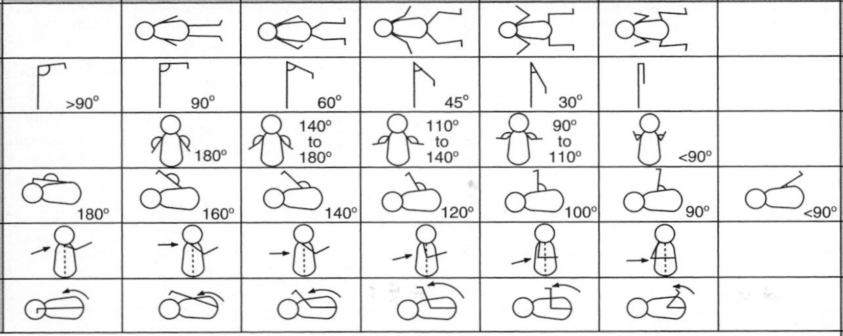

Neuromuscular maturity

Neuromuscular maturity sign	−1	0	1	2	3	4	5	Record score here
Posture								
Square window (wrist)	>90°	90°	60°	45°	30°	0°		
Arm recoil		180°	140° to 180°	110° to 140°	90° to 110°	<90°		
Popliteal angle	180°	160°	140°	120°	100°	90°	<90°	
Scarf sign								
Heel to ear								

Total neuromuscular maturity score

FIGURE 4–1. Maturational assessment of gestational age (New Ballard Score). (*Reproduced, with permission, from Ballard JL et al: New Ballard Score, expanded to include extremely premature infants.* J Pediatr 1991;119:417.)

25

Physical maturity

Physical maturity sign	Score								Record score here
	−1	0	1	2	3	4	5		
Skin	sticky friable transparent	gelatinous red translucent	smooth pink visible veins	superficial peeling &/or rash, few veins	cracking pale areas rare veins	parchment deep cracking no vessels	leathery cracked wrinkled		
Lanugo	none	sparse	abundant	thinning	bald areas	mostly bald			
Plantar surface	heel-toe 40–50 mm: −1 <40 mm: −2	>50 mm no crease	faint red marks	anterior transverse crease only	creases ant. 2/3	creases over entire sole			
Breast	imperceptible	barely perceptible	flat areola no bud	stippled areola 1–2 mm bud	raised areola 3–4 mm bud	full areola 5–10 mm bud			
Eye/ear	lids fused loosely: −1 tightly: −2	lids open pinna flat stays folded	sl. curved pinna; soft slow recoil	well curved pinna; soft but ready recoil	formed and firm, instant recoil	thick cartilage ear stiff			
Genitals (male)	scrotum flat, smooth	scrotum empty, faint rugae	testes in upper canal rare rugae	testes descending few rugae	testes down good rugae	testes pendulous deep rugae			
Genitals (female)	clitoris prominent & labia flat	prominent clitoris & small labia minora	prominent clitoris & enlarging minora	majora & minora equally prominent	majora large minora small	majora cover clitoris & minora			
							Total physical maturity score		

Gestational age (weeks)

By dates _____
By ultrasound _____
By exam _____

FIGURE 4-1. (*Continued*)

Name _____   Date of exam _____   Length _____

Hospital No. _____   Sex _____   Head circ. _____

Race _____   Birth weight _____   Gestational age _____

Date of birth _____

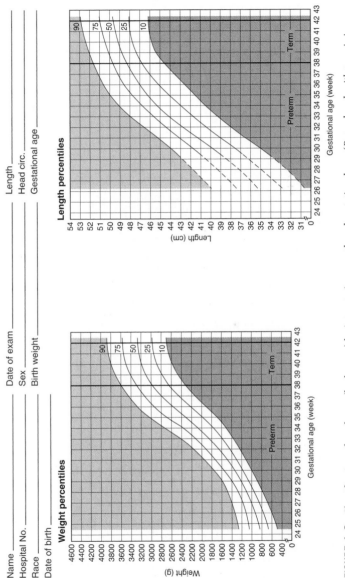

Weight percentiles

Length percentiles

FIGURE 4–2. Classification of newborns (both sexes) by intrauterine growth and gestational age. (*Reproduced, with permission, from Battagli FC, Lubchenco LO: A practical classification for newborn infants by weight and gestational age.* J Pediatr 1967;71:159; *and Lubchenco LO et al: Intrauterine growth in length and head circumference as estimated from live births at gestational ages from 26 to 42 weeks.* Pediatrics 1966;37:403. *Courtesy of Ross Laboratories, Columbus, Ohio 43216.*)

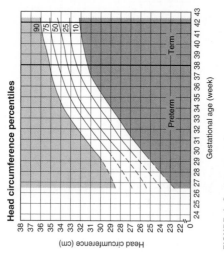

Classification of infant*	Weight	Length	Head circ.
Large for gestational age (LGA) (>90th percentile)			
Appropriate for gestational age (AGA) (10th to 90th percentile)			
Small for gestational age (SGA) (<10th percentile)			

*Place an "X" in the appropriate box (LGA, AGA, or SGA) for weight, for length, and for head circumference.

Head circumference percentiles

Head circumference (cm)

90
75
50
25
10

Preterm — Term

24 25 26 27 28 29 30 31 32 33 34 35 36 37 38 39 40 41 42 43

Gestational age (week)

FIGURE 4–2. (*Continued*)

iii. **Plantar surface.** Measure foot length from the tip of the great toe to the back of the heel. If the results are <40 mm, then give a score of −2. If it is between 40 and 50 mm, assign a score of −1. If the measurement is >50 mm and no creases are seen on the plantar surface, give a score of 0. If there are creases, score accordingly.

iv. **Breast.** Palpate any breast tissue and score.

v. **Eye and ear.** This section has been expanded to include criteria that apply to the extremely premature infant. Loosely fused eyelids are defined as closed, but gentle traction opens them. Score this as −1. Tightly fused eyelids are defined as inseparable by gentle traction. Base the rest of the score on open lids and the examination of the ear.

vi. **Genitalia.** Score according to the diagram.

C. **Direct ophthalmoscopy.** Another method for determination of gestational age uses direct ophthalmoscopy of the lens. Before 27 weeks, the cornea is too opaque to allow visualization; after 34 weeks, atrophy of the vessels of the lens occurs. Therefore, this technique allows for accurate determination of gestational age at 27–34 weeks only. This method is reliable to ±2 weeks. The pupil must be dilated under the supervision of an ophthalmologist, and the assessment must be performed within 48 h of birth before the vessels atrophy. The following grading system is used, as shown in Figure 4–3.

1. **Grade 4 (27–28 weeks):** Vessels cover the entire anterior surface of the lens or the vessels meet in the center of the lens.

2. **Grade 3 (29–30 weeks):** Vessels do not meet in the center but are close. Central portion of the lens is not covered by vessels.

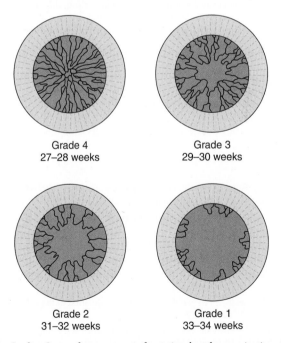

Grade 4
27–28 weeks

Grade 3
29–30 weeks

Grade 2
31–32 weeks

Grade 1
33–34 weeks

FIGURE 4–3. Grading System for assessment of gestational age by examination of the anterior vascular capsule of the lens. (*Reproduced, with permission, from Hittner HM et al: Assessment of gestational age by examination of the anterior vascular capsule of the lens. J Pediatr 1977; 91:455.*)

3. **Grade 2 (31–32 weeks):** Vessels reach only to the middle-outer part of the lens. The central clear portion of the lens is larger.
4. **Grade 1 (33–34 weeks):** Vessels are seen only at the periphery of the lens.

D. **Other methods of gestational assessment**
1. **Femur length measurement.** The shaft of the femur is imaged and measured using calipers and gestational age was estimated from tables of fetal femur length. Results found excellent correlation($r = 0.93$) when using this method for infants <1500 g without intrauterine growth restriction.
2. **Fetal foot length.** An ultrasound was done on the fetal foot, and measurements were taken from the heel to the end of the big toe. Results found a statistically significant linear correlation between the fetal foot length and gestational age.
3. **Cranial ultrasound assessment.** Anatomic features of the cerebral hemispheres were studied by ultrasound. A scoring system was devised based on anatomic and ultrasound appearance. There was a positive correlation between ultrasound score and gestational age.
4. **Cerebellar dimension assessment.** The area, circumference, and vertical length of the vermis and the area, circumference, and maximum transverse width of the cerebellar body were measured on ultrasound. All of these were found to correlate with gestational age.
5. **Fetal scapular length.** Scapular length (cm) was measured in infants between 15 and 42 weeks' gestation (infants at gestational age >26 weeks were only included if their estimated fetal weight was between the 10th and 90th percentile). Scapular length can predict gestational age in infants with normal growth.
6. **Maturational changes in skin color.** Using a tristimulus photo-colorimeter, the skin color was examined. The "L," which represents lightness or darkness, changes from black to white with maturation and can be directly correlated with gestational age.

Selected References

Amiel-Tison C: Neurological evaluation of the maturity of newborn infants. *Arch Dis Child* 1968;43:89.

Ballard JL et al: A simplified score for assessment of fetal maturation of newly born infants. *J Pediatr* 1979;95:769.

Ballard JL et al: New Ballard Score, expanded to include extremely premature infants. *J Pediatr* 1991;119:417.

Chatterjee MS et al: Fetal foot: evaluation of gestational age. www.TheFetus.net, 1994.

Dodd V: Gestational age assessment. *Neonatal Netw* 1996;15:1.

Dubowitz LM et al: Clinical assessment of gestational age in the newborn infant. *J Pediatr* 1970;77:1.

Farr V et al: The definition of some external characteristics used in the assessment of gestational age in the newborn infant. *Dev Med Child Neurol* 1966;8:657.

Fletcher MA: Ch. 3 *Assessment of Gestational Age. Physical Diagnosis of Neonatology,* 1st ed. Philadelphia: Lippincott Raven, 1998;55-66.

Hittner HM et al: Assessment of gestational age by examination of the anterior vascular capsule of the lens. *J Pediatr* 1977;91:455.

Mackanjee HR et al: Assessment of postnatal gestational age using sonographic measurements of femur length. *J Ultrasound Med* 1996;15(2):115-120.

Murphy NP et al: Cranial ultrasound assessment of gestational age in low birthweight infants. *Arch Dis Child* 1989;64:569-572.

Sherer DM et al: Fetal scapular length in the ultrasonographic assessment of gestational age. *J Ultrasound Med* 1994;13(7):523-528.

Usher R et al: Judgment of fetal age: II. Clinical significance of gestational age and objective measurement. *Pediatr Clin North Am* 1966;13:835.

Watanabe M et al: Maturational changes in skin color of Japanese newborn infants. *Neonatology* 2007;91:275-280.

5 Newborn Physical Examination

Newborns are examined after birth to check for major abnormalities and to make sure the transition to extrauterine life is without difficulty. The newborn infant should undergo a complete physical examination within 24 h of birth. It is easier to listen to the heart and lungs first when the infant is quiet. Warming the stethoscope before using it decreases the likelihood of making the infant cry.

I. **Vital signs**
   A. **Temperature.** Indicate whether the temperature is rectal (which is usually 1° higher than oral), oral, or axillary (which is usually 1° lower than oral).
   B. **Respirations.** The normal respiratory rate in a newborn is 40-60 breaths/min.
   C. **Blood pressure.** Blood pressure correlates directly with gestational age, postnatal age of the infant, and birthweight. (For normal blood pressure curves, see Appendix C.)
   D. **Pulse rate.** The normal pulse rate is 100-180 beats/min in the newborn (usually 120-160 beats/min when awake, 70-80 beats/min when asleep). In the healthy infant, the heart rate increases with stimulation.

II. **Head circumference, length, weight, and gestational age**
   A. **Head circumference and percentile.** (For growth charts, see Appendix E.) Place the measuring tape around the front of the head (above the brow [the frontal area]) and the occipital area. The tape should be above the ears. This is known as the occipitofrontal circumference, which is normally 32-37 cm at term.
   B. **Length and percentile.** For growth charts, see Appendix E.
   C. **Weight and percentile.** For growth charts, see Appendix E.
   D. **Assessment of gestational age.** See Chapter 4.

III. **General appearance.** Observe the infant and record the general appearance (eg, activity, skin color, and obvious congenital abnormalities). Are the general movements normal? Is the skin tone normal?

IV. **Skin.** See also Chapter 68.
   A. **Color**
      1. **Plethora (deep, rosy red [ruddy] color).** Plethora is more common in infants with polycythemia but can be seen in an overoxygenated or overheated infant. It is best to obtain a central hematocrit on any plethoric infant. Erythema neonatorum is a condition in which an infant has an overall blush to reddish color. It usually appears in the transition period and can occur when the infant has been stimulated. This is a normal phenomenon and lasts only several hours.
      2. **Jaundice (yellowish color if secondary to indirect hyperbilirubinemia, greenish color if secondary to direct hyperbilirubinemia).** With jaundice, bilirubin levels are usually >5 mg/dL. This condition is abnormal in infants <24 h old and may signify Rh incompatibility, sepsis, and TORCH (*t*oxoplasmosis,

*o*ther, *r*ubella, *c*ytomegalovirus, and *h*erpes simplex virus) infections. After 24 h, it may result either from these diseases or from such common causes as ABO incompatibility or physiologic causes.

3. **Pallor (washed-out, whitish appearance).** Pallor may be secondary to anemia, birth asphyxia, shock, or patent ductus arteriosus (PDA). *Ductal pallor* is the term sometimes used to denote pallor associated with PDA.

4. **Cyanosis (desaturation of 5 g of hemoglobin usually necessary for one to note a bluish color)**

    a. **Central cyanosis (bluish skin, including the tongue and lips).** Central cyanosis is caused by low oxygen saturation in the blood. It may be associated with congenital heart or lung disease.

    b. **Peripheral cyanosis (bluish skin with pink lips and tongue).** Peripheral cyanosis may be associated with methemoglobinemia, which occurs when hemoglobin oxidizes from the ferrous to the ferric form; the blood actually can have a chocolate hue. Methemoglobin is incapable of transporting oxygen or carbon dioxide. This disorder can be caused by exposure to certain drugs or chemicals (eg, nitrates or nitrites) or may be hereditary (eg, NADH-methemoglobin reductase deficiency or hemoglobin M disease [NADH is the reduced form of nicotinamide adenine dinucleotide]). Treatment for infants is with methylene blue.

    c. **Acrocyanosis (bluish hands and feet only).** Acrocyanosis may be normal for an infant who has just been born (or within the first few hours after birth) or for one who is experiencing cold stress. It can be seen up to 24 h of life. If the condition is seen in an older infant with a normal temperature, decreased peripheral perfusion secondary to hypovolemia should be considered.

5. **Extensive bruising (ecchymoses)** may be associated with a prolonged and difficult delivery and may result in early jaundice. Petechiae (pinpoint hemorrhages) can be limited to one area and are usually of no concern. If they are widespread and progressive, then they are of concern and a workup for coagulopathy should be considered.

6. **"Blue on pink" or "pink on blue."** Whereas some infants are pink and well perfused and others are clearly cyanotic, some do not fit in either of these categories. They may appear bluish with pink undertones or pink with bluish undertones. This coloration may be secondary to poor perfusion, inadequate oxygenation, inadequate ventilation, or polycythemia.

7. **Harlequin sign (coloration) (clear line of demarcation between an area of redness and an area of normal coloration).** This is a vascular phenomenon and the cause is usually unknown. The coloration can be benign and transient (lasting usually a few seconds to <30 min) or can be indicative of shunting of blood (persistent pulmonary hypertension or coarctation of the aorta). There can be varying degrees of redness and perfusion. The demarcating line may run from the head to the belly, dividing the body into right and left halves, or it may develop in the dependent half of the body when the newborn is lying on one side. The dependent half is usually deep red and the upper half is pale. This occurs most commonly in lower birthweight infants. (*Note:* This is not **Harlequin fetus;** see Section IV A, 12.)

8. **Mottling (lacy red pattern)** may be seen in healthy infants and in those with cold stress, hypovolemia, or sepsis. It can be caused by dilation of capillaries and is usually seen on the extremities but can be seen on the trunk. **Cutis marmorata,** or **persistent mottling,** is found in infants with Down syndrome, Cornelia de Lange syndrome, trisomy 13, or trisomy 18. It can also be seen in hypothyroidism, cardiovascular hypertension, and central nervous system dysfunction.

9. **Vernix caseosa.** This greasy white substance covers the skin until the 38th week of gestation. Its purpose is to provide a moisture barrier. It is completely normal.

10. **Collodion infant.** In this condition, the skin resembles parchment, and there can be some restriction in growth of the nose and ears. This may be a normal condition or can be a manifestation of another disease.

11. **Dry skin.** Most term infants do not have dry skin. Postdate or postmature infants can exhibit excessive peeling of skin. Congenital syphilis and candidiasis can present with peeling skin at birth.

12. **Harlequin fetus.** This is the most severe form of congenital ichthyosis. The infants have thickening of the keratin layer of skin that causes thick scales. Survival of these infants has improved with supportive care.

13. **Cutis aplasia.** Absence of some or all the layers of the skin. Most common is a solitary area on the scalp (70%). Excellent prognosis. If the area is large, surgical repair may be necessary.

B. **Rashes**

1. **Milia.** Milia is a rash in which tiny sebaceous retention cysts are seen. The whitish pinhead-size concretions are usually on the chin, nose, forehead, and cheeks. No erythema is seen. These benign cysts disappear within a few weeks after birth. These are seen in ~33% of infants. Pearls are large single milia that can occur on the genitalia and areola.

2. **Erythema toxicum.** In erythema toxicum, numerous small areas of red skin with a yellow-white papule in the center are evident. Lesions are most noticeable 48 h after birth but may appear as late as 7–10 days. Wright staining of the papule reveals eosinophils. This benign rash, which is the most common type, resolves spontaneously. If suspected in an infant younger than 34 weeks' gestation, it is best to rule out other causes because this rash is more common in term infants.

3. *Candida albicans* **rash.** *C. albicans* diaper rash appears as erythematous plaques with sharply demarcated edges. Satellite bodies (pustules on contiguous areas of skin) are also seen. Usually, the skinfolds are involved. Gram's stain of a smear or 10% potassium hydroxide preparation of the lesion reveals budding yeast spores, which are easily treated with nystatin ointment or cream applied to the rash four times daily for 7–10 days.

4. **Transient neonatal pustular melanosis** is a benign, self-limiting condition that requires no specific therapy. It is characterized by three stages of lesions, which may appear over the entire body:
   a. Pustules.
   b. Ruptured vesicopustules with scaling/typical halo appearance.
   c. Hyperpigmented macules.

5. **Acne neonatorum.** The lesions are typically seen over the cheeks, chin, and forehead and consist of comedones and papules. The condition is usually benign and requires no therapy; however, severe cases may require treatment with mild keratolytic agents.

6. **Herpes simplex.** One can see a pustular vesicular rash, vesicles, bullae, or denuded skin. The rash is most commonly seen at the fetal scalp monitor site, occiput, or buttocks (presentation site at time of delivery). Tzanck smear reveals multinucleated giant cells.

C. **Nevi.** Hemangiomas near the eyes, nose, or mouth that interfere with vital functions or sight may need surgical intervention.

1. **Macular hemangioma ("stork bites").** A macular hemangioma is a true vascular nevus normally seen on the occipital area, eyelids, and glabella. The lesions disappear spontaneously within the first year of life.

2. **Port-wine stain (nevus flammeus)** is usually seen at birth, does not blanch with pressure, and does not disappear with time. If the lesion appears over the forehead and upper lip, then **Sturge-Weber syndrome** (port-wine stain over the forehead and upper lip, glaucoma, and contralateral jacksonian seizures) must be ruled out.

3. **Mongolian spot.** Mongolian spots are dark blue or purple bruise-like macular spots usually located over the sacrum. Usually present in 90% of blacks and Asians, they occur in <5% of white children and disappear by 4 years of age. They are the most common birthmark.

4. **Cavernous hemangioma.** A cavernous hemangioma usually appears as a large red, cyst-like, firm, ill-defined mass and may be found anywhere on the body. The majority of these lesions regress with age, but some require corticosteroid therapy. In more severe cases, surgical resection may be necessary. If associated with thrombocytopenia, **Kasabach-Merritt syndrome** (thrombocytopenia associated with a rapidly expanding hemangioma) should be considered. Transfusions of platelets and clotting factors are usually required in patients with this syndrome.

5. **Strawberry hemangioma (macular hemangioma).** Strawberry hemangiomas are flat, bright red, sharply demarcated lesions that are most commonly found on the face. Spontaneous regression usually occurs (70% disappearance by 7 years of age).

V. **Head.** Note the general shape of the head. Inspect for any cuts or bruises secondary to forceps or fetal monitor leads. Transillumination can be done for severe hydrocephalus and hydranencephaly. Check for microcephaly or macrocephaly.

A. **Macrocephaly.** Occipitofrontal circumference is >90th percentile. May be normal or be secondary to hydrocephaly, hydrencephaly, or a neuroendocrine or chromosomal disorder.

B. **Microcephaly.** Occipitofrontal circumference is <10th percentile. Brain atrophy or decreased size in the brain can occur.

C. **Anterior and posterior fontanelles.** The anterior fontanelle usually closes at 9–12 months and the posterior fontanelle at 2–4 months. A large anterior fontanelle is seen with hypothyroidism and may also be found in infants with skeletal disorders such as osteogenesis imperfecta, hypophosphatasia, and chromosomal abnormalities and in those who are small for gestational age. A bulging fontanelle may be associated with increased intracranial pressure, meningitis, or hydrocephalus. Depressed (sunken) fontanelles are seen in newborns with dehydration. A small anterior fontanelle may be associated with hyperthyroidism, microcephaly, or craniosynostosis.

D. **Molding.** Molding is a temporary asymmetry of the skull resulting from the birth process. Most often seen with prolonged labor and vaginal deliveries, it can be seen in cesarean deliveries if the mother had a prolonged course of labor before delivery. A normal head shape is usually regained within 1 week.

E. **Caput succedaneum.** Caput succedaneum is a diffuse edematous swelling of the soft tissues of the scalp that may extend across the suture lines. It is secondary to the pressure of the uterus or vaginal wall on areas of the fetal head bordering the caput. Usually, it resolves within several days (Figure 5–1).

F. **Cephalhematoma** is a subperiosteal hemorrhage that *never* extends across the suture line. It can be secondary to a traumatic delivery or forceps delivery. Radiographs or computed tomography scans of the head should be obtained if an underlying skull fracture is suspected (<5% of all cephalhematomas). Hematocrit and bilirubin levels should be monitored in these patients. Most cephalhematomas resolve in 2–3 weeks. Aspiration of the hematoma is rarely necessary (Figure 5–1).

G. **Subgaleal hematoma/hemorrhage.** Hemorrhage bleeding occurs below the epicranial aponeurosis. It can cross over the suture line and onto the neck or ear. It can be life threatening and may be necessary to replace blood volume lost and correct coagulopathy if present. It can be caused by asphyxia, vacuum extraction, or coagulopathy (Figure 5–1).

H. **Increased intracranial pressure.** The increased pressure may be secondary to hydrocephalus, hypoxic-ischemic brain injury, intracranial hemorrhage, or subdural

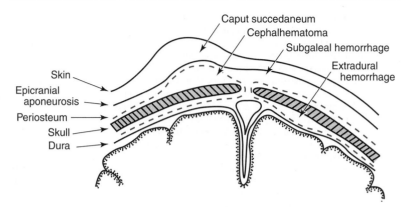

FIGURE 5–1. Types of extradural fluid collections seen in newborn infants. (*Volpe JJ: Neurology of the Newborn, 3rd ed. Philadelphia: WB Saunders, 1995; and based on data from Pape KE et al: Haemorrhage, Ischemia and the Perinatal Brain. Philadelphia: JB Lippincott,1979.*)

hematoma. The following signs are evident in an infant with increased intracranial pressure:

1. Bulging anterior fontanelle.
2. Separated sutures.
3. Paralysis of upward gaze (setting-sun sign).
4. Prominent veins of the scalp.
5. Increasing macrocephaly.

    I. **Craniosynostosis.** Craniosynostosis is the premature closure of one or more sutures of the skull. It should be considered in any infant with an asymmetric skull. On palpation of the skull, a bony ridge over the suture line may be felt, and inability to move the cranial bones freely may occur. Radiographs of the head should be performed, and surgical consultation may be necessary.

    J. **Craniotabes,** a benign condition, is a congenital softening or thinness of the skull that usually occurs around the suture lines (top and back of head) and disappears within days to a few weeks after birth. It can also be associated with rickets, osteogenesis imperfecta, syphilis, and subclinical vitamin D deficiency in utero.

    K. **Plagiocephaly.** Plagiocephaly is an oblique shape of a head, which is asymmetric and flattened. It can be seen in preemies and infants whose heads stay in the same position. Anterior plagiocephaly can be due to premature fusion of the coronal or lambdoidal sutures.

    L. **Brachycephaly.** This is caused by premature closure of the coronal suture and causes the head to have a short broad appearance. It can be seen in trisomy 21 or Apert syndrome.

    M. **Anencephaly.** The anterior neural tube does not close and the brain is malformed. Most of these infants are stillborn or die shortly after.

    N. **Acrocephaly.** The coronal and sagittal sutures close early. The skull has a narrow appearance with a cone shape at the top. This can be seen in Crouzon and Apert syndromes.

    O. **Dolichocephaly/Scaphocephaly.** The sagittal suture closes prematurely and there is a restriction of lateral growth of the skull, resulting in a long narrow head.

  VI. **Neck.** Eliciting the rooting reflex (see page 42) causes the infant to turn the head and allows easier examination of the neck. Palpate the sternocleidomastoid for a hematoma and the thyroid for enlargement, and check for thyroglossal duct cysts. A **short neck** is seen in Turner, Noonan, and Klippel-Feil syndromes. A **webbed neck** (with redundant skin) can be seen in Turner, Noonan, and Down syndromes. **A cystic hygroma is the most common neck mass.** It is a fluctuant mass that can be transilluminated and is usually found laterally or over the clavicles. A goiter or thyroglossal duct cyst is rarely seen at this age. **Torticollis** is a shortening of the sternocleidomastoid muscle that causes the head to go toward the affected side.

VII. **Face.** Look for obvious abnormalities. Note the general shape of the nose, mouth, and chin. Look for unequal movement of the mouth and lips. The presence of hypertelorism (eyes widely separated) or low-set ears should be noted.

   A. **Facial nerve injury.** Unilateral branches of the facial (eighth) nerve are most commonly involved. There is facial asymmetry with crying. The corner of the mouth droops, and the nasolabial fold is absent in the paralyzed side. The infant may be unable to close the eye or move the lip, and drools on the side of the paresis. If the palsy is secondary to trauma, most symptoms disappear within the first week of life, but sometimes resolution may take several months. If the palsy persists, absence of the nerve should be ruled out.

VIII. **Ears.** Look for an unusual shape or an abnormal position. The normal position is determined by drawing an imaginary horizontal line from the inner and outer canthi of the eye across the face, perpendicular to the vertical axis of the head. If the helix of the ear lies below this horizontal line, the ears are designated as low set. **Low-set ears** are seen with many congenital anomalies (most commonly Treacher Collins, triploidy, and trisomy 9 and 18 syndromes as well as fetal aminopterin effects). **Preauricular skin tags** (papillomas), which are benign, are common. **Hairy ears** are seen in infants of diabetic mothers. **Microtia** is a misshaped dysplastic ear that can be associated with other abnormalities such as middle ear abnormalities. **Otoscopic exam is usually not done at the first examination because the ear canals are full of amniotic debris.**

IX. **Eyes.** Check the red reflex with an ophthalmoscope. If the pupil is white, consider cataracts, glaucoma, or retinoblastoma. This requires an immediate evaluation by an ophthalmologist. If a cataract is present, opacification of the lens and loss of the reflex are apparent. Congenital cataracts require early evaluation by an ophthalmologist. The sclera, which is normally white, can have a bluish tint if the infant is premature because the sclera is thinner in these infants than in term infants. If the sclera is deep blue, **osteogenesis imperfecta** should be ruled out. A **coloboma** has a key-shaped defect in the iris.

   A. **Brushfield spots** (salt-and-pepper speckling of the iris or white or yellow spots on the iris) are often seen with Down syndrome or may be normal.

   B. **Subconjunctival hemorrhage.** Rupture of small conjunctival capillaries can occur normally but is more common after a traumatic delivery. This condition is seen in 5% of newborn infants.

   C. **Conjunctivitis.** If there is a discharge present, see Chapter 47.

   D. **Epicanthal folds.** May be normal or in Down syndrome, there is a skin fold of the upper eyelid covering the inner corner of the eye.

   E. **Leukocoria.** This is a white pupil and can be seen in cataract, retinoblastoma, vitreous hemorrhage, or retinal detachment. Further evaluation is necessary.

   F. **Nystagmus.** This is an involuntary usually rapid eye movement that can be horizontal, vertical, or mixed. Can be normal if occasional, but if persistent it needs to be evaluated.

   G. **Ptosis.** A drooping of an upper eyelid caused by third cranial nerve paralysis or weakness in the levator muscle.

X. **Nose.** If unilateral or bilateral choanal atresia is suspected, verify the patency of the nostrils with gentle passage of a nasogastric tube. **Infants are obligate nose breathers;** therefore, if they have **bilateral choanal atresia,** they will have cyanosis and severe respiratory distress at rest. Nasal flaring is indicative of respiratory distress. **Sniffling and discharge** are typical of congenital syphilis. **Sneezing** can be a response to bright light or drug withdrawal.

XI. **Mouth.** Examine the hard and soft palates for evidence of a cleft palate. A short lingual frenulum (tongue-tie) may require surgical treatment (especially if tongue mobility is limited).

   A. **Cleft lip/palate.** This is secondary to midline fusion failure.

   B. **Ranula.** A ranula is a cystic swelling in the floor of the mouth. Most disappear spontaneously.

   C. **Epstein pearls.** These keratin-containing cysts, which are normal, are located on the hard and soft palates and resolve spontaneously.

   D. **Mucocele.** This small lesion on the oral mucosa occurs secondary to trauma to the salivary gland ducts. It is usually benign and subsides spontaneously.

   E. **Natal teeth** are usually lower incisors. Radiographs are needed to differentiate the two types because management of each is different.

      1. **Predeciduous teeth.** Supernumerary teeth are found in 1 in 4000 births. They are usually loose, and the roots are absent or poorly formed. Removal is necessary to avoid aspiration.

      2. **True deciduous teeth.** These teeth are true teeth that erupt early. They occur in <1 in 2000 births. They should not be extracted.

   F. **Macroglossia.** Enlargement of the tongue can be congenital or acquired. Localized macroglossia is usually secondary to congenital hemangiomas. Macroglossia can be seen in **Beckwith syndrome** (macroglossia, gigantism, omphalocele, and severe hypoglycemia), **Pompe disease** (type II glycogen storage disease), and hypothyroidism.

   G. **Frothy or copious saliva** is commonly seen in infants with an esophageal atresia with tracheoesophageal fistula.

   H. **Thrush.** Oral thrush, common in newborns, is a sign of *C. albicans.*

   I. **Micrognathia.** This is an underdeveloped jaw that is seen in **Pierre Robin sequence**.

XII. **Chest**

   A. **Observation.** First, note whether the chest is symmetric. An asymmetric chest may signify a space or air-occupying lesion such as tension pneumothorax. Tachypnea, sternal and intercostal retractions, and grunting on expiration indicate respiratory distress.

   B. **Breath sounds.** Listen for the presence and equality of breath sounds. A good place to listen is in the right and left axillae. Absent or unequal sounds may indicate pneumothorax or atelectasis. Absent breath sounds with the presence of bowel sounds indicates a diaphragmatic hernia; an immediate radiograph and emergency surgical consultation are recommended.

   C. **Retractions.** Mild retractions usually subcostal are normal. Others are an indication of respiratory distress.

   D. **Pectus excavatum (funnel chest).** Pectus excavatum is a sternum that is depressed in shape. Usually, this condition is of no clinical concern. May be associated with Marfan and Noonan syndromes.

   E. **Pectus carinatum (pigeon chest).** This is caused by a protuberant sternum. May be associated with Marfan and Noonan syndromes.

   F. **Barrel chest.** A barrel chest occurs when there is an increased anteroposterior diameter of the chest. It can be secondary to mechanical ventilation, pneumothorax, pneumonia, or space-occupying lesions.

   G. **Breasts in a newborn** are usually 1 cm in diameter in term male and female infants. They may be abnormally enlarged (3–4 cm) secondary to the effects of maternal estrogens. This effect, which lasts <1 week, is of no clinical concern. A usually white discharge, commonly referred to as **"witch's milk,"** may be present. Supernumerary nipples (**polythelia**) are extra nipples along the mammary line ("milk line") and occur as a normal variant; the association with renal disorders is not ironclad but is supported by some studies.

XIII. Heart. Observe for heart rate (normal 110–160 beats/min awake, may drop to 80 beats/min during sleep), rhythm, quality of heart sounds, active precordium, and presence of a murmur. The position of the heart may be determined by auscultation. Abnormal situs syndromes are described in Chapter 81.

A. Murmurs may be associated with the following conditions:

1. **Ventricular septal defect (VSD)**, the most common heart defect, accounts for ~25% of congenital heart disease. Typically, a loud, harsh, blowing pansystolic murmur is heard (best heard over the lower left sternal border). Symptoms such as congestive heart failure usually do not begin until after 2 weeks of age and typically are present from 6 weeks to 4 months. The majority of these defects close spontaneously by the end of the first year of life.

2. **Patent ductus arteriosus (PDA)** is a harsh, continuous, machinery-type, or "rolling thunder" murmur that usually presents on the second or third day of life, localized to the second left intercostal space. It may radiate to the left clavicle or down the left sternal border. A hyperactive precordium is also seen. Clinical signs include wide pulse pressure and bounding pulses.

3. **Coarctation of the aorta,** a systolic ejection murmur, radiates down the sternum to the apex and to the interscapular area. It is often loudest in the back.

4. **Peripheral pulmonic stenosis (PPS).** A systolic murmur is heard bilaterally in the anterior chest, in both axillae, and across the back. It is secondary to the turbulence caused by disturbed blood flow because the main pulmonary artery is larger than the peripheral pulmonary arteries. This usually benign murmur may persist up to 3 months of age. It may also be associated with rubella syndrome.

5. **Hypoplastic left heart syndrome (HLHS).** A short midsystolic murmur usually presents anywhere from day 1 to 21. A gallop is usually heard.

6. **Tetralogy of Fallot (TOF)** typically is a loud, harsh systolic or pansystolic murmur best heard at the left sternal border. The second heart sound is single.

7. **Pulmonary atresia (PA)**
   a. **With ventricular septal defect.** An absent or soft systolic murmur with the first heart sound is followed by an ejection click. The second heart sound is loud and single.
   b. **With intact intraventricular septum.** Most frequently, there is no murmur and a single second heart sound is heard.

8. **Tricuspid atresia (TA).** A pansystolic murmur along the left sternal border with a single second heart sound is typically heard.

9. **Transposition of the great vessels (TGV)** is more common in males than females.
   a. **Isolated (simple).** Cardiac examination is often normal, but cyanosis and tachypnea are present along with a normal chest radiograph and electrocardiogram.
   b. **With ventricular septal defect.** The murmur is loud and pansystolic and is best heard at the lower left sternal border. The infant typically has congestive heart failure at 3–6 weeks of life.

10. **Ebstein disease.** A long systolic murmur is heard over the anterior portion of the left chest. A diastolic murmur and gallop may be present.

11. **Truncus arteriosus (TA).** A systolic ejection murmur, often with a thrill, is heard at the left sternal border. The second heart sound is loud and single.

12. **Single ventricle.** A loud systolic ejection murmur with a loud single second heart sound is heard.

13. **Atrial septal defects (ASDs)**
    a. **Ostium secundum defect** rarely presents with congestive heart failure in infancy. A soft systolic ejection murmur is best heard at the upper left sternal border.
    b. **Ostium primum defect** rarely occurs in infancy. A pulmonary ejection murmur and early systolic murmur are heard at the lower left sternal border. A split second heart sound is heard.

    c. **Common atrioventricular canal** presents with congestive heart failure in infancy. A harsh systolic murmur is heard all over the chest. The second heart sound is split if pulmonary flow is increased.

14. **Anomalous pulmonary venous return**
    a. **Partial anomalous pulmonary venous return (PAPVR).** Findings are similar to those for ostium secundum defect (see Section XIII, A, 13a).
    b. **Total anomalous pulmonary venous return (TAPVR).** With a severe obstruction, no murmur may be detected on examination. With a moderate degree of obstruction, a systolic murmur is heard along the left sternal border, and a gallop murmur is heard occasionally. A continuous murmur along the left upper sternal border over the pulmonary area may also be audible.

15. **Congenital aortic stenosis (AS).** A coarse systolic murmur with a thrill is heard at the upper right sternal border and can radiate to the neck and down the left sternal border. If left ventricular failure is severe, the murmur is of low intensity. Symptoms that occur in infants only when the stenosis is severe are pulmonary edema and congestive heart failure.

16. **Pulmonary stenosis (with intact ventricular septum).** If the stenosis is severe, a loud systolic ejection murmur is audible over the pulmonary area and radiates over the entire precordium. Right ventricular failure and cyanosis may be present. If the stenosis is mild, a short pulmonary systolic ejection murmur is heard over the pulmonic area along with a split-second heart sound.

B. **Palpate the pulses (femoral, pedal, radial, and brachial).** Bounding pulses can be seen with PDA. Absent or delayed femoral pulses are associated with coarctation of the aorta.

C. **Check for signs of congestive heart failure.** Signs may include hepatomegaly, gallop, tachypnea, wheezes and rales, tachycardia, and abnormal pulses.

XIV. **Abdomen.** See also Chapters 118 and 119.

A. **Observation.** Obvious defects may include an **omphalocele,** in which the intestines are covered by peritoneum and the umbilicus is centrally located; **gastroschisis,** in which the intestines are not covered by peritoneum (the defect is usually to the right of the umbilicus); or **exstrophy of the bladder,** in which the bladder protrudes out.

B. **Auscultation.** Listen for bowel sounds.

C. **Palpation.** Check the abdomen for distention, tenderness, or masses. The abdomen is most easily palpated when the infant is quiet or during feeding. In normal circumstances, the liver can be palpated 1–2 cm below the costal margin and the spleen tip at the costal margin. Hepatomegaly can be seen with congestive heart failure, hepatitis, or sepsis. Splenomegaly is found with cytomegalovirus (CMV) or rubella infections or sepsis. The lower pole of both kidneys can often be palpated. Kidney size may be increased with polycystic disease, renal vein thrombosis, or hydronephrosis. Abdominal masses are more commonly related to the urinary tract.

D. **Diastasis rectus.** This is a protrusion from the xiphoid to the umbilicus because of a separation of the muscles. It is a benign finding in newborns.

E. **Scaphoid abdomen.** A sunken abdomen that can be seen with a diaphragmatic hernia.

F. **Prune belly syndrome.** Usually seen in males (97%), unknown genetic origin, it consists of a large thin wrinkled abdominal wall, genitourinary malformations, and cryptorchidism. Surgery may be required and survival rate has improved (see Chapter 123).

G. **Patent urachus.** A communication between the bladder and the umbilicus occurs, resulting in urine coming from the umbilicus. Need to work up to rule out lower urinary tract obstruction.

XV. **Umbilicus.** Normally, the umbilicus has two arteries and one vein. The absence of one artery occurs in 5–10 of 1000 singleton births and in 35–70 of 1000 twin births. The presence of only two vessels (one artery and one vein) could indicate renal or genetic problems (most commonly trisomy 18). If there is a single umbilical artery, there is an increased prevalence of congenital anomalies (40%) and intrauterine growth restriction and a higher rate of perinatal mortality. If it occurs without any other abnormalities, it is usually benign. If the umbilicus is abnormal, ultrasonography of the abdomen is recommended. In addition, inspect for any discharge, redness, or edema around the base of the cord that may signify a patent urachus or omphalitis. The cord should be translucent; a greenish yellow color suggests meconium staining, usually secondary to fetal distress. Umbilical hernias result from a weakness in the muscle of the abdominal wall and usually require no treatment.

XVI. **Genitalia.** Any infant with a **disorder of sex development** (presence of genitalia that does not fit into a male or female classification, formerly "ambiguous genitalia") should not undergo gender assignment until a formal endocrinology and urologic evaluation has been performed (see Chapter 82). A male with any question of a penile abnormality should not be circumcised until he is evaluated by a urologist or a pediatric surgeon.

A. **Male.** Check for **hypospadias** (abnormal location of the urethral meatus on the ventral surface of the penis), **epispadias** (abnormal location of the urethral meatus on the dorsal surface of the penis), **dorsal hood** (associated with hypospadias), and **chordee** (dorsal or ventral curvature of the penis). Determine the site of the meatus. Normal penile length at birth is >2 cm. **Micropenis** is a penis two standard deviations below the mean length and width for age. **Priapism** (persistent erection of the penis) is an abnormal finding and can be seen in polycythemia. Newborn males always have a marked **phimosis.** Verify that the testicles are in the scrotum and examine for groin hernias. Undescended testicles are more common in premature infants. **Hydroceles** are common and usually disappear by 1 year of age unless associated with a hernia. Observe the color of the scrotum. A bluish color may suggest testicular torsion or trauma and requires immediate urologic/surgical consultation. Infants will have well-developed scrotal rugae at term; a smooth scrotum suggests prematurity.

B. **Female.** Examine the labia and clitoris. A **mucosal tag** is commonly attached to the wall of the vagina. **Discharge from the vagina** is common and is often blood tinged secondary to maternal estrogen withdrawal. If the labia are fused and the clitoris is enlarged, adrenal hyperplasia should be suspected. **Clitoromegaly** (a large clitoris) can be normal in a premature infant or can be associated with maternal drug ingestion (excess androgens during fetal life) or a disorder of sex development. Labia majora at term are enlarged.

XVII. **Lymph nodes.** Palpable lymph nodes, usually in the inguinal and cervical areas, are found in ~33% of normal neonates.

XVIII. **Anus and rectum.** Check for patency of the anus to rule out **imperforate anus** (absence of a normal anal opening). Check the position of the anus. Meconium should pass within 48 h of birth for term infants. Premature infants are usually delayed in passing meconium.

XIX. **Extremities.** Examine the arms and legs, paying close attention to the digits and palmar creases. (See also Chapter 106.)

A. **Syndactyly,** or abnormal fusion of the digits, most commonly involves the third and fourth fingers and the second and third toes. A strong family history exists. Surgery is performed when the neonates are older.

B. **Polydactyly** is supernumerary digits on the hands or the feet. This condition is associated with a strong family history. A radiograph of the extremity is usually obtained to verify whether any bony structures are present in the digit. If there are no bony structures, a suture can be tied around the digit until it falls off. If bony structures are present, surgical removal is necessary. Axial extra digits are associated with heart anomalies.

C. **Brachydactyly.** This is a shortening of one or more digits. It is usually benign if an isolated trait.

D. **Camptodactyly.** This usually involves the little finger and is a flexion deformity that causes it to be bent.

E. **Arachnodactyly.** This is spiderlike fingers that can be seen in Marfan syndrome and homocystinuria.

F. **Clinodactyly.** This usually involves the little finger, is usually benign, and is a radial or ulnar deviation.

G. **Arthrogryposis.** A persistent contracture of the joints of the fingers. Can be associated with oligohydramnios.

H. **Simian crease.** A single transverse palmar crease is most commonly seen in Down syndrome but is occasionally a normal variant.

I. **Talipes equinovarus (clubfoot)** is more common in males. The foot is turned downward and inward, and the sole is directed medially. If this problem can be corrected with gentle force, it will resolve spontaneously. If not, orthopedic treatment and follow-up are necessary.

J. **Metatarsus varus** is a defect where the forefoot rotates inward (adduction). This condition usually corrects spontaneously.

K. **Metatarsus valgus** is a defect where the forefoot rotates outward.

L. **Rocker bottom feet.** Usually seen with trisomy 13 and 18, it involves an arch abnormality that causes a prominent calcaneus with a rounded bottom of the sole.

M. **Tibial torsion.** This is an inward twisting of the tibia bone that causes the feet to turn in. It is most commonly caused by the position in the uterus and resolves spontaneously.

N. **Genu recurvatum.** The knee is able to be bent backward. This abnormal hyperextensibility can be secondary to joint laxity or trauma and is found in Marfan and Ehlers-Danlos syndromes.

XX. **Trunk and spine.** Check for any gross defects of the spine. Any abnormal pigmentation, swelling, or hairy patches over the lower back should increase the suspicion that an underlying vertebral or spinal abnormality exists. A sacral or pilonidal dimple may indicate a small meningocele or other anomaly. Sacral dimples below the line of the natal (gluteal) cleft are benign. If they are above the natal (gluteal) cleft, an ultrasound is indicated to check for a track to the spinal cord.

XXI. **Hips.** (See Chapter 106.) Congenital hip dislocation occurs in ~1 in 800 live births. More common in white females (9:1), this condition is more likely to be unilateral and to involve the left hip. It is also more common if there is a positive family history, if breech presentation, or in infants with a neuromuscular disorder. Two clinical signs of dislocation are asymmetry of the skinfolds on the dorsal surface and shortening of the affected leg. Evaluate for congenital hip dislocation by using the **Ortolani** and **Barlow maneuvers.** Place the infant in the frog-leg position. Abduct the hips by using the middle finger to apply gentle inward and upward pressure over the greater trochanter **(Ortolani).** Adduct the hips by using the thumb to apply outward and backward pressure over the inner thigh **(Barlow).** (Some clinicians suggest omitting the Barlow maneuver because this action may contribute to hip instability by stretching the capsule unnecessarily.) A click of reduction and a click of dislocation are elicited in infants with hip dislocation. If this disorder is suspected, imaging studies (such as ultrasound) and orthopedic consultation should be obtained.

XXII. **Nervous system.** First, observe the infant for any abnormal movement (eg, seizure activity) or excessive irritability. Then evaluate the following parameters:

A. **Muscle tone**

1. **Hypotonia.** Floppiness and head lag are seen.

2. **Hypertonia.** Increased resistance is apparent when the arms and legs are extended. Hyperextension of the back and tightly clenched fists are often seen.

B. **Reflexes.** The following reflexes are normal for a newborn infant. Primary reflexes reflect normal brainstem activity. CNS depression should be suspected if they cannot be elicited and their persistence beyond a certain age can suggest damage of cortical functioning.

1. **Rooting reflex.** Stroke the lip and the corner of the cheek with a finger and the infant will turn in that direction and open the mouth.
2. **Glabellar reflex (blink reflex).** Tap gently over the forehead and the eyes will blink.
3. **Grasp reflex (Palmar grasp).** Place a finger or object in the palm of the infant's hand and the infant will grasp the finger (flexion of the fingers will occur).
4. **Neck-righting reflex.** Turn the infant's head to the right or left, and movement of the contralateral shoulder should be obtained in the same direction.
5. **Moro reflex.** Support the infant behind the upper back with one hand, and then drop the infant back ≥1 cm to, but not on, the mattress. This should cause symmetrical abduction of both arms and extension of the fingers followed by flexion and adduction of the arms. Asymmetry may signify a fractured clavicle, hemiparesis, or brachial plexus injury.
6. **Plantar grasp.** When one strokes the ball of the foot, the toes will curl.
7. **Placing reflex.** Hold the infant upright and place the dorsum of the foot by the edge of the bed; the infant places the foot on the surface.

C. **Cranial nerves.** Note the presence of gross nystagmus, the reaction of the pupils, and the ability of the infant to follow moving objects with his or her eyes.

D. **Movement.** Check for spontaneous movement of the limbs, trunk, face, and neck. A fine tremor is usually normal. Clonic movements are not normal and may be seen with seizures.

E. **Peripheral nerves**
   1. **Brachial plexus injuries.** These involve damage to the spinal nerves that supply the arm, forearm and hand. Etiology is multifactorial.
      a. **Erb-Duchenne paralysis (upper arm paralysis)** involves injury to the fifth and sixth cervical nerves. It is the most common brachial plexus injury. There is adduction and internal rotation of the arm. The forearm is in pronation; the power of extension is retained. The wrist is flexed. This condition can be associated with diaphragmatic paralysis. The Moro reflex is absent.
      b. **Klumpke paralysis (lower arm paralysis)** involves the seventh and eighth cervical nerves and the first thoracic nerve. The hand is flaccid with little or no control. If the sympathetic fibers of the first thoracic root are injured, ipsilateral ptosis, enophthalmos and miosis (**Horner syndrome**) can occur. It occurs rarely.
      c. **Paralysis of the entire arm.** The entire arm is limp and cannot move. The reflexes are absent.
   2. **Facial nerve palsy.** Intrauterine position or forceps can cause compression of the seventh cranial nerve. This results in ptosis, unequal nasolabial folds, and asymmetry of facial movement.
   3. **Phrenic nerve injury.** This can occur secondary to a brachial plexus injury. It causes paralysis of the diaphragm leading to respiratory distress.

F. **General signs of neurologic disorders**
   1. **Symptoms of increased intracranial pressure** (bulging anterior fontanelle, dilated scalp veins, separated sutures, and setting-sun sign) (see Section V, H, 1–5).
   2. **Hypotonia or hypertonia.**
   3. **Irritability or hyperexcitability.**
   4. **Poor sucking and swallowing reflexes.**
   5. **Shallow, irregular respirations.**
   6. **Apnea.**
   7. **Apathy.**
   8. **Staring.**
   9. **Seizure activity** (sucking or chewing of the tongue, blinking of the eyelids, eye rolling, and hiccups).
   10. **Absent, depressed, or exaggerated reflexes.**
   11. **Asymmetric reflexes.**

6 Temperature Regulation

The chance of survival of neonates is markedly enhanced by the successful prevention of excessive heat loss. For that purpose, the newborn infant must be kept under a **neutral thermal environment.** This is defined as the external temperature range within which metabolic rate and hence oxygen consumption are at a minimum while the infant maintains a normal body temperature (Figures 6–1 and 6–2 and Table 6–1). The **normal skin temperature** in the neonate is 36.0–36.5°C (96.8–97.7°F). The **normal core (rectal) temperature is** 36.5–37.5°C (97.7–99.5°F). **Axillary temperature** may be 0.5–1.0°C lower (95.9–98.6°F). A normal body temperature implies only a balance between heat production and heat loss and should not be interpreted as the equivalent of an optimal and minimal metabolic rate and oxygen consumption.

I. **Hypothermia and excessive heat loss.** Preterm infants are predisposed to heat loss because they have a high ratio of surface area to body weight, little subcutaneous fat, and reduced glycogen and brown fat stores. In addition, their hypotonic ("frog") posture limits their ability to curl up to reduce the skin area exposed to the colder environment.

    A. **Mechanisms of heat loss** in the newborn include the following:

        1. **Radiation.** Radiation is heat loss from the infant (warm object) to a colder nearby (not in contact) object.

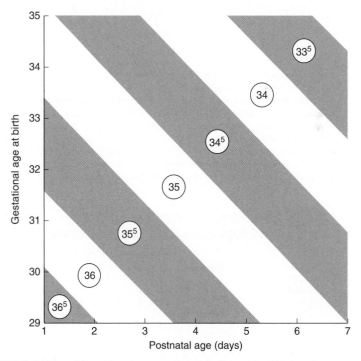

FIGURE 6–1. Neutral thermal environment during the first week of life, based on gestational age. (*Reproduced, with permission, from Sauer PJJ et al: New standards for neutral thermal environment of healthy very low birthweight infants in week one of life. Arch Dis Child 1984;59:18.*)

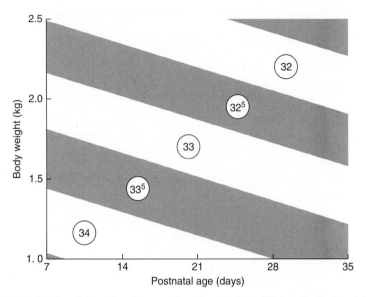

FIGURE 6–2. Neutral thermal environment from days 7 to 35 (in °C), based on body weight. (*Reproduced, with permission, from Sauer PJJ et al: New standards for neutral thermal environment of healthy very low birthweight infants in week one of life.* Arch Dis Child *1984;59:18.*)

2. **Conduction.** Conduction is direct heat loss from the infant to the surface with which he or she is in direct contact.
3. **Convection.** Convection is heat loss from the infant to the surrounding air.
4. **Evaporation.** Heat may be lost by water evaporation from the skin of the infant (especially likely immediately after delivery).

B. **Consequences of excessive heat loss.** Those related to the compensatory augmentation in heat production through the increase in metabolic rate include the following:

1. **Insufficient oxygen supply and hypoxia** from increased oxygen consumption.
2. **Hypoglycemia** secondary to depletion of glycogen stores.

Table 6–1. **APPROXIMATE NEUTRAL THERMAL ENVIRONMENT IN INFANTS WHO WEIGH >2500 g OR ARE >36 WEEKS' GESTATION[a]**

Age	Temperature (°C)
0–24 h	31.0–33.8[b]
24–48 h	30.5–33.5
48–72 h	30.1–33.2
72–96 h	29.8–32.8
4–14 d	29.0–32.6
>2 wk	Data not established[b]

[a]For infants <2500 g or <36 weeks, see Figures 6–1 and 6–2.
[b]In general, the smaller the infant, the higher the temperature.
Based on data from Scopes J, Ahmed I: Range of initial temperatures in sick and premature newborn babies. *Arch Dis Child* 1966;41:417.

3. **Metabolic acidosis** caused by hypoxia and peripheral vasoconstriction.
4. **Decreased growth.**
5. **Apnea.**
6. **Pulmonary hypertension** as a result of acidosis and hypoxia.
C. **Consequences of hypothermia.** As the capacity to compensate for the excessive heat loss is overwhelmed, hypothermia will ensue.
  1. **Clotting disorders** such as disseminated intravascular coagulation and pulmonary hemorrhage can accompany severe hypothermia.
  2. **Shock** with resulting decreases in systemic arterial pressure, plasma volume, and cardiac output.
  3. **Intraventricular hemorrhage.**
  4. **Severe sinus bradycardia.**
  5. **Increased neonatal mortality.**
D. **Treatment of hypothermia.** Rapid versus slow rewarming continues to be *controversial,* although more clinicians are leaning toward more rapid rewarming. Rewarming may induce apnea, hypotension, and rapid electrolytes shifts (Ca^{++}, K^+); therefore, the hypothermic infant should be continuously and closely monitored regardless of the rewarming method. One recommendation is to rewarm at a rate of 1°C/h unless the infant weighs <1200 g, the gestational age is <28 weeks, or the temperature is <32.0°C (89.6°F) and the infant can be rewarmed more slowly (with a rate not to exceed 0.5°C/h). Another recommendation is that, during rewarming, the skin temperature should not be >1°C warmer than the coexisting rectal temperature.
  1. **Equipment**
    a. **Closed incubator.** Incubators are usually used for infants who weigh <1800 g. Closed incubators are convectively heated (heated airflow); therefore, they do not prevent radiant heat loss unless they are provided with double-layered walls. Similarly, evaporation loss is compensated for only when additional humidity is added to the incubator. One disadvantage of incubators is that they make it difficult to closely observe a sick infant or to perform any type of procedure. Body temperature changes associated with sepsis may be masked by the automatic temperature control system of closed incubators. Such changes will hence be expressed in the variations of the incubator's environmental temperature. An infant can be weaned from the incubator when his or her body temperature can be maintained at an environmental temperature of <30.0°C (usually when the body weight reaches 1600–1800 g). Enclosed incubators maintain a neutral thermal environment by using one of the following devices:
      i. **Servocontrolled skin probe attached to the abdomen of the infant.** If the temperature falls, additional heat is delivered. As the target skin temperature (36.0–36.5°C) is reached, the heating unit turns off automatically. A potential disadvantage is that overheating may occur if the skin sensor is detached from the skin or the reverse if the infant is lying on probe-attached side.
      ii. **Air temperature control device.** With this device, the temperature of the air in the incubator is increased or decreased depending on the measured temperature of the infant. Use of this mode requires constant attention from a nurse and is usually used in older infants.
      iii. **Air temperature probe.** This probe hangs in the incubator near the infant and maintains a constant air temperature. There is less temperature fluctuation with this kind of probe.
    b. **Radiant warmer.** The radiant warmer is typically used for very unstable infants or during the performance of medical procedures. Heating is provided by radiation and therefore does not prevent convective and evaporative heat loss. The temperature can be maintained in the "servo mode" (ie, by means of a skin probe) or the "nonservo mode" (also called the "manual mode"), which maintains a constant radiant energy output regardless of the infant's temperature. Serious overheating can result from mechanical failure of the controls, from

dislodgment of the sensor probe, or from manual operation without careful monitoring. Deaths are associated with hyperthermia-induced radiant warmers. On manual mode, such as in the delivery room, they should be used only for a limited period. Insensible water loss may be extremely large in the very low birthweight (VLBW) infant (up to 7 mL/kg/h). Covering of the skin with semipermeable dressing or the use of a water-based ointment (eg, Aquaphor) may help reduce insensible transepidermal water loss.

2. **Temperature regulation in the healthy term infant (weight >2500 g).** Studies have shown that a healthy term infant can be wrapped in warm blankets and placed directly into the mother's arms without any significant heat loss.
   a. **Place the infant** under a preheated radiant warmer immediately after delivery.
   b. **Dry the infant completely** to prevent evaporative heat loss.
   c. **Cover the infant's head** with a cap.
   d. **Place the infant,** wrapped in blankets, in a crib.

3. **Temperature regulation in the sick term infant.** Follow the same procedure as for the healthy term infant, except place the infant under a radiant warmer with temperature servoregulation.

4. **Temperature regulation in the premature infant (weight 1000–2500 g):**
   a. **For an infant who weighs 1800–2500 g** with no medical problems, use of a crib, cap, and blankets is usually sufficient.
   b. **For an infant who weighs 1000–1800 g:**
      i. **A well infant** should be placed in a closed incubator with servo-control.
      ii. **A sick infant** should be placed under a radiant warmer with servo-control.

5. **Temperature regulation in the VLBW infant (weight <1000 g):**
   a. **In the delivery room.** Considerable evaporative heat loss occurs immediately after birth. Consequently, speedy drying of the infant has been emphasized as a very important aspect of the management of the VLBW infant. A more efficient and different approach has been advocated whereby the infant is placed in a plastic bag from feet to shoulder, without drying, immediately at birth.
   b. **In the nursery.** Either the radiant warmer or the incubator can be used, depending on the institutional preference. More recently hybrid devices such as the Versalet Incuwarmer (Hill-Rom Air-Shields, Batesville, IN) and the Giraffe Omnibed (Datex-Ohmeda; GE Medical Systems, Finland) have become available .They offer the combined features of radiant warmer and incubator in a single device, allowing for seamless conversion between modes as deemed clinically necessary.
      i. **Radiant warmer**
         (a) **Use servo-control** with the temperature for abdominal skin set at 36.0–36.5°C.
         (b) **Cover the infant's head** with a cap.
         (c) **To reduce convective heat loss,** place plastic wrap (eg, Saran Wrap) loosely over the infant. Prevent this wrap from directly contacting the infant's skin. Avoid placing the warmer in a drafty area.
         (d) **Maintain an inspired air temperature** of the hood or ventilator of ≥34.0–35.0°C.
         (e) **Place under the infant** a heating pad (K-pad) that has an adjustable temperature within 35.0–38.0°C. To maintain thermal protection, it can be set between 35.0 and 36.0°C. If the infant is hypothermic, the temperature can be increased to 37.0–38.0°C *(controversial).*
         (f) **If the temperature cannot be stabilized,** move the infant to a closed incubator (in some institutions).
      ii. **Closed incubator.** Excessive humidity and dampness of the clothing and incubator can lead to excessive heat loss or accumulation of fluid and possible infections.

      (a) **Use servo-control,** with the temperature for abdominal skin set at 36.0–36.5°C.

      (b) **Use a double-walled incubator** if possible.

      (c) **Cover the infant's head** with a cap.

      (d) **Keep the humidity level** at ≥40–50%.

      (e) **Keep the temperature** of the ventilator at ≥34.0–35.0°C.

      (f) **Place under the infant** a heated mattress (K-pad) that has an adjustable temperature within 35.0–38.0°C. For thermal protection, the temperature can be set between 35.0 and 36.0°C. For warming a hypothermic infant, it can be set as high as 37.0–38.0°C.

      (g) **If the temperature is difficult to maintain,** try increasing the humidity level or use a radiant warmer (in some institutions).

  II. **Hyperthermia** is defined as a temperature that is greater than the normal core temperature of 37.5°C.

    A. **Differential diagnosis**

      1. **Environmental causes.** Some causes include excessive environmental temperature, overbundling of the infant, placement of the incubator in sunlight, a loose temperature skin probe with an incubator or radiant heater on a servo-control mode, or a servo-control temperature set too high.

      2. **Infection.** Bacterial or viral infections (eg, herpes).

      3. **Dehydration.**

      4. **Maternal fever in labor.**

      5. **Maternal epidural analgesia during labor.**

      6. **Drug withdrawal.**

      7. **Unusual causes.**

        a. **Hyperthyroid crisis or storm.**

        b. **Drug effect** (eg, prostaglandin E_1).

        c. **Riley-Day syndrome** (periodic high temperatures secondary to defective temperature regulation).

    B. **Consequences of hyperthermia.** Hyperthermia, like cold stress, increases metabolic rate and oxygen consumption, resulting in tachycardia, tachypnea, irritability, apnea, and periodic breathing. If severe, it may lead to dehydration, acidosis, brain damage, and death.

    C. **Treatment**

      1. **Defining the cause of the elevated body temperature is the most important initial issue.** Mainly, one needs to determine whether the elevated temperature is the result of a hot environment or an increased endogenous production, such as is seen with infections. In the former case, one may find a loose temperature probe, an elevated incubator air temperature, and the extremities of the infant as high as the rest of the body. In the case of "true fever," one expects a low incubator air temperature as well as cold extremities secondary to peripheral vasoconstriction.

      2. **Other measures** include turning down any heat source and removing excessive clothing.

      3. **Additional measures for older infants** with significant temperature elevation:

        a. A tepid water sponge bath.

        b. **Acetaminophen** (5–10 mg/kg per dose, orally or rectally, every 4 h).

        c. **Water-filled cooling blanket** such as the **Banketrol system** (Cincinnati Sub Zero, Cincinnati, OH).

Selected References

Baumgart S: Iatrogenic hyperthermia and hypothermia in the neonate. *Clin Perinatol* 2008;35:183

Cramer K et al: Heat loss prevention: a systematic review of occlusive skin wrap for premature neonates. *J Perinatol* 2005;25:763

Sarman I et al: Rewarming preterm infants on a heated, water-filled mattress. *Arch Dis Child* 1989;64:687.

Sauer PJJ et al: New standards for neutral thermal environment of healthy very low birthweight infants in week one of life. *Arch Dis Child* 1984;59:18.

Scopes J, Ahmed I: Range of initial temperatures in sick and premature newborn babies. *Arch Dis Child* 1966;41:417.

Tafari N, Gentz J: Aspects on rewarming newborn infants with severe accidental hypothermia. *Acta Paediatr Scand* 1974;63:595.

7 Respiratory Management

The management of infants with respiratory distress is a basic function of neonatal intensive care. Skillful use of the ever-increasing range of mechanical devices and pharmacologic agents in the treatment of respiratory disease depends on a sound knowledge of respiratory physiology and pathology. Optimal treatment continues to be difficult to define and considerable variability exists in assessing the risk–benefit ratio of various management strategies. This section provides an overview of current techniques used for neonatal respiratory support.

   I. **Assessing and monitoring respiratory status**
      A. **Physical examination.** The presence of following signs may be useful in recognizing respiratory distress. The absence of signs may be secondary to neurologic depression rather than absence of pulmonary disease.
         1. **Nasal flaring.** One of the earliest signs of respiratory distress, nasal flaring may be present in intubated, ventilated patients as well.
         2. **Grunting.** Commonly seen early in respiratory distress syndrome (RDS) and transient tachypnea, grunting is a physiologic response to end-expiratory alveolar collapse. Grunting helps maintain functional residual capacity (FRC) and therefore oxygenation.
         3. **Retractions.** Intercostal, subcostal, and sternal retractions are present in conditions of decreased lung compliance or increased airway resistance and may persist during mechanical ventilation if support is inadequate.
         4. **Tachypnea.** A respiratory rate >60/min implies the inability to generate an adequate tidal volume and may persist during mechanical ventilation.
         5. **Cyanosis.** Central cyanosis indicates hypoxemia. Cyanosis is difficult to appreciate in the presence of anemia. Acrocyanosis is common shortly after birth and is not a reflection of hypoxemia.
         6. **Abnormal breath sounds.** Inspiratory stridor, expiratory wheezing, and rales should be appreciable. Unfortunately, unilateral pneumothorax may escape detection on auscultation.
      B. **Blood gases.** Management of ventilation, oxygenation, and changes of acid-base status is most accurately determined by **arterial blood gas studies.**
         1. **Arterial blood gas studies** are the most standardized and accepted measure of respiratory status, especially for the oxygenation of low birthweight infants. They are considered invasive monitoring and require arterial puncture or an indwelling arterial line. Access is now considered routine by the umbilical artery or peripherally in the radial or posterior tibial artery.
         2. **Normal arterial blood gas values** may not be the same as target values for particular patients, nor acceptable values. Table 7–1 lists examples of normal values for infants.

Table 7–1. **NORMAL RANGE OF ARTERIAL BLOOD GAS VALUES FOR TERM AND PRETERM INFANTS AT NORMAL BODY TEMPERATURE AND ASSUMING NORMAL BLOOD HEMOGLOBIN CONTENT**[a]

Gestational Age	Pao_2 (mm Hg)	$Paco_2$ (mm Hg)	pH	Hco_3 (mEq/L)	BE/BD
Term	80–95	35–45	7.32–7.38	24–26	±3.0
Preterm (30–36 wk gestation)	60–80	35–45	7.30–7.35	22–25	±3.0
Preterm (<30 wk gestation)	45–60	38–50	7.27–7.32	19–22	±4.0

Hco_3, bicarbonate; BE, base excess; BD, base deficit.

[a]Values for Pao_2, $Paco_2$, and pH are measured directly by electrodes. Hco_3 and BE/BD values are calculated from nomograms of measured values at normal (14.8–15.5 mg/dL) hemoglobin content and body temperature (37°C) and assuming hemoglobin saturation of ≥88%.

3. Calculated arterial blood gas indexes for determining progression of respiratory distress are as follows:
   a. **Alveolar-to-arterial oxygen gradient (AaDo$_2$)** of >600 mm Hg for successive blood gases over 6 h is associated with high mortality in most infants if treatment and ventilation do not become effective. The formula for **AaDo$_2$** is

$$A - aDO_2 = \left[(FIO_2)(Pb - 47) - \frac{Paco_2}{R} \right] - Pao_2$$

   where Pb = barometric pressure (760 mm Hg at sea level), 47 = water vapor pressure, $Paco_2$ is assumed to be equal to alveolar Pco_2, and R = respiratory quotient (usually assumed to be 1 in neonates).
   b. **Arterial-to-alveolar oxygen ratio (a/A ratio)** is also an index for effective respiration. The a/A ratio is the most often used index for evaluation of response to surfactant therapy and is used as an indicator for inhaled nitric oxide therapy for pulmonary hypertension. The formula for the a/A ratio is

$$a / A = Pao_2 \Bigg/ \left[(FIO_2)(Pb - 47) - \frac{Paco_2}{R} \right]$$

4. **Venous blood gases.** Determination of values is the same as for arterial blood gases, but the interpretation is different. The pH values are slightly lower, and $Pvco_2$ values are slightly higher, whereas Pvo_2 values are of no value in assessing oxygenation.
5. **Capillary blood gases.** Arterializing of capillary blood is simply warming of the infant's heel just before sampling. The pH value is usually slightly lower and the Pco_2 is usually slightly higher than arterial values, but this may vary considerably depending on the sampling technique. Po_2 data are of no value.
C. **Noninvasive blood gas monitoring.** Use of these technologies is strongly encouraged. They allow for continuous monitoring and can dramatically reduce the frequency of blood gas sampling, reducing iatrogenic blood loss and decreasing cost. Blood gas sampling is still necessary for calibrating noninvasive measures, determining acid-base status, and detecting hyperoxia.
   1. **Pulse oximetry.** The pulse oximeter measures the relative absorption of light by saturated and unsaturated hemoglobin, which absorbs light at different frequencies. The ratio changes in response to the rapid influx of arterial blood during the upstroke of the pulse. Through the detection of the peak of the ratio, the oximeter

Table 7–2. Sao$_2$ AS A FUNCTION OF PO$_2$ AND PH[a,b]

PO$_2$	pH				
	7.30	7.35	7.40	7.45	7.50
120	98	98	98	98	99
100	97	97	97	98	98
90	96	96	97	97	97
80	95	95	96	96	97
70	92	93	94	95	95
65	91	92	93	94	94
60	88	90	91	92	93
55	85	87	89	90	91
50	81	83	85	87	88
45	76	78	80	83	85
40	69	71	74	77	79
35	61	63	66	69	72
30	51	54	57	60	62
20	29	32	34	36	39
10	7	8	9	10	11

[a]Assuming a temperature of 37°C, normal levels of 2,3 diphosphoglycerate, a Paco$_2$ of 40 mm Hg, and adult hemoglobin.
[b]This table is merely a reference tool and is not to be used for deriving precise values of PO$_2$ or pH from the Ohmeda Biox saturation readings.
Courtesy of the Ohmeda Company, Boulder, CO (now GE Healthcare).

is able to determine the pulse rate and the percentage of arterial oxygen saturation. Sao$_2$ is arterial oxygen saturation by direct measurement, Spo$_2$ is arterial oxygen saturation by pulse oximetry. Table 7–2 shows Sao$_2$ as a function of Pao$_2$ and pH and is useful in the interpretation of pulse oximeter readings.

    a. Limitations include poor correlation of Sao$_2$ to Pao$_2$ at upper and lower Pao$_2$ values. Sao$_2$ of 88–93% corresponds to Pao$_2$ of 50–80 mm Hg. For infants with high or low saturations, arterial blood gas correlation is needed.

    b. Advantages include minimal damage to the skin and no required manual calibration. Sao$_2$ by pulse oximetry is less affected by skin temperature and perfusion than transcutaneous oxygen.

    c. Disadvantages include the tendency of patient movement and excessive external lighting to interfere with readings and the fact that there is no correction of Sao$_2$ for abnormal hemoglobin (eg, methemoglobin).

2. **Transcutaneous oxygen (tcPo$_2$) monitoring** measures the partial pressure of oxygen from the skin surface by an electrochemical sensor known as the Clark polarographic electrode. The electrode heats the skin to 43–44°C, and contact is maintained through a conducting electrolyte solution and an oxygen-permeable membrane.

    a. Limitations include the need for daily recalibration, relocation to different skin sites every 4–6 h, and irritation or injury to a premature infant's skin secondary to adhesive rings and thermal burns. Poor skin perfusion caused by shock, acidosis, hypoxia, hypothermia, edema, or anemia may prevent accurate measurements.

    b. Other disadvantages are related to the high cost of technician time and materials for relocation of the electrode and recalibration. Also, tcPo$_2$ has limited or no use for extremely low birthweight infants because it may result in skin injury.

    c. **Advantages** are that $tcPo_2$ is noninvasive and *may* provide indication of excessively high Pao_2 (>100 mm Hg).

3. **Transcutaneous carbon dioxide monitoring ($tcPco_2$)** is usually accomplished simultaneously by a single lead enclosed with a $tcPo_2$ electrode. The $tcPco_2$ electrode (Stowe-Severinghaus) operates by tissue CO_2 equilibration across the skin and generation of an electrical charge proportional to the change in pH of the contact electrolyte solution.

    a. **Limitations** of $tcPco_2$ include all of those associated with $tcPo_2$ monitoring. Calibration and response times are longer for $tcPo_2$.

    b. **Advantages.** $tcPco_2$ is noninvasive and relatively accurate. $tcPco_2$ determination does not require the high electrode temperatures necessary for $tcPco_2$. The combination of $tcPo_2$ and pulse oximetry can dramatically decrease the frequency of arterial blood gas sampling.

    c. **Disadvantages** include the need for frequent technical support as well as skin injury in extremely low birthweight infants.

4. **End-tidal CO_2 monitoring ($ETco_2$ or $Petco_2$).** Expired breath analysis by infrared spectroscopy for CO_2 content gives close correlation to $Paco_2$. This technique is increasingly available for neonates. It gives rapid information about changes in CO_2, unlike the slow response time of $tcPco_2$.

    a. **Limitations.** An adapter to the endotracheal tube is required, which may significantly increase the dead space of the patient's circuit. Accuracy is limited when the respiratory rate is >60 breaths/min (bpm) or if the humidity of inspired air is excessive. Current devices are of limited use for premature infants.

    b. **Advantages** are that it is a noninvasive technique that may correlate well with arterial $Paco_2$.

    c. **Disadvantages** are related to various disease states. High ventilation-perfusion mismatches such as intrapulmonary shunts, uneven ventilation, or increased dead space are conditions that would give unreliable $Petco_2$ values. Generally, a/A ratios of <0.3 negate $Petco_2$ monitoring.

D. **Monitoring mechanical ventilation.** Although there are many different types of infant ventilators, only a few devices and means for monitoring events during mechanical breath cycles are available.

1. **Inspired oxygen.** Fraction of inspired oxygen (Fio_2) is a percentage of oxygen available for inspiration. It is expressed either as a percentage (21–100%) or as a decimal (0.21–1.00). Battery-operated oxygen analyzers are a standard for monitoring oxygen therapy for infants. They consist of electrochemical cells calibrated by ambient or inspired oxygen concentrations up to 100%. During mechanical ventilation, an inline oxygen analyzer with a ventilator circuit for continuous readout of the oxygen concentration flowing to the infant is preferable. Further management of oxygen therapy requires:

    a. **Calibration of the analyzer** every 8–12 h.

    b. **Blending of air and oxygen** to ensure the least amount of oxygen required to maintain desired blood oxygen saturation.

    c. **Humidification of all inspired oxygen** and air mixtures.

    d. **Warming of inspired gases** to 34–35°C through a humidification device gives >96% water vapor saturation.

2. **Mean airway pressure ($\overline{Paw}$)** is an average of the proximal pressure applied to the airway throughout the entire respiratory cycle (Figure 7–1).

    a. **$\overline{Paw}$ correlates well with mean lung volume** for a given mode and strategy of mechanical ventilation.

    b. **$\overline{Paw}$ > 10–15 cm H_2O during conventional ventilation** is associated with an increased risk of air leaks (pneumothorax or pulmonary interstitial emphysema).

    c. **$\overline{Paw}$ of high-frequency ventilation** is *not* strictly comparable with the $\overline{Paw}$ of conventional mechanical ventilation.

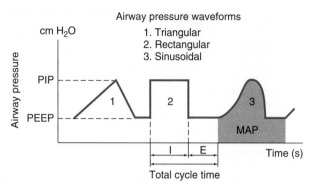

FIGURE 7–1. Graphic representation of ventilator airway pressure waveforms and other ventilator terminology. See Glossary (page 67) for explanations.

   d. **Oxygen index (OI)** is a frequently used calculation that incorporates F_{IO_2}, $\overline{Paw}$, and Pao_2. OI values of 30–40 are indicative of severe respiratory distress. If OI is found to increase steadily over a 6-h period from 30 to 40, profound respiratory failure on conventional mechanical ventilation is apparent. Mortality may exceed 80%.

3. **Pulmonary functions.** New flow sensors allow for frequent or continuous monitoring of mechanical and spontaneous breath mechanics for flow, airway pressure, and volume. With flow sensors or pneumotachographs, additional pulmonary function testing is possible. Occluded breath techniques provide passive mechanics for compliance and resistance as well as determination of time constants.

   a. **Airway pressure** $\overline{Paw}$ is determined in the proximal airway from a differential pressure transducer. Transpulmonary pressure is a measure of the difference between airway pressure and esophageal pressure taken from an indwelling esophageal catheter or balloon.

   b. **Tidal volume** (V_T), a function of peak inspiratory pressure (PIP) during mechanical ventilation, is integrated from flow (mL/s) and measured as mL/breath. By convention, V_T is expressed as breath volume adjusted to body weight as mL/kg. Several devices are now available for continuous bedside V_T monitoring. V_T varies from 5 to 7 mL/kg for most newborn infants.

   c. **Minute volume (MV).** Also known as minute ventilation, the respiratory rate and V_T combine to give MV as

$$MV = Rate \times V_T$$

   Example: 40 bpm × 6.5 mL/kg = 260 mL/kg/min.

   d. **Normal MV values for newborns are 240–360 mL.** Monitoring of V_T and MV simultaneously with $\overline{Paw}$ provides for graded adjustments of PIP, positive end-expiratory pressure (PEEP), and inspiratory time (Ti). Optimal V_T should be determined on the basis of adequate MV at the least PIP and balanced by achieving acceptable blood gases.

   e. **Pressure-volume (P-V) and flow-volume (F-V) loops** are a visualization of breath-to-breath dynamics. Flow, volume, and pressure signals combine to give P-V and F-V loops. Loops give inspiratory and expiratory limits of the breath cycle. F-V loops provide information regarding airway resistance, especially restricted expiratory breath flow. P-V loops illustrate changing lung dynamic compliance.

f. **Compliance** (C_L) values of < 1.0 cm H_2O/mL are consistent with interstitial or alveolar lung disease such as RDS. Lung compliance of 1.0–2.0 mL/cm H_2O reflects recovery, as in post–surfactant therapy.

g. **Resistance** (R_L) of >100 cm H_2O/L/s is suggestive of airway disease with restricted airflow such as in bronchopulmonary dysplasia or the need for airway suctioning.

h. **Time constant** (K_T) is the product of $C_L \times R_L$ (in seconds). Normal values are 0.12–0.15 s. K_T is a measure of how long it takes for alveolar and proximal airway pressures to equilibrate. At the end of 3 time constants, 95% of the V_T has entered (during inspiration) or left (during expiration) the alveoli. To avoid gas trapping, the measured expiratory time should be >3 times K_T (0.36–0.45 s).

E. **Chest radiographs.** Chest radiographs (Chapter 10) are essential to the diagnosis of lung disease, in the management of respiratory support and in the investigation of any acute change in respiratory status.

II. **Ventilatory support.** Infants with respiratory distress may need only supplemental oxygen, whereas those with respiratory failure and apnea require mechanical ventilatory support. This section reviews the spectrum of available means for ventilatory support, with the exception of high-frequency ventilation (see Section VI). Mechanical ventilatory support offers great benefits but also incurs significant risks. There continues to be considerable *controversy* concerning the proper use of any mode or strategy of assisted ventilation.

A. **Oxygen supplementation without mechanical ventilation.** Hypoxic infants able to maintain an adequate minute ventilation are assisted with free-flow oxygen or air-oxygen mixtures.

1. **Oxygen hoods** provide an enclosure for blended air-oxygen supply, humidification, and continuous oxygen concentration monitoring. Hoods are easy to use and provide access to and visibility of the infant. Pulse oximetry is recommended while hoods are in use.

2. **Mask oxygen** is not suitable for infants because of poor control and lack of monitoring of oxygen supply.

3. **Nasal cannulas** are well suited for infants needing low concentrations of oxygen. Delivery can be controlled by flowmeters delivering as little as 0.025 L/min. Flow rates of >1 L/min may impart distending airway pressure. Table 7–3 gives approximate percentages of nasal cannula oxygen based on flow rates of 0.25–1.0 L/min at blended FIO_2 settings of 40–100%. Pulse oximeter monitoring is recommended while nasal cannulas are in use.

B. **Continuous positive airway pressure (CPAP).** A mask, nasal prongs, or an endotracheal tube can be used to apply CPAP. It improves Pao_2 by stabilizing the airway and allowing alveolar recruitment. CO_2 retention may result from excessive distending airway pressure.

1. **Mask CPAP** is rarely used in the newborn.

Table 7–3. NASAL CANNULA CONVERSION TABLE

Flow Rate (L/min)	FIO_2			
	100%	80%	60%	40%
0.25	34%	31%	26%	22%
0.50	44%	37%	31%	24%
0.75	60%	42%	35%	25%
1.00	66%	49%	38%	27%

General guideline only; numbers are not exact.

2. **Nasal CPAP prongs** are the most commonly applied means of delivering CPAP and are used for respiratory assistance in an infant with mild RDS. The prongs are also used postextubation to maintain airway and alveolar expansion in the process of weaning from mechanical ventilation and recovery from respiratory diseases. This treatment maintains upper airway patency and, as such, is useful in infants with apnea of infancy. CPAPs may range from 2 to 8 cm H_2O, although 2–6 cm H_2O is most often used. Overdistention of the airway can lead to excessive CO_2 retention or air leak (pneumothorax). Gastric distention may be a complication of nasal CPAP, and an orogastric tube for decompression should be used. Infants can be fed by nasogastric tube during nasal CPAP therapy with close monitoring of abdominal girth.

3. **Nasopharyngeal CPAP** is an alternative to nasal prongs. An endotracheal tube is passed nasally and advanced to the nasopharynx. A ventilator or CPAP device is used to deliver continuous distending pressure as with nasal prongs. This approach is slightly more secure in active infants and may cause less trauma to the nasal septum.

4. **Nasal ventilation.** Using a ventilator for the generation of CPAP allows for the addition of a "bump rate." Breath rates of 10–15/min with peak pressures set to 10 cm H_2O above CPAP are well tolerated. Nasal ventilation seems to be particularly helpful in managing apnea. Some newer ventilators allow for synchronized nasal ventilation.

5. **Endotracheal tube CPAP** is rarely indicated in neonates.

C. **Mechanical ventilation.** The decision to initiate mechanical ventilation is complex. The severity of respiratory distress, severity of blood gas abnormalities, natural history of the specific lung disease, and degree of cardiovascular and other physiologic instabilities are all factors to be considered. Because mechanical ventilation may result in serious complications, the decision to intubate and ventilate should not be taken lightly.

1. **Bag-and-mask or bag-to-endotracheal tube handheld assemblies** allow for emergency ventilatory support. Portable manometers are always required for monitoring peak airway pressures during hand-bag ventilation. Bags may be self-inflating or flow-dependent, anesthesia-type bags. All handheld assemblies must have pop-off valves to avoid excessive pressures to the infant's airway.

2. **Conventional infant ventilators.** Conventional mechanical ventilation delivers physiologic tidal volumes at physiologic rates via an endotracheal tube. Modern microprocessor controlled ventilators provide numerous modes of ventilation, which vary in the degree to which patient effort controls the ventilator. These modes are critically dependent on the function of flow and/or pressure sensors for accurate performance. The very rapid respiratory rates and small tidal volumes encountered in some neonates may prevent the use of patient-triggered or controlled ventilator modes. Table 7–4 gives basic ventilator setting changes and expected blood gas responses.

Table 7–4. **CHANGES IN BLOOD GAS LEVELS CAUSED BY CHANGES IN VENTILATOR SETTINGS**

Variable	Rate	PIP	PEEP	IT	F_{IO_2}
To increase $Paco_2$	↓	↓	NA	NA	NA
To decrease $Paco_2$	↑	↑	NA[a]	NA[b]	NA
To increase Pao_2	↑	↑	↑	↑	↑
To decrease Pao_2	NA	↓	↓	NA	↓

PIP, peak inspiratory pressure; PEEP, positive end-expiratory pressure; IT, inspiratory time; F_{IO_2}, fraction of inspired oxygen; NA, not applicable.

[a]In severe pulmonary edema and pulmonary hemorrhage, increased PEEP can decrease $Paco_2$.

[b]Not applicable unless the inspiratory-to-expiratory ratio is excessive.

a. **PEEP (positive end-expiratory pressure)** is common to all modes of continuous mandatory ventilation (CMV). PEEP is usually generated with a continuous flow through the ventilator circuit, which allows for untriggered spontaneous ventilation. In most cases, PEEP will be set at 3–5 cm H_2O. Use of higher PEEP is often appropriate in conditions of alveolar collapse, but it must be balanced with the risk of overdistending the lung during inspiration.

b. **Ventilator modes.** Various modes of mechanical ventilation are determined by the parameters that are set by the clinician to determine the characteristics of the mechanical breath and the circumstances under which it is delivered. Not all modes are available on every ventilator, and subtle differences between the same mode may exist between different manufacturers. The characteristics of each breath are as follows:

   i. **Length of breath (T_i)**
      (a) **Time cycled.** Each mechanical breath lasts for a controlled set time.
      (b) **Flow cycled.** Each breath lasts until inspiratory flow falls below a threshold.

   ii. **Size of breath (VT)**
      (a) **Volume limited.** Each mechanical breath is the same volume; the pressure used may vary.
      (b) **Pressure limited.** A set pressure is reached with each mechanical breath, the VT delivered may vary. This mode uses a continuous flow through the ventilator circuit, allowing for spontaneous respiration to occur without ventilator action.
      (c) **Pressure control.** As in pressure-limited ventilation, the clinician specifies the desired peak pressure; however the flow rate through the circuit is variable. Ventilator action is necessary for every breath.
      (d) **Volume assurance/guarantee.** Ventilator automatically adjusts set pressure to deliver target VT.

   iii. **Frequency of mechanical breaths**
      (a) **IMV (intermittent mandatory ventilation).** Breaths are delivered at set intervals without regard to patient effort.
      (b) **SIMV (synchronized IMV).** The set rate determines time frames during which the ventilator will deliver a breath in response to a patient trigger or will deliver a mandatory breath if no trigger is sensed. The minimum and maximum ventilator rates are equal.
      (c) **A/C (assist/control).** Each patient trigger results in a ventilator breath. If no trigger is sensed, a minimum set rate is delivered. Maximum rate may be much higher than minimum. Excessive trigger sensitivity may lead to auto-cycling and much greater rates than needed.
      (d) **Support or assist.** Each patient trigger results in a breath. No mandatory backup rate.

   iv. **The preceding sets of parameters are often combined to yield the following modes:**
      (a) **IMV.** Usually refers especially to nontriggered, pressure-limited, time-cycled ventilation. **Use:** In absence of reliable patient trigger.
      (b) **SIMV.** May be either volume or pressure limited, time cycled. **Use:** Prevents hyperventilation from auto-cycling.
      (c) **Pressure control.** Pressure limited (usually with a decreasing flow rate during inspiration), time cycled, A/C. **Use:** Provides well-tolerated support in patients with easily sensed respiratory effort.
      (d) **Volume control.** Volume-limited, time-cycled, A/C. **Use:** As in pressure control, but may result in more consistent VT.
      (e) **Pressure support.** Pressure-limited, flow-cycled, support. **Use:** In addition to SIMV, especially during weaning.

v. **Patient triggers.** The advanced patient-regulated ventilation modes available with modern microprocessor-controlled ventilators depend on reliable detection of patient respiratory effort. In the smallest premature infants, it is difficult to separate flow or pressure changes due to inspiratory effort from those due to measurement error or leaks.

vi. **Flow** determinations by pneumotach or mass airflow sensors. Measurements vary with gas composition, temperature, and humidity, although not significantly. Large errors may be expected with anesthesia gases or heliox. It is also subject to error with fluid contamination or air leaks. Placement between the patient's endotracheal tube and the circuit gives greatest sensitivity.

vii. **Pressure.** Pressure triggers may be confused by ringing within the circuit, especially with rainout in the tubing.

viii. **Neural.** Using a bipolar esophageal lead placed at the level of the diaphragm, phrenic nerve impulses to the diaphragm can be detected and used to trigger mechanical breaths. This new technology is promising but not yet adequately studied in neonates.

III. **Pharmacologic respiratory support and surfactant.** Numerous medications are available for improvement of respiration. They represent a broad range of therapeutics, of which the bronchodilators and anti-inflammatory drugs are the oldest and most common. The use of mixtures of inhaled gases such as helium and nitric oxide are recent forms of treatment. Sedatives and paralyzing agents remain *controversial* in neonatal respiratory management. Finally, surfactant replacement therapy has rapidly become a major adjunct in the care of preterm infants, and its use has expanded to disease states other than RDS (hyaline membrane disease), for which it was originally intended. All medications are discussed with regard to dosage and side effects in Table 7-5, but they are briefly reviewed here for the purpose of incorporating their use into respiratory management strategies.

A. **Bronchodilators (inhaled agents).** Most of these drugs are sympathomimetic agents that stimulate β_1, β_2, or α-adrenergic receptors. They have both inotropic and chronotropic effects and provide bronchial smooth muscle and vascular relaxation. Albuterol is probably the most commonly used aerosolized bronchodilator. Other bronchodilators are presented in Table 7-5. Two anticholinergic agents (atropine and ipratropium) are also used as inhaled bronchodilators for inhibition of acetylcholine at lung receptor sites and bronchial smooth muscle relaxation. All are used to minimize airway resistance and allow decreased P$\overline{\text{aw}}$ needed for mechanical ventilation.

B. **Bronchodilators (systemic).** Aminophylline (parenteral) and theophylline (enteral) are methylxanthines with considerable bronchial dilating action. Neonatal use includes bronchodilatation and stimulation of respiratory effort.

C. **Anti-inflammatory agents**

1. **Steroid therapy** has been used to treat or prevent chronic lung disease. Although steroid therapy results in significant short-term improvement in pulmonary function, long-term benefit remains unproved. The substantial adverse effects of steroid therapy have led the American Academy of Pediatrics and the Canadian Pediatric Society to issue a joint recommendation against the routine use of steroid therapy.

2. **Cromolyn** prevents mast cells from releasing histamine and leukotriene-like substances. Its actions are slow but progressive over 2–4 weeks. Indications for its use in neonates have not been established. This agent is considered for use in infants with progressive reactive airway disease, prolonged mechanical ventilatory support, and minimal response to attempts to wean from the ventilator.

D. **Inhaled gas mixtures**

1. **Heliox** (helium, 78–80%; oxygen, 20–22%) produces an inspired gas less dense than nitrogen-oxygen mixtures or oxygen alone. Use of heliox reduces the increased

Table 7–5. **AEROSOL THERAPY IN NEONATES, INDICATING DOSING, RECEPTOR EFFECTS, AND COMMON SIDE EFFECTS**

Drug	Receptors	Side Effects
Isoproterenol (Isuprel): 0.1–0.25 mL (0.5–1.25 mg) of 0.5% solution. Dilute with NS to 3 mL. Dose: every 3–4 hours.	β_1: Chronotropic, inotropic β_2: Relax airways and vasculature, smooth muscle	Tachycardia Arrhythmias Hypertension Hyperglycemia Tolerance, tremor Excessive smooth muscle relaxation = airway collapse
Albuterol (Salbutamol, Ventolin): 0.04 mL/kg/dose of 0.5% solution. Dilute with NS to 3 mL. Dose: every 4–6 hours.	β_2: Long lasting (duration, 3–8 hours) Fewer side effects than isoproterenol or metaproterenol	Tachycardia (potentiated by methylxanthines) Hypertension Hyperglycemia Tremor
Metaproterenol: 0.1–0.25 mL (5–12.5 mg) of 5% solution. Dilute with NS to 3 mL. Dose: every 6 hours.	β_2: Less specific for airways than albuterol	Same as isoproterenol Cardiac arrhythmias potentiated by hypoxia
Cromolyn (Intal): 20 mg. Dilute with NS to 3 mL. Dose: every 6–8 hours.	Anti-inflammatory by stabilizing mast cells	Anaphylaxis Caution in patients with liver or renal disease Bronchospasm from inflammatory response Upper airway irritation
Terbutaline (Brethine): 0.01–0.02 mg/kg. Dilute IV solution with NS to 3 mL. Dose: every 2–8 hours. Minimum dose: 0.1 mg.	β_2: Peripheral dilation	Hypertension Hyperglycemia Tachycardia
Atropine: 0.03–0.05 mg/kg. Dilute IV solution with NS to 2.5 mL. Dose: every 6–8 hours.	Vagolytic	Tachycardia Arrhythmia Hypotension Ileus, airway dryness If thick secretions: Suggest use in combination with albuterol
Ipratropium (Atrovent): Neonates: 25 mcg/kg/dose. Infants: 125–250 mcg/dose. Dilute with NS to 3 mL. Dose: every 8 hours.	Antagonizes acetylcholine at parasympathetic sites	Nervousness Dizziness Nausea, blurred vision Cough, palpitations Rash, urinary difficulties

(*Continued*)

Table 7–5. **AEROSOL THERAPY IN NEONATES, INDICATING DOSING, RECEPTOR EFFECTS, AND COMMON SIDE EFFECTS (*CONTINUED*)**

Drug	Receptors	Side Effects
Epinephrine, racemic (Vaponefrin): 0.1–0.3 mL. Dilute with NS to 3 mL. Dose: every 30 minutes, maximum 4 doses. (Racemic epinephrine, 2 mg = L-epinephrine, 1 mg) L-Epinephrine 1:1000: 0.05–0.15 mL. Dilute with NS to 3 mL. Dose: every 30 minutes, maximum 4 doses.	α receptor	Tachycardia Tremor Hypertension
Levalbuterol (Xopenex) 0.31 mg–1.25 mg every 4–6 hours as needed for bronchospasm. (NHLBI asthma 2007 guidelines)	β_2: R(-)enantiomer of racemic albuterol: little effect on heart rate	Nervousness, tremor tachycardia, hypertension, hypokalemia. Paradoxical bronchospasm may occur, especially with first use

NS, Normal saline.

resistive load of breathing, improves distribution of ventilation, and creates less turbulence in narrow airways. Limited neonatal use has indicated that heliox is associated with lower inspired oxygen requirements and shorter duration of mechanical ventilatory support.

2. **Inhaled Nitric oxide (iNO)** is a potent gaseous vasodilator produced by endothelial cells. NO is rapidly bound by hemoglobin, limiting its action to the site of production or administration. Delivered in the ventilatory gas, iNO produces vasodilation only in the vascular bed of well-ventilated regions of the lung, thereby reducing intrapulmonary shunt as well as pulmonary vascular resistance. Furthermore, there is no systemic effect.

   a. **Actions.** iNO diffuses rapidly across alveolar cells to vascular smooth muscle, where it causes an increase in cyclic GMP, resulting in smooth muscle relaxation.

   b. **Dosage.** iNO is administered at low concentration, 2–80 parts per million (ppm). The dose is titrated to effect (improved oxygenation being the most common). Rarely do concentrations >20–40 ppm yield additional benefit.

   c. **Administration.** iNO is blended into the ventilatory gases, preferably close to the patient connector to avoid excessive dwell time with high oxygen concentrations, which may result in excessive NO_2 concentrations. Inline sensors are used to measure delivered NO and NO_2 concentrations. Techniques for use with high-frequency ventilators have also been developed. **Co-oximetry measurement of methemoglobin is required.** The NO dose should be decreased if methemoglobin is >4% or if the NO_2 concentration is >1–2 ppm.

   d. **Indications for use.** iNO is indicated for hypoxic respiratory failure of term and near-term newborns. Recommendations have been made by the AAP for care and referral of these infants. It is currently under investigation for use in a variety of lung diseases in which inappropriate pulmonary vascular constriction adversely affects oxygenation. The resultant vasodilation may decrease pulmonary vascular resistance in general, thereby reducing right-to-left shunting, or may result in less intrapulmonary shunt, or both. Use in cases of severe respiratory failure suggests that iNO may reduce the need for extracorporeal membrane oxygenation (ECMO) in 30–45% of eligible patients. Use of inhaled NO in premies with RDS decreases the incidence of chronic lung disease and death. Routine use of iNO early in the course of RDS in extreme premature infants may improve long-term outcome.

  e. **Adverse effects.** Systemic vascular effects are *not* seen with iNO use. NO_2 poisoning and methemoglobinemia are the most likely complications.

E. **Other medications**
  1. **Sildenafil,** an oral phosphodiesterase 5 inhibitor, reduces pulmonary vascular resistance and is approved in adults for pulmonary hypertension. Its use is attractive in patients with bronchopulmonary dysplasia (BPD), with further study required before use in newborns.
  2. **Prostacyclin (PGI$_2$)** is a potent pulmonary vasodilator given as an aerosol or intravenous drip. Hypotension may develop. Use with iNO has been reported.
  3. **Bosentan,** an oral endothelin 1 receptor blocker, reduces pulmonary vascular resistance. Its use in neonates is as yet undefined.

F. **Sedatives and paralyzing agents.** Agitation is a common problem for infant mechanical ventilation. Infants may have interrupted respiratory cycles and respond by "bucking" or "fighting" the ventilator breaths. The agitation that results is often associated with hypoxic episodes. Sedation or muscle relaxation by paralysis may be required. It should be noted, however, that with the use of ventilators with either flow-sensed or patient-triggered synchronized ventilation (SIMV), much less sedation is required and paralysis is rarely needed.
  1. **Sedatives** include lorazepam, phenobarbital, fentanyl, or morphine. Each agent has advantages and side effects. (See Chapter 69.)
  2. **Paralyzing agents** include pancuronium and vecuronium. Muscle relaxation by paralysis results in considerable third spacing of fluid, requiring added volume expanders to maintain blood pressure and urine output.

G. **Surfactant replacement therapy.** The availability of surfactant treatment has dramatically changed the care of infants with RDS (also known as hyaline membrane disease [HMD]). Surfactant administration early in the course of RDS restores pulmonary function and prevents tissue injury that otherwise results from ventilation of surfactant-deficient lungs. As a result, mortality from RDS has dropped dramatically.
  1. **Composition.** Currently available surfactants are all of animal origin: beractant (Survanta) and calfactant (Infasurf) are derived from bovine lung and lung lavage, respectively. Poractant alfa (Curosurf) is derived from porcine lung. All contain the hydrophobic surfactant proteins, SpB and SpC, although at different concentrations. Calfactant and poractant alfa contain surfactant phospholipids. In beractant, additional phospholipid is added to the minced lung extract to increase the ratio of surfactant to membrane phospholipids. Synthetic surfactants that equal the in vivo actions of the natural surfactants have been on the horizon for several years.
  2. **Actions.** All surfactant preparations are intended to replace the missing or inactivated natural surfactant of the infant. Surface tension reduction and stabilization of the alveolar air–water interface are the basic functions of surfactant compounds. Air–water interface stability imparts lower alveolar surface tension and prevents atelectasis, or alternating areas of atelectasis and hyperinflation.
  3. **Dosage and administration.** Each preparation has specific dosage and dosing procedures. Direct tracheal instillation is involved in all preparations. Surfactants are given both by continuous infusion via side port on the endotracheal tube adapter and mostly by aliquots via a catheter placed through the endotracheal tube. Changes in body position during dosing aid in more uniform delivery of

surfactant. The relative advantages of these methods of administration are currently being studied.

  a. **Prophylactic dosing at birth.** This form of treatment is used less often, and only when resuscitation and surfactant administration can be safely pursued simultaneously.

  b. **Administration of surfactant preparations after respiratory distress is established.** Currently, surfactant therapy occurs once the patient has been stabilized and the diagnosis of RDS has been established.

  c. **Repeat dosing** may follow at 6- to 12-h intervals. Repeat doses should follow loss of response after initial improvement has been seen. Repeat dosing after the second dose is ***controversial.***

  d. **Airway obstruction** may occur during surfactant administration because of the viscosity of the surfactant preparations. Increased mechanical support may be required until the surfactant is spread from the airways to the alveoli.

4. **Efficacy of surfactant treatment** can be observed for both immediate and long-term clinical conditions.

  a. **Early effects include a reduction of** FIO_2 **need** and improved PaO_2, $PaCO_2$, and a/A ratio. Likewise, improved VT and compliance should be noted with improved lung function and decreased ventilator PIPs.

  b. **Long-term effects** should result in decreased necessity for mechanical ventilation and less severe chronic lung disease of infancy. Complications of patent ductus arteriosus, necrotizing enterocolitis, and intraventricular hemorrhage have not been significantly influenced by surfactant therapy to date.

5. **Side effects**
  a. Small risk of pulmonary hemorrhage.
  b. Secondary pulmonary infections.
  c. Air leak (pneumothorax) following bolus administration of surfactant compounds. Rapid changes in VT require immediate reduction of PIPs. Failure to do so while also decreasing FIO_2 may lead to air leaks.

6. **Surfactant therapy for diseases other than RDS (hyaline membrane disease).** Encouraging preliminary reports of surfactant therapy have been noted in cases of pneumonia, meconium aspiration syndrome, persistent pulmonary hypertension, pulmonary hemorrhage, and adult respiratory distress syndrome (ARDS), but no protocols for treatment are available at this time. Dilute surfactant solutions are being studied for use as lung lavage fluids for meconium aspiration.

IV. **Strategies of respiratory support**

  A. **General approaches.** Although use of the tools and techniques discussed in this section are essential to neonatal intensive care, their use is not without peril. One general approach is to provide the minimal support necessary to support gas exchange, unless a more aggressive intervention may change the course of the pulmonary disease, such as early intubation for the delivery of surfactant in RDS. Noninvasive nasal CPAP or ventilation is preferable to intubation and mechanical ventilation. Patient-triggered ventilation modes are usually better tolerated by patients and may result in less need for support. Aggressive weaning of mechanical support in response to the resolution of the underlying disease is crucial.

  B. **Mechanisms of lung injury**

  1. **Oxygen toxicity** is a risk factor for BPD and retinopathy of prematurity (ROP) and may be reduced by careful monitoring and the setting of gestational age appropriate SpO_2 targets.

  2. **Inflammation and infection** result from intubation. Use of noninvasive ventilation and early extubation are desired.

  3. **Barotrauma/volutrauma** results from overinflation of the lung or stress from repeated reopening of collapsed lung units or from shear between adjacent lung units. Maintenance of functional residual capacity (FRC) using appropriate PEEP and the use of small VT to prevent overdistension help limit injury.

C. **Fine-tuning mechanical ventilation.** (See also Chapter 40.) Adequate gas exchange must be determined for each patient because goals vary depending on diagnosis, patient's gestational age, and level of support required.

1. **Oxygenation defects** are usually caused by poor matching of ventilation and perfusion. Support beyond the use of supplemental oxygen is directed either at improving aeration in the lung or influencing the distribution of perfusion.

   a. Prevent lung collapse at end expiration by the use of PEEP and the use of surfactant in RDS.

   b. Recruit collapsed lung by the use of adequate VT and PIP.

   c. iNO selectively decreases vascular resistance in well-ventilated regions of the lung, improving oxygenation. Extrapulmonary shunt due to persistent pulmonary hypertension may respond to prostacyclin in addition to iNO.

   d. Consider the use of HFO to maintain high mean lung volume.

2. **Ventilation defects** result from inadequate minute volume. Abnormal low lung compliance may be a result of collapsed lung and therefore be correctable by the use of nasal CPAP. If mechanical ventilation is required, overventilation should be avoided. Although *controversial,* a target Pco_2 of 45–60 torr helps prevent lung injury.

   a. Increasing VT is usually accomplished by increasing the PIP. If PIP >20–25 mm Hg is needed in a premature infant, high-frequency jet ventilation (HFJV) should be considered.

   b. When using patient-triggered ventilation modes, set the ventilator rate high enough to prevent hypoventilation should the patient become apneic.

3. **Neonatal lung disease** is rarely static, necessitating frequent adjustments to ventilatory parameters. Table 7–4 lists basic ventilator setting changes and effects.

D. **Weaning from mechanical ventilation and extubation.** As lung function improves with disease resolution, mechanical support should be decreased as quickly as tolerated. Most patients do not need to be "weaned" from mechanical support; they need support decreased to match their need. Continuous monitoring with pulse oximetry and $tcPco_2$ aids in weaning and limits the need for blood gas sampling. A reduced oxygen requirement and improved compliance (decrease in PIP to maintain VT) usually herald the weaning phase. Although *controversial,* **pretreatment of infants with aminophylline is believed by some clinicians to enhance infant response to progressive weaning efforts.** Disease state, gestational age, and caloric support influence response to weaning process.

1. **PIP** is usually weaned first because overinflation injury is more deleterious than providing a greater rate than necessary. PIP is decreased to maintain normal VT (or chest excursion).

2. Fio_2 is weaned whenever possible as determined by pulse oximetry or blood gases. Decreases in PIP decrease Paw and may transiently increase oxygen requirements during weaning.

3. **Progressive rate wean.** Rate settings should be decreased frequently. Infants ready to be weaned tolerate the rate wean and do not require more Fio_2. An infant should be able to maintain adequate minute ventilation without developing hypercarbia or apnea. When the ventilator rate is <10–15 bpm, the infant should be extubated. Some infants may require several hours to wean, whereas others need several days to a week or more.

4. **Weaning assist/control ventilation.** Because all spontaneous breaths are mechanically supported by this mode of ventilation, reduction of the rate below the patient's spontaneous rate has no effect on the level of support. Weaning is accomplished by successive decreases in PIP. When adequate ventilation is maintained with minimal pressures (10–15 cm H_2O), extubation may be attempted.

E. **Care after extubation.** Continued monitoring of blood gases, respiratory effort, and vital signs is required. Additional oxygen support is often needed in the immediate postextubation period.

1. **Supplemental oxygen** may be given by hood or by nasal cannula. The oxygen concentration should be increased by >5% over the last oxygen level obtained while the infant was on the ventilator.
2. **Nasal CPAP** may be especially helpful in preventing reintubation secondary to postextubation atelectasis.
3. **Chest physical therapy** (every 3–4 h) after extubation helps to maintain a clear airway. Postural drainage with percussion and suction procedures should be followed routinely. Chest physical therapy should be avoided in the first 1 to 3 days of life in infants at risk for intraventricular hemorrhage. Aerosol treatments with bronchodilators also help to maintain airway patency.
4. **If the infant has had an increasing oxygen requirement** or has clinically deteriorated, an anteroposterior chest radiograph should be obtained at 6 h postextubation to monitor for atelectasis.

V. **Strategies for respiratory management of certain newborn diseases**

A. **RDS (hyaline membrane disease)**

1. **Clinical presentation.** Patients are premature with immature lungs and surfactant deficiency. Blood gases reflect poor oxygenation, declining a/A ratios (< 0.5), and CO_2 accumulation. Monitoring of lung mechanics reveals poor compliance and diminished V_T but near-normal airway resistance. Progressive atelectasis resulting from surfactant deficiency worsens the compliance (lung stiffness), and the work of breathing increases to maintain minute ventilation. All of the above results in exhaustion of the infant and, ultimately, apnea.
2. **Management.** Oxygen supplementation is required to maintain Pao_2 at 50–80 mm Hg. The goal of ventilation is to increase the Pao_2 and decrease the $Paco_2$. Ventilator settings begin with PIPs to allow even movement of the chest wall and provide a V_T of 5–7 mL/kg. If V_T cannot be measured, chest radiograph for expansion to eight ribs is an estimate of adequate PIP. Rates can be determined by a decline in CO_2 or by calculating minute ventilation. For the more hypercarbic infants, rates of 50–60 bpm and V_Ts of 5–6 mL/kg will give minute ventilation of ~360. PEEP of 4–5 cm H_2O is most often required. ITs vary from 0.20 to 0.38 s. As soon as optimal lung expansion, V_T, and minute ventilation have been achieved, surfactant therapy by tracheal instillation should begin (at 2–4 h of life). This should result in a 30% reduction of Fio_2 and a 30% increase in the a/A ratio. The improvement should allow for a decreased PIP while maintaining an adequate V_T and minute ventilation.

B. **Group B β-hemolytic streptococcal (GBS) disease of the newborn with pneumonia and hypotension**

1. **Clinical presentation.** Infants may be of any gestational age but are often near term or term. The disease represents interstitial inflammation, atelectasis caused by inflammatory debris, and surfactant deficiency. Mild respiratory distress with tachypnea rapidly becomes severe, with marked cyanosis and hypoxemia. Ventilatory support is needed as soon as blood gases confirm a poor a/A ratio or $AaDo_2$. Natural surfactant production is suppressed, and alveolar surfactant is inactivated by inflammatory proteins.
2. **Management.** Following endotracheal intubation, mechanical ventilation should be at a rate that is synchronized with the infant's spontaneous rate (SIMV). Increased PIPs to achieve V_Ts of 5–8 mL/kg and minute ventilation of 300–360 mL/kg are required in larger infants. Systemic hypotension often accompanies GBS. Excessive PEEP (5–6 cm H_2O) may impede venous return. PEEP of 2–4 cm H_2O is recommended. Because GBS patients may develop severe hypoxia from persistent pulmonary hypertension, monitoring of the OI should begin early. With Fio_2 at 100%, a calculated OI of >30 suggests the need for more advanced respiratory support. High-frequency ventilation should be considered along with inhaled NO therapy. If there is no response to high-frequency ventilation and the OI is >40, ECMO may also be considered. A trial of surfactant therapy and inhaled

NO may be performed before ECMO. Additional support includes the use of vasopressors, colloid infusions, antibiotics, intravenous immune globulins, glucose, and electrolyte solutions.

C. **Chronic lung disease of infancy**

1. **Clinical presentation.** Infants are usually 2–3 weeks old, ventilator dependent, and requiring supplemental oxygen. Lung mechanics reveal marginal compliance of 0.8–1.0 mL/cm H_2O and marked increases of resistance to 120–140 cm $H_2O/L/s$. Airway resistance is most increased on expiration.

2. **Management.** Many parameters must be addressed in infants with chronic lung disease of infancy. Careful fluid management and maximal caloric intake are required. Respiratory care includes chest physical therapy and appropriate airway humidification. Hypoxia must be avoided by administering supplemental oxygen to continuously maintain SaO_2 at 92–95%. Bronchodilators, both systemic and aerosol, are helpful. Steroid therapy is associated with marked improvement in many infants. The use of dexamethasone is associated with poor long-term neurologic outcome and should be avoided. Hydrocortisone does not have the same adverse effects, but it should be used sparingly until proven safe. Ventilator management seeks to maintain adequate VT (6–8 mL/kg) delivered over longer ITs (>0.4 s). PIP is dictated by achieving adequate VT and minute ventilation. Synchronized ventilation is particularly helpful to patients with chronic lung disease of infancy. $PaCO_2$ may be accepted at higher values (55–60 mm Hg) with adequate acid-base balance from renal compensation. Ventilatory support should take into account that airway resistance and consequently respiratory time constant are markedly elevated. Slow respiratory rates are to be preferred to high rates. A short expiratory time does not allow for adequate expiratory flow and produces air trapping with cystic or bullous changes of the lungs.

VI. **Overview of high-frequency ventilation.** High-frequency ventilation refers to a variety of ventilatory strategies and devices designed to provide ventilation at rapid rates and very low VTs. The ability to provide adequate ventilation in spite of reduced VT (equal to or less than dead space) may reduce the risk of barotrauma. Rates during high-frequency ventilation are often expressed in hertz (Hz). A rate of 1 Hz (1 cycle/s) is equivalent to 60 bpm.

All methods of high-frequency ventilation should be administered with the assistance of well-trained respiratory therapists and after comprehensive education of the nursing staff. Furthermore, because rapid changes in ventilation or oxygenation may occur, continuous monitoring is highly recommended. Optimal use of these ventilators is evolving, and different strategies may be indicated for a particular lung disease.

A. **Definitive indications for high-frequency ventilation support**

1. **Pulmonary interstitial emphysema (PIE).** A multicenter trial has demonstrated HFJV to be superior to conventional ventilation in early PIE as well as in neonates who fail to respond to conventional ventilation.

2. **Severe bronchopleural fistula.** In severe bronchopleural fistula not responsive to thoracostomy tube evacuation and conventional ventilation, HFJV may provide adequate ventilation and decrease fistula.

3. **Hyaline membrane disease.** High-frequency ventilation has been used with success. It is usually implemented at the point of severe respiratory failure with maximal conventional ventilation (a rescue treatment). Earlier treatment has been advocated. No advantages have yet been demonstrated for a very early intervention (in the first hours of life) when infants are pretreated with surfactant.

4. **Patients qualifying for ECMO.** Pulmonary hypertension with or without associated parenchymal lung disease (eg, meconium aspiration, pneumonia, hypoplastic lung, or diaphragmatic hernia) can result in intractable respiratory failure and high mortality unless the patient is treated by ECMO. The prior use of high-frequency ventilation among ECMO candidates has been successful and eliminated the need for ECMO in 25–45% of cases.

B. **Possible indications.** High-frequency ventilation has been used with success in infants with other disease processes. Further study is needed to develop clear indications and appropriate ventilatory strategies before this treatment can be recommended for routine use in infants with these diseases.

1. **Pulmonary hypertension.**
2. **Meconium aspiration syndrome.**
3. **Diaphragmatic hernia with pulmonary hypoplasia.**
4. **Postoperative Fontan procedures.**

C. **High-frequency ventilators, techniques, and equipment.** Three types of high-frequency ventilators in the United States are high-frequency jet ventilators (HFJVs), high-frequency oscillatory ventilators (HFOVs), and high-frequency flow interrupters (HFFIs).

1. **High-frequency jet ventilators.** The HFJV injects a high-velocity stream of gas into the endotracheal tube, usually at frequencies between 240 and 600 bpm and VTs equal to or slightly greater than dead space. During HFJV, expiration is passive. The only FDA-approved HFJV is the Life Pulse (Bunnell, Inc., Salt Lake City, UT) ventilator, discussed here.

   a. **Indications.** Mostly used for PIE, the Life Pulse HFJV has been used for the other indications described for all types of high-frequency ventilation.

   b. **Equipment**

      i. **Bunnell Life Pulse ventilator.** The inspiratory pressure (PIP), jet valve "on time," and respiratory frequency are entered into a digital control panel on the jet. PIPs are servo-controlled by the Life Pulse from the pressure port. The ventilator has an elaborate alarm system to ensure safety and to help detect changes in pulmonary function. It also has a special humidification system.

      ii. **Conventional ventilator.** A conventional ventilator is needed to generate PEEP and sigh breaths. PEEP and background ventilation are controlled with the conventional ventilator.

   c. **Procedure**

      i. **Initiation. Close observation** is required at all times, especially during initiation.

         (a) **Replace the endotracheal tube adapter with a jet adapter.**

         (b) **Settings on the jet ventilator**
            (i) **Default jet valve "on time":** 0.020 s.
            (ii) **Frequency of jet:** 420/min.
            (iii) **PIP on the jet:** 2–3 cm H_2O below what was on the conventional ventilator. Frequently, infants require considerably less PIP during high-frequency jet ventilation.

         (c) **Settings on the conventional ventilator**
            (i) **PEEP.** Maintained at 3–5 cm H_2O.
            (ii) **Rate.** As the jet ventilator comes up to pressure, the rate is decreased to 5–10 bpm.
            (iii) **PIP.** Once at pressure, the PIP is adjusted to a level 1–3 cm H_2O below that on the jet (low enough not to interrupt the jet ventilator).

   d. **Management.** Management of high-frequency jet ventilation is based on the clinical course and radiographic findings.

      i. **Elimination of CO_2.** Alveolar ventilation is much more sensitive to changes in VT than in respiratory frequency during high-frequency ventilation. As a result, the **delta pressure** (PIP minus PEEP) is adjusted to attain adequate elimination of CO_2, whereas jet valve "on time" and respiratory frequency are usually not readjusted during HFJV.

      ii. **Oxygenation.** Oxygenation is often better during HFJV than during conventional mechanical ventilation in neonates with PIE. However, if oxygenation is inadequate and if the infant is already on 100% oxygen, an increase in Paw usually results in improved oxygenation. It can be accomplished by:

(a) **Increasing PEEP.**

(b) **Increasing PIP.**

(c) **Increasing background conventional ventilator** (either rates or pressure).

   iii. **Positioning of infants.** Positioning infants with the affected side down may speed resolution of PIE. In bilateral air leak, alternating placement on dependent sides may be effective. Diligent observation and frequent radiographs are necessary to avoid hyperinflation of the nondependent side.

e. **Weaning.** When weaning, the following guidelines are used.

   i. **PIP is reduced as soon as possible** ($Paco_2$ <35–40 mm Hg). Because elimination of CO_2 is very sensitive to changes in V_T, PIP is weaned 1 cm H_2O at a time.

   ii. **Oxygen concentration** is weaned if oxygenation remains good (Pao_2 >70–80 mm Hg).

   iii. **Jet valve "on time" and frequency are usually kept constant.**

   iv. **Constant attention is paid to the infant's clinical condition** and radiographs to detect early atelectasis or hyperinflation.

   v. **Air leaks are resolved.** Continuation of HFJV occurs until the air leak has been resolved for 24–48 h, which often corresponds to a dramatic drop in ventilator pressures and oxygen requirement.

   vi. **If no improvement in the condition occurs,** a trial of conventional ventilation is used after 6–24 h on jet ventilation.

f. **Special considerations**

   i. **Airway obstruction.** This problem can usually be recognized quickly. Chest wall movement is decreased, although breath sounds may be adequate. The servo pressure (driving pressure) is usually very low.

   ii. **Inadvertent PEEP (air trapping).** In larger infants, the flow of jet gases may result in inadvertent PEEP. Decreasing the background flow on the conventional ventilator may correct the problem, or it may be necessary to decrease the respiratory frequency to allow more time for expiration.

g. **Complications**

   i. **Tracheitis.** Necrotizing tracheobronchitis was a frequent complication in the early days of jet ventilation. This problem is much less frequent with the recognition of the critical importance of proper humidification of the jet gases. If tracheitis occurs, emergent bronchoscopy may be indicated. The clinical signs include the following:

   (a) **Increased airway secretions.**

   (b) **Evidence of airway obstruction (including air trapping).**

   (c) **Acute respiratory acidosis.**

   ii. **Intraventricular hemorrhage.** There has been no increase in the incidence or severity of intraventricular hemorrhage with the use of the HFJV.

   iii. **Bronchopulmonary dysplasia.** There has been no apparent decrease in the incidence of bronchopulmonary dysplasia with the use of the HFJV.

2. **High-frequency oscillatory ventilators.** The HFOV generates V_T less than or equal to dead space by means of an oscillating piston or diaphragm. This mechanism creates active exhalation as well as inspiration. The SensorMedics 3100A HFOV (SensorMedics Inc., Yorba Linda, CA) is currently approved by the FDA for use in neonates.

a. **Indications.** Respiratory failure: High-frequency oscillatory ventilation is indicated when conventional ventilation does not result in adequate oxygenation or ventilation or requires the use of very high airway pressures. Like other forms of high-frequency ventilation, success is more likely when increased airway resistance is not the dominant pulmonary pathophysiology. Best results are seen when parenchymal disease is homogeneous. Some clinicians advocate high-frequency oscillatory ventilation as the primary method of assisted ventilation in premature infants with RDS.

    b. Equipment. The SensorMedics HFOV (Cardinal Health, Dublin, OH) has a piston oscillator and is not used in conjunction with a conventional ventilator. The user-defined parameters are frequency, $\overline{Paw}$, and power applied for piston displacement.

    c. Procedure

      i. Initiation

        (a) **Conventional ventilator is discontinued.**

        (b) **Settings**

          (i) **Frequency** is usually set at 15 Hz for premature infants with RDS. Larger infants, or those with a significant component of increased airway resistance (meconium aspiration), should be started at 5–10 Hz.

          (ii) $\overline{Paw}$ is set higher (2–5 cm H_2O) than on the previous conventional ventilation. If overdistention or air leaks were present prior to initiation of high-frequency oscillatory ventilation, a lower $\overline{Paw}$ should be considered.

          (iii) **Amplitude** (analogous to PIP on conventional ventilation) is regulated by the power of displacement of the piston. This power is increased until there is visible chest wall vibration.

        (c) **After high-frequency oscillatory ventilation has been initiated, careful and frequent assessment of lung expansion and adequate gas exchange are necessary.** Air trapping is a continuous potential threat in this form of treatment. Signs of overdistention, such as descended and flat diaphragms and small heart shadow, are monitored with frequent chest radiographs.

    d. Management

      i. If Pao_2 is low, an increase in $\overline{Paw}$ may be necessary. Chest radiographs may be helpful in determining the adequacy of lung expansion.

      ii. If $Paco_2$ is high:

        (a) **If oxygenation is also poor,** the $\overline{Paw}$ may be too high or too low, resulting in either hyperinflation or widespread collapse, respectively. Again, chest radiographs are necessary to differentiate between these two conditions.

        (b) **If oxygenation is adequate,** the amplitude (power) should be increased.

    e. Weaning

      i. In the absence of hyperinflation, Fio_2 is weaned prior to $\overline{Paw}$ for adequate Pao_2. Below 40% Fio_2, wean $\overline{Paw}$ exclusively.

      ii. $\overline{Paw}$ should be weaned as the lung disease improves with the goal of maintaining optimal lung expansion. Excessively aggressive early weaning of $\overline{Paw}$ may result in widespread atelectasis and the need for significant increases in $\overline{Paw}$ and Fio_2.

      iii. Amplitude should be weaned for acceptable $Paco_2$.

      iv. Frequency is usually not adjusted during weaning. A decrease in frequency is necessary when signs of lung overdistention cannot be eliminated by a reduction in $\overline{Paw}$.

      v. The neonate may be switched to conventional ventilation at a low level of support or may be extubated directly from an HFOV.

    f. Complications. See Section VI, C, 1g.

   3. High-frequency flow interupters. The Infant Star (Infrasonics Inc., San Diego, CA) is no longer supported. The Bronchotronflow interrupter (Percussionaire Corp., Sandpoint, ID) is being used at some institutions, but published safety data and efficacy are not yet available.

VII. Liquid ventilation. Liquid ventilation uses perfluorocarbon (PFC) liquids (inert, colorless, and odorless liquids that provide gas exchange) instilled in the lungs. The liquid provides gas exchange with even inflation of the lungs, decreases inflammatory

injury, and improves lung compliance. Two methods are described: **total liquid ventilation (TLV)** (completely filled lungs) and **partial liquid ventilation (PLV)** (where the
lungs are filled to functional residual capacity while conventional ventilation is maintained). Studies have been done on evaluation of PLV and perfluorocarbon induced lung
growth (PILG) in newborns with CDH on ECMO. This study showed that PILG can be
performed safely, and the results were encouraging. Another study addressed the addition of a low dose of PFC with HFO showing it was effective in achieving adequate oxygenation with a reduction in further lung injury. Studies need to be done to see if HFO
and perfluorocarbons together would improve outcomes. **At the present time liquid
ventilation is only used for investigational purposes, and perfluorocarbon is not available in the United States for routine use.**

GLOSSARY OF TERMS USED IN RESPIRATORY MANAGEMENT

Arterial to alveolar ratio (a/A ratio). See Section I, B, 3b.
Assist. A setting at which the infant initiates the mechanical breath, triggering the ventilator
to deliver a preset V_T or pressure.
Assist/control. The same as assist, except that if the infant becomes apneic, the ventilator deliv-
ers the number of mechanical breaths per minute set on the rate control.
Continuous positive airway pressure (CPAP). A spontaneous mode in which the ambient
intrapulmonary pressure that is maintained throughout the respiratory cycle is increased.
Control. A setting at which a certain number of mechanical breaths per minute is delivered.
The infant is unable to breathe spontaneously between mechanical breaths.
End-tidal CO_2 (Etco$_2$ or Petco$_2$). A measure of the P_{CO_2} of end expiration.
Expiratory time (ET). The amount of time set for the expiratory phase of each mechanical
breath.
Flow rate. The amount of gas per minute passing through the ventilator. It must be sufficient
to prevent rebreathing (ie, 3 times the minute volume) and to achieve the PIP during Ti.
Changes in the flow rate may be necessary if changes in the airway waveform are desired. The
normal range is 6–10 L/min; 8 L/min is commonly used.
Fraction of inspired oxygen (FiO_2). The percentage of oxygen concentration of inspired gas
expressed as decimals (room air = 0.21).
I:E ratio. Ratio of inspiratory time to expiratory time. The normal values are 1:1, 1:1.5, or 1:2.
Inspiratory time (Ti). The amount of time set for the inspiratory phase of each mechanical breath.
Intermittent mechanical ventilation. Mechanical breaths are delivered at intervals. The infant
breathes spontaneously between mechanical breaths.
Minute ventilation. V_T (proportional to PIP) multiplied by rate.
Oxygen index (OI). See Section I, D, 2d.
Oxyhemoglobin dissociation curve. A curve showing the amount of oxygen that combines
with hemoglobin as a function of Pa_{O_2} and Pa_{CO_2}. The curve shifts to the right when oxygen
takeup by the blood is less than normal at a given PO_2, and it shifts to the left when oxygen
takeup is greater than normal.
Pa_{O_2}. Partial pressure of arterial oxygen.
PAP. The total airway pressure. In the Siemens Servo 900-C, it is the PIP plus the PEEP.
$P\overline{a}w$. The average proximal pressure applied to the airway throughout the entire respiratory cycle.
Pco_2. Carbon dioxide partial pressure.
Peak inspiratory pressure (PIP). The highest pressure reached within the proximal airway
with each mechanical breath. *Note:* In the Siemens Servo 900-C, the PIP is defined as the inspi-
ratory pressure above the PEEP.
PO_2. Partial pressure of oxygen.
Positive end-expiratory pressure (PEEP). The pressure in the airway above ambient pressure
during the expiratory phase of mechanical ventilation.
Rate. Number of mechanical breaths per minute delivered by the ventilator.
Sa_{O_2}. Oxygen saturation of arterial blood measured by direct measurement (arterial blood gas).
Tidal volume (V_T). The volume of gas inspired or expired during each respiratory cycle.

Suggested References

Goldsmith JP, Karotkin E: *Assisted Ventilation of the Neonate*, 4th ed. Philadelphia: WB Saunders, 2004.

Cochrane Neonatal Group: http://neonatal.cochrane.org.

Donn SM, Sinha SK: *Neonatal Respiratory Care,* 2nd ed. Philadelphia: Mosby, 2006.

Tobin M: *Principles and Practice of Mechanical Ventilation.* New York: McGraw-Hill, 2006.

8 Body Water, Fluid, and Electrolytes

An assessment of body water metabolism and electrolyte balance plays an important role in the early medical management of preterm infants and sick term infants coming to neonatal intensive care. Intravenous or intra-arterial fluids given during the first several days of life are a major factor in the development, or prevention, of morbidities such as intraventricular hemorrhage, necrotizing enterocolitis, patent ductus arteriosus, and bronchopulmonary dysplasia. Therefore it is crucial that an infant's clinician pay close attention to the details of maintaining and monitoring body water and serum electrolytes, and the management of fluid infusion therapies.

Bodily fluid balance is a function of the distribution of water in the body, water intake, and water losses. **Body water distribution gradually changes with increasing gestational age of the fetus, from the very immature fetus with 90% of body weight as water, to the late preterm fetus with 75–80% body weight as water.** At birth these gestational changes in body water are reflected in the developing maturity of renal function, transepidermal insensible water losses, and neuroendocrine adaptations. A clinician must account for these variables when deciding the amount of infusion fluids to administer to an infant.

I. **Body water**
   A. **Total body water (TBW).** Water accounts for nearly 75% of the body weight in term infants and as much as 85–90% of body weight of preterm infants. TBW is divided into two basic body water compartments: intracellular water (ICW) and extracellular (ECW). ECW is composed of intravascular and interstitial water. For the fetus there is a gradual decrease in ECW to 53% at 32 weeks' gestation and a gradual increase in ICW. Thereafter the proportions remain fairly constant until 38 weeks' of gestation when increasing body mass of protein and fat stores reduce ECW further by approximately 5%.

   At birth there begins a further contraction of the ECW as a function of the normal transition from intrauterine to extrauterine life. A diuresis occurs that reduces body weight proportionally to gestational age. For the very low birthweight preterm infant body, weight losses of 10–15% can be expected, whereas full-term infants usually lose 5% of body weight. These losses are largely accounted for as water and, to a lesser extent, body fat stores.

   B. **TBW balance in the newborn**
      1. **Renal.** Fetal urine flow steadily increases from 2–5 mL/h to 10–20 mL/h at 30 weeks' gestation. At term, fetal urine flow reaches 25–50 mL/h and then drops to 8–16 mL/h (1–3 mL/kg/h). These volume changes illustrate the large exchange of body water during fetal life and the abrupt changes forcing physiologic adaptation at birth. Despite marked fetal urine flow in utero, glomerular filtration rates

(GFR) are low. At birth, GFR remains low but steadily increases in the newborn period under the influence of increasing systolic blood pressure, increasing renal blood flow, and increasing glomerular permeability. Infant kidneys are able to produce dilute urine within limits dependent on GFR. The low GFR of preterm infants is the result of low renal blood flow but increases considerably after 34 weeks' postconceptual age. Term infants can concentrate urine up to 800 mOsm/L compared to 1500 mOsm/L of older children and adults. The preterm infant kidney is less able to concentrate urine secondary to a relatively low interstitial urea concentration, an anatomically shorter loop of Henle, and a distal tubular and collecting system that is less responsive to antidiuretic hormone (ADH). In extreme prematurity, urine osmolarity can be as low as 90 mOsm/L and with urine flows up to 7 mL/h. Although limitations exist, healthy preterm infants with constant sodium intake, but variable fluid infusion between 90 and 200 mL/kg/day, are able to concentrate or dilute urine to maintain a balance of body water.

Against the backdrop of changing GFR and variable urine concentrating ability, all infants undergo a diuresis and a natriuresis in the days immediately following birth. Newborn diuresis is a contraction of the ECW and the initiation of body water conservation as the adaptation from an aquatic intrauterine existence to the less humid near-arid and free water dependent newborn state. The diuresis is facilitated by limited ADH responsiveness but diminished by increasing serum osmolality (>285 mOsm/kg) and decreasing intravascular volume. Natriuresis is the result of increasing levels of atrial natriuretic peptide and decreased renal sodium absorption; infant kidneys have decreased secretion of bicarbonate, potassium, and hydrogen ion.

2. **Insensible water loss (IWL).** Evaporation of body water occurs largely through the skin and mucous membranes (two thirds), and the respiratory tract (one third). A most important variable influencing IWL is the maturity of the infants' skin. The greater IWL in preterm infants results from body water evaporation through an immature epithelial layer. The stratum corneum is not well developed until 34 weeks' gestation. Throughout the third trimester the stratum corneum and epidermis thicken. Keratinization of the stratum corneum forms the principal barrier to water loss. Keratinization begins early in the second trimester and continues until birth. Additionally, IWL is related to a larger skin surface area-to-body weight ratio in preterm infants and relatively greater skin vascularity.

IWL through the respiratory tract is related to the respiratory rate and the water content of the inspired air or air-oxygen mix (humidification). Table 8–1 lists other factors for IWL in newborn infants.

In general, for healthy premature infants weighing 800–2000 g cared for in double walled incubators, IWL increases linearly as body weight decreases.

Table 8–1. FACTORS IN THE NICU ENVIRONMENT THAT AFFECT INSENSIBLE WATER LOSS

Body weight	Inversely proportional to maturity
Radiant warmer use	IWL increase by 50–100% over incubator care. See also Chapter 16
Phototherapy	IWL controversial; may be minimal for term infants, but appreciable for preterm
Ambient humidity and temperature	High ambient humidity and a thermal neutral environment conserve TBW
High body temperature	May increase loss by 30–50%
Tachypnea	Variable depending on respiratory support
Skin breakdown	Most often from adhesives denuding skin areas
Congenital absence of normal skin covering	Large omphaloceles, neural tube defects, or skin losses in epidermolysis bullosa

Table 8–2. **ESTIMATES OF INSENSIBLE WATER LOSS IN PRETERM INFANTS DURING FIRST WEEK OF LIFE IN A THERMAL NEUTRAL ENVIRONMENT**

Birth weight (g)	IWL (mL/kg/day)
<750	100–200
750–1000	60–70
1001–1250	50–60
1251–1500	30–40
1501–2000	20–30
>2000	15–20

(Based on data from Dell KM, Davis ID: Fluid and electrolyte management. In *Fanaroff and Martin's Neonatal-Perinatal Medicine: Diseases of the Fetus and Infant.* Philadelphia: Mosby Elsevier, 2006;695–703.)

However, for sick infants of similar weight cared for in a radiant warmer and undergoing ventilator respiratory support, IWL increases exponentially as body weight decreases. See Table 8–2.

Phototherapy may increase IWL by way of increasing body temperature and increasing peripheral blood flow. Generally recommended fluid increases for preterm infants have been 10–20 mL/kg/day. This may not be necessary with newer phototherapy lights using light emitting diodes (LEDs) because they generate very little heat. Moreover, term infants receiving adequate fluid intake and with no increased body water loss may not need added fluid intake. Occasionally, phototherapy induces loose stools and IWL would need to be reconsidered.

3. **Neuroendocrine.** TBW balance is also influenced by hypothalamic osmoreceptors and carotid baroreceptors. Serum osmolarity >285 mOsm/kg stimulates the hypothalamus and vasopressin (antidiuretic hormone [ADH]) is released to affect free water retention. Additionally, volume diminution affects carotid bodies and baroreceptors to further stimulate ADH secretion to retain free water at the level of the collecting ducts of the distal nephrons. Collectively the osmoreceptors and the baroreceptors seek to maintain TBW with adequate intravascular volume at normal serum osmolarity. Vasopressin (ADH) secretion can be demonstrated in the fetus from midgestation. Fetal and neonatal animal models have specific triggers for ADH secretion (ie, serum hyperosmolarity, hypoxia, intracranial hemorrhage, and trauma). In the neonate, hypoxia with acidemia and hypercarbia are potent stimulators of ADH. An excessive secretion of ADH can follow one or more of the insults just described in the absence of hyperosmolarity or volume depletion. Thus a syndrome of inappropriate ADH secretion can occur (SIADH). It is manifested as hyponatremia, hypo-osmolar serum, dilute urine, and low blood urea nitrogen. Because ADH (vasopressin) secretion begins early in fetal development, SIADH can occur as readily in preterm infants as in term infants.

C. **Monitoring TBW balance**
   1. **Body weight.** Using in-bed scales, body weight should be recorded daily for all infants undergoing intensive care, and twice daily for very low birthweight and extremely low birthweight infants. **Expected weight loss during the first 3–5 days of life is 5–10% of birthweight for term infants, and 10–15% of birthweight for preterm infants.** A loss of >15% of birthweight during the first week of life should be considered excessive and body water balance carefully reevaluated. If weight loss is <2% in the first week of life, maintenance infusion fluid administration may be excessive.
   2. **Physical examination.** Edema or loss of skin turgor, moist or dry mucous membranes, sunken or puffy periorbital tissues, and full or sunken anterior fontanel have been time-honored sites to examine for dehydration or overhydration. They may be helpful when observing newborn infants but are unreliable in low birthweight

infants. They must be observed within the context of all other TBW points of monitoring.

3. **Vital signs**
   a. **Blood pressure** can be an indicator of altered intravascular volume, but usually is later rather than early. But pressure changes and trend are needed in the overall assessment of TBW balance.
   b. **Pulse volumes,** decreased in dehydration with tachycardia, are fairly sensitive indicators of early intravascular volume loss.
   c. **Tachypnea** may be an early sign of metabolic acidosis accompanying inadequate intravascular volume.
   d. **Capillary refill time (CRT)** has been a reliable and time-honored observation. CRT of >3 s in term infants is suspect for decreased intravascular volume, whereas a CRT of barely 3 s in a preterm infant should be equally suspect.

4. **Hematocrit (Hct).** Increases or decreases of central Hct (venous or arterial) from accepted normal values strongly suggest significant changes in intravascular volume as it relates to TBW. Apart from obvious hemorrhage, overhydration, or dehydration during infusion fluid management in the first week of life must be accounted for TBW assessment.

5. **Serum chemistries**
   a. **Sodium** values of 135–140 mEq/L are indicative of TBW and natremic balance. Values above or below are suggestive of hyper- or hypo-osmolarity. A sodium value of ≤130 mEq/L strongly suggests that SIADH may be a factor.
   b. **Serum osmolarity** of 285 mOsm/L (±3 mOsm) is the standard for TBW balance; values above or below must be considered indicative of over- or under-hydration. If serum osmolarity is <280 mOsm/L, SIADH must also be considered in any preterm or sick full-term infant.

6. **Acid-base status**
   a. **Hydrogen ion (pH).** A less than normal pH (7.28–7.35) is indicative of metabolic acidosis and will be accompanied by other factors, suggesting a contracted intravascular volume and hyperosmolarity.
   b. **Base deficit (BD).** An increasing BD (ie, metabolic acidosis with BD >5.0) with decreased urine output, decreased blood pressure, and a prolonged CRT strongly suggests dehydration.
   c. **Chloride ion, carbon dioxide (CO_2) content, and bicarbonate (HCO_3)** determinations are important for calculating anion gap.
   d. **Anion gap.** The anion gap is a unifying determination for identifying metabolic acidosis in the face of dehydration. It is the sum of the serum sodium and potassium ions *minus* the sum of the serum chloride and bicarbonate ions. The normal range for anion gap is 5–15. Values for an anion gap >15 are indicative of an organic acidemia. In the face of dehydration with decreased intravascular volume, lactic acidemia follows poor tissue perfusion and is reflected as a widening anion gap.

7. **Urine**
   a. **Urine output should be 1–3 mL/kg/h by the third day of life in all newborn infants with normal kidneys.** Preterm infants have limited but some urine formation on day 1, and thereafter increasing through day 2.
   b. **Urine specific gravity of 1.005–1.012 is consistent with TBW balance.**
   c. **Urine electrolytes and urine osmolarity** offer additional information as to renal concentrating ability. Term infants can concentrate urine to 800 mOsm/kg, whereas preterm infants are limited to 600 mOsm/kg.

D. **Maintenance of TBW.** Infusion fluid therapy for newborn infants (term and preterm) must be carefully calculated to allow for normal ECW losses and body weight losses while avoiding dehydration from excessive IWL. The consequences of dehydration are hypotension, hypernatremia, and acidosis. Conversely, excessive infusion fluid therapy is associated with clinically significant patent ductus arteriosus, necrotizing enterocolitis, intraventricular hemorrhage, and bronchopulmonary dysplasia. Given careful monitoring for TBW as detailed earlier, the following infusion fluid therapy guidelines are offered for maintenance of TBW balance in term and preterm infants (with the exception of infusion fluid therapy for extremely low birthweight infants; see Chapter 16.)

1. **Term infants in need of infusion fluid therapy**
   a. **Day 1.** Give dextrose 10% in water (D10W) at a rate of 60–80 mL/kg/day. This provides 6–7 mg/kg/min of glucose in support of energy needs while providing limited hydration during the immediate postnatal adaptation period. Neither sodium nor potassium supplementation are needed unless unusual body fluid losses are known.
   b. **Days 2–7.** Once tolerance of infusion fluid therapy has been established and confirmed by TBW monitoring (eg, urine output of 1–2 mL/kg/h), the rate and composition of fluid therapy can be modified. **The goals of infusion fluid therapy include expected weight loss of 5% body weight, confirmed normal serum electrolyte values, and continued urine output of 2–3 mL/kg/h.** Specifics of fluid therapy are:
      i. **Infusion fluid volume** 80–120 mL/kg/day. May increase to 120–160 mL/kg/day by week's end as tolerated or to meet needs per monitoring.
      ii. **Glucose** to be provided to maintain serum glucose values >60 mg/dL; may increase to 8–9 mg/kg/min infusion as D10W or D12.5W.
      iii. **Sodium requirement daily** is 2–4 mEq/kg/day per monitoring of serum (target values, 135–140 mEq/L).
      iv. **Potassium daily requirements** are 1–2 mEq/kg/day per monitoring of serum (target values, 4.0–5.0 mEq/L). Potassium supplementation is not begun until the second or third day, and only when normal renal function is confirmed by adequate urine output and normal serum electrolyte values have been established.
      v. **Nutrition.** Infusion fluid glucose does not meet all energy needs for basal metabolism, growth, and activity. Enteral feeds must be started as soon as possible; however, if patient unable to take formula by mouth or only in limited amounts, then total parenteral nutrition (TPN) becomes necessary. **As enteral feeds increase, infusion fluids or TPN can be progressively decreased, but keeping total volume intake at 120–160 mL/kg/day.**

2. **Preterm infants**
   a. **Day 1.** During the immediate postnatal period, critically ill premature infants may require volume resuscitation for shock or acidosis. Fluids administered during stabilization should be considered when planning subsequent fluid management.
   b. **Days 1–3.** Infusion fluid therapy is aimed at allowing a 10–15% body weight loss through the first week while maintaining TBW balance and electrolyte balance.
      i. **Infusion fluid volumes.** Preterm low birthweight infants (>1500 g) require 60–80 mL/kg/day. Preterm very low birthweight infants (1000–1500 g) require 80–100 mL/kg /day. Preterm extremely low birthweight infants (<1000 g) require a range of fluid volumes from100–200 mL/kg/day (see Table 16–1 for breakdown into 100-g birthweight increments).
      ii. **Glucose supplementation** is best achieved by using D5W or D7.5W infusion fluids to minimize hyperglycemia. Because of the high fluid requirements in the smallest infants, glucose utilization may not be sufficient to prevent buildup of serum glucose and a hyperosmolar state secondary to hyperglycemia. Insulin may be required to control hyperglycemia in some of the very small infants.
      iii. **Sodium.** During the first week of life, fluid therapy should be managed by increments or decrements of 20–40/mL/kg/day depending on weight

changes and serum sodium values, while attempting to keep serum sodium at 135–140 mEq/L. Sodium supplementation is not usually required in the first 3 days of life. Sodium supplementation is begun on the basis of body weight losses (postnatal isotonic contraction of ECW compartment, a physiologic diuresis). Usually by day 3–5, weight loss and a slight serum sodium decrease from baseline dictate the need to start sodium supplementation by way of the infusion fluids. Judicious restriction of sodium intake during the first 3–5 days of life facilitates a trend for normal serum osmolarity throughout the first week of life for preterm infants.

    iv. **Potassium** supplementation follows that of term infants, meaning that well-established renal function with good urine output is required before supplementation at 1–2 mEq/kg/day.

    v. **Nutrition.** Caloric needs to provide for the relative hypermetabolic state of low birthweight infants can be met through TPN fluid therapy. Initiation of TPN after the first 24 h of life is desirable. (See Chapters 9 and 16.)

  c. **Days 3–7.** Infusion fluid and electrolyte management is dictated by the monitoring parameters as already given. Infusion fluids should be advanced or decreased as the transition period progresses. Excessive weight loss suggests increased IWL losses and the threat of dehydration. Likewise, edema and minimal or no weight loss suggests excessive fluid administration or decreasing renal function and decreased urine output. All preterm infants should be cared for whenever possible in double-walled incubators for a more stable humidity control and less IWL.

3. **Other infusion fluid calculations and considerations**
  a. **Environmental**
    i. **Radiant warmers.** Infusion fluid volume recommendations as outlined earlier are for assumed double-walled incubator care. If radiant warmer exposure is to be maintained, fluid therapy must be increased by 50–100%. Plastic sheeting limits increased needs to 30–50%.
    ii. **Phototherapy.** If infant is full term, increased fluid therapy may not be needed. If infant is low birthweight, most likely 10–20 mL/kg/day will be needed to minimize IWL while phototherapy lights are in use.
  b. **Glucose. The normal glucose requirement is 6–8 mg/kg/min, and intake can be slowly increased to 10–12 mg/kg/min as needed, but with careful monitoring for hyperglycemia and glucosuria as an osmotic diuresis.**

Glucose requirements (mg/kg/min) =

$$\frac{(\text{Percentage of glucose} \times \text{Rate[mL/h]} \times 0.167)}{\text{Weight (kg)}}$$

The alternate method is

Glucose requirement (mg/kg/min) =

$$\frac{(\text{Amount of glucose/mL [from Table 8–3]} \times \text{Total fluids})}{\text{Weight (kg)/(60 min)}}$$

  c. **Sodium. The normal sodium requirement for infants is 2–3 mEq/kg/day.** The following calculations can be used to determine the amount of sodium ($Na+$) per day that an infant will receive from a given saline infusion fluid:

Amount of Na^+/mL (from Table 8–4) × Total fluids/day = Amount of Na^+/day

$$\frac{\text{Amount of Na}^+\text{/day}}{\text{Weight (kg)}} = \text{Amount of Na}^+ \text{ (kg/day)}$$

Table 8–3. GLUCOSE CONCENTRATION IN COMMONLY USED
INTRAVENOUS INFUSION FLUIDS

Solution (%)	Glucose Concentration (mg/mL)
Dextrose 5% water	50
Dextrose 7.5% water	75
Dextrose 10% water	100
Dextrose 12.5% water	125
Dextrose 15% water	150

   d. **Potassium. The normal potassium requirement for infants is 1–2 mEq/kg/day.**
      Potassium supplementation should not begin until adequate urine output is
      established.
II. **Electrolyte disturbances**
   A. **Sodium.** Serum values of 135–145 mEq/L represent homeostatic sodium balance.
      The wide range of 131–149 mEq/L is the lower and upper limit for sodium (Na^+) bal-
      ance. Values above or below are clinical indicators of either hyper- or hyponatremia.
      1. **Hypernatremia**
         a. **Decreased ECW with Na^+ of ≥150 mEq/L**
            i. **Causes** include increased renal free water losses and/or increased IWL, pri-
               marily through skin, especially very low birthweight and extremely low
               birthweight infants.
            ii. **Clinical findings** are weight loss, low blood pressure, tachycardia, decreased
               or absent urine output, and increased urine specific gravity.
            iii. **Treatment** of hypernatremic dehydration requires careful infusion fluid
               management. **Replacing free water is the first goal, and maintaining Na^+
               balance is the second goal.** Both goals need to be accomplished without
               precipitating rapid ICW and ECW shifts of water or sodium; especially
               within the central nervous system (CNS). **Excessively rapid correction of
               hypernatremia can result in seizures.** Hypernatremic dehydration does
               not represent a deficit of body sodium. Infusion therapy should be guided
               to reduce serum Na^+ by not more than 0.5 mEq/L/kg/h, or less, with a tar-
               get of total correction time of 24–48 h. Consider using D5%W 0.25 NS as
               an initial infusion fluid for correction.
         b. **Increased ECW and hypernatremia**
            i. **Causes** include excessive administration of normal saline or sodium
               bicarbonate, as in resuscitation efforts or postresuscitation treatment for
               perinatal asphyxia with metabolic acidosis and hypotension.

Table 8–4. **SODIUM CONTENT OF COMMONLY USED INFUSION FLUIDS**

Solution	Sodium Concentration (mEq/L)
3% normal saline	0.500
Normal saline	0.154
0.50% normal saline	0.075
0.25% normal saline	0.037
0.125% normal saline	0.019

ii. **Clinical findings** are increased weight gain and edema. If cardiac output has been compromised, findings of edema and weight gain increase. Depending on cardiac status heart rate, blood pressure and urine output will be within normal limits or decreased.

iii. **Treatment** involves identification of cardiac status. Identification of infusion fluid excesses and establishing maintenance infusion fluid limits; thereafter sodium restriction until serum Na^+ values return to normal range.

2. **Hyponatremia** See also Chapter 57.

  a. **Increased ECW as increased intravascular water and increased third space interstitial water.**

   i. **Causes** are increased ECW with serum Na^+ >130 mEq/L most likely represents excessive infusion fluid administration, and increased third space (interstitial) water secondary to sepsis, shock, and capillary leakage. It may also be secondary to cardiac failure or pharmacologic neuromuscular paralysis during mechanical ventilation. More frequently it occurs in newborn infants as SIADH following CNS trauma, intracranial hemorrhage, meningitis, perinatal asphyxia, or pneumothorax.

   ii. **Clinical findings** result from inadvertent excessive infusion fluid administration: body weight is increased with edema, serum Na^+ is decreased, urine output is increased with decreased urine osmolarity and specific gravity. Conversely, if SIADH is the root cause of increased ECW and hyponatremia, the clinical findings reveal increased body weight, variable presence of edema, decreased serum Na^+, **decreased urine output, and increased urine specific gravity.** Some cases of SIADH do not reflect increased ECW but rather manifest simply as hyponatremia with decreased urine output and urine specific gravity.

   iii. **Treatment** in both situations is free water restriction allowing serum Na^+ to concentrate to normal levels. **If serum Na^+ is <120 mEq/L and neurologic symptoms are present, consider titrating with infusion of 3% saline solution boluses.** Consultation by a nephrologist is recommended.

  b. **Decreased ECW with hyponatremia**

   i. **Causes** include excessive diuretic therapy, glycosuria with an osmotic diuresis, vomiting, diarrhea, and third spaced fluid with necrotizing enterocolitis.

   ii. **Clinical findings** include decreased body weight, signs of dehydration with sunken fontanel, loss of skin turgor, dry mucous membranes, increased blood urea nitrogen (BUN), metabolic acidosis, decreased urine output, and increased urine specific gravity.

   iii. **Treatment** involves replacing sodium and water while minimizing any ongoing sodium losses.

  c. **Isotonic losses may occur and present as hyponatremia.** Such losses may be cerebrospinal fluid from drainage procedures, thoracic as in chylothorax, nasogastric drainage, or peritoneal fluid (ascites).

   Normal saline for fluid replacement usually suffices, or normal saline plus colloid as fresh-frozen plasma or human albumin may facilitate intravascular volume and restore serum saline.

B. **Potassium**

 1. **Hyperkalemia** is represented by serum K^+ values >5.5 mEq/L. Some infants do not manifest symptoms until serum levels reach 7–8 mEq/L. Hyperkalemia can be caused by or related to renal failure, hemolysis, blood transfusions, exchange transfusions, or inadvertent excessive administration of a potassium solution (KCl). Cardiac conduction is the most immediate concern, and electrocardiographic monitoring is essential until treatment corrects serum K^+ levels. For a detailed discussion of hyperkalemia and treatment, see Chapter 53.

2. **Hypokalemia.** Potassium levels <4.0 mEq/L suggest impending hypokalemia, and values <3.5 mEq/L require treatment to correct. Meanwhile cardiac conduction abnormalities may occur, and monitoring electrocardiographically, as in hyperkalemia, is essential until hypokalemia is corrected. For a detailed discussion of hypokalemia and treatment, see Chapter 56.

C. **Chloride**

1. **Hypochloremia.** Serum values of 97–110 mEq/L are taken as normal in most newborn infants. Serum values <97 are indicative of low chloride and suggest either inadequate supplementation during infusion fluid therapy, or more commonly they reflect chloride ion losses. Typically, chloride ion accompanies Na^+ and K^+ as NaCl or KCl solutions in maintenance infusion solutions. Chloride losses independent of Na^+ or K^+ occur usually from excessive gastrointestinal fluid losses, particularly gastric hydrochloric acid losses. Chloride losses lead to increased bicarbonate reabsorption and metabolic alkalosis.

2. **Hyperchloremia** is uncommon in the newborn period but may be found when inadvertent concentrations of Cl^- ion are given in parenteral nutrition solutions. Occasionally increased Cl^- ion is reflective of excessive renal conservation of Cl^- during correction of alkalosis when forming alkaline urine.

Selected References

Baumgartner S: Fluid, electrolyte and glucose maintenance in the very low birth weight infant. *Clin Pediatr* 1982;4:199-204.

Brion LP, Satlin LM: Clinical significance of developmental renal physiology. In Polin RA, Fox WW (eds): *Fetal and Neonatal Physiology*, 2nd ed. Philadelphia, PA: WB Saunders, 1998:1677–1683.

Costarino AT, Baumgartner S: Controversies in fluid and electrolyte therapy for the premature infant. *Clin Perinatol* 1988;15:863-878.

Costarino AT et al: Sodium restriction versus daily maintenance replacement in very low birth weight premature neonates: A randomized, blind therapeutic trial. *J Pediatr* 1992;120:99–106.

Dell KM, Davis ID: Fluid and electrolyte management. In Martin RJ et al (eds): *Fanaroff and Martin's Neonatal-Perinatal Medicine: Diseases of the Fetus and the Infant*, 8th ed. Philadelphia, PA: Elsevier Mosby, 2006:695-703.

Gawlowski Z et al: Hypernatremia in preterm infants born at less than 27 weeks' gestation. *J Paediatr Child Health* 2006;42:771-774.

Hartnoll G: Basic principle and practical steps in the management of fluid balance in the newborn. *Semin Neonatol* 2003;8:307-313.

Leake RD: Fetal and neonatal neurohypophyseal hormones. In Polin RA, Fox WW (eds): *Fetal and Neonatal Physiology*, 2nd ed. Philadelphia, PA: WB Saunders, 1998:2442–2446.

Maisels MJ, McDonagh AF: Phototherapy for neonatal jaundice. *N Engl J Med* 2008;358:920-928.

Meyer MP et al: A clinical comparison of radiant warmer and incubator care for preterm infants from birth to 1800 grams. *Pediatrics* 2001;108:395-401.

Modi N: Management of fluid balance in the very immature neonate. *Arch Dis Child Fetal Neonatal Ed* 2004;89:F108-F111.

9 Nutritional Management

GROWTH ASSESSMENT OF THE NEONATE

I. **Anthropometrics.** Serial measurements of weight, length, and head circumference allow for evaluation of growth patterns.
   A. **Weight.** During the first week of life, weight loss of 10–20% of birthweight is expected because of changes in body water compartments. Preterm infants lose more weight and regain birthweight slower than term infants. Weight gain generally begins by the second week of life. Average daily weight gain based on normal intrauterine growth is 10–20 g/kg/day (1–3% of body weight/day). Infants should be weighed daily.
   B. **Length.** Length is a better indicator of lean body mass and long-term growth and is not influenced by fluid status. Weekly assessment is recommended. Average length gain in preterm infants is 0.8–1.0 cm/week, whereas term infants average 0.69–0.75 cm/week.
   C. **Head circumference.** Intrauterine head growth is 0.5–0.8 cm/week. This is used as an indicator of brain growth. Premature infants exhibit catchup growth in head circumference that may exceed normal growth rate, but an increase in head circumference >1.25 cm/week may be abnormal and associated with hydrocephalus or intraventricular hemorrhage.
   D. **Weight for length** can be used to determine symmetry of growth. Current weight expressed as a percentage of ideal weight for length can identify infants at risk for under- or overnutrition. Catchup growth occurs faster if only weight is lagging compared to length and head circumference. Weight gain is slower in large for gestational age infants.
II. **Classification**
   A. **Measurements** of weight, length, and head circumference are plotted on growth charts to facilitate comparison to established norms. This can help to identify special needs.
   B. **Growth charts** provide longitudinal assessment of an infant's growth. Growth charts for term boys and girls are available from the Centers for Disease Control (www.cdc.gov/growthcharts). Two types of charts exist for very low birthweight (VLBW) infants: those based on intrauterine growth or those based on postnatal growth. Assessment of postnatal growth failure is better reflected on postnatal growth charts. Variations exist in the reference populations for the various growth charts. **Normal growth** customarily falls between the 10th and 90th percentiles when adjusted for gestational age. Intrauterine growth is classified as **appropriate for gestational age; large for gestational age** (eg, infants of diabetic mothers, postmature infants, or infants with Beckwith-Wiedemann syndrome) or **small for gestational age.**

NUTRITIONAL REQUIREMENTS IN THE NEONATE

I. **Calories**
   A. **To maintain weight,** give 50–60 kcal/kg/day (60 nonprotein kcal/kg/day).
   B. **To induce weight gain,** give 100–120 kcal/kg/day to a term infant (gain: 15–30 g/day) and 110–140 kcal/kg/day to a premature infant (70–90 nonprotein kcal/kg/day). Growth in premature infants is assumed to be adequate when it approximates the intrauterine rate (ie, 15 g/kg/day).
II. **Carbohydrates.** Approximately 10–30 g/kg/day (7.5–15g/kg/day) are needed to provide 40–50% of total calories. Lesser amounts of carbohydrates should provide total energy requirements in infants with chronic lung disease.

III. **Proteins.** Adequate protein intake has been estimated at 2.25–4.0 g/kg/day (7–16% of total calories, or 2–3 g/100 kcal for efficient utilization). Protein intake in low birthweight infants should not exceed 4.0 g/kg/day.

IV. **Fats.** Fat requirements are 5–7 g/kg/day (limit: 40–55% of total calories or ketosis may result). To meet essential fatty acid requirements, 2–5% of nonprotein calories should be in the form of linoleic acid and 0.6% in the form of linolenic acid (together comprising 3% of total energy requirements). Linoleic and linolenic acids are precursors for arachidonic acid (AA) and docosahexanoic acid (DHA), important in neural and retinal maturation. Breast milk contains long-chain polyunsaturated fatty acids (LCPUFAs), but concentrations vary over the world (0.1–1.4%). LCPUFAs are transferred transplacentally predominantly in the third trimester. LCPUFA-enriched formulas are associated with improved retinal sensitivity and visual acuity but have no effect on short-term morbidities like bronchopulmonary dysplasia (BPD), necrotizing enterocolitis (NEC), and retinopathy of prematurity (ROP). The optimal dose for supplementation has not been determined. The effect on growth and anthropometric parameters is conflicting, although some long-term benefits in development are reported in preterm infants.

V. **Vitamins and minerals.** Vitamin requirements for preterm infants are not clearly established. Guidelines are provided in Tables 9–1 to 9–3 for low birthweight infants. Caution is required with vitamin supplementation because toxicity may occur with both water- and fat-soluble vitamins as a result of immature renal and hepatic function. Vitamin supplementation may be needed with certain types of infant formulas (see Table 9–4).

   A. **Vitamin A** may be useful in attenuating chronic lung disease in VLBW infants at a dose of 5000 IU intramuscularly three times/week for 12 doses.

   B. **In infants with osteopenia of prematurity,** various amounts of calcium, phosphorus, and vitamin D may be supplemented.

   C. **For infants receiving recombinant human erythropoietin therapy (rhEPO),** additional iron supplementation is necessary. Although recommended doses vary, it is generally agreed that a dose in excess of maintenance therapy is needed. These doses may approach 6–10 mg/kg/day. Iron can also be added to parenteral nutrition. For infants on high doses of iron, monitoring for hemolytic anemia is important, and vitamin E supplementation (15–25 IU/day) may be required. rhEPO use is associated with increased risk of ROP.

   D. **Iron deficiency** is associated with short-term and long-term neurodevelopmental deficits, delayed maturation of the auditory brainstem responses, and abnormalities of memory and behavior. Iron supplementation of term infants at risk of iron deficiency is associated with improved neurodevelopmental outcomes. Preterm infants are more susceptible to iron deficiency due to small iron stores at birth, high growth velocity, and phlebotomy losses. However, blood transfusions provide a rich source of iron. Preterm infants should receive iron supplementation (2–4 mg/kg/day; maximum 15 mg/day) by 2 months of age or when birthweight is doubled, whichever comes first. All term infant formulas have supplemental iron.

VI. **Fluids.** See Chapter 8 for fluid requirements.

PRINCIPLES OF INFANT FEEDING

I. **Criteria for initiating infant feeding.** Term healthy infants should be breast-fed as soon as possible within the first hour. The following criteria should usually be met before initiating infant feedings.

   A. **No history of excessive oral secretions,** vomiting, or bilious-stained gastric aspirate.

   B. **Nondistended, soft abdomen,** with normal bowel sounds. If the abdominal examination is abnormal, an abdominal radiograph should be obtained.

   C. **Respiratory rate** <60 breaths/min for oral feeding and <80 breaths/min for gavage feeding. Tachypnea increases the risk of aspiration.

   D. **Prematurity.** Considerable controversy surrounds the timing of initial enteral feeding for the preterm infant. However, it is now believed that feedings should

Table 9–1. **DAILY ENTERAL VITAMIN AND MINERAL REQUIREMENTS FOR TERM AND STABLE PRETERM LBW INFANTS**

Nutrient	Term Infant (per day)	Stable Preterm Low Birthweight Infant (dose/kg)
Vitamins		
Vitamin A (with lung disease)	700 mcg	700–1500 mcg
Vitamin D	400 IU	400 IU
Vitamin E	7 IU	6–12 IU
Vitamin K	200 mcg	8–10 mcg
Vitamin C	80 mg	18–24 mg
Thiamine	1.2 mg	0.18–0.24 mg
Riboflavin	1.4 mg	0.25–0.36 mg
Niacin	17 mg	3.6–4.8 mg
Pyridoxine	1.0 mg	0.15–0.20 mg
Vitamin B_{12}	1.0 mcg	0.3 mcg
Folic acid	140 mcg	25–50 mcg
Biotin	20 mcg	3.6–6.0 mcg
Pantothenate	5 mg	1.2–1.7 mg
Minerals		
Calcium	250 mg	120–330 mg
Phosphorus	150 mg	60–140 mg
Magnesium	20 mg	7.9–15 mg
Sodium	1–2 mEq/kg	2.0–3.0 mEq
Potassium	2–3 mEq/kg	2.0–3.0 mEq
Iron	1 mg/kg	2–3 mg
Copper	20 mcg/kg	120–150 mcg
Zinc		1000 mcg
Manganese	5 mcg/100 kcal	0.75–7.5 mcg
Molybdenum	0.75–7.5 mcg	0.3 mcg
Selenium	2 mcg/kg	1.3–3.0 mcg
Chromium	0.20 mcg/kg	0.1–0.5 mcg
Iodide	1 mcg/kg	30–60 mcg

be initiated as soon as clinically possible. Early enteral feedings are associated with better endocrine adaptation, enhanced immune functions, and earlier discharge. Institutional practices may vary; however, enteral feeding may be started in the first 3 days of life with the objective of reaching full enteral feeding in 2–3 weeks. Parenteral nutrition, including amino acids and lipids, should be initiated within 1–3 days to provide adequate protein and caloric intake. Early parenteral nutrition is also associated with better weight gain.

1. For the **stable, larger premature neonate** (>1500 g), the first feeding may be given within the first 24 h of life. Early feeding may allow the release of enteric hormones, which exert a trophic effect on the intestinal tract.

2. Caution should be exercised in the presence of perinatal asphyxia, hemodynamic instability, sepsis, absent end-diastolic flow, indomethacin therapy, and hemodynamically significant patent ductus arteriosus due to apprehension about **NEC in extremely low birthweight (ELBW) and low birthweight (LBW) infants.**

E. **Term infants** with perinatal depression, polycythemia, and congenital heart disease are also at risk of developing NEC.

Table 9–2. **DAILY PARENTERAL REQUIREMENTS FOR VITAMINS AND MINERALS IN TERM, PRETERM, AND STABLE PRETERM INFANTS**

Nutrient	Term infant (per day)	Preterm infant (dose/kg)	Stable Preterm Infant (dose/kg)
Vitamins			
Vitamin A	700 mcg	500 mcg	700–1500 mcg
(with lung disease)			
Vitamin D	400 IU	160 IU	40–160 IU
Vitamin E	7 mg	2.8 mg	3.5 mg
Vitamin K	200 mcg	80 mcg	8–10 mcg
Vitamin C	80 mg	25 mg	15–25 mg
Thiamine	1.2 mg	0.35 mg	0.2–0.35 mg
Riboflavin	1.4 mg	0.15 mg	0.15–0.20 mg
Niacin	17 mg	6.8 mg	4.0–6.8 mg
Pyridoxine	1.0 mg	0.18 mg	0.15–0.20 mg
Vitamin B_{12}	1.0 mcg	0.3 mcg	0.3 mcg
Folic acid	140 mcg	56 mcg	56 mcg
Biotin	20 mcg	6 mcg	5–8 mcg
Pantothenate	5 mg	2 mg	1–2 mg
Minerals			
Calcium		75–90 mcg	
Phosphorus		48–67 mcg	
Magnesium		6–10.5 mcg	
Sodium	1–2 mEq/kg	2.5–3.5 mEq	
		<1.5 kg: 4–8 mEq	
Potassium	2–3 mEq/kg	2–3 mEq	
Iron		2–4 mcg	
		(after 6–8 wk)	
Copper[a]	20 mcg/kg	20 mcg	
Zinc	250 mcg/kg	1200–1500 mcg	
Manganese	1 mcg/kg	10–20 mcg	
Molybdenum	0.25 mcg	0.3 mcg	
Selenium[b]	2 mcg/kg	2 mcg	
Chromium	0.20 mcg/kg	0.2 mcg	
Iodide	1 mcg/kg	1 mcg	

[a]Omit in cholestatic jaundice.
[b]Start supplementation at 2–4 weeks. Omit in renal dysfunction.

Table 9–3. **CONDITIONALLY ESSENTIAL NUTRIENTS**

Nutrients*	Supplementation/100 kcal
Cystine	225–395 mmol/100 kcal
Taurine	30–60 mmol/100 kcal
Tyrosine	640–800 mmol/100 kcal
Inositol	150–375 mmol/100 kcal
Choline	125–225 mmol/100 kcal

*Nutrients normally synthesized by humans but for which premature infants may have a reduced synthetic capability to produce.

Table 9–4. INFANT FORMULA INDICATIONS AND USES

Formula	Indications	Vitamins and Mineral Supplement[a]
Human milk	All infants	MV; iron if >1500 g; fluoride at 40 wk; folate until 2000 g
Breast milk fortifiers	Preterm infant (<1500 g and <34 wk)	
Term formulas iso-osmolar		
Enfamil LIPIL 20	Full-term infants: as supplement to breast milk	MV if <32 oz/d
Similac 20	Preterm infants >1800–2000 g	
Preterm iso- and hyperosmolar		
Enfamil Premature 24 Similac Special Care 24 and 30	Preterm infants: for infants on fluid restriction or who cannot handle required volumes of 20-cal formula to grow	
Soy formulas (*Note:* Soy formulas not recommended in infants <1800 g.)		
ProSobee (lactose and sucrose free)	Term infants: milk sensitivity, galactosemia, carbohydrate intolerance	MV if <32 oz/d
Isomil (lactose free)	*Do not use in preterm infants. Phytates can bind calcium and cause rickets.*	
Protein hydrolysate formulas Casein predominant		
Nutramigen	Term infants: gut sensitivity to proteins, galactosemia, multiple food allergies, persistent diarrhea	MV if <32 oz/d
Pregestimil	Preterm and term infants: disaccharidase deficiency, diarrhea, GI defects, cystic fibrosis, food allergy, celiac disease, transition from TPN to oral feeding	
Alimentum	Term infants: protein sensitivity, pancreatic insufficiency, diarrhea, allergies, colic, carbohydrate, and fat malabsorption	
Protein hydrolysate formulas Whey predominant		
	Partially hydrolyzed to small peptides. Not truly hypoallergenic, but less expensive and more available; iron fortified	

(Continued)

Table 9–4. INFANT FORMULA INDICATIONS AND USES (*CONTINUED*)

Formula	Indications	Vitamins and Mineral Supplement[a]
Carnation Good Start	Term infants: whey protein; moderate mineral content; may be more palatable	
Enfamil Gentlelease LIPIL	Term infants	
Free amino acid elemental formulas	100% amino acids as protein source (not hydrolyzed), hypoallergenic. Used in cow's milk allergy, food protein intolerance, short bowel, eosinophilic esophagitis	
Neocate	Term infants: cow's milk protein allergies; contains 100% free amino acids (elemental formula)	
EleCare	Elemental formula containing amino acids indicated for malabsorption, protein maldigestion, short bowel syndromes	
Special formulas		
Similac PM 60/40	Preterm and term infants: problem feeders on standard formula; infants with renal, cardiovascular, or digestive diseases that require decreased protein and mineral levels; breast-feeding supplement, initial feeding	MV and Fe if standard formula weight >1500 g
Similac Sensitive (previously called Lactose Free)	Preterm and term infants: lactose free, milk sensitivity	
Enfamil AR	Rice starch added for thickening after ingestion (pH sensitive). Used for simple reflux.	Not indicated for preterm infants
Premature formulas **Low osmolality**		
Similac Special Care 20 Enfamil Premature 20	Premature infants (<1800–2000 g) who are growing rapidly. These formulas promote growth at intrauterine rates. Vitamin and mineral concentrations are higher to meet the needs of growth. Usually started on 20 cal/oz and advanced to 24 cal/oz as tolerated.	
Iso-osmolar		
Similac Special Care 24	Same as for low-osmolality premature formulas	
Enfamil Premature 24	Preterm infants >1800 g. Promotes catchup growth and improved bone	

Table 9–4. **INFANT FORMULA INDICATIONS AND USES (*CONTINUED*)**

Formula	Indications	Vitamins and mineral supplement[a]
Discharge or transitional formulas		
EnfaCare LIPIL NeoSure Advance	Preterm infants; increased protein, calcium, phosphorous, Vitamins A and D, promotes better mineralization. Can also be used to fortify human milk feedings	

Fe, iron; GI, gastrointestinal; MV, multivitamin; TPN, total parenteral nutrition.
[a]Such as Poly-Vi-Sol (Mead Johnson).

II. **Feeding guidelines and choice of formula.** Human milk is preferred for feeding term, preterm, and sick infants. If a commercial infant formula is chosen, generally no special considerations apply to healthy, full-term newborn infants. Preterm infants may require more careful planning. Many different, highly specialized formulas are available. Iron-fortified formula has become the formula of choice for term infants because its use has contributed to a decreased rate of anemia. Table 9–4 outlines indications for various formulas. The compositions of commonly used infant formulas and breast milk can be found in Table 9–5.
   A. **Formulas**
      1. **Hypo or iso-osmolar formulas (<300 mOsm/kg water).** The majority of term and preterm infant formulas are iso-osmolar or mildly hypo-osmolar to improve tolerance and decrease risk of NEC in preterm infants. Premature formulas that contain 24 cal/oz are also iso-osmolar.
      2. **Hyperosmolar formulas (>300 mOsm/kg water)** are 30 cal/oz formulas. Formulas such as Similac 30 are hypercaloric formulas designed to provide a greater percentage of the calories as protein and to provide increased mineral concentrations. They are used to provide nutritional needs for infants on fluid restriction.
      3. **Transitional formulas.** Preterm infants continue to need nutritional supplementation after discharge. These have higher protein and mineral contents than term formulas. Infants discharged on special formulas (eg, NeoSure, EnfaCare; see Table 9–5) have better somatic growth, weight gain, and bone mineralization. Supplementation should be continued until a corrected age of 9 months.
   B. **General guidelines**
      1. **Initial feedings.** Use maternal breast milk for initiating feedings. In the absence of maternal breast milk, donor breast milk (see later discussion of breast milk) may be used in VLBW infants (after obtaining parental consent) to initiate feeds. The use of formula feeds is associated with a 6–10 times higher incidence of NEC in preterm LBW infants than breast milk and 3 times higher when breast milk and formulas are used together versus breast milk alone.
      2. **Subsequent feedings.** Feedings should be advanced gradually if the initial feeds are tolerated. There are no fixed guidelines. Feedings are advanced once to twice a day. Increments range between 10 and 35 mL/kg/day in various studies. Caution should be exercised when advancing rapidly, particularly with formula feeds, due to risk of NEC. Some clinicians advance feeds in small volumes with each feeding. Particular care should be taken in intrauterine growth retardation (IUGR) infants, those with absent end-diastolic flow on antenatal Doppler ultrasonography, and those at risk for NEC (see prior discussion of NEC). Formula or breast milk should not be diluted.

Table 9–5. COMPOSITION OF INFANT FORMULAS

Characteristics	Mature Human Breast Milk	Enfamil 20, Enfamil 20 with Iron	Similac 20 with Low Iron[a] Similac with Iron, Similac Advance
Calories/100 mL	68	67	67.6
Osmolality (mOsm/kg H_2O)	290	300	300
Osmolarity (mOsm/L)	255	270	270
Protein			
Grams/100 mL	1.05	1.41	1.4
% Total calories	6	8.5	8
Source		Nonfat milk, whey whey : casein = 60:40)	Nonfat milk, whey protein
Fat			
Grams/100 mL	3.9	3.55	3.65
% Total calories	52	48	49
Source		Palm olein, soy, coconut, high-oleic sunflower, DHAI- and ARA-rich oil blend	High-oleic safflower, soy, and coconut oils (0.15% DHA, 0.40% ARA)
Oil ratio		44:19.5:19.5:14.5:2.5	40:30:29
Linoleic acid (mcg)	374	576.2	675.7
Linolenic acid (mg)		56.6	
DHA (mg)		11.3	
ARA (mg)		22.7	
Carbohydrates			
Grams/100 mL	7.2	7.3	7.3
% Total calories	42	43.5	43
Source	Lactose	Lactose	Lactose
Minerals (mg/100 mL)			
Calcium (mg) (mEq)	28	52.3	52.8 (2.63)
Phosphorus (mg)	14	28.8	28.4
Iodine (mcg)	11	6.7	4.1
Iron (mg)	0.03	1.20	1.2
Magnesium (mg)	3.5	5.36	4.1
Sodium (mg) (mEq)	18	18	16.2 (7.1)
Potassium (mg) (mEq)	52	72.3	71 (1.82)
Chloride (mg) (mEq)	42	42.2	44 (1.24)
Zinc (mg)	0.12	0.68	0.51
Copper (mcg)	25	50.2	60.9
Manganese (mcg)	0.6	10	3.4
Selenium (mcg)	1.5	1.87	1.22
Vitamins/100 mL			
Vitamin A (IU)	223	200	202
Vitamin D (IU)	2	40	40.6
Vitamin E (IU)	0.3	1.34	1.0
Vitamin K (mcg)	0.2	5.36	5.4
Thiamine/B_1 (mcg)	21	53.6	67.6
Riboflavin/B_2 (mcg)	35	93.8	101.4
Niacin/B_3 (mcg)	150	676	710.1
Vitamin B_6 (mcg)	20	40	40.6
Vitamin B_{12} (mcg)	0.05	0.20	0.17
Folic acid (mcg)	5	10.7	10.1
Vitamin C (mg)	4.1	8.0	6.1
Pantothenic acid (mcg)	180	335	304.3
Biotin (mcg)	0.4	2.0	2.9
Choline (mg)	9.2	16	10.8
Inositol (mg)	15	4.0	3.2
Carnitine (mg)		1.34	
Taurine (mg)		4.0	

[a]Similac products: C. cohnii oil, source of DHA; M. Alpina oil, source of ARA.
Enfamil LIPIL is also available as a 24 cal/oz formula.

(Continued)

Table 9–5. COMPOSITION OF INFANT FORMULAS (*CONTINUED*)

Characteristics	Similac Organic (organic iron-fortified formula)	Similac Special Care 20 (low iron/ with iron)	Enfamil Premature LIPIL (without/with iron)
Calories/100 mL	67.6	67.6	68
Osmolality (mOsm/kg H$_2$0)	225	235	240
Osmolarity (mOsm/L)		211	220
Protein			
Grams/100 mL	1.4	2.02	2
% Total calories	8	12	12
Source	Organic nonfat dry milk	Nonfat milk, whey concentrate	Nonfat milk, whey concentrate
Fat			
Grams/100 mL	3.71	3.67	3.4
% Total calories	49	47	44
Source	Organic high-oleic sunflower, soy, and coconut oils (0.15% DHA, 0.40% ARA)	MCTs, soy, and coconut oils (0.25% DHA, 0.40% ARA)	MCTs, soy, high-oleic vegetable oils, single-cell oil blend rich in DHA and ARA
Oil ratio	40:29:29		
Linoleic acid (mcg)	581.6	473	550
Linoleic acid (mg)			60
Arachidonic acid (mg)			23
DHA (mg)			11.5
ARA (mg)			23
Carbohydrates			
Grams/100 mL	7.14	6.97	7.4
% Total calories	42	41	44
Source	Organic maltodextrin, lactose, sugar (46:27;27)	Lactose, corn syrup solids (50:50)	Lactose, corn syrup solids
Minerals (mg/100 mL)			
Calcium (mg) (mEq)	52.8 (2.63)	121.7 (6.0)	112
Phosphorus (mg)	28.4	67.6	56
Iodine (mcg)	4.1	4.1	16.9
Iron (mg)	1.22	0.25/1.2	0.34/1.22
Magnesium (mg)	4.1	8.1	6.1
Sodium (mg) (mEq)	16.2 (7.1)	29.1 (1.26)	39
Potassium (mg) (mEq)	71 (1.81)	87.2 (2.23)	66
Chloride (mg) (mEq)	43.9 (1.24)	54.8 (1.55)	61
Zinc (mg)	0.51	1.01	1.01
Copper (mcg)	60.9	8.1	4.3
Manganese (mcg)	3.4	169.1	81
Selenium (mcg)	1.22	1.2	1.89
Vitamins/100 mL			
Vitamin A (IU)	202	845	850
Vitamin D (IU)	40.6	101	162
Vitamin E (IU)	1.0	2.7	4.3
Vitamin K (mcg)	5.4	8.1	5.4
Thiamine/B$_1$ (mcg)	67.6	169	135
Riboflavin/B$_2$ (mcg)	101.4	419	200
Niacin/B$_3$ (mcg)	710.1	3381	2700
Vitamin B$_6$ (mcg)	40.6	169	101
Vitamin B$_{12}$ (mcg)	0.17	0.37	0.17
Folic acid (mcg)	10.1	25	27
Vitamin C (mg)	6.1	25	13.5
Pantothenic acid (mcg)	304.3	1285	810
Biotin (mcg)	2.9	25	2.7
Choline (mg)	10.8	6.8	13.5
Inositol (mg)	3.2	27	30
Carnitine (mg)			1.62

(*Continued*)

Table 9–5. COMPOSITION OF INFANT FORMULAS (*CONTINUED*)

Characteristics	Similac Special Care 24 (low iron/ with iron)	Enfamil Premature LIPIL 24 (without/ with iron)	Similac Special Care 30 (with iron)
Calories/100 mL	81.2	81	101.4
Osmolality (mOsm/kg H_2O)	280	300	325
Osmolarity (mOsm/L)	246	260	
Protein			
Grams/100 mL	2.43	2.4	3.0
% Total calories	12	12	12
Source	Nonfat milk, whey concentrate	Nonfat milk, whey concentrate	Nonfat milk, whey concentrate
Fat			
Grams/100 mL	4.40	4.1	6.7
% Total calories	47	44	57
Source	MCTs, soy, and coconut oils (0.25% DHA, 0.40% ARA)	MCTs, soy, high-oleic vegetable oils, single-cell oil blend rich in DHA and ARA	MCTs, soy, and coconut oils (0.21% DHA, 0.33% ARA)
Oil ratio	50:30:18.3		50:30:18.3
Linoleic acid (mcg)	568.1	660	710.1
Arachidonic acid (mg)		28	
DHA (mg)		13.8	
Carbohydrates			
Grams/100 mL	8.36	8.9	7.8
% Total calories	41	44	31
Source	Lactose, corn syrup solids (50:50)	Lactose, corn syrup solids	Lactose, corn syrup solids (50:50)
Minerals/100 mL			
Calcium (mg) (mEq)	146.1 (7.3)	134	182.6 (9.1)
\Phosphorus (mg)	81.2	67	101.4
Iodine (mcg)	4.9	20	6.1
Iron (mg)	0.3/1.46	0.41/1.46	1.83
Magnesium (mg)	9.7	7.3	12.2
Sodium (mg) (mEq)	34.9 (1.52)	47	43.6 (1.9)
Potassium (mg) (mEq)	104.7 (2.7)	80	130.8 (3.35)
Chloride (mg) (mEq)	65.7 (1.8)	73	82.1 (2.32)
Zinc (mg)	1.21	1.22	1.52
Manganese (mcg)	9.7	5.1	12.2
Copper (mcg)	202.9	97	253.6
Selenium (mcg)	1.46	2.3	1.83
Vitamins/100 mL			
Vitamin A (IU)	1014	1010	1268.1
Vitamin D (IU)	121.7	195	152.2
Vitamin E (IU)	3.2	5.1	4.06
Vitamin K (mcg)	9.7	6.5	12.2
Thiamine/B_1 (mcg)	202.9	162	253.6
Riboflavin/B_2 (mcg)	503.2	240	629.0
Niacin/B_3 (mcg)	4057.8	3200	5072.2
Vitamin B_6 (mcg)	202.9	122	253.6
Vitamin B_{12} (mcg)	0.44	0.20	0.56
Folic acid (mcg)	30	32	37.5
Vitamin C (mg)	30	16.2	37.5
Pantothenic acid (mcg)	1541.9	970	1927.4
Biotin (mcg)	30	3.2	37.5
Choline (mg)	8.1	16.2	10.1
Inositol (mg)	32.5	36	40.6
Carnitine		1.95	

(*Continued*)

Table 9–5. **COMPOSITION OF INFANT FORMULAS (*CONTINUED*)**

Characteristics	Isomil 20/ Isomil Advance	Enfamil ProSobee LIPIL 20 cal/oz	Enfamil LactoFREE LIPIL 20 cal/oz
Calories/100 mL	67.6	68	68
Osmolality (mOsm/kg H_2O)	200	200	200
Osmolarity (mOsm/L)		180	182
Protein			
Grams/100 mL	1.65	1.69	1.42
% Total calories	10	10	8.5
Source	Soy protein isolate, L-methionine	Soy protein isolate	Milk protein isolate
Fat			
Grams/100 mL	3.69	3.6	3.6
% Total calories	49	48	48
Source	High-oleic safflower, soy, and coconut oils (41:30:29)	Palm olein, soy, coconut, and high-oleic sunflower oils, single-cell oil blend rich in DHA and ARA	Palm olein, soy, coconut, and high-oleic sunflower oils, single-cell oil blend rich in DHA and ARA
Linoleic acid (mcg)	**675/676.3**	580	580
Arachidonic acid (mg)		23	23
DHA (mg)		11.5	11.5
Carbohydrates			
Grams/100 mL	6.9	7.2	7.4
% Total calories	41	42	42
Source	Corn syrup solids, sugar (80:20)	Corn syrup solids	Corn syrup solids
Minerals/100 mL			
Calcium (mg) (mEq)	71 (3.54)	71	55
Phosphorus (mg)	50.7	56	37
Iodine (mcg)	10.0	10.1	10.1
Iron (mg)	1.22	1.22	1.22
Magnesium (mg)	5.1	7.4	5.4
Sodium (mg) (mEq)	29.8 (1.29)	24	20
Potassium (mg) (mEq)	73 (1.87)	81	74
Chloride (mg) (mEq)	41.9 (1.18)	54	45
Zinc (mg)	0.50	0.81	0.68
Manganese (mcg)	50.7	56	51
Copper (mcg)	16.9	16.9	10.1
Selenium (mcg)	1.22	1.89	1.89
Vitamins/100 mL			
Vitamin A (IU)	202.9	200	200
Vitamin D (IU)	40.6	41	41
Vitamin E (IU)	1.01	1.35	1.35
Vitamin K (mcg)	7.4	5.4	5.4
Thiamine/B_1 (mcg)	40.6	54	54
Riboflavin/B_2 (mcg)	60.9	61	95
Niacin/B_3 (mcg)	913	680	680
Vitamin B_6 (mcg)	40.6	41	41
Vitamin B_{12} (mcg)	0.3/0.60	0.2	0.2
Folic acid (mcg)	10.1	10.8	10.8
Vitamin C (mg)	6.1	8.1	8.1
Pantothenic acid (mcg)	507.2	340	340
Biotin (mcg)	3	2	2
Choline (mg)	8.1	8.1	8.1
Inositol (mg)	3.38	4.1	4.1
Carnitine		1.35	1.35

(*Continued*)

Table 9–5. **COMPOSITION OF INFANT FORMULAS (*CONTINUED*)**

Characteristics	Isomil DF 20 cal/oz	NeoSure 22	EnfaCare LIPIL 22 cal/oz
Calories/100 mL	67.6	74.4	74
Osmolality (mOsm/kg H$_2$O)	240	250	250 (liquid); 260 (powder)
Osmolarity (mOsm/L)	220	224	220 (liquid); 230 (powder)
Protein			
Grams/100 mL	1.8	2.08	21.0
% Total calories	11	11	11
Source	Soy protein isolate, L-methionine	Nonfat milk, whey concentrate	Nonfat milk, whey concentrate
Fat			
Grams/100 mL	3.69	4.1	3.9
% Total calories	49	49	47
Source	Soy and coconut oils	Soy, coconut, MCT oils (45.3:29.4:25.3) (01.5% DHA, 0.40% ARA)	MCT, high-oleic vegetable, soy coconut, single-cell oil blend rich in DHA and ARA
Oil ratio	60:40		20:34:14:29:3
Linoleic acid (mcg)	879	557.9	700
Linoleic acid (mg)			63.3
Arachidonic acid (mg)			25
DHA (mg)			12.6
Carbohydrates			
Grams/100 mL	6.8	7.51	7.7
% Total calories	40	40	42
Source	Corn syrup solids, sugar (60:40)	Lactose, corn syrup solids (50:50)	Maltodextrin, lactose, corn syrup solids
Minerals/100 mL			
Calcium (mg) (mEq)	71 (3.54)	78.1 (3.9)	89
Phosphorus (mg)	51	46.1	49
Iodine (mcg)	10	11.2	15.5
Iron (mg)	1.22	1.34	1.33
Magnesium (mg)	5.07	6.7	5.9
Sodium (mg) (mEq)	29.8 (1.29)	24.5 (1.07)	26
Potassium (mg) (mEq)	73 (1.87)	105.6 (2.7)	78
Chloride (mg) (mEq)	41.9 (1.18)	5.58 (1.57)	58
Zinc (mg)	0.50	0.89	0.92
Copper (mcg)	50.7	89.3	89
Manganese (mcg)	16.9	7.4	11.1
Selenium (mcg)	1.22	1.7	2.1
Vitamins/100 mL			
Vitamin A (IU)	202.9	342.2	330
Vitamin D (IU)	40.6	52.1	59
Vitamin E (IU)	1.01	2.68	3
Vitamin K (mcg)	7.4	8.18	5.9
Thiamine/B$_1$ (mcg)	40.6	163.7	148
Riboflavin/B$_2$ (mcg)	60.9	111.6	148
Niacin/B$_3$ (mcg)	913	1450.6	1480
Vitamin B$_6$ (mcg)	40.6	74.4	74
Vitamin B$_{12}$ (mcg)	0.3	0.29	0.22
Folic acid (mcg)	10.1	18.6	19.2
Vitamin C (mg)	6.1	11.2	11.8
Pantothenic acid (mcg)	507.2	595.1	630
Biotin (mcg)	3	6.7	4.4
Choline (mg)	8.1	11.9	17.8
Inositol (mg)	3.38	26.0	22
Carnitine (mg)			1.48

(*Continued*)

Table 9–5. **COMPOSITION OF INFANT FORMULAS (*CONTINUED*)**

Characteristics	Similac PM 60/40	EleCare[b]	Alimentum
Calories/100 mL	67.6	67.6	67.6
Osmolality	280	350	370
(mOsm/kg H$_2$0)			
Osmolarity	250		
(mOsm/L)			
Protein			
Grams/100 mL	1.5	2.0	1.86
% Total calories	9	15	11
Source	Whey, sodium caseinate	Free L-amino acids	Casein hydrolysate, L-cysteine, L-tyrosine, L-tryptophan
Fat			
Grams/100 mL	3.79	3.2	3.75
% Total calories	50	42	48
Source	High-oleic safflower, soy, and coconut oils (41:30:29)	High-oleic safflower oil, MCTs, soy oil (39:33:28)	Safflower, MCTs, soy oil (0.15% DHA, 0.40% ARA) (38:33:28)
Oil ratio			
Linoleic acid (mcg)	676.3	562.8	1285
Linolenic acid (mg)		56.2	
Carbohydrates			
Grams/100 mL	6.9	7.16	6.9
% Total calories	41	43	41
Source	Lactose	Corn syrup solids	Sugar, modified tapioca starch
Minerals/100 mL			
Calcium (mg) (mEq)	37.9 (1.89)	77.7 (3.9)	71 (3.54)
Phosphorus (mg)	18.9	56.4	50.7
Iodine (mcg)	4.1	5.6	10.1
Iron (mg)	0.47	1.0	1.2
Magnesium (mg)	4.06	5.6	5.1
Sodium (mg) (mEq)	16.2 (7.1)	30.1 (1.3)	29.8 (1.29)
Potassium (mg) (mEq)	54.1 (1.38)	100 (2.5)	79.8 (2.03)
Chloride (mg) (mEq)	39.9 (1.13)	40 (1.1)	54.1 (1.55)
Zinc (mg)	0.51	0.5	0.5
Copper (mcg)	60.9	70.3	50.7
Manganese (mcg)	3.4	56.2	5.4
Selenium (mcg)	1.22	1.54	1.22
Vitamins/100 mL			
Vitamin A (IU)	202.9	182.9	202.9
Vitamin D (IU)	40.6	28.1	30.4
Vitamin E (IU)	1.01	1.4	2.03
Vitamin K (mcg)	5.4	4	10.1
Thiamine/B$_1$ (mcg)	67.6	140.7	40.6
Riboflavin/B$_2$ (mcg)	101.4	70.3	60.9
Niacin/B$_3$ (mcg)	710	1125.6	913
Vitamin B$_6$ (mcg)	40.6	56.2	40.6
Vitamin B$_{12}$ (mcg)	0.17	0.26	0.30
Folic acid (mcg)	10.1	19.7	10.1
Vitamin C (mg)	6.1	6	6.1
Pantothenic acid (mcg)	304.3	282.07	507.2
Biotin (mcg)	3.0	2.8	3.0
Choline (mg)	8.1	6.4	8.1
Inositol (mg)	16.2	3.4	3.4

[b]Contains molybdenum and chromium.

(*Continued*)

Table 9–5. COMPOSITION OF INFANT FORMULAS (*CONTINUED*)

Characteristics	Good Start Supreme	Enfamil A.R. LIPIL 20 cal/oz	Enfamil Nutramigen LIPIL 20 cal/oz
Calories/100 mL	67	68	68
Osmolality (mOsm/kg H_2O)		240 (liquid); 230 (powder)	270 (liquid); 300 (powder)
Osmolarity (mOsm/L)		220 (liquid); 210 (powder)	240 (liquid); 270 (powder)
Protein			
Grams/100 mL	1.47	1.69	1.89
% Total calories		10	11
Source	Whey protein concentrate	Nonfat milk	Casein hydrolysate, amino acids
Fat			
Grams/100 mL	3.42	3.4	3.6
% Total calories		46	48
Source	Palm olein, soy, high-oleic safflower, coconut	Palm olein, soy, coconut, and high-oleic sunflower oils, single-cell blend rich in DHA and ARA	Palm olein, soy, coconut, and high-oleic sunflower oils, single-cell blend rich in DHA and ARA
Linoleic acid (mcg)	603	580	580
Linolenic acid (mg)	67	56.6	56.6
Arachidonic acid (mg)		23	23
DHA (mg)		11.5	11.5
Carbohydrates			
Grams/100 mL	7.5	7.4	7
% Total calories		44	41
Source	Lactose, corn maltodextrin	Lactose, rice starch, maltodextrin	Corn syrup solids, modified corn starch
Minerals/100 mL			
Calcium (mg)	44.9	53	64
Phosphorus (mg)	25.5	36	43
Iodine (mcg)	8.04	6.8	10.1
Iron (mg)	1.01	1.22	1.22
Magnesium (mg)	4.69	5.4	7.4
Sodium (mg)	18.1	27	32
Potassium (mg)	72.4	73	74
Chloride (mg)	43.6	51	58
Zinc (mg)	0.54	0.68	0.68
Copper (mcg)	53.6	51	51
Manganese (mcg)	10.1	10.1	16.9
Selenium (mcg)	2.01	1.89	1.89
Vitamins/100 mL			
Vitamin A (IU)	201	200	200
Vitamin D (IU)	40.2	41	34
Vitamin E (IU)	1.34	1.35	1.35
Vitamin K (mcg)	5.36	5.4	5.4
Thiamine/B_1 (mcg)	67	54	54
Riboflavin/B_2 (mcg)	93.8	95	61
Niacin/B_3 (mcg)	703.5	680	680
Vitamin B_6 (mcg)	50.3	41	41
Vitamin B_{12} (mcg)	0.22	0.2	0.2
Folic acid (mcg)	10.1	10.8	10.8
Vitamin C (mg)	6.03	8.1	8.1
Pantothenic acid (mcg)	301.5	340	340
Biotin (mcg)	2.95	2	2
Choline (mg)	16.1	8.1	8.1
Inositol (mg)	4.02	4.1	11.5
Nucleotides	3.4		
Carnitine		1.35	1.35

(*Continued*)

Table 9–5. **COMPOSITION OF INFANT FORMULAS (*CONTINUED*)**

Characteristics	Pregestimil 20 cal/oz	Pregestimil 24 cal/oz
Calories/100 mL	68	81
Osmolality (mOsm/kg H$_2$0)	280 (liquid); 330 (powder)	330
Osmolarity (mOsm/L)	250 (liquid); 300 (powder)	290
Protein		
Grams/100 mL	1.89	2.3
% Total calories	11	11
Source	Casein hydrolysate, amino acids	Casein hydrolysate, amino acids
Fat		
Grams/100 mL	3.8	4.5
% Total calories	48	48
Source	MCT, soy, and high-oleic safflower oils	MCT, soy, and high-oleic safflower oils
Oil ratio	55:35:7.5 and 2.5% oil rich in DHA and ARA (liquid) 55:25:10^c: 7.5 and 2.5% oil rich in DHA and ARA (powder)	
Linoleic acid (mcg)	626.6	746.0
Linolenic acid (mg)	80 (liquid)/63.3 (powder)	95.2
DHA (mg)	11.3	13.4
ARA (mg)	22.6	26.8
Carbohydrates		
Grams/100 mL	6.9	8.3
% Total calories	41	41
Source	Corn syrup solids, modified corn starch, dextrose	Corn syrup solids, modified corn starch
Minerals/100 mL		
Calcium (mg)	78	93
Phosphorus (mg)	51	61
Iodine (mcg)	10.1	8.9
Iron (mg)	1.22	1.53
Magnesium (mg)	7.4	9.7
Sodium (mg)	32	38
Potassium (mg)	74	89
Chloride (mg)	58	70
Zinc (mg)	0.68	0.89
Copper (mcg)	51	89
Manganese (mcg)	16.9	24
Selenium (mcg)	1.89	2.3
Vitamins/100 mL		
Vitamin A (IU)	260	310
Vitamin D (IU)	34	41
Vitamin E (IU)	2.7	3.1
Vitamin K (mcg)	8.1	15.3
Thiamine/B$_1$ (mcg)	54	65
Riboflavin/B$_2$ (mcg)	61	73
Niacin/B$_3$ (mcg)	680	810
Vitamin B$_6$ (mcg)	41	49
Vitamin B$_{12}$ (mcg)	0.2	0.24
Folic acid (mcg)	10.8	13
Vitamin C (mg)	8.1	9.7
Pantothenic acid (mcg)	340	410
Biotin (mcg)	2	2.4
Choline (mg)	8.1	9.7
Inositol (mg)	11.5	13.8
Carnitine (mg)	1.35	1.62

^{c} Corn oil.

3. **Continuous versus bolus feeds.** Although no clear advantage has been shown for either method, infants with short gut syndromes or gastroesophageal reflux and ELBW infants may benefit from continuous feeds. Institutional practices may vary. If using breast milk, the infusion syringe should be placed vertically to allow fats to be delivered.

4. **Minimal enteral feedings ("trophic feeding").** Trophic feeds are subnutritional quantities of milk feeds, based on the concept of minimal enteral feedings. This practice—also called hypocaloric, trophic, trickle feedings, low-volume enteral substrate, or gastrointestinal priming—is characterized by a small-volume feeding to supplement parenteral nutrition. Studies have focused on use in infants <1500 g at birth. This method has been accepted because of benefits such as improved feeding tolerance, prevention of gastrointestinal atrophy, and facilitation of gastrointestinal tract maturation leading to a shorter time required for attaining full enteral feedings. Other benefits include decreased incidences of cholestasis, nosocomial infections, metabolic bone disease, and decreased hospital stay without an increase in the incidence of NEC. There is no standard method of minimal enteral feeding, and a wide variety of feeding techniques and formulas exist. Mother's breast milk should be preferred over donor breast milk or preterm formula for trophic feedings. Start trophic feeds as soon as possible if infant is clinically stable.

   a. **Type of feeds.** Breast milk is the preferred feeding; however, positive results have been achieved using preterm infant formulas. Enteral solution patterned after human amniotic fluid have also been used.

   b. **Feeding method.** Orogastric or nasogastric routes are used for feeding. Nasogastric tubes in small infants may increase airway resistance. Both continuous and bolus feedings have been used. The most effective method remains to be identified, but a trend exists toward bolus feedings. Enteral feedings should be advanced as clinically tolerated.

   c. **Volume.** Volumes studied have varied from 0.1–24 mL/kg/day.

   d. **Minimal enteral feedings for ELBW infants (<1000 g, <28 weeks)** should start at 10–20 mL/kg/day divided as every 2–3 h feeds, advanced as tolerated. Alternatively, start at 0.5–2 mL every 6 h; advance to every 4 h and then every 2 h. If continuous feeds are used, up to 0.5–1 mL/kg/h volume may be used.

4. **Weight-specific guidelines are based on birthweight and gestational age** as presented in this section. For an infant presumed to be at risk for NEC, the rate of enteral feeding advancement should not exceed 20 mL/kg/day and 10 cal/kg/day. Protocols vary by institution.

   a. **VLBW infants <1000 g. Gavage feeding** through an orogastric or nasogastric tube is appropriate. Gavage feeding typically involves passing a 5F (<1000 g) to 8F feeding tube into the abdomen and verifying its position by injecting a few milliliters of air and listening for a characteristic "whoosh" (Chapter 30). The stomach contents are aspirated and if <20% of previous feed or <2 mL, the contents may be fed again. Small amounts of feeding are placed in the tube under gravity using the open end of the syringe. Typically 2–3 mL/min are infused.

      i. **Initial feeding.** Breast milk or donor breast milk (see prior discussion); preterm infant formulas.

      ii. **Maintenance feeding.** Breast milk (with or without human milk fortifier; see indications presented later) or preterm formulas (20 or 24 cal/oz). Donor breast milk should not be used for maintenance because it does not provide adequate proteins and minerals for long-term growth. Our practice is to transition to formula feeds once infant is between 1000 and 1200 g.

      iii. **Subsequent feedings**

         (a) **Volume.** Bolus feeds, 10–20 mL/kg/day in divided volumes every 2–3 h. Advance feeds by 10–20 mL/kg/day. Alternatively, give

0.5–1.0 mL/h continuously and increase by 0.5–1.0 mL every 12–24 h. When 10 mL/h is tolerated, change feedings to every 2 h and advance as tolerated.

   (b) **Strength.** Use expressed breast milk or preterm formula. Once full feedings of 20 cal/oz are tolerated, consider advancing to 24 cal/oz feedings or adding human milk fortifier to breast milk. Some institutions start with 24 cal/oz formulas.

  b. **LBW <1500 g.** Gavage feeding (see earlier) through a nasogastric tube should be used.

    i. **Initial feeding.** Give breast milk or preterm formula every 2 to 3 h.

    ii. **Subsequent feedings**

      (a) **Volume.** Bolus feeds, 10–20 mL/kg/day in divided volumes, every 3 h. Advance feeds by 10–20 mL/kg/day. Alternatively, give 2 mL/kg every 2 h, and increase by 1 mL every 12 h up to 20 mL every 2 h. Then change to feedings every 3 h.

      (b) **Strength.** Use breast milk or preterm formulas. Once full feedings of 20 cal/oz formula are tolerated, advance to 24 cal/oz if desired or add human milk fortifier (22 or 24 cal/oz). Some institutions start with 24 cal/oz formulas.

  c. **Weight: 1500 to 2500 g.** Use gavage feeding through an orogastric or nasogastric tube. Breast-feeding or bottle-feeding can be attempted if the infant is >1600 g, >34 weeks' gestation, and neurologically intact. Initiation of early nursing is associated with earlier time to achieve full enteral feeds.

    i. **Initial feeding.** Use expressed breast milk or preterm infant formulas. For infants >1800 g (35–36 weeks), term infant formulas are frequently used. Breast milk or preterm infant formula should be used. In stable infants, starts feeds at 80 mL/kg/day, and then advance 10–20 mL/kg/day.

  d. **Weight: >2500 g.** Breast-feed or use a bottle if the infant is neurologically intact. Stable infants can be fed *ad libitum* with breast milk or term formula.

III. **Management of feeding intolerance.** If feeding is initiated but not tolerated, a complete abdominal examination should be performed. Preterm infants <32 weeks may not establish antegrade peristalsis. In the absence of other clinical symptoms and signs, bilious aspirate by itself is not a contraindication for feedings in VLBW infants. Increasing feeding volume or continuing feeds may be helpful in improving tolerance. Presence of bilious aspirates, emesis, blood in stool, abdominal distension, or other systemic signs and symptoms like apnea and bradycardia should be closely evaluated. Aspirate volumes >2 mL in infants <750 g and >3 mL in infants 751 to 1000 g (or greater than a fifth of the feed volume) in the absence of other signs and symptoms should not limit feeding. Consider abdominal radiographs if the physical findings are suspicious. If the abdominal evaluation is normal:

  A. **Attempt continuous feedings** with a nasogastric or orogastric tube. Check the gastric aspirate, and follow the recommendations presented in Chapter 48.

  B. **Use breast milk preferably or special formula** (eg, Pregestimil) because they may be better tolerated.

IV. **Nutritional supplements.** Supplements are sometimes added to feedings, primarily to increase caloric intake (Table 9–6). They provide additional energy supplies with no concomitant increase in fluid volume. Protein supplementation results in an increase in short-term weight gain, linear growth, and head growth. Long-term effects on growth and neurodevelopment are not conclusive. There are insufficient data to evaluate the effects of carbohydrate or fat supplementation on long-term growth and development in preterm infants.

    Some clinicians strongly believe that any necessary caloric supplementation should be given as a high-calorie formula (ie, 24 kcal/oz) instead of as a supplement because all nutrients in such a formula are in proportion to one another and allow maximum

Table 9–6. NUTRITIONAL SUPPLEMENTS USED IN INFANTS

Supplement	Nutrient Content	Calories	Indications and Contraindications	Amount to Use
Carbohydrate				
Polycose	Glucose polymers from hydrolyzed cornstarch	3.8 kcal/g powder; 2 kcal/mL liquid	Calorie supplementation[a] (lactose and gluten free) Contains Na, K, Ca, Cl, and P	**Powder:** 0.5 g/oz of 20-cal formula = 22 cal/oz; 1 g/oz of 20-cal formula = 24 cal/oz **Liquid:** 1 mL to 1 oz of 20-cal formula =22 cal/oz 1 tsp/4 oz of formula or milk
Infant rice cereal	Rice	15 cal/tbsp	Thickens feedings	
Fat				
Medium-chain triglyceride	Lipid fraction of coconut oil	8.3 kcal/g, 7.7 cal/mL	Limit to 50% calories from fat to prevent ketosis; may cause diarrhea; do not use in BPD because of risk of aspiration pneumonia[b]	0.5 mL/4 oz of formula = 21 cal/oz; 1 mL/4 oz of formula = 22 cal/oz; 1 mL/2 oz of formula = 22 cal/oz
Vegetable oil	Soy, corn oil	9.0 cal/g (120 cal/tbsp)	To increase calories if fat absorption is normal[c]	0.5 mL/4 oz of formula = 21 cal/oz; 1 mL/4 oz of formula = 22 cal/oz
Microlipid	Safflower oil Soy lecithin Ascorbic acid Linoleic acid	4.5 cal/mL 5.9 g/tbsp	To increase caloric density, fluid restriction[d]	1 mL/2 oz of formula = 22 cal/oz
Protein				
Beneprotein	Whey protein isolate/ soy lecithin	4.1 cal/g (6 g of protein/packet[e]) Calcium = 30 mg/scoop Sodium = 15 mg/scoop Potassium = 35 mg/scoop Phosphorus = 15 mg/scoop Calories = 25/scoop	Useful for protein and calorie supplementation	Clinical experience is limited

BPD, bronchopulmonary dysplasia.

[a]Limiting formula intake while increasing calories may compromise protein, vitamin, and mineral intake, which may also lead to hyperglycemia and diarrhea.

[b]Always mix with formula to avoid the possibility of lipid aspiration or pneumonia.

[c]Vitamin E may need to be increased to at least 1 IU/g of linoleic acid.

[d]See text.

[e]1 packet = 1 scoop = 1 1/2 tablespoon = 7 g.

absorption. Nutritional supplements are often used in infants with BPD who are not gaining weight and need additional calories with no increase in protein, fat, or water intake.

Microlipid can induce the formation of hydroxyperoxides when mixed with human milk. Preterm milk with Microlipid can abolish the enterocyte barrier function and can result in degradation of enterocyte transepithelial electrical resistance, suggesting that stored milk mixed with Microlipid may increase the risk of gut infections.

Attempts have been made to supplement milk with immunoglobulins to decrease incidence of NEC with no significant benefits. Some benefit, however, has been noted with arginine supplementation.

V. **Postnatal growth failure and catchup growth in preterm infants.** Preterm birth deprives the fetus of nutrient transfer that takes place in the third trimester, particularly of amino acids, fats, and minerals. Preterm birth is therefore associated with significant nutritional deficits a priori. Postnatally, low amino acid and high glucose intake and delayed enteral feedings result in poor weight gain and extrauterine growth failure by as much as 20% by the time of discharge. Many infants remain at <10th percentile of the intrauterine growth charts at time of discharge that can persist for up to 18 months. A longer time to regain birthweight and total protein intake influences long-term neurodevelopmental outcomes.

Attempts have been made to reduce postnatal growth failure and to provide "catchup" growth by 2–3 months of age in VLBW and LBW infants by initiating early parenteral and enteral nutrition. The use of aggressive parenteral nutrition including high proteins and lipids has been found to be safe, and it is associated with a shorter time to regain birthweight and a trend toward lower risks of late onset-sepsis without any increased risk of NEC or BPD. Protein intake of 3 g/kg/day results in weight gain similar to intrauterine weight gain. Use of specialized preterm formulas can also help in catchup growth and can overcome mineral deficits.

However, caution must be exercised in promoting aggressive growth in the form of weight gain because rapid growth results predominantly in fat deposition and may be associated with subsequent development of obesity, insulin resistance, diabetes, and cardiovascular disease. Improvement in lean body mass and use of maternal milk results in better outcomes.

BREAST-FEEDING

I. Advantages
   A. **Protein quality.** The predominance of whey and the mixture of amino acids are compatible with the metabolic needs of LBW infants.
   B. **Digestion and absorption** are improved with breast milk.
   C. **Immunologic benefits.** Breast-feeding provides immunologic protection against bacterial and viral infections (particularly upper respiratory tract and gastrointestinal infections). Studies of infants breast-fed for >6 months show that they have a decreased incidence of cancer.
   D. **Promotion of bonding** between the mother and her infant.
   E. **Lower renal solute load,** which facilitates better tolerance.
   F. **Other advantages.** Breast-feeding in preterm infants is associated with a decreased risk for NEC and a significantly higher intelligence quotient (IQ) at the age of 8 years. The risk of breast and ovarian cancers in the mother also appears to be lower. Human milk feedings are associated with beneficial effects on visual, cognitive, psychomotor, and neurodevelopmental outcomes that persist in childhood. Breast milk contains omega-3 fatty acids, that is, α-linolenic acid (ALA), from which other essential LCPUFAs, DHA, and AA are produced. These play an important role in retinal and neurologic development. Most formulas are now supplemented with DHA and AA. Partial breast milk (>50 mL/kg) feedings are associated with decreased risk of late-onset sepsis and NEC in preterm infants.

II. **Contraindications and disadvantages**

   Note: Temporary problems in the mother, such as sore or cracked nipples that resolve with treatment or mastitis treated with antibiotics, do not preclude nursing.

   A. **Active tuberculosis** in the mother.

   B. **Certain viral and bacterial infections** in the mother. For specific recommendations, see Appendix F.

   C. **Use of medications** that are passed in significant amounts in the breast milk, which may harm the infant. For the effects of drugs and substances on lactation and breast-feeding, see Chapter 133.

   D. **Galactosemia**

   E. **An infant with a cleft lip or palate** may have difficulty in nursing. Expressed breast milk can be fed to the infant using specially designed bottles (relative contraindication).

   F. **IUGR infants (<1500 g)** may require greater amounts of protein, sodium, calcium, phosphorus, and vitamin D than unfortified breast milk contains. These requirements should be monitored routinely and supplemented as necessary.

III. **Donor breast milk (http://www.hmbana.org).** The use of donor breast milk is both regional and ***controversial.*** Historically, donor breast milk was used for centuries; however, current practice tends toward limited use. In recent years, concerns regarding the transmission of infections, such as HIV, cytomegalovirus, and tuberculosis, have led to questions regarding the safety of its use. If donor breast milk or milk banks are to be used, donor screening, heat treatment (pasteurization) of the milk, and parental counseling on these potential risks are recommended.

   Pasteurization and refrigeration result in loss of milk components. Donor milk is deficient in protein, minerals, and calories to meet long-term requirements of preterm infants for growth and development. A recent meta-analysis showed that formula feeds compared to donor milk is associated with increased weight gain and growth but also with increased risk of NEC (relative risk, 95% CI = 2.5, 1.2–5.1). Use of fortified donor milk versus formula is associated with slower weight gain. When compared to mother's own milk, donor breast milk does not appear to offer an advantage over formula in decreasing risks of infections or length of stay. At our institution, we initiate enteral feedings with donor milk in infants <1000 g if no maternal milk is available and subsequently transition to formula.

IV. **Storage.** Breast milk can be stored frozen at –20°C for up to 6 months and refrigerated at 4°C for up to 24 h.

V. **Breast milk fortifiers (supplements).** The breast milk fortifiers (Table 9–7) are designed as a supplement to mother's milk for rapidly growing premature infants. Use of human milk beyond the second and third weeks in preterm infants may provide insufficient amounts of protein, calcium, phosphorus, and possibly copper, zinc, and sodium. Clinical experience has shown that the addition of human milk fortifier to a preterm mother's milk resulted in nitrogen retention, increased blood urea levels, and increased somatic and linear growth related to increased protein and energy intake. There is no effect on serum alkaline phosphatase levels. Effect on bone mineral content beyond 1 year of age is not known. Periodic monitoring of urine osmolality, serum blood urea nitrogen, creatinine, and calcium is required. Table 9–7 shows some of the fortifiers currently available in the United States.

   A. **Indications.** Breast milk fortifiers are indicated for those premature infants who tolerate unfortified human milk at full feedings, usually at 2–4 weeks of age, up to the time of discharge or at a weight of 3600 g. Criteria for use include <34 weeks' gestation at birth and <1500 g at birth. In addition, breast milk fortifiers are indicated for fluid-restricted infants who require an increase in calories. Fortifiers can be added when 100 mL/kg/day of enteral feeding is reached, although practices may vary. Iron-enriched fortifiers are well tolerated and may decrease the need for late blood transfusions. Fortification of fresh breast milk is not associated with increased bacterial growth for up to 6 hours. The fortifiers available in the United States are shown on the next page.

Table 9–7. **COMPOSITION OF PRETERM HUMAN MILK[a] AND COMMERCIALLY AVAILABLE BREAST-MILK FORTIFIERS**

Variable	Preterm Human Milk[a]	Enfamil HMF[b]	Similac HMF[c]
Volume	100 mL	4 packets/100 mL	4 packets/ 100 mL
Total calories	67	81	79 (24 cal/oz)
Osmolality (mOsm/kg H_2O)	290	325	385
Osmolarity	255		
Calories	67	81	79
Protein (g)	1.4	2.5	2.3
Fat (g)	3.9	4.9	4.1
Linoleic acid (mg)	369	140	359
Linolenic acid (mg)		17	
Carbohydrates (g)	6.6	<0.4	8.2
Minerals /100 mL			
Calcium (mg)	24.8	90	138
mEq	1.24		6.9
Chloride (mg)	55	13	90
mEq	1.6		2.5
Copper (mcg)	64.4	44	228
Iron (mg)	0.12	1.44	0.45
Magnesium (mg)	3.1	1	9.8
Phosphorus (mg)	12.8	50	77
Potassium (mg)	57	29	116
mEq	1.5		2.9
Sodium (mg)	24.8	16	38
mEq	1.1		1.7
Zinc (mg)	0.34	0.72	1.3
Iodine (mcg)	10.7		10.5
Manganese (mcg)	0.6	10	7.6
Selenium (mcg)	1.5		1.9
Vitamins/100 mL			
Vitamins A (IU)	389	950	984
Vitamin B_1 (mcg)	20.8	150	247
Vitamin B_2 (mcg)	48.3	220	453
Vitamin B_6 (mcg)	14.8	115	219
Vitamin B_{12} (mcg)	0.04	0.18	0.67
Vitamin C (mcg)		12	34
Vitamin D (IU)	2	150	118
Vitamin E (IU)	1.1	4.6	4.1
Vitamin K (mcg)	0.2	4.4	8.3
Folic acid (mcg)	3.3	25	25
Niacin (mcg)	150.3	3000	3622
Pantothenic acid (mcg)	180.5	730	1636
Biotin (mcg)	0.4	2.7	25
Choline (mg)	9.4		10
Inositol (mg)	14.7		18

[a]Represents mature preterm human milk.
[b]Enfamil HMF: Data provided per 4 packets.
[c]4 packets per 100 mL human milk provides 24 cal/oz.

1. **Enfamil human milk fortifier (EHMF)**
   a. **Composition.** The predominant source of energy is fat. The fat is 70% medium-chain triglyceride (MCT) and 30% soy with linoleic and linolenic acid providing 1 g/4 packets. Fats also reduce the osmolar load. The protein is 60% whey protein and 40% casein, which is similar to breast milk. Four packets provide 1.1 g of protein. The carbohydrate is corn syrup solids, mineral salts, and trace amounts of lactose and galactose. This fortifier comes in powder form.
   b. **Calories.** One packet of fortifier added to 50 mL of human milk provides an additional 2 cal/fl oz. The same amount of fortifier added to 25 mL of human milk supplies an additional 4 cal/fl oz. Once the powder is added to the milk, the container should be capped and mixed well. It can be covered and stored under refrigeration (2–4°C) but should be used within 24 h. It should be used within 4 h after mixing at room temperature. Do not reuse if it is not refrigerated for >2 h after mixing. Agitate before each use. *Do not microwave* for heating.
   c. **Hypercalcemia** has been reported in some ELBW (<1000 g) infants receiving fortified breast milk. For these infants, serum calcium must be monitored. Fortification of breast milk should start beyond 2 weeks' postnatal age at a ratio not exceeding 1 packet/25 mL of breast milk.
2. **Similac human milk fortifier (SHMF)**
   a. **Composition.** The protein is from nonfat milk, whey protein concentrate. There is <2% soy lecithin. The carbohydrate is lactose and corn syrup solids. The fat is predominantly coconut oil (MCT).
   b. **Calories.** The fortifier provides 24 kcal/fl oz, when added in the ratio of 1 packet/25 mL of breast milk.
   c. Use until infant reaches a weight of 3600 g or as directed.
3. **Human milk fortifier.** Recently, a human milk fortifier has become commercially available (ProlactaPlus H^2MF) that is made from 100% pasteurized donor human breast milk. Concentrated up to 2–10 times, it is fortified with essential minerals and offers protein delivery up to 2.3 to 3.7 g/100mL and an additional 4 to10 cal/oz of fortified milk, respectively (www.prolacta.com). However, clinical experience with this fortifier is currently limited.

VI. **Probiotics and milk.** Recent studies have shown a beneficial effect of supplementing milk with bifidobacter and other probiotics in decreasing the risk of NEC. Beneficial effects have also been reported on decreasing intestinal permeability, improvements in growth and head circumference, and improved feeding tolerance. Bifidobacter is present in human milk. Routine supplementation with probiotics is as yet not established in the United States.

VII. **Organic formulas.** Several organic milk formulas are available that are produced without the use of pesticides, antibiotics, or growth hormones. They are fortified with vitamins, minerals, choline, and DHA and ARA. The sources for DHA and ARA include vegetarian sources, fish oil, algae, and eggs. Organic soy formulas are also available. Concerns have been raised about the presence of high sugar content in some of these formulas and the risk for later childhood obesity and for injury to developing tooth enamel. The increased cost of organic formulas is considerable. There are currently no clinical trials comparing benefits, or lack of, for organic formulas to proprietary infant formulas.

VIII. **Feeding in short gut syndrome.** Short gut syndrome is a frequent complication following bowel resection in infants following NEC and other congenital malformations. The loss of the ileocecal valve, bacterial overgrowth, deconjugation of bile salts, cholestatic liver disease, and vitamin B_{12} and mineral deficiency can occur. Total parenteral nutrition (TPN) toxicity can be a complication due to excess lipids (phytosterols causing liver damage), excess amino acids, and manganese and copper toxicity *(controversial)*.

Adequate zinc supplementation is needed to compensate for losses through stomas. Careful attention should also be placed on fluid and electrolyte balance. Refeeding through mucous fistulas, continuous feeds, pectin, elemental amino acid formulas, and initiating early enteral feedings postoperatively have all been tried in an attempt to decrease liver disease.

TOTAL PARENTERAL NUTRITION

TPN is the intravenous administration of all nutrients (fats, carbohydrates, proteins, vitamins, and minerals) necessary for metabolic requirements and growth. Parenteral nutrition (PN) is supplemental intravenous administration of nutrients. Enteral nutrition (EN) is oral or gavage feedings. The optimal amount of energy intake remains unclear, but no additional benefit in protein balance has been shown with energy intake beyond 70–90 kcal/kg/day. Protein accretion is improved with increasing protein intake at energy intakes of 30–50 kcal/kg/day.

I. **Intravenous routes used in PN**
   A. **Central PN.** Central PN is usually reserved for patients requiring long-term (>2 weeks) administration of most calories. Basically, this type of nutrition involves infusion of a hypertonic nutrient solution (15–25% dextrose, 5–6% amino acids) into a vessel with rapid flow through an indwelling catheter whose tip is in the vena cava just above or beyond the right atrium. Disadvantages include increased risk of infection and complications from placement. Two methods are commonly used for placement.
      1. **A percutaneous inserted central catheter,** positioned in the antecubital, temporal, external jugular vein, or saphenous vein, is advanced into the superior or inferior vena cava. This technique avoids surgical placement and results in fewer complications (see Chapter 36).
      2. **A central catheter (Broviac)** can be placed through a surgical cutdown in the internal or external jugular, subclavian vein, or femoral vein. The proximal portion of the catheter (which has a polyvinyl cuff to promote fibroblast proliferation for securing the catheter) is tunneled subcutaneously to exit some distance from the insertion site, usually the anterior chest. This protects the catheter from inadvertent dislodgement and reduces the risk of contamination by microorganisms. The anesthesia and surgery needed for placement of the catheter are disadvantages to this method.
      3. **Photoprotection of parenteral nutrition** may help decrease vitamin loss and oxidative damage to amino acids, decrease generation of hydrogen peroxides and free radicals, limit alterations in vasomotor tone via generation of lipid peroxides and decreased nitric oxide production, and improve tolerance to minimal EN.
   B. **Peripheral PN.** The use of a peripheral vein may also be used in the neonatal intensive care unit and is usually associated with fewer complications. The concentration of the amino acids and the dextrose solution limit the amount of solution that can be infused. The maximum concentration of dextrose that can be administered is 12.5%; the maximum concentration of amino acids, 3.5%.
   Note: PN can be given through an umbilical artery catheter, a route that has been used in some centers; however, the umbilical artery is not a preferred site and should be used with caution. The maximum dextrose concentration that can be administered using this method is 15%.
II. **Indications.** PN is used as a supplement to enteral feedings or as a complete substitution (TPN) when adequate nourishment cannot be achieved by the enteral route. Common indications in neonates include congenital malformation of the gastrointestinal tract, gastroschisis, meconium ileus, short bowel syndrome, NEC, paralytic ileus, respiratory distress syndrome, extreme prematurity, sepsis, and malabsorption. PN, particularly amino acids, should be started on the first day of life, and as soon as possible

in sick infants. In preterm ELBW and VLBW infants, 1.5–2.5 g/kg/day of amino acids should be started on day 1 and is associated with better linear growth and neurodevelopmental outcomes.

III. **Caloric concentration.** Caloric densities of various energy sources are as follows.
   A. **Dextrose (anhydrous): 3.4 kcal/g.**
   B. **Protein: 4 kcal/g.**
   C. **Fat: 9 kcal/g.**
IV. **Composition of PN solutions**
   A. **Carbohydrates**
      1. **The only commercially available carbohydrate source is dextrose (glucose).** A solution of 5.0–12.5 g/dL is used in peripheral PN and up to 25 g/dL in central PN. Dextrose concentrations should be calculated as milligrams per kilograms per minute. Dextrose is provided to maintain blood sugar between 45 mg/dL and 125 mg/dL (see also Chapter 55). Providing glucose alone in the absence of proteins results in negative nitrogen balance that can be reversed by providing 1.1–2.5 g/kg/day of protein with energy intake as low as 30 kcal/kg/day (see Proteins later).
      2. **To allow for an appropriate response of endogenous insulin** and to prevent the development of osmotic diuresis secondary to glucosuria, neonates should not routinely be started on >6–8 mg/kg/min of dextrose. Infusion rates can be increased by 0.5–1 mg/kg/min each day as tolerated up to10–12 mg/kg/min to achieve adequate caloric intake in the presence of stable blood sugar levels. This also allows adequate glucose for protein deposition. Endogenous glucose requirements decrease with increasing gestational age. In the presence of hyperglycemia, glucose infusion rate should not be reduced below 4 mg/kg/min. Insulin may be required to maintain adequate blood glucose levels. See Chapter 8 for the formula used to calculate the amount of glucose(mg/kg/min) an infant is receiving.
   B. **Proteins.** Inadequate protein intake may result in failure to thrive, hypoalbuminemia, and edema. Excessive protein can cause hyperammonemia, serum amino acid imbalance, metabolic acidosis, and cholestatic jaundice. Early addition of amino acids to PN may also stimulate endogenous insulin secretion. Postnatal protein loss is inversely proportional to gestational age. LBW infants lose 1% of endogenous protein daily unless supplemented.
      1. **Crystalline amino acid** solutions are available as nitrogen sources. The standard solutions originally designed for adults are not ideal because they contain high concentrations of amino acids (eg, glycine, methionine, and phenylalanine) that are potentially neurotoxic in premature infants. Pediatric crystalline amino acid solutions (eg, TrophAmine, Aminosyn PF) are available that contain less of those potentially neurotoxic amino acids as well as additional tyrosine, cystine, and taurine. These pediatric solutions also have a lower pH to allow for the addition of sufficient quantities of calcium (2 mEq/dL) and phosphorus (1–2 mg/dL) to meet daily requirements.
      2. **Amino acids.** Early protein intake of 3 g/kg/day within the first 24 h is safely tolerated in VLBW infants and improves nitrogen balance because of an increased ability to synthesize protein (see earlier). Early amino acid supplementation may help decrease hyperglycemia and hyperkalemia in the ELBW infants by promoting insulin secretion. In term infants, the starting rate can be 1.5 g, with increases of 1 g/kg/day. To avoid hyperammonemia and acidosis, total proteins should not exceed 4 g/kg/day in preterm infants. At most institutions, amino acid solutions are prepared in 1%, 2%, and 3% concentrations.
      3. **Cysteine hydrochloride** is often added to TPN solutions because cysteine is unstable over time and is omitted from amino acid solutions. The premature infant lacks the ability to convert methionine to cysteine; thus it is conditionally

essential. Cysteine is also converted to cystine and to glutathione, an antioxidant. Addition of cysteine into TPN lowers the pH of the solution, resulting in acidosis. Additional acetate may be required. It may also decrease hepatic cholestasis. The recommended dose is 40 mg of cysteine per gram of protein (72–85 mg/kg/day).

4. **Glutamine** has been identified as a key amino acid, as respiratory fuel for rapidly proliferating cells like enterocytes and lymphocytes, in acid-base balance, and as a nucleotide precursor. Glutamine may play a role in maintaining gut integrity and may decrease the incidence of sepsis. It also attenuates gut atrophy in fasting states. Vernix is a rich source of glutamine. However, glutamine supplementation does not have significant effect on mortality or neonatal morbidities including invasive infection, NEC, time to achieve full enteral nutrition, or duration of hospital stay.

C. **Fats.** Fats are essential for normal body growth and development, in cell structure and function, and in retinal and brain development. Because of their high caloric density, intravenous fat solutions (eg, Intralipid, Liposyn II, Nutrilipid, Soyacal) provide a significant portion of daily caloric needs. Most intravenous fat solutions are isotonic (270–300 mOsm/L), and therefore they are not likely to increase the risk of infiltration of peripheral lines. Delay in initiating lipids can result in biochemical and clinical evidence of essential fatty acid deficiency within 3 days and increase susceptibility to oxidant injury. When administering fat solutions to neonates with unconjugated hyperbilirubinemia, caution may be needed because of the competitive binding between bilirubin and nonesterified fatty acids on albumin, which may increase significantly with high infusion rates. Increased risk of coagulase-negative staphylococci, release of thromboxanes and prostaglandins, and increased pulmonary vascular resistance have also been noted.

1. **Concentrations.** Lipid emulsions are usually supplied either as 10% or 20% solutions providing 10 g or 20 g of triglyceride, respectively. Starting lipids at 0.5–1 g/kg/day within 24–30 h of birth is safe. Advance by 0.5–1.0 g/kg/day as tolerated up to 3.0–3.5 g/kg/day. The infusion is given continuously over 20 to 24 h, and the rate should not exceed 0.12 g/kg/h. Use of 20% lipid emulsion is associated with decreased levels of cholesterol, triglycerides, and phospholipids because of its lower phospholipids-to-triglycerides ratio and lower liposomal contents than 10% lipid emulsions.

2. **Complications.** Fat intolerance (hyperlipidemia) may be seen. Periodic determination of blood triglyceride levels is recommended. Levels should be <150 mg/dL when the infant is jaundiced and <200 mg/dL otherwise. The infusion of fats should be decreased or stopped when these levels are exceeded. Advance cautiously in infants with respiratory distress due to risk of hypoxemia and increased pulmonary vascular resistance.

3. **Carnitine supplementation** *(controversial).* Carnitine synthesis and storage are not well developed in infants <34 weeks' gestation. Carnitine is a carrier molecule necessary for oxidation of long-chain fatty acids. An exogenous source of carnitine is available from human milk and infant formulas; however, studies have shown that preterm infants on TPN become deficient in 6–10 days. Carnitine can be added to TPN solutions at a safe initial dose of 10 mg/kg/day. Carnitine-deficient infants may experience hypotonia, nonketotic hypoglycemia, cardiomyopathy, encephalopathy, and recurrent infections.

D. **Vitamins.** Vitamins are added to intravenous solutions in the form of a pediatric multivitamin suspension (MVI Pediatric) based on recommendations by the Nutritional Advisory Committee of the American Academy of Pediatrics. The dose of parenteral vitamins for preterm infants should be 2 mL/kg of the 5-mL reconstituted MVI Pediatric sterile lyophilized powder. Vitamin A delivery is hampered by binding to plastic tubing.

Table 9–8. **RECOMMENDATIONS FOR TRACE ELEMENT SUPPLEMENTATION IN TPN SOLUTIONS FOR NEONATES**

Element (mcg/kg/d)	Full Term	Premature
Zinc	250	400
Copper	20	20
Chromium[a]	0.2	0.2
Manganese[a]	1	1
Fluoride	500[b]	—
Iodine	1	1
Molybdenum[a]	0.25	0.25
Selenium	2.0	2.0

TPN, total parenteral nutrition.
[a]For TPN > 4 weeks.
[b]Not well defined in the premature infant. Indicated only in prolonged TPN therapy (eg, >3 months).

E. **Trace elements.** Trace elements are added to the solution based on weight and total volume: 0.5 mL/kg/wk for infants on short-term TPN and 0.5 mL/kg/day for those on long-term TPN. Increased amounts of zinc (1–2 mg/day) are often given to help promote healing in patients who require gastrointestinal surgery. At many institutions, a prepared solution is available. For recommended doses of trace elements, see Table 9–8.

F. **Electrolytes.** Electrolytes can be added according to specific needs, but for LBW infants, requirements are usually satisfied by standard amino acid solution formulations that contain electrolytes (Table 9–9).

G. **Heparin.** Heparin should be added to PN (0.5–1 units/mL TPN) to maintain catheter patency. In addition, there is a decreased risk for phlebitis and an increase in lipid clearance as a result of release of lipoprotein lipase.

V. **Monitoring of PN.** Hyperalimentation can cause many alterations in biochemical function. Thus compulsive anthropometric and laboratory monitoring is essential for all patients. Recommendations are given in Table 9–10.

VI. **Complications of PN.** Most complications of PN are associated with the use of central hyperalimentation and primarily involve infections and catheter-related problems. Metabolic difficulties can occur with both central and peripheral TPN. The major complication of peripheral hyperalimentation is accidental infiltration of the solution, which causes sloughing of the skin.

A. **Infection.** Sepsis can occur in infants receiving central hyperalimentation. The most common organisms include coagulase-positive and coagulase-negative *Staphylococcus*, *Streptococcus viridans*, *Escherichia coli*, *Pseudomonas* spp, *Klebsiella* spp, and *Candida albicans*. Contamination of the central catheter can occur as a result of infection at the insertion site or use of the catheter for blood sampling or administration of blood. It is best not to open the catheter.

B. **Catheter-associated problems.** Complications associated with placement of central catheters (specifically in the subclavian vein) occur in ~4–9% of patients. Complications include pneumothorax, pneumomediastinum, hemorrhage, and chylothorax (caused by injury to the thoracic duct). Thrombosis of the vein adjacent to the catheter tip, resulting in "superior vena cava syndrome" (edema of the face, neck, and eyes), may be seen. Pulmonary embolism may occur secondary to thrombosis. Malpositioned catheters may result in collection of fluid in the pleural cavity, causing hydrothorax, or the pericardial space causing tamponade.

Table 9–9. COMPOSITION OF AMINO ACID SOLUTIONS FOR LOW BIRTHWEIGHT INFANTS (STANDARD FORMULATION)

Electrolytes (mEq/L)	Amino Acid Concentration					
	1.0%		2.0%		3.0%	
	A	T	A	T	A	T
Na^+	20	20	20	20	20	20
Cl^-	20	20	20	20	20	20
K^+	15	15	15	15	15	15
Mg^{2+}	11	11	11	11	11	11
Ca^{2+}	15	15	15	15	15	15
Acetate	7.6	9.3	15.3	18.6	22.8	27.9
Phosphorus (mmol/L)	10	10	10	10	10	10

A, Aminosyn PF; T, TrophAmine.

Table 9–10. SUGGESTED MONITORING SCHEDULE FOR NEONATES RECEIVING PARENTERAL NUTRITION

Measurement	Baseline Study	Frequency of Measurement
Anthropometric		
Weight	Yes	Daily
Length	Yes	Weekly
Head circumference	Yes	Weekly
Intake and Output	Daily	Daily
Metabolic		
Glucose	Yes	2–3 times/d initially; then as needed
Calcium, phosphorus, and magnesium	Yes	2–3 times/wk initially; then every 1–2 wk
Electrolytes (Na, Cl, K, CO_2)	Yes	Daily initially, then 2–3 times/wk. More frequently in ELBW infants <1000 g
Hematocrit	Yes	Every other day for 1 week; then weekly
BUN and creatinine	Yes	2–3/ wk; then every 1–2 wk
Bilirubin	Yes	Weekly
Ammonia	Yes	Weekly if using high protein
Total protein and albumin	Yes	Every 2–3 wk
AST/ALT	Yes	Every 2–3 wk
Triglycerides	Yes	1–2 weekly
Vitamins and trace minerals		As indicated
Urine		
Specific gravity and glucose	Yes	1–3 times/d initially; then as needed (*controversial*)

ALT, alanine aminotransferase; AST, aspartate aminotransferase; BUN, blood urea nitrogen; ELBW, extremely low birthweight; VLBW, very low birthweight.

C. Metabolic complications

1. **Hyperglycemia** resulting from excessive intake or change in metabolic rate, such as infection or glucocorticoid administration.

2. **Hypoglycemia** from sudden cessation of infusion (secondary to intravenous infiltration).

3. **Azotemia** from excessive protein (nitrogen) uptake; however, aggressive protein intake is safe (see earlier).

4. **Hyperammonemia.** All currently available amino acid mixtures contain adequate arginine (>0.05 mmol/kg/day). Therefore, if there is an increase in blood ammonia, symptomatic hyperammonemia does not occur.

5. **Abnormal serum and tissue amino acid pattern.**

6. **Mild metabolic acidosis.**

7. **Cholestatic liver disease.** With prolonged administration of intravenous dextrose and protein and absence of enteral feeding, cholestasis usually occurs. The incidence ranges from as high as 80% in VLBW infants receiving TPN for >30 days (with no enteral feeding) to ≤15% in neonates weighing >1500 g receiving TPN for >14 days. Monitoring for abnormalities in liver function and the development of direct hyperbilirubinemia is important in long-term TPN. IUGR infants are at high risk of developing cholestasis. Fish oil based lipids have recently been associated with reversal of cholestasis.

   a. **Bacterial infection** may play a significant role in the occurrence of cholestatic liver disease.

   b. **The use of amino acid mixtures** designed to maintain normal plasma amino acid patterns and early starting (as soon as possible) of enteral feedings in small amounts may help alleviate this problem.

   c. **TPN may be cycled over 10–18 hours as opposed to a continuous 24-hours infusion.** This facilitates a short period of decreased circulating insulin levels, which in turn facilitates mobilization of fat and glycogen stores, decreasing the risk of fatty infiltration of the liver and hepatic dysfunction. This practice is reserved for infants who are stable on TPN and who are expected to remain in need of long-term TPN.

   d. **The trace elements copper and manganese** should be withheld in the presence of hepatic dysfunction.

8. **Complications of fat administration.** Infusion of fat emulsion is associated with several metabolic disturbances, hyperlipidemia, platelet dysfunction, acute allergic reactions, deposition of pigment in the liver, and lipid deposition in the blood vessels of the lung. Most metabolic problems apparently occur with rapid rates of infusion and are not seen at infusion rates of <0.12 g/kg/h.

   Exposure of lipids to light, especially phototherapy, may cause increased production of toxic hydroperoxides. Steroids cause elevated triglyceride levels. In sepsis, there is decreased peripheral use of lipids. Free fatty acids produced from lipid breakdown compete with bilirubin for binding with albumin, resulting in elevated free bilirubin. Lipid infusion should not exceed 0.5–1 g/kg/day with plasma bilirubin >8–10 mg/dL and albumin levels 2.5–3.0 g/dL. Additional complications include thrombocytopenia, increased risk of sepsis, alteration in pulmonary functions, and hypoxemia.

9. **Deficiency of essential fatty acids (EFAs)** is associated with decreased platelet aggregation (thromboxane A_2 deficiency), poor weight gain, scaling rash, sparse hair growth, and thrombocytopenia. EFA deficiency can occur within 72 h in preterm infants if exogenous fatty acids are not supplemented. Use of only safflower oil to provide lipid emulsions may result in deficiency omega-3 LCPUFAs. EFAs are essential to the developing eyes and brain of the human neonate.

10. **Mineral deficiency.** Most minerals are transferred to the fetus during the last trimester of pregnancy. The following problems may occur.

    a. **Osteopenia, rickets, and pathologic fractures** (see Chapter 107).

    b. **Zinc deficiency** occurs if zinc is not added to TPN after 4 weeks. Cysteine and histidine in TPN solution increases urinary losses. Infants with this deficiency can have poor growth, diarrhea, alopecia, increased susceptibility to infection, and skin desquamation surrounding the mouth and anus (acrodermatitis enteropathica). Zinc losses are increased in patients with an ileostomy or colostomy.

    c. **Infants with copper deficiency** have osteoporosis, hemolytic anemia, neutropenia, and depigmentation of the skin.

    d. **Deficiency** of manganese, copper, selenium, molybdenum, and iodine may occur if not supplemented after 4 weeks.

CALORIC CALCULATIONS

An infant should receive 100–120 kcal/kg/day for growth. (Infants require fewer calories [70–90 cal/kg/day] if receiving TPN only.) Some hypermetabolic infants may require >120 kcal/kg/day. For maintenance of a positive nitrogen balance, oral intake of 70–90 nonprotein kcal/kg/day is necessary. Equations for calculating the caloric intake for oral formula and TPN follow (see also Table 9–11).

   I. **Infant formulas.** Most standard infant formulas are 20 cal/oz and contain 0.67 kcal/mL. Specific caloric concentrations of formulas are given in Table 9–5. To calculate total daily calories, use the following equation:

$$\text{kcal/kg/day} = \frac{\text{Total mL of formula} \times \text{kcal/mL}}{\text{Wt (kg)}}$$

  II. **Carbohydrates.** If only dextrose infusion is given, the total daily caloric intake is calculated as follows. (For caloric concentration of common solutions, see Table 9–12.)

$$\text{kcal/kg/day} = \frac{\text{mL of solution/h} \times 24\text{ h} \times \text{kcal in solution}}{\text{Wt (kg)}}$$

Table 9–11. TPN CALCULATIONS

Amino acids:	$\%\text{ Amino acids} = \dfrac{\text{Wt(kg)} \times (\text{g/kg/d}) \times 100}{\text{vol in 24 h}}$
Dextrose: Glucose utilization rate (mg/kg/min):	$\dfrac{\text{Rate(mL/h)} \times \%\text{ dextrose}}{\text{Wt(kg)} \times 6}$
Lipids:	$\text{Rate(mL/h)}: \dfrac{\text{g/kg/d} \times 5 \times \text{Wt(kg)}}{24}$
Nonprotein calories/kg/d:	$(\text{mL lipid/24 h} \times 2\text{ Cal/mL}^{a}) + \dfrac{\text{mL TPN/24 h} \times \%\text{ dextrose} \times 0.034}{\text{kg}}$

TPN, total parenteral nutrition.
^{a}For 20% lipids only.

Table 9–12. CALORIC CONCENTRATIONS OF VARIOUS PARENTERAL SOLUTIONS

Dextrose solutions (anhydrous)	% Concentration	Caloric Concentration (kcal/mL)
D_5	5	0.17
$D_{7.5}$	7.5	0.255
D_{10}	10	0.34
$D_{12.5}$	12.5	0.425
D_{15}	15	0.51
D_{20}	20	0.68
D_{25}	25	0.85
Protein Solutions (g/d)		
0.5	0.5	0.02
1.0	1	0.04
1.5	1.5	0.06
2.0	2.0	0.08
2.5	2.5	0.10
3.0	3.0	0.12

A 0.5% solution, if given 100 mL/d; = 0.5 g of protein/d.

III. **Proteins.** Use the prior formula given for carbohydrates and the caloric concentrations given in Table 9–12.

IV. **Fat emulsions.** A 10% fat emulsion (Intralipid) contains 1.1 kcal/mL; a 20% emulsion, 2 kcal/mL. Use the following formula to calculate daily caloric intake supplied by Intralipid 20%.

$$\text{kcal/kg/day} = \frac{\text{Total mL/day of solution} \times 2 \text{ kcal/mL}}{\text{Wt (kg)}}$$

Selected References

Alfaleh K, Bassler D: Probiotics for prevention of necrotizing enterocolitis in preterm infants. *Cochrane Database Syst Rev* 2008;1:CD005496.

Auestad N et al: Visual, cognitive, and language assessments at 39 months: a follow-up study of children fed formulas containing long-chain polyunsaturated fatty acids to 1 year of age. *Pediatrics* 2003;112:77-83.

Berseth CL et al: Growth, efficacy, and safety of feeding an iron-fortified human milk fortifier. *Pediatrics* 2004;114:699-706.

Bonner CM et al: Effects of parenteral L-carnitine supplementation on fat metabolism and nutrition in premature infants. *J Pediatr* 1995;126:287.

Chan GM et al: Effects of a human milk-derived human milk fortifier on the antibacterial actions of human milk. *Breastfeeding Med* 2007;2:205-208.

Darlow BA, Graham PJ: Vitamin A supplementation to prevent mortality and short and long-term morbidity in very low birth weight infants. *Cochrane Database Syst Rev* 2007;4:CD000501.

Denne SC, Poindexter BB: Evidence supporting early nutritional support with parenteral amino acid infusion. *Semin Perinatol* 2007;31:56.

Denne SC et al: Nutrition and metabolism in the high-risk neonate: enteral nutrition. In Fanaroff AA, Martin RJ (eds): *Neonatal-Perinatal Medicine—Diseases of the Fetus and Infant,* Vol. 1, 7th ed. St. Louis, MO: Mosby-Year Book, 2002;578-598.

Diehl-Jones WL, Askin DF: Nutritional modulation of neonatal outcomes. *AACN Clinical Issues* 2004;15:83-96.

Ehrenkranz RA: Early, aggressive nutritional management of very low birth weight infants: what is the evidence? *Semin Perinatol* 2007;31:48-55.

Fenton TR: A new growth chart for preterm babies: Babson and Benda's chart updated with recent data and a new format. *BMC Pediatrics* 2003;3:13.

Greer FR: Post-natal discharge nutrition: what does the evidence support? *Semin Perinatol* 2007;31:89-95.

Groh-Wargo S, Thompson M, Cox J (eds): *Nutritional Care for the High Risk Newborns.* Chicago, IL: Precept Press, 2000.

Gura KM et al: Reversal of parenteral nutrition–associated liver disease in two infants with short bowel syndrome using parenteral fish oil: implications for future management. *Pediatrics* 2006;118:197-201.

Hay WW: Early postnatal nutritional requirements of the very preterm infants based on a presentation at the NICHD-AAP workshop on research in neonatology. *J Perinatol* 2006;26:S13-S18.

Heiman H, Schanler RJ: Benefits of maternal and donor human milk for premature infants. *Early Hum Dev* 2006;82:781-787.

Heiman H, Schanler RJ: Enteral nutrition for premature infants: the role of human milk. *Semin Perinatol* 2007;12:26-34.

Henderson G et al: Formula milk versus maternal breast milk for feeding preterm or low birth weight infants. *Cochrane Database Syst Rev* 2007;4:CD002972.

Kalhan SC, Edmison JM: Effect of intravenous amino acids on protein kinetics in preterm infants. *Curr Opin Clin Nutr Metab Care* 2007;10:69-74.

Kashyap S: Enteral intake for the very low birth weight infants: what should the composition be? *Semin Perinatol* 2007;31:74-82.

Katrine KF: Anthropometric assessment. In Groh-Wargo S, Thompson M, Cox JH (eds): *Nutritional Care for the High Risk Newborns.* Chicago, IL: Precept Press, 2000:9-14.

Khashu M et al: Photoprotection of parenteral nutrition enhances advancement of minimal enteral nutrition in preterm infants. *Semin Perinatol* 2007;31:139-145.

Morales Y, Schanler RJ: Human milk and clinical outcomes in VLBW infants: how compelling is the evidence of benefit? *Semin Perinatol* 2007;31:83-88.

Moyer-Mileur LJ: Anthropometric and laboratory assessment of very low birth weight infants: the most helpful measurements and why. *Semin Perinatol* 2007;31:96-103.

Ohlsson A, Aher SM: Early erythropoietin for preventing red blood cell transfusion in preterm and/or low birth weight infants. *Cochrane Database Syst Rev* 2006;3:CD004863.

Poindexter BB et al: Early provision of parenteral amino acids in extremely low birth weight infants: relation to growth and neurodevelopmental outcome. *J Pediatr* 2006;148:300-305.

Reynolds RM, Thureen PJ: Special circumstances: trophic feeds, necrotizing enterocolitis and bronchopulmonary dysplasia. *Semin Fetal Neo Med* 2007;12:64-70.

Sherry B et al: Evaluation of and recommendations for growth references for very low birth weight (≤1500 grams) infants in the United States. *Pediatrics* 2003;111:750.

Smithers et al: Long chain polyunsaturated fatty acid (LCPUFA) supplementation in infants born preterm. *NeoReviews* 2007;4:143-150.

Steinmacher J et al: Randomized trial of early versus late enteral iron supplementation in infants with a birth weight of less than 1301 grams: neurocognitive development at 5.3 years' corrected age. *Pediatrics* 2007;120:538-546.

Stratiki Z et al: The effect of a bifidobacter supplemented bovine milk on intestinal permeability of preterm infants. *Early Hum Dev* 2007;83:575-579.

Tsang RC et al (eds): *Nutrition of the Preterm Infant: Scientific Basis and Practical Guidelines.*
Cincinnati, OH: Digital Education Publishing, 2005.

Tubman TRJ, Thompson TW: Glutamine supplementation for prevention of morbidity in
preterm infants. *Cochrane Database Syst Rev* 2001;4:CD001457.

Tyson JE, Kennedy KA: Trophic feedings for parenterally fed infants. *Cochrane Database Syst
Rev*2005;3:CD000504.

Tyson JE et al: Vitamin A supplementation for extremely low birth weight infants. *N Engl J
Med* 1999;340:1962-1968.

Vohr BR et al: Persistent beneficial effects of breast milk ingested in the neonatal intensive care
unit on outcomes of extremely low birth weight infants at 30 months of age. *Pediatrics*
2007;120:953-959.

Wessel JJ, Kocoshis SA: Nutritional management of short bowel syndrome. *Semin Perinatol*
2007;31:104-111.

10 Neonatal Radiology

COMMON RADIOLOGIC TECHNIQUES

I. **Radiographic examinations.** The need for radiographs must always be weighed against the
risks of exposure of the neonate to radiation (eg, 3–5 mrem per chest radiographic view). The
infant's gonads should be shielded as much as possible, and any person holding the infant
during the x-ray procedure should also wear a protective shield. For the usual vertically ori-
ented radiographic exposure, personnel need to be only 1 ft outside the zone of exposure.

   A. **Chest radiographs**

   1. **The anteroposterior (AP) view** is the single best view for identification of heart
      or lung disease, verification of endotracheal tube and other line positions, and
      identification of air leak complications of mechanical ventilation, such as
      pneumothorax.

   2. **The cross-table lateral view** is of limited diagnostic value except to determine
      whether a pleural chest tube is positioned anteriorly (best for drainage of a pneu-
      mothorax) or posteriorly (best for drainage of a pleural fluid collection).

   3. **The lateral decubitus view** is best at evaluating for a small pneumothorax or a
      small pleural fluid collection as either can be difficult to identify on the AP view.
      For example, if a pneumothorax is suspected on the left, a right lateral decubitus
      view of the chest should be obtained, with the infant placed right side down (con-
      tralateral decubitus). An air collection between lung and chest wall will be visible
      on the side on which the pneumothorax is present. By contrast, for pleural fluid
      identification, the same side should be placed down (ipsilateral decubitus). The
      disadvantages of the lateral decubitus view are that it is sometimes difficult to per-
      form in unstable infants and more time consuming than a regular AP supine view.

   4. **The upright view,** which is rarely used in the neonatal intensive care unit (NICU),
      can identify abdominal perforation by showing free air under the diaphragm.

B. Abdominal radiographs
   1. **The AP view** is the single best view for diagnosing abdominal disorders such as intestinal obstruction or mass lesions and checking placement of support lines such as umbilical arterial and venous catheters and intestinal tubes.
   2. **The cross-table lateral view** helps diagnose abdominal perforation, but the left lateral decubitus view is better for this purpose. Abdominal perforations may be missed on the AP and cross-table lateral views if the amount of intraperitoneal air is limited or if the segment of perforated bowel contains only fluid.
   3. **The left lateral decubitus view** (with the infant placed left side down) is best for diagnosis of intestinal perforation. Free intra-abdominal air resulting from bowel perforation will be visible as an air collection between the liver and right lateral abdominal wall.
C. Barium contrast studies (barium swallow or barium enema). Barium sulfate, an inert compound, is not absorbed from the gastrointestinal (GI) tract and results in little or no fluid shift.
   1. **Indications.** The use of barium as a contrast agent is recommended for the following:
      a. **GI tract imaging.** Barium enema is used to rule out lower intestinal tract obstruction from a variety of causes.
      b. **Suspected H-type tracheoesophageal fistula (TEF) without esophageal atresia (type E).** Most esophageal atresias can be diagnosed by inserting a radiopaque nasogastric tube; the tube curls up in the blind-ending proximal esophageal pouch. If additional confirmation is required, air can be injected under fluoroscopy to distend the pouch. Barium or other contrast agent injection is rarely required. However, evaluation for the rare H-type TEF requires contrast injection, such as barium, into the esophagus.
      c. **Suspected esophageal perforation.** Barium swallow is used only if previous studies using low-osmolality water-soluble contrast agents were negative.
      d. **Suspected gastroesophageal reflux.** Barium swallow is used as the first-line study.
   2. **Contraindications.** Barium contrast studies are not recommended in infants with suspected abdominal perforation because barium is irritating to the peritoneum and can result in "barium peritonitis."
D. High-osmolality water-soluble contrast studies
   1. **Advantages** of these agents (eg, Hypaque or Gastrografin) over barium include the following:
      a. **These materials are not toxic to the peritoneum** if they leak from the GI tract, and they are absorbed and cleared from the body.
      b. **Because these agents draw water into the bowel lumen,** they may be used therapeutically to relieve some cases of bowel obstruction or to treat meconium ileus.
   2. **Disadvantages**
      a. **Significant fluid shift may occur.** Thus, to avoid inducing hypovolemic shock, fluid and electrolyte status must be monitored closely if these agents are used.
      b. **These materials are very irritating to the lungs if aspirated.**
      c. **Necrotizing enterocolitis** resulting in death has been reported. Bowel necrosis has rarely occurred after the use of these agents for meconium ileus.
   3. **Indications**
      a. **Evaluation** of the bowel if perforation is suspected.
      b. **Differentiation** of ileus from obstruction.
      c. **Treatment** of meconium obstruction syndromes.
E. Low-osmolality water-soluble contrast agents. These agents have many advantages over barium and the high-osmolality contrast agents.
   1. **Advantages**
      a. **These agents do not cause fluid shifts.**

b. **If bowel perforation is present**, these substances are nontoxic to the peritoneal cavity. In addition, they do not damage the bowel mucosa.

c. **If aspirated, there is limited irritation (if any) to the lungs.**

d. **Unlike high-osmolality water-soluble contrast agents, low-osmolality water-soluble contrast agents have very limited absorption** from the normal intestinal tract and thus maintain good opacification throughout the intestinal tract on delayed imaging.

2. **Disadvantages** include a higher cost than barium and other water-soluble agents.

3. **Indications**
   a. **Suspected H-type TEF.**
   b. **Suspected esophageal perforation.**
   c. **Evaluation of the bowel if perforation is suspected.**
   d. **Unexplained pneumoperitoneum.**
   e. **Evaluation of "gasless abdomen"** in a neonate >12 h of age.

F. **Radionuclide studies.** Radionuclide studies provide more physiologic than anatomic information and usually involve a lower radiation dose to the patient compared with radiographic examinations.

1. **The reflux scintiscan (also called "milk scan" if formula or milk is used)** is used for documenting and quantitating gastroesophageal reflux. This procedure is comparable to the pH probe examination and superior to the barium swallow. Technetium-99m-labeled pertechnetate in a water-based solution is instilled into the stomach. The patient is then scanned in the supine position for 1–2 h with a gamma camera.

2. **The radionuclide cystogram** is used for documenting and quantitating vesicoureteral reflux. Advantages over the radiographic voiding cystourethrogram (VCUG) is a much lower radiation dose (by 50–100 times) and a longer monitoring period (1–2 h). Disadvantages include much poorer anatomic detail; bladder diverticula, posterior urethral valves, or mild reflux cannot be reliably identified. This technique should not be the initial examination for evaluation of the lower urinary tract, especially in boys.

3. **The radionuclide bone scan** is used for evaluation of possible osteomyelitis. This procedure involves a three-phase study (blood flow, blood pool, and bone uptake) after intravenous injection of technetium-99m-labeled methylene diphosphonate.
   a. **Advantages** include a sensitivity to bony changes earlier than with the radiograph.
   b. **Disadvantages** are several. Such a bone scan may not identify the acute phase of osteomyelitis (ie, the first 24–48 h), requires absence of patient motion, gives poorer anatomic detail than radiographs, and has resultant areas of positive uptake ("hot spots") that are nonspecific.

4. **The HIDA (hepatobiliary) scan** is used in certain types of neonatal jaundice to assist in differentiating biliary atresia (surgical disorder) from neonatal hepatitis (medical disorder).

II. **Ultrasonography**

A. **Ultrasonography of the brain** is performed primarily to rule out intraventricular hemorrhage, ischemic change (periventricular leukomalacia [PVL]), hydrocephalus, and developmental anomalies. It can be performed in any NICU with a portable ultrasound unit. No special preparation is needed. However, an open anterior fontanelle must be present, and no intravenous catheters should be placed in the scalp. The classification of intraventricular hemorrhage (IVH) based on ultrasonographic findings, is demonstrated in Figures 10–1 through 10–4. Figure 10–5 shows a posterior fossa hemorrhage, and Figure10–6 demonstrates ischemic changes of PVL. Grading of IVH in the neonate by sonography as developed by Papile (see Dolfin et al, 1983) is as follows:

1. **Grade I:** Subependymal, germinal matrix hemorrhage.
2. **Grade II:** Intraventricular extension without ventricular dilatation.
3. **Grade III:** Intraventricular extension with ventricular dilatation.
4. **Grade IV:** Intraventricular and intraparenchymal hemorrhage.

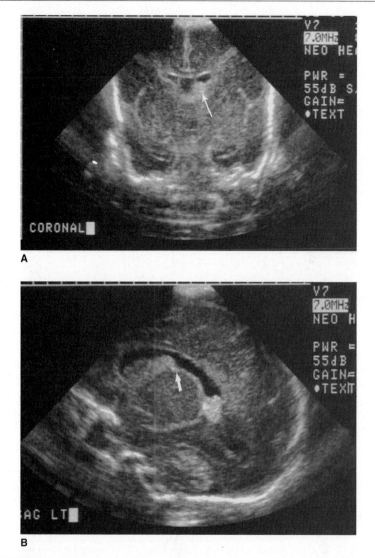

FIGURE 10–1. Ultrasonogram of the brain. Coronal (A) and left sagittal (B) views show a left germinal matrix hemorrhage (grade I intraventricular hemorrhage or subependymal hemorrhage at arrow).

   B. **Abdominal ultrasonography** is useful in the evaluation of abdominal distention, abdominal masses, and renal failure. Abdominal sonography can be performed portably. The addition of duplex and color Doppler evaluation of regional vessels is a supplementary procedure that can identify vascular occlusion resulting from thrombosis.
   C. **Power Doppler sonography** better demonstrates amplitude of blood flow compared with color Doppler but does not define direction of blood flow and is very motion sensitive.

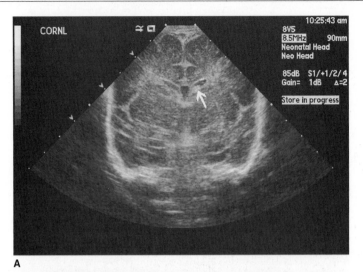

A

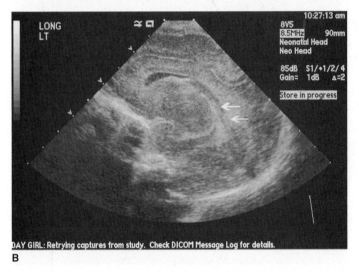

B

FIGURE 10–2. Ultrasonogram of the brain. Coronal (A) and left sagittal (B) views show a limited intraventricular hemorrhage (IVH) with minimal ventricular enlargement at arrow (grade II IVH).

III. **Computed tomographic (CT) scanning**

    A. **CT scanning of the head** is more complicated than ultrasonography because the patient must be moved to the CT unit and be adequately sedated. However, as CT scanning times progressively decrease due to technical improvements, the need for sedation is decreasing. CT scanning provides more global information than ultrasonography of the head, particularly at the periphery of the brain.

    B. **This technique can be used to diagnose intraventricular, subdural, or subarachnoid bleeding and cerebral edema or infarction.** To diagnose cerebral infarction,

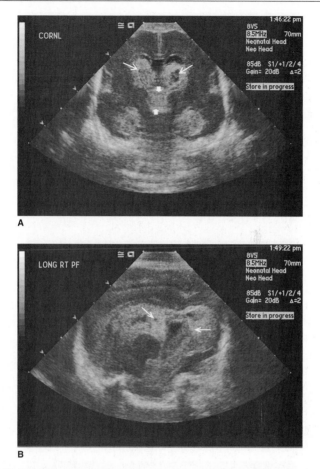

FIGURE 10–3. Ultrasonogram of the brain. Coronal (A) and right parasagittal (B) views demonstrate severe dilatation of both lateral (small arrows) as well as the third (large arrows) ventricles, which are filled with clots (grade III intraventricular hemorrhage).

infusion of contrast medium is necessary. If contrast is used, blood urea nitrogen and creatinine levels must be obtained before the CT test to rule out renal impairment, which may be a contraindication to the use of intravenous contrast media. An intravenous catheter must be placed, preferably not in the head.

IV. **Magnetic resonance imaging (MRI)** is now an acceptable mode of imaging in the neonate, and its use is expanding. MRI is superior to CT for imaging the brainstem, spinal cord, soft tissues, and areas of high bony CT artifact. Supplemental magnetic resonance arteriography and magnetic resonance venography are now available to improve vascular anatomy and flow.

   A. **Advantages** are the absence of ionizing radiation and visualization of vascular anatomy without contrast agents.

   B. **Disadvantages** are as follows: it cannot always be performed on critically ill infants requiring ventilator support, the scanning time is longer, and sedation is usually required.

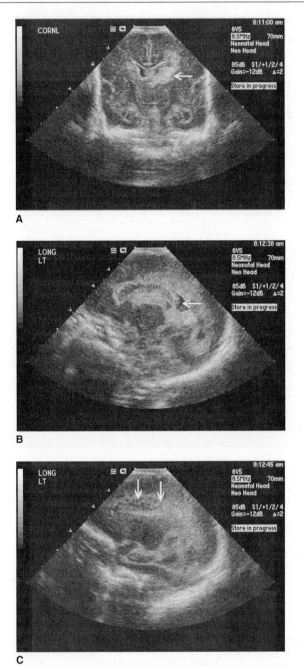

FIGURE 10–4. Ultrasonogram of the brain. Coronal (A) and left sagittal (B, C) demonstrate left intraventricular hemorrhage (IVH) with ventricular dilatation and localized left intraparenchymal hemorrhage (grade IV IVH) (arrows). (See next page for follow-up sonography.)

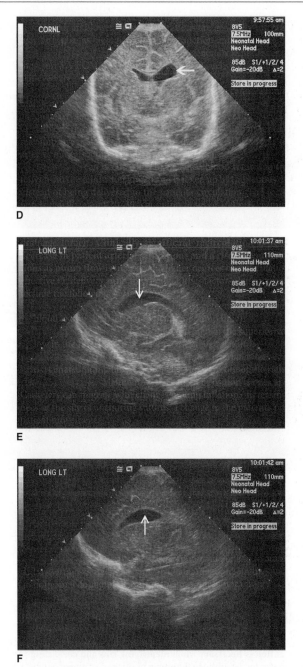

FIGURE 10–4. Ultrasonogram of the brain. Follow-up sonogram 3 months later (coronal view, D and left sagittal, E and F, views) shows resolution of clot, residual mild ventriculomegaly, and focal porencephaly (arrow) at the site of previous parenchymal hemorrhage.

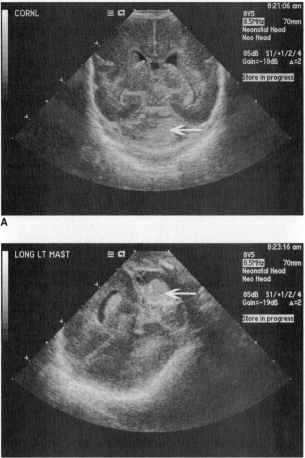

FIGURE 10–5. Ultrasonogram of the brain. Coronal (A) and mastoid (B) views demonstrate focal hemorrhage into the left cerebellar hemisphere (posterior fossa hemorrhage, arrow).

COMMON RADIOLOGIC PREPARATIONS

See Table 10–1 for guidelines for common radiographic studies. Institutional guidelines may vary slightly from these.

RADIOGRAPHIC EXAMPLES

Invasive life support and monitoring techniques depend on proper positioning of the device being used. **Caution is necessary when identifying ribs** and correlating vertebrae in the newborn as a means for determining the proper position of a catheter or tube. Errors are occasionally made because it is assumed that infants have 12 ribs, as do older children and adults. In fact, it is not uncommon for infants to have a noncalcified 12th rib; thus the 11th rib is mistaken for the 12th rib, and an incorrect count of the lumbar vertebrae follows.

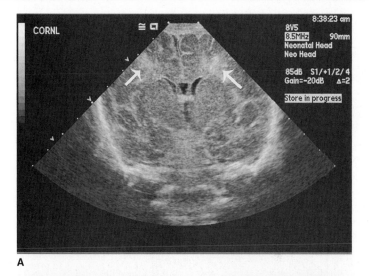

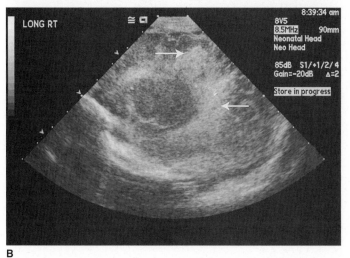

FIGURE 10–6. Ultrasonogram of the brain. Periventricular leukomalacia (PVL). Coronal (A) and right sagittal (B) views demonstrate increased periventricular echogenicity (PVE) suggesting ischemic white matter disease (arrows). (See next page for follow-up sonography.)

I. **Endotracheal intubation**
   A. **The preferred location of the endotracheal tube (ETT) tip** is halfway between the thoracic inlet (the medial ends of the clavicles) and the carina. Correct tube placement is shown in Figure 10–7.
   B. **If the ETT is placed too low,** the tip usually enters the right main bronchus, a straighter line than with the left main bronchus. The chest film may show asymmetric aeration with both hyperinflation and atelectasis. If the tube extends below the carina or does

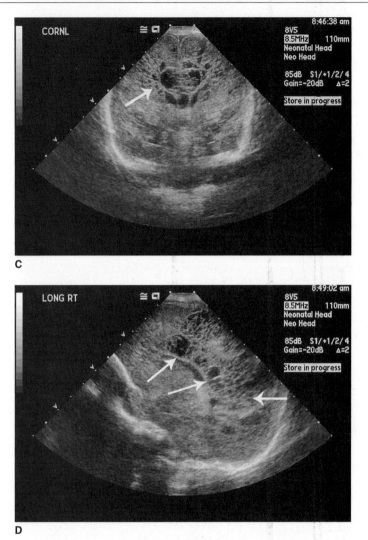

FIGURE 10–6. Ultrasonogram of the brain. Follow-up sonography of the brain 1 month later (C, coronal, and D, sagittal, views) shows extensive periventricular cystic change reflecting PVL.

not match the tracheal air column in position, suspect esophageal intubation. Increased proximal intestinal air may also reflect esophageal intubation. An ETT placed too high has the tip above the clavicle, and the x-ray film may show diffuse atelectasis.

II. **Umbilical vein catheterization (UVC).** The catheter tip should be at the junction of the inferior vena cava and right atrium, projecting just above the diaphragm on the AP chest radiograph. Degree and direction of patient rotation affect how the UVC appears positioned on the radiograph. **Due to its more anterior location, the UVC deviates more from the midline with patient rotation than will the umbilical artery catherization (UAC).** Figure 10–8 shows correct UVC tip placement.

Table 10–1. **PREPARATORY PROCEDURES FOR PREMATURE AND NEWBORN INFANT RADIOLOGIC STUDIES***

Neonatal Study	Preparation
Upper GI series	NPO for 1–2 h (neonates and infants; NB to 2 y), 3–4 h (children 2–10 y), 6 h (>10 y)
Contrast enema	No preparation needed for evaluation of bowel obstruction or to rule out Hirschsprung disease
Renal sonography	No preparation
Abdominal sonography	NPO for 1 h, for filling of gallbladder
HIDA (hepatobiliary) scan	Oral phenobarbital (5mg/kg/d) for 5 d prior to the examination
CT of abdomen/pelvis	Oral contrast beginning 2 h prior to scanning
Voiding cystourethrogram (VCUG)	No preparation required

CT, computed tomography; GI, gastrointestinal; HIDA, hepatoiminodiacetic acid; NPO, nothing by mouth; VCUG, voiding cystourethrogram.
*Review your institutional-specific recommendations before ordering.

III. **Umbilical artery catheterization (UAC).** The use of high versus low UAC placement depends on institutional preference. High catheters were once thought to be associated with a higher risk of vascular complications, but a recent analysis showed a decreased risk of vascular complications and no increased risk of hypertension, necrotizing enterocolitis (NEC), IVH, or hematuria. Low catheters are associated with an increased risk of vasospasms.

   A. **If high UAC placement is desired,** the tip should be between thoracic vertebrae 6 and 9 (above the origin of the celiac axis) (Figure 10–9).

   B. **For low UAC placement,** the tip should be below the third lumbar vertebra, optimally between L3 and L5 (Figure 10–10). A catheter placed below L5 usually does not function well and carries a risk of severe vasospasm in small arteries. Note that the catheter turns downward and then upward on an abdominal x-ray film. The upward turn is the point at which the catheter passes through the internal iliac artery (hypogastric artery).

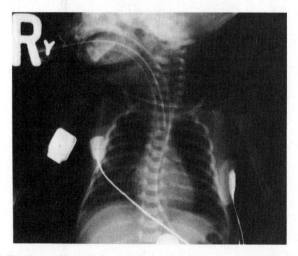

FIGURE 10–7. Chest radiograph showing proper placement of an endotracheal tube.

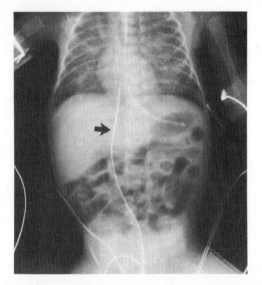

FIGURE 10–8. Abdominal radiograph showing correct placement of an umbilical venous catheter with tip at arrow. The tip of the nasogastric tube is properly positioned in the stomach.

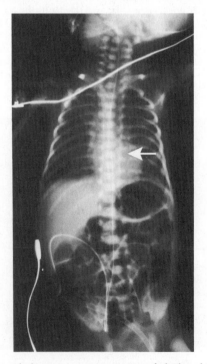

FIGURE 10–9. Radiograph showing correct positioning of a high umbilical artery catheter.

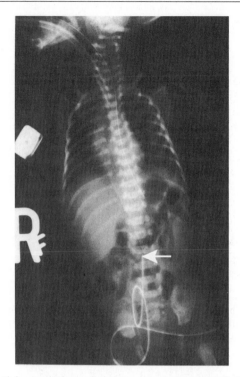

FIGURE 10–10. Abdominal radiograph showing correct positioning of a low umbilical artery catheter.

Note: If both a UAC and a UVC are positioned and an x-ray study is performed, it is necessary to differentiate the two so that line placement can be properly assessed. **The UAC turns downward and then upward on the x-ray film, whereas the UVC takes only an upward or cephalad direction.**

IV. **Extracorporeal membrane oxygenation (ECMO).** ECMO is a type of external life support using a membrane oxygenator that can be applied to a neonate in severe but reversible respiratory or cardiac failure (Chapter 13). Desaturated blood is removed by a jugular venous cannula (arrows in Figure 10–11) while oxygenated blood is returned to the neonate by a carotid arterial cannula (arrowhead in Figure 10–11).

RADIOGRAPHIC PEARLS

I. **Pulmonary diseases**
   A. **Hyaline membrane disease (HMD).** A fine, diffuse reticulogranular pattern is seen secondary to microatelectasis of the alveoli. The chest radiograph reveals radiolucent areas known as air bronchograms, produced by air in the major airways and contrasted with the opacified, collapsed alveoli (Figure 10–12).
   B. **Meconium aspiration syndrome.** Bilateral, patchy, coarse infiltrates and hyperinflation of the lungs are present (Figure 10–13).
   C. **Pneumonia.** Diffuse alveolar or interstitial disease that is usually asymmetric and localized. Group B streptococcal pneumonia can appear similar to HMD. Pneumatoceles

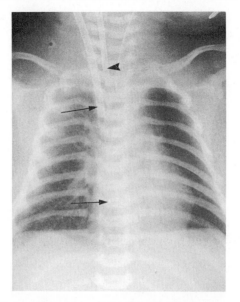

FIGURE 10–11. Chest radiograph showing well-positioned extracorporeal membrane oxygenation venous (arrows) and arterial (arrowhead) cannulas in the right atrium and the aortic arch, respectively, in a patient on extracorporeal membrane oxygenation life support.

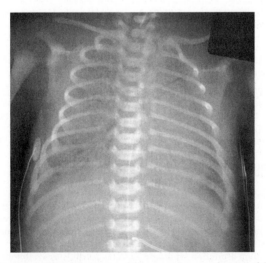

FIGURE 10–12. Chest radiograph showing diffuse granular opacification of the lungs with air bronchograms. In the premature neonate, this would almost always represent respiratory distress syndrome or hyaline membrane disease (HMD).

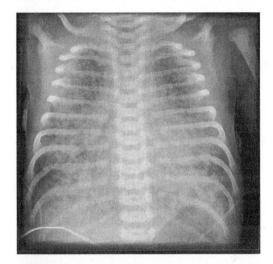

FIGURE 10–13. Chest radiograph showing diffuse coarse increase in lung markings accompanied by hyperinflation, typical for MAS (meconium aspiration syndrome). Pneumothorax is common in MAS (not seen in this example).

(air-filled lung cysts) can occur with staphylococcal pneumonia. Pleural effusions or empyema may occur with any bacterial pneumonia (Figure 10–14).
  D. **Transient tachypnea of the newborn.** Hyperaeration with symmetric perihilar and interstitial streaky infiltrates are typical. Pleural fluid may occur as well, appearing as widening of the pleural space or as prominence of the minor fissure (Figure 10–15).
  E. **Bronchopulmonary dysplasia.** Now more commonly referred to as **chronic lung disease (CLD)**, the radiographic appearance is highly variable, from a fine, hazy appearance to the lungs to mildly coarsened lung markings to a coarse, cystic lung pattern (Figure 10–16). Typically occurring in ventilated premature neonates,

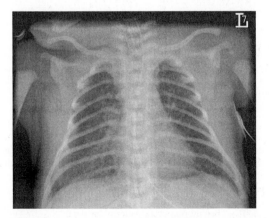

FIGURE 10–14. Diffuse increase in interstitial lung markings is typical with neonatal pneumonia but could also be produced by transient tachypnea of newborn.

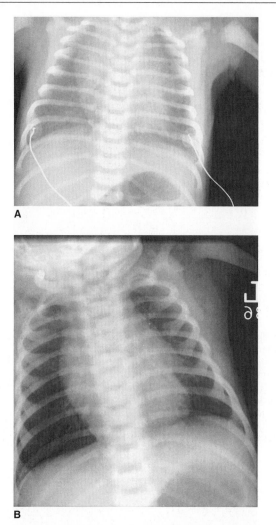

FIGURE 10–15. Chest radiograph (A) showing diffuse, mild increase in interstitial lung markings, consistent with transient tachypnea of newborn. The findings had typically resolved by the following day (B).

CLD usually requires a minimum of 7–10 days to develop. Many centers no longer rely on the following grading system for this condition, but it is included for historical purposes.

1. **Grade I:** X-ray findings are similar to those of severe HMD.
2. **Grade II:** Dense parenchymal opacification is seen.
3. **Grade III:** A bubbly, fibrocystic pattern is evident.
4. **Grade IV:** Hyperinflation is present, with multiple fine, lacy densities spreading to the periphery and with areas of lucency similar to bullae of the lung.

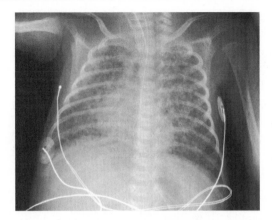

FIGURE 10–16. Chest radiograph showing a diffuse, moderately coarse increase in lung density, which in a 2-month old ventilated ex-premie is most consistent with chronic lung disease (CLD)/bronchopulmonary dysplasia.

   F. **Air leak syndromes**
      1. **Pneumopericardium.** Air surrounds the heart, including the inferior border (Figure 10–17).
      2. **Pneumomediastinum**
         a. AP view. A hyperlucent rim of air is present lateral to the cardiac border and beneath the thymus, displacing the thymus superiorly away from the cardiac silhouette ("angel wing sign") (Figure 10–18, left panel).
         b. Lateral view. An air collection is seen either substernally (anterior pneumomediastinum) or in the retrocardiac area (posterior pneumomediastinum) (Figure 10–18, right panel).
      3. **Pneumothorax.** The lung is typically displaced away from the lateral chest wall by a radiolucent zone of air. The adjacent lung may be collapsed with larger pneumothoraces (as in Figure 10–19). The small pneumothorax may be very difficult

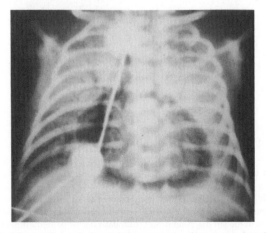

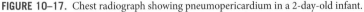

FIGURE 10–17. Chest radiograph showing pneumopericardium in a 2-day-old infant.

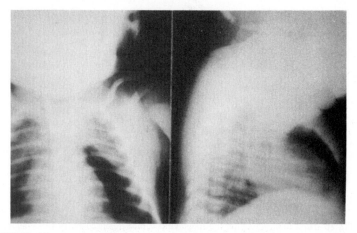

FIGURE 10–18. Pneumomediastinum on anteroposterior (left panel) and cross-table lateral (right panel) radiograph, demonstrating central chest air and elevation of the lobes of the thymus.

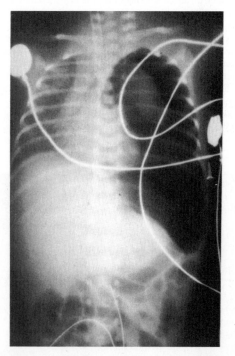

FIGURE 10–19. Left tension pneumothorax as shown on an anteroposterior chest radiograph in a ventilated infant on day 2 of life. Note the accompanying collapse of the left lung, depression of the left diaphragm, and contralateral shift of mediastinal structures, all signs of increased pressure within a pneumothorax.

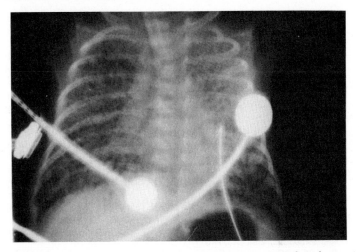

FIGURE 10–20. Chest radiograph showing bilateral pulmonary interstitial emphysema in a 7-day-old ventilated infant.

to identify, with only a subtle zone of air peripherally, a diffusely hyperlucent hemithorax, unusually sharply defined cardiothymic margins, or a combination of these.

4. **Tension pneumothorax.** The diaphragm on the affected side is depressed, the mediastinum is shifted to the contralateral hemithorax, and collapse of the ipsilateral lobes is evident (Figure 10–19).

5. **Pulmonary interstitial emphysema (PIE).** Single or multiple circular radiolucencies with well-demarcated walls are seen in a localized or diffuse pattern. The volume of the involved portion of the lung is usually increased, often markedly so (Figure 10–20). PIE usually occurs in ventilated premies with respiratory distress syndrome (RDS), within the initial few days of life.

G. **Atelectasis.** A decrease in lung volume or collapse of part or all of a lung is apparent, appearing as areas of increased opacity. The mediastinum may be shifted toward the side of collapse. Compensatory hyperinflation of the opposite lung may be present.

1. **Microatelectasis.** See Chapter 89.

2. **Generalized atelectasis.** Diffuse increase in opacity ("whiteout") of the lungs is visible on the chest film. It may be seen in severe RDS, airway obstruction, if the endotracheal tube is not in the trachea, and hypoventilation.

3. **Lobar atelectasis.** Lobar atelectasis is atelectasis of one lobe. The most common site is the right upper lobe, which appears as an area of dense opacity ("whiteout") on the chest film. In addition, the right minor fissure is usually elevated. This pattern of atelectasis commonly occurs after extubation.

H. **Pulmonary hypoplasia.** Small lung volumes and a bell-shaped thorax are seen. The lungs usually appear radiolucent.

I. **Pulmonary edema.** The lungs appear diffusely hazy with an area of greatest density around the hilum of each lung. Heart size is usually increased.

II. **Cardiac diseases.** The cardiothoracic ratio, which normally should be <0.6, is the width of the base of the heart divided by the width of the lower thorax. An index >0.6 suggests cardiomegaly. The pulmonary vascularity is increased if the diameter of the descending branch of the right pulmonary artery exceeds that of the trachea.

A. **Cardiac dextroversion.** The cardiac apex is on the right, and the aortic arch and stomach bubble are on the left. The incidence of congenital heart disease associated with this finding is high (>90%).

B. **Congestive heart failure.** Cardiomegaly, pulmonary venous congestion (engorgement and increased diameter of the pulmonary veins), diffuse opacification in the perihilar regions, and pleural effusions (sometimes) are seen.

C. **Patent ductus arteriosus.** Cardiomegaly, pulmonary edema, ductal haze (pulmonary edema with a patent ductus arteriosus), and increased pulmonary vascular markings are evident.

D. **Ventricular septal defect.** Findings include cardiomegaly, an increase in pulmonary vascular density, enlargement of the left ventricle and left atrium, and enlargement of the main pulmonary artery.

E. **Coarctation of the aorta**
   1. **Preductal coarctation.** Generalized cardiomegaly, with normal pulmonary vascularity, is seen.
   2. **Postductal coarctation.** An enlarged left ventricle and left atrium and a dilated ascending aorta are present.

F. **Tetralogy of Fallot.** The heart is boot shaped. A normal left atrium and left ventricle is associated with an enlarged, hypertrophied right ventricle and small or absent main pulmonary artery. There is decreased pulmonary vascularity. A right aortic arch occurs in 25% of patients.

G. **Transposition of the great arteries.** The chest film may show cardiomegaly, with an enlarged right atrium and right ventricle, narrow mediastinum, and increased pulmonary vascular markings, but in most cases the chest film appears normal.

H. **Total anomalous pulmonary venous return (TAPVR).** Pulmonary venous markings are increased. Cardiomegaly is minimal or absent. Congestive heart failure and pulmonary edema may be present, especially with type 3 (subdiaphragmatic) TAPVR.

I. **Hypoplastic left heart syndrome.** The chest film can be normal at first but then may show cardiomegaly and pulmonary vascular congestion, with an enlarged right atrium and ventricle.

J. **Tricuspid atresia.** Heart size is usually normal or small, the main pulmonary artery is concave, and pulmonary vascularity is decreased.

K. **Truncus arteriosus.** Characteristic findings include cardiomegaly, increased pulmonary vascularity, and enlargement of the left atrium. A right aortic arch occurs in 30% of patients.

L. **Atrial septal defect.** Varying degrees of enlargement of the right atrium and ventricle are seen. The aorta and the left ventricle are small, and the pulmonary artery is large. Increased pulmonary vascularity is also evident.

M. **Ebstein's anomaly.** Gross cardiomegaly and decreased pulmonary vascularity are apparent. The right heart border is prominent as a result of right atrial enlargement.

N. **Valvular pulmonic stenosis.** Heart size and pulmonary blood flow are usually normal unless the stenosis is severe. Dilatation of the main pulmonary artery is the typical chest film finding.

III. **Abdominal disorders**
   A. **Changes in the following normal patterns** should raise suspicion of GI tract disease.
      1. **Air in the stomach** should occur within 30 min after delivery.
      2. **Air in the small bowel** should be seen by 3–4 h of age.
      3. **Air in the colon and rectum** should be seen by 6–8 h of age.
   B. **Intestinal obstruction.** Gaseous intestinal distention is present. Gas may be decreased or absent distal to the obstruction. Air-fluid levels are seen proximal to the obstruction.
   C. **Ascites.** Gas-filled loops of bowel, if present, are located in the central portion of the abdomen. The abdomen may be distended, with relatively small amounts of gas (**"ground-glass" appearance**). A uniform increase in the density of the abdomen, particularly in the flank areas, may be evident.

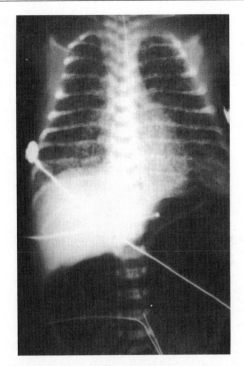

FIGURE 10–21. Abdominal radiograph showing pneumoperitoneum in a 3-day-old infant.

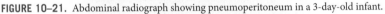

D. **Calcification** in the abdomen is most often seen secondary to meconium peritonitis, which may also cause calcifications in the scrotum in male infants. Calcifications in the abdomen may also be seen in infants with neuroblastoma or teratoma or may signify calcification of the adrenals after adrenal hemorrhage.

E. **Pneumoperitoneum**
   1. **Supine view.** Free air is seen as a central lucency, usually in the upper abdomen (Figure 10–21).
   2. **Upright view.** Free air is present in a subdiaphragmatic location.
   3. **Left lateral decubitus view.** Air collects over the lateral border of the liver, separating it from the adjacent abdominal wall.

F. **Pneumatosis intestinalis.** Intraluminal gas in the bowel wall (produced by bacteria that have invaded the bowel wall) may appear as a string or cluster of bubbles (submucosal) or a curvilinear lucency (subserosal). It is most frequently seen in infants with NEC (Figure 10–22).

G. **Situs inversus (complete).** The stomach, aortic arch, and cardiac apex all are right sided. There is only a limited increased incidence of congenital heart disease.

H. **Ileus.** Distended loops of bowel are present. Air-fluid levels may be seen on the upright or cross-table lateral abdominal film.

I. **Absence of gas in the abdomen.** Absence of gas in the abdomen may be seen in patients taking muscle-paralyzing medications (eg, pancuronium) because they do not swallow air. It may also be evident in infants with esophageal atresia without tracheoesophageal fistula and in cases of severe cerebral anoxia resulting in central nervous system depression and absence of swallowing.

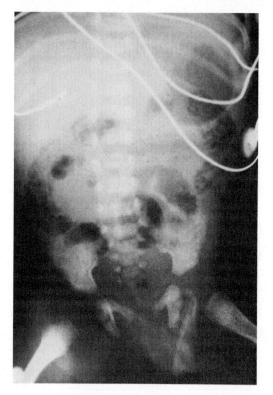

FIGURE 10–22. Abdominal radiograph showing pneumatosis intestinalis in a 4-day-old infant. It is most frequently seen in infants with NEC.

J. **Portal venous air.** Air is demonstrated in the portal veins (often best seen on a lateral view). This finding may indicate bowel necrosis, which can occur in an advanced degree of NEC, intestinal infarction secondary to mesenteric vessel occlusion, and iatrogenically introduced gas into the portal vein, which can occur during umbilical vein catheterization or exchange transfusion.

Selected References

Agrons GA et al: Lung disease in premature neonates: radiologic-pathologic correlation. *Radiographics* 2005;25:1047-1073.

Breysem L et al: Bronchopulmonary dysplasia: correlation of radiographic and clinical findings. *Pediatr Radiol* 1997;17:642-646.

Dinger J et al: Radiologic changes after therapeutic use of surfactant in infants with respiratory distress syndrome. *Pediatr Radiol* 1997;27:26-31.

Dolfin T et al: Incidence, severity and timing of subependymal and intravascular hemorrhages in preterm infants born in a prenatal unit as detected by serial real-time ultrasound. *Pediatrics* 1983;71:541.

Donnelly LF, Frush DP: Localized radiolucent chest lesions in neonates: causes and differentiation. *AJR* 1999;172:1651-1658.

Donoghue V: *Radiological Imaging of the Neonatal Chest.* Berlin, Germany: Springer, 2002.

Ferguson EC et al: Classical imaging signs of congenital cardiovascular abnormalities. *Radiographics* 2007;27:1323-1324.

Greenspan JS et al: Partial liquid ventilation in critically ill infants receiving extracorporeal life support. *Pediatrics* 1997;99:1.

Gross GW et al: Thoracic complications of extracorporeal membrane oxygenation: findings on chest radiographs and sonograms. *AJR Am J Roentgenol* 1992;158:353.

Gross GW et al: Bypass cannulas utilized in extracorporeal membrane oxygenation in neonates: radiographic findings. *Pediatr Radiol* 1995;25:337.

Kirks DR: *Practical Pediatric Imaging,* 3rd ed. Philadelphia, PA: Lippincott-Raven, 1998.

Swischuk LE: *Imaging of the Newborn, Infant and Young Child,* 3rd ed. Philadelphia, PA: Williams & Wilkins, 1989.

Veyrac C et al: Brain ultrasonography in the premature infant [symposium]. *Pediatr Radiol* 2006;36:626-635.

11 Infant Transport

The goal of an infant transport is to provide early stabilization and initiation of advanced care at a referring institution with continuation of critical care therapies and monitoring during transport to ensure safety and a positive neonatal outcome. Transport of infants who need a higher level of care from a referring hospital to a level III neonatal intensive care unit (NICU) enables each patient to benefit from the regionalization and specialization of critical care personnel, capabilities, and services. A great deal of planning must take place for a specialized transport team to function effectively, and clear guidelines must be established regarding personnel, procedures, and equipment needed. A preplanned transport algorithm is essential to organize a smooth transition of care. Ideally, the mother would be transferred to the level III center before delivery of a high-risk infant, but this is not always possible.

I. **Transport team**
   A. **Personnel.** The team may include physicians, nurses, neonatal nurse practitioners or advanced practice nurses, respiratory therapists, and perhaps emergency medical technicians. Limited research supports similar outcomes from transport teams with and without the direct presence of a transport physician. Team members should have received special training in the care of sick infants and have the ability to contact the attending neonatologist at any time during transport. Appropriate insurance coverage is necessary for team members, and questions of liability must be worked out with legal consultation among hospitals, ambulance services, and aircraft services.
   B. **Procedures.** Policies and procedures reflect the unique characteristics of each region (size, geography, economics, and sophistication of medical services). Lines of communication must always be open between the referring hospital and the NICU at all levels (ie, administrators, physicians, nurses) and with ambulance or air services. At the referring hospital, team members should conduct themselves as professional representatives of the NICU, avoiding situations of conflict or criticism with the staff.
II. **Equipment.** Each transport team should be self-sufficient. Special emphasis is placed on having all of the necessary equipment to enable stabilization of the infant at the referring hospital to optimize an uneventful transport instead of a "swoop and scoop" mentality. Medications and equipment can be chosen according to published lists. Special considerations are maintaining thermal neutrality (eg, plastic swaddling or heated,

humidified inspired air mixtures) and noise and vibration, which often compromise auditory and visual monitoring. Well-calibrated blood pressure and transcutaneous monitors may be useful. An instant camera is a "must" because pictures of the infant may be the mother's only psychological support for days.

III. **Protocol for stabilization and transfer.** The mobile environment has risks and limitations that can be balanced by pretransport stabilization, qualified professionals, and equipment and monitoring devices adapted for use during transport.

   A. **General procedures.** Unless active resuscitation is underway, the team's first task at the referring hospital is to listen to the history and assessment of the infant's status. The vital signs are then obtained. A complete physical assessment should be performed as well as review of all laboratory values and radiographic studies. Obtain copies of the medical record and radiographic studies if possible. At this point, a precise diagnosis of all the infant's problems may be less important than predicting what the infant will need during transport. Problems that may occur during transport should be anticipated. The level III NICU should be given an expected arrival time. During transport, vigilant monitoring of respiratory rate, heart rate, blood pressure, and oxygen levels should continue for unexpected changes in the infant's status.

   B. **General stabilization.** Attention to the details of stabilization is important! In most cases, an infant is not ready for transport until basic neonatal needs are met: acceptable cardiac and respiratory function, thermal stabilization, intravenous access, and blood glucose levels in the normal range. Vital signs must be stable, and catheters and tubes should be appropriately placed. Infants at risk for sepsis and those with indwelling catheters should probably receive antibiotic therapy after blood cultures are obtained.

   C. **Gastric intubation.** If the infant has a gastrointestinal disorder (including ileus accompanying critical illness or a diaphragmatic hernia) or if positive airway pressure is administered through the nose or a mask, venting of the stomach with a nasogastric or orogastric tube is indicated, especially if air transport is used. Venting should be performed before transport because the air trapped in the gastrointestinal tract will expand in volume as atmospheric pressure decreases (see Section VI, B).

   D. **Temperature control and fluid balance.** Special attention to temperature and fluid balance is required for infants with open lesions (eg, myelomeningocele or omphalocele). A dry or moist protective dressing over the lesion can be covered by thin plastic wrap to reduce radiant heat loss.

   E. **Family support.** Keep parents updated by outlining the initial medical concerns and potential hospital course. The parents should be allowed to see and touch the infant before transport and if possible provided with pictures. Contact information and directions to the accepting hospital should be supplied. After transfer is completed, the team should talk with the parents and, if possible, with the referring physician.

IV. **Evaluation of transport.** Each transport should have a scoring system that reflects the "before" and "after" status of the infant. For example, vital signs and blood glucose measurements taken when the team first arrives at the referring hospital should be compared with the same measurements taken on admission to the NICU. This system provides quality control of transports and is useful in outreach education to convey constructive criticism to referring hospitals. It is also important to review regularly team response time, referring hospital satisfaction, difficult transports, safety updates, team credentialing, medical protocols, and so on as part of quality assurance and safety evaluation.

V. **Outreach education.** Transport team members should meet with professionals from each referring hospital. Such a forum for discussion of transport issues and specific transported patients provides mutual feedback and stimulates interhospital protocol decision making as well as quality improvement processes.

VI. **Special considerations in air transport.** The most critical factor in determining mode of transport is the safety of the team and patient. Each region should develop protocols for choosing ground or air transport, based on distance, time of day, geography, weather, location of landing sites, and patient severity and stability.

A. **Safety guidelines.** Clear guidelines should be established regarding air transport. Decisions regarding flight safety should be made according to weather and other flight conditions and not influenced primarily by patient status. Controlled landing sites familiar to the pilot should be used. Loading and unloading of the aircraft should not take place while engines are running; an idling helicopter is dangerous.

B. **Dysbarism.** In helicopters and unpressurized aircraft, dysbarism (imbalance between air pressure in the atmosphere and the pressure of gases within the body) causes predictable problems. Partial pressures of inspired gases decrease as altitude increases, so infants require an increased concentration of inspired oxygen. Trapped free air in the thorax or intestines expands in volume and may cause significant pulmonary compromise. A cuffed tube or catheter should be evacuated before takeoff. *Note:* Because blood pressure varies with changing gravitational force, fluctuations noted during climbing or descent should not be cause for alarm.

Selected References

American Academy of Pediatrics Task Force on Inter-hospital Transport: Guidelines for Air and Ground Transport of Neonatal and Pediatric Patients, 3rd ed. Elk Grove, IL: American Academy of Pediatrics, 2007.

Das UG, Leuthner SR: Preparing the neonate for transport. *Pediatr Clin N Am* 2004;51(3):581-598.

Horowitz R, Rozenfeld RA: Pediatric critical care interfacility transport. *Clin Pediatr Emerg Med* 2007;8(3):190-202.

King BR et al: Pediatric and neonatal transport teams with and without a physician: a comparison of outcomes and interventions. *Pediatr Emerg Care* 2007;23(2):77-82.

Lee SK et al: Transport risk index of physiologic stability: a practical system for assessing transport care. *J Pediatr* 2001;139(2):220-226.

12 Blood Component Therapy

I. **Blood banking procedures**
   A. **Type and screen.** Whenever possible, samples from both mother and infant should be obtained for initial ABO group and Rh (D) type determination.
      1. **Investigations on the maternal sample should include:**
         a. ABO group and Rh (D) type.
         b. Screen for atypical red cell antibodies by an indirect antiglobulin technique (IAT).
      2. **Investigations on the infant (or umbilical cord) sample:**
         a. ABO group and Rh (D) type.
         b. Direct antiglobulin test performed on neonatal red cells.
         c. In the absence of maternal serum, infant's serum is screened for atypical antibodies by an IAT.
   B. **Type and cross-match.** In addition to ABO group and Rh (D) type, this includes mixing donor red blood cells (RBC) and maternal or infant serum (or both) to inspect for any reaction. Infants rarely make alloantibodies in the first 4 months of life so there is no need to repeat cross-matching during that period unless the patient has been exposed to exchange transfusion or repeated plasma infusions.

II. **Routine blood donation**
   A. **Voluntary blood donations** are from screened donors with a negative history for potentially blood transmissible diseases. All blood donors are tested using serological enzyme immunoassays (EIAs) and nucleic amplification testing for viral risks that include:
      1. **HIV: types 1 and 2.**
      2. **Hepatitis viruses B and C (HBV and HCV).**
      3. **Human T-cell lymphotrophic viruses (HTLV-I/II).**
      4. **West Nile virus (WNV).**
      5. **Trypanosoma cruzi EIA antibodies.** Cause of Chagas disease.
      6. *Treponema pallidum* (syphilis) **EIA or microhemagglutination testing is still required.**
      7. **Testing for the following bloodborne viruses is *not* routinely done:** cytomegalovirus (CMV), hepatitis A virus, hepatitis G virus (HGV; also known as GB virus-C [GBV-C]; no proven disease association), Torque teno virus (TTV or transfusion-transmitted virus; no proven disease association), Epstein-Barr virus (EBV), and human herpes virus 8 (HHV8 or KSHV; associated with Kaposi sarcoma and with multicentric Castleman disease and primary effusion lymphoma in HIV-infected patients).
   B. **The residual risks of transfusion per unit transfused are estimated to be:**
      1. **HIV and HCV: 1 in 1,800,000 units.**
      2. **HBV: 1 in 220,000 units.**
      3. **WNV: 1 in 350,000 units** (during mosquito-borne community outbreaks).
      4. **For perspective, selected comparative mortality odds ratios are anesthesia:** 1/7,000–1/340,000; flood: 1/455,000; and lightning strike: 1:10,000,000.
III. **Donor-directed blood products.** Blood provided by a relative or friend of the family for a specified infant. This technique cannot be used in the emergency setting because it takes up to 48 h to process the blood for use. No evidence indicates that donor-directed transfusion is safer than blood provided by routine donation. Mothers may not be ideal donors because maternal plasma frequently contains a variety of antibodies (against leukocyte and platelet antigens) that could interact with antigens expressed on neonatal cells. Similarly, transfusions from paternal donors present a risk because the neonate may have been passively immunized against paternal blood cellular antigens (by transplacental transfer of maternal antibodies against paternal antigens).
IV. **Autologous blood donation**
   In adults, safety of transfusion is markedly enhanced with the use of autologous blood collected preoperatively.
   A. **The fetoplacental blood reservoir contains a blood volume of approximately 110 mL/kg and 30–50% of this volume is contained in the placenta. Thus placental blood is autologous blood.** Approximately 20 mL/kg can be harvested at birth and used for future transfusion. The potential for bacterial contamination coupled with the additional expense of collection have limited the widespread adoption of placental autologous blood transfusion.
   B. **As an alternative, delayed cord clamping for 30–45 s after birth allows the transfer of a significant amount of blood from the placenta to the infant.** The blood volume of newborn subjected to delayed cord clamping is 15–30 mL/kg larger than that of neonates with early cord clamping. Beneficial effects from this procedure are: reduction in transfusions needed, decreased iron deficiency at a later age, and possibly decreased risk of intraventricular hemorrhage in preterm infants.
V. **Irradiated/Filtered blood components**
   A. **The following adverse reactions to blood transfusion are caused by passenger contaminant leukocytes (WBC) whose numbers are maximal when fresh blood is used.**
      1. Sensitization to human leukocyte antigens (HLA).
      2. Febrile transfusion reactions.

3. Immunomodulation, which may increase the risk of postoperative infection.
4. CMV transmission.
5. Transfusion-associated graft-versus-host disease (TA-GVHD) from engraftment of donor T lymphocytes.

B. **HLA sensitization and febrile transfusion reactions are unusual in infants, whereas transfusion-transmitted CMV and TA-GVHD can be life threatening.**
   1. **At greatest risk** of severe CMV infection are preterm infants (<1200 g) born to CMV-seronegative mothers.
   2. **Patients at risk** for TA-GVHD include recipients of donor-directed units from first-degree blood relatives, HLA-matched platelets, intrauterine transfusions, massive fresh blood transfusions or exchange transfusions, as well as patients with suspected immunodeficiency states (eg, DiGeorge syndrome).

C. **For these high-risk patients, transfused blood components must be processed to remove passenger WBC.**
   1. **Leukoreduction (removal of passenger WBC)** is almost always performed by filtration of the blood component through proprietary hollow-fiber filters to which intact WBC adhere. (Centrifugation-based techniques are outdated.) Leukocyte counts can be reduced from 10^9 to 4–6×10^5 per RBC unit (4 log unit reduction) with fourth-generation filters.
   2. **Leukoreduction is effective in reducing** HLA alloimmunization and transmission of cell-associated viruses (especially herpes viruses [such as CMV and HHV8] and EBV) as well as preventing some febrile transfusion reactions.
   3. **Gamma irradiation** of cellular blood components delivers a dose of 25 Gy and prevents subsequent WBC mitoses and, thereby, TA-GVHD.

VI. **Emergency transfusions.** Uncross-matched (or "emergency release") blood is rarely transfused because most blood banks can do a complete cross-match within 1 hour. In cases of massive, exsanguinating hemorrhage, "type-specific" blood (ABO and Rh (D)-matched only), usually available in 10 min, can be used. If this delay is too long (as in severe fetomaternal transfusion), type O Rh (D)-negative RBC should be used.

VII. **Blood bank products**
A. **Red blood cells**
   1. **Packed red blood cells (PRBC)**
      a. **Indications.** RBC transfusions are given to maintain the hematocrit (Hct) at a level judged best for the clinical condition of the baby. The selected target Hct is *controversial* and varies greatly among neonatal units. General guidelines are as follows:
         i. Hct >35–40% in the presence of severe cardiopulmonary disease.
         ii. Hct >30–35% for moderate cardiopulmonary disease or major surgery.
         iii. Hct >20–25% for infants with stable, so-called asymptomatic anemia.
         iv. **The severity of cardiopulmonary disease** is assessed based on the level of respiratory support (IPPV, CPAP, Fio_2) required, symptoms of unexplained apnea and/or tachycardia, and/or poor growth.
      b. **Administration** is 10–20 mL/kg given over 1–3 h (4 h maximum). Use the following formula as a guide:

      $$\text{Volume PRBC to transfuse (mL)} = 1.6 \times \text{weight (kg)} \times \text{desired rise in Hct (\%)}$$

   2. **Adsol PRBC.** The traditional use of relatively fresh RBC (<7 days' storage) has been largely replaced by the practice of transfusing aliquots of RBC from a dedicated unit of PRBC stored for up to 42 days. This requires a sterile connecting device and is done to diminish the number of donor exposures among infants expected to require numerous transfusions during their stay in the NICU (infants whose birthweight is <1500 g). PRBC are suspended in a citrate-anticoagulated storage solution at a Hct of 55–60% stored at 1–6°C. The storage or additive solutions (AS or Adsol-1, 3, or 5) contain various combinations of preservatives (dextrose, sodium chloride, phosphate, adenine, and mannitol).

3. **CPD (citrate phosphate dextrose) PRBC.** Because of concern about potential hepatorenal toxicity of adenine and mannitol, units of RBC without extended storage medium are used for large volume transfusions such as exchange transfusion and transfusions for major surgical procedures. PRBC units (CPDA-1 and CPDA-2) with only small amounts of adenine and devoid of mannitol have a hematocrit of 65–80% and a shelf life of 35 days. PRBC units (CPD) lacking both adenine and mannitol also have a hematocrit of 65–80% but a shelf life of only 21 days. Washed PRBC Adsol units are an alternative if these other PRBC units are unavailable.

4. **Washed PRBC.** During storage, potassium is progressively released from RBC so that, by the end of the storage period, extracellular (plasma) potassium levels approximate 50 and 80 mEq/L for Adsol and CPD units, respectively. This leakage is increased in irradiated blood. For small-volume transfusions the amount of infused K is, in general, of little clinical significance (0.3–0.4 mEq/kg per 15 mL/kg RBC transfusion). But it may become hazardous for larger transfusion volumes such as in exchange transfusion. In such an event and in the absence of fresh whole blood (<2–3 days old), RBC washed free of their potentially hyperkalemic supernatant using normal saline and then reconstituted to an hematocrit of 50–55% with fresh-frozen plasma ("reconstituted whole blood") can be used. Irradiated reconstituted whole blood should be used for total exchange transfusion.

B. **Other transfusion products**

1. **Plasma: fresh-frozen plasma (FFP), thawed plasma.** Plasma is removed after centrifugation of donated whole blood is used to separate RBC and frozen for later use. It contains albumin, immune globulins, and clotting factors, some of which retain much of their activity after thawing (vWF and factors V, VII, and VIII may have their activity reduced during processing before freezing).

   a. **Indications**

      i. Correction of coagulopathy due to inherited deficiencies of some clotting factors.

      ii. Vitamin K deficiency (hemorrhagic disease of the newborn).

      iii. DIC.

      iv. Inherited clotting factor deficiency. When available, clotting factor concentrates are preferred over the use of FFP. There are no single factor concentrates available for factors II, V, and X. Prothrombin complex concentrates containing factors II, IX, and X are used for factor II and X deficiencies.

      v. Prophylaxis for dilutional coagulopathy associated with massive blood transfusion administered for replacement of blood loss in excess of half of the blood volume.

      vi. Preparation of reconstituted whole blood from washed PRBC for total exchange transfusion.

      vii. Although FFP provides excellent colloid volume support, it is not recommended for volume expansion or antibody replacement because safer components are available for these purposes.

   b. **Administration**

      i. Transfused plasma should be ABO compatible with the patient's blood group. Incompatible antibodies in the donor plasma (such as anti-A or -B antibodies in group O plasma) may rarely, if given in sufficient volume, result in an acute hemolytic reaction in the transfused patient.

      ii. Dose 10–20 mL/kg over 1–2 h (4 h maximum).

      iii. Rapid transfusion may result in transient hypocalcemia due to the sodium citrate that is added to the original donated blood. If rapid infusion of FFP is needed, a small bolus of calcium chloride (3–5 mg/kg) may be considered.

2. **Cryoprecipitate** is prepared from FFP by thawing it at 1–6°C. In this range, a cryoprecipitate forms and is separated from so called cryo-poor supernatant plasma by centrifugation. The pellet is then frozen as cryoprecipitate. Prior to use, it must again be thawed and dissolved off the interior surface of its plastic bag with normal saline (with total volume of 10–15 mL). **Cryoprecipitate is a concentrated source of the following blood clotting proteins: factor VIII, von Willebrand factor vWF), fibrinogen, and factor XIII (with some other proteins, eg, fibronectin).**
   a. Indications
      i. To restore fibrinogen levels in patients with acquired hypofibrinogenemia (as occurs in DIC and massive transfusion).
      ii. Factor XIII in deficient patients.
   b. Administration
      i. Like FFP, it should be ABO compatible with the recipient's blood group.
      ii. Dose 10 mL/kg (0.1–0.2 units/kg raises fibrinogen by 60 to 100 mg/dL). Infusion should be completed within 6 h of thawing.
3. **Platelets.** Platelets are prepared from whole blood donations by centrifugation (termed "random donor") or by automated apheresis (termed "single donor" or "platelets pheresis"). Each random donor unit contains 5.5×10^{10} platelets in 50–70 mL of anticoagulated plasma. Each single donor unit contains 3×10^{11} platelets, typically in 300–350 mL of anticoagulated plasma. Both are stored at room temperature (20–24°C) with agitation for a maximum of 5 days. Because of room temperature storage, bacterial contamination of platelet units is actively sought, typically by culture of each component. Increased mortality and morbidity have been described among preterm infants receiving multiple platelet transfusions.
   a. **Indications.** There are no absolute guidelines regarding platelet counts that necessitate transfusion.
      i. In general, platelet transfusion is indicated for platelet counts <50,000 μL.
      ii. In the presence of active bleeding or prior to surgery, this "transfusion trigger" may be raised to 100,000 μL, whereas in a nonbleeding, stable neonate, platelet counts as low as 20,000–30,000 μL may be tolerated.
      iii. In septic patients, platelet increments after transfusion may only be transient.
   b. Administration
      i. Infant and donor should be ABO identical if possible. When ABO identical platelets are unavailable, use group A platelets for group B recipients and vice versa. Group O platelets are the least suitable for non-Group-O infants because passively transfused anti-A or anti-B antibodies may lead to hemolysis.
      ii. Rh (D) negative platelets should be given whenever possible to Rh (D) negative patients, especially female infants.
      iii. For infants with alloimmune thrombocytopenia, platelets lacking human platelet-specific antigens (HPA) to which antibodies are directed are required. If such platelets are unavailable, then HPA 1a,5b negative platelets may be given because these will be compatible in 95% of cases. If anti-HPA antibodies are not demonstrated, then anti-HLA antibodies may be alternatively present requiring HLA-matched platelets.
      iv. **Intravenous dosage:** 10–20 mL/kg should raise neonatal platelet counts by 60,000–100,000 μL.
VIII. **Transfusion reactions**
   A. **Acute intravascular hemolysis** is due to incompatibility of donor RBC with antibodies in the patient plasma. Most common antibodies responsible for complement-mediated acute hemolysis are isohemagglutinins (anti-A, anti-B). Newborns do not all make isohemagglutinins in high titer until 4–6 months of age.

1. However, transfusion of ABO-incompatible donor RBC (mostly due to clerical error) may result in hemolysis if isoagglutinin titers are high enough. Accordingly, some neonatal units may transfuse all neonates with O Rh (D) negative PRBC (if the blood bank can support this policy).
2. Incompatible isoagglutinins are more often found in the neonatal circulation due to transfusion of the ABO-incompatible plasma in platelet units.
3. Transplacental passage of Group O maternal isohemagglutinins to non-Group-O fetus may also cause hemolysis of neonate's own RBC in the absence of transfusion (typically mild; "ABO hemolytic disease of the fetus and newborn [HDFN]").
4. Red cell T-antigen is present on all human erythrocytes but expressed only after exposure to neuraminidase produced by a variety of infectious organisms, in particular streptococcus, clostridia, and influenzae viruses. Anti-T antibodies are present in almost all adults but are not present in the plasma of infants until 6 months of age. Anti-T may be associated with hemolysis in patients whose red cells are "activated" (eg, infants with NEC or sepsis). When intravascular hemolysis occurs and T-activation of neonatal RBC is identified through peanut lectin testing, donor RBC and platelets should be washed prior to use.
5. Possible symptoms of intravascular hemolysis include hypotension, fever, tachycardia, hematuria, and hemoglobinuria. Diagnosis may be confirmed by an elevated free serum hemoglobin, absent haptoglobin (if it is not congenitally absent as in ~10% of African American infants), as well as the presence of schistocytes on a peripheral blood smear.

B. **Nonhemolytic febrile reactions.** Usually mild, due to transfusion of cytokines released from donor WBC during storage or of fragmented donor WBC.

C. **Allergic transfusion reactions.** Allergic reactions are due to antibodies in the plasma reacting to epitopes on donor plasma proteins. **Unusual in neonatal transfusion recipients.**

D. **Transfusion-associated acute lung injury.** Typically due to antibodies in donor plasma that react with the patient's HLA antigens. More likely to occur with blood components containing large amounts of plasma such as FFP or platelets.

E. **Bacterial contamination.** There is a small, but potentially fatal, risk of bacterial infection on the order of 1 in 8–13 million for PRBC but of 1/300,000 for platelets (because of room temperature storage). *Escherichia coli, Pseudomonas, Serratia, Salmonella,* and *Yersinia* are the most commonly implicated bacteria.

F. **Hypothermia.** Large volume transfusions of either reconstituted whole blood (exchange transfusion) or PRBC (major surgery; large fetomaternal hemorrhages) that are stored at 1–6°C result in hypothermia unless a blood warmer is used.

G. **Hyperkalemia.** At risk are infants receiving large transfusions of RBC, such as in exchange transfusion, major surgery, or ECMO. Reconstituted whole blood (washed PRBC [<14 days old] with Hct adjusted using FFP) is recommended. In some neonatal units, fresh whole blood (<2–3 days) may be available.

Selected References

Baer VL et al: Do platelet transfusions in the NICU adversely affect survival? Analysis of 16000 thrombocytopenic neonates in a multihospital healthcare system. *J Perinatol* 2007;27:790-796.

Bonnar J et al: Summary of the national blood users group guideline for the transfusion of blood components to preterm infants. Blood banking and transfusion issues. *Irish Med J* 2007;100(6):1-33.

Nordmeyer D et al: Advances in transfusion medicine. *Adv Anesthesia* 2007;25:11-58.

Strauss RG: How I transfuse red blood cells and platelets to infants with anemia and thrombocytopenia of prematurity. *Transfusion* 2008;48:209-217.

13 Extracorporeal Membrane Oxygenation of the Newborn

I. **Introduction.** Extracorporeal membrane oxygenation (ECMO) is a mechanical means of providing oxygen (O_2) delivery and carbon dioxide (CO_2) removal for patients who have cardiac and/or respiratory failure. It is accomplished by draining blood from the right atrium with the aid of a roller or centrifugal blood pump that propels blood through an oxygenator where gas exchange occurs. From there it is warmed in a heat exchanger and then transfused back to the patient into the aorta (venoarterial [VA]) or into the right atrium (venovenous [VV]) (Figures 13–1 and 13–2). Uniform guidelines have been established to describe essential equipment, procedures, personnel, and training required for neonatal ECMO.

II. **Indications.** ECMO is used primarily for critically ill term and late preterm newborns with reversible respiratory and/or cardiac failure who have failed appropriate maximal medical management with ventilator support (conventional and/or high frequency), inhaled nitric oxide, volume expansion, as well as vasopressor and inotropic support. **Neonatal conditions treated using ECMO support include meconium aspiration syndrome, congenital diaphragmatic hernia, persistent pulmonary hypertension of the newborn, respiratory distress syndrome, sepsis, pneumonia, and cardiac failure due to cardiomyopathies or severe rhythm disturbances.** ECMO can also be used as a bridge to cardiac surgery or transplantation and after open heart surgery.

III. **Relative ECMO entrance criteria**

   A. **Weight ≥ 1.8 kg; gestational age ≥ 34 weeks.** (The cannula size is limited by the infant's weight.)

   B. **Respiratory criteria**

      1. **Oxygenation index (OI) >30–40 for 0.5–4 h**

$$OI = \frac{FIO_2 \times MAP \times 100}{PaO_2}$$

      (Fio$_2$, fraction of inspired O_2; MAP, mean airway pressure; Pao$_2$, partial pressure of oxygen, arterial)

      2. **Acute deterioration with intractable hypoxemia.** For example, a Pao$_2$ <30–40 mm Hg or preductal Sao$_2$ <70% not responding to conventional support.

      3. **Barotrauma.** Severe air leak not responsive to low tidal volume conventional ventilation and/or high-frequency oscillatory or jet ventilation.

   C. **Cardiovascular/oxygen delivery criteria**

      1. **Plasma lactate >45 mg/dL or 5 mmol/L** with a metabolic acidosis that is not improving or escalating despite volume expansion and inotropic support.

      2. **Mixed venous saturation <55–60% for 0.5–1 h.**

      3. **Cardiac arrest.**

IV. **Relative contraindications to ECMO**

   A. **Gestational age <32–34 weeks and/or a birthweight <1800 g** due to the risk of intracranial hemorrhage and surgical difficulties with vessel cannulation. Lower birthweight is associated with increased mortality and morbidity.

   B. **Mechanical ventilation >10–14 days** due to likely irreversible lung disease.

   C. **Intracranial hemorrhage greater than grade I** due to higher risk of bleeding. Patients with an intracranial hemorrhage greater than grade I may be considered a candidate for ECMO, but these decisions are institutionally and individually based.

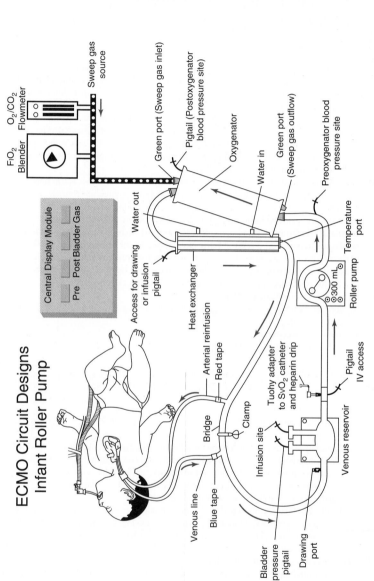

ECMO Circuit Designs
Infant Roller Pump

FIGURE 13–1. ECMO circuit with membrane gas exchange and roller pump. (*Courtesy of Cheryl Ziegler, Children's Hospitals and Clinics of Minnesota, Minneapolis.*)

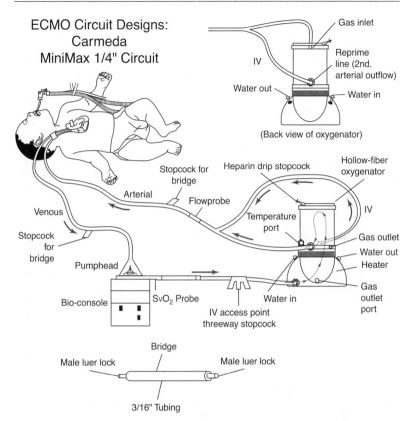

FIGURE 13–2. ECMO circuit with hollow fiber gas exchange and centrifugal pump. (*Courtesy of Cheryl Ziegler, Children's Hospitals and Clinics of Minnesota, Minneapolis.*)

D. **Coagulopathy** unlikely to resolve with transfusion therapy.

E. **Severe congenital anomalies** incompatible with long life.

F. **Cardiac lesions** that cannot be corrected or palliated.

G. **Congenital diaphragmatic hernia patients** whose best OI >45, or who never have a preductal saturation >85% (varies per institution).

H. **Marked perinatal asphyxia**

   1. **Severe neurologic syndrome persisting after respiratory and metabolic resuscitation** (stuporous, flaccid, and absent primitive reflexes) (varies per institution).

   2. **Plasma lactate >225 mg/dL (25 mmol/L)**

     a. **Lactate levels >225 mg/dL (25 mmol/L)** are highly predictive of death.

     b. **Lactate levels >135 mg/dL (15 mmol/L)** are highly predictive of adverse neurologic outcome.

   3. **Base deficit >30 on two ABGs.**

V. **Transfer of patients possibly needing ECMO.** Patients with the potential need for ECMO should be transferred early in their course. It must be remembered that an OI of >25 suggests significant hypoxic respiratory failure. This equates to a patient requiring a mean airway pressure of 15 on 100% oxygen who is able to achieve a Pao_2 of only 60 mm Hg. Any patient requiring 100% oxygen without signs of improvement on high-frequency and/or inhaled nitric oxide within 2–3 h or those who have persistent hypotension, acidosis, and/or lactic acidosis despite vasopressor or inotropic therapy should be considered a candidate for transport on their current therapy to an ECMO center.

VI. **Parental Consent.** Several potential complications can occur during ECMO, and parents need to be fully informed of these. Difficulties can arise with cannulation (such as a venous web or valve) that may result in the inability to achieve adequate venous drainage or infusion if VV or VA ECMO is attempted. Rupture of the right atrium can occur during venous cannulation attempts causing pericardial tamponade, cardiopulmonary failure, and subsequent death. Because of the need for heparin use during ECMO, hemorrhage (the most common problem) can occur in any organ, most significantly the brain. Blood can also accumulate in the pericardium, abdomen, retroperitoneum, or chest resulting in decreased pulse pressure, low SvO_2 (central venous hemoglobin oxygen saturation) levels and hypotension, making it impossible to maintain ECMO flow. The risk of bleeding can be decreased by monitoring the clotting time and treating with fresh-frozen plasma (FFP) and cryoprecipitate or using a Carmeda (heparin-bonded) circuit and decreasing or discontinuing heparin. If there is significant bleeding, ECMO may need to be discontinued. Due to potential clotting or emboli in the circuit, there is an increased risk for an infarction or stroke in the brain. Other complications that should be addressed include the potential for a pneumothorax, hemolysis, renal failure, myocardial stun, accidental decannulation, arrhythmias (due to the venous catheter being positioned in the atrium), and mechanical problems (raceway rupture, oxygenator failure, and centrifugal pump head failure).

Parents also need to know that their newborns could have significant neurologic problems as they grow and develop resulting from the disease process and/or therapy used to treat them (see Section XVIII). Some infants have decreased tone and poor feeding, which could lengthen their hospital stay. Some children may develop long-term complications, resulting in the need for rehabilitative services and require special support in school. Hearing loss can occur due to the underlying disease process, ECMO, or conventional support or medications used to treat the infant. Blindness is also a possibility. Because of the disease process, ventilatory support, and/or inflammation, chronic lung changes can develop as well causing children to require hospitalizations throughout subsequent years. Despite the multitude of potential complications and risks, many children go on to lead happy, productive lives.

VII. **Pre-ECMO studies.** Before initiating ECMO, patients should be evaluated for a congenital heart defect and intracranial hemorrhage with a cardiac echo and head ultrasound, respectively.

VIII. **Pretreatment with glucocorticoids.** During ECMO, the patient's blood is exposed to plastic and silicone in the circuit. This results in activation of the human immune system involving inflammatory mediators (complement, leukotrienes, cytokines, and leukocytes). The coagulation cascade is activated, as is the fibrinolytic system. Adding to this problem is the consumption of platelets by the membrane oxygenator. These responses can result in a massive capillary leak. This process can possibly be minimized somewhat by pretreating the patient with a glucocorticoid and/or using a heparin-bonded circuit.

IX. **Gas exchange.** Gas exchange through the **oxygenator** or **artificial lung** mimics pulmonary respiration (Figures 13–1 and 13–2). Blood flows on one side of a semipermeable membrane or hollow fibers and gas flows on the other side. Gas molecules diffuse across the membrane based on partial pressure gradients, allowing O_2 delivery and CO_2 removal. Two settings are adjusted to achieve this. To provide different oxygen concentrations, the **gas blender** is used. CO_2 removal is regulated by adjusting the **flow meter,** which provides gas flow, known as "sweep gas," through the oxygenator. Gas exchange also depends on the flow of blood through the oxygenator.

A. O$_2$ delivery is influenced by the following:
   1. O$_2$ content of blood after it passes through the oxygenator.
   2. Rate of blood flow through the ECMO circuit.
   3. O$_2$ uptake through the patient's lung.
   4. Cardiac output through the patient's heart.
B. With regard to the oxygenator, oxygenation depends on:
   1. The amount of O$_2$ in the blood and gas phases (the driving diffusion gradient).
   2. The ease with which O$_2$ crosses the membrane or fiber (permeability).
   3. The ability of O$_2$ to diffuse through the blood layer (its solubility in plasma). Because there is so much more O$_2$ in the sweep gas than in the blood, there is always a large gradient that never achieves equilibrium as long as the gradient is maintained; thus the flow of the sweep gas is not important to oxygen exchange as long as it is greater than zero. The flow of blood, however, is important. If the blood flows faster than the time it takes to achieve complete saturation of the hemoglobin with oxygen, blood will leave the membrane incompletely saturated. The "rated flow" is the pump blood flow rate at which maximal O$_2$ delivery is achieved. Above that flow rate, oxygenation decreases.
C. CO$_2$ exchange is affected by three factors:
   1. The relative concentration of CO$_2$ on either side of the oxygenator membrane or fibers (which is usually ~45–50 mm Hg in the venous blood and zero in the sweep gas of the oxygenator, allowing very efficient transfer of CO$_2$).
   2. The movement of air through the oxygenator or sweep gas flow (which constantly refreshes the pressure gradient by moving air through the oxygenator).
   3. The surface area of the membrane or hollow fibers. Because the diffusion of CO$_2$ through blood and the membrane or fibers is so rapid (six times faster than O$_2$), it is independent of blood flow through the device. Factors that decrease the functional surface area, however, will limit CO$_2$ transfer before affecting oxygenation.
X. Comparison of VA and VV ECMO
   A. Advantages and disadvantages of VA and VV ECMO
      1. VA ECMO
         a. Advantages
            i. Can provide full cardiac and respiratory support for nonfunctional heart and lungs.
            ii. Can unload the work of the heart, allowing it to rest.
         b. Disadvantages
            i. Results in ligation of the carotid artery (although some surgeons reconstruct the carotid artery after decannulation).
            ii. Higher incidence of central nervous system (CNS) hemorrhage and infarcts.
            iii. Potential for emboli to enter the arterial circulation.
            iv. Lack of pulsatility of flow may compromise organ tolerance to hypoxia (especially brain and kidneys).
      2. VV ECMO
         a. Advantages
            i. Lower mortality. (This may in part be due to patient selection because patients with cardiac and pulmonary failure and those who have sustained a cardiac arrest usually go on to VA ECMO. As a consequence, the mortality in the VA ECMO group may be higher.)
            ii. Carotid artery is preserved.
            iii. Pulsatile flow may better preserve organ function.
            iv. Lungs are still able to serve as filters for emboli.
         b. Disadvantages
            i. Provides no circulatory support other than improved myocardial oxygenation.

      ii. May not provide full oxygen delivery if the cannula is small. In this case some native lung function may be necessary to sustain appropriate gas exchange.

      iii. Difficulties with cannula position can arise.

XI. Cannulation guidelines

    A. Neonatal vascular access is usually through the right internal jugular vein and right common carotid artery for venoarterial ECMO. Venovenous ECMO uses only the internal jugular vein and a dual lumen cannula.

    B. Patient positioning. Patients should be positioned with the head turned to the left and the neck hyperextended using a neck roll. The right side is preferred.

    C. Medications. To provide comfort and surgical readiness, patients need to be treated with a narcotic and a neuromuscular blocking agent before the surgical procedure. Sedatives and narcotics are usually provided throughout the ECMO course; however, most patients do not require ongoing therapy with neuromuscular blocking agents.

    D. X-ray placement. An x-ray cassette should be placed under the patient before initiation of surgical placement of the cannula(s).

    E. Heparin for anticoagulation. Patients previously not heparinized should have an activated clotting time (ACT) drawn and receive a heparin bolus of 50–100 units/kg prior to cannulation to prevent clot formation in the cannulas. To assure appropriate anticoagulation, a continuous heparin drip is subsequently initiated at 25 units/kg/h and adjusted per institutional protocol.

    F. Appropriate cannula positions. See Figure 10–11, page 122.

      1. For VA cannulation the arterial cannula tip should be in the brachiocephalic artery, at or just above the junction of the aortic arch. Optimal positioning is achieved when the cannula tip is at T3-4 (just above the carina) after the neck roll is removed. The tip of the venous cannula should be in the right atrium.

      2. For VV cannulation the cannula tip should be well into the right atrium at T 7-8 or about 1–2 cm above the diaphragm after removal of the neck roll. Of special note, taking out the neck roll may advance the catheter up to 1 cm. VV cannulas can kink and limit ECMO flow, so no sutures should be placed around the thin-walled portion of the cannula. Proper cannula position is critical in VV ECMO to maintain flows. Flows of 120 mL/kg/min should be obtainable following volume expansion and removal of the neck roll. It is imperative to assess for signs of significant recirculation after VV cannulation. In this situation venous saturations may be >85% and arterial saturations may be <85%. At any time during the ECMO course the patient's lung volumes can change, resulting in the need to reposition the cannulas to maintain adequate flow and minimize recirculation.

    G. Volume. During connection of the ECMO cannulas to the circuit, extra volume may be needed to prevent hypotension in the patient.

    H. Ongoing heparin therapy. ACTs are monitored and generally **kept in ranges between 180 and 210 s** but vary dependent on patient circumstances. The ACT is affected by heparin concentration, factor levels, ATIII level, fibrinogen concentration, and platelet count. Reduced heparin protocols are institution specific. Any time ECMO flow is interrupted for circuit changes or modifications and the ACT is <180 s, a heparin bolus may be necessary. ECMO flow should be maintained at high levels such as >80 mL/kg/min whenever ACT levels are <170 s. If the ACT is on the low end of the range when platelets or cryoprecipitate are given, a bolus of heparin (5 to 10 units/kg) may be needed. Furosemide often prompts a brisk diuresis, increasing heparin clearance.

    I. Management of coagulopathy. Site-specific guidelines are kept in individual institutional ECMO references. Coagulopathies should be corrected immediately after ECMO is initiated.

      1. Fibrinogen levels are kept >150 mg/dL with cryoprecipitate.

      2. INR levels are kept ≤1.4 by treating with FFP and/or cryoprecipitate.

3. **Platelet** counts are generally maintained >100,000 μL.
4. **Some centers follow antithrombin III activity** and treat with ATIII concentrate or FFP to keep levels >60–80% in ECMO patients.
5. **An unfractionated heparin level (anti-Xa)** is very helpful in determining if a prolonged ACT is due to a heparin effect or a coagulopathy.

XII. **Monitoring during ECMO**

A. **Thromboses in the artificial lung** can be detected by the difference in the circuit pressures before and after the membrane lung, noted as a rise of the premembrane pressure and a fall in the postmembrane pressure (Figure 13–1).

B. **Gas pressure** is monitored or controlled in the sweep gas line to avoid air embolism if a leak occurs in the membrane.

C. **When CO_2 clearance is decreased,** the sweep gas flow rate can be briefly increased to evaporate the water droplets on the oxygenator surface.

D. **SvO_2 levels** during ECMO reflect the degree of O_2 extraction and should normally be in the 70–80% range. SvO_2 levels <50% indicate an increased rate of oxygen extraction and suggest that the rate of tissue metabolism is exceeding the rate of oxygen delivery. Once this occurs, cells use a less efficient anaerobic metabolism producing lactic acid. SvO_2 levels are a useful parameter to follow in VA ECMO, but due to the recirculation phenomenon in VV ECMO they are more difficult to interpret (see Tables 13–1 and 13–2).

XIII. **Lung rest during ECMO.** Generally patients who reach ECMO criteria already have a fair amount of ventilator-associated lung inflammation and injury. The best therapy once on ECMO is to provide "resting" ventilator settings. Although centers vary in their ventilator settings, for VA ECMO patients, most choose a low rate of 10 breaths/min (10–20), a modest to high positive end-expiratory pressure (PEEP) of 5–14 cm H_2O, a low peak inspiratory pressure (PIP) in the 12–20 cm H_2O range, and a low FIO_2 of ~40%. **The ventilator FIO_2 is generally kept around 40% because coronary blood is primarily oxygenated by blood from native lung perfusion ejected from the left ventricle.** Higher settings may be necessary on VV ECMO with a rate of 20–30 breaths/min, PIP of 15–25 cm H_2O, PEEP of 5–10 cm H_2O, and FIO_2 from 30–50%. Some centers use high-frequency oscillatory ventilation for lung rest, usually with a mean airway pressure of 10 to 14 cm H_2O and low amplitudes.

XIV. **Flow dynamics during ECMO.** During VA ECMO, a sufficient blood flow rate is necessary to provide adequate oxygen delivery to all tissues. The kidneys may be sensitive to the nonpulsatile flow resulting in a decrease in renal function. ECMO patients frequently require diuretic therapy. For those patients who develop ongoing renal failure, a hemofiltration or dialysis system may be added in parallel to the ECMO circuit via a small shunt. This system allows for removal of excess fluid and stabilizes electrolyte abnormalities.

Table 13–1. DECREASED SvO_2 LEVELS DURING ECMO

O_2	Causes	Etiologies
↓ O_2 supply	↓ CO	Heart failure, cardiac depressants, arrhythmias, ↑ PEEP, ↓ preload
	↓ SaO_2	↓ Respiratory function, suctioning
	↓ Hb	Anemia
		↓ ECMO blender FIO_2
		Insufficient ECMO flow
↑ O_2 demand	↑ VO_2	Fever, shivering, agitation, pain, seizures, infection
	↑ CO	↑ Work of breathing

ECMO, extracorporeal membrane oxygenation; PEEP, positive end-expiratory pressure.

Table 13–2. **INCREASED SvO$_2$ LEVELS DURING ECMO**

O$_2$	Causes	Etiologies
↑ O$_2$ supply	↑ CO	Improved heart function
	↑ SaO$_2$	Improved lung function
	↑ Hb	↑ FiO$_2$, blood transfusion
		Excess ECMO flow
↓ O$_2$ demand	↓ VO$_2$	Hypothermia, anesthesia, paralysis, relaxation
	↓ Utilization	Sepsis, cyanide toxicity (from sodium nitroprusside)

ECMO, extracorporeal membrane oxygenation; PEEP, positive end-expiratory pressure.

XV. **Practical considerations for ECMO management**
  A. **VA ECMO**
    1. **VA ECMO blood flows.** After cannulation, bypass flow is slowly increased. The ECMO pump creates nonpulsatile flow, and as more blood is routed through the circuit, the systemic arterial pulse contour becomes dampened and then flat if total bypass is reached. Usually ECMO flow is maintained at ~60–80% (80–120 mL/kg/min) of total blood flow and the pulse pressure is 10–20 mm Hg if the heart has reasonable contractility.
    2. **Hematocrit levels.** Generally patients are transfused to maintain a hematocrit of around 35–45, and the ECMO blood flow is adjusted to achieve an adequate oxygen delivery as reflected by appropriate central venous saturations.
    3. **SvO$_2$ levels.** A SvO$_2$ of 70–80% reflects adequate tissue oxygen supply.
    4. **Medications and nutrition.** Patients can be treated with medications and total parenteral nutrition into the bypass circuit, but because of an increased volume of distribution (ECMO circuit volume), higher doses are frequently required. Patient venous access locations can also be used.
    5. **Factors that increase oxygen delivery:**
      a. Increased hematocrit.
      b. Increased ECMO blood flow/Increased ECMO blender FiO$_2$.
      c. Increased native cardiac output.
      d. Increased native pulmonary function.
    6. **Factors that decrease oxygen delivery:**
      a. Decreased hematocrit.
      b. Decreased ECMO blood flow.
      c. Decreased ECMO blender FiO$_2$.
      d. Decreased biologic cardiac output.
      e. A failing oxygenator (results in reduced surface area).
      f. Exceeding the "rate flow" of the oxygenator (the blood moves too fast to pick up the oxygen).
    7. **Factors that decrease carbon dioxide content of blood:**
      a. Increased sweep gas flow rate.
      b. Decreasing CO$_2$ added to the sweep gas, if previously added.
    8. **Factors that increase carbon dioxide:**
      a. Decreased sweep gas flow rate.
      b. Adding CO$_2$ to the sweep gas from an exogenous CO$_2$ tank.
      c. A failing oxygenator with condensation or a clot.
    9. **Trialing off VA ECMO.** Once pulmonary function improves, as demonstrated by continuous venous saturation measurements from the circuit, chest radiographs and lung compliance, and the disease process has subsided, patients are ready to be weaned off VA ECMO.
      a. **The ECMO blood flows are decreased slowly** and ventilator settings adjusted as needed based on blood gases.

    b. **Patients are weaned to 10% of their cardiac output (20 mL/kg/min or "idling" flow) for a few hours.** Trials off are usually limited to 1 h if conducted by clamping and unclamping ("flashing") the cannulas. Trials done with an open bridge technique may be extended.

    c. **If parameters remain within the acceptable ranges,** patients are permanently discontinued from ECMO and decannulated.

B. VV ECMO

  1. **VV ECMO flows.** As with VA ECMO, bypass flow is gradually increased to 100–120 mL/kg/min. Blood is simultaneously withdrawn from the right atrium and continuously reinfused back into the right atrium so there is no net effect on right atrial volume, intracardiac flow, or aortic blood flow. Ideally the output from the return port is directed toward the tricuspid valve. The native cardiac output propels oxygenated blood forward to the arterial system and tissues. O_2 delivery can be augmented by increasing the O_2 content of the venous blood in the right atrium. Because oxygenator blood is always mixed with desaturated venous blood in the right atrium, the final O_2 content of the blood reaching the aorta and tissues is limited by the amount of blood that can be drained into the EMO circuit, oxygenated, and returned to the venous system. The optimal pump flow rate is one that provides the highest effective pump flow at the lowest revolutions per minute of the pump, resulting in the highest O_2 delivery and causing the least degree of tubing wear and hemolysis.

  2. **PaO_2 levels.** Patients usually have arterial saturation levels between 85% and 95% with Pao_2 levels of 50–80 mmHg. With VV ECMO, only partial support is achieved, and lower oxygen saturations are generally tolerated. Pao_2 levels may be higher as biologic pulmonary function improves.

  3. **Hematocrit levels.** Hematocrit levels are generally kept higher (40–45%) than those on VA ECMO to provide adequate O_2 delivery because O_2 saturations achieved are generally lower.

  4. **Ventilator strategies.** When the size of the venous cannula limits ECMO flow, maintenance of native pulmonary gas exchange may be necessary to achieve adequate oxygenation. In this situation, using higher PEEP levels may facilitate O_2 delivery. Indirectly VV ECMO allows for reduction in ventilator needs that may improve preload and cardiac output. Improved O_2 supply to the coronary arteries may also improve myocardial function.

  5. **Recirculation** can occur when oxygenated blood returning from the circuit flows from the reinfusion lumen and is taken up by the venous drainage lumen instead of being delivered to the patient's circulation. The recirculation fraction is usually about 20–30% at pump flows of 100 mL/kg/min. If the pump flow is increased beyond optimal flow, the percentage of recirculation increases as oxygenated blood from the ECMO circuit streams back into the venous drainage lumen. **Clinically significant recirculation is recognized by a decrease in patient arterial saturations and a rise in central venous saturations as pump flow is increased.** Higher degrees of recirculation decrease the effective O_2 delivery from the circuit. Other factors that increase recirculation include the following:

    a. **Decreased right atrial volume** (a higher percentage of returned oxygenated blood is drained back out to maintain pump flow).

    b. **Catheter malposition** (a position too high in the superior vena cava or too low in the inferior vena cava increases recirculation).

    c. **Poor cardiac output** (which leads to more recirculation because less of the oxygenated pump blood is propelled forward out of the right atrium).

  6. **Catheter position.** Maintaining the catheter position is critical in VV ECMO. Catheters can migrate with changes in lung inflation, increasing edema of the neck at the site of anchoring sutures; a change in the patient's position; or with patient movement.

7. **Factors that improve oxygen delivery from the EMCO circuit:**
   a. Increased ECMO flow.
   b. Increased hematocrit.
   c. Increased native cardiac output.
   d. Decreased percentage of recirculated pump flow.
8. **Factors that decrease O_2 delivery:**
   a. Decreased ECMO flow.
   b. Decreased hematocrit.
   c. Decreased cardiac output.
   d. Increased percentage of recirculated pump flow.
9. **Weaning the patient from VV ECMO:**
   a. **ECMO blood flow is left at a constant amount** (usually 60–100 mL/kg/min or ~200 mL/min) followed by weaning the FIO_2 of the sweep gas to room air.
   b. **The sweep gas flow rate is reduced to zero** (or the artificial lung is "capped off," which functionally removes the patient from ECMO). At this point blood draining from the right atrium returns to the right atrium unchanged.
   c. **Once patients have tolerated being capped off** for 1 to 2 h, the cannula is removed. Ventilator settings are adjusted as necessary.

XVI. **Circuit changes.** Clots in the circuitry may necessitate the need for a circuit change. During these times a large percentage of blood volume is exchanged and there can be electrolyte imbalances, arrhythmias, and cardiac stun. Blood drug levels may need to be adjusted as well. Clots in the cannulas themselves can be challenging to manage because removal of these clots requires temporary discontinuation of ECMO.

XVII. **Complications of ECMO**
   A. **Patient complications of ECMO** in order of frequency per the Extracorporeal Life Support Organization (ELSO) data as of January 2008:
      1. Acute renal failure (hemofiltration required, 13.9%, dialysis required, 3.4%).
      2. Hypertension requiring vasodilators, 12.6%.
      3. Hemolysis,11.3%.
      4. Seizures, 10.2%.
      5. Hypotension requiring inotropics, 8.4%.
      6. CNS infarction, 8.1%.
      7. Intracranial hemorrhage, 6.3%.
      8. Culture-proven infection, 6.3%.
      9. Surgical bleeding, 6.2%.
      10. Pulmonary hemorrhage, 4%.
      11. Disseminated intravascular coagulation, 1.9%.
      12. Brain death, 1%.
   B. **Mechanical problems,** listed in order of frequency, include the following:
      1. Clots, 17.9%.
      2. Cannula problems, 11.4%.
      3. Oxygenator failure, 6%.
      4. Air in the circuit, 5.1%.
      5. Pump failure, 1.7%.
      6. Raceway rupture, 0.3%.

XVIII. **Prognosis.** The Neonatal ECMO Registry (established 1985), as of January 2008, lists nearly 21,916 neonatal patients, the first of whom was treated in 1975. Currently, the overall cumulative neonatal survival rate is 76%, but survival in 2007 alone was 64%. The drop in survival reflects a larger proportion of patients treated with high mortality diagnoses. The registry also tracks cumulative survival rates for specific diseases, and these data are as follows: meconium aspiration syndrome, 94%; pulmonary hypertension, 78%; hyaline membrane disease, 84%; sepsis, 75%; pneumonia, 58%; and congenital diaphragmatic hernia, 51%. Congenital diaphragmatic hernia and lower birthweight status in those patients treated for respiratory failure are variables associated with increased mortality and morbidity.

XIX. **Neurodevelopmental outcomes.** Results of the randomized study comparing patients treated with ECMO versus conventional support done by Dr. Helena McNally and the United Kingdom Collaborative ECMO Trial Group published in 2006 suggest that the underlying disease process appears to be the major influence on morbidity at 7 years of age in former newborns with severe respiratory failure. When comparing the ECMO group to the conventionally treated group, a higher respiratory morbidity and increased risk of behavioral problems was noted in the group of children treated conventionally. There were no cognitive differences between the two trial groups (76% of the children available for follow-up testing in both groups were within the normal range, although they fell below population norms). Both groups demonstrated difficulties with spatial and processing tasks; learning problems were believed to be similar in the two groups. Overall 40% of the children had normal neuromotor development (43% of the children in the ECMO group and 35% in the conventionally treated group). Parental and teacher reports of behavioral problems, particularly hyperactivity, were more common in the conventionally treated children. Progressive sensorineural hearing loss was found in both groups and could be late onset and progressive. Some of the neurologic outcomes are difficult to discern with regard to inciting causes. However, it was felt that cannulation itself, causing disruption of the cerebral circulation, was not responsible for subsequent neurologic or behavioral consequences; rather the underlying disease process was considered to be the major influence. The increased survival among children randomized to ECMO (67% compared with conventional survival at 41%) was not offset by disability among survivors.

Selected References

Bahrami KR, Van Meurs KP: ECMO for neonatal respiratory failure. *Semin Perinatol* 2005;29(1):15-23.

Bennett CC et al: A comparison of clinical variables that predict adverse outcome in term infants with severe respiratory failure randomized to a policy of extracorporeal membrane oxygenation or to conventional neonatal intensive care. *J Perinat Med* 2002;30(3):225-230.

Cheung Po-Yin et al: Use of plasma lactate to predict early mortality and adverse outcome after neonatal extracorporeal membrane oxygenation: a prospective cohort in early childhood. *Crit Care Med* 2002;3(9):2135-2139.

Extracorporeal Life Support Organization: *Registry Report, International Summary.* Extracorporeal Life Status Support Organization, January 2008.

Hansell DR: ECLS equipment and devices. In Van Meurs K et al (eds): *ECMO Extracorporeal Cardiopulmonary Support in Critical Care,* 3rd ed. Ann Arbor, MI: Extracorporeal Life Support Organization, 2005:108.

Hardart GE: Intracranial hemorrhage in premature neonates treated with extracorporeal membrane oxygenation correlates with conceptional age. *J Pediatr* 2004;145:184-189.

Hustead V, Orton L: *ECMO Training Manual.* Children's Hospitals and Clinics, Minneapolis, MN, 2007. Available upon request.

McNally H et al: United Kingdom collaborative randomized trial of neonatal extracorporeal membrane oxygenation; follow-up to age 7 years. *Pediatrics* 2006;117(5):e845-e854.

Van Meurs K: *ECMO Specialist Training Manual,* 2nd ed. Ann Arbor, MI: Extracorporeal Life Support Organization, 1999.

14 Newborn Screening

I. **Introduction.** Newborn screening is a population-based system for the identification and early treatment of potentially devastating medical conditions. In the United States, this screening is mandated in every state, but the disorders included in the screening panels vary. A list of the screening tests provided by each state can be found on the "Peristats" section of the March of Dimes website at http://marchofdimes.com/peristats or at the National Newborn Screening and Genetics Resource Center website at http://genes-r-us. uthscsa.edu. An expert panel commissioned by The American College of Medical Genetics has recommended 29 conditions on newborn screening panels (Table 14–1).

Screening of infants cared for in the neonatal intensive care unit (NICU) can present special challenges. Underlying medical conditions, including prematurity, can impact the validity of the screening results, as can some of the therapies provided in the NICU. Regulations related to follow-up of screening specimens vary from one state to another, and information on optimal methodology and timing of screening is incomplete for many disorders.

II. **Timing.** It is recommended practice to obtain a specimen prior to blood transfusion if a specimen has not already been sent; otherwise an initial specimen is typically drawn between the third and fifth days of life. Any results judged to be invalid by the performing laboratory or any results that are reported as positive must have a repeat specimen. This chapter addresses selected disorders included in most state newborn screen panels, as well as special considerations related to discharge planning and follow-up.

III. **Selected disorders included in newborn screening panels**

   A. **Amino acid metabolism disorders**

   1. **Phenylketonuria (PKU)**

      a. **Screening process.** Increased concentrations of phenylalanine in the blood can be detected using the Guthrie bacterial inhibition assay (BIA), fluorometric analysis, and tandem mass spectrometry (sometimes referred to as MS/MS). It is important to note that antibiotic administration interferes with validity of test results only if the Guthrie BIA is the testing modality used.

      b. **Follow-up.** Children diagnosed with PKU should receive diets with reduced phenylalanine. Subspecialty follow-up should be arranged with a nutritionist as well as with a pediatrician who specializes in metabolic disorders.

   2. **Maple syrup urine disease (MSUD)**

      a. **Screening process.** Tandem mass spectrometry is the screening tool of choice.

      b. **Follow-up.** Positive screen results should be followed by plasma amino acid analysis. Diagnostic findings include elevated branched-chain amino acids, low levels of alanine, and the presence of alloisoleucine. Children with MSUD should receive follow-up care by a pediatrician who specializes in metabolic disorders, as well as a nutrition consultant.

   3. **Homocystinuria (HCY)**

      a. **Screening process.** HCY is multifactorial and involves interference in the pathway that converts methionine into cysteine. If untreated, the disease manifests with recurrent thromboembolic events and can lead to mental retardation, as well as ocular and skeletal problems. Screening may be done by a bacterial inhibition assay or tandem mass spectrometry. There may be an increase in false-negative screening results if protein intake via feedings is not adequate.

      b. **Follow-up.** Increased levels of methionine on screening require follow-up with serum or plasma amino acid levels to check for elevations of methionine and homocystine, decreased levels of cystine, and absent cystathionine. Genetic counseling is advised for family members because carriers are at risk for thromboembolic events.

Table 14–1. **ESTIMATED INCIDENCE OF 29 DISORDERS RECOMMENDED BY ACMG FOR INCLUSION ON NEWBORN SCREENING PANELS**

	Estimated Incidence
Amino Acid Metabolism Disorders	
Phenylketonuria (PKU)	1:12,000
Argininosuccinic acidemia (ASA)	1: 70,000
Tyrosinemia type I (TYR I)	<1:100,000
Citrullinemia (CIT)	1:100,000
Maple syrup urine disease (MSUD)	1: 100,000–300,000
Homocystinuria (HCY)	1:300,000
Organic Acid Metabolism Disorders	Rare: 1:20,000–200,000
	Incidence unknown for many
Glutaric acidemia type I (GA I)	>1:75,000
Methylmalonic acidemia due to mutase deficiency (MMA)	>1:75,000
3-Methylcrotonyl-CoA carboxylase deficiency (3MCC)	>1:75,000
Propionic acidemia (PROP)	>1:75,000
Beta-ketothiolase deficiency (BKT)	<1:100,000
Hydroxymethylglutaric aciduria (HMG)	<1:100,000
Isovaleric acidemia (IVA)	<1:100,000
Methylmalonic acidemia cblA and cblB (Cbl A, B)	<1:100,000
Multiple carboxylase deficiency (MCD)	<1:100,000
Fatty Acid Oxidation Disorders	
Medium-chain acyl-CoA dehydrogenase deficiency (MCAD)	1:10,000–20,000
Long-chain 3-OH acyl-CoA dehydrogenase deficiency (LCHAD)	1:100,000
Very long-chain acyl-CoA dehydrogenase deficiency (VLCAD)	1:100,000
Trifunctional protein deficiency (TFP)	Unknown
Carnitine uptake defect (CUD)	Unknown
Hemoglobinopathies	
Sickle cell anemia (Hb SS)	1:5,000
Hb S/C disease (Hb S/C)	>1:25,000
Hb S/ Beta-Thalassemia (Hbs/βTh)	>1:50,000
Others	
Hearing loss (HEAR)	2–3:1,000
Congenital hypothyroidism (CH)	1:3,500–5,000
Cystic fibrosis (CF)	>1:5,000
Congenital adrenal hyperplasia (CAH)	1:15,000
Classical galactosemia (GALT)	1:60,000
Biotinidase deficiency (BIOT)	1:110,000

ACMG, American College of Medical Genetics.

B. Organic acid metabolism disorders
  1. Methylmalonic acidemia (MMA)
    a. **Screening.** Elevated levels of propionylcarnitine are detected by tandem mass spectrometry.
    b. **Follow-up.** Abnormal screening results should be followed with plasma and/or urine organic acid analysis, which can establish the presence or absence of methylmalonic acid. A high level of methylmalonic acid is diagnostic. Treatment

includes the institution of a low-protein diet. Follow-up care should be arranged with a pediatrician who specializes in metabolic disorders, as well as with a nutritionist. MMA has an autosomal recessive inheritance pattern. Genetic counseling should be provided.

C. **Fatty acid oxidation disorders**
   1. **Medium-chain acyl-CoA dehydrogenase deficiency (MCAD)**
      a. **Screening.** Tandem mass spectrometry is the screening tool of choice for MCAD. Levels of octanoylcarnitine are higher during the first three days of life, so screening is best performed in the newborn period. Prematurity, immaturity of hepatic function, and total parenteral nutrition can result in abnormal amino acid results necessitating a repeat specimen.
      b. **Follow-up.** Diagnostic testing is done though plasma acylcanitine analysis and urinary organic acid analysis. Molecular analysis to determine the particular gene involved provides prognostic information.

D. **Hemoglobinopathies**
   1. **Sickle cell anemia/disease**
      a. **Screening.** Hemoglobin variants are detected using isoelectric focusing, high-performance liquid chromatography (HPLC) or cellulose acetate electrophoresis. Retesting of abnormal screen samples is usually done by electrophoretic technique, HPLC, immunologic testing, or DNA assays. Blood transfusions that include red cell components can invalidate the screen results, so initial screening should be done prior to transfusion. (Plasma, platelets, and albumin transfusions do not affect screening results.)
      b. **Follow-up.** The majority of states require follow-up screening on normal screens 90 days after the last transfusion. Confirmatory testing should be done on abnormal screens before 2 months of age. A pediatric hematologist should be involved in follow-up care.

E. **Other**
   1. **Congenital hypothyroidism**
      a. **Screening.** Most screens measure T4 with a thyrotropin (TSH) level if the T4 is low. False-positive elevations in TSH may occur in infants screened at <48 h of age due to a thyrotropin surge after birth. This surge may be delayed in preterm infants. Likewise preterm infants with hypothyroidism have delayed elevation of TSH levels, presumably due to immaturity of the hypothalamic-pituitary-thyroid axis. Therefore it may be prudent to consider a second routine screening on preterm infants between 2 and 6 weeks of age. Preterm infants also typically have lower T4 levels resulting in more false-positive results. Screening of hypothyroidism is unaffected by diet and transfusion, except in the case of total exchange transfusion.
      b. **Follow-up.** Abnormal screening results should be immediately followed up with serum T4 and TSH testing, as well as T3 or free T4. Etiology of hypothyroidism can be determined using thyroid ultrasound or thyroid uptake and scan, thyrotropin-binding inhibitor immunoglobulin (in cases of suspected transient hypothyroidism related to maternal autoimmune thyroid disease), or urinary iodine (if iodine exposure or deficiency is suspected). Diagnostic testing to determine etiology is optional but does not alter treatment, and it should never delay treatment.
   2. **Biotinidase deficiency (BIOT)**
      a. **Screening.** Filter paper spotted with whole blood is assessed for biotinidase activity by a semiquantitative colorimetric method. Up to 20% of patients with symptomatic biotinidase can be missed if screened with tandem mass spectrometry, so this methodology should not be used.
      b. **Follow-up.** Some states require a repeat specimen between 1 week to 4 months after the last red blood cell transfusion. A serum specimen for quantitative measurement of biotinidase activity should be obtained if the screening results

were positive. Children with BIOT should be followed by a pediatric endocrinologist for biotin therapy.

3. **Galactosemia (GALT)**
   a. **Screening.** Three different enzyme deficiencies may result in GALT. **Classic galactosemia,** which is the most common form, results from the deficiency of galactose 1-phospate (GALT). **Galactokinase (GALK) deficiency** and **galactose-4-epimerase (GALE) deficiency** also result in galactosemia but are very rare. Screening tests vary by state but may measure galactose, galactose 1-phosphate plus galactose, and/or GALT enzyme deficiency. Tandem mass spectrometry may be used. The GALT enzyme test is performed using red blood cells and is diagnostic only for classic galactosemia. It is not affected by the infant's diet but rather by red blood cell transfusions. Test results of galactose and galactose 1-phosphate are influenced by the infant's diet, so the infant should receive a galactose-containing formula or breast milk prior to screening.
   b. **Follow-up.** A false-negative result may persist for 3 months after a red blood cell transfusion, so a repeat test is needed 90 days after the last transfusion. All infants with positive screening results should receive a nutrition consultation and be placed on a galactose-restricted diet pending definitive diagnostic testing. Breast-milk feedings are contraindicated for infants with galactosemia, and soy-based formulas are commonly used. Quantitative analysis of galactokinase (GALK) and galactose-4-epimerase (GALE) identifies these less common types of galactosemia.

4. **Congenital adrenal hyperplasia (CAH)**
   a. **Screening.** Measurement of 17-hydroxyprogesterone (17-OHP)is performed through a variety of reagents/immunoassays or tandem mass spectrometry. A high rate of false-positive results occurs in samples taken at <1 day of age. Normal 17-OHP levels are affected by birthweight and gestational age; thus prematurity and illness can result in false-positive screen results. Preterm infants tend to have higher levels. Levels are not affected by transfusions if they are drawn several hours after the transfusion. However some states require a repeat specimen with the timing of the repeat screen varying from 72 hours to 4 months after transfusion.
   b. **Follow-up.** Abnormal screening results should be followed with a serum 17-OHP level. Serum electrolytes and serum 17-OHP levels should be obtained in neonates with a disorder of sex development. A adrenocorticotropic hormone stimulation test is useful for ruling out nonclassic CAH in infants with mild elevations of 17-OHP levels. Infants with CAH should be followed by a pediatric endocrinologist.

5. **Hearing loss**
   a. **Screening.** Universal screening should be done before 1 month of age and/or prior to initial hospital discharge. Although automated auditory brainstem response (ABR) and otoacoustic emission are the primary methods used, ABR is the recommended screening tool for infants with NICU stays >5 days because of high risk of neural hearing loss.
   b. **Follow-up.** Audiologic testing and medical follow-up should be performed prior to 3 months of age for all infants who do not pass the initial screen. Rescreening of both ears is recommended. Infants who have one or more risk factors for hearing loss should be reassessed by an audiologist no later than 24–30 months of age regardless of initial screening results. **Risk factors include the following:**
      i. **A family history of sensorineural hearing loss.**
      ii. **TORCH (*t*oxoplasmosis, *o*ther infections, *r*ubella, *c*ytomegalovirus, and *h*erpes simplex) infections.**
      iii. **Craniofacial anomalies.**

  iv. Birthweight <1500 g.
   v. Hyperbilirubinemia necessitating exchange transfusion.
  vi. Ototoxic medications including chemotherapy.
 vii. Treatment with extracorporeal membrane oxygenation.
viii. Bacterial meningitis.
  ix. One-minute Apgar score of 0–4.
   x. Five-minute Apgar score of 0–6.
  xi. Mechanical ventilation for ≥5 days.
 xii. Neurodegenerative disorders.
xiii. Syndromes known to include hearing loss.
 xiv. Trauma.
  xv. Caregiver concern.

Infants with confirmed hearing loss should receive evaluation by a pediatric oto-laryngologist, evaluation by a pediatric ophthalmologist for assessment of visual acuity, and early intervention services as soon as possible but no later than 6 months of age. A genetic consultation should also be considered.

Selected References

California Department of Health Services: California Newborn Screening Program, Sacramento, CA, 2004. Available at: http://www.dhs.ca.gov/pcfh/gdb/html/NBS/.

Fernhoff PM: Muddling the water: factors that affect NBS results. Paper presented at: Association of Public Health Laboratories Newborn Screening and Genetics Testing Symposium; May 3, 2004; Atlanta, GA. Available at: http://www.aphl.org/conferences/2004_conferences/newborn_screening_genetics_2004/Pages/default.aspx.

Genetics Home Reference: Genetic conditions. Bethesda, MD; 2007. Available at: http://ghr.nlm.nih.gov.

Hooper PF et al: A national survey of newborn screening policies concerning samples submitted post-transfusion—the 50 states and the District of Columbia. Paper presented at: Association of Public Health Laboratories Newborn Screening and Genetics Testing Symposium; May 3, 2004; Atlanta, GA. Available at: http://www.aphl.org/conferences/2004_conferences/newborn_screening_genetics_2004/Pages/default.aspx.

Illinois Department of Public Health Newborn Screening Program: Springfield, IL; 2005. Available at: http://www.idph.state.il.us/home.htm.

Joint Committee on Infant Hearing: Year 2007 position statement: principles and guidelines for early hearing detection and intervention programs. *Pediatrics* 2007;120(4): 898-921.

Kaye CI & The Committee on Genetics: Newborn screening fact sheets. *Pediatrics* 2006;118(3):934-963.

Lockwood C et al (eds): *Guidelines for Perinatal Care*, 6th ed. Elk Grove, IL: American Academy of Pediatrics & The American College of Obstetricians and Gynecologists, 2007:223-224.

March of Dimes: Newborn screening. White Plains, NY; 2007. Available at: http://www.marchofdimes.com/.

National Institute on Deafness and Other Communication Disorders: Statistics about hearing disorders, ear infections, and deafness. Bethesda, MD; 2007. Available at: http://www.nidcd.nih.gov/health/statistics/hearing.asp.

State Newborn Screening and Short Term Follow-up Working Group Public Health Infrastructure Cluster; Region 4 Genetics Collaborative 2005–07: Newborn screening in the neonatal intensive care unit (Attachment 10 Agenda Item V E, VE1 & VE2). Paper presented at: Advisory Group Meeting; June 11, 2007; Okemos, MI. Available at: http://www.region4genetics.org/resources/advisorygroup_materials.aspx.

University of Texas Health Science Center at San Antonio: National Newborn Screening and Genetics Resource Center. Austin, TX; 2007. Available at: http://genes-r-us.uthscsa.edu.

U.S. Department of Health and Human Services Administration Maternal and Child Health Bureau: Newborn screening: toward a uniform screening panel and system—report for public comment. Rockville, MD; 2005. Available at: http://mchb.hrsa.gov/screening.

Venditti CP: Methylmalonic acidemia. Seattle, WA, 2007. Available at: http://www.genetests.org.

---

15 Studies for Neurologic Evaluation

Although recent improvements in neuroimaging and neuromonitoring have added insight into the developing brain and have brought information to the bedside to help the clinician identify infants at risk for poor neurologic outcome, available techniques continue to be limited in their ability to predict future intelligence and motor, language, and problem-solving skills accurately. Moreover, given the enormous plasticity of the neonate's brain, even significant defects detectable with these tests may result in "normal" neurodevelopmental outcomes. Nevertheless, these modalities hold future promise in assisting clinicians to better identify and refer patients at risk.

I. **Neuroimaging**

A. **Ultrasonography**

1. **Definition.** By using the bone window of a fontanelle, sound waves are directed into the brain and reflected according to the echodensity of the underlying structures. The reflected waves are used to create two- and three-dimensional images.

2. **Indication.** Ultrasonography is the preferred tool for identification and observation of germinal matrix/intraventricular hemorrhage and hydrocephalus and is valuable in detecting midline structural abnormalities, hypoxic-ischemic injury, subdural and posterior fossa hemorrhage, ventriculitis, tumors, cysts, and vascular abnormalities. Ultrasonography of the developing cingulate sulcus has been suggested to reflect gestational age (see sample studies in Chapter 10).

3. **Method.** A transducer is placed over the anterior fontanelle, and images are obtained in coronal and parasagittal planes. The posterior fontanelle is the preferred acoustic window for the imaging of the infratentorium, including brainstem and cerebellum. Advantages of this technique include high resolution, convenience (performed at the bedside), safety (no sedation, contrast material, or radiation), noninvasiveness, and low cost compared with other imaging studies. Disadvantages include the lack of visualization of nonmidline structures, especially in the parietal regions, and the lack of differentiation between gray and white matter.

4. **Results.** The integrity of the following structures may be evaluated with ultrasonography: all four ventricles, the choroid plexus, caudate nuclei, thalamus, septum pellucidum, and corpus callosum.

B. **Doppler ultrasonography**

1. **Definition.** Like regular ultrasonography, this technique uses a bone window to direct sound waves into the brain. Moving objects (eg, red blood cells) reflect sound waves with a shift in frequency (Doppler shift) that is proportional to their speed. These changes are measured and expressed as the pulsatility index. The angle of the probe in relation to the flow affects the Doppler shift and requires exact standards for serial measurements.

2. **Indication.** Knowing the cross section of the vessel (area), Doppler ultrasonography can provide information on cerebral blood flow (CBF) and resistance.

$$\text{CBF (cm}^3/\text{time)} = \text{CBF velocity (cm/time)} \times \text{Area (cm}^2)$$

Changes in CBF and resistance have been noted in a variety of pathologic states. Doppler ultrasonography is of clinical value in states of cessation of CBF (eg, brain death or cerebrovascular occlusion), states of altered vascular resistance (eg, hypoxic-ischemic encephalopathy, hydrocephalus, or arteriovenous malformation), and ductal steal syndrome.

3. **Method.** Combined with conventional ultrasonography to identify the blood vessel, Doppler ultrasonography produces a color image indicating flow (red, toward the transducer; blue, away from the transducer). CBF velocity is measured as the area under the curve of velocity waveforms. Small body weight and low gestational ages negatively influence the success rate in visualizing intracranial vasculature.

4. **Results.** Doppler ultrasonography measurements can be compared with age-adjusted norm values for systolic, end-diastolic, and mean flow velocity. Although this technique is not a standard bedside tool, it might also prove useful to evaluate the need for ventriculoperitoneal shunts in progressive hydrocephalus (decreased CBF secondary to increased intracranial pressure).

C. **Computed tomography (CT)**

1. **Definition.** Using computerized image reconstruction, CT produces two- and three-dimensional images of patients exposed to ionizing radiation.

2. **Indication.** CT is the preferred tool for evaluation of the posterior fossa and non-midline disorders (eg, blood or fluid collection in the subdural or subarachnoid space) as well as parenchymal disorders. It is also helpful in the diagnosis of skull fractures.

3. **Method.** The patient is placed into the scanner and advanced in small increments, and images (cuts) are obtained. Cerebral white matter (more fatty tissue in myelin sheaths around the nerves) and inflammation appear less dense (blacker) than gray matter. Calcifications and hemorrhages appear white. If a patient receives contrast material, blood vessels and vascular structures (eg, falx cerebri and choroid plexus) appear white. Spaces containing cerebrospinal fluid are clearly shown in black, making it easy to identify diseases that alter their size and shape. Bones also appear white but are poorly defined, and details are better evaluated in a "bone window." Disadvantages include the need for transportation of the neonate, the need for sedation (see Chapter 69), the potential for hypothermia, and radiation exposure.

4. **Results.** CT provides detailed information on brain structures not accessible by ultrasonography and is superior to magnetic resonance imaging (MRI) in the diagnosis of intracranial calcifications. Caution should be exerted when considering the use of multiple diagnostic CT studies in infants given the recent literature suggesting that exposure to ionizing radiation in infancy can play a role in future development of malignancies.

D. **Magnetic resonance imaging (MRI)**

1. **Definition.** Inside a strong magnetic field, atomic nuclei with magnetic properties (hydrogen protons being most common) align themselves and emit an electromagnetic signal when the field is terminated and the nuclei return to their natural state. Computers reconstruct the signal into 2D image cuts. A variety of contrasts can be obtained in MRI and include T1- and T2-weighted imaging, (reflecting two relaxation time constraints, longitudinal and transverse respectively), diffusion-weighted imaging (DWI), blood-oxygen-level-dependent (BOLD) imaging, and proton-density weighted imaging. In functional MRIs (fMRI), such as BOLD and DWI, underlying brain physiology is reflected in the created images.

2. **Indication.** MRI is the preferred tool for a number of brain disorders in the neonate that are difficult to visualize by CT, such as disorders of myelination or neural migration, ischemic or hemorrhagic lesions, agenesis of the corpus callosum, arteriovenous malformations, and lesions in the posterior fossa and the spinal cord. Diffusion-based MRI is the most sensitive to acute brain injury in the first week after injury. After 1 week following the injury, conventional T1- and T2-weighted MRI are preferred. Conventional MRI has been used at term equivalent or at the time of discharge from the hospital to predict neurologic outcome.

3. **Method.** The patient is placed into the scanner, advanced in small increments, and images (cuts) are obtained. Gray matter appears gray, and white matter, white. Cerebrospinal fluid and bones appear black; however, the fat content in the bone marrow and the scalp appear white. In T1 and T2 MRI, fluid may appear dark or bright depending on the type of weighted image. Advantages of MRI include the ability to identify normal and pathologic anatomy without the use of ionizing radiation and the ability to provide insight into neurological prognosis. Disadvantages include the need for transportation of the neonate, the need for sedation, the potential for hypothermia, difficulties in monitoring the infant during the procedure, and the need for removal of all ferromagnetic objects. Because of the need for a ferromagnetic-free environment, ventilated infants pose a special problem. MRI incubators have been developed and used to help prevent motion artifact, provide improved cardiorespiratory monitoring, maintain temperature and fluid status, and improve image quality by using built-in head coils. They hold promise as MRI use becomes more widespread in neonatology.

4. **Results.** MRI provides high-resolution images of the brain with exquisite anatomic detail and allows diagnosis of a number of illnesses easily missed by CT. The temporal development of the prenatal brain, including the emergence of sulci and gyri and the myelination process, has been described, allowing for a more meaningful interpretation of MRI in premature infants. Quantitative volumetric MRI has been used to demonstrate the effects of postnatal dexamethasone on cortical gray matter volume and to help provide long-term prognosis for neurologic outcome. Diffusion-weighted MRI can be used in the early diagnosis of perinatal hypoxic-ischemic encephalopathy at *any* stage of development. fMRI promises new insights into the functional reorganization of the brain after injury. Newer magnetic resonance spectroscopy allows the study of metabolic mechanisms through quantitative measurements of certain metabolites.

E. **Near-infrared spectroscopy (NIRS)**

1. **Definition.** Light in the near-infrared range can easily pass through skin, thin bone, and other tissues of the neonate. At selected wavelengths, light absorption depends on oxygenated and deoxygenated hemoglobin as well as oxidized cytochrome aa_3, allowing for qualitative measurements of oxygen delivery, cerebral blood volume, and brain oxygen availability and consumption.

2. **Indication.** Although NIRS is not widely used, it has potential as a bedside tool to follow cerebral oxygen delivery or CBF. It is a useful technique to assess the effects of new treatments and common interventions (eg, endotracheal suction, continuous positive airway pressure) on cerebral perfusion and oxygenation.

3. **Method.** A fiberoptic bundle applied to the scalp transmits laser light. Another fiberoptic bundle collects light and transmits it to a photon counter.

4. **Results.** NIRS allows qualitative determination of oxygen delivery, cerebral blood volume, and oxygen consumption. In intubated infants, NIRS has been used to identify pressure-passive cerebral circulation, a condition associated with a fourfold increase in periventricular leukomalacia and severe intraventricular hemorrhage.

II. **Electrographic studies**
  A. **Electroencephalogram (EEG)**
    1. **Definition.** An EEG continuously captures the electrical activity between reference electrodes on the scalp. In the neonatal period, cerebral maturation and development result in significant EEG changes during different gestational ages that must be considered when interpreting results.
    2. **Indication.** Indications include documented or suspected seizure activity, events with potential for cerebral injury (eg, hypoxic-ischemic, hemorrhagic, traumatic, or infectious), central nervous system (CNS) malformations, metabolic disorders, developmental abnormalities, and chromosomal abnormalities.
    3. **Method.** Several electrodes are attached to the infant's scalp, and the electrical activity is amplified and measured. Recordings can be traced on paper or can be saved electronically. EEG waves are classified into different frequencies: delta (1–3/s), theta (4–7/s), alpha (8–12/s), and beta (13–20/s).
    4. **Results.** EEGs are sensitive to a number of external factors, including acute and ongoing illness, medications or drugs, position of the electrodes, and state of arousal. A number of abnormal findings can be documented on the EEG of the term and preterm infant, including the following:
      a. Abnormal pattern of development.
      b. Depression or lack of differentiation.
      c. Electrocerebral silence ("flat" EEG).
      d. Burst suppression pattern (depressed background activity alternating with short periods of paroxysmal bursts). Burst suppression patterns are associated with especially high morbidity and mortality and poor prognosis.
      e. Persistent voltage asymmetry.
      f. Sharp waves (multifocal or central).
      g. Periodic discharges.
      h. Rhythmic alpha-frequency activity.
  B. **Cerebral function monitor (CFM)/Amplitude-integrated EEG (aEEG)**
    1. **Definition.** CFM or aEEG records a single EEG channel for each hemisphere. The range of the signal amplitude is displayed in microvolts. Discontinuity in the EEG results in a wider trace amplitude and a decreased lower margin.
    2. **Indication.** The cerebral function monitor allows for the fast identification of infants at risk for hypoxic-ischemic encephalopathy (HIE) and for assistance in the identification of clinical and subclinical seizure activity. In addition, it has been used to select patients for neuroprotective measures such as head or total-body cooling and has been useful in providing information on neurodevelopmental outcome in cases of HIE and intraventricular hemorrhages. Not available in all institutions, the aEEG has also been used in other conditions including metabolic disorders, congenital anomalies, extracorporeal membrane oxygenation, and postoperative monitoring.
    3. **Method.** Electrodes are attached to the scalp, and the aEEG channel is recorded at a speed of 6 cm/h. CFM cannot provide information on aEEG frequency or focal lesions. Unlike standard EEG, this technique requires fewer operating and interpreting skills, making it more readily available. The aEEG should be used in conjunction with the standard EEG to provide clinical information.
    4. **Results.** The aEEG provides information on the background pattern of electrical activity of the brain (Table 15–1), the presence or absence of the sleep-wake cycle (SWC) (Table 15–1), and/or the presence of epileptiform activity (Figure 15–1). After asphyxia, the occurrence of a moderately or severely abnormal aEEG trace has a positive predictive value >70% for abnormal neurologic outcome. For instance, burst suppression, low voltage, and flat trace in the first 12–24 h after injury is associated with a poor prognosis. SWC returning before 36 h is associated with good outcome and after 36 h is associated with bad outcome.

Table 15–1. **SUMMARY OF NORMAL SINGLE-CHANNEL aEEG FEATURES IN NEWBORNS AT DIFFERENT GESTATIONAL/POSTCONCEPTIONAL AGES**

Gestational or Postconceptional Age (wk)	Dominating Background pattern	SWC	Minimum Amplitude (mcV)	Maximum Amplitude (mcV)	Burst/h
24 through 25	DC	(+)	2 to 5	25 to 50 (to 100)	>100
26 through 27	DC	(+)	2 to 5	25 to 50 (to 100)	>100
28 through 29	DC/(C)	(+)/+	2 to 5	25 to 30	>100
30 through 31	C/(DC)	+	2 to 6	20 to 30	>100
32 through 33	C/DC in QS	+	2 to 6	20 to 30	>100
34 through 35	C/DC in QS	+	3 to 7	15 to 25	>100
36 through 37	C/DC in QS	+	4 to 8	17 to 35	>100
38 +	C/DC in QS	+	7 to 8	15 to 25	>100

Sleep-wake cycling; SWC (+) = imminent/immature; SWC + = developed SWC; QS = quiet/deep sleep; DC = discontinuous background pattern, (C) = continuous.
Reproduced from Hellstrom-Westas L, et al: Amplitude-integrated EEG classification and interpretation in preterm and term infants. *NeoReviews* 2006;7:e76.

    C. **Peripheral nerve conduction velocity**
        1. **Definition.** Nerve conduction velocity allows the diagnosis of a peripheral nerve disorder by measuring the transmission speed of an electrical stimulus along a peripheral (median, ulnar, peroneal) nerve. Because of smaller nerve fiber diameters affecting the nerve transmission speed, neonates have a lower nerve conduction velocity than adults.
        2. **Indication.** In the workup of the weak and hypotonic neonate, nerve conduction velocity is an important tool in diagnosing a peripheral nerve disorder.
        3. **Method.** A peripheral nerve is stimulated with a skin electrode, and the corresponding muscle action potential is recorded with another skin electrode. To determine

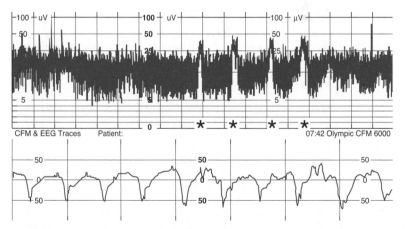

FIGURE 15–1. Repetitive epileptic discharges on a CNV background pattern in a child who has a middle cerebral artery infarction. CNV, continuous normal voltage. Reproduced from De Vries LS, Toet MC: Amplitude integrated electroencephalography in the full-term newborn. *Clin Perinatol* 2006;33:619.

the nerve conduction alone (as opposed to nerve conduction, synaptic transmission, and muscle reaction), the nerve is stimulated at two points and the resulting muscle response times are subtracted. The distance between the two points of stimulation divided by the time difference equals the nerve conduction velocity.

4. **Results.** Nerve conduction velocities are prolonged in disorders of myelination and in axon abnormalities and may have potential clinical value in combination with other tests (eg, muscle biopsy or electromyogram) in these disorders. Initially, infants with anterior horn cell disorders (eg, Werdnig-Hoffmann paralysis) have normal nerve conduction but may demonstrate decreased velocity later in the course. Neuromuscular junction and muscle disorders do not alter nerve conduction velocity. This test is also used for gestational age assessment.

D. **Evoked potentials.** An evoked potential is an electrical response by the CNS to a specific stimulus. Evoked potentials are used to evaluate the intactness and maturity of *ascending* sensory pathways of the nervous system and are relatively unaffected by state, drug, or metabolic effects.

1. **Auditory evoked potential (AEP)**

a. **Definition.** An AEP is an electrical response by the CNS to an auditory stimulus.

b. **Indication.** Brainstem AEPs may be used to detect abnormalities in threshold sensitivities, conduction time, amplitudes, and shape and may be useful as a hearing screen in high-risk infants.

c. **Method.** Although neonates respond to an auditory stimulus with brainstem as well as cortical evoked responses, the latter are variable, depending on the state of arousal, and thus difficult to interpret. As a result, AEPs (generated by a rapid sequence of clicks or pure tones) traveling along the eighth nerve to the diencephalon are recorded by an electrode over the mastoid and vertex as brainstem AEPs, amplified and digitally stored. The shape (a series of waves) and latency of brainstem AEPs depend on gestational age. This technique is sensitive to movement and ambient noise.

d. **Results.** Injuries in the peripheral pathway (middle ear, cochlea, and eighth nerve) result in an increased sound threshold and an increase in latency of all waves, whereas central lesions cause only increased latency of waves originating from distal (in relation to the lesion) structures. Brainstem AEPs are used to demonstrate disorders of the auditory pathways caused by hypoxia-ischemia, hyperbilirubinemia, bacterial meningitis, and other infections (eg, cytomegalovirus), intracranial hemorrhage, trauma, systemic illnesses, drugs (eg, aminoglycoside or furosemide), or a combination of these.

When used as a screening procedure in low birthweight infants, brainstem AEPs have a high false-positive rate secondary, in all likelihood, to known gestational differences (longer latency, decreased amplitude, and increased threshold in preterm infants). Up to 20–25% of infants in the neonatal intensive care unit have abnormal (failed) tests, and most have normal tests at 2–4 months. In asphyxiated infants, abnormal brainstem AEPs are associated with neuromotor impairments. Because infants with congenital infection and persistent pulmonary hypertension may experience progressive hearing loss, they require serial hearing evaluations even if results are normal.

2. **Visual evoked potential (VEP)**

a. **Definition.** A VEP is an electrical response by the CNS to a visual stimulus.

b. **Indication.** A VEP may provide information on disorders of the visual pathway and has been used as an indicator for cerebral malfunctioning (eg, hypoxia).

c. **Method.** An electrical response to a visual stimulus (eg, light flash in neonates or checkerboard pattern reversal in older children) is measured via a surface electrode. The electrical response is complex and undergoes significant developmental changes in the preterm infant.

   d. Results. When corrected for conceptual age, visual evoked responses allow the detection of various visual pathway abnormalities. Although generalized insults such as severe hypoxemia may result in temporary loss of visual evoked responses, local abnormalities may have similar results (eg, compression of the pathway in hydrocephalus). Persistent visual evoked response abnormalities in postasphyxiated infants have been strongly correlated with poor neurologic outcomes. Although VEPs may aid in the prognosis of long-term neurodevelopmental outcomes, they may not be helpful in predicting blindness or loss of vision. Improvements in visual evoked responses have also been applied to determine the success of interventions such as a ventricular-peritoneal shunt. The prognostic value in preterm infants is ***controversial.***

3. **Somatosensory evoked potential (SEP)**
   a. Definition. A SEP is an electrical response by the CNS to a peripheral sensory stimulus.
   b. Indication. SEPs allow insight into disorders of the sensory pathway (peripheral nerve, plexus, dorsal root, posterior column, contralateral nucleus, medial lemniscus, thalamus, and parietal cortex).
   c. Method. SEPs have been recorded over the contralateral parietal scalp after providing an electric stimulus to the median or the posterior tibial nerve. SEPs are technically more difficult to obtain than auditory brainstem evoked potentials and are age dependent, with significant changes occurring in the first months of life.
   d. Results. SEPs may allow evaluation of peripheral lesions such as spinal cord trauma and myelodysplasia as well as cerebral abnormalities such as hypoxia-ischemia, hemorrhage, hydrocephalus, hypoglycemia, and hypothyroidism. SEP abnormalities in term infants have a high positive predictive value for neurologic sequelae and abnormal neurodevelopmental outcome. Current studies are applying SEP to the evaluation, characterization, and pain in newborn infants. The significance of SEP remains ***controversial*** in the preterm infant.

III. **Clinical neurodevelopmental examination**
   A. Definition. The clinical neurodevelopmental examination combines the assessment of posture, movement, extremity and axial muscle tone, deep tendon reflexes, pathologic reflexes, primitive (or primary) reflexes, cranial nerve and oromotor function, sensory responses, and behavior by an experienced clinician.
   B. Indication. All infants should undergo a brief neurologic examination, including tone and reflex assessment, as part of their initial physical examination. A more detailed neurodevelopmental examination should be performed on high-risk infants. Important risk factors include prematurity, hypoxic-ischemic encephalopathy, congenital infection, meningitis, significant abnormalities on neuroimaging studies (eg, intraventricular hemorrhage, ventricular dilatation, intraparenchymal hemorrhage, infarct, or cysts), and feeding difficulties.
   C. Method. The experienced clinician should examine the infant when stable, preferably during the recovery phase. However, the examination may also be quite useful when performed serially, as with hypoxic-ischemic encephalopathy. The infant's state of alertness may affect many responses, including sensory response, behavior, tone, and reflexes. Normal findings change according to age (actual and postconceptional).
   1. **The full-term neonate.** The normal full-term neonate has flexor hypertonia, hip adductor tone, hyperreflexia (may have unsustained clonus), symmetric tone and reflexes, good trunk tone on ventral suspension, some degree of head lag on pulling to a sitting from a supine position with modulation of forward head movement, presence of pathologic (eg, Babinski sign) and primitive reflexes (eg, Moro, grasp, and asymmetric tonic neck reflexes), alerting to sound, visual fixation, and a fixed focal length of 8 in.
   2. **The preterm neonate.** Before 30 weeks' postconceptional age, the infant is markedly hypotonic. Extremity flexor and axial tone and the reflexes emerge in a

caudocephalad (ie, lower to upper extremity) and centripetal (ie, distal to proximal) manner. Visual attention and acuity improve with postconceptional age. The extremely preterm infant can suck and swallow, but coordination of suck with swallow occurs at ~32–34 weeks' postconceptional age. Flexor tone peaks at term and then becomes decreased in a caudocephalad manner. In comparison to fullterm neonates, preterm infants at term have less flexor hypertonia, more extensor tone, more asymmetries, and mild differences in behavior.

D. **Results.** Abnormalities on neurodevelopmental examination include asymmetries of posture or reflexes (especially significant if marked or persistent), decreased flexor or extremity tone or axial tone for postconceptional age, cranial nerve or oromotor dysfunction, abnormal sensory responses, abnormal behavior (eg, lethargy, irritability, or jitteriness), and extensor neck, trunk, or extremity tone. A normal neonatal neurodevelopmental examination is reassuring, but an abnormal examination cannot be used to diagnose disability in the neonatal period. The more abnormalities that are found on examination and the greater the degree of abnormality (eg, marked neck extensor hypertonia), the higher the incidence of later disability, including cerebral palsy and mental retardation.

Selected References

Allen MC: The neonatal neurodevelopmental examination. In Capute AJ, Accardo PJ (eds): *Developmental Disabilities in Infancy and Childhood*, Vol. 1, 2nd ed. Baltimore, MD: Paul H. Brookes, 1996a.

Allen MC: Preterm development. In Capute AJ, Accardo PJ (eds): *Developmental Disabilities in Infancy and Childhood*, Vol. 2, 2nd ed. Baltimore, MD: Paul H. Brookes, 1996b.

Allen MC, Capute AJ: Neonatal neurodevelopmental examination as a predictor of neuromotor outcome in premature infants. *Pediatrics* 1989;83:498.

Bode H, Wais U: Age dependence of flow velocities in basal cerebral arteries. *Arch Dis Child* 1988;63:606.

Brenner DJ, Hall EJ: Computed tomography—an increasing source of radiation exposure. *N Engl J Med* 2007;357(22):2277-2284.

De Vries LS, Toet MC: Amplitude integrated electroencephalography in the full-term newborn. *Clin Perinatol* 2006;33:619-632.

Di Salvo DN: A new view of the neonatal brain: clinical utility of supplemental neurologic US imaging windows. *Radiographics* 2001;21:943.

Hellstrom-Westas L et al: Amplitude-integrated EEG classification and interpretation in preterm and term infants. *NeoReviews* 2006;7(2):e76.

Holmes GL, Lombroso CT: Prognostic value of background patterns in the neonatal EEG. *J Clin Neurophysiol* 1993;10:323.

Huppi PS, Inder TE: Magnetic resonance techniques in the evaluation of the perinatal brain: recent advances and future directions. *Semin Neonatol* 2001;6:195.

Majnemer A et al: Prognostic significance of multimodality response testing in high-risk newborns. *Pediatr Neurol* 1990;6:367.

Muttitt SC et al: Serial visual evoked potentials and outcome in term birth asphyxia. *Pediatr Neurol* 1991;7:86.

Neil JJ, Iner TE: Imaging perinatal brain injury in premature infants. *Semin Perinatol* 2004;28:433-443.

Osredkar D et al: Sleep-wake cycling on amplitude-integrated EEG in full-term newborns with hypoxic-ischemic encephalopathy. *Pediatrics* 2005;115(2):327-332.

Panigrahy A, Bluml S: Advances in magnetic resonance neuroimaging techniques in the evaluation of neonatal encephalopathy. *Top Magn Reson Imaging* 2007;18(1):3-29.

Robertson CM, Finer NN: Long-term follow-up of term infants with perinatal asphyxia. *Clin Perinatol* 1993;20:483.

Smyth MD et al: Cumulative diagnostic radiation exposure in children with ventriculoperitoneal shunts: a review. *Childs Nerv Syst* 2008;4:493-497.

Stapells DR, Kurtzberg D: Evoked potential assessment of auditory system integrity in infants. *Clin Perinatol* 1991;18:497.

Volpe JJ: *Neurology of the Newborn,* 4th ed. Philadelphia, PA: WB Saunders, 2001.

Willis J et al: Somatosensory evoked potentials predict neuromotor outcome after periventricular hemorrhage. *Dev Med Child Neurol* 1989;31:435.

16 Management of the Extremely Low Birth-Weight Infant During the First Week of Life

This chapter addresses the initial care of premature infants of <1000 g birthweight. Many aspects of the care of extremely low birthweight (ELBW) infants are ***controversial,*** and each institution must develop its own philosophy and techniques for management. It is of utmost importance to follow the practices of your own institution. This chapter offers guidelines that the authors have found useful for stabilizing and caring for extremely small infants.

I. **Delivery room management**

   A. **Ethics.** (See also Chapter 20.) The neonatologist and other health-care team members should make every effort to meet with the family before delivery to discuss the treatment options for the ELBW infant. Counseling should include discussions with the parents regarding survival rate and both short- and long-term complications. Moreover, counseling regarding treatment options for the 22–24 week gestation infant is crucial.

   B. **Resuscitation**

   1. **Thermoregulation.** A polyethylene wrap or bag used immediately after birth prevents heat loss at delivery in very preterm infants. The wrap is removed and infant dried after being placed in a thermal neutral environment in the neonatal intensive care unit (NICU).

   2. **Respiratory support.** Oxygen (O_2) use in resuscitation has been challenged in recent years. It takes 7–10 min for oxyhemoglobin saturations to rise to 90% after delivery. The Neonatal Resuscitation Program recommends availability of pulse oximetry and blended O_2 for resuscitation and low saturation protocol. For infants who require intubation, prophylactic surfactant is recommended; however, for infants breathing spontaneously it remains ***controversial***. If the infant is breathing spontaneously and has a heart rate >100, continuous positive airway pressure (CPAP) of 4–6 cm of H_2O should be initiated to prevent atelectasis. CPAP cannot be delivered with a self-inflating bag.

   3. **Transport.** As soon as possible the infant should be transported to the NICU. Transport must be in a prewarmed portable incubator equipped with blended O_2 and CPAP availability. Occlusive wrap should remain in place, and the infant should be placed under warmed blankets with a knit hat. Infants transported from referring hospitals should be handled in a similar manner with the addition of an underlying thermal mattress.

II. **Temperature and humidity control.** Because the tiny infant has a relatively large skin surface area and minimal energy reserves, a constant neutral thermal environment is essential (environmental temperature that minimizes heat loss without increasing O_2 consumption or incurring metabolic stress). To maintain minimal evaporative heat loss, it is best if the environmental humidity is 60–90%. Lower ambient humidity requires higher ambient temperatures to maintain infant skin temperature.

A. **Incubators or radiant warmers.** ELBW infants should be admitted into prewarmed **double-walled incubators or under radiant warmers with polyethylene covers.** Radiant warmers allow accessibility to the infant but cause large evaporative heat with water losses and slightly higher basal metabolic rates than the incubator. Use of the radiant warmer is dictated by the infant's clinical status and medical needs.

B. **Humidification.** ELBW infants have increased insensible water loss secondary to large body surface area and a greater proportion of body water to body mass. Transcutaneous water loss is enhanced by their thin epidermis and underdeveloped stratum corneum. Increased environmental humidity can minimize these losses. **Warm humidification within the incubator or the area beneath the protective plastic cover of a radiant warmer is recommended.** Double-walled incubators provide the best control for monitoring humidity levels.

1. **Use a respiratory care humidification unit,** the same as used with O_2 hoods. The fluids used for humidification in these systems should be changed every 24 h.

2. **Minimize nosocomial infection in humidified environments** by not allowing stuffed toys or other nonmedical items inside the incubator or radiant warmer and by changing linens regularly if the infant's condition is stable. Change bed every 7–10 days per manufacturer's recommendation.

C. **Monitoring and maintenance of body temperature.** Infants weighing <1000 g have poor mechanisms for regulation of temperature and depend on environmental support.

1. **Maintain axillary skin temperature of 36.0–36.5°C.** If skin temperature is outside the range, you may need to change from servo- to non-servo-control (manual) to warm the smallest infants. Use extreme caution while in the manual temperature mode because the danger of hyperthermia does exist. Rectal thermometers are not to be used for tiny infants. Electronic thermometers are readily available and eliminate concerns for mercury toxicity or accidental glass breakage.

2. **Using a servo-control skin probe,** record skin temperature and environmental temperature every hour until the skin temperature is stable (36.0–36.5°C) and follow up thereafter with recordings at 2-h intervals.

3. **Record the incubator humidity** every hour until it is stable (60–90%) and then every 2 h for maintenance.

4. **Low birthweight infants must be weighed** at least once daily for management of fluids and electrolytes. The incubator should be equipped with an **in-bed scale for continuous weighing of the infant to minimize handling and loss of the thermal-controlled environment.**

5. **Other heat-conserving practices** include the use of knit hats, fetal positioning, and occlusive port sleeves on incubators.

6. **Accessory items for infant care must be prewarmed.** These items may include intravenous fluids, stethoscope, saline lavages, and any other items that come in direct contact with the infant. Placement of these items in the infant's incubator 30 min before use warms them to avoid heat loss by conduction from the infant.

D. **Slow warming or cooling of infants.** Warming of infants who become hypothermic must be gradual.

1. **Warming.** If the infant's temperature is <36.0°C, set the warmer temperature 0.4°C higher than the infant's temperature. Continue this procedure until the

desired temperature is achieved. Frequent observations of environmental and skin temperatures are essential to evaluate warming efforts. **Do not rewarm faster than 1°C/h.** When skin temperature of 36.5°C is achieved, rewarming efforts should be gradually discontinued and temperature maintenance by servo-control should be monitored. Rapid rewarming of ELBW infants must be avoided because core body temperatures >37.5°C causes increased insensible water losses, increased O_2 consumption, increased incidence of intraventricular hemorrhage, deviations in vital signs, and a detrimental effect on neurodevelopment.

2. **In case of hyperthermia** skin temperature >37.0°C, set the warmer temperature control to 0.4°C lower than the infant's skin temperature. Continue to reduce the warmer temperature until desired temperature is achieved. If increased temperature persists, consider evaluation for pathologic conditions such as sepsis, intraventricular hemorrhage, or mechanical overheating by exterior lamps. Do not turn off the warmer because this may cause a sudden decrease in the infant's temperature.

E. **Infants on mechanical ventilation**

1. **For all ELBW infants receiving mechanical ventilation, humidification and warming of administered ventilatory gases** are important to minimize insensible fluid losses.

2. **In-line warming of ventilatory gas circuits** minimizes "rainout" of the humidified air and O_2 and maintains airway temperature as close as possible to 35°C.

3. **Infants on high-flow nasal cannula need heated humidification.**

III. **Fluids and electrolytes.** Because of increased insensible water loss and immature renal function, these infants have greater fluid requirements, necessitating intravenous fluid therapy. (See Chapter 8.)

A. **Intravenous fluid therapy**

1. **Insensible water loss** increases with the use of radiant warmers and low ambient humidity. Under these circumstances one should provide additional fluids. However, be aware that excessive fluid intake may contribute to the development of a hemodynamically significant patent ductus arteriosus (PDA); see Table 16–1.

2. **First day of life.** Table 16–2 gives guidelines for total fluids per kilogram of body weight for the first day of life. The table gives suggested volumes (including catheter flushes and medications) for infants in incubators.

3. **Second and subsequent days of life.** Fluid management on the second and subsequent days depends on changes in body weight, renal function (blood urea nitrogen, creatinine, urine output), and serum electrolyte concentrations (see Chapter 8).

4. **Additional fluid may be required if phototherapy is used.** The fluid volume should be increased by 10–20 mL/kg/day.

Table 16–1. **ADMINISTRATION RATES FOR THE FIRST DAY OF LIFE FOR INFANTS ON RADIANT WARMERS**

Birthweight (g)	Gestational Age (wk)	Fluid Rate (mL/kg/d)
500–600	23	140–200
601–800	24	120–150
801–1000	25–27	100–120

Fluid rates may be decreased with the addition of a humidity tent.

Table 16–2. **ADMINISTRATION RATES FOR THE FIRST DAY OF LIFE FOR INFANTS IN INCUBATORS**

Birthweight (g)	Gestational Age (wk)	Fluid Rate (mL/kg/d)
500–600	23	60–80
601–800	24	60–80
801–1000	25–27	50–70

Fluid rates based on 80% or higher humidity; fluids should be increased incrementally with decreasing environmental humidity.

B. **Infusion of fluids.** Confirm appropriate line placement and document prior to infusion.

1. **Umbilical artery catheter.** Use only for laboratory and hemodynamic monitoring if other intravenous access is available. Infuse $1/_2$ normal saline (NS) + $1/_2$ unit heparin/mL. Our institution uses $1/_2$ (NS) + $1/_2$ Sodium acetate + $1/_2$ unit heparin/mL. Sodium acetate aids in the acid-base balance.

2. **Umbilical venous catheter.** Fluids containing glucose and amino acids add 0.5 unit heparin/mL to maintenance fluids.

3. **Broviac or percutaneous infusion catheters.** Add 0.5 unit heparin/mL to maintenance fluids.

4. **Radial arterial line/posterior tibial arterial line.** Add 2 unit heparin/mL to 0.5 NS.

5. **Heparin use** not necessary when infusion rate is >2 mL/h.

C. **For catheter flushing, use the same fluids as those infused as intravenous fluids.** Avoid NS as a flush solution because of excessive sodium. In addition, avoid hypotonic solutions (<0.45 NS or <5% dextrose); these solutions may cause red blood cell hemolysis.

D. **Monitoring of fluid therapy.** The infant's fluid status should be evaluated at least twice daily during the first few days of life and the fluid intake adjusted accordingly. Fluid status is monitored via measurement of body weight, urine output, blood pressure measurements, serum sodium, hematocrit, and physical examination.

1. **Body weight.** The most important method of monitoring fluid therapy is the measurement of body weight. If an in-bed scale is used, weigh the infant daily. If an in-bed scale is not available, weighing may have to be delayed to every 24–48 h, depending on the stability of the tiny infant, to prevent excessive handling and cold stress. A weight loss of up to 15% of birthweight may be experienced by the end of the first week of life. Greater weight loss is considered excessive, and environmental controls for insensible fluid losses and fluid management must be carefully reviewed.

2. **Urine output.** Monitoring urine output is the second most important method of monitoring fluid therapy. For greatest accuracy, diapers should be weighed before use and immediately after urination.

   a. **First 12 h.** Any amount of urine output is acceptable.

   b. **12–24 h.** The minimum acceptable urine output is 0.5 mL/kg/h.

   c. **Day 2 and beyond.** Normal urine output for the second day is 1–2 mL/kg/h. After the second day of life and during a diuretic phase, urine output may increase to 3.0–5.0 mL/kg/h. Values outside this range warrant reevaluation of fluid management.

3. **Hemodynamic monitoring** is a valuable tool in assessing fluid status in the infant.

   a. **Heart rate.** The accelerated heart rate of the tiny infant, which averages 140–160 beats/min, is generally considered within normal limits. Tachycardia, with a heart rate >160 beats/min, may be a sign of hypovolemia, pain, inadequate ventilation, anemia, sepsis, or hyperthermia. Low heart rate (<100 beats/min) may be related to hypoxia and medication.

b. **Arterial blood pressure.** The most accurate measurement of arterial blood pressure is via an indwelling arterial catheter and transducer. Cuff pressures may be difficult to obtain because of the infant's small size and lower systemic pressures. A recognized standard is to maintain the infant's mean arterial pressure at or equal to the gestational age during the first 48 h. Thereafter, mean blood pressure increases with chronological age with a goal > 30 mm Hg. It is necessary to evaluate the infant's perfusion, urine output, and acid-base balance continuously.

4. **Electrolyte values.** Serum electrolyte levels should be monitored at least twice daily or every 8 h for the most immature infants. Sodium is added as diuresis begins, and potassium is added after urination is established.

a. **Sodium.** Initially, tiny infants have a sufficient sodium level (132–138 mEq/L) with no ongoing loss and require no additional sodium; however, when the serum sodium level begins to decrease postdiuretic phase (usually on the third to fifth days of life), sodium should be added to the intravenous fluids (3–8 mEq/kg/day of sodium). Hyponatremia in the prediuretic phase usually indicates fluid overload, and hypernatremia during the same period usually indicates dehydration. *Note:* Hypernatremia in the prediuretic phase is due to excessive insensible water loss. This can be effectively treated with sterile water intragastric drip. This avoids use of hyposmolar intravenous fluids. In subsequent monitoring of the serum sodium levels:

   i. **Hypernatremia Na^+ >150 mEq/L,** differential diagnosis:
      (a) Premature addition of sodium in the prediuretic phase.
      (b) Dehydration.
      (c) Excessive Na^+ intake.

   ii. **Hyponatremia Na^+<130 mEq/L,** differential diagnosis:
      (a) Fluid overload.
      (b) Inadequate Na^+ intake.
      (c) Excessive Na^+ loss.

b. **Potassium**

   i. **During the first 48 h after birth,** tiny infants are prone to the development of increased serum potassium levels of ≥5 mEq/L (range, 4.0–8.0 mEq/L). The increase is mostly a result of the following:
      (a) Relative hypoaldosteronism
      (b) Shift of intracellular potassium to the extracellular space due to an immature Na^+, K^+-ATPase pump
      (c) Immature renal tubular function
   Most clinicians recommend that no potassium be given during the prediuretic phase.

   ii. **K^+ >6 mEq/L mandates close monitoring of the infant's electrocardiography (ECG) for T-wave changes and rhythm disturbances along with electrolyte trends, acid-base status, and urine output.** Acidosis should be aggressively treated because this tends to cause intracellular potassium to leak out. Use of a Kayexalate enemas is *controversial* in this age group. Albuterol metered-dose inhaler (MDI) (4 puffs every 2 h; 1 puff = 90 mcg) are successful in decreasing potentially high levels. K^+ >7 could be treated with insulin, $NaHCO_3$, and calcium gluconate.

   iii. **3–6 days after birth.** Usually by this time, the initially elevated serum potassium level begins to decrease. When potassium levels approach 4 mEq/L, add supplemental potassium to intravenous fluids. Begin with 1–2 mEq/kg/day. Measure serum potassium every 6–12 h until the level is stabilized.

IV. **Blood glucose.** As with larger high-risk infants, ELBW infants should be supported with 4–6 mg/kg/min glucose infusion. This support can usually be achieved by starting with a 5–10% dextrose solution, depending on glucose needs. Amino acid used immediately after birth along with glucose solutions achieves better glucose homeostasis. Glucose levels should be monitored frequently until blood glucose level (50–90 mg/dL) has been established. Abnormal values should be confirmed with serum glucose.

A. **Hypoglycemia < 40mg/dL** could be because of inadequate glucose infusion rate because they lack glycogen stores. Pathologic states such as sepsis, cold stress, or hyperinsulinemia need to be considered.

B. **Hyperglycemia >150 mg/dL** can cause osmotic glycosuria, resulting in excessive fluid loss. Hyperglycemia may be secondary to increased glucose infusion rate, or pathologic causes such as sepsis, necrotizing enterocolitis (NEC), intraventricular hemorrhage (IVH), or a stress response. It is important to find the underlying etiology and recalculate glucose administration. Treatment with insulin infusion is indicated if the blood sugar is persistently >200 mg/dL while maintaining glucose infusion at 4 mg/kg/min.

V. **Calcium.** Serum calcium and ionized calcium should be monitored daily. Hypocalcemia is considered in preterm infants when serum calcium <6 mg/dL and ionized calcium <4.4 mg/dL. However, in our institution we provide maintenance calcium along with total parenteral nutrition soon after birth, and asymptomatic hypocalcemia is not treated with additional calcium because it resolves with time. Symptomatic hypocalcemia is treated with calcium salts (for dosage, see Chapter 132). This decrease usually happens on the second day of life. Although a few infants may not require calcium therapy, some centers routinely institute daily maintenance calcium supplementation in their intravenous solutions (eg, 2 mg of calcium gluconate/mL intravenous solution).

VI. **Nutrition.** If the infant is metabolically stable, in our institution:

A. **Parenteral nutrition** is started on admission and continues until the infant is receiving sufficient enteral feeding to promote growth.

B. **Intravenous lipids** (20%) should be started by 24 h of age; one should start with perhaps 0.5 g/kg/day and increase by 0.5 g/kg/day every 24–48 h up to 2 g/kg/day while monitoring triglyceride levels. Septic and thrombocytopenic infants require caution before advancing lipids. Most centers have arbitrarily taken 100–200 mg/dL as a safe triglyceride level.

C. **Early feeds of small amounts of breast milk or premature formulas** (0.5–1.0 mL/h by bolus or continuous drip intragastrically) can promote gut development, characterized by increased gut growth, villous hypertrophy, digestive enzyme secretion, and enhanced motility. This approach is called **minimal enteral feedings.** The decision to either advance or maintain minimal enteral feedings at a constant level should take into account the clinical status of the infant. Minimal enteral feeding should be started with maternal or donor breast milk. The incidence of infection, NEC, and retinopathy of prematurity is decreased when breast milk is used. Mothers should be provided information regarding the benefits of breast milk and should be encouraged to pump their breasts regularly. Once feedings are established, the breast milk can be fortified with supplements. If breast milk is not available, premature formulas can be used.

D. **Controversy exists** with regard to feeding in infants with PDA and undergoing pharmacologic management for closure.

VII. **Respiratory support.** The smaller the infant, the weaker are the muscles of ventilation. Many of these infants initially require mechanical ventilation; others, if vigorous, may be supported with CPAP.

A. **Endotracheal intubation**

1. **Type of endotracheal tube (ETT).** When possible, use an ETT with 1-cm markings on the side. The internal diameter (ID) of the tube should routinely be 2.5 or 3.0 mm, according to body weight:

   a. <500 g: 2.0–2.5 mm ID (suctioning may be difficult with 2.0).

   b. 500–1000 g: 2.5-mm ID.

   c. 1000–1250 g: 3.0-mm ID.

  2. **ETT placement.** The procedure for ETT placement is described in detail in Chapter 28. Confirm proper placement by a chest radiograph study, performed with the infant's head in the midline position, noting the marking at the gum. **Note:** In ELBW infants the carina tends to be slightly higher than T4. As a means of subsequently checking proper tube position, on every shift the nurse responsible for the infant should check and record the numbers or letters at the gum line.

B. **Mechanical ventilation.** With the advancement of ventilation technology, various modes are available, including volume ventilation, pressure support, and high-frequency ventilation. Ventilation applied appropriately assists the clinician in avoiding overexpansion of the lung or atelectasis.

  1. **Conventional ventilation.** Tiny infants respond to a wide range of ventilator settings. Some do relatively well on 20–30 cycles/min; others require 50–60 cycles/min, with inspiratory times ranging from 0.25–0.35 s. The goal is to use minimal pressure and tidal volume for optimal expansion of the lung avoiding volutrauma and atelectasis. Seek to maintain mechanical breath tidal volumes of 4–6 mL/kg; this often may be achieved with as little as 8–12 cm inspiratory pressure and 3–5 cm positive end-expiratory pressure. In our institution, we have found that pressures can be kept to a minimum by allowing permissive hypercapnia (pH 7.25–7.32; Pco_2, 45–60 mm Hg). The following conventional ventilatory support guidelines are offered for the initiation of respiratory care. Each tiny infant requires frequent reassessment and revision of settings and parameters. Recommended initial settings for pressure-limited time-cycled ventilators in tiny infants are as follows.

   a. **Rate:** 20–60 (usually 30) breaths/min.

   b. **Inspiratory time:** 0.25–0.35 s.

   c. **Peak inspiratory pressure (PIP):** Select PIP allowing optimal expansion of lungs.

   d. **Fio_2:** As required to maintain O_2 saturation 85–92%.

   e. **Flow rate:** 6–8 L/min.

   f. **Synchronized intermittent mandatory ventilation (SIMV) and volume/pressure control ventilators** have the internal controls that adjust flow delivery. Current ventilators have incorporated enhancements for pressure support, resulting in increased triggering sensitivity, shortened response times, reduced flow acceleration, and improved breath termination parameters.

  2. **High-frequency ventilation** uses small (less than dead space) tidal volumes and extremely rapid rates. The advantage of delivering small tidal volumes is that it can be done at relatively low pressures, reducing the risk of barotrauma. A small disadvantage is that infant positioning is restricted.

  3. **Nasal CPAP (NCPAP).** Some ELBW infants may not require mechanical ventilation, whereas others may require ventilation for a short period of time for surfactant replacement. NCPAP has become a mainstay of respiratory management in these infants initiating soon after birth. Infants requiring intubation and mechanical ventilation should be transitioned to NCPAP as clinical condition allows. Nasal intermittent positive pressure ventilation may facilitate in this transition. NCPAP helps maintain lung expansion and improves oxygenation without causing significant barotrauma. Care should be taken to use nasal prongs appropriately to prevent nasal injuries.

  4. **High-flow nasal cannula (HFNC).** Nasal flows >1 L using blended gases are used as an alternative to NCPAP in the management of respiratory distress and apnea of prematurity. Newer equipment delivering >2 L of flow are available, but the efficacy and safety has not been established in this population. Appropriate heated humidification should be used with all HFNCs.

C. **Monitoring of ventilatory status**
   1. **Oxygenation**
      a. **Blood gas sampling.** Arterial catheterization (See Chapter 22 for percutaneous arterial catheterization or Chapter 23 for umbilical arterial catheterization) should be performed for frequent blood gas sampling. As the infant becomes clinically stable, frequency of laboratory testing should be decreased to minimize phlebotomy loss and the need for blood replacement.
         i. **Desirable arterial blood gas values**
            (a) Pao_2: 45–60 mm Hg.
            (b) $Paco_2$: 45–60 mm Hg. A slightly higher $Paco_2$ is acceptable if the pH remains acceptable.
            (c) **pH:** 7.25–7.32 is acceptable.
         ii. **Abnormal blood gas values** indicate the need for assessment including ETT placement, chest wall movement, effectiveness of ventilation, assessment for pneumothorax, and need for suction. Actions may include immediate chest radiographs (see Section VII, C, 2), chest wall transillumination (see Chapter 26), and repeat blood gas determinations.
      b. **Continuous O_2 monitoring** should also be performed, preferably by pulse oximetry. To prevent skin breakdown, pulse oximetry should be changed every 8 h and a protective barrier placed under the probe site. The O_2 mixture should be adjusted to maintain the pulse oximeter reading between 85% and 92% hemoglobin O_2 saturation. Excess oxygenation must be avoided in this group of infants. Failure to regulate the administration of O_2 can contribute to the development of retinopathy of prematurity and bronchopulmonary dysplasia.
   2. **Chest radiograph study**
      a. **Indications**
         i. Abnormal change in blood gas values.
         ii. Adjustment of the ETT (to confirm proper positioning).
         iii. Sudden change in the infant's status.
         iv. Significant increase in O_2 requirement or frequent desaturations.
      b. **Technique.** A chest radiograph should be taken with the infant's head in the midline position to check for ETT placement.
      c. **Radiograph evaluation.** Check the chest radiograph for expansion of the lung, chest wall, and diaphragm. Overexpansion (exhibited by hyperlucent lungs and diaphragm below the ninth rib) must be avoided. If overexpansion is present, differentiate between volutrauma and air trapping based on the age of the infant and underlying disease process. Consider decreasing the peak airway pressure if volutrauma is suspected. Some tiny infants may do very well with peak inspiratory pressures as low as 8 cm H_2O.
D. **Suctioning.** Suctioning should be done on an as-needed basis. The need for suctioning can be determined with the use of flow-loop monitoring, which indicates restricted airflow caused by secretions.
   1. **Assessment of the need for suctioning.** To assess the need for suctioning, the nurse or physician should consider the following:
      a. **Breath sounds.** Wet or diminished breath sounds may indicate secretions obstructing the airways and the need for suctioning.
      b. **Blood gas values.** If significant increase in $Paco_2$, consider ETT malposition, secretions blocking the airway passages, inadequate ventilation, prior bicarbonate/acetate administration, or pain. Suctioning should be considered to clear the airways and avoid the "ball-valve" effect of thick secretions.
      c. **Airway monitoring.** By using airflow sensors and continuous computer graphic screen displays, abnormal waveforms indicative of accumulating secretions or airway blockage can be easily seen, and immediate steps can be taken to clear the airway.

      d. Visible secretions in the ETT.

      e. Loss of chest wall movement.

   2. Technique

      a. **In-line suctioning is recommended to minimize airway contamination.** Suctioning should be done only to the depth of the ETT. Use a suctioning guide or a marked (1-cm increments) suction catheter.

      b. **Suctioning without lavage solution is recommended.** An exception may be the use of warm sterile normal saline lavage for thick secretions.

      c. **Suction should be regulated** at 80–100 mm Hg for in-line suction (closed system) and 60–80 mm Hg (open system).

E. Extubation

   1. **Pre-extubation.** Consider use of caffeine. Current information indicates that caffeine citrate loading improves respiratory drive and reduced length of time on mechanical ventilation.

   2. **Indications.** When an infant has been weaned to a mean airway pressure of 6 cm H_2O and a low (30%) FIO_2, extubation should be considered. Most infants >26 weeks and 800 g birthweight can be extubated in the first 72 h. These are the other indications for extubation:

      a. Ventilator rate ≤10 breaths/min.

      b. Regular spontaneous respiratory rate.

   3. **Postextubation care.** Frequent observation of breathing patterns, respiratory effort, auscultation of the chest, monitoring of vital signs, and blood gas analysis are necessary. After extubation, the infant is placed on HFNC with blended O_2 or CPAP. Some experts suggest that extubation to nasal prong or mask CPAP has beneficial effects on respiratory function and the prevention of atelectasis.

F. Vitamin A. Vitamin A as a mode of therapy for decreasing chronic lung disease in ELBW infants is well established in clinical trials. Dosing should begin the first week of life, 5000 IU intramuscularly (IM) three times per week for 4 weeks. Some institutions are reluctant in using this therapy because of the frequency of IM injections. Vitamin A delivery via intravenous fluids is not effective because it binds to the tubing.

VIII. Surfactant. (See Chapter 7). Most centers administer surfactant replacement to ELBW infants. Evidence-based medicine indicates early administration of surfactant during the first 4 h of life decreases chronic lung disease in these infants. Several surfactants are available; some have the advantage of smaller volume and dosing intervals. It should be administered according to the protocol provided with the specific surfactant replacement product.

IX. PDA. Incidence of persistent PDA is inversely proportional to gestational age. Infants should be monitored clinically for signs and symptoms of PDA. An echocardiogram is recommended to rule out other structural heart defects and confirmation of PDA prior to treatment. Efforts should be made to minimize the risk of PDA. Overhydration must be avoided. If the infant shows any sign of a hemodynamically significant PDA, medical treatment with either indomethacin or ibuprofen is generally accepted. (For dosages, see Chapter 132.) Renal and gastrointestinal adverse effects are less with administration of ibuprofen or with slower infusion rates of indomethacin. Indomethacin can be considered for IVH prophylaxis.

X. Transfusion. These infants usually have low red blood cell volume, with a hematocrit <40, and they are subjected to frequent phlebotomies. Most centers keep the hematocrit between 35% and 40%. Lower values may be acceptable if the infant is asymptomatic. A cumulative record of blood drawn is also a useful indicator in the decision to transfuse blood. The public is increasingly aware of transfusion issues, and parents should be encouraged to participate in a directed-donor program. Epogen and iron therapy is being used in many centers to stimulate production of red blood cells and to try to limit the use of transfusions. Each institution should have transfusion guidelines established to minimize donor exposure and the number of transfusions.

XI. **Skin care.** Maintenance of intact skin is the tiny infant's most effective barrier against infection, insensible fluid loss, protein loss, and blood loss and provides for more effective body temperature control. Minimal use of tape is recommended because the infant's skin is fragile, and tears often result with removal. Hypak zinc-based tape can be used. Alternatives to tape include the use of Op-Site Flexigrid or a hydrogel adhesive, which removes easily with water. Hydrogel adhesive infant care products include electrodes, temperature probe covers, and Bili-Masks. In addition, the very thin skin of the tiny infant allows absorption of many substances. Skin care must focus on maintaining skin integrity and minimizing exposure to topical agents. Tegaderm can be used over areas of bony prominence, such as the knees or elbows, to prevent skin friction breakdown or under monitoring devices (ie, temperature probe, saturation monitor, or SIMV probe). Use of humidity helps maintain skin integrity until skin is mature (2–3 weeks). Humidity can be weaned as tolerated after 2 weeks.

Note: **When the skin appears dry, thickened, and no longer shiny or translucent (usually in 10–14 days), these skin care recommendations and procedures may be modified or discontinued.**

A. **Use a hydrogel skin probe or cut servo-control skin probe covers to the smallest size possible** (try a 2-cm diameter circle) to reduce skin damage resulting from the adhesive.

B. **Monitoring of O_2 therapy is best accomplished by use of a pulse oximeter** for hemoglobin O_2 saturation. The probe must be placed carefully to prevent pressure sores. The site should be rotated a minimum of every 8 h. Alternative means of O_2 monitoring include umbilical catheter blood sampling.

C. **Urine bags and blood pressure cuffs should not be used routinely** because of adhesives and sharp plastic edge cuts. For urine collection, turn the diaper plastic side up. Bladder aspirations are discouraged.

D. **Eye ointment for gonococcal prophylaxis should be applied** per routine admission plan. If the eyelids are fused, apply along the lash line.

E. **When the infant requires a procedure** (eg, placement of an umbilical artery or venous catheter or chest tube), measure 1 mL of povidone-iodine solution. One milliliter is sufficient to disinfect 50–60 cm² of skin area effectively. After the procedure is completed, the solution should be sponged off immediately with warm sterile water. The use of chlorhexidine in the ELBW infant is *controversial* and should be used per institution guidelines.

F. **Attach ECG electrodes using as little adhesive as possible.** Options include the following:
   1. Consider using limb electrodes.
   2. Consider water-activated gel electrodes.
   3. Use electrodes that have been trimmed down and secured with a flexible dressing material (e.g., Kling or Coban).

G. **An initial bath** is not necessary, but if HIV is a consideration, those infants should receive a mild soap bath such as Neutrogena when the infant's temperature has stabilized. Warm sterile water baths are given only when needed during the next 2 weeks of life.

H. **Avoid the use of anything that dries out the skin,** such as soaps and alcohol. Bonding agents such as skin prep and Mastisol should be avoided. Solvents such as Detachol should not be used.

I. **Sterile water-soaked cotton balls** are helpful for removing adhesive tape, probe covers, and electrode covers.

J. **Environmental.** Use of sheepskins, mattress covers, or blankets in humidified environments helps prevent skin breakdown.

K. **Treatment of skin breakdown**
   1. Clean skin breakdown/excoriated area with warm sterile water.
   2. Apply topical antibiotic over broken-down infected areas, leaving open to air.
   3. Apply transparent dressings (eg, Tegaderm) over excoriated areas.
   4. Administer intravenous antibiotics if necessary.

XII. **Other special considerations for the ELBW infant**
  A. **Infection**
    1. **Cultures.** Many of these infants are born infected or are from an infected environment. If the infant is delivered from an infected environment, all body fluids should be cultured including blood and urine. Spinal fluid may be deferred if unstable. Surveillance skin cultures may be necessary on admission if methicillin-resistant staphylococcus aureus strains are a threat.
    2. **Antibiotics.** If the infant has a septic risk after obtaining cultures, start on **ampicillin** and **cefotaxime** or **aminoglycoside.** Drug levels must be monitored if using aminoglycosides and the dose adjusted accordingly (see Chapter 132).
    3. **Intravenous gamma globulin therapy.** Studies have suggested that prophylactic treatment with intravenous gamma globulin may prevent infections in ELBW infants. This therapy remains *controversial;* consult your individual institution for guidelines (see Chapter 132).
    4. **Nosocomial infection.** The ELBW infant is at higher risk for nosocomial infection because of immature immune system, poor skin integrity, and extended hospitalization. Hand hygiene is extremely important in the prevention and containment of infection. All caregivers/visitors should be instructed in appropriate hand hygiene. Nosocomial infections should be contained by cohorting infants and the use of dedicated equipment and staff.
  B. **Central nervous system hemorrhage.** Cranial ultrasonography maybe indicated during the first 7 days for possible intracranial hemorrhage.
  C. **Hyperbilirubinemia**
    1. **Risk.** Efforts should be made to keep the serum bilirubin <10 mg/dL. Serum bilirubin may need to be monitored twice daily. An exchange transfusion should be considered when the bilirubin approaches or exceeds 12 mg/dL (see Chapters 51 and 92).
    2. **Phototherapy.** Phototherapy to reduce the serum bilirubin level may be needed and can be used to minimize the need for exchange transfusion. Some centers start phototherapy immediately after birth; others when approaching 5 mg/dL. If the infant is treated with phototherapy, reassess fluid needs.
  D. **Pain.** Even the smallest of infants have shown response to painful stimuli. Several multidimensional pain assessment tools are available that include both physiological (heart rate, O_2 saturation, respiratory rate, blood pressure) and behavioral indicators (facial expression, vocalization, and motor activity). ELBW pain assessment is very difficult, and none of these tools have been standardized. Our unit uses a pain assessment tool that allows for gestational age adjustment. Pain should be assessed as the fifth vital sign and more often as indicated by pain scores. Methods for pain management include both nonpharmacologic (swaddling, facilitated tucking, kangaroo care, pacifiers, 24% sucrose solution, decreased environmental stimuli) and pharmacologic interventions (morphine, fentanyl, topical anesthetic).
  E. **Social problems.** Many families have great difficulty in coping with the issues related to their infant's extreme prematurity and the loss of the idealized infant. Participation in a parent-to-parent support group appears to improve maternal–infant relationships. Experienced nurses and the use of a primary nurse together with ongoing communication from the medical team can decrease the parents' stress and keep them up to date on their infant's medical problems. Parents should be invited to participate in the infant's care from the beginning. A social service consultation is mandatory for all of these families. Parent conferences involving the physician, social worker, and primary nurse help the family understand the complex extended care of their infant. Parent–infant bonding should be promoted, and parents should be encouraged to assist in caring for their child. Additional discussions may include quality of life, death, dying, withholding and withdrawal of support, and parental religious or spiritual beliefs.

F. **Developmental issues**
   1. **Minimal stimulation.** These tiny infants do not tolerate handling and medically necessary procedures. Other stressors include noise, light, and activity such as moving the incubator. Routine tasks should be clustered to allow the infant undisturbed and prolonged periods of rest.
   2. **Positioning.** The fetus is maintained in a flexed position. Care should be taken to simulate this positioning in the extremely premature infant. A flexed side-lying or prone posture with supportive boundaries is preferred. A change in position is recommended every 4 h or at the infant's cue. Many positioning aids are available and should be used per institution guidelines.
   3. **Kangaroo care** has been defined as "intrahospital maternal infant skin-to-skin contact" (see Chapter 19 for details). It promotes behavioral state organization, increased parental attachment/confidence, and nurturing behaviors that support growth and development. Temperature, heart rate, respiratory rate, and O_2 saturation remain within normal limits during kangaroo care. It also is a safe practice for intubated infants with central catheters when skilled nurses support and educate parents.
   4. **Environmental issues.** Infants are unable to control their own environment, so efforts must be made to decrease ambient noise and provide cyclic lighting to support their circadian rhythms.
   5. **Parental education.** Family-centered care should be encouraged on admission. Parents should be educated about behavioral cues that invite interaction or signal overstimulation. Parents should be instructed on containment techniques and calming interactions.

Selected References

Ambalavanan N et al: A comparison of three vitamin A dosing regimens in extremely-low-birth-weight infants. *J Pediatr* 2003;142:656-661.

American Academy of Pediatrics, Committee on Fetus and Newborn and Section on Surgery, and the Canadian Paediatric Society, Fetus and Newborn Committee: Prevention and management of pain in the neonate: an update. *Pediatrics* 2006;118:2231-2241.

American Heart Association, American Academy of Pediatrics: 2005 American Heart Association (AHA) guidelines for cardiopulmonary resuscitation (CPR) and emergency cardiovascular care (ECC) of pediatric and neonatal patients: neonatal resuscitation guidelines. *Pediatrics* 2006;117:e1029-e1038.

Chow LC et al: Can changes in clinical practice decrease the incidence of severe retinopathy of prematurity in very low birth weight infants? *Pediatrics* 2003;111:339.

Darlow BA et al: Vitamin A supplementation to prevent mortality and short and long-term morbidity in very low birthweight infants. *Cochrane Database Syst Rev* 2007;4:CD000501.

Finer N: To intubate or not-that is the question: continuous positive airway pressure versus surfactant and extremely low birth weight infants. *Arch Dis Child Fetal Neonatal Ed* 2006;91:F392-F394.

Gaylord M et al: Improved fluid management utilizing humidified incubators in extremely low birth weight infants. *J Perinatol* 2001;21:438-443.

Hummel P et al: Clinical reliability and validity of the N-PASS: neonatal pain, agitation and sedation scale with prolonged pain. *J Perinatol* 2008;28:55-60.

Kaempf JW et al: Medical staff guidelines for periviability pregnancy counseling and medical treatment of extremely premature infants. *Pediatrics* 2006;117:22-29.

Malloy CA et al: A randomized trial comparing beractant and poractant treatment in neonatal respiratory distress syndrome *Acta Paediatr* 2005;94:779-784.

McClure RJ, Newell SJ: Randomised controlled study of clinical outcome following trophic feeding. *Arch Dis Child Fetal Neonatal Ed* 2000;82:F29-F33.

Modi N: Management of fluid balance in the very immature neonate. *Arch Dis Child Fetal and Neonatal Ed* 2004;89:F108.

Schmidt B et al: Long-term effects of caffeine therapy for apnea of prematurity. *N Engl J Med* 2007;357:1893-1902.

Seri I: Management of hypotension and low systemic blood flow in the very low birth weight neonate during the first postnatal week. *J Perinatol* 2006;26:S8-S13.

Sreenan C et al: High-flow nasal cannulae in the management of apnea of prematurity: a comparison with conventional nasal continuous positive airway pressure *Pediatrics* 2001;107:1081-1083.

Teixeira LS, McNamara PJ: Enhanced intensive care for the neonatal ductus arteriosus. *Acta Paediatrica* 2006;95:394–403.

The STOP-ROP Multicenter Study Group: Supplemental therapeutic oxygen for prethreshold retinopathy of prematurity: a randomized, controlled trial: I. Primary outcomes. *Pediatrics* 2000;105:295-310.

Verder H: Nasal CPAP has become an indispensable part of the primary treatment of newborns with respiratory distress syndrome. *Acta Paediatr* 2007;96:482-484.

Vohra S et al: Heat loss prevention in the delivery room: a randomized controlled trial of polyethylene occlusive skin wrapping in very preterm infants. *J Pediatrics* 2004;145:750-753.

17 Management of the Late Preterm Infant

I. **Introduction.** The increased number of infants who deliver between 34 and 37 weeks is a vexing problem for pediatric and obstetric practitioners alike. It has been the subject of growing interest and concern that has generated new research into the causation as well as the appropriate management of these patients.

   The most agreed-on **definition of late preterm infants are those born between 34 0/7 and 36 6/7 weeks' gestation.** Older literature refers to these infants as "near term," suggesting they are equivalent to term infants. **Recently, the consensus is to refer to these infants as "late preterm," which conveys an appropriate sense of their vulnerability.**

   Between 1992 and 2002, late preterms increased from 7.3–8.5% of all births, a 16% increase. They now represent about three quarters of all preterm births. Davidoff demonstrated the median gestational age at delivery for singletons born in the United States is now 39 weeks. Another study showed that infants born at 34 weeks were 4.6 times more likely to die than those at 40 weeks, which contributes significantly to the neonatal mortality rate.

II. **Potential etiologies.** Although the exact causation of increased late preterm delivery remains elusive, the rate must be rising due to increased medical interventions at or beyond 34 weeks.

   A. **Preeclampsia** is the most common complication of pregnancy occurring in between 6% and 10% of pregnancies and is rising. Studies are conflicting as to whether the increase in late preterm deliveries is due to preeclampsia.

   B. **Preterm labor and premature rupture of membranes** may lead to late preterm delivery but are not currently preventable.

   C. **Multifetal gestations** are rising due to advanced parental age from delayed childbearing and artificial reproductive technology (ART). Multiples contribute to late preterm delivery by virtue of earlier gestation at delivery, unique obstetric complications, and an increased risk of intrauterine growth restriction and preeclampsia. Interventions to prevent preterm delivery in multiples have been ineffective. Refinement in

ART leading to decreased numbers of multifetal gestation may help decrease their contribution to late preterm deliveries.

D. **Stillbirths** have declined from 14 to 6.7 per 1000 live births since 1970. There were 27,000 stillborns in 1998 equivalent to the annual deaths from prematurity and sudden infant death syndrome (SIDS) combined. Current research does not support stillbirth prevention as a cause of late preterm delivery.

III. **Complications of late preterm birth**

A. **Respiratory distress syndrome (RDS).** In one large study, 21% of infants born at 33 weeks, 7.3% at 35–36 weeks, and 0.6% at 37–42 weeks had RDS. Late preterm infants are deprived of the normal hormonal changes that occur at term and promote the clearance of lung fluid. In the United States, 17,000 infants >34 weeks are admitted to neonatal intensive care units (NICUs) annually, accounting for up to a third of NICU admissions. In another review, 11% of late preterm infants with respiratory failure developed chronic lung disease and 5% died.

B. **Length of stay.** Wang et al found that late preterm infants had a similar median length of stay as term infants but with wider variability. **The most common causes of delayed discharge were jaundice and poor feeding.** Late preterm delivery triples the cost of the infant's initial hospital stay.

C. **Jaundice.** Late preterm infants are at increase risk of hyperbilirubinemia secondary to hepatic immaturity. Late preterm may have an increased risk of bilirubin-induced neurologic dysfunction due to decreased bilirubin binding as evidenced by the 25% of babies in the Kernicterus Registry who were born late preterm.

D. **Poor feeding and necrotizing enterocolitis (NEC).** Most late preterm infants with poor feeding require a prolonged initial hospitalization. Suck-swallow coordination and intestinal motility remain immature, which impacts their feeding capability. Late preterm infants are also at increased risk of NEC.

E. **Temperature instability.** Hypothermia is more common in late preterm infants due to an immature epidermal barrier, higher surface area to body weight ratios, and more frequent delivery room interventions.

F. **Hypoglycemia.** Hypoglycemia occurs in 10–15% of late preterm infants. This is due to a delay in the activity of hepatic glucose 6 phosphatase, which is needed in the final step of gluconeogenesis exacerbated by poor intake. Hypoglycemia can occur anytime in the first 24 h.

G. **SIDS and apnea.** Immaturity of the autonomic nervous system in late preterm infants elevates the risk of apnea, bradycardia, and acute life-threatening events. Infants born between 33 and 36 weeks are twice as likely to die from SIDS as those born ≥37 weeks.

H. **Readmission.** Late preterms are almost twice as likely to require readmission. Jaundice and infection are the most common diagnoses. The strongest risk factor for readmission was breast-feeding at discharge. Two recent studies demonstrated that early follow-up visits or home nursing visits were effective at reducing readmission.

I. **Long-term outcomes.** By comparison, moderately low birthweight infants (1500–2500 g) are more likely than infants >2500 g to have a special health-care needs, a chronic condition, a learning disability, or attention deficit hyperactivity disorder (ADHD). Moderately low birthweight infants are at increased risk for poor health outcomes. A 2008 study by Petrini and associates indicated that infants born at 34–36 weeks (late preterm) are three times more likely to be diagnosed with cerebral palsy than those born at term. The study also noted increased rates of developmental delays, mental retardation, and seizures.

IV. **Recommendations for management.** Iatrogenic prematurity should be prevented by prolonging pregnancy whenever feasible. Because late preterm infants are at risk for certain medical problems previously outlined, specific management strategies should be developed for both their initial hospitalization as well as their care after discharge. Early monitoring of respiratory status, temperature, feeding ability, bilirubin, and glucose levels are critical. Long-term strategies should include closer follow-up of issues such as weight gain and development, as well as good family support. More studies are needed to address both the safety and efficacy of common neonatal interventions that have only been studied in smaller infants, as well as the long-term outcomes of this population.

V. **Conclusion.** It is clear that the number of late preterm infants is on the rise, but the reasons for this phenomenon are not. Infants born from 34–37 weeks have an increased risk of short-term health problems and long-term health, behavioral, and learning issues. Research is needed to ascertain the reasons for the increased number of late preterm deliveries. Close monitoring of the health status of the late preterm infant is needed to ensure optimal outcomes for this at-risk population.

Selected References

Bhutani VK, Johnson L: Kernicterus in late preterm infants cared for as term healthy infants. *Semin Perinatol* 2006;30:89-97.

Clark RH: The epidemiology of respiratory failure in neonates born at an estimated gestational age of 34 weeks or more. *J Perinatol* 2005;25:251-257.

Davidoff MJ et al: Changes in gestational age distribution among US singleton birth: impact on rates of preterm birth 1992–2002. *Semin Perinatol* 2006;30:8-15.

Escobar GJ et al: Short term outcomes of infants born at 35 and 36 weeks gestation: we need to ask more questions. *Semin Perinat* 2006;30:28-33.

Escobar GJ et al: Rehospitalisation after birth hospitalisation: patterns among infants of all gestation. *Arch Dis Child* 2005;90:125-131.

Hankins GDV, Longo M: The role of stillbirth prevention and late preterm (near term) births. *Semin Perinatol* 2006;30:20-23.

Hauth JC et al: Pregnancy outcome in healthy nulliparous women who subsequently developed hypertension. *Obstet Gynecol* 2000;95:24-28.

Hauth JC: Spontaneous preterm labor and premature rupture of membranes at late preterm gestations: to deliver or not to deliver. *Semin Perinatol* 2006;30:98-102.

Hunt CE: Ontogeny of autonomic regulation in late preterm infants born at 34–37 weeks postmenstrual age. *Semin Perinatol* 2006;30:73-76.

Jain L, Easton DC: Physiology of fetal lung fluid clearance and effect of labor. *Semin Perinatol* 2006;30:34-43.

Knuist M et al: Intensification of fetal and maternal surveillance in pregnant women with hypotensive disorders. *Int J Gynecol Obstet* 1998;61:127-134.

Laptook A, Jackson GL: Cold stress and hypoglycemia in the late preterm (near term) infant: impact on nursery of admission. *Semin Perinatol* 2006;30:24-27.

Lee YM et al: Multiple gestation and late preterm (near-term) deliveries. *Semin Perinatol* 2006;30:103-112.

Malloy MH, Freeman DH: Birthweight and gestational age specific sudden infant death syndrome mortality: United States 1991 versus 1995. *Pediatrics* 2000;105(6):90:1227-1231.

Meara E et al: Impact of early newborn discharge legislation and early follow-up visits on infant outcomes in state Medicaid population. *Pediatrics* 2004;113:1619-1627.

Medoff-Cooper B et al: The AWHONN Near Term Initiative: a conceptual framework for optimizing health for near-term infants. *JOGNN* 2005;34(6):666-671.

Neu J: Gastrointestinal maturation and feeding. *Semin Perinatol* 2006;30:77-80.

Petrini, JR et al: Increased risk of adverse neurologic development for late preterm infants. *J Pediatr* 2009;154:169-176.

Raju TN et al: Optimizing care and outcome for late-preterm (near-term) infants: a summary of the workshop sponsored by the NICHD. *Pediatrics* 2006;118:1207-1214.

Sibai BM: Preeclampsia as a cause of preterm and late preterm (near term) births. *Semin Perinatol* 2006;30:16-19.

Sibai BM et al: Hypertensive disorders in twin versus singleton pregnancies. *Am J Obstet Gynecol* 2000;182:934-942.

Stein REK et al: Are children of moderately low birth weight at increased risk for poor health? A new look at an old question. *Pediatrics* 2006;118(1):217-223.

Tomashek KM et al: Early discharge among late preterm and term newborns and risk of neonatal morbidity. *Semin Perinatol* 2006;30:61-68.

Wang ML et al: Clinical outcomes of near term infants. *Pediatrics* 2004;114(2):372-376.

Young PC et al: Mortality of late preterm (near-term) newborns in Utah. *Pediatrics* 2007; 119(3):659-665.

18 Follow-Up of High-Risk Infants

Whenever an infant requires neonatal intensive care, initial concerns about survival are followed by concerns about the infant's quality of life. Follow-up clinics are an important and necessary adjunct to neonatal intensive care because they provide feedback regarding the child's ongoing health and development to families and to their neonatologists and obstetricians.

I. **Goals of the neonatal follow-up clinic**
    A. **Early identification of developmental disability.** These infants need to be referred for further diagnostic multidisciplinary evaluation or community services.
    B. **Parent counseling.** Parents of children who do well can be reassured by positive feedback. If their child demonstrates signs of developing disability, parents need to know as soon as possible, and they must get honest, caring support during this period of high anxiety. Physical and occupational therapists provide valuable suggestions regarding positioning, handling, and feeding of infants. All parents of high-risk infants need anticipatory guidance for recognizing early signs of school or behavior problems and the need for further comprehensive neurodevelopmental evaluation at that time.
    C. **Identification and treatment of medical complications.** Some disorders may not be anticipated at the time of discharge from the neonatal intensive care unit.
    D. **Referral for comprehensive evaluations and community services as indicated.**
    E. **Feedback from neonatologists, pediatricians, obstetricians, and pediatric surgeons** regarding developmental progress, medical status, and unusual or unforeseen complications in these infants is essential.
II. **Staff of the neonatal follow-up clinic.** Pediatricians, neurodevelopmental pediatricians, and neonatologists make up the regular staff of the clinic, and many clinics include neuropsychologists and physical or occupational therapists. Some infants may need to be referred for consultation with audiologists, ophthalmologists, occupational therapists, speech-language specialists, neuropsychologists, social workers, respiratory therapists, nutritionists, pediatric surgeons, orthopedic surgeons, or other subspecialists.
III. **Risk factors for developmental disability.** It is virtually impossible to diagnose developmental disability with certainty in the neonatal period, but a number of perinatal risk factors have been identified for selecting high-risk infants for close follow-up.
    A. **Preterm birth.** Although the majority of preterm infants do not develop cerebral palsy or intellectual disability, they all have a higher incidence of neurodevelopmental disability than full-term neonates. The risk of disability, especially cognitive impairments, is highest in survivors born at the limit of viability (at or before 25 weeks' gestation). All preterm infants are at greater risk than full-term infants for disorders of higher cortical function, including language disorders, visual perception problems,

attention deficits, and learning disabilities. The risk of disability decreases with increasing gestational age at birth but is higher than full-term infants even in late preterm infants, born at 33–36 weeks' gestation. Besides gestational age, predictors of neurodevelopmental disability include poor growth (especially head growth), asphyxia, sepsis (especially meningitis), chronic lung disease, and retinopathy of prematurity. Risk is highest in infants with signs of brain injury, including abnormal neonatal neurodevelopmental assessments and neuroimaging abnormalities, such as severe intraventricular hemorrhage, intraparenchymal hemorrhage, porencephaly, and signs of white matter injury (intraparenchymal cysts, periventricular leukomalacia, and ventriculomegaly).

B. **Intrauterine growth restriction (IUGR).** Full-term infants who are small for gestational age (SGA) have a higher risk of motor or cognitive impairments, attention deficits, specific learning disability, and school and behavior problems than appropriate for gestational age infants. The etiology and severity of their IUGR, timing of the insult, and subsequent perinatal complications (eg, asphyxia, hypoglycemia, or polycythemia) influence their degree of risk. **Preterm SGA infants have the combined risks of IUGR and preterm birth.** After 30 weeks' gestation, compensatory mechanisms for adverse intrauterine circumstances include accelerated maturation. The survival advantage in the event of a preterm birth comes at the cost of their intellectual development.

C. **Neonatal encephalopathy (NE)** is a clinical syndrome characterized by a constellation of findings, including seizures and abnormalities of consciousness, muscle tone, reflexes, respiratory control, and feeding. Etiologies include infection, inflammation, metabolic errors, drug exposures, brain malformations, stroke, as well as hypoxia, ischemia, or any combination of these conditions. Etiology, severity of clinical symptoms, an abnormal electroencephalogram pattern (especially low voltage or burst-suppression patterns), and patterns of brain injury (especially basal ganglia/thalamus pattern) are much stronger predictors of neurodevelopmental disability than signs of fetal distress, cord pH, or Apgar scores. **Many infants with mild or moderate NE do not develop major disability but may have more subtle disorders, including attention deficit, specific learning disability, or school problems. Infants with severe NE have a high mortality rate, and survivors generally develop severe multiple disabilities, including intellectual disability, spastic quadriplegia, microcephaly, seizures, and sensory impairment.** The efficacy of emerging therapies (eg, induced hypothermia) to improve neurodevelopmental outcomes needs further study.

D. **Respiratory failure.** In addition to preterm infants with respiratory distress syndrome, many late preterm and fullterm infants require neonatal intensive care for respiratory support. Respiratory failure can be due to pulmonary hypoplasia (eg, with congenital diaphragmatic hernia), infection, meconium aspiration, and/or persistent pulmonary hypertension. **Outcome studies for randomized controlled trials of treatments for severe respiratory failure (eg, inhaled nitric oxide, extracorporeal membrane oxygenation) report that 25–30% of survivors have cognitive impairments, 6–13% develop cerebral palsy, 6–30% develop hearing impairments, and when followed to school age, many had problems with attention deficit, specific learning disability, minor neuromotor dysfunction, and behavior problems.** Health sequelae include poor growth and reactive airway disease. Evidence of progressive hearing loss in some survivors emphasize the need for serial hearing testing during the first 5 years after birth.

E. **Infection and/or inflammation.** Maternal, fetal, and neonatal infection or inflammation has been implicated as etiologies of preterm birth, brain injury (eg, white matter injury), cerebral palsy, and cognitive impairments.

F. **Other risk factors.** Other perinatal factors are less common but are associated with or can contribute to a high risk of disability.

1. **Congenital infections (TORCH: *t*oxoplasmosis, *o*ther, *r*ubella, *c*ytomegalovirus, and *h*erpes simplex virus).** Infants with congenital cytomegalovirus infection,

toxoplasmosis, or rubella who are symptomatic at birth have a high incidence (60–90%) of neurodevelopmental disability. Asymptomatic infants are at risk for sensory impairment and learning disability.

2. **In utero exposures.** Intrauterine exposure to narcotics can result in neonatal abstinence syndrome and later attention and behavior problems. Fetal alcohol syndrome includes poor growth, dysmorphic features or anomalies, cognitive impairment, hyperactivity, and fine motor dysfunction. Other maternal drugs reported to influence fetal development include **cocaine, phenytoin, trimethadione, valproate, warfarin, aminopterin, and retinoic acid.** There are concerns that environmental toxicants influence preterm birth and neurodevelopment.

IV. **Parameters requiring follow-up**

A. **Growth.** Growth parameters (**height, weight, and head circumference**) should be assessed at each follow-up visit (**see Appendix E**). Most preterm infants "catch up" in growth, but some infants with IUGR, extremely preterm birth, or severe chronic lung disease may remain smaller than their peers. Poor head growth is associated with lower cognitive scores.

B. **Blood pressure.** A silent sequela of neonatal intensive care with potentially serious long-term consequences is high blood pressure. Follow-up assessments should include periodically monitoring blood pressure.

C. **Breathing disorders**

1. **Apnea.** For infants discharged home on monitors, there is often uncertainty as to when it is safe to discontinue the monitor. (See Chapter 76.)

2. **Chronic lung disease.** Infants with chronic lung disease are at high risk for ongoing health problems, poor growth, rehospitalization, respiratory infections, reactive airway disease, and neurodevelopmental disability. They may continue to need supplemental oxygen, monitoring, diuretics, and other medications after hospital discharge, as well as subspecialty consultations. These children need to be protected from secondhand smoke and discouraged from ever smoking themselves.

D. **Hearing.** Because hearing is essential for the acquisition of language, it is important to diagnose hearing impairment as early as possible. All neonates should be screened for hearing impairment (eg, **brainstem auditory evoked potentials and transient evoked otoacoustic emissions**). Infants who fail neonatal hearing screens need comprehensive audiologic evaluations because hearing aids, cochlear implants, and other treatment strategies can have a profound effect on language acquisition. Infants with a family history of childhood hearing impairment, congenital perinatal (eg, TORCH) infection, congenital malformations of the head or neck, respiratory failure (eg, persistent pulmonary hypertension of the newborn), or chronic otitis warrant serial hearing tests.

E. **Vision. Retinopathy of prematurity (ROP)** is a disease of the developing retina in preterm infants. An indirect ophthalmoscopic examination should be performed by a skilled ophthalmologist at 31 weeks' postmenstrual age for infants born before 28 weeks' gestation and at 4 weeks' chronological age for infants born at 28–32 weeks' gestation. **Infants born before 30–32 weeks' gestation, with birthweights <1500 g, or after 30 weeks if they had unstable neonatal courses should have serial eye examinations until their retinas are fully vascularized.** Infants with congenital infection, congenital anomalies, and neonatal encephalopathy may also benefit from an ophthalmologic examination. All high-risk infants should have an assessment of visual acuity by 1–5 years of age. (See Chapter 84.)

F. **Language and motor skills.** Developmental progress can be assessed during clinic visits with a history and observation of language and motor milestones. Infants with persistent delay, dissociation, or deviance should be further evaluated by a neurodevelopmental pediatrician, neuropsychologist, or multidisciplinary team.

1. **Delay** is late acquisition of milestones, compared with age-based norms.

2. **Dissociation** is delay in one area of development compared with other areas and can help diagnose disability. For example, delay in gross and fine motor development with

normal language development suggests cerebral palsy, whereas delay in language acquisition with normal motor development suggests intellectual disability, language disorder, or hearing impairment.

3. **Deviance** is acquisition of milestones out of normal sequence (eg, the child is able to stand but does not sit well). This is a more subtle sign of brain dysfunction.

G. **Developmental screening and assessment tests.** A number of standardized tests are available for developmental screening or assessment, and many of them are easy to learn and administer.

H. **Neurologic development** is a dynamic process, and what is typical at one specific age may be abnormal at another. The examiner must know typical development at each age and the significance of deviations from the norm. For example, extremely preterm infants are hypotonic at birth and develop flexor tone in a caudocephalad direction. Preterm infants at term and full-term newborns have flexor hypertonia in both arms and legs. This flexor hypertonia is then suppressed by higher cortical function in the months following term (ie, 40 weeks' gestational or postmenstrual age).

1. **The neurodevelopmental examination** includes an assessment of the following:
   a. **Posture.**
   b. **Muscle tone in the extremities.**
   c. **Axial (neck and trunk) muscle tone.**
   d. **Deep tendon reflexes.**
   e. **Pathologic reflexes (eg, Babinski reflex).**
   f. **Primitive reflexes (eg, Moro or asymmetric tonic neck reflex).**
   g. **Postural reactions (eg, head control, righting or equilibrium responses).**

2. **Neuromotor abnormalities.** Many high-risk infants have abnormalities during the first year of life that resolve by 1 year of age. Even if they disappear or do not cause significant functional impairment, these early neuromotor abnormalities may signal more subtle brain dysfunction, including problems with balance, attention, learning, or behavior. Persistent multiple abnormalities in conjunction with motor delay suggests cerebral palsy. A comprehensive multidisciplinary evaluation is indicated because infants with motor impairment often have more debilitating associated deficits (eg, cognitive, sensory, or learning problems). Common neuromotor abnormalities include the following:

   a. **Hypotonia** (generalized or axial hypotonia for age) is common in preterm infants and infants with chronic lung disease.
   b. **Hypertonia** is most common at the ankles and hips. Persistent hypertonia (especially extensor) and hyperreflexia indicate spasticity.
   c. **Asymmetry** of function, tone, posture, or reflexes. Encourage infant to look to each side and use both hands.
   d. **Neck, trunk, and lower extremity extensor hypertonia and shoulder retraction** can interfere with head control, hand use, rolling, sitting, and getting in and out of a sitting position. Encourage family to hold infant with head midline and shoulders forward. Avoid standing activities.
   e. **Involuntary movements, grimacing, and poor coordination** suggest extrapyramidal involvement.
   f. **Feeding problems.** Tube-fed infants need ongoing oromotor stimulation programs because they can develop oral aversion.

I. **Cognitive development.** Language and visual attention are good early predictors of cognition. Encourage families to talk often to their infant, reinforce their vocalizations, and after a few months, read books and identify objects by name. Formal cognitive assessments of infants can be difficult, but high-risk children benefit from neuropsychology evaluations at 1–3 years and preschool age to identify their strengths and weaknesses. An audiologic evaluation by 6–12 months ensures normal hearing.

V. **Correction for degree of prematurity.** Although most agree that when assessing preterm infants, one should correct for degree of prematurity for 1–2 years, but correction beyond that is ***controversial.*** The older a child becomes, the less important this issue is: By the time a child is 5, arithmetically 3 months' difference (eg, 60 vs 57 months) matters little. Motor milestone attainment up to independent walking proceeds according to age corrected for degree of prematurity, but some data suggest that for cognitive scores, correction is an issue for children born extremely preterm up to age 8.

VI. **Multidisciplinary evaluation.** The presence of one disability is an indication for careful evaluation of other areas of function. Brain damage is seldom focal and often diffuse. Referral for a comprehensive multidisciplinary evaluation helps recognize areas of strength, develop strategies for intervention, provide realistic data for parent counseling, and identify community programs and resources.

Selected References

Accardo PJ, Capute AJ: *The Capute Scales.* Baltimore, MD: Paul H. Brookes, 2005.

Accardo PJ: *Capute & Accardo's Neurodevelopmental Disabilities in Infancy and Childhood,* 3rd ed. Baltimore, MD: Paul H. Brookes, 2008.

Allen MC: Risk assessment and neurodevelopmental outcomes. In Taeusch HW et al (eds): *Avery's Diseases of the Newborn.* Philadelphia, PA: WB Saunders, 2004.

Allen MC: Outcomes of preterm and fullterm infants. In Rudolph C et al (eds): *Rudolph's Pediatrics.* New York, NY: McGraw-Hill, 2008.

Chyi LJ et al: School outcomes of late preterm infants: special needs and challenges for infants born at 32 to 36 weeks gestation. *J Pediatr* 2008;153:25-31.

Council on Children with Disabilities; Section on Developmental Behavioral Pediatrics; Bright Futures Steering Committee; Medical Home Initiatives for Children with Special Needs Project Advisory Committee: Identifying infants and young children with developmental disorders in the medical home: an algorithm for developmental surveillance and screening. *Pediatrics* 2006;118:405-420.

Ferriero DM: Neonatal brain injury. *N Engl J Med* 2004;351(19):1985-1995.

Institute of Medicine Committee on Understanding Premature Birth and Assuring Healthy Outcomes: *Preterm Birth. Causes, Consequences, and Prevention.* Washington, DC: The National Academies Press, 2007.

19 Complementary and Alternative Medical Therapies in Neonatology

I. **Introduction.** The wave of complementary/alternative care sweeping the country has virtually bypassed neonatal intensive care units (NICUs). But if we listen, we find families asking for complements to traditional care in many aspects of medicine. The consciousness that patients wanted around their deathbeds wasn't even on the radar screen of the health-care profession when the hospice movement was developed. Today, we find a similar perception in the freestanding birthing center movement. In the neonatal unit, a new sense of nurturant care is struggling to take shape. **Complementary and alternative medical (CAM)** therapies may be one adjunct to help soften the high-tech environment of an NICU by imbuing the nurturing elements one would expect to find around newborns.

Early exposure to the ex utero environment, long before development is capable of handling it, has myriad sequelae. Although we have seen a marked decrease in the mortality in preterm infants this decade, we've seen little or no reduction in the problematic outcomes among the smallest survivors. We know now, too well, the outcomes of living in an NICU. Follow-up studies continue to show that preterm infants have long-term problems with self-regulation, as well as difficulty in concentration and problems with attention. CAM therapies may provide balance to support the amazing technological advances we have made in decreasing preterm infant mortality rates. Proponents of complementary therapies believe that physiologic manipulations and brain development are not separate and thus require a simultaneous focus to minimize some of the well-known complications associated with prematurity.

Preterm infants are fetuses with extremely vulnerable nervous systems developing in extrauterine settings at a time when brain development is more rapid than any other time in their life. During the period from 24 weeks to term, the human cortex is particularly vulnerable as its neurons undergo significant structural and functional transformations. The process of cortical cell migration and cell death that is sculpting the developing cortex is much more dynamic than previously imagined. Taking into consideration what we know about brain development and because this is such a crucial period of cortical development, we must give this stage the focus and support it deserves. CAM therapies give us some options that might help ameliorate some of the routinely expected morbidities.

Once we appreciate that infants are amazingly responsive organisms, we are faced with the realization that these infants require developmental care equal to their acute and chronic medical care. We also can't escape the realization of how much the environment influences the development of the immature brain.

This chapter briefly describes some of the most popular and promising CAM therapies, explores how these options are used in the NICU, provides some evidence-based support of CAM therapies, and presents ideas on potential future CAM expansions.

The four divisions of CAM therapies addressed come from the standard categorization of these modalities from the National Center of Complementary Medicine:
A. Lifestyle therapies (called "developmental care" in neonatology). Examples included are light and color therapies, sound and music therapies, aromatherapy, kangaroo care, and co-bedding.
B. Biomechanical therapies. Massage, reflexology, osteopathy/craniosacral, and chiropractic care.
C. Bioenergetic therapies. Acupuncture, healing touch, Reiki, energy workers.
D. Biochemical therapies. Homeopathy and herbal medicine.
II. Lifestyle therapies. Many complementary or alternative practices currently implemented in neonatal units are categorized under lifestyle therapies, but they are more commonly referred to in the NICU as developmental care intervention. CAM therapies attempt to create an environment in the NICU that is reflective of the intrauterine environment. Research shows that the environment of a newborn is an important influence on sensory, neural, and behavioral development.
A. Developmental care includes many interventions, both on the macro- and microenvironmental level. Many neonatal units have made tremendous efforts to modify existing nurseries or have designed new units with environmental modifications that include particular attention to noise levels, light exposure, organization of care, and family-centered care.
1. Noise. Adverse environmental auditory stimuli are a common concern. Noise levels both in the unit and in the incubator have been addressed. We know one of the drawbacks of incubators are their approximate 77-decibel noise level and their minimal vestibular stimulation, which differs markedly from in utero acoustics or the sound of soothing music. Ambient noise in the NICU may cause distress, and attempts have been made to cover the noise using ear plugs or using sound to negate other sounds, called sonic acoustic masking. Most who have worked in the NICU have a hard enough time locating alarms with the constant confusing barrage of sounds and couldn't even imagine trying to sleep in that environment.
2. Light. Regulation of ambient light in the NICU is also an important concern. Constant exposure to light can result in disorganization of an infant's state. Unit lighting

is now designed or modified to regulate light and to include developmentally supportive circadian dark/light cycling. Focused lighting for procedures and the use of eye covers or incubator drapes, used to shield infants in incubators from direct light, are all great adjuncts.

3. **Care organization.** Infant-specific care plans help better regulate the myriad intrusions of intensive care. Positioning, handling, and interactions should be coordinated when possible with cues of readiness from the infant. This is felt to help the infant minimize energy losses and allow for more optimal conditions for neurodevelopment maturation. This more holistic understanding is quite different from the medical thinking of decades past. Educated families now want this more conscious care for their infants when the situation allows.

4. **Family involvement.** In treating disease, practitioners of CAM look at many factors, including the nature of relationships, such as the relationship between parents and infants, and the dynamic between the healer and patient. For years parents have expressed a feeling of helplessness when given little opportunity to be involved in the care of their sick child. Many complementary therapies have the benefit of encouraging early participation by family members, encouraging parent–neonate interactions, and enhancing bonding. Many professionals, who wouldn't otherwise even consider some of the complementary therapies that follow, now look at these for no other reason than having something that allows more parental participation and connection. Parents tend to be a greatly underused resource in NICU care, and we are just beginning to see how they can be included in our expanded focus on the developmental aspects of care.

   Parents are certainly more exquisitely attuned to the emotional needs of an infant. For example, often on rounds, an infant crying elicits the response, "That baby has good lungs." Rounds continue, often walking right past a crying baby. Attuned to the emotional needs of an infant, a parent would rarely respond this way. Parents can create a loving environment that can help instill a sense of security and a trusting responsiveness more so than any professionally consistent behavior. However, when they are met with "You can't touch your baby" or some other fear, based on a feeling of overstimulation of the infant, they can feel pushed aside and confused.

   At this point, what parents need is a context for their interactions—for someone to teach them how to titrate interactions while becoming more aware of their infant's signals. The parents need to be taught the range of states and how their infant's cues demonstrate them. Some of the typical states are sleeping, alert wakefulness, transitional, active, and crying states. These can be detected by reading the infant's sign language or state-related behaviors such as finger splaying, frequent fisting, trunk arching, gaze aversion, or more typical behaviors such as cooing, babbling or fussing with a frowning face. Awareness of these states has changed our understandings from thinking of an infant as a passive organism to an active partner in a feedback system of rich human interactions.

   Reading the preterm infant's behavior moves traditional newborn intensive care delivery into a collaborative, relationship-based neurodevelopment framework. The Newborn Individualized Developmental Care and Assessment Program (NIDCAP) has been especially influential in encouraging awareness of the use of infants' communications as a basis for individualized care delivery. NIDCAP results indicate that increased support of behavioral self-regulation improves developmental outcome, perhaps by preventing the active inhibition of central nervous system pathways that can be caused by inappropriate inputs during a highly sensitive period of brain development.

5. **Kangaroo care (KC)** is usually used to promote bonding and attachment between the infant and the parent (the infant is usually wearing nothing more than a diaper while held on the parent's bare chest). KC was originally developed for a different purpose. Preterm infants in the maternity hospital in Bogota, Colombia, were dying of infection caused by cross-contamination from shared bedding space

and equipment in the nursery. In the late 1970s, Colombian physicians decided to try something new: having the mothers stay in the hospital and incubate their infants next to their bodies until the babies were stable enough to go home. This resulted in a greatly reduced rate of infant mortality, decreased infection rates, fewer apnea and bradycardia spells, increased rates of lactation, and, most interestingly, vastly decreased rates of abandonment.

KC has many cogent reasons for support. It supports the growing consumer interest in participation in the care of hospitalized infants. A significant feeling of autonomy can arise in the parent's recurrent use of KC.

Engler et al conducted a survey of 1133 NICUs in the United States to determine what percentage of those NICUs used KC. They found 82% of the units practiced some form of skin-to-skin care. As with many CAM therapies, there is a significant complexity in initiating these additions to neonatal care. Studies show that with KC, nurses with five or more years of experience seem to be more agile in their allowance of parental participation, whereas nurses with less experience are less receptive to this level of participation.

When a parent holds the infant against his or her skin, the infant's breathing, oxygen saturation, heart rate, and tone improved. It has also been shown that skin-to-skin care results in less episodes of apnea, less disorganized sleep states, and a doubling in the periods of quiet regular sleep. Various body positions also seem to affect gastric emptying and reflux. Mounting evidence in favor of KC to promote physiologic stability has encouraged expanded studies with very immature, unstable, and ventilated infants.

6. **Co-Bedding.** Co-bedding of twins and higher-order multiples is considered a developmentally supportive care strategy. One completed study demonstrated that a co-bedded group had a more positive growth rate in both weight and in head circumference than controls. No difference in infection rates or thermal needs were noted between the two groups. Studies are underway that examine the effects of co-bedding on physiologic stability, soothing, motoric organization, proprioceptive stimulation, and enhanced growth.

7. **Aromatherapy.** Several recent articles address the role of olfaction as a tool in preterm infants. The most illustrative was a French study that appeared in *Pediatrics* in 2005, demonstrating a 36% reduction in apnea with the introduction of the aroma vanillin (used because of its weak trigeminal nerve activation) when used in the treatment of apnea unresponsive to caffeine and doxapram.

Researchers have reported that newborns have an acute sense of smell. Odor forms part of the complex bonding process. Sugano, from Japan, has demonstrated that when used and unused breast pads are placed on either side of the newborn's head, the newborn turns more often to the side of the used pad and that within a week after birth, the newborn can discern its mother's milk on a breast pad from the milk of other mothers.

The soothing effects of a mother's odor are in stark contrast to the noxious odors of alcohol, skin cleansers, and adhesives normally found in an NICU. In some cultures familiar odors are often left in a newborn's crib to calm an infant in the mother's absence. One article assessed the effects of familiar odors (maternal breast milk, amniotic fluid, etc.) used on healthy preterm infants during routine blood draws (heelstick and venipuncture) noting a decrease in crying and grimacing compared with baseline in infants given various types of odorization.

Through the use of aromas, neurotransmitters are released that calm, sedate, and decrease painful sensations or can be used for stimulation. Lavender has been the most studied. In adults, lavender is placed on pillows to alleviate insomnia, as well as to help patients in the intensive care unit cope with stress.

Questions that arise include these: Could we use lavender rather than sedatives for sleep or use it to calm infants during procedures such as computerized tomography or magnetic resonance scans? Could chamomile help regulate sleep-wake cycles?

As in the French study, could other aromatic stimulants like peppermint be used in incubators as "olfactory caffeine" to minimize apnea and bradycardia? Is it possible to manipulate scents to use them as anxiolytics or to enhance attachment? Would allowing a premature infant to smell its mother's breast milk when being fed by gavage reinforce the mother's smell with feedings, thus fostering the formation of the neural pathways between smell/taste and feeding? Could olfaction be used in helping minimize deleterious effects of neonatal pain?

Aroma therapy could be helpful for NICU staff as well. In a study from Japan, keypunch operators were monitored 8 hours per day for 1 month. When the office air was scented with jasmine, error rates decreased 33%, and the scent was found to increase efficiency and relieve stress among employees. Could NICU staff use this anxiety-relief and stress reduction technique as well?

A variety of aromatherapy oils are also used for diaper rashes, such as lavender sitz baths, almond oils, and beeswax. Another oil, Brazilian guava, was found to have analgesic effects and is being investigated for use in infants.

8. **Sound and music therapy.** Lullabies have been linked with infants throughout history; music therapy carries this tradition over into the NICU. In the first meta-analysis of music therapy in premature infants, Standley reported heart and respiratory rates, oxygen saturations, weight gain, length of stay, feeding rate, and rates of nonnutritive sucking as all being positively influenced.

Leonard and Kaminski have shown significant improvement in agitation after music therapy interventions that allowed infants to develop more organized states and sleep more deeply. It has been theorized that music therapy during nursing interventions may even alleviate some of the distress infants sustain with suctioning and heelsticks. Others document improvements in feedings and weight gain and enhanced development and parental bonding.

Recent literature on the pacifier-activated lullaby (a pacifier fitted with a pressure transducer that activates music) coordinates the infants sucking with music. Sucking rates during the periods of contingent music were 2.43 times greater than baseline (silence) sucking rates. Music reinforcement for nonnutritive sucking seems to aid in the development of nipple feeding.

A few studies seek to mimic in utero noises and movements by using waterbeds and vibroacoustic stimulation. Some music therapies are used for stimulation, whereas others are used to mask over stimulation—a sonic camouflage, all attempting to enhance a neonate's neurodevelopment environment. Music promotes both neurologic development and language development.

There are still many unanswered questions about the potential for sound therapy in our nurseries. Should we use it? Which types of music are best in particular situations? Is it Shostakovich, Vivaldi, or the nurses' favorite radio station? Is there a sonic caffeine—a music or sound pattern that could ameliorate apnea and bradycardia in preterm infants?

9. **Color and light therapy.** Health-care workers tend to dismiss color and light therapy as something from the distant annals of medicine, but certainly neonatologists could expand awareness in this area due to the near omnipresent use of phototherapy in neonatal units. Research on phototherapy has shown the biological significance of light exposure. Aside from the classically recognized effects of diminishing bilirubin and activation of vitamin D, numerous studies have shown phototherapy's effect on thyroid stimulation alterations in renal and vascular parameters, increased gut-transit times, and a host of other metabolic alterations. Could it be such an intellectual challenge to think that other wavelengths of light might have other physiologic effects? This is the basis for the field of color and light therapy.

The current focus on light therapy in the NICU has less emphasis on the effect of different wavelengths (colors) on an infant's metabolic milieu than on the generalized lighting in the unit. Establishing circadian rhythmicity by varying light cycles in the infant's environment seems to ablate endocrine alterations as well as the states of disorganization that come from constant light stimulation. We can only postulate the potential long-term neurologic dysfunction that could come from constant light stimulation. Prior to 28 weeks, when not using incubator covers or eye patches, it has been suggested that overexposure to light may also interfere with the development of other senses.

III. **Biomechanical therapies**

A. **Massage therapy** has been used in the care of premature infants for many years, and a significant body of research has already shown its effectiveness. Tiffany Fields has conducted infant massage research since the 1970s, much of which has focused on the premature infant. Fields reported that massaged infants have improved weight gain and better organized sleep states; moreover, they are more responsive to social stimulation, have more organized motor development, and are commonly discharged 6 to 10 days earlier from the hospital. One of Fields's studies suggests that massage increases vagal activity, which in turn releases gastrin and insulin, which may explain the weight gain in the premature infant. Physical activity when combined with infant massage seems to stimulate bone growth and mineralization in premature infants.

The amount of massage or stimulation applied should be altered according to the infant's maturation, acuity, engagement cues, and response to touch. The various types of massage may include stroking, gentle touch without stroking, therapeutic touch, kinesthetic (bicycling) stimulation, or even confinement holds mimicking the womb. Being aware of the infant and his or her receptivity and alertness is important in determining the best time for a massage rather than relying on a predetermined time. Seemingly just as important as the technologies of intensive care medicine is the supportive touch of a parent in helping activate an optimal neurodevelopment milieu. Data suggest benefits to the "massager" as well—such as lower stress hormone levels and decreased postnatal depression and anxiety.

A significant emphasis has been placed on fathers performing massage as a bonding tool similar to what breast-feeding would be for the mother. It can also be a great way to get other family members, such as grandparents, involved.

Although there are numerous replicated studies, infant massage is not yet a mainstay of neonatal care. Concerns as to whether infant massage can produce overstimulation and therefore adverse effects have been raised. Further research is needed through controlled trials to determine the benefits as well as the risks of this therapy. However many CAM therapists feel this is a classic example of the difficulties of integrating CAM therapies in an NICU. If the extensive research in massage doesn't translate into a change in practice, many wonder what hope is there for other therapies? They believe that in the current medical milieu, if a drug were developed that had the same effects, it would surely be used.

B. **Osteopathy/Craniosacral therapy.** Osteopaths believe that many problems begin at birth. Labor is seen as quite traumatic, and an infant may be altered both physically and psychologically by the experience. Cranial-sacral therapists feel that misalignment of structure that is not corrected can lead to potential alterations in function. Problems such as sucking/swallowing difficulties and recurrent reflux after birth are so common that many mothers and doctors consider them to be normal; however, in osteopathy, they are believed to be based in craniosacral abnormalities. Recognition and treatment of these dysfunctions in the immediate postpartum period is considered an essential preventive measure. According to cranial-sacral theory, these can be easily rectified.

The occipital area is thought to sustain most of the trauma at delivery. A complex study by Viola Frymann, DO, explores the relationship between symptomatology in the newborn and anatomic disturbances. The study suggests that strains within the unfused fragments of the occipital bones produce problems in the nervous system, such as vomiting, reflux, hyperactive peristalsis, tremor, hypertonicity, and irritability. Frymann notes that compression of the hypoglossal nerve's egress can cause an infant to suck ineffectively. Symptoms left untreated may result in tongue thrust, deviant swallowing, speech problems, and, in later life, malocclusion. Decompress the condylar parts of the occiput, and the vomiting stops. In temporal bone development, misalignment may cause recurrent otitis media. If the sphenoid sinuses are involved, the child may have headaches. When the vagus nerve is compressed, recurrent vomiting or reflux can occur.

Osteopaths believe that every child should be structurally evaluated after any type of trauma, especially birth. Until the structural cause of a problem is recognized and addressed, the underlying pathophysiology will not change. A practitioner of this discipline gently realigns cranial bones, bringing them into proper relationship.

C. **Chiropractic therapy.** Chiropractic adjustments have been used on pregnant women, newborns, and infants for more than a century. The specialization of chiropractic pediatrics has emerged in the past decade. The need for spinal care immediately after birth is a focus of the chiropractic profession, particularly if there is any history of birth trauma.

A neonatal chiropractic examination consisting of observation, static and range of motion palpation, and spinal percussion is used to detect fixation or aberrant movement in the vertebral column. Gentle and precise chiropractic adjustment is used to correct any detected abnormalities.

IV. **Bioenergetic therapies**

A. **Acupuncture** is part of the traditional system of Chinese medicine. The main concept behind this system is that of chi (body energy not currently measurable by current instrumentation in Western science), which underlies and supports all aspects of the physical body. This chi/energy circulates throughout the body along specific pathways called meridians. Obstructions in the flow of chi may cause disease. By gently placing thin, solid, disposable, metallic needles into the skin along the meridians where chi is blocked, acupuncturists rebalance the flow of energy.

Acupuncture has shown promising results in use for anesthesia, postoperative pain, and addiction recovery. Auricular acupuncture has been used since the early 1970s for various forms of maternal addiction and withdrawal prenatally. It is also used to help reduce the effects of neonatal drug withdrawal.

Currently in China, acupuncture is used to treat infants with jaundice (augmenting hepatic chi), skin problems, teething, ear infections, constipation, conjunctivitis, and peripheral nerve injury. Researchers are currently considering whether acupuncture can help treat colic, constipation, diminished postoperative urine output, apnea, and bradycardia. It is used also in intraoperative and postoperative pain control.

B. **Healing touch (HT)** is an energy-based therapy based on clearing, aligning, and balancing the human energy system through touch. It was developed by Janet Mentgen and the American Holistic Nurses Association in the late 1980s and is currently offered at over 100 U.S. hospitals. Healing touch is an energy therapy that uses gentle hand techniques purported to help reconfigure a patient's energy field and accelerate healing.

HT consists first of a full-body scan assessment done by slowly moving the practitioner or trained parent hands, from head to toe ~6 in above the infant's body to detect changes in the energy field. Once the assessment is completed, a variety of methods are used to balance the infant's energy field.

One HT technique that can empower parents to feel like they are actively participating in care of their infant is called comfort infusion and used to relieve pain. Parents are taught to place their left palm over the infant, encouraging any pain the infant may be having, to move up from the infant to the parent's palm and then through their body to drain out of their right hand. When parents no longer sense pain, the right hand is placed over the infant and the left one turned upward to infuse healing energy. This is a great technique to teach parents. When the parents are at a point of feeling totally helpless in their infant's plight, this can restore a feeling of energetic connection with no touch involved at all. Most are already familiar with the concept, and they can do this no matter how ill their infant may be.

C. **Reiki** is a form of noninvasive energy healing, similar to HT, in which energy is transferred from the hands of a Reiki master to a patient using a sequence of hand positions above the body. Reiki relaxes and heals by clearing energy meridians and chakras (vortices of energy along the spine). Energy blockages are dissolved allowing the vibration frequency of the body to increase, thus restoring balance. As a calming balance occurs, respirations slow, blood pressure normalizes, and pain is relieved—all of which are felt to accelerate the healing process.

D. **Reflexology** is an ancient form of healing, somewhat similar to traditional acupuncture. In this modality, chi is restored by manipulation of reflex points in the hands and feet that have specific correlates to organs, glands, and body parts. Reflexology may benefit infants by increasing blood flow to specific organs such as increasing perfusion to the kidneys or increasing cardiac output.

Imagine the distress to a newborn brought about by a heelstick; the affects of reflexology are just the opposite. Instead of a painful stick, this modality is thought to provide a grounding for a patient—a balancing and soothing of their bioenergies.

E. **Energy workers.** Energy-based healing is growing in popularity. Energy workers are a contemporary twist on some of the ancient traditions working with chi. Their ability to "read" energy patterns can provide some novel ideas in caring for infants. They stress an infant's energetic receptivity early in life. A wide-open crown chakra at the site of the cranial soft spot is noted to be a physical and psychospiritual vulnerability in the newborn. The chakras are described as open at birth, meaning there are no protective filters available, allowing unimpeded exposure to different positive and negative energies. Many cultures honor this openness: Muslims whisper at birth, "there is no God but Allah." Hispanics want to protect a child from the "evil eye." Scientologists also are known to have a ritual protective practice at birth along with their well-known "silent birth" technique. In addition to the energy receptivity, there are other numerous energetic observations made around birthing and bonding. One is known as "psychic umbilica," a persistent energetic connection between the mother and infant after delivery. This connection is felt to diminish over the course of time, such that if breast-feeding duration is left to the infant's natural instincts, a child stops breast-feeding exactly when this energetic connection can no longer be seen or felt by a practitioner. Energy workers mention the striking alterations they feel in this energetic connection depending on the birth method (ie, medicated vs nonmedicated vaginal deliveries or cesarean section deliveries).

Another interesting concept is one from India, where it is felt that along with the standard corporeal nutrition of breast milk, there are small energetic openings (or "chakras") in the mother's nipples that supply the infant with energetic nourishment.

V. **Biochemical interventions**

A. **Homeopathy.** The basic idea behind homeopathy is that the body's internal wisdom will defend and heal itself by choosing the most beneficial response. Homeopathy is based on the "like cures, like principle": a symptom in a patient is treated with a remedy that causes this same symptom, thus further stimulating the body's natural responses (similar in philosophy to a vaccine). Homeopathy can be considered a catalyst to jump-start the body's healing process. Homeopathic remedies are an enigma to those unaware of the concept of the memory of water and the potentiating successions that are believed to enhance that memory.

Homeopaths prescribe medicine that is very patient specific, and they base these prescriptions on past health history, past medical treatments, genetic inheritance, and a constellation of physical, emotional, mental, and spiritual symptomatology. Apparently, titrating individualized medicine(s) for newborns is not always easy.

Chubby infants require different constitutional remedies than small or low birthweight infants, as do infants who sleep through the night compared to those who do not.

Some examples of therapies: infants that endure traumatic labors with bruising or other injuries (ie, postnatal intravenous infiltrates) are considered to benefit from a remedy called **arnica** and **hypericum perforatum,** which are thought to optimize the body's attempts to heal wounds, both physical and psychological. It is hypothesized that homeopathic remedies such as these, as well as **staphysagria** and **calendula,** can help circumcised newborns heal from the physical and psychological trauma of the procedure.

In Europe, where homeopathic remedies are much more commonly used, **carbovege** is used for apnea and bradycardia. **Aethusa** is used for milk intolerance as well as for reflux. **Nux vomica** and **chamomilla** are used for colic. **Magnesium phosphorica** is used to relieve symptoms of gas, bloating, and burping. **Topical calendula** is used for diaper dermatitis.

B. **Herbal medicine.** The World Health Organization estimates that ~ 75% of the world population relies on botanical medicines; indeed, 30% of Americans also use botanical remedies, and the practice is growing in popularity. It behooves health-care professionals to be familiar with the expanding field of herbal medicine. Many mothers use herbal remedies during pregnancy. They are especially popular among breastfeeding women. Knowing what, if any, herbal remedies nursing mothers use is essential because the substances can be passed through breast milk to children. **Galactogogue herbs** have gained a reputation for increasing breast milk. **Domperidone, fenugreek, teas, herbal extracts, blessed nettle, anise, dill,** and **fennel seed** are some common options. **Sage** and **parsley** can dry up milk supply. **St. John's wart** is commonly used for postpartum depression. It has been speculated that the increased incidence of neonatal unconjugated hyperbilirubinemia in Asians may result from maternal ingestion of certain ethnically characteristic herbal medications or foods. Some of these herbal remedies can cause hemolysis in infants with glucose-6-phosphate dehydrogenase deficiency.

Caffeine is probably the herbal medicine most used in neonatal care. Many credit the use of probiotics, a hot topic in neonatology for prevention of necrotizing enterocolitis, as originating from the field of herbal medicine. **Digitalis** is also an herbal remedy. Many others are herbal folk remedies. **Aloe vera** is used as a skin protectant or for burns and skin irritations. Creams made from **comfrey, plantain,** or **marigolds** are used for treatment of rashes and cradle cap. **Calendula** is used in Russia for conjunctivitis. **Tree tea oil** is used as an antifungal. Dandelion is used as a diuretic. **Peppermint** stimulates bile flow and decreases lower esophageal sphincter pressure. **Tripola** increases intestinal peristalsis. **Milk thistle** increases enterohepatic circulation. In China, **artemisia, Scutellaria, rheum officinale, glycyrrhiza,** and **coptis shinesis** are prescribed to jaundiced infants often in combination with phototherapy. **Kava** can be used to induce oral numbness, which would be helpful with endotracheal tube discomfort.

VI. **Supportive care**
A. **Hospice/Palliative care.** Another CAM focus, increasingly prevalent in the NICU setting, is hospice care. Many NICUs are developing stronger links with palliative and hospice care teams to address the process of dying, pain management, and the stages of grief.

Hospice has even extended its philosophical trajectory to the prenatal arena, so that families not opting to abort infants with known lethal anomalies receive support services while the child is in utero.

B. **Emotional care.** Another complementary area of focus is the myriad of options that address the emotional and spiritual needs of parents. Support groups can help parents gain perspective on their situation. These groups may help to obviate the emotional trauma parents may feel about having such a vulnerable infant, or they may address the extreme disruption families experience in the usual stages of pregnancy, which may influence their preparation for nurturing their child. The same idea can be used to meet the often overlooked needs of siblings.

VII. **Conclusion.** As neurodevelopmental care emerges as neonatology's new frontier, CAM therapies challenge us to think of the many options for supporting and nurturing the complexities of health and healing in infants. Because mainstream medicine has traditionally viewed CAM therapies with suspicion, research will be needed to demonstrate the efficacy of many of these therapies as well as to assess the short- and long-term benefits and burdens.

Selected References

Ackerman RW: *Auricular acupuncture treatment for chemical dependency.* Paper presented at: National Acupuncture Detoxification Association; 1992; Vancouver, WA.

Als H et al: Early experience alters brain function and structure. *Pediatrics* 2004;113:846-857.

Altimier L, Lutes L: Co-bedding multiples. *Newborn Infant Nursing Rev* 2001;1(4):205-206.

Aly H et al: Physical activity combined with massage improves bone mineralization in premature infants: a randomized trial. *J Perinatol* 2004;24(5):305-309.

Anderson GC: The mother and her newborn: mutual caregivers. *J Obstet Gynecol Neonatal Nurs* 1977;6(5):50-57.

Ballard KL: Meeting the needs of siblings of children with cancer. *Pediatric Nurs* 2004; 30(5):394-401.

Barrett B et al: Assessing the risks and benefits of herbal medicine: an overview of scientific evidence. *Alternative Ther Health Med* 1999;5(4):40-49.

Brennan BA: *Hands of Light: A Guide to Healing Through the Human Energy Field.* New York, NY: Bantam Books, 1988.

Bullock ML et al: Controlled trial of acupuncture for severe recidivistic alcoholism. *Lancet* 1989;1:1435-1439.

Butt ML, Kisilevsky BS: Music modulates behavior of premature infants following heel lance. *J Can Nurs Res* 2000;31(4):17-39.

Caine J: The effects of music on the selected stress behaviors, weight, caloric and formula intake, and length of hospital stay of premature and low birth weight neonates in a neonatal intensive care unit. *J Music Ther* 1991;28:180-192.

Chamberlain D: *The Mind of Your Newborn Baby*, 3rd ed. New York, NY: North Atlantic Books, 1998.

Chou LL et al: Effects of music therapy on oxygen saturation in premature infants receiving endotracheal suctioning. *J Nurs Res* 2003;11(3):209-216.

Conover E, Buehler BA: Use of herbal agents by breastfeeding women may affect infants. *Pediatric Ann* 2004;33(4):210.

Engler AJ et al: Kangaroo care in the United States: a national survey. *J Invest Med* 1999;47:175A.

Fields TM: *Touch in Early Development.* Mahwah, NJ: Erlbaum, 1995.

Fok TF: Neonatal jaundice-traditional Chinese medicine approach. *Perinatology* 2001;21(suppl 1): S98-S100; discussion S104-S107.

Frymann VM: *The Collected Papers of Viola M. Frymann, DO: Legacy of Osteopathy to Children.* Ann Arbor, MI: Edward Brothers, 1998.

Glover V et al: Benefits of infant massage for mothers with postnatal depression. *Semin Neonatol* 2002;7(6):495-500.

Goubet N et al: The olfactory experience mediates response to pain in preterm newborns. *Dev Psychobiol* 2003;42:171-180.

Goubet N et al: Familiarity breeds content? Soothing effect of a familiar odor on full-term newborns. *J Dev Behav Pediatr* 2007;28(3):189-194.

Klaus MH: Bach, Beethoven, or rock—and how much? *J Pediatr* 1976;88(2):300.

Kramer LI, Pierpont ME: Rocking waterbeds and auditory stimuli to enhance growth of preterm infants. *J Pediatr* 1976;88(2):297-299.

Lorenz JM et al: A quantitative review of mortality and developmental disability in extremely premature newborns. *Arch Pediatr Adolesc Med* 1998;152:425-435.

Ludington SM, Engler A: Kangaroo care congress report. *Neonatal Netw*1999;18(4):55-56.

Ludington-Hoe SM: Randomized controlled trial of kangaroo care: Cardiorespiratory and thermal effects on healthy preterm infants. *Neonatal Netw* 2004;23(3):39-48.

Marlier L et al: Olfactory stimulation prevents apnea in premature newborns. *Pediatrics* 2005;115(1):83-88.

Morton J: Guava. In *Fruits of Warm Climates*. Miami, FL: Flair Books, 1987:356-363.

Pearson J, Anderson K: Evaluation of a program to promote positive parenting in the neonatal intensive care unit. *Neonatal Netw* 2001;20(4):43-48.

Rivkees SA: Developing circadian rhythmicity. *Pediatric Endocrinol* 1997;44 (2):467-487.

Rosch PJ: Stress reduction effects of smells and sounds. *Health and Stress, The Newsletter of the American Institute of Stress* 1997;4:4-5.

Standley JM: The effect of music and multimodal stimulation on responses of premature infants in neonatal intensive care. *Pediatr Nurs* 1998;24:532.

Standley JM: The effect of contingent music to increase non-nutritive sucking of premature infants. *Pediatric Nurs* 2000;26(5):493-499.

Standley JM: Music therapy for the neonate. *Newborn Infant Nurs Rev* 2001;1:211.

Standley JM: A meta-analysis of the efficacy of music therapy for premature infants. *J Pediatric Nurs* 2002;17(2):107-113.

Tan KL et al: Effect of phototherapy on thyroid stimulatory hormone and free thyroxine levels. *J Pediatr Child Health* 1996;32:508-511.

Wong RJ et al: Neonatal jaundice and liver disease. In Fanaroff AA et al (eds): *Neonatal-Perinatal Medicine*, 8th ed. Philadelphia, PA: Mosby Elsevier, 2006:1427.

20 Neonatal Bioethics

I. **Introduction. Ethics** is a term to describe "doing good." The study of bioethics as a field separate from medicine itself is a recent phenomenon. Physicians have historically set and maintained policies concerning ethical behavior in medical practice. During the last 30 years, the distinct study of bioethics has come into being. The obligation to act in an ethical manner in medical practice requires that we know something about how we should act and what internal and external guidelines should be followed to accomplish that end. Bioethical issues should be examined from the perspectives of the patient and family, the physician, and society as a whole.

II. **Bioethics perspectives**
   A. **The patient.** Patient-centered bioethics deals with basic principles in which every interaction should be filtered. This protects patients in their more vulnerable position and allows equal treatment. The principles that govern physician–patient interaction are **respect of autonomy, nonmaleficence, beneficence, and justice.**
   B. **The physician.** Despite an increasing public distrust of physicians' motives, the practice of medicine requires physicians to perform in an exceptionally professional

manner. Indeed, the very idea of "professional" is closely linked to good conduct and virtuous behavior. Several important virtues make the practice of medicine a profession as opposed to everyday work.

1. **Fidelity to trust.** Trust is an important virtue in any human relationship. This involves not only truth telling but also aspects of consistency, integrity, and confidence. The medical relationship between physician and patient extends even further into this idea of trust. The relationship between professionals such as physicians, lawyers, and ministers is termed a **fiduciary relationship.** In such a relationship, the patient trusts the physician to help the patient, and the physician is expected to provide this help to the best of his or her ability. In other words, as physicians, we should always be found trustworthy.

2. **Compassion.** If there is one aspect of a physician's character most scrutinized by patients, it is compassion. Compassion, although difficult to define precisely, is the quality most associated with ethical behavior. The word **compassion** (*com* meaning "with" and *passion* meaning "suffering") literally means to "suffer with" your patient.

3. **Phronesis.** The term **phronesis** was used by Aristotle for the virtue of practical wisdom, the capacity for moral insight, the capacity, in a given set of circumstances, to discern what moral choice or course of action is most conducive to the good of the agent or the activity in which the agent is engaged. In short, *phronesis* can be defined as "common sense."

4. **Justice. Justice** is defined as "the rendering to one what is due." As physicians, we have a specific obligation to render to our patients what is due: the patient's healing. The virtue of justice also indicates an unfailing quality. This quality is linked to the rule of nonmaleficence or the avoidance of doing harm to the patient.

5. **Fortitude. Fortitude** describes not only physical but also mental and emotional courage. We tend to think of courage in terms of a soldier in battle, but physicians display courage in a variety of ways: caring for patients with HIV infection, continuing in our care long past any hour that reasonable jobs would require, and facing the emotional wear and tear of dealing with families in crisis situations.

6. **Temperance. Temperance**, or **prudence**, is usually thought of in terms of social activities or moral life. The physician also would be wise to consider this; however, temperance in medicine deals with our use of technology.

7. **Integrity.** To **integrate** is to "bring all parts together." In the same sense, physicians need to have all the parts together. Our outward presentation to patients and families should be that of consistency and predictability. This virtue is important in developing trust in our physician–patient relationships. True integrity, as opposed to a facade of self-confidence, requires ongoing self-examination and reflection.

8. **Self-effacement. Self-effacement** is avoiding the elevation of oneself above another. Although physicians are highly trained and skilled in the art of medicine, it is important to remember our place; we are to help the parents (or guardians) in caring for the patient. Self-effacement also involves attitudes toward patients in research studies and protocols.

9. **Society.** In some instances, the good of **society** outweighs individual rights. In cases of quarantine for infectious diseases or mandatory treatment to prevent epidemics, we must understand that the temporary loss of rights is for the greater good of all people. This perspective should always be thought of in health-care decisions but should not have primacy in that unjust loss of rights might result.

III. **Pediatric issues**

A. **The best-interest standard.** When physicians work with patients who cannot talk, either because of age or because of mental incapacity, we cannot obtain direct consent for treatment and procedures. In these cases, we must decide which treatment options the patient would choose. This is called the "best interest standard," which describes what we should do as physicians: provide care that is in the patient's best interest. In the case of young children, we normally assume that the parents have the best idea of what constitutes the child's best interest. In other cases, the patient's best interests are decided by a guardian, or legal appointee. Physicians sometimes assume this role in emergencies when there is not enough time to contact other responsible family members.

B. **Parents as patient advocates**

1. **Parental rights.** In the care of infants and children, the parents are uniformly thought to represent the patient's best interests. They are intimately involved in the child's situation and will be long after the physician is out of the picture. Unless imminent harm will come to the child, the parents should be permitted to make all decisions concerning the welfare of their child.

2. **Exception cases.** There are a few cases in which parental rights are not maintained. The widest known of these concerns blood transfusions in children of families who belong to the Jehovah's Witness sect. The parent's right to refuse potentially lifesaving therapy, however, commonly does not extend to the children. The reasoning is that this particular request is outside of what is "normal and usual" in American society, and thus the parental right to refuse this therapy is challenged. Normally, a physician can seek a court order that will place the child in the custody of the state, which then consents to blood transfusion. This same standard has been applied to other parental requests that are outside what would be reasonably expected. Refusal of surgery for a correctable anomaly or demand for treatments that have no effectiveness are cases in which parental rights may be refused.

C. **Minors as parents.** Increasingly, we see teenagers—minors themselves—now giving birth to children. In most circumstances, the minor parent is treated with adult status. In many cases, there may be an overseer figure, such as a grandparent, who helps in this decision process. Note, however, that the parent does have final say in issues of consent and treatment unless that minor parent is otherwise incapacitated.

D. **Child abuse.** Normally, we think of child abuse as occurring after birth when we see a number of injuries and problems associated with this, such as physical and emotional abuse, neglect, or sexual abuse. Several states, however, have made proposals to prosecute prenatal child abuse by mothers who act in a harmful or neglectful manner toward their unborn infants. Continued intravenous or cocaine drug abuse is considered directly harmful to the fetus and, in some instances, has been prosecuted. In these cases, the child becomes a ward of the state after birth.

IV. **Specific issues in neonatology**

A. **Informed consent. Informed consent** is a recent term. It implies the two components required for proper treatment of patients. First, they must be informed completely of the disease and its short- and long-term ramifications. Additionally, the treatment or procedures should be performed in a like manner. Potential major complications, long-term side effects, and indications and benefits of the treatment or procedure must be explained to the understanding of the parents. Possible alternative treatment should also be presented. As physicians, we also need to evaluate the consent that is given. Do the parents have a good understanding of the child's disease, prognosis, and therapeutic options? Are the parents capable of acting in the child's best interest and thus capable of giving consent? Obviously, it is impossible to discuss every complication or ramification of the operation; however, some mention should be made that other complications exist, and the major complications should be listed. These should be explained more fully if the parent desires. The consent obtained should always be durable and written, not assumed merely because the parent voices no dissenting opinion. Emergency and life-threatening situations complicate our ability to obtain informed consent. It is prudent, therefore, to try to discuss potential problems before they develop.

B. **Withholding care.** There is sometimes a feeling among physicians that, to provide optimal care, patients should be offered every technological treatment or procedure possible. In many cases, however, the application of highly technical procedures is not in the best interest of the patient. Frequently, critically ill infants who are not responding to present therapy should have further or more advanced therapy withheld. The decision in these cases rests on whether further therapy will:

1. Have its intended effect.
2. Reverse the process.
3. Restore the quality of life that is acceptable to the patient or the caregivers.

With these goals in mind, one can see that it is as important to obtain informed consent for withholding care as it is for the application of procedures. The physician should not withhold care without discussing this course of action with the parents. Likewise, the decision to withhold care should be discussed with the other physicians and nursing staff involved. The indications for and benefits of withholding care should be clearly defined.

C. **Withdrawing care.** In some cases, care can and should be withdrawn for a number of reasons.

1. The care or treatment rendered no longer accomplishes its intended purpose (ie, futility of care).
2. Ongoing evaluations or tests reveal information changing the diagnosis or prognosis of the patient. In these cases, reevaluation and discussion with the patient's parents are required to provide for the patient's best interest with this new information.
3. Care given in an emergency should be withdrawn if it is contrary to the parents' wishes when they are informed. As noted, there are a few legal exceptions to this rule. Overall, the withdrawal of care hinges on the idea of futility. Does the patient benefit from such care? Can we expect the therapy to accomplish both short- and long-term goals? As an example, the use of pressor agents in a moribund infant may reach the point of futility. If the short-term goal (ie, raising the blood pressure) is not accomplished and neither is the long-term goal (ie, restoring health), then therapy is no longer useful and should be withdrawn. The difficulty with withdrawing care rests on the definition of **futility**. This may depend on the healthcare worker's perspective. The ability of a physician to use the virtues of compassion, phronesis, and temperance comes into play when discussing these issues. At every step, the patient's parents should be clearly informed of the decisions and possible outcomes.

D. **Nutrition and patient comfort. Nutrition** has been classified as a therapy, that is, as a medicine that could potentially be withdrawn or, in other instances, as one of the basic patient's rights for comfort. In any discussion of ethics and patient care, there is consensus that the patient should be provided some basic comforts despite what other circumstance may be in question. The comfort of nursing care, cleanliness, pain relief, and mere presence are factors considered to be basic to human life and not subject to diminution or withdrawal, secondary to end-of-life issues. In most cases, nutrition (ie, food and water) is classified as one of these basic comfort cares. This has been contested in the legal system in a variety of cases, with a broad spectrum of varying opinions. With this in mind, it is probably wise to assume nutrition and feeding to be basic rights for patient care and to challenge this position only in extreme circumstances. The parents' understanding of nutrition as therapy or as a basic right is important. Agreement among the parents, caregivers, administration, and legal authorities must be obtained if the withdrawal of nutrition is contemplated. The activation and opinion of the institution's bioethics committee may be very helpful in resolving these issues.

E. **Delivery room issues.** Neonatal care in the delivery room requires rapid assessment and quick decision making. In infants with severe congenital anomalies or extreme prematurity, these first few moments of life are critical. In these instances, the pediatrician is called on to make critical decisions within seconds concerning viability, quality of life, and prognosis. Care during this period should be guided by the following general principles.

1. **Discuss as fully as possible** with the parents their wishes and expectations before actual delivery of the child. Coordination between the pediatricians and obstetricians can facilitate this dialogue.

2. **Err on the side of life.** If the mother is unable to express her wishes, then emergency therapy must be performed. It is much better to err on the side of life-sustaining therapy than to withhold such therapy. If in the aftermath of this crisis it is discovered that the parents wish no such therapy, then it is appropriate to withdraw therapy. This, however, gives the parents the opportunity to form their own opinion and exercise their right in protecting the child's best interest.

3. **Noninitiation of resuscitation** in the extremely immature infant or in cases of severe congential anomaly is a challenging problem in neonatology. According to guidelines from the American Heart Association and American Academy of Pediatrics, noninitiation of resuscitation appears appropriate in confirmed gestation of <23 weeks or birthweight <400 g, anencephaly, or confirmed trisomy 13 or 18. In these cases, all data suggest that resuscitation of these infants is highly unlikely to result in survival or survival without severe disability. In cases in which the antenatal information may be unreliable or with uncertain prognosis, options include a period of resuscitation with the option of discontinuation of the resuscitation if assessment of the infant after delivery does not support the continued efforts. Initial resuscitation and subsequent withdrawal of support may allow time to gather key clinical information and to counsel the family appropriately.

4. **Discontinuation of resuscitation** may be appropriate if the infant fails to have return of spontaneous circulation within 15 min. This is based on strong data suggesting that after a period of 10 min of asystole, survival or survival without severe disability is highly unlikely. The Guideline Committee of the American Academy of Pediatrics and American Heart Association recommends that each institution develop local discussions of these issues based on the availability of resources and outcome data.

V. **Conflict resolution**

   A. **Identifying conflict. Conflict** is any dispute or disagreement of opinion. This may occur between the physician and the patient or the patient's guardian. Alternatively, conflicts can arise between the physician and the nursing staff, health-care workers, and administrative staff or any combination of these. Most ethical issues arise as conflict between differing values or moral ideals. Therefore, the identification of conflict is a key or essential ingredient in bioethical decisions. Conflict is best identified by ongoing communication. Normally, we think of this as communication between physician and patient. However, this is just the first step. Continued communication among members of the health-care team, parents, family members, and others involved in the case will uncover unvoiced concerns and opinions. These should be dealt with in an open and honest fashion to obtain consensus about ethical issues.

   B. **Putting virtue into practice.** Section II of this chapter describes various virtues or attributes that will assist a physician in making ethical decisions. Many of these virtues are common for all humans. Others, however, apply specifically to the obligations and responsibilities of a physician. If used, many of these virtues will help the physician defuse or avoid completely many ethical issues. Careful attention to the physician's responsibility and behavior creates an environment in which open dialogue and an exchange of ideas and values can occur between the patient and the physician. This ongoing dialogue automatically corrects many of the miscommunications or conflicts that lead to ethical crises.

   C. **The bioethics consult: obtaining an outside perspective.** Many institutions have standing bioethics committees or departments that can aid in resolving bioethical conflicts. Despite our best intentions, we are sometimes unable to resolve conflict with patients or cannot fully explain the necessity of action to patients, causing confusion. In these instances, an outside perspective may be of value. A consultation from the bioethics committee is simply an outside review of the facts and values associated with a particular crisis. This outside observer may be a physician, another health-care worker, or a member of the clergy. The purpose of the consult is not to render a "more expert" opinion but to uncover differing moral values and miscommunication that lead to conflict. In many instances, this is all that is needed to resolve these problems. If consensus cannot be obtained in this manner, further interventions are warranted.

D. **The bioethics committee.** A bioethics committee is usually multidisciplinary in membership. Composed of administrators, lawyers, physicians, nursing staff, and clergy, the committee reviews ethical dilemmas put before it. Many bioethics committees also have a standing role in monitoring the ethical behavior of physicians and health-care workers at their institution. Activation of the bioethics committee, as opposed to a consult, is a more involved process. The committee's purpose is to not only resolve conflict in particular instances but also provide policy and general guidelines for ethical behavior at that institution. Because of the potential legal ramifications, this body may routinely consult the judiciary system for further advice. It is the usual policy of most committees that the body may be queried by physicians or other health-care workers, family members, clergy, or other interested parties. These queries can be put forth without fear of retribution or chastisement from other staff members. The procedure for activating the bioethics committee should be posted in the residents' or physicians' handbook or nursing manual for that patient unit.

E. **The legal system.** On occasion, conflict arises that cannot be resolved by the physician, bioethics consult, or committee opinion. In these instances, outside judiciary opinions should be sought. The bioethics committee can usually be helpful in obtaining this legal opinion. Not only does the committee have familiarity with accessing the judiciary system, but they should also be able to frame the question in such a way to provide the most concise legal response. Activation of the legal system in this way also protects the physician from direct consequence from legal action.

Selected References

Barber B: *The Logic and Limits of Trust.* New Brunswick, NJ: Rutgers University Press, 1983.

Beauchamp TL et al: *Principles of Biomedical Ethics,* 4th ed. New York, NY: Oxford University Press, 1994.

Kattwinkel J: *Textbook of Neonatal Resuscitation,* 5th ed. Elk Grove, IL: American Heart Association/American Academy of Pediatrics, 2006.

Pellegrino ED: Socrates at the bedside. *Pharos Alpha Omega Alpha Honor Medical Society* 1983;46(1):38

Pellegrino ED, Thomasma DC: *The Virtues in Medical Practice.* New York, NY: Oxford University Press, 1993.

Standard precautions integrate and expand the elements of the previously adopted **universal precautions** and are designed to protect both health-care workers and patients. **Standard precautions** apply to contact with blood, all body fluids, secretions, and excretions except sweat, nonintact skin, and mucous membranes. **Standard precautions** must be used in the care of all patients, regardless of their infection status.

In the case of a known transmissible infection, additional precautions known as **expanded or transmission-based precautions** are recommended. These are used to interrupt the spread of diseases that are transmitted by airborne, droplet, or contact transmission. Most bedside procedures incorporate principles of **standard precautions**.

Standard Precautions Key Components

- Handwashing before and after patient contact.
- Gloves for contact with blood, body fluids, secretion, contaminated items, mucous membranes, and nonintact skin.
- Personal protection equipment (masks, goggles, face masks) when contact with blood and body fluids is likely.
- Gowns for blood or body fluid contact and to prevent soiling of clothing.
- Sharps precautions avoid recapping used needles, avoid bending, breaking, or manipulating used needles by hand, and place used sharps in puncture-resistant containers. Use self-shielding needle devices whenever possible.

There is a growing concern over latex exposure in the hospital. Certain pediatric populations are at higher risk for **latex allergies** such as in spina bifida. Many hospitals are converting to a latex-free environment. Latex-free equipment is recommended when available in the neonatal unit.

---

21 Arterial Access: Arterial Puncture (Radial Artery Puncture)

I. **Indications**
   A. To obtain arterial blood for blood gas measurements.
   B. When blood is needed and venous or capillary blood samples cannot be obtained.

II. **Equipment.** A 23- to 27-gauge scalp vein needle or a 23- to 25-gauge venipuncture needle (self-shielding safety type recommended), a 1- or 3-mL syringe, povidone-iodine and alcohol swabs, a 4×4 gauze pad, gloves, and 1:1000 heparin.

III. **Procedure**
   A. **For a blood gas sample,** most hospitals already have 1-mL syringes coated with heparin. If this is not available, draw a small amount of heparin (concentration 1:1000) into the syringe to be used for submitting the blood gas sample and then discard the excess heparin from the syringe. The small amount of heparin coating the syringe is sufficient to prevent coagulation of the sample. Excessive heparin may interfere with laboratory results, causing a falsely low pH and $Paco_2$. If any other laboratory test is to be performed, do not use heparin.
   B. **The radial artery is the most frequently used puncture site and is described here.** Alternative sites are the posterior tibial or the dorsalis pedis artery. Femoral arteries should be reserved for emergency situations. Brachial arteries should not be used

because there is minimal collateral circulation and a risk of median nerve damage. Temporal arteries should not be used because of the high risk of neurologic complications.

C. Check for collateral circulation and patency of the ulnar artery by means of the **Allen test**. Elevate the arm and simultaneously occlude the radial and ulnar arteries at the wrist; rub the palm to cause blanching. Release pressure on the ulnar artery. If normal color returns in the palm in <10 s, adequate collateral circulation from the ulnar artery is present. If normal color does not return for >15 s or does not return at all, the collateral circulation is poor and it is best not to use the radial artery in this arm. The radial and ulnar arteries in the other arm should then be tested for collateral circulation.

D. Use of topical local anesthetic agents may diminish pain from arterial puncture. Oral sucrose given 2 min prior to the procedure (0.1–1.5 mL of a 24% solution depending on gestational age) and/or pacifier are preferred. (See Chapter 69.)

E. To obtain the sample, take the patient's hand in your left hand (for a right-handed operator) and extend the wrist. Hyperextension can occlude the vessel. Palpate the radial artery with the index finger of your left hand (Figure 21–1). Transillumination with a high-intensity fiberoptic light or marking the puncture site with a fingernail imprint may be helpful.

F. Clean the puncture site with a povidone-iodine swab (preferred for blood cultures) and then with an alcohol swab.

G. Puncture the skin at about a 30-degree angle, and slowly advance the needle with the bevel up until blood appears in the tubing (see Figure 21–1). With arterial blood samples, little aspiration is usually needed to fill the syringe. If there is no return of blood, withdraw the needle slowly because the artery may have been punctured through and through. Using the bevel down can be useful in very superficial arteries or in the extremely low birthweight infant.

H. Collect the least amount of blood needed. The volume of blood taken should not exceed 3–5% of the total blood volume (the total blood volume in a neonate is ~80 mL/kg). As an example, if 4 mL of blood is drawn from an infant weighing 1 kg, this represents 5% of the total blood volume.

I. Withdraw the needle and apply firm, but not occlusive, pressure to the site for ≥5 min with a 4 × 4 gauze pad to ensure adequate hemostasis. Shield and dispose needle in appropriate container.

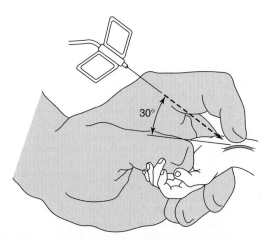

FIGURE 21–1. Technique of arterial puncture in the neonate.

J. Before submitting an arterial blood gas sample, expel air bubbles from the sample and tightly cap the syringe. Failure to do this can lead to errors in testing. (See the following discussion of inaccuracy of blood gas results.)

K. Place the syringe in ice, and take it to the laboratory immediately. Note the collection time and the patient's temperature and hemoglobin on the laboratory slip.

IV. **Complications**

A. **Hematoma.** To minimize hematoma risk, use the smallest gauge needle possible. Immediately after withdrawing the needle, apply pressure for ~5 min. Hematomas usually resolve spontaneously.

B. **Arteriospasm, thrombosis, and embolism.** These can be minimized by using the smallest gauge needle possible. With thrombosis, the vessel usually recanalizes over a period of time. Arteriospasm usually resolves spontaneously.

C. **Infection.** The infection risk is rare and can be minimized by using strict sterile technique. Infection is commonly caused by gram-positive organisms such as *Staphylococcus epidermidis*, which should be treated with nafcillin or vancomycin and gentamicin (see Chapter 132). Drug sensitivities at the specific hospital should be checked. Osteomyelitis has been reported.

D. **Inaccuracy of blood gas results.** Excessive heparin in the syringe may result in a falsely low pH and $Paco_2$. Remove excess heparin before obtaining the blood sample. Air bubbles caused by failure to cap the syringe may falsely elevate the Pao_2 and falsely lower the $Paco_2$. Crying during arterial puncture can decrease $Paco_2$, decrease HCO_3, and oxygen saturation.

E. **Arteriovenous fistula.** This can occur after multiple arterial punctures and is treated surgically.

F. **Nerve damage.** Nerve damage has been reported after brachial artery puncture.

22 Arterial Access: Percutaneous Arterial Catheterization

I. **Indications**

A. When frequent arterial blood samples are required and an umbilical arterial catheter cannot be placed or has been removed because of complications.

B. When intra-arterial blood pressure monitoring is required.

II. **Equipment.** A 22- or 24-gauge needle with a 1-in catheter encasement. A 24-gauge is recommended for infants <1500 g. An arm board (or two tongue blades taped together), adhesive tape, sterile drapes, povidone-iodine and alcohol swabs, gloves, antiseptic ointment, a needle holder, suture scissors, 4–0 or 5–0 silk sutures, 0.5 normal saline or 0.25 normal saline solution (the latter preferred in premature infants to decrease hypernatremia risk) in a 1- or 3-mL syringe with heparinized saline solution (1 unit of heparin/mL saline) in a pressure bag, and connecting tubing. Pressure transducer for continuous blood pressure monitoring.

III. **Procedure.** Two methods are described here; both use the radial artery, the most common site, and can be adapted to other arteries. Another common site is the posterior tibial artery. Ulnar and dorsalis pedis arteries are alternative sites but not routinely recommended. The temporal artery and femoral arteries are not recommended. Axillary artery cannulation is very difficult and also not recommended. **Lateral or posterior wrist transillumination may be helpful in locating the artery in premature infants.** Arterial catheterization requires a great deal of patience.

A. **Method 1**
   1. Verify adequate collateral circulation in the hand using the Allen test. (See Chapter 21.)
   2. Place the infant's wrist on an armboard; some prefer to use an intravenous bag. Hyperextend the wrist by placing gauze underneath it. Tape the arm and hand securely to the board (Figure 22–1). Put on gloves, and place sterile drapes around the puncture site. Cleanse the site, first with povidone-iodine swabs and then with alcohol swabs.
   3. Use of topical local anesthetic agents may diminish pain. Oral sucrose (0.1–1.5 mL, amount depending on gestational age, of a 24% solution) and/or pacifier are preferred. (See Chapter 69.)
   4. Puncture both the anterior and posterior walls of the artery at a 30- to 45-degree angle. Remove the stylet. There should be little or no backflow of blood.
   5. Pull the catheter back slowly until blood is seen; this signifies that the arterial lumen has been entered.
   6. Advance the catheter after attaching the syringe and flush the catheter. Never use hypertonic solutions to flush an arterial catheter.
   7. Secure the catheter with 4–0 or 5–0 silk sutures in two or three places. Occasionally, it is not possible to suture the catheter, and it should be securely taped instead.
   8. Connect the tubing from the heparinized saline pressure bag to the catheter.
   9. Place povidone-iodine ointment on the area where the catheter enters the skin and cover the area with gauze taped securely in place.
B. **Method 2 (alternative method, preferred for premature infants)**
   1. Perform steps 1, 2, and 3 as described earlier.
   2. Puncture the anterior wall of the artery until blood return is seen. At this point, the catheter should be in the lumen of the artery. Vasospasm is common, and the procedure should be performed slowly.

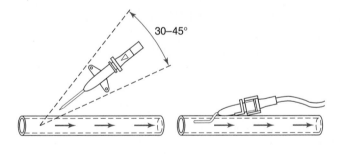

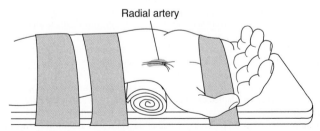

FIGURE 22–1. When placing an indwelling arterial catheter, the wrist should be secured as shown. The catheter assembly is introduced at a 30- to 45-degree angle.

3. Advance the catheter into the artery while simultaneously withdrawing the needle. The blood should be flowing freely from the catheter if the catheter is properly positioned.
4. Attach the syringe and flush the catheter.
5. Secure the line as in method 1.

IV. Complications
 A. **Arteriospasm.** The risk of arteriospasm can be minimized by using the smallest gauge catheter possible and performing as few punctures as possible. If prolonged arteriospasm occurs, the catheter must be removed until the spasm resolves.
 B. **Embolism or thrombosis.** To prevent these, make certain that air is not introduced into the catheter and the catheter is flushed with heparinized saline.
 C. **Skin ischemia/necrosis or gangrene.** Adequate collateral circulation decreases the risk of this complication. Always perform the Allen test to verify collateral flow for radial puncture. (See Chapter 21.)
 D. **Hematoma.** See Chapter 21.
 E. **Blood loss.** Accidental loss of catheter position, resulting in hemorrhage, can occur.
 F. **Infection.** Local infection and sepsis have been reported.
 G. **Infiltration of solution.**
 H. **Pseudoaneurysm.**
 I. **Skin ulcers.**
 J. **Nerve damage.** Median, ulnar, posterior tibial, and peroneal nerve damage have all been reported based on the catheter site.

23 Arterial Access: Umbilical Artery Catheterization

I. Indications
 A. When frequent or continuous measurements of arterial blood gases are required.
 B. For continuous arterial blood pressure monitoring.
 C. To provide access for exchange transfusion.
 D. For angiography.
 E. For emergency resuscitation (umbilical vein preferred).
 F. Infusion of maintenance solutions (glucose/electrolyte) and/or medications.
II. **Equipment.** Prepackaged umbilical artery catheterization trays usually include sterile drapes, a tape measure, a needle holder, suture scissors, a hemostat, a forceps, a scalpel, and a blunt needle. Also needed are a three-way stopcock, an umbilical artery catheter (3.5F for an infant weighing <1.2 kg, 5F for an infant weighing >1.2 kg; newer double-lumen catheters are also available to provide an additional access), umbilical tape, silk tape (eg, Dermicel), 3–0 silk suture, gauze pads, antiseptic solution, gloves, a mask and a hat, a 10-mL syringe, 0.5 normal or 0.25 normal saline flush solution (saline with heparin 1–2 units/mL; to decrease thrombotic complications, it is recommended to use a continuous infusion with heparin), and a 22-gauge needle. Calibrated pressure transducer for gauge pressure monitoring.
III. Procedure
 A. Place the patient supine. Wrap a diaper around both legs and tape the diaper to the bed. This stabilizes the patient for the procedure and allows observation of the feet for vasospasm.

B. Put on sterile gloves, a mask, a hat, and a sterile gown.

C. Prepare the umbilical catheter tray by attaching the stopcock to the blunt needle and then attaching the catheter to the blunt needle. Fill the 10-mL syringe with flush solution, and inject it through the catheter.

D. Clean the umbilical cord area with antiseptic solution. Place sterile drapes around the umbilicus, leaving the feet and head exposed. Observe the infant closely during the procedure for vasospasm in the legs or signs of distress.

E. Tie a piece of umbilical tape around the base of the umbilical cord tightly enough to minimize blood loss but loosely enough so that the catheter can be passed easily through the vessel (ie, snug but not tight). Cut off the excess umbilical cord with scissors or a scalpel, leaving a 1-cm stump (Figure 23-1A). A scalpel usually makes a cleaner cut, so that the vessels are more easily seen. There are *usually* two umbilical arteries and one umbilical vein. The arteries are smaller and are usually located at the 4- and 7-o'clock positions. The vein usually has a floppy wall (Figure 23–1B).

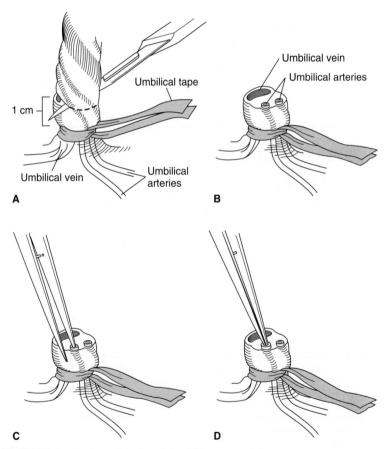

FIGURE 23–1. (**A**) The umbilical cord should be amputated, leaving a 1-cm stump. (**B**) Identification of the umbilical cord vessels. (**C** and **D**) A forceps is used to gently dilate the umbilical artery.

F. Using the curved hemostat, grasp the end of the umbilicus to hold it upright and steady.

G. Use the forceps to open and dilate the umbilical artery. First, place one arm of the forceps in the artery, and then use both arms to gently dilate the vessel (Figure 23–1C and D).

H. Once the artery is sufficiently dilated, insert the catheter.

I. Be certain you know the correct length of catheter to be inserted. The catheter is positioned in one of two ways. In "**low catheterization**," the tip of the catheter lies below the level of L3 or L4. In "**high catheterization**," the tip lies above the diaphragm at the level of T6-T9. Positioning is usually determined by the routine at a given institution. A recent meta-analysis recommends high catheters over low because of the fewer vascular-related complications. High positioning is associated with a decreased incidence of vascular complications, and studies have revealed there is no statistically significant increase in hypertension, intraventricular hemorrhage, necrotizing enterocolitis, or hematuria. High positioning is also associated with a lower incidence of blanching and cyanosis of the extremities. Low positioning has been associated with more episodes of vasospasm of the lower extremities. The length of catheter needed can be obtained from the **umbilical catheter measurements** (Figure 23–2). A rapid method for determining the length needed for low catheterization is to measure two thirds of the distance from the umbilicus to the midportion of the clavicle.

J. Once the catheter is in position, aspirate to verify blood return.

K. There are multiple ways to secure the catheter.

  1. **Method 1.** Secure the catheter as shown in Figure 23–3. The silk tape is folded over part of the way, the catheter is placed, and the remaining portion of the tape is folded over. Suture the silk tape to the base of the umbilical cord (through the Wharton jelly, not the skin or vessels) using 3–0 silk sutures. Connect the tubing to the monitor and flush it. No special dressing is needed. The umbilical stump with the catheter in place is left open to the air. Once the catheter is secure, loosen the umbilical tape.

  2. **Method 2.** Place a purse string suture around the base of the cord (not the skin or vessels). Lightly tighten the suture, and then you can sew the ends through a piece of tape (as in method 1).

  3. **Method 3.** Place a purse string around the base of the cord, and then you can wrap the ends of the suture around the catheter and tie.

  4. **Method 4.** Secure the catheter with a tape bridge.

L. Obtain an abdominal radiograph to verify the position of a low catheter or a chest radiograph to check the position of a high catheter. Figure 23–4 shows landmarks and the relationship of umbilical arteries to the other major abdominal arteries. Radiographs showing positioning can be found in Chapter 10.

IV. **Complications**

  A. **Infection.** Infection can be minimized by using strict sterile technique. No attempt should be made to advance a catheter once it has been placed and sutured into position; instead, the catheter should be replaced.

  B. **Vascular accidents.** Thrombosis, embolism, or infarction may occur. Vasospasm may lead to loss of an extremity. **Hypertension** is a long-term complication caused by stenosis of the renal artery as a result of improper catheter placement near the renal arteries. Loss of any extremity is rare but can occur. Air embolism has also been reported. Congestive heart failure from aortic thrombosis and paraplegia can also occur.

  C. **Hemorrhage.** Hemorrhage may occur if the catheter or tubing becomes disconnected. The tubing stopcocks must be securely fastened. If hemorrhage occurs, blood volume replacement may be necessary.

  D. **Vessel perforation.** The catheter should never be forced into position. If the catheter cannot be easily advanced, use of another vessel should be attempted. If perforation occurs, surgical intervention may be necessary.

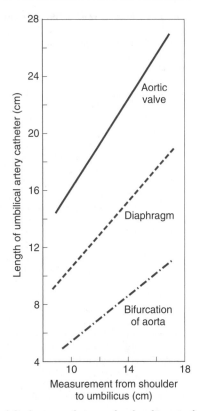

FIGURE 23–2. The umbilical artery catheter can be placed in one of two positions. The low catheter is placed below the level of L3 to avoid the renal and mesenteric vessels. The high catheter is placed between the thoracic vertebrae from T6 to T9. The graph is used as a guide to help determine the catheter length for each position. The low line corresponds to the aortic bifurcation in the graph, whereas a high line corresponds to the diaphragm. To determine catheter length, measure (in centimeters) a perpendicular line from the top of the shoulder to the umbilicus. This determines the shoulder-umbilical length. Plot this number on the graph to determine the proper catheter length for the umbilical artery catheter. Add the length of the umbilical stump to the catheter length. (*Based on data from Dunn PM: Localization of the umbilical catheter by postmortem measurement.* Arch Dis Child *1966;41:69.*)

    E. **Necrotizing enterocolitis.** Intestinal necrosis or perforation has been reported.
    F. **Improperly placed catheter.** This can cause perforation of a vessel, false aneurysm, perforation of the peritoneum, sciatic nerve palsy, and refractory hypoglycemia.
    G. **Other complications that can occur.** Injury and rupture of the bladder, urinary ascites, Wharton jelly or cotton fiber embolus, hypernatremia, and factitious hypernatremia or hyperkalemia.

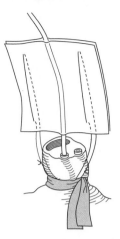

FIGURE 23–3. The umbilical artery catheter is secured with silk tape, which is attached to the base of the cord (through the Wharton's jelly, not the skin or vessels).

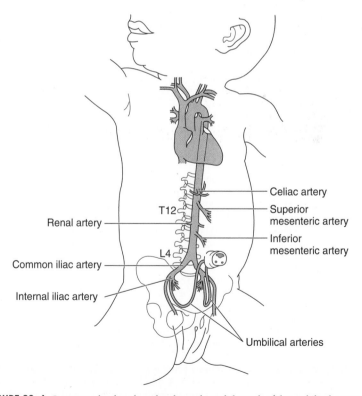

FIGURE 23–4. Important landmarks, related vessels, and the path of the umbilical artery. The internal iliac artery is also called the hypogastric artery.

24 Bladder Aspiration (Suprapubic Urine Collection)

I. **Indications.** To obtain urine for culture when a less invasive technique is not possible. It is the most accurate and preferred culture source for infants when compared with urethra catheterization and bag urine specimens. Any bacteria or growth on a suprapubic culture is considered abnormal and requires treatment.

II. **Equipment.** Sterile gloves, povidone-iodine solution, a 23- or 25-gauge 1-in needle (a 21- to 22-gauge $1^1/_2$-in needle can be used in a larger infant) with a 3-mL syringe attached, 4 × 4 gauze pads, gloves, and a sterile container. Transillumination or ultrasound may also be used.

III. **Procedure**

    A. Bladder aspiration is contraindicated in thrombocytopenia, bleeding disorders, cellulitis at the site, after recent lower abdominal or urologic surgery or if the bladder is empty.

    B. Verify that voiding has not occurred within the previous hour so there will be enough urine in the bladder to make collection worthwhile. Transillumination or ultrasound of the bladder can help determine the size and location of the bladder. Ultrasound significantly improves diagnostic yield; a minimum volume on ultrasound of 10 mL is associated with a 90% successful bladder aspiration. If the cephalocaudal diameter of the bladder (sagittal view) was >20 mm and the anteroposterior diameter was >15 mm, the success rate approaches 100%.

    C. An assistant should hold the infant in a supine position with the legs in the frog-leg position.

    D. Locate the site of bladder puncture, which is ~1–2 cm above the pubic symphysis, in the midline of the lower abdomen. In neonates the bladder is located predominantly intra-abdominally.

    E. Put on sterile gloves, and clean the skin at the puncture site with antiseptic solution three times. Local anesthesia often turns this from a "one-stick" to a "two-stick procedure." Lidocaine or topical anesthetic agents may be used. (See Chapter 69.)

    F. Palpate the pubic symphysis. Insert the needle 1–2 cm above the pubic symphysis at a 90-degree angle (Figure 24–1).

    G. Advance the needle while aspirating ~2–3 cm. Once urine is seen in the syringe, do not advance the needle >1–2 cm; this helps prevent perforation of the posterior wall of the bladder. Use gentle suction when aspirating to prevent the needle from suctioning the bladder wall and preventing the collection of urine.

    H. Withdraw the needle, maintain pressure over the site of puncture, and apply a bandage.

    I. Place a sterile cap on the syringe or transfer the specimen to a sterile urine cup, and submit the specimen to the laboratory.

IV. **Complications**

    A. **Bleeding.** Microscopic hematuria is common and rarely causes concern. Gross hemorrhage is more likely if there is a bleeding disorder. With thrombocytopenia, the procedure should not be performed. Hematomas (abdominal wall, pelvic and bladder wall) are rare.

    B. **Infection (rare).** Infection is not likely to occur if strict sterile technique is used. Sepsis, abdominal wall abscess, and osteomyelitis of the pubic bone have all been reported but are very rare.

    C. **Perforation of the bowel or other pelvic organs.** With careful identification of the landmarks, this complication is rare. If the bowel is perforated (indicated by the aspiration of bowel contents), close observation is recommended, and intravenous antibiotics should be considered. Surgical consultation may be obtained.

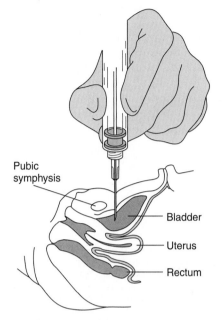

FIGURE 24–1. Technique of suprapubic bladder aspiration.

25 Bladder Catheterization

I. **Indications**
   A. To collect a urine specimen when a clean-catch specimen cannot be obtained or is unsatisfactory or suprapubic aspiration cannot be performed.
   B. To monitor urinary output, relieve urinary retention, or to instill contrast to obtain a cystogram or voiding cystourethrogram.
   C. To determine a bladder residual.
II. **Equipment.** Sterile gloves, cotton balls, povidone-iodine solution, sterile drapes, lubricant, a sterile collection bottle (often packaged together as a commercial set), urethral catheters (3.5, 5.0, 6.5, and 8F urinary catheters). A 5F feeding tube and a 3.5 or 5F umbilical catheter may be used as an alternative to a urethral catheter. General guidelines are: 3.5F, infants <1000 g; 5F, infants weighing 1000–1800 g; 8F, infants weighing >1800 g). Try to use the smallest catheter possible to avoid trauma.
III. **Procedure**
   Bladder catheterization is an acceptable alternative to suprapubic aspiration but is not the method of first choice.
   A. **Males**
      1. Place the infant supine, with the thighs abducted (frog-leg position).
      2. Cleanse the penis with povidone-iodine solution, starting with the meatus and moving in a proximal direction.
      3. Put on sterile gloves, and drape the area with sterile towels.

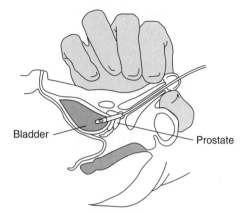

FIGURE 25–1. Bladder catheterization in the male.

4. Place the tip of the catheter in sterile lubricant.
5. Hold the penis approximately perpendicular to the body to straighten the penile urethra and help prevent false passage. Advance the catheter until urine appears. A slight resistance may be felt as the catheter passes the external sphincter, and steady, gentle pressure is usually needed to advance past this area. Never force the catheter (Figure 25–1).
6. Collect the urine specimen. If the catheter is to remain in place, some physicians believe it should be taped to the lower abdomen rather than to the leg in males to help decrease stricture formation caused by pressure on the posterior urethra.
B. **Females**
1. Place the infant supine, with the thighs abducted (frog-leg position).
2. Separate the labia, and cleanse the area around the meatus with povidone-iodine solution. Use anterior-to-posterior strokes to prevent fecal contamination.
3. Put on sterile gloves, and drape sterile towels around the labia.
4. Spread the labia with two fingers. See Figure 25–2 for landmarks used in the catheterization of the bladder in females. Lubricate the catheter, and advance it in

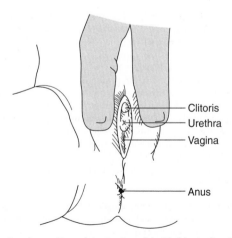

FIGURE 25–2. Landmarks used in catheterization of the bladder in females.

the urethra until urine appears. Tape the catheter to the leg if it is to remain in position.

IV. **Complications**
  A. **Infection.** The risk of introducing bacteria into the urinary tact and then the bloodstream is common. Sterile technique is necessary to help prevent infection. "In-and-out" catheterization carries a small (<5%) risk of urinary tract infection. The longer a catheter is left in place, the greater is the infection risk. Infections that can occur include sepsis, cystitis, pyelonephritis, urethritis, and epididymitis.
  B. **Trauma to the urethra ("false passage") or the bladder.** Urethral tear, erosion, stricture, meatal stenosis or perforation, or bladder injury (perforation) is more common in males. Minimize by adequately lubricating the catheter and stretching the penis to straighten the urethra. Never force the catheter if resistance is felt. Use the smallest catheter possible and advance only until urine is obtained.
  C. **Hematuria.** Hematuria is usually transient but may require irrigation with normal saline solution. Gross hematuria on insertion may indicate a false passage.
  D. **Urethral stricture.** Stricture is more common in males. It is usually caused by a catheter that is too large or by prolonged or traumatic catheterization. In males, taping the catheter to the anterior abdominal wall helps decrease the pressure on the posterior urethra.
  E. **Urinary retention** secondary to urethral edema.
  F. **Catheter knot** can happen if the catheter advances too far. Insert only enough to obtain urine and never force a catheter. Using appropriate lengths based on age and sex may help prevent this complication (6 cm for male and 5 cm for female term newborns). Using a feeding tube may increase the risk of a catheter knot because these tubes are softer and coil more easily.

26 Chest Tube Placement

I. **Indications**
  A. Tension pneumothorax causing respiratory compromise and decreased venous return to the heart, resulting in decreased cardiac output and hypotension. **This is an emergency that should be handled by immediate needle aspiration before tube placement.** (See Chapter 63.)
  B. Pneumothorax compromising ventilation and causing increased work of breathing, hypoxia, and increased $Paco_2$.
  C. Drainage of significant pleural fluid (pleural effusion, empyema, chylothorax, hemothorax).
  D. Postsurgical drainage after repair of a tracheoesophageal fistula or esophageal atresia.
II. **Equipment.** Prepackaged chest tube tray (sterile towels, 4×4 gauze pads, 3–0 silk suture, curved hemostats, a no. 11 or 15 scalpel, scissors, a needle holder, antiseptic solution, antibiotic ointment, 1% lidocaine, 3-mL syringe, and a 25-gauge needle); chest tube 10F for infants <2000 g, 12F for infants >2000 g. Sterile gloves, a mask, eye protection, hat, and gown, and a suction-drainage system (eg, the Pleur-Evac system) are also needed.
III. **Procedure**
  A. The site of chest tube insertion is determined by examining the anteroposterior and cross-table lateral or lateral decubitus chest films. Air collects in the uppermost areas of the chest, and fluid in the most dependent areas. For air collections, place the tube anteriorly. For fluid collections, place the tube posteriorly and laterally. **Transillumination**

of the chest may help detect pneumothorax. With the lights in the room turned down, a strong light source is placed on the anterior chest wall above the nipple and in the axilla. The affected side usually appears hyperlucent and "lights up" compared with the unaffected side. Transillumination may not reveal a small pneumothorax. Unless the infant's status is rapidly deteriorating, a chest radiograph should be obtained to confirm pneumothorax before the chest tube is inserted. See Figure 10–19 for a radiograph showing a left tension pneumothorax.

B. Position the patient so the site of insertion is accessible. The most common position is supine, with the arm at a 90-degree angle on the affected side.

C. Select the appropriate site (Figure 26–1). For anterior placement, the site should be the second or third intercostal space at the midclavicular line. For posterior placement, use the fourth, fifth, or sixth intercostal space at the anterior axillary line. The nipple is a landmark for the fourth intercostal space.

D. Put on a sterile gown, mask, hat, and gloves. Cleanse the area of insertion with povidone-iodine solution, and drape.

E. Infiltrate the area superficially with 0.5–1% lidocaine (see dose in Chapter 69) and then down to the rib. Infiltrate into the intercostal muscles and along the parietal pleura. Make a small incision (approximately the width of the tube, usually ≤0.75 cm) in the skin over the rib just below the intercostal space where the tube is to be inserted (Figure 26–2A).

F. Insert a closed curved hemostat into the incision, and spread the tissues down to the rib. Using the tip of the hemostat, puncture the pleura just above the rib and spread gently. The intercostal vein, artery, and nerve lie below the ribs (see Figure 26–2A). This creates a subcutaneous tunnel that aids in closing the tract when the tube is removed.

G. When the pleura has been penetrated, a rush of air is often heard or fluid appears.

H. Insert the chest tube through the opened hemostat (see Figure 26–2B). Be certain that the side holes of the tube are within the pleural cavity. The presence of moisture

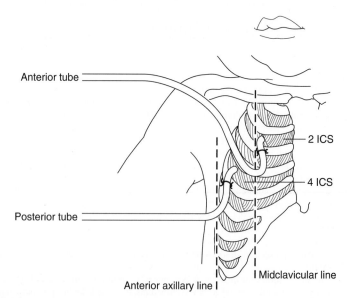

FIGURE 26–1. Recommended sites for chest tube insertion in the neonate: 2 ICS and 4 ICS (second and fourth intercostal space.)

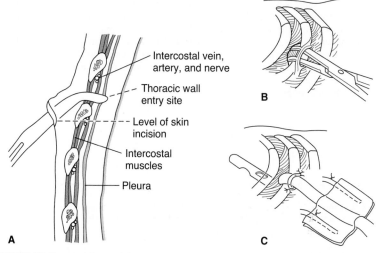

FIGURE 26–2. Procedures of chest tube insertion. (**A**) Level of skin incision and thoracic wall entry site in relation to the rib and the neurovascular bundle. (**B**) Opened hemostat, through which the chest tube is inserted. (**C**) The chest tube is then secured to the skin with silk sutures.

in the tube usually confirms proper placement in the intrapleural cavity in a pneumothorax. Use of a trocar guide is usually unnecessary and may increase the risk of complications such as lung perforation. **The chest tube should be inserted 2–3 cm for a small preterm infant and 3–4 cm for a term infant.** (These are guidelines only; the length of tube to be inserted varies based on the size of the infant.) An alternative approach to tube insertion is to measure the length from the insertion site to the apex of the lung (approximately the midclavicle) and tie a silk suture around the tube the same distance from the tip. Position the tube until the silk suture is just outside the skin.

I. Hold the tube steady first and then allow an assistant to connect the tube to a water-seal vacuum drainage system (eg, the Pleur-Evac system). Five to 10 cm of suction is usually used. Start at the lower level of suction and increase as needed if the pneumothorax or effusion does not resolve. Systems such as the Pleur-Evac provide both continuous suction and water seal. A water seal prevents air from being drawn back into the pleural space.

J. Secure the chest tube with 3–0 silk sutures and silk tape (see Figure 26–2C). Close the skin opening with sutures if necessary. Obtain an immediate chest radiograph to verify placement and check for residual fluid or pneumothorax. Positioning of the tube must always be verified by a chest radiograph.

IV. **Complications**

A. **Infection.** Strict sterile technique helps minimize infections. Cellulitis is common. Intrapleural inoculation of Candida has been reported after chest tube placement. Many institutions recommend prophylactic antibiotics (eg, nafcillin [see Chapter 132]) when a chest tube is placed (**controversial**).

B. **Bleeding.** Bleeding may occur if one of the major vessels (intercostal, axillary, pulmonary, or internal mammary) is perforated or if the lung is damaged during the procedure. This complication can be avoided if landmarks are properly identified. Bleeding is less likely if a trocar is not used. Bleeding may stop during suctioning; however, if significant bleeding continues, immediate surgical consultation is necessary.

C. Nerve damage. Passing the tube over the top of the rib helps avoid injury to the intercostal nerve running under the rib. Horner syndrome, and diaphragmatic paralysis or eventration from phrenic nerve injury has been reported.

D. Trauma. Lung trauma (perforation or laceration) can be minimized by never forcing the tube into position. Trauma can also occur to the breast tissue.

E. Subcutaneous emphysema secondary to a leak through the pleural opening.

F. Chylothorax.

G. Cardiac tamponade.

27 Defibrillation and Cardioversion

Defibrillation and cardioversion are used for rapid termination of a tachyarrhythmia (a fast abnormal rhythm originating either in the atrium or ventricle) that is unresponsive to baseline treatment or is causing the patient to have cardiovascular compromise (inadequate systemic perfusion). Baseline treatment consists of correction of a metabolic problem, use of vagal maneuvers (bag of ice water over the eyes and face of the infant without obstructing the airway, putting pressure on closed eyelids), use of medications (adenosine, digoxin, propranolol, verapamil, amiodarone, procainamide, lidocaine, or magnesium sulfate), or transesophageal pacing. It is best to try these maneuvers or medical therapy if intravenous access is available. **Neonatal arrhythmias are rare, and the majority of them can be treated with these initial measures.**

Current defibrillators are capable of delivering two modes of shock: synchronized and unsynchronized. Synchronized shocks are lower dose and used for cardioversion. Unsynchronized shocks are higher dose and used for defibrillation. **Pediatric cardiology consultation is recommended for all infants with a tachyarrhythmia.**

I. Indications

A. **Cardioversion.** Synchronized cardioversion is used for:

1. Unstable patients with tachyarrhythmias who have a perfusing rhythm but evidence of poor perfusion, heart failure, or hypotension (signs of cardiovascular compromise). Examples of tachyarrhythmias are:

a. Tachycardia (supraventricular tachycardia [SVT] or ventricular tachycardia [VT]) with a pulse and poor perfusion.

b. Supraventricular tachycardia with shock and no vascular access.

c. Atrial flutter with shock.

d. Atrial fibrillation with shock (very rare in infants).

2. Elective cardioversion in infants with **stable** SVT, VT, or atrial flutter (good tissue perfusion and pulses) unresponsive to other treatments. This is always done under the close supervision of a pediatric cardiologist. Sedation and a 12-lead electrocardiogram are recommended prior to cardioversion.

B. **Defibrillation (asynchronized)** is used in pulseless arrest with a shockable rhythm (VT and ventricular fibrillation). It is used in between cardiopulmonary resuscitation (CPR) and **not used in asystole or pulseless electrical activity.** The most common cause of a ventricular arrhythmia in a neonate is electrolyte imbalance. Defibrillation will not stop the arrhythmia in these patients. **Defibrillation is the most effective treatment** for:

1. Ventricular fibrillation.

2. Pulseless ventricular tachycardia.

II. Equipment

A. External standard defibrillator (manual or semiautomated) and two paddles of the correct sizes with conductive pads. For infants, use the smallest size. It is important to be familiar with the institution's equipment because there are many different types and models of machines. Pediatric-capable automatic external defibrillators have been approved by the U.S. Food and Drug Administration but are not readily available yet.

B. Other equipment includes a heart rate monitor, airway equipment, resuscitation medications, antiarrhythmic medications, and equipment used in basic and advanced life support.

III. Procedure

A. Adequate sedation (may not be possible in emergency situations) and preoxygenation are essential. Emergency airway equipment should be readily available. Continuous heart monitoring should be done during the procedure.

B. Wipe any cream or soap off the chest.

C. Place the paddles firmly on the chest wall. To prevent skin burns, be sure the conductive pad totally covers the paddle and that the skin is not in contact with any non-insulated part of the paddle. There are two different positions for pad placement (Figures 27–1 and 27–2).

1. Anterior-lateral positioning (Figure 27–1). The anterior pad is placed to the right of the upper sternum, and the posterior pad placed below the left nipple toward the axilla.

2. Anterior–posterior positioning (Figure 27–2). This may be preferred in atrial tachycardia. The anterior pad is placed on the midsternal border and the posterior pad is placed between the scapulae. The paddles or pads should not be in contact with one another. **With dextrocardia, the pads need to be placed across the right chest.**

D. Charge the defibrillator.

1. Cardioversion uses lower energy. Charge the defibrillator to **0.5 J/kg** and synchronize. **The SYNC button must be activated each time because the default setting on a defibrillator is on the asynchronized setting.**

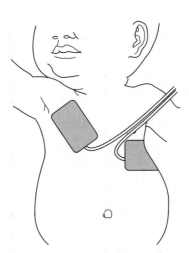

FIGURE 27–1. Anterior-lateral pad and paddle placement.

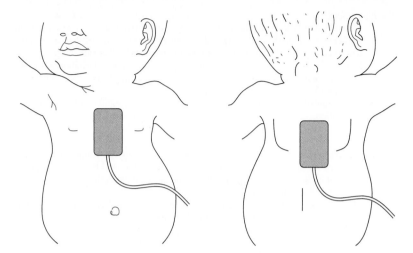

FIGURE 27–2. Anterior-posterior pad and paddle placement.

2. **Defibrillation** uses higher energy. **Charge the defibrillator to 2J/kg.**
3. **Once charged, make sure everybody is clear of the patient, including the person holding the oxygen.** Ask if everyone is clear and visually check while they answer. Use the phrase **"I'm clear, you're clear, oxygen clear."** Verify that oxygen is not flowing across the area. It is best to disconnect the bag and verify that no one is touching the endotracheal tube or any part of the ventilation circuit. The machine will indicate that it is charged and ready for discharge with an audible signal and/or a flashing red light either on the machine or the end of the paddle based on the model.
   E. **Deliver the shock** by pressing both buttons together.
      1. **Cardioversion.** If the first attempt does not work, additional attempts should be made. **Repeat steps C–E using 1 J/kg, then up to a max of 2 J/kg.**
      2. **Defibrillation.** In pulseless infants, continue CPR with appropriate compressions, ventilation, and medications between attempts. Additional attempts should be made by repeating steps C–E. **The second and any subsequent shock should have a dose of 4 J/kg.** Acidosis and hypoxia decrease the success of defibrillation, and correction increases the likelihood of success.
IV. **Complications**
   A. **Altered skin integrity.** Soft tissue injury, chest wall lesions, skin burns, bruising, and pain can occur.
   B. **Embolic phenomenon.** Atrial or ventricular thrombus can dislodge and travel to the lungs or systemically, resulting in stroke or organ damage. This is most common in atrial fibrillation.
   C. **Pulmonary edema** is a rare complication.
   D. **Respiratory arrest.**
   E. **Neurologic impairment.**
   F. **Cardiac arrhythmia.**
   G. **Profound bradycardia/asystole** can occur after cardioversion, and it may not respond to medication or temporary pacing.

H. **Myocardial damage.** When excessive energy is delivered, heart tissue can be damaged.
I. **Cardiogenic shock.**
J. **Fire (rare).** A case report of a fire that resulted from sparks in the presence of oxygen and cotton. The infant's stocking cap and part of the sheet caught on fire.
K. **Electrical shock to health-care providers.**

28 Endotracheal Intubation

I. **Indications**
   A. To provide mechanical respiratory support.
   B. To obtain aspirates for culture.
   C. To assist in bronchopulmonary hygiene ("pulmonary toilet").
   D. To alleviate upper airway obstruction (subglottic stenosis).
   E. To clear the trachea of meconium.
   F. Selective bronchial ventilation.
   G. Diaphragmatic hernia.
   H. To administer medications in the emergency setting before intravenous access is established.
II. **Equipment.** A correct endotracheal tube (Table 28–1), a pediatric laryngoscope handle with a Miller blade ("00" blade for extremely preterm infants, "0" blade for preterm infants, 1 blade for full-term infants; straight blades are preferred over curved blades), a bag-and-mask apparatus, an endotracheal tube adapter, a suction apparatus, tape, scissors, a malleable stylet (*optional*), personal protection equipment, and tincture of benzoin. A bag-and-mask apparatus with 100% oxygen should be available at the bedside. The mechanical ventilator should be checked and ready. Monitoring with electrocardiogram and pulse oximetry is essential if time permits.
III. **Procedure**
   A. Oropharyngeal intubation is more commonly performed emergently and is described here. Nasotracheal intubation is more commonly performed in the elective setting or if anatomy precludes the oral route. The endotracheal tube should be precut to

Table 28–1. GUIDELINES FOR ENDOTRACHEAL TUBE SIZE AND DEPTH OF INSERTION BASED ON WEIGHT AND GESTATIONAL AGE

Weight (g)	Gestational Age (wk)	Endotracheal Tube Size, Inside Diameter (mm)	Depth of Insertion (cm from upper lip)
<1000	<28	2.5	6 (if < 750 g)–7
1000–2000	28–34	3.0	7–8
2000–3000	34–38	3.5	8–9
>3000	>38	3.5–4.0	9–10

Based on guidelines from Kattwinkel J: *Textbook of Neonatal Resuscitation*, 5th ed. EIK Grove, IL: American Heart Association/American Academy of Pediatrics, 2006.

eliminate dead space (cut to 15 cm). Some newer tubes are marked "oral" or "nasal" and should be cut appropriately.

B. Be certain that the light source on the laryngoscope is working before beginning the procedure. Place the stylet (if used) in the endotracheal tube. Flexible stylets are optional but may help guide the tube into position more efficiently. Be sure the tip of the stylet does not protrude out of the end of the endotracheal tube.

C. Place the infant in the "sniffing position" (with the neck slightly extended); a small roll behind the neck may help with positioning. Hyperextension of the neck in infants may cause the trachea to collapse. The infant's head should be at the same level as the operator.

D. Cautiously suction the oropharynx as needed to make the landmarks clearly visible.

E. Preoxygenate the infant with a bag-and-mask device, and monitor the heart rate, color, and pulse oximeter. **To limit hypoxia, limit each intubation attempt to <20 sec before reoxygenation.**

F. Hold the laryngoscope with your left hand. Insert the scope into the right side of the mouth, and sweep the tongue to the left side. Some practitioners move the tongue to the left by using the index finger of the right hand placed alongside the head. To perform this maneuver, stabilize the head and hold the mouth open.

G. Advance the blade a few millimeters, passing it beneath the epiglottis.

H. Lift the blade vertically to elevate the epiglottis and visualize the glottis (Figure 28–1). *Note:* The purpose of the laryngoscope is to lift the epiglottis vertically, not to pry it open. To better visualize the vocal cords, an assistant may place gentle external pressure on the thyroid cartilage.

I. Pass the endotracheal tube along the right side of the mouth and down past the vocal cords during inspiration. It is best to advance the tube *only* 2–2.5 cm into the trachea to avoid placement in the right main stem bronchus (no more than 1–2 cm below the vocal cords).

J. It may be helpful to tape the tube at the lip when the tube has been advanced 7 cm in a 1-kg infant, 8 cm in a 2-kg infant, 9 cm in a 3-kg infant, or 10 cm in a 4-kg infant (**the rule of "1, 2, 3, 4, 7, 8, 9, 10"**). Infants weighing <750 g may only require a 6-cm insertion (see Table 28–1). **Another way to remember suggested depth is 6 plus the patient's weight in kilograms.** This rule does not work in infants with congenital anomalies of the neck such as Pierre Robin syndrome. The stylet should be removed gently while the tube is held in position.

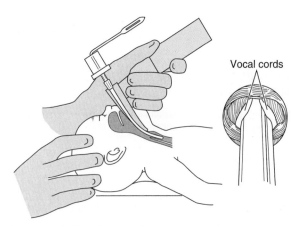

Vocal cords

FIGURE 28–1. Endotracheal intubation in the neonate.

K. Confirm the position of the tube. The resuscitation bag is attached to the tube using the adapter, and an assistant provides mechanical breaths while the operator listens for equal breath sounds on both sides of the chest. Auscultate the stomach to be certain that the esophagus was not intubated. End tidal carbon dioxide detectors are commercially available that rapidly confirm proper endotracheal placement.

L. Paint the skin with tincture of benzoin. Tape the tube securely in place.

M. Obtain a chest radiograph to confirm proper placement of the tube. Figure 10–7 shows proper placement of an endotracheal tube.

N. **Certain emergency medications can be given through the endotracheal tube.** These medications are lidocaine, atropine, naloxone, and epinephrine. These can be remembered by the mnemonic "LANE" or "NEAL."

IV. Complications

A. **Tracheal perforation and trauma.** Tracheal perforation is a rare complication requiring surgical intervention. It can be prevented by careful use of the laryngoscope and the endotracheal tube.

B. **Esophageal perforation** is usually caused by traumatic intubation, and treatment depends on the degree of perforation. Most injuries can be managed by use of parenteral nutrition until the leak seals, use of broad-spectrum antibiotics, and observation for signs of infection. A barium swallow contrast study may be necessary after several weeks to evaluate healing or rule out stricture formation.

C. **Laryngeal edema.** is usually seen after extubation and may cause respiratory distress. A short course of steroids (eg, dexamethasone) can be given intravenously before and just after extubation. However, systemic dexamethasone has no effect in reducing acute postextubation stridor in neonates.

D. **Improper tube positioning (esophageal intubation, right main stem bronchus).** Signs of esophageal intubation include poor chest movement, zero mist in the tube, continued cyanosis, gastric distension, and air heard over the stomach. Signs of right main stem bronchus intubation include breath sounds heard over the right chest and none heard over the left and no improvement in color.

E. **Tube obstruction or kinking.** Try suctioning or possibly reintubation.

F. **Infection.**

G. **Palatal grooves.** Palatal grooves are usually seen in cases of long-term intubation and typically resolve with time.

H. **Subglottic stenosis.** Subglottic stenosis is most often associated with long-term (>3–4 weeks) endotracheal intubation. Surgical correction is usually necessary. With prolonged intubation, consideration may be given to surgical tracheostomy to help prevent stenosis.

29 Exchange Transfusion

Exchange transfusion is a technique used most often to maintain serum bilirubin at levels below neurotoxicity. Serum levels of bilirubin for which to begin an exchange transfusion are currently under considerable debate (for more details, see Chapters 51 and 92). Exchange transfusions are also used to control other conditions, such as polycythemia or anemia. Three types of exchange transfusion are commonly used: (1) 2-volume exchange, (2) isovolumetric 2-volume exchange, and (3) partial exchange (<2 volumes) with normal saline, 5% albumin in saline, or plasma protein fraction (Plasmanate). These procedures are used primarily in sick newborn infants but may also be used for intrauterine exchanges in fetuses at high risk for central nervous system toxicity (eg, erythroblastosis fetalis) by percutaneous umbilical blood sampling and umbilical vein catheterization under ultrasound guidance.

I. **Indications**

A. **Hyperbilirubinemia.** Exchange transfusions are used in infants with hyperbilirubinemia of any origin when the serum bilirubin level reaches or exceeds a level that puts the infant at risk for central nervous system toxicity (eg, kernicterus) if left untreated (see Table 51–1 and Table 92–3). Two-volume exchange transfusions taking 50–70 min are usually recommended for removal and reduction of serum bilirubin. Efficiency of bilirubin removal is increased in slower exchanges because of extravascular and intravascular bilirubin equilibration.

B. **Hemolytic disease of the newborn** results from destruction of fetal red blood cells (RBCs) by passively acquired maternal antibodies. Exchange transfusion aids in removing antibody-coated RBCs, thereby prolonging intravascular RBC survival. It also removes potentially toxic bilirubin from an increased bilirubin load resulting from RBC breakdown and provides plasma volume and albumin for bilirubin binding. Repeated 2-volume exchange transfusions may be needed when RBC destruction is rapid.

C. **Sepsis.** Neonatal sepsis may be associated with shock caused by bacterial endotoxins. A 2-volume exchange may help remove bacteria, toxins, fibrin split products, and accumulated lactic acid. It may also provide immunoglobulins, complement, and coagulating factors.

D. **Disseminated intravascular coagulation (DIC) from multiple causes.** A 2-volume exchange transfusion is preferred; however, depending on the sick infant's condition, any one of the exchange methods may help provide necessary coagulation factors and help reduce the underlying cause of the abnormal coagulation. Repletion of clotting factors by transfusion of fresh-frozen plasma (10–15 mL/kg) may be all that is necessary in less severe cases of DIC.

E. **Metabolic disorders causing severe acidosis (eg, aminoaciduria with associated hyperammonemia).** Partial exchanges are usually acceptable. Peritoneal dialysis may also be useful for treating some progressive metabolic disorders.

F. **Severe fluid or electrolyte imbalance (eg, hyperkalemia, hypernatremia, or fluid overload).** Isovolumetric partial exchanges are recommended to prevent large electrolyte fluctuations with each aliquot of blood exchanged. Transfusions with blood products may bind calcium; therefore, calcium gluconate should be available. Fresh blood products should be used to prevent contribution of the by-products of older blood, such as excess potassium.

G. **Polycythemia.** It is usually best to give a partial exchange transfusion using normal saline. Plasma protein fraction (eg, Plasmanate) or 5% albumin in saline may also be used; however, normal saline is preferred because it reduces both the polycythemia and the hyperviscosity of the infant's circulating blood volume. Either plasma protein fraction or 5% albumin may leave viscosity unchanged despite reductions in circulating red cell mass.

H. **Severe anemia (normovolemic or hypervolemic) causing cardiac failure,** as in hydrops fetalis, is best treated with a partial exchange transfusion using packed RBCs.

I. **Any disorder requiring complement, opsonins, or gammaglobulin.** Infants with these conditions may require frequent exchanges, and their fluid status must be carefully managed. Partial exchanges are recommended.

II. **Equipment**

A. Radiant warmer.

B. Equipment for respiratory support and resuscitation (eg, oxygen and a suctioning device). This equipment and medications used in resuscitation should be immediately available.

C. Equipment for monitoring the heart rate, blood pressure, respiratory rate, temperature, Pao_2, $Paco_2$, and Spo_2 must be utilized. Immediate access to blood gas determinations is also needed.

   D. Equipment for umbilical artery and umbilical vein catheterization (see Chapters 23 and 38).
   E. Disposable exchange transfusion tray.
   F. Nasogastric tube for evacuating the stomach before beginning the transfusion.
   G. A temperature-controlled device must be used for warming of the blood before and during the transfusion. The device should have an internal disposable coil and connectors to the donor blood bag and the exchange transfusion circuit. The blood should be warmed to 37°C. Use of makeshift water baths or heaters is not advised because blood that is too warm may hemolyze.
   H. An assistant to help maintain a sterile field, monitor and assess the infant, and record the procedure and exchanged volumes.
III. **Blood transfusion**
   A. **Blood collection**
      1. **Homologous blood.** Blood donated by an anonymous donor with a compatible blood type is most commonly used. Donor-directed blood (blood donated by a selected blood type–compatible person) is another option.
      2. **Cytomegalovirus (CMV).** Seronegative donor blood is preferred. White blood cells harboring CMV can be removed using leukodepletion filters during blood preparation. The use of frozen deglycerolized RBCs, reconstituted with fresh-frozen plasma, is another means of using seropositive blood free of viable CMV.
      3. **Hemoglobin S (sickle cell trait).** Precautions should be taken to avoid exchange transfusion with donor blood from a carrier. If the donor blood with sickle trait becomes acidic, sickling can occur with expected complications to the patient.
      4. **Graft-versus-host disease.** Consideration should be given for using irradiated donor blood to avoid graft-vs-host disease in known immune-compromised infants and low birthweight infants. Preterm infants who have been transfused in utero or who have received >50 mL of transfused blood are candidates for irradiated blood.
   B. **Blood typing and cross-matching**
      1. **Infants with Rh incompatibility.** The blood must be type O, Rh-negative, low-titer anti-A, anti-B blood. It must be cross-matched with the mother's plasma and RBCs.
      2. **Infants with ABO incompatibility.** The blood must be type O, Rh-compatible (with the mother and the infant) or Rh-negative, low-titer anti-A, anti-B blood. It must be cross-matched with both the infant's and mother's blood.
      3. **Other blood group incompatibilities.** For other hemolytic diseases (eg, anti-Rh-c, anti-Kell, anti-Duffy), blood must be cross-matched to the mother's blood to avoid offending antigens.
      4. **Hyperbilirubinemia, metabolic imbalance, or hemolysis not caused by isoimmune disorders.** The blood must be cross-matched against the infant's plasma and RBCs.
   C. **Freshness and preservation of blood.** In newborn infants, it is preferable to use blood or plasma that has been collected in citrate phosphate dextrose (CPD). The blood should be <72 h old. These two factors ensure that the blood pH is >7.0. For disorders associated with hydrops fetalis or fetal asphyxia, it is best to use blood that is <24 h old.
   D. **Hematocrit (Hct).** Most blood banks can reconstitute a unit of blood to a desired Hct of 50–70%. The blood should be agitated periodically during the transfusion to maintain a constant Hct.
   E. **Potassium levels in donor blood.** Potassium levels in the donor blood should be determined if the infant is asphyxiated or in shock and renal impairment is suspected. If potassium levels are >7 mEq/L, consider using a unit of blood that has been collected more recently or a unit of washed RBCs.
   F. **Temperature of the blood.** Warming of blood is especially important in low birthweight and sick newborn infants.

IV. **Procedure**
   A. Simple 2-volume exchange transfusion is used for uncomplicated hyperbilirubinemia.
      1. **The normal blood volume in a full-term newborn infant is 80 mL/kg.** In an infant weighing 2 kg, the volume would be 160 mL. Twice this volume of blood is exchanged in a 2-volume transfusion. Therefore, the amount of blood needed for a 2-kg infant would be 320 mL. Blood volume of low birthweight and extremely low birthweight newborns (which may be up to 95 mL/kg) should be taken into account when calculating exchange volumes.
      2. **Allow adequate time for blood typing and cross-matching** at the blood bank. The infant's bilirubin level increases during this time, and this increase must be taken into account when ordering the blood.
      3. **Perform the transfusion in an intensive care setting.** Place the infant in the supine position. Restraints must be snug but not tight. A nasogastric tube should be passed to evacuate the stomach and should be left in place to maintain gastric decompression and prevent regurgitation and aspiration of gastric juices.
      4. **Scrub and put on a sterile gown and gloves.**
      5. **Perform umbilical vein catheterization** and confirm the position by radiograph (see Figure 10–8) If an isovolumetric exchange is to be performed, then an umbilical artery catheter must also be placed and confirmed by radiograph (see Figure 10–9 for correct positioning of a high umbilical artery catheter and Figure 10–10 for correct positioning of a low umbilical artery catheter).
      6. **Have the unit of blood prepared.**
         a. **Check the blood types** of the donor and the infant.
         b. **Check the temperature** of the blood and warming procedures.
         c. **Check the Hct.** The blood should be agitated regularly to maintain a constant Hct.
      7. **Attach the bag of blood to the tubing and stopcocks according to the directions on the transfusion tray.** The orientation of the stopcocks for infusion and withdrawal must be double-checked by the assistant.
      8. **Establish the volume of each aliquot** (Table 29–1).
   B. **Isovolumetric 2-volume exchange transfusion.** Isovolumetric 2-volume exchange transfusion is performed using a double setup, with infusion via the umbilical vein and withdrawal via the umbilical artery. This method is preferred when volume shifts during simple exchange might cause or aggravate myocardial insufficiency (eg, hydrops fetalis). Two operators are usually needed: one to perform the infusion and the other to handle the withdrawal.
      1. **Perform steps 1–6** as in simple 2-volume exchange transfusion. In addition, perform umbilical artery catheterization.
      2. **Attach the unit of blood to the tubing and stopcocks attached to the umbilical vein catheter.** If the catheter is to be left in place after the exchange transfusion (usually to monitor central venous pressure), it should be placed above the diaphragm, with placement confirmed by chest radiograph.

Table 29–1. **ALIQUOTS USUALLY USED IN NEONATAL EXCHANGE TRANSFUSION**

Infant Weight	Aliquot (mL)
>3 kg	20
2–3 kg	15
1–2 kg	10
850 g–1 kg	5
<850 g	1–3

3. **The tubing and the stopcocks of the second setup** are attached to the umbilical artery catheter and to a sterile plastic bag for discarding the exchanged blood.
4. **If isovolumetric exchange is being performed because of cardiac failure,** the central venous pressure can be determined via the umbilical vein catheter; it should be placed above the diaphragm in the inferior vena cava.
C. **Partial exchange transfusion.** A partial exchange transfusion is performed in the same manner as 2-volume exchange transfusion. If a partial exchange is for poly-cythemia (using normal saline or another blood product) or for anemia (packed RBCs), the following formula can be used to determine the volume of the transfusion.

$$\text{Volume of exchange (mL)} =$$

$$\frac{\text{Estimated blood volume (mL)} \times \text{Weight (kg)} \times (\text{Observed Hct} - \text{Desired Hct})}{\text{Observed Hct}}$$

D. **Isovolumetric partial exchange transfusion** with packed RBCs is the best proce-dure in cases of severe hydrops fetalis.
E. **Ancillary procedures**
   1. **Laboratory studies.** Blood should be obtained for laboratory studies before and after exchange transfusion.
      a. **Blood chemistry studies** include total calcium, sodium, potassium, chloride, pH, $Paco_2$, acid-base status, bicarbonate, and serum glucose.
      b. **Hematologic studies** include hemoglobin, Hct, platelet count, white blood cell count, and differential count. Blood for retyping and cross-matching after exchange is often requested by the blood bank to verify typing and re-cross-matching and for study of transfusion reaction, if needed.
      c. **Blood culture** is recommended after exchange transfusion (**controversial**).
   2. **Administration of calcium gluconate.** The citrate buffer binds calcium and tran-siently lowers ionized calcium levels. Treatment of suspected hypocalcemia in patients receiving transfusions is **controversial**. Some physicians routinely admin-ister 1–2 mL of 10% calcium gluconate by slow infusion after 100–200 mL of exchange donor blood. Others maintain that this treatment has no therapeutic effect unless hypocalcemia is documented by electrocardiogram showing a change in the QT interval.
   3. **Phototherapy.** Begin or resume phototherapy after exchange transfusion for dis-orders involving a high bilirubin level.
   4. **Monitoring of serum bilirubin levels.** Continue to monitor serum bilirubin lev-els after transfusion at 2, 4, and 6 h and then at 6-h intervals. A rebound of biliru-bin levels is to be expected 2–4 h after the transfusion.
   5. **Remedication.** Patients receiving antibiotics or anticonvulsants need to be remed-icated. Unless the cardiac status is deteriorating or serum digoxin levels are too low, patients receiving digoxin should not be remedicated. The percentage of lost medications is extremely variable. As little as 2.4% of digoxin is lost, but up to 32.4% of theophylline may be lost during a 2-volume exchange transfusion. Deter-mination of drug levels after exchange transfusion is advisable
   6. **Antibiotic prophylaxis** after the transfusion should be considered on an individ-ual basis. Infection is uncommon but is the most frequent complication.
V. **Complications**
   A. **Infection.** Bacteremia (usually caused by a Staphylococcus organism), hepatitis, CMV infection, malaria, and AIDS have been reported.
   B. **Vascular complications.** Clot or air embolism, arteriospasm of the lower limbs, thrombosis, and infarction of major organs may occur.
   C. **Coagulopathies.** Coagulopathies may result from thrombocytopenia or diminished coagulation factors. Platelets may decrease by >50% after a 2-volume exchange transfusion.

D. **Electrolyte abnormalities.** Hyperkalemia and hypocalcemia can occur.
E. **Hypoglycemia.** Hypoglycemia is especially likely in infants of diabetic mothers and in those with erythroblastosis fetalis. Because of islet cell hyperplasia and hyperinsulinism, rebound hypoglycemia may result in these infants in response to the concentrated glucose (300 mg/dL) contained in CPD donor blood.
F. **Metabolic acidosis.** Metabolic acidosis from stored donor blood (secondary to the acid load) occurs less often in CPD blood.
G. **Metabolic alkalosis.** Metabolic alkalosis may occur as a result of delayed clearing of citrate preservative from the donated blood by the liver.
H. **Necrotizing enterocolitis.** An increased incidence of necrotizing enterocolitis after exchange transfusion has been suggested. For this reason, the umbilical vein catheter should be removed after the procedure unless central venous pressure monitoring is required. Also, we recommend that feedings be delayed for at least 24 h to observe the infant for the possibility of postexchange ileus.

30 Gastric Intubation

I. **Indications**
   A. **Enteric feeding.** Gastric intubation for enteric feeding in the following situations:
      1. **High respiratory rate.** At some institutions, enteric feedings are used if the respiratory rate is >60 breaths/min to decrease the risk of aspiration pneumonia (**controversial**).
      2. **Neurologic disease** if it impairs the sucking reflex or the infant's ability to feed.
      3. **Premature infants** may have immature sucking and swallow mechanisms and tire before they can take in enough calories to maintain growth.
   B. **Gastric decompression** may be required in infants with necrotizing enterocolitis, bowel obstruction, or ileus.
   C. **Administration of medications.**
   D. **Analysis of gastric contents.**
II. **Equipment.** Infant feeding tube (3.5 or 5F if <1000 g or 5 to 8F if ≥1000 g), stethoscope, sterile water (to lubricate the tube), a syringe (5–10 mL), 2-in adhesive tape, gloves, suctioning equipment, bag-and-mask ventilation with 100% oxygen.
III. **Procedure**
   A. Monitor the patient's heart rate and respiratory function throughout this procedure.
   B. Place the infant in the supine position, with the head of the bed elevated.
   C. The insertion distance is determined by using minimum insertion lengths (Table 30–1) or by measuring the distance from the corner of the mouth or nose to the earlobe and to the point halfway between the umbilicus and end of the xiphoid. (**This measurement proved to be the most accurate in one study.**) Mark the length on the tube. Table 30–1 has recommendations for infants ≤1500 g.
   D. Moisten the end of the tube with sterile water.
   E. The tube can be placed in one of two positions.
      1. **Nasal insertion. Avoid nasal insertion in very low birthweight infants because of increased incidence of respiratory compromise.** One study revealed infants <2 kg demonstrated significant pulmonary compromise with nasogastric tube placement. Flex the neck, push the nose up, and insert the tube, directing it straight back. Advance the tube the desired distance.
      2. **Oral insertion.** Push the tongue down with a tongue depressor and pass the tube into the oropharynx. Slowly advance the tube the desired distance.

Table 30–1. **GUIDELINES FOR MINIMUM OROGASTRIC TUBE INSERTION LENGTH TO PROVIDE ADEQUATE INTRAGASTRIC POSITIONING IN VERY LOW BIRTHWEIGHT INFANTS**

Weight (g)	Insertion Length (cm)
< 750	13
750–999	15
1000–1249	16
1250–1500	17

Data from Gallaher KJ et al: Orogastric tube insertion length in very low birth weight infants. *J Perinatol* 1993;13:128.

    F. Continue to observe the infant for respiratory distress or bradycardia.

    G. Determine the location of the tube. One method is to inject air into the tube with a syringe and listen for a rush of air in the stomach. One study found this method unreliable because a rush of air can occur when the tip is in the distal esophagus. Some clinicians recommended either palpating the tube in the abdomen or aspirating the contents to determine the acidity by pH tape. Gastric pH should be <6. If the pH is >6, placement should be questioned. If the location is still uncertain, obtain a radiograph. If feedings are to be initiated, the position should be verified by plain radiograph. See Figure 10–8 which shows the tip of the nasogastric tube properly positioned in the stomach.

    H. Aspirate the gastric contents and secure the tube to the face with benzoin and 2-in tape.

IV. **Complications**

    A. **Apnea and bradycardia** are usually mediated by a vagal response and resolve without specific treatment.

    B. **Perforation of the esophagus, posterior pharynx, stomach, or duodenum.** The tube should never be forced during insertion.

    C. **Hypoxia.** Always have bag-and-mask ventilation with 100% oxygen available to treat this problem.

    D. **Aspiration** can occur if feeding has been initiated in a tube that is accidentally inserted into the lung or if the gastrointestinal tract is not passing the feedings out of the stomach. Periodically check the residual volumes in the stomach to prevent overdistention and aspiration. (See Chapter 48.)

31 Heelstick (Capillary Blood Sampling)

I. **Indications.** Capillary blood sampling is the most common procedure done in neonatal intensive care nurseries.

    A. Collection of blood samples when only a small amount of blood is needed or when there is difficulty obtaining samples by venipuncture.

    B. Capillary blood gas sampling.

    C. Blood cultures when venous access is not possible.

    D. Newborn metabolic screen.

II. **Equipment.** Sterile lancet (2-mm lancet if <1500 g or 4-mm lancet in larger infants). Automated self-shielding lancets are associated with fewer complications and decreased pain (BD Quickheel Preemie and Tenderfoot Preemie are 1.75 mm for >1000 g; BD Quickheel Infant and Tenderfoot Newborn are 2.5 mm for term up to 6 months; Tenderfoot Micro-Preemie are for <1000 g); alcohol swabs, 4 × 4 sterile gauze pads, a capillary tube (for rapid hematocrit and bilirubin tests) or larger BD Microtainer collection tubes (if more blood is needed [eg, for blood chemistry determinations]), filter paper card for newborn screening (if appropriate), clay to seal the capillary tube, a warm washcloth, gloves, and a diaper.

III. **Procedure**

    A. Wrap the foot in a warm washcloth and then in a diaper for 5 min. Although not mandatory, it will produce hyperemia which increases vascularity, making blood collection easier. It is mandatory when collecting a sample for a blood gas or pH determination. A warming pad may be used, but its temperature should not exceed 40°C. Commercial packs are now available to heat the heel, and these should be applied for 5 min.

    B. Eutectic mixture of lidocaine and prilocaine (EMLA) was not found to be effective in heelsticks. Automated devices cause less pain. Oral sucrose, swaddling, and a pacifier can also be used for pain reduction. (See Chapter 69.)

    C. Choose the area of puncture (Figure 31–1A). Avoid the center of the heel because this area is associated with an increased incidence of osteomyelitis. Heelsticks are contraindicated with local infection, significant edema, or poor perfusion.

    D. Wipe the area with an alcohol swab, and let it dry. If the area is wet with alcohol, hemolysis may occur, altering the results of blood testing.

    E. Using a **standard heel lancet,** encircle the heel with the palm of your hand and index finger (see Figure 31–1A). Make a quick deep (<2.5-mm) puncture.

        1. Wipe off the first drop of blood with gauze. Gently squeeze the heel, and place the collection tube at the site of the puncture. The capillary tubes should automatically fill by capillary action. It may be necessary to gently "pump" the heel to continue the blood flow to collect drops of blood in a larger tube. Allow enough time for capillary refill of the heel, and apply pressure so the incision is opened with each pumping maneuver.

        2. Avoid excessive squeezing, which may cause hemolysis and give inaccurate results. Seal the end of the capillary tube with clay; collect the larger samples in the BD Microtainer or similar tubes.

        3. Always do the blood gas sample first and send it to the lab at once.

        4. For filter paper newborn screening, the paper can be directly applied to the heel or the blood can be transferred to a capillary tube and then applied to the filter paper.

        5. Maintain pressure on the puncture site with a dry sterile gauze pad until the bleeding stops; elevate the foot. A 4 × 4 gauze pad can be wrapped around the heel and left on to provide hemostasis; adhesive bandages are not recommended.

    F. **Using an automated lancet** (eg, BD Quickheel Infant or others), hold the device 90 degrees to the surface. The device can be oriented perpendicular or at 90 degrees to the long axis of the foot (see Figure 31–1B). Depress the trigger to activate the device and automatically make the puncture. Immediately discard the device and follow the steps just outlined (see Section III, E, 1–5).

IV. **Complications**

    A. **Cellulitis** risk can be minimized with the proper use of sterile technique. A culture of tissue from the affected area should be obtained and the use of broad-spectrum antibiotics considered.

    B. **Osteomyelitis** usually occurs in the calcaneus bone. Avoid the center area of the heel, and do not make the puncture opening too deep. If osteomyelitis occurs, tissue should be obtained for culture, and broad-spectrum antibiotics should be started until a specific organism is identified. Infectious disease and orthopedics consultation is usually obtained.

    C. **Other infections** reported include abscess and perichondritis.

    D. **Scarring of the heel** occurs when there have been multiple punctures in the same area. If extensive scarring is present, consider another technique of blood collection, such as central venous sampling.

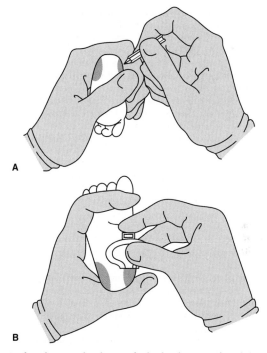

FIGURE 31–1. Preferred sites and technique for heelstick in an infant. **(A)** Use the shaded area when performing a heelstick in an infant. Standard lancet technique is shown. **(B)** Use of an automated self-retracting lancet (BD Quickheel) for heelstick in an infant is illustrated. The automated lancet is held 90 degrees to the axis of the foot and activated. (*Reproduced with permission from Gomella LG, Haist SA [eds], Clinician's Pocket Reference, 11th ed. New York: McGraw-Hill, 2007.*)

    E. Pain caused by heelsticks in premature infants can cause declines in hemoglobin oxygen saturation as measured by pulse oximetry.

    F. **Calcified nodules** usually disappear by 30 months of age.

    G. **Inaccurate results.** Falsely elevated Dextrostix, potassium, hematocrit, and inaccurate blood gas values (slightly lower pH and slightly higher Pco_2) can occur with heelstick sampling.

32 Lumbar Puncture (Spinal Tap)

I. **Indications**

    A. Obtaining cerebrospinal fluid (CSF) for the diagnosis of central nervous system (CNS) disorders such as meningitis/encephalitis. Infections that can be diagnosed are bacterial, viral, fungal and TORCH (**T**oxoplasmosis, **O**ther infections[usually syphilis], **R**ubella, **C**ytomegalovirus, and **H**erpes simplex).

B. To aid in the diagnosis of intracranial hemorrhages. CSF studies are indicative but not diagnostic for intracranial hemorrhage. Can see large number of RBC's, xanthochromia, increased protein content, and hypoglycorrhachia (abnormally low CSF glucose content).

C. To diagnose an inborn error of metabolism. CSF amino acid analysis can be obtained to rule out nonketotic hyperglycinemia. Postmortem CSF (1–2 mL frozen specimen) is recommended when an inborn error of metabolism is suspected.

D. Draining CSF in communicating hydrocephalus associated with intraventricular hemorrhage. (Serial lumbar punctures for this are *controversial*.)

E. Administration of intrathecal medications or contrast material.

F. Monitoring efficacy of antibiotics used to treat CNS infections by examining CSF fluid.

II. **Equipment.** Lumbar puncture kit (usually contains three sterile specimen tubes; four sterile tubes are often necessary, sterile drapes, sterile gauze, 20-to 22-gauge 1-in spinal needle with stylet, 1% lidocaine), gloves, povidone-iodine solution, 1-mL syringe.

III. **Procedure.** Normal CSF values are listed in Table 32–1.

A. **Contraindications** include increased intracranial pressure (risk of CNS herniation), uncorrected bleeding abnormality, infection near puncture site, and lumbosacral abnormalities that may interfere with identification of key structures.

B. An assistant should restrain the infant in either a **sitting or a lateral decubitus position**, depending on personal preference. An intubated, critically ill infant must be treated in the lateral decubitus position. Some advocate that if CSF cannot be obtained in the lateral decubitus position, the sitting position should be used. In the lateral decubitus position, the spine should be flexed (knee-chest position). The neck should not be flexed because of an increased incidence of airway compromise; maintain airway patency. Supplemental oxygen used before the procedure or increasing oxygen if the infant is already on it can prevent hypoxemia. Monitor vital signs and pulse oximetry during the procedure.

C. Once the infant is in position, check for landmarks (Figure 32–1). Palpate the iliac crest and slide your finger down to the L4 vertebral body. Then use the L4-L5 interspace (preferred) as the site of the lumbar puncture. Make a nail imprint at the exact location to mark the site.

D. Prepare the materials (open sterile containers, pour antiseptic [povidone-iodine] solution into the plastic well located in the lumbar puncture kit).

Table 32–1. **NORMAL CEREBROSPINAL FLUID VALUES IN NEONATOLOGY**

	WBC (mm³)	Protein (mg/dL)	Glucose (mg/dL)
Term	0–32 (mean 61% PMN)	20–170	34–119
Preterm (970–2500 g)	0–29 (mean 57% PMN)	65–170	24–63
VLBW (550–1500 g)	0–44 (range 0–66% PMN)	45–370	29–217

PMN, polymorphonuclear neutrophils.
Based on data from Rodriguez AF et al: Cerebrospinal fluid values in the very low birth weight infant. *J Pediatr* 1990;116(6):971–974; Sarff LD et al: Cerebrospinal fluid evaluation in neonates: comparison of high-risk infants with and without meningitis. *J Pediatr* 1976;88(3):473–477; and Martín-Ancel A et al: Cerebrospinal fluid leucocyte counts in healthy neonates. *Arch Dis Child Fetal Neonatal Ed* 2006;91(5): F357–F358.

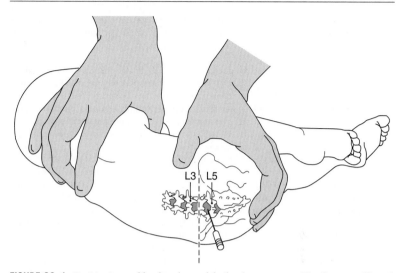

FIGURE 32–1. Positioning and landmarks used for lumbar puncture. The iliac crest (dotted line) marks the approximate level of L4.

E. Put gloves on and clean the lumbar area with antiseptic solution, starting at the interspace selected. Prep in a widening circle from that interspace up and over the iliac crest.
F. Drape the area with one towel under the infant and one towel covering everything but the selected interspace. Keep the infant's face exposed.
G. Palpate again to find the selected interspace. At this time, 0.5–1% lidocaine (dose in Chapter 69) can be injected subcutaneously for pain relief (optional and usually not done in neonates.). *Note:* Physiologic instability is not reduced with lidocaine use during the procedure. EMLA (topical lidocaine and prilocaine) or other topical agents may be used (***controversial***).
H. Insert the needle in the midline with steady pressure aimed toward the umbilicus. Advance the needle slowly and then remove the stylet to check for appearance of fluid. One usually does not feel a "pop" as the ligamentum flavum and dura are penetrated, as is the case with older children and adults. Therefore, remove the stylet frequently to keep from going too far and getting a bloody specimen. Rotate the needle if no fluid is seen.
I. Collect ~1 mL of CSF in each of the four sterile specimen tubes by allowing the fluid to drip into the tubes. For routine CSF examination, send four tubes of CSF to the laboratory in the following recommended order:
  • **Tube 1:** For Gram stain, culture, and sensitivity testing.
  • **Tube 2:** For glucose and protein levels.
  • **Tube 3:** For cell count and differential.
  • **Tube 4:** Is optional and can be sent for rapid antigen tests for specific pathogens (eg, group B streptococcus) or PCR (polymerase chain reaction) (eg, herpes).
J. If a bloody specimen is obtained in the first tube, observe for clearing in the second and third tubes.
  1. If bleeding clears, the tap was traumatic.
  2. If blood does not clear but forms clots, a blood vessel has probably been punctured. Because CSF has not been obtained, a repeat tap must be done.
  3. If blood does not clear and does not clot in the container, the infant probably has had intraventricular bleeding.

K. Replace the stylet before removing the needle to prevent trapping the spinal nerve roots and withdraw the needle. Maintain pressure on the site, and clean off the antiseptic solution.

IV. Complications

A. **Infection.** Use sterile technique to reduce the risk. Bacteremia may result if a blood vessel is punctured after the needle has passed through contaminated CSF. Abscess (spinal and epidural) and vertebral osteomyelitis have been reported.

B. **Intraspinal epidermoid tumor** results from performing a lumbar puncture with a needle that does not have a stylet and is caused by the displacement of a "plug" of epithelial tissue into the dura. Note that the incidence of traumatic lumbar puncture is not reduced by the use of a needle without a stylet.

C. **Herniation of cerebral tissue through the foramen magnum** is not a common problem in neonatal intensive care units because of the open fontanelle in infants.

D. **Spinal cord and nerve damage.** To avoid this complication, use the L4-L5 interspace.

E. **Apnea and bradycardia** sometimes occur from respiratory compromise caused by the infant being held too tightly during the procedure.

F. **Hypoxia.** Increasing the oxygen during the procedure may help prevent transient hypoxia. Preoxygenation of the patient may also decrease hypoxia.

G. **Bleeding.** Spinal epidural, subdural, and subarachnoid hematomas have been reported.

H. **Cardiopulmonary arrest.**

I. **Cerebrospinal fluid leakage.** Frequent complication seen on sonograms.

J. **Intramedullary hemorrhage resulting in paraplegia.** Important to consider the location of the conus medullaris in a preterm infant.

33 Paracentesis (Abdominal)

I. Indications

A. **To obtain peritoneal fluid for diagnostic tests** to determine the cause of ascites. Ascites can be caused by or associated with necrotizing enterocolitis with perforation; biliary, urinary, chylous, or meconium peritonitis; iatrogenic or congenital infections; or inborn errors of metabolism.

B. **As a therapeutic procedure,** such as removal of peritoneal fluid or air from a pneumoperitoneum to aid in ventilation in a patient with cardiorespiratory compromise.

II. **Equipment.** Sterile drapes, sterile gloves, povidone-iodine solution, sterile gauze pads, sterile tubes for fluid, a 10-mL syringe, and a 22- or 24-gauge catheter-over-needle assembly (24 gauge for infants weighing <2000 g, 22–24 gauge for infants weighing >2000 g).

III. Procedure

A. The infant should be supine with both legs restrained. To restrict all movements of the legs, a diaper can be wrapped around the legs and secured in place.

B. Choose the site for paracentesis. The area between the umbilicus and the pubic bone is not generally used in neonates because of the danger of perforating the bladder or bowel wall. The sites most frequently used are the right and left flanks. A good rule is to draw a horizontal line passing through the umbilicus and select a site between this line and the inguinal ligament (Figure 33–1).

C. Prepare the area with povidone-iodine in a circular fashion, starting at the puncture site.

D. Put on sterile gloves, and drape the area.

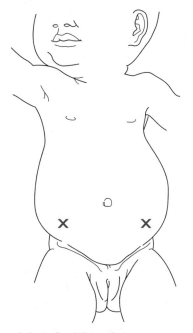

FIGURE 33–1. Recommended sites for abdominal paracentesis.

E. Infiltrate the area with anesthesia (lidocaine 0.5–1%) (see Chapter 69).
F. Insert the needle at the selected site. A "Z-track" technique is usually used to prevent persistent leakage of fluid after the tap. Insert the needle perpendicular to the skin. When the needle is just under the skin, move it 0.5 cm before puncturing the abdominal wall.
G. Advance the needle, aspirating until fluid appears in the barrel of the syringe. Then remove the needle and aspirate the contents slowly with the catheter. It may be necessary to reposition the catheter to obtain an adequate amount of fluid. Once the necessary amount of fluid is taken (usually 3–5 mL for specific tests or enough to aid ventilation), remove the catheter. If too much fluid is removed or if it is removed too rapidly, hypotension may result.
H. Cover the site with a sterile gauze pad until leakage has stopped.

IV. Complications
   A. **Hypotension.** Hypotension is caused by removing too much fluid or removing fluid too rapidly. To minimize this possibility, take only the amount needed for studies or what is needed to improve ventilation. Always remove fluid slowly.
   B. **Infection.** The risk of peritonitis is minimized by using strict sterile technique.
   C. **Perforation of the intestine.** To help prevent perforation, use the shortest needle possible and take careful note of landmarks (see Section III, B). If perforation occurs, broad-spectrum antibiotics may be indicated with close observation for signs of infection.
   D. **Perforation of the bladder.** Perforation of the bladder is normally self-limited and requires no specific treatment.
   E. **Persistent fluid leak.** The Z-track technique (see Section III, F) usually prevents the problem of persistent leakage of fluid. Persistent fluid leaks may have to be bagged to quantify the volume.

F. **Pneumoperitoneum.** Observation is usually required. (See Figure 10–21 for radiograph of a pneumoperitoneum.)

G. **Bleeding.** Bleeding from the liver or vessels can be severe and may require emergency surgery consultation and surgery.

34 Pericardiocentesis

I. **Indications**

A. Treatment of cardiac tamponade caused by pneumopericardium or pericardial effusion. (**Note:** Pericardial effusions are a rare but life-threatening complication of central venous catheters including umbilical venous catheters. Keep a high index of clinical suspicion in a neonate who has a central line and suddenly has cardiovascular collapse.

B. To obtain pericardial fluid for diagnostic studies in infants with pericardial effusion.

II. **Equipment.** Equipment includes povidone-iodine solution, sterile gloves and gown, a 22-or 24-gauge 1-in catheter-over-needle assembly, sterile drapes, a 10-mL syringe, a connecting tube, and an underwater seal for use if the catheter is to be left indwelling.

III. **Procedure**

A. **Ideally, pericardiocentesis is done with the help of echocardiography.** This guides needle insertion to decrease the incidence of complications. With pneumopericardium, thoracic transillumination may be helpful. With sudden cardiovascular collapse, time does not allow these tests, and immediate aspiration is necessary. (See Figure 10–17 for a radiograph of pneumopericardium.)

B. **Monitor electrocardiogram and vital signs.** Prep the area (xiphoid and precordium) with antiseptic solution. Put on the sterile gloves and gown and drape the area, leaving the xiphoid and a 2-cm circular area around it exposed.

C. Local anesthesia can be administered (0.5–1% lidocaine subcutaneously). See Chapter 69 for dose.

D. Prepare the needle by attaching the syringe to it. If you want to leave an indwelling catheter in, a three-way stopcock and tubing should be attached to the needle in addition to the syringe.

E. Identify the area where the needle is to be inserted. The area most commonly used is ~0.5 cm to the left of and just below the infant's xiphoid (Figure 34–1).

F. Insert the needle at about a 30-degree angle, aiming toward the midclavicular line on the left (see Figure 34–1). Apply constant suction on the syringe while advancing the needle.

G. Once air or fluid is obtained (depending on which is to be evacuated), remove the needle from the catheter. Withdraw the necessary amount of air or fluid, that is, enough to relieve symptoms or to obtain sufficient fluid for laboratory studies.

H. If an indwelling catheter is to be left in place, secure it with tape and attach the tubing to continuous suction.

I. Obtain a chest radiograph to confirm the position of the catheter and the effectiveness of drainage.

IV. **Complications**

A. **Puncturing the heart.** Perforation of the right ventricle can be avoided by advancing the needle only far enough to obtain fluid or air. Ultrasound guidance is recommended if time permits. Another technique to avoid puncturing the heart is to attach the electrocardiogram anterior chest lead to the needle with an alligator clip. If changes

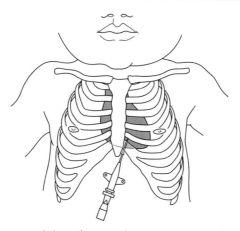

FIGURE 34–1. Recommended sites for pericardiocentesis.

are seen on the ECG (eg, ectopic beats, changes in the ST segment, increase in the QRS voltage), the needle has contacted the myocardium and should be withdrawn. Avoid leaving a metal needle indwelling for continuous drainage. Most needle perforations heal spontaneously.

B. **Pneumothorax or hemothorax** can occur if landmarks are not used and "blind" punctures are done. If this complication has occurred, a chest tube on the affected side is usually needed.

C. **Infection.** Strict sterile technique minimizes the risk of infection.

D. **Arrhythmias** are usually transient. Repositioning the needle is usually effective, but with persistent arrhythmia, treatment may be necessary.

E. **Bleeding.** Bleeding is usually superficial and controlled with pressure. Hepatic puncture can occur.

F. **Hypotension** may occur if a significant amount of fluid is drained. A fluid bolus may be necessary.

G. **Pneumomediastinum.** Observation is only required.

---

35 Venous Access: Intraosseous Infusion

I. **Indications.** Intraosseous infusion can be used for emergency vascular access (for administration of fluids and medications) when other methods of vascular access have been attempted and have failed. Many agents have been infused by this technique in the literature, including intravenous (IV) solutions (eg, Ringer's lactate or normal saline), blood and blood products, and a wide variety of medications. See Table 35–1 for a complete list.

II. **Equipment.** Needed are povidone-iodine solution, 4 × 4 sterile gauze pads, a syringe, sterile towels, gloves, an 18-gauge disposable iliac bone marrow aspiration needle (preferred), an intraosseous needle, or an 18- to 20-gauge short spinal needle with a stylet, a short (18- to 20-gauge) hypodermic needle or a butterfly (16- to 19-gauge) needle, a

Table 35–1. **AGENTS ADMINISTERED BY THE
INTRAOSSEOUS ROUTE REPORTED IN THE LITERATURE**

Fluids
Crystalloids (normal saline, lactated Ringer's, others)
Glucose (dilute if possible when using D50)

Blood and Blood Products
Medications

Anesthetic agents	Ephedrine
Antibiotics	Epinephrine
Atropine	Heparin
Calcium gluconate	Insulin
Dexamethasone	Isoproterenol
Diazepam	Lidocaine
Diazoxide	Morphine
Dobutamine	Phenytoin
Dopamine	Sodium bicarbonate
	(dilute *if possible*)

Contrast Material

From MacDonald MG, Ramasethu J (eds), *Procedures in Neonatology*, 4th ed. Baltimore, MD: Lippincott Williams & Wilkins, 2007. Reproduced with permission.

sterile drape, and a syringe with saline flush. Specific devices for the newborn are now available (Bone Injection Gun; Waismed, Houston, TX, and the EZ-IO Pediatric; Vidacare, San Antonio, TX), but lack of studies prevents the use in premature infants.
III. **Procedure.** The proximal tibia is the preferred site and is described here (Figure 35–1). Other sites are the distal tibia and the distal femur.
  A. Restrain the patient's lower leg.
  B. Place a small sandbag or IV bag behind the knee for support.
  C. Select the area in the midline on the flat surface of the anterior tibia, 1–3 cm below the tibial tuberosity.

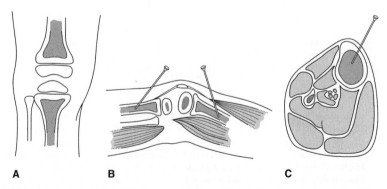

A   **B**   **C**

FIGURE 35–1. Technique of intraosseous infusion. (**A**) Anterior view of sites on the tibia and the fibula. (**B**) Sagittal view. (**C**) Cross-section through the tibia. (*Reproduced with permission from Hodge D: Intraosseous infusion: a review.* Pediatr Emerg Care 1985;1:215.)

D. Clean the area with povidone-iodine solution. Sterile drapes can be placed around the area.

E. Lidocaine (0.5–1%) can be used for pain management. Inject into the skin and soft tissue. See Chapter 69 for dosage (optional because this procedure is used for emergency access and time may not allow for pain management).

F. Insert the needle at an angle of 10–15 degrees toward the foot to avoid the growth plate.

G. Advance the needle until a lack of resistance is felt (usually no more than 1 cm is necessary), at which point entry into the marrow space should have occurred.

H. Remove the stylet. (*Note:* At this point, aspiration of bone marrow for laboratory studies can be done, if needed. Bone marrow aspirates can be sent for blood chemistry values, carbon dioxide level, pH, hemoglobin level, culture and sensitivity, and blood type and cross-match.) Secure the needle to the skin with tape to prevent it from dislodging.

I. Attach the needle to IV fluids. Hypertonic and alkaline solutions should be diluted 1:2 with normal saline.

J. Withdraw the needle, and apply pressure over the puncture site.

K. To avoid the risk of infectious complications, this method of vascular access should optimally be used for <2 h.

IV. **Complications**

A. **Fluid infiltration of subcutaneous tissue** (most common).

B. **Subperiosteal infiltration of fluid.**

C. **Localized cellulitis/Abscess.**

D. **Formation of subcutaneous abscesses.**

E. **Clotting of bone marrow,** resulting in loss of vascular access.

F. **Osteomyelitis** (rare).

G. **Fracture of the bone.** Radiograph confirmation of the needle should be done to confirm position and rule out fracture.

H. **Compartment syndrome.**

I. **Blasts in the peripheral blood.** Blasts in the peripheral blood have been noted after intraosseous infusions in two patients who have no malignant, infectious, or infiltrative disease of the bone marrow.

J. **Sepsis** is minimized by the use of sterile technique.

K. **Fat embolism** is less likely in children than adults.

L. **Bone growth concerns** have been ruled out.

36 Venous Access: Percutaneous Central Venous Catheterization

I. **Indications.** Percutaneous central venous catheterization (peripherally inserted central catheter, or PICC) involves inserting a long small-gauge catheter into a peripheral vein and threading it into a central venous location. The catheter is placed peripherally but is longer than the usual intravenous (IV) device, and hence its tip lies in a more central location. The catheter can be placed in large vessels such as the cephalic and basilic veins in the arm or the saphenous vein in the leg.

A. When it is anticipated that an infant will need IV access for several weeks.

B. In low birthweight infants when it is anticipated that full enteral feedings will not be achieved within a short period.

C. For the delivery of fluids, nutritional solutions, and medications when other venous access is not acceptable (eg, hypertonic IV solutions).

II. **Equipment.** Cap and mask, sterile gloves, a sterile gown, and a neonatal percutaneous catheter device are needed. Two types of devices are available: **Silastic catheters,** which generally do not have an introducer wire, and **polyurethane catheters,** which contain an introducer wire. Several sizes are available, ranging from 24 gauge to as small as 28 gauge in diameter, which is useful in infants <1000 g. Double-lumen catheters are also available. Transparent dressing (for stabilization of the catheter), a sterile tray (multipurpose tray or one used for umbilical artery catheter placement may be used), povidone-iodine solution, a sterile tourniquet (or a rubber band), saline flush solution, a T-connector, and sterile tape strips (Steri-Strips) for catheter stabilization.

III. **Procedure.** There are two commonly used types of catheters, and some of the smaller ones come with guidewires. The procedure varies if a guidewire is or is not present because the guidewire needs to be removed before blood is withdrawn or the catheter is flushed. **It is suggested that the person placing the catheter should be familiar with the specific manufacturer's guidelines for placement of the catheters used.** A review of the National Association of Neonatal Nurses (NANN) *Guideline for Peripherally Inserted Central Catheters* is also suggested (Pettit J, Wyckoff MM: *Peripherally Inserted Central Catheters: Guideline for Practice.* Glenview, IL: National Association of Neonatal Nurses, 2007).

A. Obtain informed consent. Gather the equipment and assemble the tray with the catheter using sterile technique.

B. Select a suitable vein in the arm, such as the cephalic or basilic vein, or use the saphenous vein in the leg (see Figure 37–1). Position the infant so that the selected vessel is accessible. Restrain the infant to prevent contamination of the sterile field with the other extremities. It is helpful to have a second person available to help stabilize the infant's position, to help maintain sterility, and to offer a pacifier and comfort measures.

C. Determine the length of the catheter by measuring the distance between the insertion site and the desired catheter tip location. (For catheters placed in the upper extremities, measure to the level of the superior vena cava or the right atrium; for catheters placed in the lower extremities, measure to the inferior vena cava.) Catheters are typically marked at 5-cm increments to assist with placement.

D. Put on the cap and mask, wash your hands, and then put on the sterile gown and gloves.

E. Prepare the area of insertion with a triple preparation of povidone-iodine solution, and allow the solution to dry. Some catheters warn against using alcohol due to degradation of the catheters. (Consult your manufacturer's guidelines regarding preparation solutions.) **Note:** Catheters that do not contain a guidewire require flushing with heparinized saline before being inserted into the vessel. Consult the package insert for instructions specific to the type of catheter.

F. Have an assistant apply the tourniquet if using a nonsterile tourniquet.

G. Place sterile drapes around the area of insertion.

H. Remove the plastic protector from the introducer needle.

I. Insert the introducer needle into the vein. Confirm entry into the vein by observing for a flashback of blood in the needle. Do not advance the introducer needle once the flashback (or the blood) has been noted, or you may puncture through the other side of the vessel (Figure 36–1).

J. Release the tourniquet.

K. Hold the introducer needle to maintain the position in the vein, and slowly advance the catheter through the introducer needle with a pair of smooth forceps or fingers into the vein. (**Do not use a hemostat or ridged forceps because it may damage the catheter.**) (See Figure 36–2.)

L. Once the catheter has been advanced to the premeasured location, stabilize the catheter by placing a finger over the vessel where the catheter has been introduced

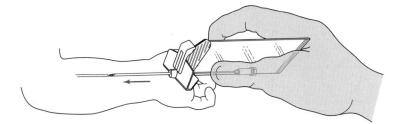

FIGURE 36–1. Technique for insertion of the introducer needle into the vein.

(~1–2 cm above the tip of the introducer needle). Then carefully withdraw the introducer needle completely out of the skin. The area may bleed around the catheter. Hold sterile gauze to the area until the bleeding resolves. (See Figure 36–3.)

M. Separate the introducer needle from the catheter by using the technique specified by the manufacturer of the needle. Grasp the opposite halves of the introducer needle, and carefully peel each half apart until the needle splits completely. (See Figure 36–4.)

N. While removing the needle, occasionally the catheter also partially pulls out of the vein and has to be readvanced to the desired location.

O. If a guidewire is present, remove the wire slowly and steadily from the catheter (do not attempt to reintroduce the wire once it has been removed from the catheter).

P. As the introducer wire is withdrawn, a blood return may or may not be observed in the catheter, depending on the size of catheter. Smaller catheters are less likely to have blood return. Using a 3-mL syringe, aspirate the blood through the catheter until the blood reaches the hub. (Slightly more pressure is necessary to withdraw blood through the very small diameter of the catheter; however, if blood is returning, the catheter is patent and in the intravascular system.) Once the blood has been aspirated back to the catheter hub, place a T-connector and flush the catheter with normal saline. (Because of the small diameter of the catheter, it will take slightly more pressure on the syringe to aspirate the blood and to flush solution through the catheter; however, do not use excessive pressure when flushing the catheter because it can cause catheter rupture or fragmentation with possible embolization.)

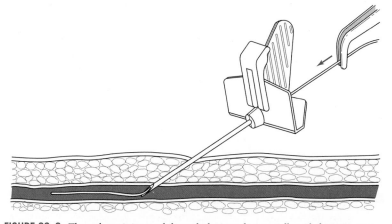

FIGURE 36–2. The catheter is inserted through the introducer needle with forceps.

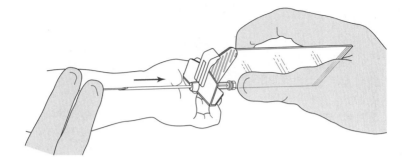

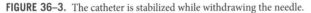

FIGURE 36–3. The catheter is stabilized while withdrawing the needle.

> *Note:* Practice the flushing technique on another catheter before attempting insertion and flushing of a catheter in a patient if you are unfamiliar with this type of catheter.

Q. Secure the catheter to the extremity by placing a sterile tape strip over the catheter at the insertion site to anchor the catheter. Curl the remaining external catheter, making sure there are no kinks, and cover with a sterile transparent dressing. (Do not suture the catheter in place.)

R. Connect the IV fluid. Fresh IV fluids should be connected to the new catheter.

S. Obtain a radiograph to verify the central catheter tip location. The catheter is radiopaque and can be seen on radiograph; however, because of its small size, it may be difficult to assess the location of the tip. Most catheters are radiopaque and visualized on x-ray. Some manufacturers suggests injecting contrast medium (~0.3–1 mL) through the catheter just before the radiograph to assess catheter tip placement.

> *Note:* Ideally, the position of the catheter tip should be in a central location. However, if the catheter has a blood return and is patent but could not be advanced to a

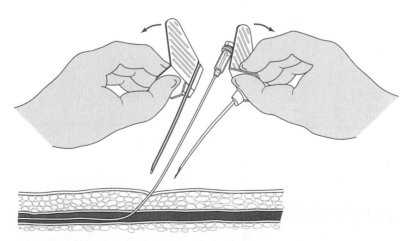

FIGURE 36–4. Technique for removing the needle wing assembly of most catheters.

central location, it may still be used as a peripheral venous access catheter. Hypertonic solutions should be infused with caution in this case.

T. Chart the size and the length of catheter that has been inserted and the position of the catheter on radiograph.

U. **Precautions**

1. Do not measure the infant's blood pressure on the extremity containing the percutaneous catheter. Doing so could cause occlusion or damage to the catheter.

2. Do not trim the catheter before placement unless specified by the manufacturer. Doing so may increase the incidence of thrombus formation because of a roughly cut end.

3. Do not use a hemostat or ribbed forceps to advance the catheter because it could damage the catheter.

4. When inserting the catheter through the introducer needle, do not pull the catheter back through the introducer needle. Doing so could sever the catheter.

5. Do not suture the catheter itself. The catheter is very small, and a suture would occlude it.

6. Do not attempt to infuse blood products or viscous solutions through the catheter; this could cause the catheter to become occluded.

7. Take care when flushing the catheter. Excessive pressure could rupture it. Do not use a syringe <3 mL to the flush line.

IV. **Complications.** Only the most common complications are listed. Refer to the manufacturer's enclosures for a list of further complications.

A. **Infiltration.** As with any intravascular device, infiltration is a risk and the area will swell. Because the catheters are longer than peripheral IV catheters, it is necessary to assess for swelling in the area where the tip of the catheter is located, not just at the insertion site.

B. **Catheter occlusion.** This catheter is extremely small, fragile, and easily occluded during taping or if the infant bends the extremity containing the catheter. When securing the catheter with the dressing and tape, avoid kinking the catheter; doing so could create an occlusion. If resistance is met when flushing the catheter, do not attempt to flush it any further. Doing so could result in catheter rupture with possible embolization.

C. **Infection or sepsis.** Infants requiring this type of catheter are at increased risk for nosocomial infections for many reasons, such as poor skin integrity, an immature immune system, multiple invasive procedures, and exposure to multiple pieces of equipment. Infection specifically related to this type of catheter appears to be related to the length of time the catheter remains in place. Infants who have catheters indwelling for >3 weeks appear to be at greater risk for catheter-related sepsis. The catheter should only be accessed when necessary to change fluids to limit the breaks in the line.

D. **Air embolism.** Because these catheters are in a central location, air embolism is a risk. The catheter should be cared for like a central catheter. Special precautions should be taken to avoid air in the line.

E. **Catheter embolus.** Do not pull the catheter back through the introducer needle, which could cause the catheter to sever.

V. **Maintenance of the catheter**

A. The transparent dressing should remain in place over the catheter. Routine dressing changes are not recommended because of the risk of tearing or dislodging the catheter. The dressing should be changed, using sterile technique, only if the current dressing has drainage under it or is no longer occlusive.

B. Examine the site and extremity or area where the catheter is located frequently for inflammation (erythema) or tenderness (as per unit's specific IV protocol).

C. Fluids running through the catheter should be heparinized according to hospital or unit protocol for central catheters.

D. Limit the number of times the catheter is accessed to decrease infection.

VI. Removal of the catheter. The catheter can remain in place for several weeks. Several studies have shown an increase in the infection rate after ~2–3 weeks. When ready to remove the catheter, follow the procedure presented here.

    A. Gently remove the occlusive dressing from the extremity and the catheter, being careful not to tear the dressing from the catheter.

    B. Grasp the catheter tubing near the insertion site, and gently pull the catheter in a continuous movement. If resistance is met, do not apply force and do not stretch the catheter. Doing so could cause the catheter to rupture.

    C. Apply a moist, warm compress to the area above the catheter tract for several minutes, and then reattempt removal of the catheter. If catheter is still resistant, consult NANN Practice Guidelines. It may take several hours to days to remove some catheters.

    D. Once the catheter is removed, inspect and measure it to make sure the entire catheter was removed from the vein. Compare this length with the initial measurement at the time of placement.

    E. Cover the area with a sterile dressing.

37 Venous Access: Percutaneous Venous Catheterization

I. Indications

    A. Administration of intravenous (IV) medications and fluids.

    B. Administration of parenteral nutrition.

    C. Administration of blood and blood products.

    D. Emergency vascular access.

II. Equipment. Armboard, adhesive tape, a tourniquet, alcohol swabs, normal saline for flush ($^1/_2$ normal saline if concerned about hypernatremia), povidone-iodine solution, a needle (a 23- or 25-gauge scalp vein needle or a 22-to 24-gauge catheter-over-needle; self-shielding safety types preferred; at least a 24-gauge for blood transfusion); transparent dressing material; appropriate IV fluid and connecting tubing.

III. Procedure

    A. Scalp vein needle

        1. Select the vein to use. Neonatal sites are shown in Figure 37–1. It is useful to select the "Y" or crotch region of the vein, where two veins join together for the insertion.

            a. Scalp. Supratrochlear, superficial temporal, or posterior auricular vein.

            b. Back of the hand. Dorsal arch vein.

            c. Forearm. Median antebrachial or accessory cephalic vein.

            d. Foot. Dorsal arch vein.

            e. Antecubital fossa. Basilic or cubital vein.

            f. Ankle. Greater saphenous vein.

        2. Shave the area if a scalp vein is to be used.

        3. Restrain the extremity on an armboard, or have an assistant help hold the extremity or the head.

        4. Apply a tourniquet proximal to the puncture site. If a scalp vein is to be used, a rubber band can be placed around the head, just above the eyebrows.

        5. Clean the area with povidone-iodine solution, allow to dry, and wipe off with sterile water or saline.

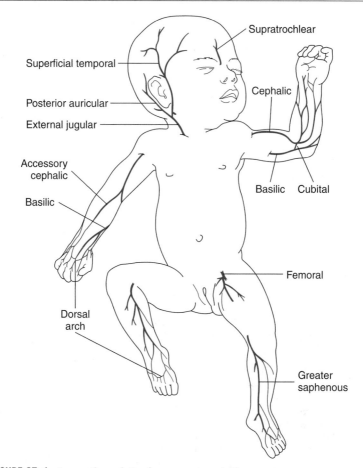

FIGURE 37–1. Frequently used sites for venous access in the neonate.

6. **Fill the tubing with flush** and detach the syringe from the needle.
7. **Grasp the plastic wings** and, using your free index finger, **pull the skin taut** to help stabilize the vein.
8. **Insert the needle** through the skin in the direction of the blood flow and advance ~0.5 cm before entry into the side of the vessel. Alternatively, the vessel can be entered directly after puncture of the skin, but this often results in the vessel's being punctured "through and through" (Figure 37–2).
9. **Advance the needle** until blood appears in the tubing.
10. **Gently inject some of the flush** to ensure patency and proper positioning of the needle.
11. **Connect the IV tubing and fluid,** and tape the needle into position.

B. **Catheter-over-needle assembly**
 1. **Follow steps 1–5** for the scalp vein needle.
 2. **Fill the needle and the hub with flush** via syringe; then remove the syringe.
 3. **Pull the skin taut** to stabilize the vein.

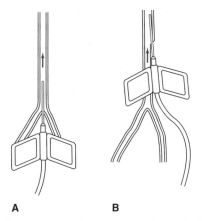

A   **B**

FIGURE 37–2. Two techniques for entering the vein for IV access in the neonate. (**A**) Direct puncture. (**B**) Side entry.

4. **Puncture the skin,** then enter the side of the vein in a separate motion. Alternately, the skin and the vein can be entered in one motion.
5. **Carefully advance the needle** until blood appears in the hub.
6. **Withdraw the needle** while advancing the catheter.
7. **Remove the tourniquet,** and gently inject some normal saline into the catheter to verify patency and position.
8. **Connect the IV tubing and fluid,** and tape securely in place using transparent dressing.

IV. **Complications**
   A. **Hematoma** (most common complication) at the site can often be managed effectively by gentle manual pressure and is the most common complication.
   B. **Phlebitis** risk increases the longer a catheter is left in place, especially if >72 h. Heparinized solutions may decrease this risk.
   C. **Vasospasm** rarely occurs when veins are accessed and usually resolves spontaneously.
   D. **Infection** risk can be minimized by using sterile technique, including antiseptic preparation. The risk of infection rises after 72 h.
   E. **Embolus (air or clot).** Never allow the end of the catheter to be open to the air, and make sure that the IV catheter is flushed free of air bubbles before it is connected.
   F. **Infiltration of subcutaneous tissue.** IV solution may leak out into the subcutaneous tissue as a result of improper catheter placement or damage to the vessel. To help prevent this, confirm placement of the catheter with the flush solution before the catheter is connected to the IV solution. Infiltration often means that the catheter needs to be removed. Avoid hyperosmolar solutions for peripheral infusion. Sloughing of the skin may result, rarely requiring skin grafts.
   G. **Calcification of subcutaneous tissue** secondary to infusion of a calcium-containing solution.

38 Venous Access: Umbilical Vein Catheterization

I. **Indications**
  A. Immediate, primarily postnatal access for intravenous (IV) fluids or emergency medications.
  B. Central venous pressure monitoring.
  C. Exchange transfusion or partial exchange transfusion.
  D. Long-term central venous access in extremely low birthweight infants.
  E. Other frequently reported indications are general venous access, intravenous fluids, total parenteral nutrition, and medications.
II. **Equipment.** Identical to umbilical artery catheterization (see page 203), except use a 5F catheter for infants <3.5 kg and 8F catheter for >3.5 kg.
III. **Procedure**
  A. Place the infant supine with a diaper wrapped around both legs to help stabilize the infant.
  B. Prepare the area around the umbilicus with povidone-iodine solution. Use a gown, gloves, and mask.
  C. Prepare the tray as you would for the umbilical artery catheterization (Chapter 23, page 204).
  D. Place sterile drapes, leaving the umbilical area exposed.
  E. Tie a piece of umbilical tape around the base of the umbilicus.
  F. Cut the excess umbilical cord with a scalpel or scissors, leaving a stump of ~0.5–1.0 cm. Identify the umbilical vein. The umbilical vein is thin walled, larger than the two arteries, and close to the periphery of the stump (see Figure 23–1B).
  G. Grasp the end of the umbilicus with the curved hemostat to hold it upright and steady (Figure 38–1A).

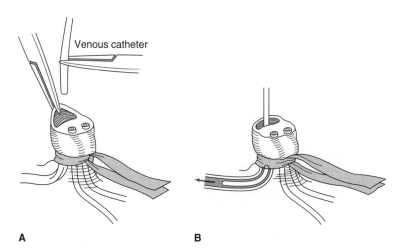

A   **B**

FIGURE 38–1. Umbilical vein catheterization. (**A**) The umbilical stump is held upright before the catheter is inserted. (**B**) The catheter is passed into the umbilical vein.

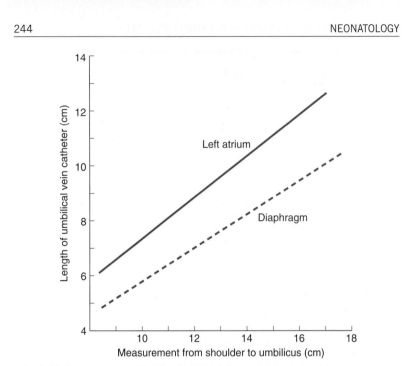

FIGURE 38–2. The umbilical venous catheter is placed above the level of the diaphragm. Determine the shoulder-umbilical length as for the umbilical artery catheter. Use this number and determine the catheter length using the graph. Remember to add the length of the umbilical stump to the length of the catheter. *(Based on data from Dunn PM: Localization of the umbilical catheter by post-mortem measurement.* Arch Dis Child 1966;41:69.)

> H. Open and dilate the umbilical vein with the forceps. Once the vein is sufficiently dilated, insert the catheter (Figure 38–1B).
>
> I. To determine the specific length of catheter needed, see Figure 38–2. Another method is to measure the length from the xiphoid to the umbilicus and add 0.5–1.0 cm. This number indicates how far the venous catheter should be inserted.
>
> J. Connect the catheter to the fluid and tubing. Place a piece of silk tape on the catheter, and secure it to the base of the umbilicus with silk sutures (see Figure 23–3, page 207). You can also place a pursestring suture at the base of the cord, not the skin or vessels, and sew it through the tape on two sides. Another way is to place a pursestring suture at the base of the cord and lightly tighten it, and then wrap it three times around the cord and tie.
>
> K. Obtain a radiograph (includes abdomen and chest, the imaging study of choice for catheter placement) to confirm the position (see Figure 10–8). The correct position for an umbilical venous catheter (UVC) is with the catheter tip 0.5–1.0 cm (some units use 0–1cm, 1–2 cm) above the diaphragm. (UVC tip at thoracic vertebrae 8 or 9 corresponding to the junction of the right atrium and inferior vena cava.) Recently, some centers have used ultrasound combined with radiography for catheter placement and to verify position. Real time ultrasound has been shown to reduce complications during catheter insertion.
>
> L. Never advance a catheter once it is secured in place.
>
> M. Occasionally, a catheter enters the portal vein (Figure 38–3). You should suspect that you have entered the portal vein if you meet resistance and cannot advance the

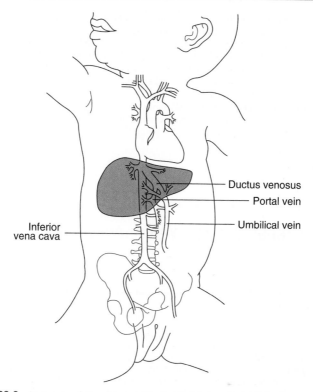

FIGURE 38-3. Anatomic relationships used in the placement of an umbilical venous catheter.

catheter the desired distance or if you detect a "bobbing" motion of the catheter. Several options are available to correct this.

1. Withdraw the catheter 2–3 cm, rotate it, and try to reinsert it.
2. Try injecting flush as you advance the catheter. Sometimes this makes it easier to pass the catheter through the ductus venosus.
3. Pass another catheter through the same opening. Sometimes this allows one catheter to go through the ductus venosus while the other enters the portal system. The one in the portal system can then be removed.
4. Apply mild manual pressure in the right upper quadrant over the liver.

IV. **Complications**
   A. **Infection.** Most common reported adverse effect. Minimize the risk of infection through the use of strict sterile technique, and never advance a catheter that has already been positioned.
   B. **Cardiac complications.** Pericardial effusion is the second most common complication. Cardiac arrhythmias are usually caused by a catheter that is inserted too far and irritates the heart. Cardiac tamponade, cardiac perforation, pneumopericardium, and thrombotic endocarditis have also been reported.
   C. **Thrombolic or embolic phenomenon.** Never allow air to enter the end of the catheter. A nonfunctioning catheter should be removed. Never try to flush clots from the end of the catheter.

D. **Necrotizing enterocolitis.** It is thought to be a complication of umbilical vein catheters, especially if left in place for >24 h.

E. **Fungal infections of the right atrium.** Reported complication of 13%.

F. **Portal vein hypertension.** It is caused by a catheter positioned in the portal system.

G. **Hepatic necrosis (rare).** Do not allow a catheter to remain in the portal system. In case of emergency placement, the catheter should be advanced only 3 cm (just until blood returns) to avoid hepatic infusion.

H. **Other rare complications that have been reported.** Portal vein thrombosis, hydrothorax, hepatic cyst, digital ischemia, perforation of the peritoneum, hemorrhagic infarction of the lungs, colon perforation, and pulmonary complications.

39 Venous Access: Venipuncture (Phlebotomy)

I. **Indications**

A. **To obtain a blood sample for routine analysis or culture.** (See also Chapter 31.) Venipuncture typically allows a larger volume of blood to be collected. It is the method of choice for obtaining blood cultures and preferred for certain blood levels (drug levels, hematocrit, karyotype, cross-matching blood).

B. **To obtain a central hematocrit.**

C. **Administer medications.**

II. **Equipment.** A 23- or 25-gauge scalp vein needle (23 gauge preferred to reduce risk of hemolysis or clotting), alcohol and povidone-iodine swabs, appropriate specimen containers (eg, red-top tube), a tourniquet or rubber band (for the scalp), 4 × 4 sterile gauze pads, syringe.

III. **Procedure**

A. Decide which vein to use. Use Figure 37–1 as a guide. The antecubital fossa or the dorsum of hand or foot are most preferred.

B. Have an assistant restrain the infant. If an assistant is not available, restrain the specific area selected for venipuncture by taping the extremity on an armboard. Oral sucrose or a pacifier can help calm the infant. See Chapter 69.

C. "Tourniquet" the extremity to occlude the vein. Use a rubber band (for the head), a tourniquet, or an assistant's hand to encircle the area proximal to the vein.

D. Prepare the site with antiseptic solution. Wipe at least three times in concentric circles starting at the puncture site for blood cultures.

E. With the bevel up, puncture the skin, and then direct the needle into the vein at a 45-degree angle.

F. Once blood enters the tubing, attach the syringe and collect the blood slowly (or administer the medication).

G. Remove the tourniquet, and next remove and shield the needle. Apply gentle pressure on the area until hemostasis has occurred (usually 2–3 min). Distribute blood samples to the appropriate containers; gently mix tubes with additives.

IV. **Complications**

A. **Infection** is rare complication that can be minimized by using sterile technique.

B. **Venous thrombosis** is often unavoidable, especially when multiple punctures are performed on the same vein.

C. **Hematoma or hemorrhage** is avoided by applying pressure to the site long enough after the needle is removed to ensure hemostasis.

This section outlines common problems encountered in the neonatal intensive care unit or newborn nursery. Guidelines for rapid diagnosis and treatment are given. Clinical situations and institutional guidelines may vary extensively, and recommendations for treatment should be modified based on these factors. If a treatment approach is designated *controversial*, the approach has been useful at some institutions but may not have been confirmed in randomized trials or other reviews.

40 Abnormal Blood Gas

I. **Problem.** An abnormal blood gas value for a neonate is reported by the laboratory.
II. **Immediate questions**
  A. **What component of the blood gas is abnormal?** Accepted normal values for an arterial blood gas sample are pH, 7.35–7.45 (pH varies with age, a pH >7.30 is generally acceptable), $Paco_2$, 35–45 mm Hg (slightly higher values accepted if the blood pH remains normal), and PaO_2 between 55 and 65 mm Hg on room air. Blood gas measures pH, Pco_2, and oxygen (O_2), and all the other components (base deficit and bicarbonate) are calculated based on the three levels measured. If one of the components is low (eg, falsely low carbon dioxide [CO_2]), this falsely elevates the base deficit.
  B. **Is this blood gas value very different from the patient's previous blood gas determination?** This is a key question. If the patient has had metabolic acidosis on the last five blood gas measurements and now has metabolic alkalosis, it might be best to repeat the blood gas measurements before initiating treatment. Do not treat the infant on the basis of one abnormal gas value, especially if the infant's clinical status has not changed.
  C. **How was the sample collected?** Blood gas measurements can be reported on arterial, venous, or capillary blood samples. Arterial blood samples are the best indicator of pH, $Paco_2$, and PaO_2. Venous blood samples give a lower pH value and a higher Pco_2 than arterial samples. Capillary samples give a fair assessment of the infant's pH and Pco_2 but do not give an accurate PaO_2. Capillary samples give a lower pH value (not as low as venous pH) and a slightly higher Pco_2 than arterial samples. An accurate capillary blood gas measurement cannot be obtained on an infant who is hypotensive or in shock.
  D. **Is the infant on ventilatory support?** Management of abnormal blood gas levels is approached differently in an intubated infant than in a patient breathing room air.
III. **Differential diagnosis**
  A. **Metabolic acidosis** is defined as a pH <7.30–7.35 with a normal CO_2 value and a base deficit >5.
    1. **Common causes**
      a. Sepsis.
      b. Necrotizing enterocolitis (NEC).
      c. Hypothermia or cold stress.
      d. Asphyxia.
      e. Periventricular-intraventricular hemorrhage.
      f. Patent ductus arteriosus (PDA).
      g. Shock.

  h. Factitious acidosis (excessive heparin in the syringe). Air contamination can give a large base deficit.

  i. Drugs (eg, acetazolamide), benzyl alcohol in doxapram, and topical carbonic anhydrase inhibitors (eg, dorzolamide) have been reported to cause metabolic acidosis.

  j. Parenteral nutrition.

2. Less common causes

  a. Renal tubular acidosis is a defect in the reabsorption of bicarbonate or the secretion of hydrogen ion and can present in three forms: proximal, distal, or mixed.

  b. Inborn errors of metabolism. See Table 93–1 for those diseases that present with metabolic acidosis.

  c. Maternal use of salicylates and maternal acidosis.

  d. Renal failure and renal bicarbonate losses.

  e. Congenital lactic acidosis.

  f. Gastrointestinal losses such as frequent loose stools and short bowel syndrome.

B. **Metabolic alkalosis** is defined as a pH value >7.45 with a base excess of >5. It is usually iatrogenic and is uncommon.

1. Common causes

  a. Excess alkali administration (eg, sodium bicarbonate, citrate, acetate, or lactate infusion).

  b. Potassium depletion.

  c. Prolonged nasogastric suction.

  d. Diuretic therapy (eg, in patients with bronchopulmonary dysplasia).

2. Less common causes

  a. Pyloric stenosis (vomiting loss of gastric contents with a high acid concentration).

  b. Bartter syndrome.

  c. Primary hyperaldosteronism.

C. **Low CO_2, high O_2**

1. Overventilation.

2. Air bubble in the blood gas collection syringe.

3. Hyperventilation therapy, as used in persistent pulmonary hypertension.

D. **High CO_2, normal or high O_2**

1. Obstructed endotracheal tube (eg, mucus plug).

2. Endotracheal tube down the right main stem bronchus or at the carina.

3. Pneumothorax.

4. PDA. Suspect a PDA if the infant has a systolic murmur, active precordium, bounding pulses, and increased pulse pressure. Other clinical signs and symptoms may include congestive heart failure, deteriorating blood gases with an increase in the ventilator settings, and a possible large heart with increased pulmonary vascularity on chest radiograph.

5. Ventilator malfunction.

6. Permissive hypercapnia. Studies have shown an association between low P_{CO_2} and development of chronic lung disease and cystic periventricular leukomalacia. One study showed decreased risk of chronic lung disease with permissive hypercapnia keeping P_{CO_2} >52 mm Hg. Recent studies have been on the impact on autoregulation of cerebral blood flow on P_{CO_2} >45 in infants <1250 g in the first week of life in which autoregulation worsens as P_{CO_2} increases. Use caution with permissive hypercapnia until further studies are done.

E. **High CO_2, low O_2**

1. Pneumothorax.

2. Improper endotracheal tube position. An endotracheal tube positioned in the oropharynx causes this type of blood gas result.

3. Increasing respiratory failure.

4. PDA.

5. Insufficient respiratory support.
6. Atelectasis.
7. Lung disease (intrapulmonary shunt).

F. **Normal CO_2, low O_2**
1. Agitation.
2. Pneumothorax.
3. Improper endotracheal tube position.
4. Atelectasis.
5. Pulmonary hypertension.
6. Pulmonary edema.

IV. **Database**
A. **Physical examination.** Evaluate for signs of sepsis (eg, hypotension or poor perfusion). Check for equal breath sounds; asymmetric breath sounds suggest pneumothorax or poor ET (endotracheal) tube placement. Observe for chest wall movement. Listen for breath sounds over the chest versus the epigastric region, which may help determine whether the ET tube is malpositioned. Listen to the heart for any murmur, and palpate for cardiac displacement.

B. **Laboratory studies**
1. **Repeat blood gas measurement** if the result is unexpected. If a major clinical decision is to be made on the basis of venous or capillary blood gas values, an arterial blood sample should be obtained.
2. **Complete blood count with differential** if sepsis is being considered.
3. **Serum potassium level.** Severe metabolic alkalosis can cause hypokalemia.

C. **Radiologic and other studies**
1. **Pulmonary mechanics.** Check the tidal volume (V_T) delivered on the ventilator. The normal V_T is 5–6 mL/kg. If the V_T is low, it could mean that not enough pressure is given or there is an obstruction in the ET tube.
2. **Transillumination of the chest** should be done if pneumothorax is suspected (see Chapter 26).
3. **Chest radiograph** should be performed if an abnormal blood gas value is reported, unless there is an obvious cause. An anteroposterior view should be obtained to check ET placement (see Figure 10–7), rule out air leak (eg, pneumothorax, see Figure 10–19), check heart size and pulmonary vascularity (increased or decreased), and determine whether the infant is being hypoventilated or hyperventilated.
4. **Abdominal radiograph** if NEC is suspected in a patient with **severe metabolic acidosis.** See Figure 10–22 for a radiograph of NEC with pneumatosis intestinalis.
5. **Ultrasonography of the head** to diagnose intraventricular hemorrhage. See Figures 10–1 to 10–4 for examples of intraventricular hemorrhages on ultrasound.
6. **Echocardiography** may detect PDA or other cardiac abnormality.

V. **Plan**
A. **Overall plan.** Verify the blood gas result, find the cause of the problem, and provide treatment for the specific cause. First, examine the infant. If the infant's clinical status has not changed, repeat blood gas measurements to verify the report. If the clinical status has changed, the abnormal report is probably correct; repeat blood gas measurements and begin further evaluation of the infant.

B. **Specific management:**
1. **Metabolic acidosis**
a. **Key points in the treatment of neonatal metabolic acidosis:**
i. The use of sodium bicarbonate is *controversial* during resuscitation. A lack of evidence supports its use, and it is not recommended early on in resuscitation. If used later in resuscitation or during a prolonged resuscitation not responding to therapy, **make sure the lungs are adequately ventilated.**
ii. **No evidence supports or refutes rapid correction of metabolic acidosis in the first 24 h of life in a low birthweight infant,** when compared with a slow correction or no correction.

    iii. There is insufficient evidence to say that infusion of a base reduces mor-
bidity and mortality in a preterm infant with metabolic acidosis.

    iv. **Research has shown that sodium bicarbonate had no beneficial effect
on arterial acid-base status in the first 24 h of life.**

    v. Some institutions only do 24-hour corrections in patients with profound
postasphyxia acidosis (*controversial*).

    vi. One study found no difference between bicarbonate-treated and control
groups (not treated) for intraventricular hemorrhage, incidence of neonatal
seizures, incidence of abnormal neurologic exam at discharge, incidence
of encephalopathy, and survival to discharge.

  b. **General measures.** Most institutions treat acidosis with an alkali infusion if
the base excess is >−5 to −10 or if the pH is ≤7.25 (*controversial*). The alkali
can be given as IV push, one dose over 30 min or can be given as an 8 to 24 h
correction. If the acidosis is mild, usually only one dose is given and repeat
blood gas measurements are obtained. If the acidosis is severe, a dose is given
and correction is started at the same time. One of three medications is used.

    i. **Sodium bicarbonate** can be used if the infant's serum sodium and P_{CO_2}
are not high.

      (a) **One time dose:** 1–2 mEq/kg/dose, given as a 4.2% solution (0.5
mEq/mL); infuse at 1 mEq/kg/min max over at least 30 min.

      (b) **IV push (for cardiac arrest, routine use not recommended; IV push,**
controversial): 1 mEq/kg slow IV push, given as 0.5 mEq/mL (4.2%
concentration). Maximum rate in neonates and infants is 10 mEq/min.
May repeat with a 0.5 mEq/kg dose in 10 min one time as indicated
by patient's unstable acid-base status. Not often recommended because
data suggest potential neurodevelopmental effects of rapid injections
of bicarbonate.

      (c) **Slow correction** should be given over 8–24 h in IV fluids. The total
dose required to correct the base deficit is as follows:

Method 1. HCO_3^- dose (mEq) = Base deficit (mEq/L) × weight (kg) × 0.3

Method 2. HCO_3^- dose (mEq) = 0.5 × weight × (24−serum HCO_3^-)

    ii. **Tromethamine (THAM)** can be used in infants who have metabolic
acidosis but have a high serum sodium (>150 mEq/L) or high P_{CO_2}
(>65 mm Hg). It does not increase CO_2 as bicarbonate does in neonates
with respiratory failure. **Use only in infants with good urine output
(hyperkalemia risk) and monitor for hypoglycemia.** (See also Chapter
132.) (*Controversial:* Many institutions do not use THAM because of side
effects: higher osmolar load, risk of hypoglycemia, severe vasospasm, apnea,
arterial vasodilatation, and decreased aortic diastolic pressure that can
lower coronary artery perfusion.)

    iii. **Polycitrate (Polycitra).** This alkali, useful in patients receiving acetazo-
lamide (Diamox), consists of 1 mEq Na$^+$, 1 mEq K$^+$, and 2 mEq citrate.
Each 1 mEq citrate equals 1 mEq bicarbonate. The dose is 2–3 mEq/kg/day
polycitrate in three to four divided doses; adjust dose to maintain a normal pH.

  c. **The underlying cause should be treated as outlined:**

    i. **Sepsis.** Initiate a septic workup and consider broad-spectrum antibiotics.
(See Chapter 117.)

    ii. **NEC.** See Chapter 104.

    iii. **Hypothermia or cold stress.** See Chapter 6.

    iv. **Periventricular-intraventricular hemorrhage.** Weekly ultrasonographic
examinations of the head and daily head circumferences are indicated.
Monitor the infant for signs of increased intracranial pressure (convulsions,
vomiting, and/or hypotension) (see Chapter 96).

v. **PDA.** The patient who has a hemodynamically significant PDA should be treated. Treatment includes furosemide, decreased fluid intake, and a course of indomethacin or ibuprofen. Ibuprofen is being used at some institutions. Recent reviews found no statistically significant difference in ibuprofen compared with indomethacin in closing the PDA. A recent study showed that neither continuous indomethacin infusion nor ibuprofen showed any adverse renal effects or peripheral vasoconstrictive effects. The data support either drug and do not make a recommendation of the drug of choice until further long-term studies are done. Physicians need to evaluate the patient, institutional guidelines, and the risks of side effects in deciding which medication to use. (See Chapter 109 on PDA and Chapter 132 for dosing information.)

vi. **Renal tubular acidosis** is treated with sodium bicarbonate (see Section III, A, 2a).

vii. **Inborn errors of metabolism.** Rare cause (see Chapter 93).

viii. **Maternal use of salicylates.** Acidosis usually resolves without treatment.

ix. **Renal failure.** See Chapter 113.

x. **Congenital lactic acidosis.** Correction of the metabolic acidosis (see Section V, b) and megavitamin therapy are indicated.

xi. **Parenteral hyperalimentation.** Preterm infants usually need acetate supplementation in hyperalimentation to correct for ongoing bicarbonate losses.

2. **Metabolic alkalosis** treatment depends on the cause.

a. **Excess administered alkali.** Adjust or discontinue the dose of THAM, sodium bicarbonate, or polycitrate; reduce acetate in hyperalimentation.

b. **Hypokalemia can cause a shift** of hydrogen ions into cells as potassium is lost. The infant's potassium level should be corrected (see Chapter 56).

c. **Prolonged nasogastric suction** is treated with IV fluid replacement, usually with 1/2 normal saline with 20 mEq KCl, replaced milliliter for milliliter each shift.

d. **Diuretics** can cause mild alkalosis; no specific treatment is usually necessary.

e. **Bartter syndrome** is treated with indomethacin and potassium supplements.

f. **Primary hyperaldosteronism** is treated with dexamethasone. (See Chapter 132 for dose.)

3. **Other causes of abnormal blood gases**

a. **ET problems.** Determine if there are any changes on the pulmonary function test measurements on the ventilator that may indicate a problem with the ET tube. Colorimetric CO_2 detectors (eg, Pedi-Cap; Nellcor) can be used to determine airway patency with a color change from purple to yellow if there is exhaled CO_2 gas. If no color change, there is airway obstruction and possible ET tube problem. A useful technique is to know and chart the specific mark on the ET tube when it is in the correct position to determine quickly if the tube is out of position.

i. **Mucus plug.** If an infant has decreased breath sounds on both sides of the chest and has retractions, a plugged ET tube is possible. Pulmonary function measurements on specific ventilators may also define this if the V_T is low. The infant can be suctioned, and, if clinically stable, repeat blood gas measurements can be obtained. If the infant is in extreme distress, replace the tube.

ii. **ET placement problems.** An infant with a tube placed down the right main stem bronchus has breath sounds on the right only. An infant with a tube that has dislodged has decreased or no breath sounds on chest auscultation.

b. **Ventilator issues.** Changes in blood gas levels based on changes in ventilator setting can be found in Chapter 7, Table 7–4, page 54).

i. **Overventilation.** If the blood gas levels reveal overventilation, the ventilation parameters need to be adjusted. If the oxygen level is high, the following parameters can be decreased: oxygen, positive end-expiratory pressure (PEEP), peak inspiratory pressure (PIP), or inspiratory time.

If the patient's CO_2 level is low, the following parameters can be decreased: rate, PIP, or expiratory time. Deciding which parameter to wean depends on the patient's lung disease and the disease course. See Table 7–4 for changes in blood gas levels caused by changes in ventilator settings.

ii. **Insufficient respiratory support.** If the infant's chest is not moving, the PIP is not high enough and adjustment of the ventilator setting is needed. Also check the V_T; if it is low, it could mean not enough pressure is given.

iii. **Ventilator malfunction.** Notify respiratory therapy to check the ventilator and replace it if necessary.

c. **Agitation** may cause the infant to drop in oxygenation and need sedation (***controversial***) or have ventilator settings changed. See also Chapter 69.

i. *Note:* **agitation can be a sign of hypoxia, so a blood gas level should be obtained before ordering sedation.** If there is documented hypoxia, attempts to increase oxygenation should be used.

ii. **Sit by the bedside** and try different ventilator rates to see whether the infant fights less.

iii. **Routine sedation is usually not recommended** because in very low birthweight infants and premature infants it is associated with an increase in severe intraventricular hemorrhage (IVH), delay in diuresis, and ileus.

iv. **If sedation is chosen,** phenobarbital, diazepam, lorazepam, midazolam, fentanyl, chloral hydrate, or morphine may be used. (See Chapters 69 and 132 for doses.) Use the preferred agent at your institution.

d. **Acute change in clinical pulmonary status**

i. **Pneumothorax.** See Chapter 63.

ii. **Atelectasis.** Treatment consists of percussion and postural drainage and possibly increased PIP or PEEP. Avoid percussion in small preterm infants; a study showed a strong link between IVH and porencephaly with chest physiotherapy in extremely premature infants.

iii. **Pulmonary edema.** Diuretics (eg, furosemide) (see Chapter 132) are the primary treatment with mechanical ventilation as indicated.

iv. **Pulmonary hypertension.** See Chapter 111.

---

41 Apnea and Bradycardia ("A's and B's")

I. **Problem.** An infant has just had an apneic episode with bradycardia. **Apnea is the absence of breathing for >20 s or a shorter pause (>10 s) associated with oxygen desaturation or bradycardia (<100 beats/min). Central apnea** is the complete absence of respiratory effort. **Obstructive apnea** occurs when an infant breathes but no airflow is present because of an obstruction. **Mixed apnea** is both central and obstructive apnea. **Periodic breathing** is three or more respiratory pauses lasting >3 s separated by normal respiratory intervals not longer than 20 s. This is not associated with bradycardia. **Apnea of prematurity (AOP)** is most prevalent in premature infants <36 weeks' gestation and is most commonly central or mixed apnea. Apnea is very common: >50% of infants <1500 g and 90% of infants <1000 g have it.

II. **Immediate questions**

A. **What is the gestational age of the infant?** Apnea and bradycardia are common in premature infants. In term infants, they are uncommon and usually associated with a serious disorder in the infant or a maternal condition such as magnesium treatment or maternal exposure to narcotics. **Apnea in a term infant is never physiologic; it requires a full workup to determine the cause.**

B. Was significant stimulation needed to return the heart rate to normal? An infant requiring significant stimulation (eg, oxygen by bag-and-mask ventilation) needs immediate evaluation and treatment. An infant who has had one episode of apnea and bradycardia not requiring oxygen supplementation may not need a full evaluation unless the infant is term.

C. If the patient is already receiving medication (eg, methylxanthine) for apnea and bradycardia, is the dosage adequate? Determine the serum drug level.

D. Did the episode occur during or after feeding? It was felt that gastroesophageal reflux (GER) caused apnea and bradycardia because it was observed when regurgitation of formula into the pharynx occurred after feeding. This has been a source of much debate with recent studies showing no temporal relationship. Consider aspiration in an infant who has been doing well and feeding. Insertion of a nasogastric tube may cause a vagal reflex, resulting in apnea and bradycardia.

E. How old is the infant? Apnea and bradycardia in the first 24 h are usually pathologic. The peak incidence of apnea of prematurity occurs between 5 and 7 days postnatal age but can occur earlier.

III. **Differential diagnosis.** Causes of apnea and bradycardia can be classified according to diseases and disorders of various organ systems, gestational age, or postnatal age.

A. **Diseases and disorders of various organ systems**

1. **Head and central nervous system**
   a. Perinatal asphyxia.
   b. Intraventricular or subarachnoid hemorrhage.
   c. Meningitis.
   d. Hydrocephalus with increased intracranial pressure.
   e. Cerebral infarct with seizures.
   f. Seizures.

2. **Respiratory system**
   a. Hypoxia.
   b. Airway obstruction.
   c. Lung disease.
   d. Inadequate ventilation or performing extubation too early.

3. **Cardiovascular system**
   a. Congestive heart failure.
   b. Patent ductus arteriosus.
   c. Cardiac disorders such as congenital heart block, hypoplastic left heart syndrome, and transposition of the great vessels.

4. **Gastrointestinal (GI) tract**
   a. **Necrotizing enterocolitis (NEC).** Apnea has been associated with the onset of NEC.
   b. **Gastroesophageal reflux (GER)** is thought by some investigators to be related to AOP; however, to date, no research has shown a relationship between the two. Some studies suggest antireflux surgery can reduce apnea in preterm infants at highest risk. Additional studies are needed. It is a rare cause of apnea in a full-term infant.
   c. **Feeding intolerance.**

5. **Hematologic system**
   a. **Anemia.** There is no specific hematocrit at which apnea and bradycardia occur. They have been seen in infants with anemia of prematurity. These infants show significant improvement after transfusion. Studies have shown liberal blood transfusion significantly reduced apnea as compared with more restrictive blood transfusion.
   b. **Polycythemia,** which is more common in term infants.

6. **Other diseases and disorders**
   a. **Temperature instability,** especially hyperthermia but also hypothermia, can cause apnea and bradycardia. Note the incubator temperature; the infant may have a normal body temperature but may have a rise in incubator temperature (the infant is hypothermic) or may require a lower incubator temperature (the infant is hyperthermic). Any rapid fluctuation of temperature can cause apnea. Cold stress can occur after birth or during transport or a procedure, and it may produce apnea.
   b. **Infection (sepsis).** Check for bacterial, fungal, and viral infections. Respiratory syncytial virus and apnea are common in preterm infants with urea plasma urealyticum infection.
   c. **Metabolic or electrolyte imbalance.** Hypoglycemia, hyponatremia, hypernatremia, hypermagnesemia (during parenteral nutrition), hyperkalemia, hyperammonemia, and hypocalcemia can cause apnea and bradycardia.
   d. **Vagal reflex** may occur secondary to nasogastric tube insertion, feeding, and suctioning.
   e. **Drugs/Drug withdrawal.** High levels of phenobarbital or other sedatives, such as diazepam and chloral hydrate, may cause apnea and bradycardia. Oversedation from maternal drugs such as magnesium sulfate, opiates, and general anesthesia can cause apnea in the newborn. Topical eye drops for routine eye examinations can sometimes cause changes in apnea pattern. Apnea can be seen in drug withdrawal of infants born to drug-addicted mothers.
   f. **Immunization.** Apnea increases in hospitalized preterm infants after immunization with the whole cell pertussis component. New studies have shown an increase in apnea/bradycardia/desaturation after the DTaP-IPV-HIb and DTaP-IPV-HIb-HBV in premature infants with chronic disease. It is recommended to give these at 8 weeks if still hospitalized with close observation.
   g. **Kangaroo care.** Studies have shown conflicting results as to whether apnea has been associated with kangaroo care. Early studies showed a relationship, but recent studies have found no adverse effects. Observe head positioning during holding.
   h. **Surgery** can cause postoperative apnea in premature infants.
B. **Gestational age.** See Table 41–1.
   1. **Full-term infants** usually do not have apnea and bradycardia from physiologic causes; the disease or disorder must be identified.

Table 41–1. MORE COMMON CAUSES OF APNEA AND BRADYCARDIA ACCORDING TO GESTATIONAL AGE

Premature Infant	Full-Term Infant	All Ages
Apnea of prematurity	Cerebral infarction	Sepsis
PDA	Polycythemia	NEC
HMD		Meningitis
Respiratory insufficiency of prematurity		Aspiration
PV-IVH		GER
Anemia of prematurity		Pneumonia
Posthemorrhagic hydrocephalus		Cardiac disorder
		Postextubation atelectasis
		Seizures
		Cold stress
		Asphyxia

HMD, hyaline membrane disease; GER, gastroesophageal reflux; NEC, necrotizing enterocolitis; PDA, patent ductus arteriosus; PV-IVH, periventricular-intraventricular hemorrhage.

2. **Preterm infants.** (See Table 41–1.) The most common cause is AOP, usually presenting between the day 2 and 7 of life (usually <34 weeks' gestation, <1800 g, and no other identifiable cause) and is a diagnosis of exclusion.

C. **Postnatal age can be a clue to cause**

1. **Onset within hours after birth:** Oversedation from maternal drugs, asphyxia, seizures, hypermagnesemia, or hyaline membrane disease.

2. **Onset <1 week:** Postextubation atelectasis, patent ductus arteriosus, periventricular-intraventricular hemorrhage, or AOP.

3. **Onset >1 week of age:** Posthemorrhagic hydrocephalus with increased intracranial pressure or seizures.

4. **Onset at 6–10 weeks:** Anemia of prematurity.

5. **Variable onset:** Sepsis, necrotizing enterocolitis (NEC), meningitis, aspiration, GER, cardiac disorder, pneumonia, cold stress, or fluctuations in temperatures.

IV. **Database.** Determine whether there has been any prenatal risk of sepsis. The cord pH should be obtained to rule out birth asphyxia. A history of feeding intolerance increases the suspicion of NEC.

A. **Complete physical examination** with attention to the following signs:

1. **Head.** Signs of increased intracranial pressure.

2. **Heart.** Listen for a murmur or gallop.

3. **Lungs.** Check for adequate movement of the chest if mechanical ventilation is being used.

4. **Abdomen.** Check for abdominal distention, one of the earliest signs of NEC. Other signs of NEC are decreased bowel sounds and visible bowel loops.

5. **Skin.** An infant with polycythemia has a ruddy appearance. Pallor is associated with anemia.

B. **Laboratory studies**

1. **Complete blood cell count with differential.** Findings may suggest infection, anemia, or polycythemia.

2. **Cultures of the blood, urine, and cerebrospinal (CSF) fluid** if infection is suspected. A C-reactive protein level at 48 h after birth may be useful as an infection screen. PCR analyses and viral cultures are appropriate if a viral infection is suspected.

3. **Serum electrolyte, calcium, magnesium, and glucose levels** to rule out metabolic abnormality.

4. **Serum phenobarbital and methylxanthine levels** if indicated.

5. **Arterial blood gas levels** to rule out hypoxia and acidosis.

6. **If an inborn error of metabolism is suspected,** test for organic acid levels, amino acid profiles, ammonia, pyruvate, and lactate. Ketones in the urine may indicate an organic academia.

C. **Radiologic and other studies**

1. **Chest radiograph** should be performed immediately if there is any suspicion of heart or lung disease.

2. **Electrocardiography** if cardiac disease is suspected.

3. **Echocardiography and cardiac consultation.**

4. **Abdominal radiograph** should be performed immediately if indicated. It may detect signs of NEC (see Figure 10–22).

5. **Ultrasonography of the head** to rule out periventricular-intraventricular hemorrhage or hydrocephalus.

6. **Computed tomography of the head** to detect cerebral infarction and subarachnoid hemorrhage. Use adjusted scanning protocol to limit radiation exposure; magnetic resonance imaging is indicated because of the concern for radiation exposure.

7. **Barium swallow** to rule out GER (only in cases of apnea and bradycardia associated with feeding). It is helpful if the infant has a swallowing dysfunction or you suspect tracheoesophageal fistula or esophageal web.

8. **Lumbar puncture and CSF analysis** if meningitis is suspected or if increased intracranial pressure from hydrocephalus is causing apnea and bradycardia.

9. **Esophageal pH probe testing (acid reflux test of Tuttle and Grossman)** is useful in determining whether acidic GER is present. A small-caliber tube with a pH electrode is passed into the distal esophagus. Continuous monitoring can be carried out over 4–24 h. If the pH is acidic, acidic GER is occurring. Most reflux in infants is not acidic. pH monitoring is of limited use in premies because their gastric pH is >4 ~90% of the time.

10. **Reflux scintiscan (termed "milk scan" if used with milk or formula).** This test is used to document GER. It is comparable to the pH probe and superior to the barium swallow. Technetium-99m-labeled pertechnetate is put in a water-based solution or milk (milk scan) and is instilled in the stomach. The patient is scanned in the supine position for 2 h with the gamma camera.

11. **Electroencephalography.** Apnea and bradycardia may be a manifestation of seizure activity.

12. **Pneumography, thermistor pneumography, and polysomnography.** See Chapter 76.

13. **Abdominal sonography or gastric emptying study** is useful where GI motility disorder is suspected.

V. **Plan** (See also Chapter 76.)

A. **Determine the cause of apnea and bradycardia, and treat if possible.**

B. **Sepsis is a cause that cannot be overlooked because antibiotics need to be started.** Rule out sepsis before treating other causes.

C. **Research does not support prophylactic methylxanthines or carnitine supplementation for apnea.**

D. **Kinesthetic stimulation (oscillating mattress) is not effective in clinically significant apnea.**

F. **Apnea of prematurity (AOP)**

1. **General measures**
   a. Maintain adequate oxygen saturation with supplemental oxygen.
   b. Keep the environmental temperature stable.
   c. Make sure the position of the infant does not compromise respiration.
   d. Avoid triggers such as vigorous suctioning.
   e. Provide tactile stimulation (eg, rubbing the skin, stroking the back, patting the infant, tapping or tickling the feet).
   f. Olfactory stimulation. One study found that introducing a pleasant odor (vanillin) into the incubator decreased apnea unresponsive to caffeine or doxapram. (See Chapter 19.)

2. **Specific treatment**
   a. **Continuous positive airway pressure (CPAP)** via nasal prongs reduces apneic spells. (**Note:** Different sources cite different CPAP parameters. Some sample ranges reported: 2–4, 3–6, 4–6, and 5–8 cm H_2O. Use the settings recommended by your institution. An alternative to nasal CPAP is to use a **high-flow nasal cannula** (rates from 1–6 L/min). This method may prevent apnea through nasal irritation causing arousal. CPAP can be used in conjunction with medication (after a therapeutic level has been obtained).
   b. **Theophylline, aminophylline, or caffeine is used initially. Caffeine** seems to have fewer side effects than theophylline and is the most preferred. Recent data suggest that caffeine therapy is associated with improved neurodevelopmental outcome and survival at 18–21 months in infants 500–1250 g. The drug of choice depends on institutional preference and availability. (See Chapter 132.) Therapy can usually be discontinued by postconceptional age, usually 35–37 weeks, depending on the weight of the infant (usually 1800–2000 g) or if the infant has been free of apnea for 5–7 days. It is important to remember that the more immature infant will probably require treatment longer. One study found that

the incidence of apnea persisting beyond 38 weeks' postconceptional age was significantly higher in the 24- to 27-week infant than in the ≥28-week infant.
  c. **If apnea persists, begin doxapram** (*controversial*). Doxapram appears to be efficacious when theophylline and caffeine have failed; it can reduce apnea within 48 h after other methods have failed. There are concerns with doxapram (risk of reduced cerebral blood flow with mental delay later; increased QTc interval >440 ms, a life-threatening threshold); doxapram contains benzyl alcohol preservative with metabolic acidosis risk. If acidosis occurs, consider stopping the medication. This medication should be used only if other treatments have failed. (For pharmacologic information, see Chapter 132.)
  d. **Mechanical ventilation** should be used if apnea and bradycardia cannot be controlled by drug therapy or nasal CPAP. Low pressures are used at the rate necessary to prevent apnea. (See Chapter 7.)
  3. **Long-term monitoring of respiratory function.** For home apnea monitoring. See Chapter 76.
G. **Anemia.** Most institutions do not treat anemia if the infant is asymptomatic, is feeding and growing, and the reticulocyte count indicates that red blood cells are being made (>5–6%). If the hematocrit is low (usually <21–25%, based on institutional guidelines), or the infant is symptomatic or not feeding well, and the reticulocyte count is not appropriate for the low hematocrit (ie, reticulocyte count <2–3%), frequent transfusion is indicated (*controversial*). If the infant is on oxygen or respiratory support, frequent transfusion is indicated to maintain a higher hematocrit. A recent study found that liberal versus restrictive blood transfusion significantly reduced apnea. Many institutions are now using recombinant human erythropoietin (rHuEPO) with iron for anemia of prematurity, decreasing the need for transfusions. A recent review noted that early or late administration of rHuEPO is not recommended. rHuEPO increased the incidence of retinopathy of prematurity (ROP) and possibly the progression of ROP. rHuEPO was a significant independent risk factor for the development of ROP.
H. **GER** is common in premature infants. Apnea is unrelated to GER in most studies. Most institutions treat GER because there may be an association (even though infrequent). Treatment options include the following:
  1. **Feedings.** Overfeeding can aggravate reflux so small volumes more frequently are recommended. Continuous tube feedings may help. Thickened feedings are recommended but *controversial* because randomized trials are inconclusive. A change in formula may be necessary if a food allergy is suspected. A diet change for the mother with a breast-feeding infant may be necessary.
  2. **Position.** Hold the infant upright in your arms at least 30 min after feeding. Complete upright and prone position is beneficial. Head-elevated prone position was preferred in infants with GER but it has become *controversial* because of its association with sudden infant death syndrome (SIDS). Infants with GER should sleep on their backs.
  3. **Medications.** If needed, the following can be used. Some clinicians advocate a prokinetic agent (eg, metoclopramide). If there is true acid reflux (documented by esophageal pH probe studies), then an H_2 blocker or proton pump inhibitor is used.
     a. **Prokinetic agents**
        i. **Metoclopramide (Reglan)** improves GI motility and reduces feeding intolerance. In GER of prematurity it is commonly used but *controversial.* (See Chapter 132 for dosing and other information.) The effectiveness of metoclopramide is inconclusive in the current literature. One of the main concerns is side effects (eg, drowsiness, restlessness, extrapyramidal symptoms). A large randomized trial is needed.
        ii. **Erythromycin** is a prokinetic agent and increases gastric motility. It has been used in GER. A recent study found that low-dose erythromycin in premature infants did not decrease the symptoms of reflux when compared with a placebo. (See Chapter 48, Section V, A, 2.)

b. **Antacids.** Maalox or Mylanta are sometimes recommended. The use of antacids increases the risk of infection and feeding intolerance in infants receiving gavage feedings. There is also a concern for the risk of concretion formation. Side effects include diarrhea or constipation. If used, the dosage is 0.5–1 mL/kg by mouth every 4 h by nasogastric tube.

c. **H_2 blockers inhibit gastric acid production in neonates and are usually recommended.** Of the four H_2 blockers available, ranitidine (Zantac) and cimetidine are most commonly used in infants. Ranitidine is preferred because of fewer side effects. H_2 blocker therapy is associated with higher rates of NEC in very low birthweight infants and an increased risk of candidal infections with H_2 blockers (predisposes to gastric colonization and increases the risk of bacteremia).

d. **Proton pump inhibitors** are being studied and look promising, but they are not approved in children. Lansoprazole and omeprazole have been used the most in infants. Like the H_2 blockers, they also increase the risk of Candida infections.

42 Arrhythmia

I. **Problem.** An infant has an abnormal tracing on the heart rate monitor.
II. **Immediate questions**
   A. **What is the heart rate?** The heart rate in newborns varies from 70–190 beats/min. It is normally 120–140 beats/min but may decrease to 70–90 beats/min during sleep and increase to 170–190 beats/min with increased activity such as crying. See Table 42–1 for normal heart rate values.
   B. **Is the abnormality continuous or transient?** Transient episodes of sinus bradycardia, tachycardia, or arrhythmias (usually lasting <15 s) are benign and do not require further workup. Episodes lasting >15 s usually require full electrocardiogram (ECG) assessment.
   C. **Is the infant symptomatic?** A symptomatic infant may need immediate treatment. Signs and symptoms of some pathologic arrhythmias include tachypnea, poor skin perfusion, lethargy, hepatomegaly, and rales on pulmonary examination. All of these signs and symptoms may signify congestive heart failure (CHF), which may accompany arrhythmias. CHF resulting from rapid cardiac rhythms is unusual with heart rates <240 beats/min.

Table 42–1. **MINIMUM AND MAXIMUM HEART RATES IN NORMAL NEWBORNS**

Age	Minimum	Mean	Maximum	SD
0–24 h	85	119	145	16.1
1–7 d	100	133	175	22.3
8–30 d	115	163	190	19.9

SD, standard deviation.
Reproduced with permission from Hastreiter AR, Abella JE: The electrocardiogram in the newborn period: I. The normal infant. *J Pediatr* 1971;78:146.

III. Differential diagnosis
   A. Heart rate abnormalities
      1. **Tachycardia** is a heart rate >2 standard deviations (SD) above the mean for age (see Table 42–1).
         a. **Benign causes**
            i. Postdelivery.
            ii. Heat or cold stress.
            iii. Painful stimuli.
            iv. Medications (eg, atropine, theophylline [aminophylline], epinephrine, intravenous glucagon, pancuronium bromide, tolazoline, and isoproterenol) can cause tachycardia.
         b. **Pathologic causes**
            i. **More common.** Fever, shock, hypoxia, anemia, sepsis, patent ductus arteriosus, and CHF.
            ii. **Less common.** Hyperthyroidism, metabolic disorders, cardiac arrhythmias, and hyperammonemia.
      2. **Bradycardia.** Bradycardia is a heart rate >2 SD below the mean for age (see Table 42–1). Transient bradycardia is fairly common in newborns; rates range from 60–70 beats/min.
         a. **Benign causes**
            i. Defecation.
            ii. Vomiting.
            iii. Micturition.
            iv. Gavage feedings.
            v. Suctioning.
            vi. Medications (eg, propranolol, digitalis, atropine, and infusion of calcium, long-acting β-blockers to treat hypertension given within 24 h of delivery).
         b. **Pathologic causes**
            i. **More common.** Hypoxia, apnea, convulsions, airway obstruction, air leak (eg, pneumothorax), CHF, intracranial bleeding, severe acidosis, and severe hypothermia.
            ii. **Less common.** Hyperkalemia, cardiac arrhythmias, pulmonary hemorrhage, diaphragmatic hernia, hypothyroidism, and hydrocephalus.
   B. Arrhythmias
      1. **Benign arrhythmias** include any transient episode (<15 s) of sinus bradycardia and tachycardia and any of the benign causes of sinus tachycardia and bradycardia noted in Section III, A, 1 and 2. Sinus arrhythmia, a phasic variation in the heart rate often associated with respiration, is also benign.
         a. **Premature atrial beats** can occur in the newborn and are usually benign. The QRS is narrow, and the T waves are often discordant. (See the example in Figure 42–1C.) They tend to decrease in number or go away entirely in the first few months of life. A workup is usually not indicated unless the infant has the premature atrial beats in association with structural cardiac disease.
         b. **Unifocal premature ventricular beats** are fairly frequent in the newborn. The QRS is wide, and the T wave is discordant with the sinus T wave. (See Figure 42–1D.) If seen in a newborn, obtain a 12-lead ECG. Do not treat unless the infant is symptomatic. Sometimes premature ventricular contractions (PVCs) become less frequent when the sinus rate increases. PVCs tend to decrease in number or go away entirely in the first few months of life.
         c. **Benign bradycardia** is unusual but not rare.
      2. **Pathologic arrhythmias**
         a. **Supraventricular tachycardia (SVT)** is the most common type of cardiac arrhythmia seen in the neonate (see Figure 42–1A).
         b. **Atrial flutter** is difficult to distinguish from other SVTs, unless the block is >2:1.
         c. **Atrial fibrillation** is less common than SVT or atrial flutter.

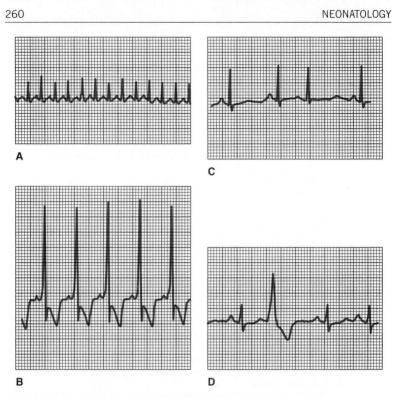

Figure 42–1. (**A**) Supraventricular, narrow QRS tachycardia with a rate of 300 beats/min. The PR interval is long for this rate. (**B**) Wolff-Parkinson-White syndrome with a short PR interval and a delta upstroke on the QRS complex. The T waves are often discordant. (**C**) A premature atrial beat. The QRS is narrow, and the T wave is concordant with sinus T waves. (**D**) A premature ventricular beat. The QRS is wide, and the T wave is discordant with the sinus T wave.

    d. Wolff-Parkinson-White syndrome (WPW) (a short PR interval and delta wave and slow upstroke of the QRS complex) is difficult to identify when the rate is fast (see Figure 42–1B).

    e. Ectopic beats.

    f. Ventricular tachycardia.

    g. Atrioventricular (AV) block, with symptoms occurring in newborns with complete AV block and ventricular rates <55 beats/min.

3. Secondary to extracardiac disease

    a. Sepsis (usually tachycardia).

    b. Diseases of the central nervous system (usually bradycardia).

    c. Hypoglycemia.

    d. Drug toxicity.

        i. Digoxin potentiated by hypokalemia, alkalosis, hypercalcemia, and hypomagnesemia.

        ii. Theophylline, but it is less frequently used now in neonatal intensive care units.

    e. Adrenal insufficiency.

   f. Electrolyte abnormalities such as potassium, sodium, magnesium, or calcium.

   g. Metabolic acidosis or alkalosis.

IV. Database

A. Physical examination. Perform a complete physical examination. Check for signs of CHF (ie, tachypnea, rales on pulmonary examination, enlarged liver, and cardiomegaly). Vomiting and lethargy may be seen in patients with digoxin toxicity. Hypokalemia can cause ileus.

B. Laboratory studies

1. **Electrolyte, calcium, and magnesium levels.**

2. **Blood gas** may reveal acidosis or hypoxia.

3. **Drug levels** to evaluate for toxicity.

   a. Digoxin. Normal serum levels are 0.5–2.0 mcg/mL (sometimes up to 4 mcg/mL). Elevated levels of digoxin alone are not diagnostic of toxicity; clinical and ECG findings consistent with toxicity are also needed, and many neonates have naturally occurring substances that interfere with the radioimmunoassay test for digoxin.

   b. Theophylline. Normal levels are 4–12 mcg/mL. Toxicity is associated with levels >15–20 mcg/mL.

C. Radiologic and other studies

1. **ECG** should be performed in all infants who have an abnormal ECG that lasts >15 s or is not related to a benign condition. Diagnostic features of the common arrhythmias are listed next.

   a. Supraventricular tachycardia (see Figure 42–1A)

   i. A ventricular rate of 180–300 beats/min.

   ii. No change in heart rate with activity or crying.

   iii. An abnormal P wave or PR interval.

   iv. A fixed R-R interval.

   b. Atrial flutter

   i. The atrial rate is 220–400 beats/min.

   ii. A sawtooth configuration seen best in leads V_1–V_3 but often difficult to identify when a 2:1 block or rapid ventricular rate is present.

   iii. The QRS complex is usually normal.

   c. Atrial fibrillation

   i. Irregular atrial waves that vary in size and shape from beat to beat.

   ii. The atrial rate is 350–600 beats/min.

   iii. The QRS complex is normal, but ventricular response is irregular.

   d. Wolff-Parkinson-White syndrome (see Figure 42–1B)

   i. A short PR interval.

   ii. A widened QRS complex.

   iii. Presence of a delta wave.

   e. Ventricular tachycardia

   i. Ventricular premature beats at a rate of 120–200 beats/min.

   ii. A widened QRS complex.

   f. Ectopic beats

   i. An abnormal P wave.

   ii. A widened QRS complex.

   g. Atrioventricular block

   i. **First-degree block**

   (a) A prolonged PR interval (normal range, 0.08–0.12 s).

   (b) Normal sinus rhythm.

   (c) A normal QRS complex.

   ii. **Second-degree block**

   (a) **Mobitz type I**

   • A prolonged PR interval with a dropped ventricular beat.

   • A normal QRS complex.

   (b) **Mobitz type II.** A constant PR interval with dropped ventricular beats.

        iii. **Third-degree block**
          (a) A regular atrial beat.
          (b) A slower ventricular rate.
          (c) Independent atrial and ventricular beats.
          (d) The atrial rate increases with crying and level of activity. The ventricular rate usually stays the same.
   h. **Hyperkalemia**
      i. Tall, tented T waves.
      ii. A widened QRS complex.
      iii. A flat and wide P wave.
      iv. Ventricular fibrillation and late asystole.
   i. **Hypokalemia**
      i. Prolonged QT and PR intervals.
      ii. A depressed ST segment.
      iii. A flat T wave.
   j. **Hypocalcemia.** A prolonged QT interval.
   k. **Hypercalcemia.** A shortened QT interval.
   l. **Hypomagnesemia.** Same as for hyperkalemia.
   m. **Hyponatremia**
      i. A short QT interval.
      ii. Increased duration of the QRS complex.
   n. **Hypernatremia**
      i. A prolonged QT interval.
      ii. Decreased duration of the QRS complex.
   o. **Metabolic acidosis**
      i. Prolonged PR and QRS intervals.
      ii. Increased amplitude of the P wave.
      iii. Tall, peaked T waves.
   p. **Metabolic alkalosis.** An inverted T wave.
   q. **Digoxin**
      i. Therapeutic levels: A prolonged PR interval and a short QT interval.
      ii. Toxic levels: Most common are sinoatrial block, second-degree AV block, and multiple ectopic beats; also seen are AV block and bradycardia.
   r. **Theophylline**
      i. Therapeutic levels: No effect.
      ii. Toxic levels: Tachycardia and conduction abnormality.
  2. **Chest radiograph** in all infants with suspected heart failure or air leak.
V. **Plan**
  A. **General management.** First, decide whether the arrhythmia is benign or pathologic, as noted. If it is pathologic, full ECG evaluation must be performed. Any acid-base disorder, hypoxia, or electrolyte abnormality needs to be corrected.
  B. **Specific management**
    1. **Heart rate abnormalities**
      a. **Tachycardia**
        i. **Benign.** No treatment is necessary because the tachycardia is usually secondary to a self-limited event.
        ii. **Medications.** With certain medications, such as theophylline, order a serum drug level to determine whether it is in the toxic range. If it is, lowering the dosage may restore normal rhythm. Otherwise, a decision must be made to accept the tachycardia, if the medication is needed, or to discontinue the drug.
        iii. **Pathologic conditions.** The underlying disease should be treated.
      b. **Bradycardia**
        i. **Benign.** No treatment is usually necessary.
        ii. **Drug related.** Check the serum drug level if possible, and then consider lowering the dosage or discontinuing the drug unless it is necessary.

    iii. Pathologic
      (a) Treat the underlying disease.
      (b) In severe hypotension or cardiac arrest, check the airway and initiate breathing and cardiac compressions.
      (c) Administer atropine, epinephrine, or isoproterenol to restore normal rhythm. (See Chapter 132 for dosing.)
  2. Arrhythmias. For dosages and other pharmacologic information, see Chapter 132; for cardioversion, see Chapter 27.
    a. Benign. Only observation.
    b. Pathologic. Treat any underlying acid-base disorders, hypoxia, or electrolyte abnormalities.
      i. Supraventricular tachycardia
        (a) **If the infant's condition is critical,** electrical cardioversion is indicated, with digoxin started for maintenance therapy.
        (b) **If the infant's condition is stable,** vagal stimulation (an ice-cold washcloth applied to the infant's face for a few seconds) can be tried. Adenosine, 100 mcg/kg, IV push into a central vein, converts SVT to sinus rhythm. It may be necessary to double the dose to 200 mcg/kg (300 mcg/kg maximum). **Never use verapamil in infants.** Digoxin should be started as a maintenance drug. Another drug that may be used instead of or in addition to digoxin is propranolol. SVT refractory to digoxin and propranolol may be treated with flecainide or amiodarone.
      ii. Atrial flutter
        (a) **If the infant's condition is critical** (severe CHF or unstable hemodynamic state), perform electrical cardioversion, with digoxin started for maintenance.
        (b) **If the infant is stable,** start digoxin, which slows the ventricular rate. A combination of digoxin and propranolol may be used instead of digoxin alone.
        (c) **If rate is rapid and 2:1 block present,** atrial flutter may be hard to identify on EKG. May give adenosine (see above) to increase block to 3 or 4:1.
      iii. Recurrent atrial flutter management is the same as that for atrial flutter.
      iv. Atrial fibrillation (unusual in infants). Management is the same as that for atrial flutter.
      v. Wolff-Parkinson-White syndrome. Treat any symptomatic arrhythmias that may occur; often accompanied by SVT. β-Blockers are preferred because digoxin may promotes 1:1 conduction and demise.
      vi. Ventricular tachycardia. Perform electrical cardioversion (except in digitalis toxicity), with lidocaine started for maintenance therapy. Although lidocaine is the drug of choice, other drugs that may be used are procainamide or phenytoin.
  3. Ectopic beats
    a. Asymptomatic. No treatment is necessary.
    b. Symptomatic. With underlying heart disease with ectopic beats that are compromising cardiac output, suppress with phenytoin, propranolol, or quinidine.
  4. Atrioventricular block
    a. First degree. No specific treatment necessary.
    b. Second degree. Treat the underlying cause.
    c. Third degree (complete). If the infant is asymptomatic, observe. Generally, if the rate is ≥70 beats/min, no problems develop. If the rate is <50 beats/min, the patient usually needs emergency transvenous pacing, with the need for subsequent permanent pacing. Between 50 and 70 beats/min is the gray zone. Check the mother for SAA or SSA antinuclear antibodies because there is an association with complete heart block.

5. **Arrhythmias secondary to an extracardiac cause**
   a. **Pathologic conditions.** Treat the underlying disease.
   b. **Digoxin toxicity.** Check the PR interval before each dose, obtain a stat serum digoxin level, and hold the dose. Consider digoxin immune Fab (Digibind) (see Chapter 132).
   c. **Theophylline toxicity.** Reduce the dosage or discontinue medication.
6. **Electrolyte abnormalities**
   a. **Check serum electrolyte levels with repeat determinations.**
   b. **Treat electrolyte abnormalities accordingly.** See Chapter 8.
VI. **Technique of defibrillation/Cardioversion** is presented in Chapter 27.

43 Bloody Stool

I. **Problem.** A newborn infant has passed a bloody stool. This is generally a benign and self-limiting disorder. In a large majority of patients, the cause is unknown.

II. **Immediate questions**
   A. **Is it grossly bloody?** This finding is usually an ominous sign; **an exception is a bloody stool as a result of swallowed maternal blood, which is a benign condition.** A grossly bloody stool usually occurs in infants with a lesion in the ileum or the colon or with massive upper gastrointestinal tract bleeding. Necrotizing enterocolitis (NEC) is the most common cause of bloody stool in premature infants and should be strongly suspected. It is seen in 25% of patients with NEC.
   B. **Is the stool otherwise normal in color but with streaks of blood?** This is more characteristic of a lesion in the anal canal, such as anal fissure. Anal fissure is the most common cause of bleeding in well infants.
   C. **Is the stool positive only for occult blood?** Occult blood often signifies that the blood is from the upper gastrointestinal tract (proximal to the ligament of Treitz). Nasogastric trauma and swallowed maternal blood are common causes. Microscopic blood as an isolated finding is usually not significant. Tests for occult blood are very sensitive and can be positive with repeated rectal temperatures.
   D. **Was the infant given vitamin K at birth?** Hemorrhagic disease of the newborn or any coagulopathy may present with bloody stools.
   E. **What medications are the mother and infant on?** Certain medications can cause bleeding. If the mother was on aspirin, cephalothin, or phenobarbital, these can cross the placenta and cause coagulation abnormalities in the infant. If the infant has been given nonsteroidal anti-inflammatory drugs, heparin, tolazoline, indomethacin, or dexamethasone, these are all associated with bleeding.

III. **Differential diagnosis**
   A. **Occult blood only, no visible blood**
      1. **Swallowing of maternal blood (accounts for 30% of bleeding)** during delivery or breast-feeding (secondary to cracked nipples) may be the cause. Swallowed blood usually appears in the stool on the second or third day of life.
      2. **Nasogastric tube trauma.**
      3. **Necrotizing enterocolitis.**
      4. **Formula intolerance.** Milk protein sensitivity is secondary to cow's milk or soybean formula, and symptoms of blood in the stool usually occur in the second or third week of life. One study found that cow's milk allergy was diagnosed in 18% of patients with rectal bleeding.
      5. **Gastritis or stress ulcer (common cause and can be secondary to certain medications).** Erosions of the esophageal, duodenal, and gastric mucosa are a common

cause of bleeding. Stress ulcers may occur in the stomach or the duodenum and are associated with prolonged, severe illness. Steroid therapy, especially prolonged, is associated with ulcers. Hemorrhagic gastritis can occur from tolazoline and theophylline therapy.

     6. Unknown cause. Many cases of bloody stool in an infant have no identifiable cause.

  B. Streaks of visible blood in the stool

     1. Anal fissure (tear) can be secondary to straining.

     2. Rectal trauma is often secondary to temperature probes.

  C. Grossly bloody stool

     1. Necrotizing enterocolitis.

     2. Disseminated intravascular coagulation (DIC). There is usually bleeding from other sites and may be secondary to an infection.

     3. Hemorrhagic disease of the newborn occurs from vitamin K deficiency and can be prevented if it is administered at birth. Bloody stools typically appear on the second or third day of life.

     4. Bleeding diathesis. Platelet abnormalities and clotting factor deficiencies can cause bloody stools.

     5. Other surgical diseases, such as malrotation with midgut volvulus, Meckel diverticulum, Hirschsprung enterocolitis, intestinal duplications, incarcerated inguinal hernia, arteriovenous malformations, and intussusception (rare in the neonatal period; incidence is greatest in infants 3 months to 1 year of age).

     6. Colitis can be secondary to the following:

       a. Intestinal infections, causing colitis such as *Shigella, Salmonella, Campylobacter, Yersinia,* enterohemorrhagic strains of *Escherichia coli, rotavirus, adenovirus,* and *enterovirus. Astrovirus* infection causes hemorrhagic diarrhea and has been reported as an outbreak in a neonatal unit. Intestinal infections can cause a temporary lactose intolerance that can cause blood in a stool.

       b. Dietary/formula intolerance factors, including allergy and dietary protein-induced colitis. The top allergens are cow's milk products and soy. Allergic enterocolitis can present with massive bloody diarrhea.

       c. Neonatal transient eosinophilic colitis. There are reported cases of infants with this with no known allergic component involved (no prior feeding had occurred).

     7. Severe liver disease.

     8. Other infections, such as cytomegalovirus, toxoplasmosis, syphilis, and bacterial sepsis.

IV. Database. The age of the infant is important. If the infant is <7 days old, swallowing of maternal blood is a possible cause; in older infants, this is an unlikely cause.

  A. Physical examination

     1. Examination of peripheral perfusion. Evaluate the infant's peripheral perfusion. An infant with NEC can be poorly perfused and may appear to be in early or impending shock. Bruising may suggest a coagulopathy.

     2. Abdominal examination. Check for bowel sounds and tenderness. Hyperactive bowel sounds are more common in upper gastrointestinal bleeding. If the abdomen is soft and nontender and there is no erythema, a major intra-abdominal process is unlikely. If the abdomen is distended, rigid, or tender, an intra-abdominal pathologic process is likely. Abdominal distention is the most common sign of NEC. Abdominal distention may also suggest intussusception or midgut volvulus. If there are red streaks and erythema on the abdominal wall, suspect NEC with peritonitis.

     3. Anal examination. If the infant's condition is stable, perform a visual examination of the anus to check for anal fissure or tear.

  B. Laboratory studies

     1. Fecal occult blood testing (Hemoccult test) to test for the presence of blood.

     2. Complete blood count (CBC) with differential to document the amount of blood loss. If a large amount of blood is lost acutely, it takes time for it to be evident on hemoglobin or hematocrit results. An increased white blood count suggests infection; platelet count may reveal thrombocytopenia.

3. **Apt test** to differentiate maternal from fetal blood if swallowed maternal blood is suspected. Submit the specimen to the laboratory. A positive test indicates that the blood is either due to gastrointestinal or pulmonary bleeding from the neonate. A negative test would indicate that the blood is of maternal origin, suggesting the infant swallowed or aspirated maternal blood.

4. **Stool culture.** Certain pathogens cause bloody stools, but they are rare in the neonatal nursery.

5. **Coagulation studies** should be performed to rule out DIC or a bleeding disorder. The usual studies are partial thromboplastin time, prothrombin time, fibrinogen level, and platelet count. Thrombocytopenia can also be seen with cow's milk protein allergy. An elevated abnormal prothrombin time can indicate a coagulopathy. A prolonged partial thromboplastin time may indicate hemophilia.

6. **Allergic enterocolitis diagnosis** is difficult because there is no laboratory test. Eosinophilia is usually negative on the differential. Serum radioallergosorbent tests for cow's milk protein are usually negative. Serum eosinophilic cationic protein and platelet-activating factor levels can confirm involvement of eosinophilia. A rectal mucosal punch biopsy can show eosinophilic infiltration that can suggest an allergic origin.

7. **If NEC is suspected, the following studies should be performed:**
   a. **CBC with differential** to establish an inflammatory response and to check for thrombocytopenia and anemia.
   b. **Serum potassium levels.** Hyperkalemia secondary to hemolysis may occur.
   c. **Serum sodium levels.** Hyponatremia can be seen secondary to third spacing of fluids.
   d. **Blood gas levels** to rule out metabolic acidosis, which is often associated with sepsis or NEC.

C. **Radiologic and other studies.** A plain radiograph of the abdomen is useful if NEC or a surgical abdomen is suspected. Look for an abnormal gas pattern, a thickened bowel wall, pneumatosis intestinalis, or perforation. Pneumatosis can appear as a "soap bubble" area (see Figure 10–22). If a suspicious area appears on the abdominal radiograph in the right upper quadrant, it is usually not stool. With perforation, one can see the "football sign" on an anteroposterior (AP) film, an overall lucency of the abdomen secondary to free intraperitoneal air. Because of the abnormal interface between free air and the peritoneum, the shape resembles a football. A left lateral decubitus view of the abdomen may show free air if perforation has occurred and it cannot be seen on a routine AP film. Surgical conditions usually show signs of intestinal obstruction.

V. **Plan. The initial plan is to address the loss of volume and give aggressive volume replacement if hypotension is present.** Individual plans are as follows:

A. **Swallowed maternal blood.** Observation only is indicated.

B. **Anal fissure and rectal trauma.** Observation is indicated. Petroleum jelly applied to the anus may promote healing.

C. **Necrotizing enterocolitis.** See Chapter 104.

D. **Nasogastric trauma.** In most cases of bloody stool involving nasogastric tubes, trauma is mild and requires only observation. If the tube is too large, replacing it with a smaller one may resolve the problem. If there has been significant bleeding, **gastric lavages** are helpful; it is *controversial* whether tepid water or normal saline is best. Then, if possible, removal of the nasogastric tube is recommended.

E. **Formula intolerance.** This diagnosis is difficult to document, so it is usually made if the patient has remission of symptoms when the formula is eliminated.

F. **Gastritis or ulcers.** Treatment usually consists of ranitidine (preferred because of less side effects) or cimetidine (for dosages and other pharmacologic information, see Chapter 132). Use of antacids in neonates is *controversial*; some clinicians believe that concretions may result from the use of antacids. Use of antacids increases the risk of infection and increases the risk of feeding intolerance in infants receiving gavage feedings. (See also Chapter 49.)

G. Unknown cause. If no cause is found, the infant is usually closely monitored. In the majority of the cases, the bleeding subsides.

H. Intestinal infections. Antibiotic treatment and isolation are standard treatment. (See Chapter 132 and Appendix F.)

I. Hemorrhagic disease of the newborn. Intravenous vitamin K is usually adequate therapy. (See Chapter 132.)

J. Surgical conditions (eg, NEC, perforation, volvulus) all require immediate surgical evaluation.

44 Counseling Parents Before High-Risk Delivery

I. Problem. The nurse calls to notify you of a pending high-risk delivery. You are on delivery room duty, and are asked to speak with the parents.

II. Immediate questions

A. Are both parents and other important family members available? Is a translator needed?

B. Is the mother too sick or uncomfortable to be able to participate adequately in the discussion? In this situation, it is essential to include other family members in the discussion.

C. How well do they understand their current situation? Review the chart.

D. What do they know about neonatal intensive care units (NICUs), pregnancy and neonatal complications, chronic health problems, and neurodevelopmental disability?

III. Differential diagnosis. Although a neonatologist can be called on to counsel expectant parents in a variety of circumstances, the following are common problems that are discussed with parents before delivery.

A. Preterm delivery.

B. Intrauterine growth restriction (IUGR).

C. Maternal drug use.

D. Fetal distress.

E. Congenital anomaly.

IV. Database

A. Maternal/paternal data. Obtain the following information: age of both parents, obstetric history, history of the current pregnancy, medication history, pertinent laboratory and sonographic data, family history, social background and supports, and communication ability.

B. Fetal. Review current fetal information with the obstetrician: findings on prenatal ultrasounds, accuracy of gestational age dating, abnormalities of fetal heart rate tracing, biophysical profile, fetal scalp pH (if done), and any other pertinent tests.

V. Plan

A. General approach to parent counseling. Parent counseling before delivery is often performed under less than ideal circumstances. Every effort should be made to communicate effectively, explaining all medical terms and avoiding abbreviations and percentages as much as possible. Expectations for what will happen at delivery, possible complications, and the range of possible outcomes should be covered in addition to the infant's chances of survival. Uncertainties regarding outcome should be acknowledged. Most important, repetition may be necessary for parents to comprehend all this information, and an opportunity to review the information should be provided. If NICU admission is anticipated, an opportunity to tour the NICU (and to see other infants hooked up to monitoring and life support equipment) should be offered. Specific and detailed survival and outcome statistics are beyond the scope of this book but are contained in neonatal and obstetric textbooks.

B. **Specific counseling issues**

1. **Preterm delivery.** The more immature the infant, the greater the risk of death, complications of prematurity, health sequelae, and neurodevelopmental disability. Current data, drawn from many published outcome studies, are presented in Table 44–1, although quoting percentages to parents should be avoided (because it is confusing to many people).

   a. **Immediate questions**

   i. **What is the infant's gestational age?** This is the most important question because morbidity and mortality are so closely tied to maturity. Both gestational age and birthweight have been used as proxies for maturity in predicting survival and outcome. However, only gestational age is available when counseling parents in labor and delivery.

   ii. **What is the reason for the preterm delivery?** The reason for preterm delivery affects infant outcome and the likelihood of delaying delivery (eg, delay is contraindicated with suspected chorioamnionitis).

   iii. **Are there signs of fetal distress?** Signs of fetal distress may signal either ongoing or impending insult to the fetus.

   b. **Specific issues to address with the parents**

   i. **Mortality.** The current lower limit of viability is 23–24 weeks' gestation, with occasional survival reported at 21–22 weeks' gestation. Survival at the lower limit of viability requires intubation and mechanical ventilation, but these efforts may merely prolong death. Survival is improved with antenatal steroids but compromised by loss of amniotic fluid before 24 weeks' gestational age.

   ii. **Complications of prematurity.** All the complications of prematurity are most common in infants born at the lower limit of viability, and their frequency decreases with increasing gestational age. Complications of prematurity include respiratory distress syndrome, metabolic problems, infection, necrotizing enterocolitis, patent ductus arteriosus,

Table 44–1. ESTIMATES OF MORBIDITY AND MORTALITY USEFUL IN COUNSELING PARENTS

Risk Factor	Mortality (%)	Cerebral Palsy (%)	Intellectual Disability (%)	Sensory Impairment (%)
None	0.2–0.3%	0.1–0.4%	1%	0.1–0.2%
Prematurity	3–4%			
GA 33–36 wk	1–1.4%	1%	1%	0.1–0.2%
GA 29–32 wk	4–5%	4–11%	2–3%	0.4–2%
GA ≤ 28 wk	10%	12–17%	10–30%	1–4%
GA ≤ 25 wk	49–60%	20–40%	21–52%	3–6%
Severe neonatal encephalopathy	50–60%	100	100	Increased
Severe persistent pulmonary hypertension	10–59%	6–13%	24–30%	6–30%

GA, completed weeks of gestation at birth (birthweight data not known for prenatal counseling).

intraventricular hemorrhage and other signs of brain injury, and apnea and bradycardia. Chronic complications include chronic lung disease, periventricular leukomalacia or intraparenchymal cysts, hydrocephalus, poor nutrition, retinopathy of prematurity, and hearing impairment.

    iii. Long-term outcome. Although the risk of disability is higher in preterm children than in the general population, the majority of preterm children do not develop a major disability (see Table 44–1) such as cerebral palsy or intellectual disability. The frequency of neurodevelopmental disability is highest at the lower limit of viability. However, even late preterm infants born at 32 to 36 weeks' gestation are at higher risk for cerebral palsy, cognitive impairments, and school problems than full-term infants. Learning disability, attention deficit disorder, minor neuromotor dysfunction, and behavior problems are more frequent in school-age preterm children than in full-term controls.

2. Intrauterine growth restriction (IUGR)

    a. Immediate questions. What is the cause of the IUGR? When was it detected? Are there signs of fetal decompensation?

    b. Specific issues to address with parents

        i. IUGR outcome. The most important determinant of IUGR outcome is its cause. Infants with chromosomal disorders and congenital infections (eg, toxoplasmosis or cytomegalovirus) experience early IUGR, often do not tolerate labor and delivery well, and commonly have a disability. The normal fetus initially compensates for fetal deprivation of supply, but when these compensatory mechanisms are overwhelmed, progressive damage to fetal organs occurs, and if there is no intervention, it results in fetal death.

        ii. Complications of IUGR. IUGR infants are more vulnerable to perinatal complications, including perinatal asphyxia, cold stress, hyperviscosity (polycythemia), and hypoglycemia.

        iii. Long-term outcome. Full-term IUGR infants with fetal deprivation of supply have an increased risk of motor and cognitive impairments including minor neuromotor dysfunction, learning disability, and attention deficits, which can lead to persistent school and behavior problems. Preterm IUGR infants have increased risk of complications of both IUGR and preterm delivery, including cerebral palsy, intellectual disability, as well as school and behavior problems.

3. Maternal use of drugs

    a. Immediate questions. Which drugs did the mother use? When? How much?

    b. Specific issues to address with parents

        i. IUGR. Infants exposed in utero to opiates, cocaine, alcohol, cigarettes, and some prescription drugs can demonstrate IUGR.

        ii. Specific syndromes and risks. Fetal alcohol and fetal hydantoin syndromes are well defined but often difficult to diagnose in the neonatal period. Both carry an increased risk of intellectual disability.

        iii. Neonatal withdrawal syndrome. Infants exposed in utero to opiates or cocaine may demonstrate neonatal withdrawal syndrome. These infants have to be closely observed and may require medications to help them through the withdrawal period. Later, these infants have an increased incidence of school and behavior problems. (See Chapter 95.)

        iv. Cocaine exposure and risks. Infants with central nervous system infarctions resulting from cocaine exposure are at risk for cerebral palsy, especially hemiplegia, as well as cognitive impairments. (See Chapter 95.)

4. Signs of fetal distress

    a. Immediate questions. Which signs of fetal distress are evident and for how long? What intervention is planned?

    b. Specific issues to address with parents

    i. **Types of fetal distress.** The many different signs of fetal distress include changes in fetal heart rate patterns, fetal reactivity, meconium staining of amniotic fluid, and decreased fetal movements as well as composite fetal measures (eg, biophysical profile; see Chapter 1). The type, severity, and duration of insult are important for prognosis, but these cannot be accurately determined.

    ii. **Accurate predictors of mortality and morbidity.** The most accurate predictors are those related to signs of brain injury on neuroimaging studies, electroencephalogram, and on neurodevelopmental assessment. Infants with chronic intrauterine hypoxia are at an increased risk for persistent pulmonary hypertension and neurodevelopmental disability (whether or not they require extracorporeal membrane oxygenation); see Table 44–1. Severity of neonatal encephalopathy is predictive of both mortality and neurodevelopmental outcomes: infants with severe encephalopathy often die, and survivors tend to have severe multiple disabilities. The majority of infants who demonstrate signs of fetal distress or *acute* perinatal depression do not develop encephalopathy, persistent pulmonary hypertension of the newborn, or neurodevelopmental disability.

45 Cyanosis

I. **Problem.** During a physical examination, an infant appears blue. **Cyanosis becomes visible when there is >3g of desaturated hemoglobin/dL.** Therefore, the degree of cyanosis depends on both oxygen saturation and hemoglobin concentration. Cyanosis is visible with much less degree of hypoxemia in the polycythemic compared with the anemic infant. Cyanosis can be a sign of severe cardiac, respiratory, or neurologic compromise.

II. **Immediate questions**

    A. **Does the infant have respiratory distress?** If the infant has increased respiratory effort with increased rate, retractions, and nasal flaring, respiratory disease should be high on the list of differential diagnoses. Cyanotic heart disease usually presents without respiratory symptoms but can have effortless tachypnea (rapid respiratory rate without retractions). Blood disorders usually present without respiratory or cardiac symptoms.

    B. **Does the infant have a murmur?** A murmur usually implies heart disease. Transposition of the great vessels can present without a murmur (~60%).One study revealed that in infants with congenital heart malformation, <50% have a murmur in the newborn period. Unfortunately, murmurs are not any more common in more severe heart defects.

    C. **Is the cyanosis continuous, intermittent, sudden in onset, or occurring only with feeding or crying?** Intermittent cyanosis is more common with neurologic disorders; these infants may have apneic spells alternating with periods of normal breathing. Continuous cyanosis is usually associated with intrinsic lung disease or heart disease. Cyanosis with feeding may occur with esophageal atresia and severe esophageal reflux. Sudden onset of cyanosis may occur with an air leak, such as pneumothorax. Cyanosis that disappears with crying may signify choanal atresia. Infants with Tetralogy of Fallot may have clinical cyanosis only with crying.

    D. **Is there differential cyanosis?** Cyanosis of the upper or lower part of the body only usually signifies serious heart disease. The more common pattern is cyanosis restricted to the lower half of the body, which is seen in patients with patent ductus arteriosus with a left-to-right shunt. Cyanosis restricted to the upper half of the body is seen occasionally in patients with pulmonary hypertension, patent ductus arteriosus, coarctation of the aorta, and D-transposition of the great arteries.

E. **What is the prenatal and delivery history?** An infant of a diabetic mother has an increased risk of hypoglycemia, polycythemia, respiratory distress syndrome, and heart disease. Infection, such as that which can occur with premature rupture of membranes, may cause shock and hypotension with resultant cyanosis. Amniotic fluid abnormalities, such as oligohydramnios (associated with hypoplastic lungs) or polyhydramnios (associated with esophageal atresia), may suggest a cause for the cyanosis. Cesarean section is associated with increased respiratory distress. Certain perinatal conditions increase the incidence of congenital heart disease. Examples of these include the following:

   1. **Maternal diabetes or cocaine:** D-transposition of the great arteries.
   2. **Maternal use of lithium:** Ebstein anomaly.
   3. **Use of phenytoin:** Atrial septal defect, ventricular septal defect, Tetralogy of Fallot.
   4. **Maternal lupus:** AV block.
   5. **Maternal congenital heart disease and/or congenital heart disease in a first-degree relative:** Increased incidence of heart disease in the child.

III. **Differential diagnosis.** The causes of cyanosis can be classified as arising from respiratory, cardiac, central nervous system (CNS), or other disorders.

   A. **Respiratory diseases**
      1. **Lung diseases**
         a. **Hyaline membrane disease.**
         b. **Transient tachypnea of the newborn.**
         c. **Pneumonia.**
         d. **Meconium aspiration.**
      2. **Air leak syndrome.**
      3. **Congenital defects** (eg, diaphragmatic hernia, hypoplastic lungs, lobar emphysema, cystic adenomatoid malformation, absent pulmonary valve syndrome, and diaphragm abnormality).

   B. **Cardiac diseases**
      1. **All cyanotic heart diseases,** which include **the 5 T's.** Other cyanotic diseases include Ebstein anomaly, patent ductus arteriosus, ventricular septal defect, hypoplastic left heart syndrome, and pulmonary atresia.
         • **T**ransposition of the great arteries
         • **T**otal anomalous pulmonary venous return
         • **T**ricuspid atresia
         • **T**etralogy of Fallot
         • **T**runcus arteriosus
      2. **Persistent pulmonary hypertension of the newborn (PPHN).**
      3. **Severe congestive heart failure.**

   C. **Central nervous system diseases.** Periventricular-intraventricular hemorrhage, meningitis, and primary seizure disorder can cause cyanosis. Neuromuscular disorders such as Werdnig-Hoffmann disease and congenital myotonic dystrophy can cause cyanosis.

   D. **Other disorders**
      1. **Congenital methemoglobinemia.** May be familial. Pao_2 is within normal limits.
      2. **Polycythemia/hyperviscosity syndrome.** Pao_2 is within normal limits.
      3. **Hypothermia.**
      4. **Hypoglycemia.**
      5. **Sepsis/meningitis.**
      6. **Pseudocyanosis** caused by fluorescent lighting.
      7. **Respiratory depression** secondary to maternal medications (eg, magnesium sulfate and narcotics).

   8. **Shock.**
   9. **Upper airway obstruction.** Choanal atresia is nasal passage obstruction caused most commonly by a bony abnormality. Other causes are laryngeal web, tracheal stenosis, goiter, and Pierre Robin syndrome. Thyroglossal duct cyst causes apnea and cyanosis in a neonate. Teratoma of the palatine tonsil is also reported.
IV. **Database.** Obtain a prenatal and delivery history (see Section II, E).
   A. **Physical examination**
      1. **Assess the infant for central versus peripheral versus acrocyanosis versus differential cyanosis.**
         a. **In central cyanosis, the skin, lips, and tongue appear blue.** The Pao_2 is <50 mm Hg.
         b. **In peripheral cyanosis,** the skin is bluish but the oral mucous membranes are pink, seen in methemoglobinemia.
         c. **In acrocyanosis,** the hands and feet are blue but nothing else. This can be present in normal infants in the first 24–48 h.
         d. **Differential cyanosis.** Cyanosis of the upper or lower part of the body only. This can signify serious heart disease. (see Section II, D).
      2. **Assess the heart** for any murmurs and for heart rate and blood pressure.
      3. **Assess the lungs.** Is there retraction, flaring of the nose, or grunting? Retractions are usually minimal in heart disease. Check the nasal passage for choanal atresia.
      4. **Assess the abdomen** for an enlarged liver. The liver can be enlarged in congestive heart failure and hyperexpansion of the lungs. A scaphoid abdomen may suggest a diaphragmatic hernia.
      5. **Check the pulses.** In coarctation of the aorta, the femoral pulses are decreased. In patent ductus arteriosus, the pulses are bounding.
      6. **Consider neurologic problems.** Check for apnea and periodic breathing, which may be associated with immaturity of the nervous system. Observe the infant for seizures, which can cause cyanosis if the infant is not breathing during seizures.
   B. **Laboratory studies**
      1. **Arterial blood gas measurements on room air.** If the patient is not hypoxic, it suggests methemoglobinemia, polycythemia, or CNS disease. If the patient is hypoxic, perform the 100% hyperoxic test, described next.
      2. **Hyperoxic test.** Measure arterial oxygen on room air. Then place the infant on 100% oxygen for 10–20 min. With cyanotic heart disease, the Pao_2 most likely will not increase significantly. If the Pao_2 rises >150 mm Hg, cardiac disease can generally be excluded but not always. Failure of Pao_2 to rise >150 mm Hg suggests a cyanotic cardiac malformation, whereas in lung disease the arterial oxygen saturation should improve and go above 150 mm Hg. **In an infant with severe lung disease or PPHN, the arterial oxygen saturation may not increase significantly.** If the Pao_2 increases to <20 mm Hg, PPHN should be considered.
      3. **Right-to-left shunt test** is done to rule out PPHN. Draw a simultaneous sample of blood from the right radial artery (preductal) and the descending aorta or the left radial artery (postductal). If there is a difference of >15% (preductal more than postductal), the shunt is significant. It is sometimes easier to place two pulse oximeters on the infant (one preductal on the right hand; one postductal on the left hand or either foot). If the simultaneous difference is >10–15%, the shunt is significant.
      4. **Complete blood count (CBC) with differential** may reveal an infectious process. A central hematocrit of >65% confirms polycythemia.
      5. **Serum glucose level** to detect hypoglycemia.
      6. **Methemoglobin level.** A drop of blood exposed to air has a chocolate hue. To confirm the diagnosis, a spectrophotometric determination should be done by the laboratory.

C. **Radiologic and other studies**

1. **Transillumination of the chest** (see Chapter 26) should be done on an emergent basis if pneumothorax is suspected.

2. **Chest radiograph** may be normal. This suggests a CNS disease process or other cause for the cyanosis (see Section III, D). It can verify lung disease, air leak, or diaphragmatic hernia. It can also help diagnose heart disease by evaluating the heart size and pulmonary vascularity. The **heart size** may be normal or enlarged in hypoglycemia, polycythemia, shock, and sepsis. **Decreased pulmonary vascular markings** can be seen in tetralogy of Fallot, pulmonary atresia, truncus arteriosus, and Ebstein anomaly. **Increased pulmonary arterial markings** can be seen in truncus arteriosus, single ventricle, and transposition. **Increased venous markings** can be seen in hypoplastic left heart syndrome and total anomalous pulmonary venous return. **Shape of the heart** can be important:

   a. **Boot-shaped heart:** Tetralogy of Fallot, tricuspid atresia.

   b. **Egg-shaped heart:** Transposition of the great arteries.

   c. **Large globular heart:** Ebstein anomaly.

   d. **Dextrocardia/mesocardia:** Congenital heart disease.

3. **Electrocardiography (ECG).** The ECG is usually normal in patients with methemoglobinemia or hypoglycemia. In those with polycythemia, pulmonary hypertension, or primary lung disease, the ECG is normal but may show right ventricular hypertrophy. The ECG is usually nondiagnostic because of the normal neonatal right axis deviation and dominant right wave in the right chest leads. It is very helpful in identifying patients with tricuspid atresia; it will show left axis deviation and left ventricular hypertrophy.

4. **Echocardiography** should be performed immediately if cardiac disease is suspected or if the diagnosis is unclear.

5. **Ultrasonography of the head** can be performed to rule out periventricular-intraventricular hemorrhage.

V. **Plan**

A. **General management.** Act quickly and accomplish many of the diagnostic tasks at once.

1. **Perform a rapid physical examination.** Transilluminate the chest (see Chapter 26). If a tension pneumothorax is present, rapid needle decompression may be needed.

2. **Order immediate studies** (eg, blood gas levels, CBC, and chest radiograph).

3. **Perform the hyperoxic test.** See Section IV, B, 2.

B. **Specific management**

1. **Lung disease.** (See the appropriate disease chapter.) Respiratory depression caused by narcotics can be treated with naloxone (Narcan) (see Chapter 132 for dosing).

2. **Air leak (pneumothorax).** See Chapter 74

3. **Congenital defects.** Surgery is indicated for diaphragmatic hernia.

4. **Cardiac disease.** Prostaglandin E_1 (PGE_1) is indicated for right heart outflow obstruction (tricuspid atresia, pulmonic stenosis, and pulmonary atresia), left heart outflow obstruction (hypoplastic left heart syndrome, critical aortic valve stenosis, preductal coarctation of the aorta, and interrupted aortic arch), and transposition of the great arteries. PGE_1 is contraindicated in hyaline membrane disease, PPHN, and dominant left-to-right shunt (patent ductus arteriosus, truncus arteriosus, or ventricular septal defect). **If the diagnosis is uncertain, a trial of PGE1 can be given over 30 min in an effort to improve blood gas values.**

5. **CNS disorders.** Treat the underlying disease.

6. **Methemoglobinemia.** Treat the infant with methylene blue only if the methemoglobin level is markedly increased and the infant is in cardiopulmonary distress

(tachypnea and tachycardia). Administer intravenously 1 mg/kg of a 1% solution of **methylene blue** in normal saline. The cyanosis should clear within 1–2 h.

7. **Shock.** See Chapter 58.
8. **Polycythemia.** See Chapter 64.
9. **Choanal atresia.** The infant usually requires surgery. (See Chapter 121.)
10. **Hypothermia.** Rewarming is necessary. The technique is described in Chapter 6.
11. **Hypoglycemia.** See Chapter 55.

46 Death of an Infant

I. **Problem.** A newborn infant is dying or has just died. Recent reviews have focused on the importance of bereavement support and the profound effect health providers can have on parents who have lost an infant. Studies have shown that a health-care provider's insensitivity to a parent can contribute to difficulties in coping and may increase the risk of a complicated grief reaction. Hospitals should establish training and protocols for an infant death so they can potentially decrease the traumatic effects.

II. **Immediate questions**

A. **Has the family been prepared for the death, or was it unexpected?** It is important to prepare the family in advance, if possible, for the death of an infant and to be ready to answer questions after the event.

B. **Was this an early or late neonatal death?** Early neonatal death describes the death of a live-born infant during the first 7 completed days of life. Late neonatal death refers to the death of a live-born infant after 7 but before 28 completed days of life. After 28 days, it is considered an infant death.

C. **Which family members are present?** Usually, several immediate family members in addition to the parents are present at the hospital, which is good for emotional support. Each of the family members may adopt a special role. The family should be allowed to go through the immediate process of grieving the way they feel most comfortable (eg, on their own, with the chaplain, with their favorite nurse, or with the physician they trust) and in the location they feel most comfortable (eg, the neonatal intensive care unit [NICU] or family conference room). Attention should focus on both parents.

D. **If the family members are not present, is a telephone contact available?** It is standard practice to ensure there is a contact telephone number available for any sick infant. If the family members are not present, telephone contact must be made as soon as possible to alert the family that their infant is dying or has already passed away. In either case, urge the family to come in and be with their infant.

E. **Are there any religious needs expressed by the family?** The religious needs must be respected and the necessary support provided (eg, priest, rabbi, chaplain, or pastoral care). Every hospital has pastoral services, and it is useful to inform the chaplain in advance because some parents may request that their child be baptized before death. Remember, that a patient's culture or religion may influence the families' decision on how to handle the time of death, autopsy, and funeral.

III. **Differential diagnosis.** Not applicable.

IV. **Database.** Remember that the dying infant may continue with a gasp reflex for some time even without spontaneous respiration and movement. The heartbeat may be very faint; therefore, auscultation for 2–5 min is advisable. Legal definitions of "death" vary by state.

V. **Plan**

A. **Preparations.** A recent review has reported on the behaviors viewed most favorably by parents after their infant has died, outlined in Table 46-1.

1. **The NICU environment.** The noise level should be kept to a minimum. The staff should be sensitive to the emotions of the parents and the family. The infant and family members should be provided privacy in an isolated quiet room or a screened-off area in the NICU. Examination of the infant by the physician to determine death may be done in that same private area, with the family.

2. **The infant.** The equipment (eg, intravenous catheters and endotracheal tubes) may be removed from the infant unless an autopsy is anticipated. In that case, it is best to leave in place central catheters and possibly the endotracheal tube. The parents should be allowed to hold the infant for as long as they desire. This type of visual and physical contact is important to begin the grieving process in a healthy manner and try to relieve any future guilt. Treating the infant carelessly by staff members is not tolerated well by parents. The practice reported in the literature of placing the deceased infant on an uncovered metal table or placed into a bucket after delivery is unacceptable. Parents are acutely aware how nurses care for the deceased infant. Bathing and dressing the infant in a caring manner and treating the deceased infant with respect is appreciated by the family. Families also appreciate when nurses took special photos of the infant and gave the family special mementos so they could have some memories.

B. **Discussion of death with the family**

1. **Location.** Parents and immediate family members should be in a quiet, private consultation room, and the physician should calmly explain the cause and inevitability of death.

2. **News of the death.** The physician needs to offer condolences to the family concerning their loss. News of the infant's death can be very difficult for the physician to convey and the family to accept. The physician must be sensitive to the emotional reactions of the family. Nurses, in one review, were perceived as the health-care provider who was most likely to provide emotional support. It is important that nurses participate in this process because they can provide more

---

Table 46-1. BEHAVIORS VIEWED MOST FAVORABLY BY PARENTS AFTER PERINATAL DEATH

Offering emotional support
Stay with the family and spend extra time with them as much as practical
Talk about the baby by name
Allow parents to grieve or cry
Be sensitive to comments that could be perceived as trite or minimizing of grief
Return to see family on multiple occasions, if possible.

Attending to physical needs of parents and baby
Continue routine postpartum nursing and medical care for mother
Treat infant's body respectfully
Consider dressing, bathing, or wrapping infant as for a live baby
Be flexible about hospital policies that may not be appropriate for bereaved families
Help parents create tangible memories of their infants

Educating parents
Communicate loss to all staff to help avoid inappropriate comments or actions
Help parents anticipate what normal grieving will be like
Provide straightforward information about cause of death if known. Use lay language.
Take time to sit down with parents when discussing information

---

Reproduced with permission from Gold KJ: Navigating care after a baby dies: a systematic review of parent experiences with health providers. *J Perinatol* 2007:27:230–237.

ongoing support through this difficult time. Communicate the news of the death to all staff members who will be taking care of the mother if she is hospitalized at the time of the infant death. This includes dietary staff and housekeepers so they know the appropriate way to act.

3. **Areas of dissatisfaction from parents.** Reviews have emphasized that parents are upset by lack of communication between staff members. Staff that did not know the infant had died and made comments, staff that avoided or were silent with the family, and staff that showed insensitivity or lack of emotional support all created great stress in the families of the deceased. Treating the mother and deceased infant with respect is important.

C. **Effects on the family**

1. **Emotional (grieving).** A brief outline of the normal grieving process may be discussed: The stages Kübler-Ross identified are denial (This isn't happening to me!); anger (Why is this happening to me?); bargaining (I promise I'll be a better person if . . .); depression (I don't care anymore); and acceptance (I'm ready for whatever comes). Temes has described three particular types of behavior exhibited by those suffering from grief and loss: numbness (mechanical functioning and social insulation); disorganization (intensely painful feelings of loss); and reorganization (reentry into a more "normal" social life.) Physicians who offered specifics to the family in what to expect in the grieving process were rated as the most competent physicians.

2. **Physical.** Loss of appetite and disruption of sleep patterns.

3. **Other siblings.** It is important to discuss the impact of death on a sibling.

4. **Surviving twin.** Staff must be aware of the added stress on the parents looking in on a surviving twin.

D. **Practical aspects**

1. **Education.** Recent reviews have reported that parents appreciated education from the health-care providers. Parents want to have information as to why the infant died and also specific information on the grieving process. Parents have indicated that staff members who kept them informed and provided honest answers with consistent information were valued the most. *Hello Means Good-Bye* by Paul Kirk and Pat Schwiebert (www.griefwatch.com) is an often recommended lay book that can help the family cope with the loss of an infant.

2. **Additional support.** Family members should be asked whether they need any support for transport or funeral arrangements and whether they need a note to the employer regarding time off from work and so on. Social workers or case workers are usually available to assist in the hospital setting.

3. **Written permission** should be obtained for the following: photography, mementos, autopsy, or biopsy.

4. **Organ donation.** Occasionally, parents and immediate family members may have discussed organ donation before the death of the infant. If not, it can be brought up gently with the family, who will be given adequate time to reflect on it, taking into consideration the requirements for organ donation. Sometimes the parents may want to donate an organ, but this may not be possible because of the presence of infection or inadequate function of the organ before death. This should be explained carefully to the parents. Follow your institution's procedure for requesting organ procurement.

5. **Autopsy.** Autopsy can be a vital part of determining the cause of death and may be important in counseling the parents for future pregnancies. It is always a very sensitive issue to discuss with the parents, especially after the loss of their loved one. Parents should always be allowed adequate time to discuss this themselves and with the family if they have not already made up their minds.

6. **Documentation**

a. **Neonatal death summary note.** The physician may include a brief synopsis of the infant's history or a problem list. Then the events leading up to the infant's death that day, whether it was sudden or gradual, and the treatment or interventions performed must be noted. It is also important to note conversations with family members while the infant was dying, if not written earlier in separate notes.

    b. **Death certificate.** The physician declaring the infant dead initiates the death certificate, following strict guidelines for each county/state.

E. **Follow-up arrangements**

    1. **Family contact.** A telephone call from one of the medical team members should be arranged within the first week of death. A letter of sympathy can be sent. Another contact can be made at the end of the first month to comfort the family, share any further information, and answer questions. Some NICU teams may make contact again at the 1-year anniversary.

    2. **Counseling.** It is extremely important to discuss the arrangements for future counseling and refer the parents to high-risk obstetrics if appropriate. Genetic counseling may also be appropriate based on the specific case. Parents should be allowed to grieve for the death of their child and should be given the opportunity to contact the physician at a later date when they are more receptive emotionally.

    3. **Autopsy follow-up.** If consent for autopsy has been obtained, an autopsy follow-up conference after ~6–8 weeks is essential. The presence of a geneticist at this follow-up may be appropriate. This autopsy conference not only provides the parents with concrete information but also assists in the process of grieving.

    4. **The obstetrician, pediatrician, and family physician** involved with the care of the mother or family should be notified of the death.

47 Eye Discharge (Conjunctivitis)

I. **Problem.** A purulent eye discharge is noted in a 3-day-old infant. Conjunctivitis is the most common neonatal infection.

II. **Immediate questions**

    A. **How old is the infant?** Age is important in determining the cause of eye discharge. In the first 6–24 h of life, conjunctivitis due to ocular silver nitrate drops immediately after birth is most likely. At 2–5 days, a bacterial infection is most likely. The organisms most common in the neonatal period are *Neisseria gonorrhoeae* and *Staphylococcus aureus*. *Chlamydia trachomatis* conjunctivitis is usually seen after the first week of life (5–14 days) and often presents as late as the second or third week. Herpes conjunctivitis is seen 5–14 days after birth. *Pseudomonas aeruginosa* infections are typically seen between 5 and 18 days of life.

    B. **Is the discharge unilateral or bilateral?** Bilateral conjunctivitis is seen with infection caused by *C. trachomatis* or *N. gonorrhoeae* or by the use of silver nitrate. Unilateral conjunctivitis is most often seen with *S. aureus, P. aeruginosa,* and *herpes simplex.* Lacrimal duct obstruction causes unilateral discharge.

    C. **What are the characteristics of the discharge?** Distinguish purulent from watery discharge. Purulent discharge is more common with bacterial infection. Chlamydia infection is watery early and purulent later. Greenish discharge is more characteristic of *P. aeruginosa.* Herpes conjunctivitis usually has a nonpurulent and serosanguineous discharge. Gonorrhea has a purulent discharge. A blood-stained discharge is highly specific for Chlamydia.

    D. **Does the mother have a history of sexually transmitted diseases?** Infants that pass through the birth canal of an infected mother with gonorrhea or Chlamydia have an increased conjunctivitis risk.

III. **Differential diagnosis.** Eye discharge can be infectious or inflammatory or due to obstruction. **Other diagnoses that may mimic conjunctivitis and need to be ruled out are foreign body, lacrimal duct obstruction, eye trauma, and glaucoma.** Conjunctivitis in the neonate is either infectious (bacterial, viral, or chlamydial) or secondary to a chemical response. Conjunctivitis in the newborn is caused by: *C. trachomatis* (2–40%), *N. gonorrhoeae* (<1%), *herpes simplex* (<1% of cases), chemical (due to silver nitrate use), and other bacterial microbes (30–50%). These other microbes include *Staphylococcus* species, *S. pneumoniae, Haemophilus influenzae, Streptococcus mitis, group A and B streptococci, Enterobacter, Acinetobacter, Neisseria cinerea, Corynebacterium species, Moraxella catarrhalis, Escherichia coli, Klebsiella pneumoniae, and P. aeruginosa.* One study revealed that 56% of conjunctivitis cases were infectious (*Chlamydia* most common) and 44% were of uncertain origin.

   A. **Chemical conjunctivitis** is usually secondary to silver nitrate ocular drops and is the most common cause of conjunctivitis in underdeveloped countries. It is less common now with erythromycin ophthalmic ointment, which is less irritating. **Prophylaxis with erythromycin does not prevent neonatal chlamydial conjunctivitis.** Silver nitrate is recommended over erythromycin if the patient population has a high number of penicillinase-producing *N. gonorrhoeae.* Povidone-iodine 2.5% is being used in some underdeveloped countries now for ophthalmia neonatorum prophylaxis.

   B. **Gonococcal conjunctivitis** is most commonly transmitted from the mother during vaginal birth. The eyes are very red with a thick purulent drainage and swelling. This is an emergency because, left untreated, it can cause corneal perforation. The incidence is low because of prophylactic ocular treatment immediately after birth.

   C. **Staphylococcal conjunctivitis** is usually a nosocomial infection. It is the most frequent isolate, but it does not always cause conjunctivitis in infants who are colonized.

   D. **Chlamydial conjunctivitis** is transmitted from the mother and develops in 25–50% of infants delivered vaginally to infected mothers. Topical prophylaxis does not prevent neonatal chlamydial conjunctivitis. The eyes have a moderate drainage, redness, and conjunctival and eyelid swelling. Corneal opacification and pseudomembranes may be present.

   E. **Pseudomonal conjunctivitis** is usually a nosocomial infection and becoming more common in nurseries. It can lead to a devastating corneal perforation and death. The organism thrives in moisture-filled environments such as respiratory equipment and occurs most often in hospitalized premature infants or those with depressed immunity. It can be responsible for epidemic conjunctivitis in premature infants.

   F. **Other bacterial infections** as noted in Section III.

   G. **Herpes simplex keratoconjunctivitis.** Herpes simplex type 2 (HSV-2) can cause unilateral or bilateral conjunctivitis, optic neuritis, chorioretinitis, and encephalitis, and it is the most frequent viral cause of conjunctivitis. The conjunctivitis can be superficial or may involve the deeper layers of the cornea; vesicles may appear on the nearby skin. Most of these infections are secondary to HSV-2 (due to maternal genital tract ascending infection), but 15–20% are caused by HSV-1. Suspect herpes if the conjunctiva is not responding to antibiotic therapy.

   H. **Viral causes (other than herpes).** These are usually associated with other symptoms of respiratory tract disease due to adenovirus, enterovirus, and parechovirus. The discharge is usually watery or mucopurulent and rarely purulent. Preauricular adenopathy can also be seen.

   I. **Lacrimal duct obstruction (congenital dacryostenosis).** The nasolacrimal duct may fail to canalize completely at birth. The obstruction is usually at the nasal end of the duct and is usually unilateral. The symptoms are persistent tearing and a mucoid discharge in the inner corner of the eye.

IV. **Database**

   A. **Physical examination**

      1. **Ophthalmic examination.** Examine both eyes for swelling and edema of the eyelids, and check the conjunctiva for injection (congestion of blood vessels).

A purulent discharge, edema, and erythema of the lids as well as injection of the conjunctiva are suggestive of bacterial conjunctivitis.

2. Perform a complete physical examination to rule out signs of respiratory or systemic infection.

B. **Laboratory studies**

1. **Gram-stained smear of the discharge** to check for white blood cells (a sign of infection) and bacteria (to identify the organism). **A sample of the discharge should also be submitted for culture and sensitivity testing.**

   a. *N. gonorrhoeae* conjunctivitis. Gram-negative intracellular diplococci and white blood cells (WBCs).

   b. *S. aureus* conjunctivitis. Gram-positive cocci in clusters and WBCs.

   c. *P. aeruginosa* conjunctivitis. Gram-negative bacilli and WBCs.

   d. Conjunctivitis caused by *Haemophilus* spp. Gram-negative coccoid rods.

   e. Streptococcal or enterococci. Streptococci are Gram-positive spherical cocci, and enterococci are Gram-positive lancet-shaped encapsulated diplococci.

   f. Other Gram-positive organisms. *Streptococcus pneumoniae, Streptococcus viridans, Staphylococcus epidermidis,* group A and B streptococci, and Corynebacterium species.

   g. Other Gram-negative organisms. *E. coli, K. pneumonia, Serratia marcescens, Proteus, Enterobacter, Hemophilus influenzae, Acinetobacter, P. aeruginosa, N. cinerea,* and *Moraxella catarrhalis.*

   h. Herpes simplex. See lymphocytes, plasma cells, and multinucleate giant cells.

   i. *C. trachomatis.* See neutrophils, lymphocytes, and plasma cells on Gram stain.

   j. Chemical conjunctivitis. See neutrophils and occasionally lymphocytes.

   k. Lacrimal duct obstruction. The Gram stain is negative or normal conjunctival flora unless there is an infection.

2. If a chlamydial infection is suspected, material is gathered for Giemsa staining by scraping (*not swabbing*) the lower palpebral conjunctiva with a wire loop or blunt spatula to obtain epithelial cells. This is a specific (but not sensitive) method for detecting conjunctivitis. Cotton or Calgonite swabs have not proved to be adequate. If chlamydial infection is present, **typical cytoplasmic inclusion bodies** are seen within the epithelial cells. Rapid antigen detection assays on the scrapings can be sent to the laboratory. Direct fluorescent antibody, enzyme immunoassay, and DNA probes are all diagnostic tests for *Chlamydia.*

3. If herpes is suspected, a conjunctival scraping shows multinucleated giant cells with intracytoplasmic inclusions. Also, the conjunctiva should be swabbed and transported on special viral transport media for culture.

C. **Radiologic and other studies.** None are usually needed.

V. **Plan.** Complications (perforation of the cornea, blindness, *Chlamydia* pneumonia) can be severe, so it is important to recognize and treat as soon as possible. Based on the results of the Gram and Giemsa stains, start empirical treatment after culturing rather than waiting for the results.

A. **Important facts in the management of conjunctivitis:**

1. Infection can spread easily from one eye to another or to other people by touching the eye or drainage. Proper handwashing and wearing gloves is essential.

2. Drainage is contagious for 24–48 h after beginning treatment.

3. Irrigate eye with normal saline to remove accumulated purulent drainage.

4. Systemic treatment is required for gonococcal, staphylococcal, *Chlamydia,* pseudomonas, and herpetic conjunctivitis.

B. **Chemical conjunctivitis.** Observation only is needed because this usually resolves within 48–72 h.

C. **Gonococcal conjunctivitis**

1. Isolate the infant during the first 24 h of parenteral antibiotic therapy.

2. Evaluate for disseminated disease. Blood and cerebrospinal cultures must be obtained. Other sites should be cultured if appropriate. Appropriate cultures from the mother and partner should be obtained and treatment started.

3. **Tests for concomitant infection** with *C. trachomatis*, congenital syphilis, and HIV.
4. **For gonococcal conjunctivitis without dissemination**, administer a single dose of ceftriaxone, 25–50 mg/kg IV or IM; in low birthweight infants, the single dose is ceftriaxone sodium, 25–50 mg/kg/day IM or IV (up to a maximum of 125 mg). An alternative therapy is cefotaxime in a single dose (100 mg/kg, given IV or IM).
5. **For gonococcal conjunctivitis with dissemination**, ceftriaxone, 25–50 mg/kg IV or IM, may be given once every day for 7 days. If meningitis is present, it should be given for a total of 10–14 days. An alternate therapy is cefotaxime (recommended for hyperbilirubinemic infants) at 50–100 mg/kg/day, given IV or IM in two divided doses for 7 days or 10–14 days if meningitis is present.
7. **In healthy infants born to mothers with gonococcal infection**, topical antimicrobial therapy is inadequate. A single dose of ceftriaxone (25–50 mg/kg IV or IM) not to exceed 125 mg is given. Cefotaxime is an alternate (100 mg/kg IV or IM). Topical antimicrobial therapy is not necessary if systemic therapy has been given.
8. **Irrigate the eyes** with sterile isotonic saline solution immediately and at frequent intervals (every 1–2 h) until clear.
9. **Ophthalmologic consultation** is usually requested because gonococcal ophthalmia can lead to corneal perforation and blindness.
10. **Both mother and partner** need full medical examinations and treatment.

C. **Staphylococcal conjunctivitis**
1. **Isolate the infant** to prevent spread of infection and culture the blood and other areas if appropriate.
2. **Systemic therapy** with a penicillinase-resistant penicillin (eg, methicillin) should be used for a minimum of 7 days.
3. **Topical antibiotics are unnecessary** if the patient is on systemic therapy.

D. **Chlamydial conjunctivitis**
1. **Recommended neonatal prophylaxis will not prevent neonatal chlamydial conjunctivitis.** Topical treatment with erythromycin ophthalmic ointment alone is ineffective but may be beneficial as an adjunct therapy.
2. **Oral erythromycin** base, or ethylsuccinate, 50 mg/kg/day, in four divided doses for 14 days by mouth, is recommended. Oral sulfonamides may be used after the immediate neonatal period for infants who do not tolerate erythromycin. A second course of antibiotics is sometimes required because ~20% of cases recur after antibiotic therapy. **Infantile hypertrophic pyloric stenosis (IHPS) has been seen in infants <6 weeks treated with erythromycin.** Counsel patients about the risk and signs of IHPS. The American Academy of Pediatrics still recommends erythromycin because other treatments have not been well studied.
3. **Infants born to mothers with untreated chlamydia** are at a high risk for infection. Prophylactic antibiotic treatment is not indicated. Monitor for infection. If adequate follow-up is not possible, some clinicians advocate treatment. Mothers and sexual partners of infected infants should be treated for *C. trachomatis*.

E. **Pseudomonal conjunctivitis**
1. **Isolate the patient** and culture blood and other sites if appropriate.
2. **Treat with gentamicin** ophthalmic ointment four times/day for 2 weeks.
3. **Parenteral therapy is recommended** because *Pseudomonas* is a virulent organism. Use a β-lactam antibiotic or an appropriate cephalosporin plus an aminoglycoside (gentamicin) for a minimum of 10–14 days. For infections that include meningitis, ampicillin or cephalosporin plus an aminoglycoside is recommended for 21 days.
4. **Ophthalmology consultation** is critical because the infection may be devastating. Infectious disease consult may also be helpful, especially with *Pseudomonas* meningitis.

F. **Other bacterial infections**
  1. **Local saline irrigation.**
  2. **Topical antibiotics** for Gram-positive organisms include erythromycin and bacitracin and for Gram-negative organisms gentamicin and tobramycin. These are applied every 6 h for 7–10 days.
G. **Herpes simplex conjunctivitis**
  1. **Isolate the patient;** implement contact precautions.
  2. **Obtain a complete set of viral cultures** (blood, cerebrospinal fluid, eyes, stool or rectum, urine, mouth or nasopharynx, and any lesions). Obtain a cerebrospinal fluid (CSF) PCR.
  3. **Administer topical ophthalmic therapy** with 3% vidarabine ointment, or 1% trifluridine ointment (both proven to be effective) five times/day for 10 days.
  4. **Systemic acyclovir therapy** for a minimum of 14 days is indicated. If central nervous system disease or disseminated disease is present, treat for a minimum of 21 days. (For dosage, see Chapter 132.)
  5. **Ophthalmologic evaluation** and follow-up are necessary because chorioretinitis, cataracts, and retinopathy may develop.
H. **Lacrimal duct obstruction**
  1. **Most clear spontaneously without treatment.** Massaging the inside corner of the eye over the lacrimal sac, with expression toward the nose, may help to establish patency.
  2. **If the problem does not resolve and symptoms persist (usually after 6–7 months), the infant should be evaluated by an ophthalmologist.** Probing of the duct is indicated with a success rate of >90%.

48 Gastric Aspirate (Residuals)

I. **Problem.** The nurse alerts you that a gastric aspirate has been obtained in an infant. Gastric aspiration is a procedure by which the stomach is aspirated with an oral or nasogastric tube. The procedure is usually performed before each feeding to determine whether the feedings are being tolerated and digested.
II. **Immediate questions**
  A. **What is the volume of the aspirate?** A volume of >30% of the total formula given at the last feeding may be abnormal and requires evaluation. A gastric aspirate of >10–15 mL is considered excessive.
  B. **What is the character of the aspirate (ie, bilious, bloody, undigested, or digested)?** This is important in the differential diagnosis (see Section III, A–C).
  C. **Are the vital signs normal?** Abnormal vital signs may indicate a pathologic process, possibly an intra-abdominal process.
  D. **Is the abdomen soft, with good bowel sounds, or distended, with visible bowel loops? Has the abdominal girth increased at least 2 cm?** Absence of bowel sounds, distention, tenderness, and erythema are signs of peritonitis. Absence of bowel sounds suggests ileus. An increase in abdominal girth of ≥2 cm showed a gastric residual of ≥23% in one study. Palpation of the abdomen may reveal a pyloric "olive" (pyloric stenosis).
  E. **When was the last stool passed?** Constipation resulting in abdominal distention may cause feeding intolerance and increased gastric aspirates.
  F. **What medications is the infant on?** Cisapride can cause increased gastric aspirates. Theophylline delays gastric emptying in very low birthweight infants.

III. **Differential diagnosis.** The characteristics of the aspirate can provide important clinical clues to the cause of the problem and are outlined next.

A. **Bilious** aspirate usually indicates an obstructive lesion distal to the ampulla of Vater. This type of aspirate is usually a serious problem, especially if it occurs in the first 72 h of life.

1. **Bowel obstruction.** One study found that 30% of infants with bilious vomiting in the first 72 h of life had obstruction, of which 20% required surgery.

2. **Necrotizing enterocolitis (NEC).** This occurs mainly in premature infants. Ten percent of the cases involve term infants.

3. **Meconium plug.**

4. **Meconium ileus.**

5. **Hirschsprung disease.**

6. **Malrotation of the intestine.**

7. **Volvulus.**

8. **Ileus.**

9. **Factitious.** Passage of the feeding tube into the duodenum or the jejunum instead of the stomach can cause a bilious aspirate.

B. **Nonbilious aspirate**

1. **Problems with the feeding regimen.** Undigested or digested formula may be seen in the aspirate if the feeding regimen is too aggressive and is more likely in small premature infants who are given a small amount of formula initially and then are given larger volumes too rapidly, or after adding fortifier to breast milk.

a. **Aspirate containing undigested formula** may be seen if the interval between feedings is too short.

b. **Aspirate containing digested formula** may be a sign of delayed gastric emptying or overfeeding. Also, if the osmolarity of the formula is increased by the addition of vitamins, retained digested formula may be seen.

2. **Other**

a. **Formula intolerance** is an uncommon cause of aspirate but should be considered. Some infants do not tolerate the carbohydrate source in some formulas. If the infant is receiving a lactose-containing formula (eg, Similac or Enfamil), perform a stool pH to rule out lactose intolerance. If the stool pH is acidic (<5.0), lactose intolerance may be present. There is usually a strong family history of milk intolerance. Diarrhea is more common than gastric aspirates with lactose intolerance.

b. **Constipation.** This is a factor especially if the abdomen is full but soft and no stool has passed in 48–72 h.

c. **NEC or post-NEC stricture.**

d. **Pyloric stenosis, incarcerated hernia.** Pyloric stenosis typically presents at 3–4 weeks.

e. **Infections.**

f. **Inborn errors of metabolism.**

g. **Adrenogenital syndrome or adrenal hypoplasia.**

h. **Hypermagnesemia.** An infant with hypermagnesemia presented with increased gastric aspirates and delayed passage of meconium.

C. **Bloody aspirate** (See also Chapter 49.)

1. **Trauma from nasogastric intubation.**

2. **Swallowed maternal blood.**

3. **Bleeding disorder.** Vitamin K deficiency, disseminated intravascular coagulation, and any congenital coagulopathy can cause a bloody aspirate.

4. **Stress ulcer.** Silent abdominal distension can present as a perforated ulcer.

5. **Severe fetal asphyxia.**

6. **NEC.**

7. **Gastric volvulus or duplication.** These are rare.

8. **Medications** that can cause a bloody aspirate: tolazoline, theophylline (rare), indomethacin, and corticosteroids. Tolazoline, especially by continuous infusion, can cause massive gastric hemorrhage.

IV. **Database**

   A. **Physical examination** is performed paying particular attention to the abdomen. Check for bowel sounds (absent bowel sounds may indicate ileus or peritonitis), abdominal distention, tenderness to palpation and erythema of the abdomen (which may signify peritonitis), or visible bowel loops. Check for hernias because they may cause obstruction.

   B. **Laboratory studies**

      1. **Complete blood count with differential** to evaluate for sepsis, if suspected. The hematocrit and platelet count may be checked if bleeding has occurred.

      2. **Blood culture** if sepsis is suspected and before antibiotics are started.

      3. **Serum potassium level** if ileus is present, to rule out hypokalemia.

      4. **Stool pH.** See Section III, B, 2a. If there is a family history of milk intolerance, a stool pH should be obtained to rule out lactose intolerance (the stool pH will usually be <5.0).

      5. **Coagulation profile (prothrombin time, partial thromboplastin time, fibrinogen, and platelets).** A bloody aspirate may signify the presence of a coagulopathy. In this case, coagulation studies should be obtained.

   C. **Radiologic and other studies**

      1. **Plain radiograph (flat plate) of the abdomen** should be obtained if the aspirate is bilious, if there is any abnormality on physical examination, or if aspirates continue. The radiograph will show whether the nasogastric tube is in the correct position and will define the bowel gas pattern. Look for an unusual gas pattern, pneumatosis intestinalis, ileus, or evidence of bowel obstruction. (See Chapter 10.) A left lateral decubitus film is useful because a perforation can be easily missed on the anteroposterior film.

      2. **Upright radiograph of the abdomen.** If bowel obstruction is suspected on the flat plate, obtain an upright radiograph of the abdomen and look for air-fluid levels.

      3. **Gastroesophageal reflux scintigraphy ("milk scan").** The infant is fed liquid (or milk) mixed with a technetium-99m-labeled pertechnetate. The infant is scanned in the supine position for 1–2 h with a gamma camera to show if there is delayed emptying of the stomach or reflux.

      4. **Endoscopy** should be considered for ulcer evaluation.

V. **Plan.** The approach to management of the neonate with increased gastric aspirates is usually initially based on the nature of the aspirate.

   A. **Prokinetic agents such as metoclopramide and erythromycin** are used to stimulate gastric emptying and decrease gastric residual volume.

      1. **Metoclopramide** is widely used to treat gastroesophageal reflux and decrease gastric residual volumes in infants. The concern with this medication is the extrapyramidal symptoms, although the literature is contradictory. Larger studies need to be done to evaluate the efficacy or toxicity of this medication.

      2. **Erythromycin.** Infants can have gastrointestinal (GI) motility immaturity that causes feeding problems. Erythromycin is a motilin agonist (the GI peptide that stimulates contractility) and produces a prokinetic effect on the gut that may help with feeding problems. Trials involving **erythromycin as a prokinetic agent** are conflicting. Studies have reported erythromycin for feeding intolerance in premature infants <35 weeks' gestation that led to a shorter time to full feeds with less feeds withheld. Another study showed that low-dose erythromycin decreased gastric aspirates in ventilated neonates <32 weeks' gestation. Erythromycin administration is given at some centers in high-risk premature infants with severe feeding intolerance or with documented delay in gastric emptying by decreased motility on the milk scan. More studies are needed before recommending routine use.

B. Treatment of specific types of aspirates

1. Bilious aspirate

   a. GI problems. All are initially managed by making the infant NPO and placing an nasogastric tube to rest and decompress the gut.

     i. NEC. See Chapter 104

     ii. Ileus may be secondary to sepsis, NEC, prematurity hypokalemia, effects of maternal drugs (especially magnesium sulfate), pneumonia, and hypothyroidism.

     iii. Other surgical problems (eg, bowel obstruction, malrotation, volvulus, meconium plug). Pediatric surgical consultation should be obtained immediately.

   b. Factitious. An abdominal radiograph will confirm the position of the nasogastric tube distally in the duodenum. Replace or reposition the tube in the stomach.

2. Nonbilious aspirate

   a. Aspirate containing undigested formula. If the volume of undigested formula in the aspirate does not exceed 30% of the previous feeding or is 10–15 mL total and the physical examination and vital signs are normal, the volume can be replaced. The time interval between feedings may not be long enough for digestion to take place. If the infant is being fed every 2 h and aspirates continue, the feeding interval may be increased to 3 h. If elevated aspirates still continue, the patient must be reevaluated. An abdominal radiograph should be obtained. Continuous gavage feedings may be tried; the patient may also have to be fed intravenously to allow the gut to rest.

   b. Aspirate containing digested formula. The aspirate is usually discarded, especially if it contains a large amount of mucus. If the physical examination and vital signs are normal, continue feedings and aspiration of stomach contents. If elevated aspirates continue, the patient must be reassessed. An abdominal film must be taken, and oral feedings should be discontinued for a time to let the gut rest. The number of calories given should be calculated to make certain that overfeeding (usually >130 kcal/kg/day) is not occurring.

   c. Other

     i. Formula intolerance. A trial of lactose-free formula (eg, ProSobee or Isomil) can be instituted if lactose intolerance is verified.

     ii. NEC or post-NEC stricture. See Chapter 104.

     iii. Pyloric stenosis. See Chapter 120.

     iv. Constipation. Anal stimulation can be attempted. If this fails, a glycerin suppository can be given. (See Chapter 60.)

     v. Infections. If sepsis is likely, broad-spectrum antibiotics are started after a laboratory workup is performed. A penicillin (usually ampicillin) and an aminoglycoside (usually gentamicin) are given initially until culture results are obtained (see Chapter 132 for doses). The patient is usually not fed orally if this diagnosis is entertained; an infant with sepsis usually does not tolerate oral feedings.

     vi. Inborn errors of metabolism. See Chapter 93.

     vii. Adrenogenital syndrome.

     viii. Adrenal hypoplasia.

     ix. Hypermagnesemia. See Chapter 99.

3. Bloody aspirate

   a. Nasogastric trauma. See Chapter 30.

   b. GI hemorrhage including stress ulcer, disseminated intravascular coagulation (DIC), vitamin K deficiency, and others are discussed in detail in Chapter 49.

49 Gastrointestinal Bleeding from the Upper Tract

I. **Problem.** Vomiting of bright red blood or active bleeding from the nasogastric (NG) tube is seen.

II. **Immediate questions**

A. **What are the vital signs?** If the blood pressure is dropping and there is active bleeding from the NG tube, urgent crystalloid volume replacement is necessary.

B. **What is the hematocrit?** A spun or STAT hematocrit should be done as soon as possible. The result is used as a baseline value and to determine whether blood replacement should be performed immediately. **With an acute episode of bleeding, the hematocrit may not reflect the blood loss for several hours.**

C. **Is blood available in the blood bank should transfusion be necessary?** Verify that the infant has been typed and cross-matched so that blood will be quickly available if necessary.

D. **Is there bleeding from other sites?** Bleeding from other sites suggests disseminated intravascular coagulation (DIC) or other coagulopathy. If bleeding is coming only from the NG tube, disorders such as stress ulcer, nasogastric trauma, and swallowing of maternal blood are likely causes to consider in the differential diagnosis.

E. **How old is the infant?** During the first day of life, vomiting of bright red blood or the presence of bright red blood in the NG tube is frequently secondary to swallowing of maternal blood during delivery. Infants with this problem are clinically stable, with normal vital signs. Pyloric stenosis usually presents at 3–4 weeks of life.

F. **What medications are being given?** Certain medications are associated with an increased incidence of gastrointestinal (GI) bleeding. The most common of these medications are indomethacin (Indocin), tolazoline (Priscoline), nonsteroidal anti-inflammatory drugs (NSAIDs), theophylline, heparin, and corticosteroids. A massive gastric hemorrhage may occur during continuous drip infusion of tolazoline. Theophylline is a rare cause of GI bleeding. Some maternal medications can cross the placenta (aspirin, cephalothin, and phenobarbital) and cause coagulation disorders in the infant.

G. **Was vitamin K given at birth?** Failure to give vitamin K at birth may result in a bleeding disorder, usually at 3–4 days of life.

III. **Differential diagnosis**

A. **Idiopathic.** More than 50% of cases have no clear diagnosis and usually resolve within several days.

B. **Swallowing of maternal blood** accounts for ~10% of cases. Typically, blood is swallowed during cesarean delivery. Blood can also be from a fissure in the mother's nipple.

C. **Ulcers.** Single stress ulcers and perforation are more common in the duodenum than the stomach in the neonate. Gastric erosions often precede the ulceration.

D. **Diffuse hemorrhagic or ulcerative esophagitis, gastritis, and duodenal mucosa lesions.** This damage can be caused by an increase in gastric acid secretion in infants.

E. **Allergic colitis** caused by allergy to milk or soy after it has been introduced. Can present with upper GI or rectal bleeding.

F. **Nasogastric trauma.** Forceful insertion or too large a tube can cause trauma.

G. **Necrotizing enterocolitis (NEC).** A rare cause of upper GI tract bleeding that indicates extensive disease.

H. **Coagulopathy.** Hemorrhagic disease of the newborn and DIC account for ~20% of cases. Also, congenital coagulopathies (most commonly factor VIII deficiency [hemophilia A] and factor IX deficiency [hemophilia B]) can cause GI bleeding from the upper tract. DIC can occur after infection, shock, and severe fetal asphyxia.

I. **Drug-induced bleeding.** Indomethacin, corticosteroids, tolazoline, heparin, NSAIDS, sulindac, and other drugs may cause upper GI tract bleeding. Theophylline is a rare cause. High-dose dexamethasone is associated with stress and perforated ulcers and hemorrhage in the newborn. Maternal use of aspirin, cephalothin, and phenobarbital can cause coagulation abnormalities in neonates.

J. **Congenital defects** such as gastric volvulus, malrotation with volvulus, Hirschsprung disease with enterocolitis, intussusception, gastric duplication, and Meckel diverticulitis are rare causes of GI bleeding.

K. **Pyloric stenosis.** Patients present at the third to fourth week of life with nonbilious projectile vomiting (occasionally bloody).

L. **GI bleeding** caused by liver disease, cholestasis.

M. **Rare causes** include gastric teratoma, isolated cavernous hemangioma of the stomach, infection with *Serratia marcescens,* and arteriovenous malformations.

IV. **Database**

A. **Physical examination** should focus attention on other possible bleeding sites. Note bowel sounds, distension, and erythema.

B. **Laboratory studies**

1. **Apt test** should be performed if swallowing of maternal blood is a possible cause. This test differentiates maternal from fetal blood. The test relies on the fact that hemoglobin F is not hydrolyzed by a strong base, whereas maternal hemoglobin A hydrolyzes to a yellow brown. However, a negative test does not rule out swallowed maternal blood.

2. **Hematocrit** should be checked as a baseline and serially to gauge the extent of blood loss.

3. **Coagulation studies (prothrombin time, partial thromboplastin time, fibrinogen, and platelets)** to rule out DIC and other coagulopathies. An elevated prothrombin time and prolonged partial thromboplastin time may indicate a coagulopathy.

4. **If cholestasis is a concern,** a total and direct bilirubin and liver function tests should be done.

C. **Radiologic and other studies**

1. **An abdominal radiograph** assesses the bowel gas pattern and rules out NEC. The film also shows the position of the NG tube and indicates a possible surgical problem.

2. **Upper GI series.** (Barium contrast studies) if nonemergent bleeding can evaluate for upper GI bleed or midgut volvulus.

3. **Fiberoptic endoscopy** should be considered and can reveal the source of bleeding in 90% of patients with upper GI bleeding.

4. **Ultrasound scans** of the abdomen if pyloric stenosis is suspected.

5. **Hepatobiliary scan** will rule out biliary atresia and neonatal hepatitis.

V. **Plan**

A. **General measures.** The most important goal is to stop the bleeding in every case except those involving infants who have swallowed maternal blood. Infants with this problem are usually only a few hours old, are not sick, and have a positive Apt test result. Once stomach aspiration is performed, no more blood is obtained.

1. **Volume replacement.** If the blood pressure is low or dropping, crystalloid (usually normal saline) can be given immediately. **Blood replacement** may be indicated, depending on the result of hematocrit values obtained from the laboratory.

2. **Stop the acute episode of GI bleeding:**
   a. **Gastric lavage** with tepid water, $^1/_2$ normal saline (NS), or NS 5 mL/kg by NG tube until the bleeding has subsided. (***Note:*** There is ***controversy*** about which fluid to use. Some believe that hyponatremia may occur if water is used and hypernatremia may occur if NS is used. Follow your institution's guidelines. **Never use cold-water lavages** because they lower the infant's core temperature too rapidly.)
   b. **Epinephrine lavage** (1:10,000 solution), 0.1 mL diluted in 10 mL of sterile water, can be used if tepid water lavages do not stop the bleeding (***controversial***).
B. **Disease specific measures**
   1. **Idiopathic.** When no cause is determined, the bleeding usually subsides and no other treatment is necessary.
   2. **Swallowing of maternal blood.** No treatment is necessary.
   3. **Stress ulcer** is commonly diagnosed after an episode of GI bleeding by endoscopy. This disorder is difficult to confirm using radiologic studies; thus they are not often obtained. Remission usually occurs; recurrence is rare.
      a. **Antacids** may be used (eg, Maalox, 0.5–1 mL/kg or 0.25 mL/kg, six times/day), placed in the NG tube until bleeding has subsided. This is ***controversial*** because it may cause concretions in the GI tract. Antacids may increase the risk of infection and feeding intolerance in infants receiving gavage feedings. Calcium- and aluminum-containing antacids cause diarrhea; magnesium-containing antacids cause constipation.
      b. **H$_2$ blockers** inhibit gastric acid production in neonates and are usually recommended. **Start ranitidine or cimetidine** (see Chapter 132 for dosing). Ranitidine is preferred because it has fewer side effects. Follow your institution's guidelines. Some institutions use cimetidine first and if bleeding continues use ranitidine. H$_2$ blocker therapy is associated with higher rates of NEC in very low birthweight infants.
      c. **Proton pump inhibitors** are used if H$_2$ blockers do not work. These include esomeprazole (Nexium), omeprazole (Prilosec), Lansoprazole (Prevacid), rabeprazole (AcipHex), and pantoprazole (Protonix). Studies with these agents are promising but not approved in children.
   4. **Diffuse hemorrhagic or ulcerative esophagitis, gastritis, and duodenal mucosa lesions.** Treatment is supportive (maintain adequate oxygenation, nasogastric suction plus the use of intravenous (IV) H$_2$ blockers is recommended). Prophylactic use of acid-reducing agents are sometimes used in high-risk patients. Surgery is rarely needed.
   5. **Allergic colitis.** Eliminate the formula and change to a hypoallergenic formula.
   6. **Ulcerative esophagitis.** Treated as ulcers above.
   7. **Nasogastric trauma** may occur if the NG tube is too large or insertion is traumatic. Use the smallest NG tube possible. Observation is indicated.
   8. **Necrotizing enterocolitis.** Severe cases of NEC cause upper GI bleeding. Treatment is discussed in Chapter 104.
   9. **Coagulopathy**
      a. **Hemorrhagic disease of the newborn.** When vitamin K deficiency is suspected, vitamin K should be administered IV or subcutaneously. Intramuscular injection can result in severe hematoma. One mg of vitamin K IV stops the hemorrhage within 2 h. There are three forms of **vitamin K deficiency:**
         i. **Early form** (first day of life) is related to maternal medications affecting production of vitamin K by the neonate (barbiturates, phenytoin, rifampin, isoniazid, warfarin).
         ii. **Classic form** between day 2 and day 7 of life is more commonly seen in infants with inadequate intake of breast milk and when an infant has not received vitamin K at birth (eg, home delivery).

      iii. **Late form** occurs between 2 weeks and 6 months of age. This is secondary to inadequate vitamin K intake (breast-fed infants) or hepatobiliary disease.
    b. **DIC** is associated with bleeding from other sites. Coagulation studies are abnormal (increased prothrombin time and partial thromboplastin time and decreased fibrinogen levels). Treat the underlying condition and support blood pressure with multiple transfusions of colloid as needed. Platelets may be required. The cause of DIC (eg, hypoxia, acidosis, bacterial or viral disease, toxoplasmosis, NEC, shock, or erythroblastosis fetalis) must be investigated. Several obstetric disorders, including abruptio placentae, chorioangioma, eclampsia, and fetal death associated with twin gestation, may give rise to DIC.
    c. **Congenital coagulopathies.** The most common that present with bleeding are secondary to factor VIII deficiency (hemophilia A) and factor IX deficiency (hemophilia B). Specific laboratory testing and appropriate consultation with a pediatric hematologist are appropriate.
  10. **Drug-induced bleeding.** The drug responsible for the bleeding should be stopped if possible.
  11. **Congenital defects such as gastric volvulus, malrotation with volvulus, Hirschsprung disease with enterocolitis, gastric duplication.** Urgent surgical consultation is recommended.
  12. **Pyloric stenosis.** Hydration and surgical pyloromyotomy are necessary.
  13. **GI bleeding from liver disease, cholestasis**
    a. **Octreotide (Sandostatin).** Dosage recommended (safety and dosing not established) is 1 mcg/kg IV bolus, followed by 1 mcg/kg/h IV infusion. If no bleeding occurs in 12 h, decrease the dose by 50%. Then stop the medication when the dose is 25% of the initial dose.
    b. **Vasopressin (Pitressin)** has been used in neonates but has many adverse effects, so it not recommended.

50 Hyperbilirubinemia, Direct (Conjugated Hyperbilirubinemia)

  I. **Problem.** An infant's direct (conjugated) serum bilirubin level is 3 mg/dL. **A value >1.5–2.0 mg/dL (or a fraction >10–20% of the total serum bilirubin) is abnormal at any age.** Guidelines from the North American Society for Pediatric Gastroenterology, Hepatology and Nutrition uses the following definition for abnormal bilirubin: direct bilirubin >1 mg/dL if total bilirubin <5mg/dL or direct bilirubin is >20% of the total if the total bilirubin >5mg/dL. A persistent or increasing elevated direct bilirubin is always pathologic and must be evaluated promptly to minimize long-term sequelae. **Conjugated hyperbilirubinemia is never normal or physiologic.** It occurs in one in every 2500 infants. **Early diagnosis and treatment is essential** because it means a better outcome for the infant and can be potentially life saving. The goal is to complete the evaluation by 45 to 60 days of age (surgery for biliary atresia has its best outcome if performed before the age of 45–60 days.)
  II. **Immediate questions**
    A. **Is the urine dark and what color is the stool?** Dark urine is a nonspecific indicator of increased conjugated bilirubin. Persistent pale or clay-colored stools occur with cholestasis and obstruction needs to be ruled out.

B. **Is the infant receiving total parenteral nutrition (TPN)?** TPN may cause direct hyperbilirubinemia by an unknown mechanism and usually does not occur until the infant has been on TPN for >2 weeks. It is more common in sick premature infants.

C. **Is the infant gaining weight?** Failure to gain weight can be seen in neonatal hepatitis and some metabolic diseases.

D. **Does the infant appear sick? Is a bacterial or viral infection present?** Infants with cholestatic jaundice caused by bacterial sepsis appear acutely ill. Infection may cause hepatocellular damage, leading to increased direct bilirubin levels. Infants with galactosemia, hypopituitarism, or gallstones with cholestatic jaundice can also appear ill. These disorders require immediate diagnosis and treatment.

E. **Did direct hyperbilirubinemia occur only after feedings had been established?** This suggests a metabolic disorder such as galactosemia may be present.

F. **Have any risk factors been identified?** The most important risk factors include low gestational age, early or prolonged exposure to parenteral nutrition, lack of enteral feeding, and sepsis. Episodes of sepsis can be associated with an increase of 30% in the bilirubin level. Other risk factors include neonatal hepatitis , ABO incompatibility, and trisomy 21.

G. **Is the infant being treated for jaundice for another condition and not improving?** Any infant who is being treated for jaundice and whose jaundice does not resolve or improve needs to be retested and evaluated for cholestasis.

H. **How old is the infant?** The Guideline Committee recommends that any infant who has jaundice at 2 weeks of age be evaluated for cholestasis, except for breastfed infants who have a normal history (no light stools or dark urine) and physical examination can be monitored and evaluated at 3 weeks of age.

III. **Differential diagnosis.** See also Table 91–1. Bilirubin is the main waste product of hemoglobin breakdown when the liver breaks down old red blood cells. There are two forms of circulating bilirubin: indirect and direct. **Direct (conjugated) bilirubin** can be measured directly in blood and is a product of bilirubin metabolism within the liver **(indirect bilirubin** is conjugated in the liver to become direct bilirubin). Direct bilirubin is excreted into bile, stool, and urine.

A. **Common causes of direct hyperbilirubinemia.** Statistics vary on what are the most common causes of direct hyperbilirubinemia. Some note that biliary atresia and genetic intrahepatic cholestasis account for 50% of cases. Another source suggested that early-onset cholestatic jaundice was more common from nonhepatic reasons. Yet others state idiopathic neonatal hepatitis is the most common cause. The Guidelines committee states the most common causes are biliary atresia and neonatal hepatitis. Whatever is reported, it is generally agreed that the most common causes in a neonatal intensive care unit are as follows:

1. **Extrahepatic biliary atresia** is a progressive obliterative process involving the bile ducts and is fatal if untreated. These infants usually have clay-colored stools and dark urine.

2. **Genetic intrahepatic cholestasis** includes progressive familial intrahepatic cholestasis, Alagille syndrome, and bile acid synthetic defect.

3. **Idiopathic neonatal hepatitis.** This diagnosis is made after all other known causes have been excluded.

4. **Hyperalimentation (total parenteral nutrition induced cholestasis)** is common in very low birthweight infants.

5. **Bacterial/Viral/Parasitic infections** (sepsis or urinary tract infection). These can be secondary to group B streptococcus, *Escherichia coli*, syphilis, *Listeria*, staphylococcus, and tuberculosis. One study found that **Gram-negative infections are the most common** cause of cholestatic jaundice. Viral infections can include Epstein-Barr virus, HIV, adenovirus, coxsackie virus, hepatitis B and C, varicella zoster, and echovirus 14 and 19. Toxoplasma can also be a cause. **If the onset of jaundice occurs after 8 days of age in an asymptomatic infant, suspect a urinary tract infection.**

6. **Intrauterine infection.** TORCH [*t*oxoplasmosis, *o*ther, *r*ubella, *c*ytomegalovirus, and *h*erpes simplex virus], hepatitis B and C, and syphilis).

7. **Hemolytic disease. Inspissated bile syndrome** is excessive bilirubin that results from hemolytic disease. It can also be seen with **extracorporeal membrane oxygenation** (secondary to hemolysis) and infants with erythroblastosis fetalis who have had an intrauterine transfusion.

8. **Choledochal cyst.**

9. **α-Antitrypsin deficiency** is the most common genetic cause of cholestasis. It causes 5–15 % of cases.

10. Galactosemia is the **most well-known metabolic disorder** that presents with prolonged jaundice.

B. **Less common causes of direct hyperbilirubinemia**

1. **Perinatal hypoxia-ischemia** has been identified as an important causal factor in transient neonatal cholestasis.

2. **Bile duct stenosis.**

3. **Neoplasm.**

4. **Cholelithiasis (gallstones) or biliary sludge.**

5. **Cystic fibrosis.** Very few of these patients have liver disease in the neonatal period.

6. **Hypothyroidism.**

7. **Rotor syndrome.**

8. **Dubin-Johnson syndrome,** a genetic defect in the canalicular transport system.

9. **Storage disease (eg, Niemann-Pick disease or Gaucher disease).**

10. **Metabolic disorders (eg, tyrosinemia, fructosemia).**

11. **Trisomy 21, 18, or 13.**

12. **Drug induced.** Prolonged use of chloral hydrate.

13. **Shock.**

14. **Zellweger syndrome (cerebrohepatorenal syndrome).**

15. **Byler disease.**

16. **Porphyria.**

17. **Wolman disease.**

18. **Spontaneous perforation of the bile duct.**

19. **Neonatal hemochromatosis.**

20. **Panhypopituitarism.**

21. **Neonatal sclerosing cholangitis.**

22. **Caroli disease.**

IV. **Database.** A detailed history, including prenatal (to evaluate for intrauterine infection or hemolytic disease) and postnatal (feeding history with questions about the composition of formula, as well as the presence of any acholic stools) history, should be obtained. Specifically ask about other members of the family having this problem. This can imply genetic disease or an autosomal dominant inheritance. Is there consanguinity? If yes, then a risk of autosomal recessive inheritance exists. Was a fetal ultrasound done and what are the results? This may identify a choledochal cyst or other abnormalities. Is there excessive bleeding which could signify a coagulopathy. Is the infant lethargic or irritable? Lethargy can mean hypothyroidism. Irritability can signify a metabolic disorder. The clinical hallmarks of the disease include **icterus, acholic or pale stools, dark urine, hepatomegaly, and splenomegaly.** See Figure 91–1 for an approach to an infant with cholestasis

A. **Physical examination.** Vital signs, weight assessment, and general assessment of nutrition and observation for any signs of sepsis. Check for bruises or petechiae on the skin. Is there evidence of pneumonia on the chest exam? Is there a murmur or evidence of heart failure? Know the characteristics of the syndromes noted above in the differential. Attention should be given to examination of the abdomen. Is it distended? Palpate for an enlarged liver or spleen or for any masses. Splenomegaly is more common in neonatal hepatitis but can be a late sign in biliary atresia. Jaundice has a greenish hue compared with unconjugated jaundice that is more yellow. **"Bronze baby syndrome" (a bronze discoloration of the skin as a result of dermal accumulation** of coproporphyrins) occurs in infants with direct hyperbilirubinemia who are exposed to phototherapy. Ask the nurses about the diaper examination. Is the urine dark and what color are the stools?

B. **Laboratory studies.** It is important to evaluate the newborn screen for hypothyroidism and galactosemia. These conditions require urgent treatment to prevent or decrease serious sequelae. If it was not done, a repeat one can be sent or urine for reducing substance and serum thyroxine and serum TSH can be sent. Sepsis evaluation should also be done early in any ill infant with jaundice to improve outcome.

   1. **For the common causes,** the workup is as follows:

      a. **Bilirubin levels (total and direct).** The most important test to determine is the fractionated bilirubin levels. A **urine bilirubin** detects a substantial elevation of conjugated bilirubin. When serum levels exceed 3–4 mg/dL, bilirubin will be found in the urine.

      b. **Liver function tests** should include aspartate aminotransferase (AST [serum glutamic oxaloacetic transaminase, or SGOT]), alanine aminotransferase (ALT [serum glutamic pyruvic transaminase, or SGPT]), alkaline phosphatase, and gamma-glutamyltranspeptidase (GGTP). Elevated levels of AST and ALT signify hepatocellular damage. Elevated alkaline phosphatase levels may signify biliary obstruction (nonspecific because it is found in the liver, kidney, and bone). Elevated GGTP is a sensitive but nonspecific marker of biliary obstruction or inflammation. It was used in the past to differentiate biliary atresia from neonatal hepatitis, but variability in results make it unreliable.

      c. **Complete blood count with differential** may help determine whether infection is present.

      d. **Serum glucose levels.** Metabolic disorders may present with hypoglycemia.

      e. **Coombs test** suggests hemolytic disease.

      f. **Ammonia levels** are elevated in advanced liver failure.

      g. **Serum cholesterol, triglycerides, and albumin levels.** Cholesterol and triglycerides can be checked for assessment of liver failure and albumin for hepatic function.

      h. **Prothrombin time, partial thromboplastin time, and serum albumin level** to evaluate hepatic function.

      i. **Reticulocyte count** may be elevated (ie, >4–5%) if bleeding has occurred or hemolysis is present.

      j. **Blood and urine cultures** if sepsis is considered.

      k. **Testing for viral disease.** Determine the serum total immunoglobulin M (IgM) level. If high, test for TORCH infections (see Chapter 127). Urine is tested for cytomegalovirus, and a serum hepatitis profile is obtained (hepatitis surface antigen and IgM hepatitis A antibody). Hepatitis B markers should be tested in both the mother and the infant with PCR studies being the most specific.

      l. **Serum α_1-antitrypsin levels** to rule out α_1-antitrypsin deficiency.

      m. **Urine testing for reducing substances** should be performed if galactosemia is suspected. Galactose in the urine results in a positive reducing substance in the urine on a Clinitest, but will have a negative urine test for glucose (glucose oxidase).

   2. **For the less common causes,** perform the following:

      a. **Serum thyroxine and thyroid-stimulating hormone levels** if hypothyroidism is suspected.

      b. **Sweat chloride test** to rule out cystic fibrosis.

      c. **Urine metabolic screen.**

      d. **Serum and urine amino acid screening.** Urine organic acid and plasma amino acid are screens for inborn errors that cause liver dysfunction.

C. **Radiologic and other studies**

   1. **Chest radiograph.** To check for cardiovascular or situs anomalies that may suggest biliary atresia.

2. **Ultrasonography of the liver and the biliary tract (hepatic ultrasound)** is recommended for all infants with cholestasis. It can rule out anatomic abnormalities such as choledochal cyst, stones, tumor, and masses and also provide information on the gallbladder. The absence or finding a small gallbladder suggests, but cannot be used to rule out biliary atresia. The procedure is operator dependent.

3. **Hepatobiliary scanning (scintigraphy).** Radionuclide scans such as **hepatobiliary iminodiacetic acid (HIDA)** or **para-isopropyl iminodiacetic acid (PIPIDA)** allow evaluation of the biliary anatomy. Injected radioactive material is normally excreted into the intestine. If there is no visualization after 24 h, biliary obstruction or hepatocellular dysfunction may be present. The test has a high sensitivity for biliary atresia, but low specificity. Tests are expensive, time consuming, and have many false positive and false negative results.

4. **Endoscopic retrograde cholangiopancreatography (ERCP)** can be done for diagnosis and therapy for bile duct stones. It is not routinely done but may be useful.

5. **Percutaneous liver biopsy** is usually performed after all other laboratory tests have been performed and a definitive diagnosis is still needed. It is recommended for most infants with cholestasis of unknown etiology. Evidence indicates that this test can be performed safely in small infants. **Some studies have shown that this procedure had the greatest diagnostic accuracy and should be done before surgery to diagnose biliary atresia.** Results should be interpreted by a pathologist with pediatric liver disease expertise and experience.

6. **Duodenal aspirate.** May be useful in remote areas where other tests are not available. Fluid is obtained from the duodenum and then the aspirate is sent for bilirubin concentration. With obstruction the aspirate bilirubin concentration is not greater than the serum level.

7. **Exploratory laparotomy and operative cholangiography should be considered** if all other tests have been done and are inconclusive and biliary atresia needs to be diagnosed.

V. **Plan.** The cause of direct hyperbilirubinemia is determined and specific treatment is directed at the cause. As few conditions are treatable, care is mostly supportive. Treatment involves dietary measures, medications, and surgery. This section also discusses some of the more common causes of cholestatic jaundice with more detailed management information (see also Chapter 91.) Consultation with a pediatric gastroenterologist is recommended.

A. **Dietary.** Most of these infants require special formulas (eg, Pregestimil and Portagen) that include medium-chain triglycerides (MCT) that can be absorbed better with a bile salt deficiency. Supplemental MCT can be given to breast-fed infants. Supplemental vitamins (A, D, E, K) are needed in many of these infants. Some infants may require dietary restrictions.

B. **Medications.** Medications often used are ursodeoxycholic acid, phenobarbital, and cholestyramine and are discussed in detail in Chapter 91, page 496.

C. **Surgery.** Surgery includes the Kasai procedure and liver transplantation. (See Chapter 91.)

D. **Specific recommendations**

1. **Biliary atresia.** Evidence suggests that earlier diagnosis and surgical repair leads to a better outcome. Exploratory surgery with intraoperative cholangiography is often the initial step. Hepatic portoenterostomy (the **Kasai procedure**) is currently the initial procedure of choice in infancy, It has the greatest chance of reestablishment of bile flow and the longest term survival of the infant's liver if performed before the age of 45 to 60 days. Orthotopic liver transplantation is selectively performed for those infants or children with progressive liver failure. Hepatic transplantation offers improved survival and quality of life to those for whom the Kasai operation is not successful.

2. **Idiopathic neonatal hepatitis.** Supportive care with a fair prognosis exists.

3. **α₁-Antitrypsin deficiency.** The only curative therapy is liver transplantation.
4. **Hyperalimentation.** Consider stopping TPN completely or using partial parenteral nutrition with some enteral feedings. Most infants recover with clearing of cholestasis in 1–3 months after normal feedings have begun. The use of phenobarbital therapy is *controversial.* Studies have shown that ursodeoxycholic acid is being used in high-risk neonates with TPN-cholestasis with good results. Cholecystokinin as a treatment or prophylactic agent has less conclusively shown a beneficial effect.
5. **Bacterial infection.** If signs of sepsis are present, appropriate cultures should be performed and empirical antibiotic therapy initiated (See Chapter 117.)
6. **Intrauterine infection.** Appropriate antiviral agents or other medications should be started, if indicated.
7. **Inspissated bile** secondary to hemolytic disease is treated with supportive management. The use of phenobarbital is *controversial.*
8. **Choledochal cyst.** The treatment is surgical removal.
9. **Galactosemia.** Immediate elimination of lactose- and galactose-containing products from the diet is required.

Selected References

Guideline for the Evaluation of Cholestatic Jaundice in Infants: Recommendations of the North American Society for Pediatric Gastroenterology, Hepatology and Nutrition. *J Pediatric Gastroenterol Nutr* 2004; 39:115-128.

51 Hyperbilirubinemia, Indirect (Unconjugated Hyperbilirubinemia)

I. **Problem.** An infant's indirect (unconjugated) serum bilirubin level is 10 mg/dL. The exact definition of a physiologic range and management of indirect hyperbilirubinemia is complex and based on many factors, including gestational age (GA), postnatal age, birthweight, disease state, risk factors, degree of hydration, nutritional status, and ethnicity. **Total bilirubin (TSB)** (sum of the direct [conjugated] and indirect [unconjugated]) and direct serum bilirubin can be measured in the blood. The indirect bilirubin is calculated by subtracting the direct bilirubin from the total bilirubin. **TcB (transcutaneous bilirubin)** is a measurement of total serum bilirubin from an instrument that uses reflectance measurements on the skin and correlates well with the laboratory TSB value.

II. **Immediate questions**

   A. **How old is the infant? High indirect serum bilirubin levels during the first 24 h of life are never physiologic.** Hemolytic disease (Rh isoimmunization or ABO incompatibility), congenital infection (eg, rubella, toxoplasmosis), sepsis, occult hemorrhage, and polycythemia are likely causes. The age and gestation of the infant help determine the bilirubin level at which phototherapy should be initiated.

   B. **Is the infant being breast-fed?** Breast milk jaundice is common and may be present; the cause is unknown and there is a familial association. Peak bilirubin levels usually occur 4–10 days after birth.

C. **What is the family ethnicity?** The incidence of neonatal jaundice is increased in infants of American Indian, Greek, and Eastern Asian descent. Greeks who were born in Greece and live there have a higher incidence of hyperbilirubinemia than Greeks living in the United States. Glucose-6-phosphate dehydrogenase (G6PD) deficiency occurs more commonly in people of Mediterranean, African, Arabian Peninsula, Southeast Asian, and Middle Eastern descent. Immigration and intermarriage have increased the incidence of G6PD in the United States. It occurs in 11–13% of African Americans. There is a rapid increase in the total serum bilirubin level after 24–48 h of age.

D. **Is the infant dehydrated?** With dehydration (or weight loss from birth is >12%), fluid administration may lower the serum bilirubin level. Additional feedings should be given, if tolerated (milk-based formula is recommended in dehydrated breast-fed infants); otherwise, IV fluids should be given. It is recommended that mothers nurse their infants 8–12 times a day as a minimum for the first few days. For example, a 3-day-old infant is strictly breast-feeding, but his mother's milk has not yet "come in," so he has lost significant weight and becomes dehydrated. Remember that adequate hydration is essential, but **excess hydration will not clear the bilirubin any more quickly, prevent hyperbilirubinemia, or decrease TSB.**

E. **What is the gestational age of the infant?** The risk of unconjugated hyperbilirubinemia is inversely proportional with GA.

III. **Differential diagnosis.** Indirect (unconjugated) bilirubin is derived mainly from hemoglobin metabolism and must be conjugated in the liver before it can be excreted in the bile, stool, or urine. It can not be directly measured in the blood and is never present in urine. (See also Chapter 92.)

A. **More common causes of indirect hyperbilirubinemia**
   1. Physiologic hyperbilirubinemia.
   2. ABO incompatibility.
   3. Breast-feeding or breast milk jaundice.
   4. Infection (eg, congenital syphilis, viral, or protozoal infections). Jaundice as the only sign of underlying sepsis is rare. In one study of 171 newborns readmitted for a mean bilirubin of 18.8 mg/dL, not one case of sepsis was identified.
   5. Subdural hematoma or cephalhematoma.
   6. Excessive bruising.
   7. Infant of a diabetic mother.
   8. Polycythemia or hyperviscosity.
   9. Asphyxia.
   10. Respiratory distress syndrome.

B. **Less common causes of indirect hyperbilirubinemia**
   1. **Rh isoimmunization.** As a result of antenatal treatment of Rh-negative mothers with RhoGAM, this has become a much less frequent cause.
   2. **G6PD deficiency.** With this condition, a late-rising bilirubin is seen. This is also more common in individuals of certain ethnic backgrounds, such as Sephardic Jews and those from Greece, Turkey, Sardinia, or Nigeria.
   3. Pyruvate kinase deficiency.
   4. Congenital spherocytosis.
   5. Lucey-Driscoll syndrome (familial neonatal jaundice).
   6. Crigler-Najjar syndrome.
   7. Hypothyroidism.
   8. Hemoglobinopathy such as α- and β-thalassemia.
   9. Gilbert syndrome.
   10. Early galactosemia.
   11. **Medications.** Novobiocin, penicillin, oxytocin, sulfonamides, vitamin K, nitrofurantoin.
   12. α-Thalassemia.
   13. Disseminated intravascular coagulopathy.

IV. Database
   A. **History.** What is the infant's feeding regimen and frequency of voiding (hydration status)? Ask about jaundice in previous siblings and family ethnicity (if G6PD deficiency is suspected). Is there a familial history of significant hemolytic disease? Is there a history of light-colored stools or dark urine?
   B. **Physical examination.** Pay particular attention to signs of bruising, cephalhematoma, or intracranial bleeding. Check for hepatosplenomegaly. The accumulation of bilirubin in body tissues produces **jaundice (yellow skin)** from bili pigments deposited in the skin and sclerae. Jaundice is seen in the face first and progresses caudally to the trunk and extremities. Pressure on the skin often reveals jaundice. The TSB can be estimated by examining for jaundice (face, ~5mg/dL; upper chest, ~10mg/dL; abdomen, ~12mg/dL; palms and soles, usually >15mg/dL).
   C. **Laboratory studies.** Studies have questioned the need for extensive testing on any infant with possible hyperbilirubinemia. In normal and healthy term infants, few tests are necessary. It is useful to save cord blood for future testing if necessary.
      1. **Jaundiced infant of >35 weeks' gestational age.** These recommendations (see a–e) are based on the American Academy of Pediatrics (AAP) Subcommittee on Hyperbilirubinemia: Management of hyperbilirubinemia in infants 35 or more weeks of gestation. *Pediatrics* 2004;114(1):297-316. It is recommended that all bilirubin levels should be interpreted in infant's age in hours. See also the algorithm in Figure 51–1 for management of jaundice in the newborn nursery.
         a. **Infant is jaundiced in the first 24 h or the jaundice appears excessive for age of the infant, measure TSB and TcB.**
         b. **Infant is receiving phototherapy or TSB is rising rapidly and unexplained by history and physical examination, obtain:**
            i. **Blood type and Coombs test, if not obtained on the cord blood.**
            ii. **Complete blood count (CBC) and smear.**
            iii. **Direct (conjugated) bilirubin.**
            iv. **Reticulocyte count**
            v. **G6PD level.**
            vi. **ETCOc if available.** ETCOc (end-tidal CO corrected for ambient CO) is a measurement of the rate of heme catabolism and rate of bilirubin production. It is used to confirm hemolysis and can help identify infants at risk for developing high bilirubin levels.
            vii. **Repeat TSB in 4–24 h depending on infant's age and TSB level.**
         c. **TSB is approaching exchange levels or is not responding to phototherapy:**
            i. **Reticulocyte count if anemia or hemolytic disease is suspected.**
            ii. **G6PD level.**
            iii. **Albumin.** An albumin of <3.0g/dL is a risk factor for lowering the threshold for phototherapy. Obtaining a serum albumin will allow you to calculate the bilirubin-to-albumin (B/A) ratio, which can help determine the need for exchange transfusion (see Figure 92–3).
            iv. **ETCOc.** See above.
         d. **Direct bilirubin is elevated:**
            i. **Evaluate for sepsis including urinalysis and urine culture if indicated.**
            ii. **See Chapters 50 and 91, for more details on direct hyperbilirubinemia.**
         e. **Jaundice is present at 3 weeks or beyond, or if the infant is sick:**
            i. **Total and direct bilirubin.**
            ii. **If direct bilirubin elevated, evaluate for cholestasis.**
            iii. **Thyroid screen (hypothyroidism) and galactosemia screen.** Does the infant have signs or symptoms of hypothyroidism?
      2. **Jaundiced infant <35 weeks' of gestation with jaundice (*controversial*).** There are no formal guidelines for jaundiced infants <35 weeks. These are recommendations only. Follow institutional guidelines.
         a. **Total and direct serum bilirubin levels.** In preterm or ill infants, check levels every 12–24 h depending on the rate of rise and until stable. In term infants, direct bilirubin is indicated only if jaundice is persistent or the infant is ill.

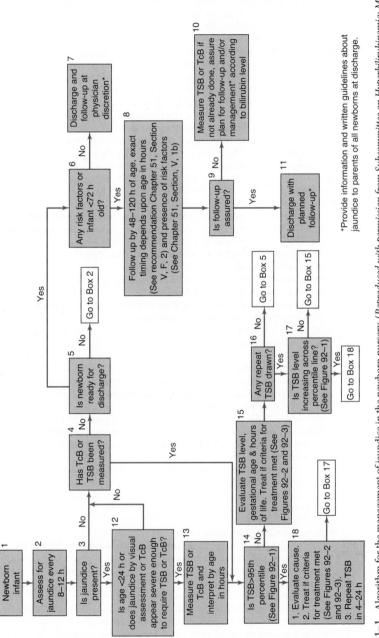

Figure 51–1. Algorithm for the management of jaundice in the newborn nursery. (*Reproduced with permission from Subcommittee on Hyperbilirubinemia: Management of hyperbilirubinemia in the newborn infant 35 or more weeks of gestation.* Pediatrics 2004;114(1):297–316.)

    b. CBC with differential if hemolytic disease, anemia, or infection is suspected.

    c. Mother's and infant's blood type with Rh determination.

    d. Direct and indirect Coombs' tests. Used to detect in vivo or in vitro antibody-antigen reactions in hemolytic anemia.

    f. Reticulocyte count if the infant is anemic or hemolytic disease is suspected.

    g. Red blood cell (RBC) smear. Fragmented RBCs should be present in hemolysis.

    h. G6PD screen. G6PD is more common in males and in infants of Mediterranean, African, Arabian, Asian, or Middle Eastern descent. The jaundice is late onset, and there is evidence of hemolysis (low hematocrit, high reticulocyte count, and a peripheral smear showing nucleated RBCs and other fragmented cells) or the response to phototherapy is poor.

    i. Hemoglobin electrophoresis. Used to rule out hemoglobinopathies (hemolytic anemia, thalassemia, sickle cell anemia, hemoglobin C disease)

    j. ETCOc.

  D. Radiologic and other studies. Usually unnecessary.

V. Plan. See also Chapter 92 for a detailed discussion.

  A. Phototherapy

    1. Phototherapy for the hospitalized infant of ≥35 weeks' gestation (see Figure 92–2). This figure is based on guidelines from the AAP. Phototherapy is started when the TSB exceeds the line (or an option is to start 2–3 levels below the line) indicated for each category. The risk factors were determined because these conditions have a negative effect on the albumin binding of bilirubin, the blood-brain barrier, and the susceptibility of the brain cells to damage by bilirubin. When following this figure it is important to remember these recommendations:

      a. Use total serum bilirubin (TSB).

      b. Measure serum albumin (optional). If it is less than 3 g/dL, it is considered a risk factor for lowering the phototherapy threshold.

      c. Risk factors are isoimmune hemolytic disease, G6PD deficiency, asphyxia, significant lethargy, temperature instability, sepsis, acidosis, or albumin <3.0 g/dL.

      d. Infants at lower risk are those ≥38 weeks and well.

      e. Infants at medium risk are those ≥38 weeks that have risk factors (see earlier). Other infants at medium risk involve those infants that are 35–37 6/7 weeks and well. It is optional if one wants to intervene at a lower TSB level for those infants that are closer than 35 weeks and at a higher level for those infants that are closer to 37 6/7 weeks.

      f. Infants at high risk are those that are 35–37 6/7 weeks with risk factors listed earlier.

    2. Phototherapy for the hospitalized infant < 35 weeks' gestation. There are no recommended guidelines from the AAP on this group of infants (see Table 51–1). The table gives recommendations for phototherapy and exchange transfusion in well and sick preterm infants and sick term infants (***controversial***). These are guidelines only, and each patient must be considered individually.

    3. If phototherapy is used, perform the following additional procedures:

      a. Increase the maintenance infusion of IV fluids by 0.5 mL/kg/h if the infant weighs <1500 g and by 1 mL/kg/h if the infant weighs >1500 g (***controversial***). Excessive fluid administration will not decrease the bilirubin level, but some infants with high bilirubin levels are dehydrated and may need extra fluid. (***Note:*** Water supplements to breast-fed infants do not reduce serum bilirubin. If supplementing breast-fed infants, it is best to use milk-based formula because it inhibits the enterohepatic circulation of bilirubin and helps decrease the level.) Maintaining adequate hydration and good urine output will help the efficacy of phototherapy because the by-products responsible for the decline in bilirubin are partially excreted in the urine.

Table 51–1. RECOMMENDATIONS FOR THE MANAGEMENT OF HYPERBILIRUBINEMIA IN PRETERM INFANTS (SICK AND WELL) AND SICK TERM INFANTS (*CONTROVERSIAL*)

	Total Serum Bilirubin (mg/dL)			
	Well Infant		Sick Infant	
Weight (g)	Phototherapy	Exchange Transfusion	Phototherapy	Exchange Transfusion
<1000	4–5	10–12	4–5	10–12
1000–1500	5–8	13–16	4–7	10–14
1500–2000	8–12	16–18	7–10	14–16
2000–2500	12–15	18–20	10–12	16–18
>2500	a	b	13–15	17–22

[a]See Table 92–2.
[b]See Table 92–3.

       b. Perform TSB testing every 6–12 h.

       c. Attempt regular feedings if possible, and feed frequently. Feeding inhibits the enterohepatic form of bilirubin and helps lower the serum bilirubin level. Studies indicate that increasing the frequency of breast-feeding will not have a significant effect on the serum bilirubin level in the first 3 days of life.

    4. Phototherapy can be safely discontinued once serum bilirubin levels have fallen >2 mg/dL below the level at which phototherapy was initiated (*controversial*). There is no standard for discontinuing phototherapy. Factors to consider when stopping phototherapy are the cause and the age at which it was initiated. A repeat TSB measurement is recommended on all infants within 24 h of stopping phototherapy. Once phototherapy is stopped, the average bilirubin rebound in infants without hemolytic disease is <1 mg/dL.

    5. If the TSB continues to rise or does not decrease on phototherapy, hemolysis may be present.

    6. If the infant has an elevated direct bilirubin level and is receiving phototherapy, some of these infants may develop bronze baby syndrome. This is not a contraindication to phototherapy. See Chapter 50 (Section IV, A).

    7. Congenital porphyria and use of medications that are photosensitizers are contraindications to phototherapy.

  B. Exchange transfusion. The procedure for exchange transfusion is presented in Chapter 29. Exchange transfusions should be performed only by trained personnel in a neonatal intensive care unit. There is considerable *controversy* concerning the exact level at which to initiate exchange transfusion.

    1. Exchange transfusion for infants >35 weeks' gestation. (See Figure 92–3.) This figure is based on guidelines from the AAP and displays the suggested levels for exchange transfusion (see lines) in jaundiced infants >35 weeks' GA despite phototherapy. There are certain factors to keep in mind when using this figure:

       a. Use total serum bilirubin (TSB). Do not subtract direct bilirubin.

       b. Risk factors. G6PD deficiency, asphyxia, sepsis, temperature instability, acidosis, isoimmune hemolytic disease, and lethargy that is significant.

       c. The first 24 h (dashed lines on Figure 92–3) represent uncertainty secondary to the wide range of clinical circumstances and a range of responses to phototherapy.

       d. Immediate exchange transfusion is indicated if the infant shows signs of bilirubin encephalopathy (hypertonia, arching, retrocollis, opisthotonos, fever, or high-pitched cry) even if the TSB is falling or if the TSB is 5 mg/dL above these lines in Figure 92–3.

    e. **Measure serum albumin and calculate B/A ratio at which exchange transfusion should be considered.** If an exchange transfusion is being considered, the serum albumin should be measured so the B/A ratio can be calculated and used with the TSB levels to help decide if an exchange transfusion needs to be done. The ratio of B/A correlates with measured unbound bilirubin in newborns, which if elevated can be associated with kernicterus in sick preterm newborns and transient abnormalities in audiometric brainstem response in infants. See Figure 92–3.

  2. **Exchange transfusion for infants <35 weeks.** (See Table 51–1.) Some general guidelines for those infants that do not fit the AAP guidelines are listed in Table 51–1. **These are guidelines only, and each patient must be considered individually.** If the infant is sick (eg, signs of hemolysis, hypoxemia, acidosis, or sepsis), has a lower GA, is on day 1 or 2 of life, or has a low birthweight, this would tend to lower the threshold used for exchange transfusion.

C. **Drug therapy**

  1. **Phenobarbital** is effective in reducing the serum bilirubin level by increasing hepatic glucuronosyltransferase activity and conjugation of bilirubin. Often used to treat Crigler-Najjar type II and Gilbert syndrome. Several studies have stated that it is effective in reducing bilirubin levels during the first week of life. It is usually not helpful in the immediate treatment because it takes a few days to become effective. Studies on the long-term effects of phenobarbital need to be done. (For dosing, see Chapter 132.)

  2. **Metal (tin and zinc) metalloporphyrins.** SnMP and ZnMP, respectively, show a dramatic decrease in the need for phototherapy in clinical trials. They work by decreasing the production of bilirubin by competitive inhibition of heme oxygenase. SnMP has been extensively studied. These drugs are not approved, and their long-term safety needs to be studied before they can be recommended.

  3. **Albumin,** given 1g/kg IV over 2 h can provide more binding sites for free bilirubin (*controversial*).

  4. **IV immunoglobulin** has been effective in infants with Rh and ABO hemolytic disease and reduces the need for exchange transfusion in limited studies. Dose is (500 mg–1g/kg) over 2 h, repeated in 12 h if necessary. **AAP recommends this in isoimmune hemolytic disease if the TSB** is rising despite phototherapy or the TSB is within 2–3 mg/dL of the exchange level. AAP also suggests its use in other types of Rh hemolytic disease (anti-C and anti-E), even though data are limited.

D. **Breast-fed infants.** The AAP does not recommend the interruption of breast-feeding in healthy term newborns with hyperbilirubinemia and encourages continued and frequent breast-feeding. The AAP feels breast-feeding in infants who require phototherapy should be continued. They recommend mothers nurse their infants at least 8–12 times per day the first several days. They do not recommend routine supplementation of nondehydrated breast-fed infants with water or sugar water. **Supplementing with water or dextrose water does not lower the bilirubin level.** Different options are available and the decision as to which treatment option to use depends on the specific infant, whether phototherapy is indicated, the physician's judgment, and the family circumstances.

  1. **If phototherapy is not recommended:**

    a. **Observation** and follow serial TSB levels.

    b. **Continue breast-feeding** but supplement with formula, while following serial TSB levels.

    c. **Interrupt breast-feeding** and substitute formula, while following serial TSB levels.

  2. **If phototherapy recommended:**

    a. **Continue breast-feeding, and administer phototherapy (AAP recommendation).** Supplementation with **expressed breast milk** is indicated if the infant's intake is inadequate, weight loss is excessive, or there is a question of dehydration.

Although phototherapy does not reduce the serum bilirubin concentration in breast-fed infants as quickly as it does in formula-fed infants, it is still effective.

   b. **Continue breast-feeding, and administer phototherapy (AAP recommendation).** Supplementation with **formula** is indicated if the infant's intake is inadequate, weight loss is excessive, or there is a question of dehydration.

   c. **Interrupt breast-feeding temporarily and substitute formula and administer phototherapy (AAP optional recommendation).** This reduces bilirubin levels and improves the efficacy of phototherapy.

E. **Breast-fed infants with persistent jaundice after 2 weeks.** About 30% of healthy term infants have persistent jaundice after 2 weeks of age. Treat as follows:

   1. Observe if the physical examination is normal and pale stools or dark-yellow urine are not present.

   2. **Check hypothyroidism screen** because congenital hypothyroidism is a cause of direct hyperbilirubinemia.

   3. **If jaundice is still present after 3 weeks,** a urine bilirubin and total and direct serum bilirubin should be obtained. If elevated, it suggests direct hyperbilirubinemia (see Chapter 50).

F. **Follow-up should be provided for all neonates** (especially those discharged <72 h of age) to monitor for bilirubin problems.

   1. **Perform a risk assessment of all infants prior to discharge.** The AAP recommends two clinical options used individually or in combination: the predischarge TSB or TcB and or a thorough evaluation of clinical risk factors. Recent studies state that combining these two offers the best estimate for predicting the risk of later hyperbilirubinemia.

      a. **Predischarge measurement of serum TSB or TcB level** can then be plotted on the nomogram on Table 92–1. This predicts subsequent significant hyperbilirubinemia. This table is for risk in well newborns at 36 weeks' GA with birthweight ≥2000 g or 35 weeks GA with BW >2500 g.

         i. TSB at discharge in the low-risk zone: 0% risk of developing a TSB level >95th percentile.

         ii. TSB at discharge in the low intermediate-risk zone: 12 % risk of developing a TSB level >95th percentile.

         iii. TSB at discharge in the high intermediate-risk zone: 46% risk of developing a TSB level >95%.

         iv. TSB at discharge in the high-risk zone: 68% risk of developing a TSB level >95%.

      b. **Risk factors based on AAP recommendations in order of importance.** The greater the number of risk factors present, the greater the risk of significant hyperbilirubinemia. Certain risk factors before discharge were noted to be more frequently associated with hyperbilirubinemia: breast-feeding, significant jaundice in a previous sibling, GA <38 weeks, and jaundice noted before discharge.

         i. **Decreased risk.** TSB or TcB in low-risk zone, gestational age ≥41 weeks, bottle feeding, black race, discharge after 72 h.

         ii. **Minor risk factors.** Predischarge TSB or TcB in the high intermediate-risk zone, GA 37–38 weeks, jaundice before discharge, previous sibling with jaundice, macrosomic infant of a diabetic mother, maternal age ≥25 years, and male gender.

         iii. **Major risk factors.** Predischarge TSB or TcB in the high-risk zone, jaundice in the first 24 h, blood group incompatibility with positive direct antiglobulin test (other known hemolytic disease, elevated ETCOc), GA 35–36 weeks, previous sibling who received phototherapy, cephalohematoma or significant bruising, exclusive breast-feeding(especially if nursing is not going well, with weight loss), east Asian race.

    c. **Key points**
      i. **Some newborns may require two follow up visits,** especially if the infant was discharged before 48 h. These can be between 24 and 72 h and 72 and 120 h.
      ii. **If an infant has risk factors for hyperbilirubinemia,** earlier and more frequent follow-ups are recommended.
      iii. **If there is elevated risk and follow-up cannot be guaranteed,** then it may be necessary to delay discharge.
  2. **Follow-up as follows:**
    a. Infant discharged before age 24 h: office follow up by 72 h.
    b. Infant discharged between 24 and 47.9 h: office follow-up by 96 h.
    c. Infant discharged between 48–72 h: office follow-up by 120 h.
  3. **Follow-up assessment should include** weight, intake, voiding and stooling pattern, and presence of jaundice. Use clinical judgment in deciding if a TSB should be obtained.

52 Hyperglycemia

  I. **Problem.** The nurse reports an infant has a blood glucose level of 240 mg/dL. **Hyperglycemia is defined as a whole blood glucose level >120–125 mg/dL or a plasma glucose concentration >145–150 mg/dL regardless of gestational or postnatal age or weight.** One review also suggests that a blood glucose of ≥216 mg/dL in extremely low birthweight (ELBW) infants as a definition of neonatal hyperglycemia due to the risk of osmotic diuresis.. There is an association between hyperglycemia and increased morbidity and mortality.

  II. **Immediate questions**
    A. **What is the serum glucose value on laboratory testing?** Dextrostix values are often inaccurate because the procedure is performed incorrectly or the strips are old and no longer reliable. Chemstrip-bG values are thought to be more reliable by some, but it is best to obtain a serum glucose level from the laboratory before initiating treatment.
    B. **Is glucose being spilled in the urine?** A trace amount of glucose in the urine is accepted as normal. If the urinary glucose level is +1, +2, or greater, the renal threshold has been reached with an increased chance of osmotic diuresis. Some institutions accept a urinary glucose level of +1 without treating the patient (***controversial***). Others feel that the presence of >1% of glucosuria suggests osmolar changes and will treat. ***Note:*** Each 18-mg/dL rise in blood glucose causes an increase in serum osmolarity of 1 mOsm/L. Normal osmolarity is 280–300 mOsm/L.
    C. **How much glucose is the patient receiving?** Normal initial maintenance glucose therapy in infants not being fed orally is 5–7 mg/kg/min (see Chapter 8).
    D. **Are there signs of sepsis?** Sepsis may cause hyperglycemia by inducing a stress response (catecholamine mediated).
    E. **What is the birthweight of the infant?** Low birthweight is the most significant risk factor for hyperglycemia at any gestational age. The incidence is ~2% in infants >2000 g, 45% in infants <1000 g, and 80% in infants <750 g.
    F. **Does the infant have any of the high-risk factors for hyperglycemia?** Risk factors include gestational age <37 weeks, postnatal age <72 h, weight <2500 g, hypoxia, and infection. These infants should have frequent monitoring of their blood sugars.
  III. **Differential diagnosis.** Hyperglycemia is very common in ELBW premature infants (60–80%) and is associated with increases in mortality, intracranial hemorrhage, stage

II/III NEC, risk of sepsis (if hyperglycemia occurs in the first few days after birth), ROP (in ELBW infants), and developmental delay. Etiologies include excess administration or production, inadequate insulin secretion or insulin resistance, glucose intolerance, and defective glucoregulatory hormone control. **The main concern with hyperglycemia is it can cause hyperosmolarity, osmotic diuresis, and subsequent dehydration and is associated with intraventricular hemorrhage.**

A. **Excess glucose administration** has a major role in hyperglycemia. Incorrect calculation of glucose levels or errors in the formulation of intravenous (IV) fluids may cause hyperglycemia.

B. **Inability to metabolize glucose** may occur with prematurity or secondary to sepsis or stress. Most commonly, a tiny infant on total parenteral nutrition becomes hyperglycemic because of glucose intolerance.

C. **Extremely low birth weight infants** (<1000 g) have greater fluid requirements because of their immature renal function and increased insensible water loss. This often leads to a high volume of fluid and administering too much glucose. They also may have insulin resistance, an immature insulin response, and are unable to stop gluconeogenesis when IV glucose is given.

D. **Sepsis** can cause hyperglycemia.

E. **Hyperosmolarity** may be secondary to a hyperosmolar formula. Ask how the formula was made. An inappropriate dilution can lead to a hyperosmolar formula, which in turn can cause transient neonatal glucose intolerance. Severe dehydration from gastroenteritis can lead to hypernatremia and hyperglycemia.

F. **Lipid infusion.** Infants who receive lipid infusion even with low rates of glucose administration may develop hyperglycemia. Lipids are emulsified in a Dextran solution. The lipid component may also cause a glycemic response, decrease peripheral glucose utilization, and may inhibit insulin's effect. One study found that giving lipid infusion increased plasma glucose concentrations by 24% over baseline values.

G. **Transient neonatal diabetes mellitus** is rare (1 in 400,000). The majority of infants are small for gestational age and present from 2 days to 6 weeks of age (most common at 12 days). It usually persists for more than 2 weeks. The most common findings are hyperglycemia, dehydration, glycosuria, polyuria, progressive wasting, hypoinsulinism, and acidosis. Ketonuria is absent. A family history is found in ~33% of cases. The C-peptide levels can be normal or transiently low in the serum or urine. The infants usually require insulin therapy. About half of these cases go on to develop insulin-dependent diabetes.

H. **Medications** such as maternal use of diazoxide can cause hyperglycemia in the infant. Drugs used in infants that have been associated with hyperglycemia include caffeine, theophylline, corticosteroids, and phenytoin. Prostaglandin E1 has been associated in a case report.

I. **Insulin-dependent diabetes mellitus** is very rare. Insulin is required throughout life. Laboratory tests reveal low to absent C-peptide levels.

J. **Stress** (pain, surgical procedures, hypoxia, respiratory distress, etc.) causes hyperglycemia secondary to increased cortisol. During surgery, infants show elevated glucose levels. Premature infants who are very sick are stressed and can have hyperglycemia.

K. **Insulin resistance** (*controversial*). Preterm infants receiving a glucose challenge show variable increases in insulin levels, consistent with a decreased sensitivity to insulin. This resistance may be related to immaturity or downregulation of peripheral receptors.

L. **Seizures** can produce hyperglycemia secondary to catecholamine release.

M. **Hyperadrenocorticism** may present with hyperglycemia secondary to increased cortisol levels.

N. **46, XXDq deletion on chromosome 13** has associated hyperglycemia.

O. **Idiopathic.**

IV. **Database**

    A. **Physical examination and history.** Infants with hyperglycemia usually have no symptoms. Perform a physical examination looking for subtle signs of sepsis (eg, temperature instability, changes in peripheral perfusion) or changes in gastric aspirates if the infant is feeding. Determine if there is a family history of diabetes and ask about maternal and infant medications.

    B. **Laboratory studies**

        1. **Serum glucose level.** Confirm any rapid paper-strip test (Dextrostix or Chemstrip-bG) result with a serum glucose level.

        2. **Urine dipstick testing for glucose.** High levels are a warning sign for osmotic diuresis.

        3. **Complete blood count (CBC) with differential** as a screening test for sepsis.

        4. **Blood and urine cultures** if sepsis is suspected and if antibiotics are to be started.

        5. **Serum electrolytes.** Hyperglycemia may cause osmotic diuresis, which may lead to electrolyte losses and dehydration. Monitor serum electrolyte levels in hyperglycemic patients.

        6. **Serum insulin level** is low to low normal in transient neonatal diabetes mellitus and normal to high in sepsis.

        7. **Serum or urine C-peptide levels** are low to absent in insulin-dependent diabetes mellitus.

    C. **Radiologic and other studies.** None are usually required; however, a chest radiograph may be useful in the evaluation of sepsis.

V. **Plan.** The standard treatment of hyperglycemia is to either decrease the amount of glucose given or give insulin or a combination of both. **While treating hyperglycemia, it is important to maintain adequate nutrition for optimal postnatal growth because this relates to morbidity.**

    A. **Excess glucose administration**

        1. **Positive urinary glucose level.** The presence of ≥1% of glucosuria may suggest a risk of osmolar changes. Decrease the amount of glucose administered by decreasing the concentration of dextrose in IV fluids or by decreasing the infusion rate gradually. Most infants who are not feeding initially require 5–7 mg/kg/min of glucose to maintain normal glucose levels. Use Dextrostix or Chemstrip-bG testing every 4–6 h, and check for glucose in the urine with each voiding.

        2. **Negative urinary glucose level.** If glucose is being given to increase the caloric intake, it is acceptable to have a higher serum glucose level as long as glucose is not being spilled in the urine. Perform Dextrostix and urinary glucose testing every 4–6 h.

    B. **Inability to metabolize glucose.** Sepsis should always be considered in an infant with hyperglycemia. If the CBC is suspicious or there are clinical signs of sepsis, it is acceptable to treat the infant for 3 days with antibiotics and stop if cultures are negative. Ampicillin and an aminoglycoside are usually given initially (for doses, see Chapter 132). Treatment of infants unable to metabolize glucose for any reason is described next.

        1. **Decrease the concentration of glucose or the rate of infusion until a normal serum glucose level is present.** Do not use a solution that has a dextrose concentration of <4.7%. Such a solution is hypo-osmolar and could cause hemolysis, with resulting hyperkalemia.

        2. **Feed as early if possible,** either with hyperalimentation or enteral; both are associated with a decreased incidence of hyperglycemia. If the clinical situation is severe, feeding may not be possible.

        3. **Insulin.** If hyperglycemia persists (usually levels >250 mg/dL or less if urine glucose is positive), insulin may be necessary. Guidelines are institution dependent and ***controversial.*** Insulin administration has been used in premature infants with

success and has allowed more energy intake, promotes glucose tolerance, and promotes weight gain in these infants. Long-term studies have not been done on this practice. If insulin is used, it can be given in the following ways:

   a. **Bolus infusion.** 0.05 to 0.1 unit/kg/dose over 15–20 min every 4–6 h as needed.
   b. **An insulin infusion (most common and preferred method).** Give a loading dose of 0.1 unit/kg/dose IV over 15–20 min, then maintenance 0.02–0.1 unit/kg/h by continuous IV infusion. Albumin added to the bag to prevent insulin from adhering to the plastic tubing is now considered unnecessary. By flushing the tubing with an adequate amount (>25 mL) of the insulin-containing solution, all sites in the tubing will be saturated satisfactorily before beginning the infusion. Potassium should be added to the solution to limit hypokalemia. Dextrostix testing must be performed every 30–60 min until the glucose is stable.
   c. **Insulin subcutaneously** 0.05–0.1 unit/kg every 6 h. Continuous IV insulin is preferred. Chemstrip-bG or Dextrostix testing must be performed every 60 min until the glucose level is stable.
   d. **Potassium levels need to be monitored** when giving insulin therapy.
C. **Transient neonatal diabetes mellitus**
   1. **Give IV or oral fluids,** and monitor the urine output, blood pH, and serum electrolyte levels.
   2. **Give insulin** either by constant infusion or subcutaneously (see Section V, B, 3). Monitor glucose levels with Chemstrip-bG or Dextrostix testing every 4–6 h. This disease usually resolves in days to months.
   3. **Consult a pediatric endocrinologist.**
   4. **Repeat serum insulin values** to rule out permanent diabetes mellitus.
D. **Medications**
   1. **If the infant is receiving theophylline,** the serum theophylline level should be checked to detect possible toxicity, with resulting hyperglycemia. Other signs of **theophylline toxicity** include tachycardia, jitteriness, feeding intolerance, and seizures. If the level is high, the dosage must be altered or the drug discontinued.
   2. **With maternal use of diazoxide,** the infant may have tachycardia and hypotension as well as hyperglycemia. Toxicity in the infant is usually self-limited, and only observation is usually necessary.
   3. **Caffeine and phenytoin** if possible should be discontinued.
   4. **Steroids.** Prolonged courses and pharmacologic dosing of corticosteroids are being used frequently for infants with chronic lung disease. When steroid use is deemed necessary, reducing the dose or frequency may limit the hyperglycemic effects.
E. **Hyperosmolarity.** Rehydration is necessary. If it is secondary to a hyperosmolar formula, stop the formula and give detailed instructions on how to make formula using powder or concentrated formula.

53 Hyperkalemia

I. **Problem.** The serum potassium level is >6 mEq/L. Normal potassium levels vary with the technique used by the laboratory and are generally between 3.5 and 5.5 mEq/L. Hyperkalemia is common in infants <1000g (~30%). If **electrocardiogram (ECG) changes relating to hyperkalemia are present, this is an emergency situation (see Section V, A).**

II. **Immediate questions**
   A. **How was the specimen collected? What is the central serum potassium level? Is it a true level or factitious?** Blood obtained by heelstick or drawn through a tiny needle may yield falsely elevated potassium levels secondary to hemolysis. Clot formation can also cause falsely elevated potassium. The blood should not be obtained from a heparin-coated umbilical catheter (release of benzalkonium from a heparin-coated umbilical catheter can elevate the potassium reading).
   B. **Does the ECG show cardiac changes characteristic of hyperkalemia? This may be the first indication of hyperkalemia.** In neonates, serum potassium >6.7 mEq/L is associated with ECG changes. Early cardiac changes include tall, peaked, "tented" T waves, followed by loss or flattened P wave, widening QRS, ST-segment depression, bradycardia, sine wave QRS-T, first-degree atrioventricular (AV) block, ventricular tachyarrhythmias, and finally cardiac arrest if the potassium levels continue to increase.
   C. **How much potassium is the infant receiving?** Normal amounts of potassium given for maintenance are 1–3 mEq/kg/day.
   D. **What are the blood urea nitrogen and creatinine levels? What is the urine output and body weight?** Elevated blood urea nitrogen (BUN) and creatinine suggest renal insufficiency. Another indication of renal failure is decreasing or inadequate urine output with weight gain.
   E. **Is there associated hyponatremia, hypoglycemia, and hypotension?** With low sodium and glucose, high potassium, and hypotension, consider adrenal insufficiency.
   F. **Does the infant have any of the common characteristics of premature newborns prone to hyperkalemia?** These include small for gestational age, female gender, more severe respiratory distress syndrome, very low birthweight, requirement of exogenous surfactant, need for inotropic medications, and delayed feeding.
III. **Differential diagnosis**
   A. **Falsely elevated potassium level** can be due to hemolysis or clot formation during phlebotomy or heelstick or by drawing the sample proximal to an IV site infusing potassium.
   B. **Excess potassium administration** from IV fluids. Potassium supplements usually are not necessary on the first day of life and often are not necessary until day 3, with the typical requirement of 1–2 mEq/kg/day.
   C. **Pathologic hemolysis of red blood cells** may be secondary to intraventricular hemorrhage, use of a hypotonic glucose solution (<4.7% dextrose), sepsis (most commonly, *Pseudomonas*), cephalohematoma, trauma, asphyxia, hypothermia, or Rh incompatibility.
   D. **Renal failure** can lead to hyperkalemia. Oliguria can cause decreased potassium clearance and hyperkalemia.
   E. **Immaturity.** Nonoliguric hyperkalemia occurs in almost half of extremely low birthweight infants and is defined as a potassium level >6.5 mmol/L in the absence of acute renal failure. This occurs without potassium intake or oliguria and can result from a shift of potassium from intracellular to extracellular space associated with decreased sodium- and potassium-activated adenosine triphosphate (Na^+, K^+-ATPase) activity or from immature renal tubular and glomerular functions. Hyperkalemia is often associated with hyperglycemia as a result of insulin resistance and intracellular energy failure.
   F. **Metabolic or respiratory acidosis** causes potassium to move out of cells, resulting in hyperkalemia. For every 0.1-unit decrease in pH, the serum potassium increases ~0.3–1.3 mEq/L.
   G. **Tissue necrosis.** In certain disease states, such as necrotizing enterocolitis (NEC), tissue necrosis can occur and hyperkalemia may result.
   H. **Medications** containing potassium may elevate the serum potassium level. Digoxin therapy can lead to hyperkalemia secondary to redistribution of potassium. K^+-sparing

diuretics cause decreased potassium losses. Both propranolol and phenylephrine are associated with hyperkalemia. High glucose load can lead to hyperkalemia secondary to increases in plasma osmolality. Other medications, including THAM, indomethacin, and angiotensin-converting enzyme inhibitors, are associated with hyperkalemia.

I. **Adrenal insufficiency** can be seen in congenital adrenal hyperplasia and bilateral adrenal hemorrhage. In salt-losing congenital adrenal hyperplasia, the infants have low serum sodium, chloride, and glucose, elevated levels of potassium, and hypotension. In bilateral adrenal hemorrhage, anemia, thrombocytopenia, and jaundice are seen and bilateral adrenal masses are palpable.

J. **Decreased insulin levels** are associated with hyperkalemia.

K. **Rare causes of hyperkalemia** included cases of selective hypoaldosteronism, secondary pseudohypoaldosteronism, and sacrococcygeal teratoma with spontaneous tumor lysis-induced hyperkalemia.

IV. **Database**

A. **Physical examination.** The infant may exhibit no symptoms or can have bradycardia, tachyarrhythmias, or shock. Pay special attention to the abdomen for signs of NEC (ie, abdominal distention, decreased bowel sounds, and visible bowel loops).

B. **Laboratory studies**

1. **Serum potassium level** measured by a clean venous sample.

2. **Serum ionized and total calcium levels.** Because hypocalcemia may potentiate the effects of hyperkalemia, maintain normal serum calcium concentrations.

3. **Serum pH** to rule out acidosis, which may potentiate hyperkalemia.

4. **BUN and serum creatinine levels** may reveal renal insufficiency.

5. **Urine specific gravity** to assess renal status.

C. **Radiologic studies**

1. **Abdominal radiograph** if NEC is suspected.

2. **ECG** may reveal the cardiac changes characteristic of hyperkalemia and provides a baseline study (see Section II, B).

V. **Plan.** First, confirm the potassium level through a STAT serum sample. **Document whether there are ECG changes and if present, this is a medical emergency and needs to be treated immediately (see later discussion). Stop all potassium intake.** Check the calculation of potassium in the IV fluids, and verify that excess potassium was not being given. Stop any potassium-containing medications. Correct hypovolemia using isotonic saline to promote tubular secretion of potassium. Treat the specific cause. Renal failure can be treated with fluid restriction. If adrenal insufficiency exists, replacement therapy is indicated. **Monitor ECG changes during therapy.** The combination of insulin and glucose is more immediate and preferred over the treatment with Kayexalate for preterm infants.

A. **Hyperkalemia with ECG changes.** See Section II, B.

1. **Give calcium gluconate (0.5–1 mEq/kg over 5–10 min) or calcium chloride (0.25–0.5 mEq/kg over 5–10 min) immediately.** Observe the ECG while infusing the medication. Once the arrhythmia disappears, the bolus can be stopped. This only decreases myocardial excitability and will not decrease the potassium concentration. It is necessary to give a medication immediately that will begin to decrease potassium.

2. **Medications to reduce potassium levels.** Both glucose and insulin and sodium bicarbonate cause cellular intake of potassium. Deciding which one to use depends on your unit's preference. One has not been shown to be superior. Most units choose glucose and insulin, especially in a very tiny infant.

a. **Sodium bicarbonate.** Correct the base deficit by using the following formula:

$$\text{NaHCO}_3 \text{ (mEq)} = 0.3 \times \text{weight (kg)} \times \text{base deficit (mEq/L)}$$

or give 1–2 mEq/kg over 10–30 min intravenously. Inducing alkalosis drives potassium ions into the cells. In very tiny infants, sodium bicarbonate may have associated risks. Avoid rapid infusion of sodium bicarbonate to decrease the risk of intraventricular hemorrhage.

b. **Glucose and insulin** drive potassium into the cells. The usual dose is 0.1–0.2 Units/kg/h insulin diluted in 10% dextrose in water. The amount of glucose needed is variable depending on blood glucose levels. Monitor the glucose levels.

c. **Sodium polystyrene sulfonate** (Kayexalate) (see Section V, B, 4) or calcium polystyrene sulfonate. Administered orally, it lowers the potassium level slowly and therefore is of limited value acutely.

d. **Inhaled albuterol** (*controversial*) (helps move potassium from the blood to the body cells; likely mediated through β-adrenergic receptors on Na$^+$ K$^+$-ATPase) can be used to lower blood potassium. One study with 19 infants showed that potassium decreased at 4 and 8 h. Another study compared albuterol with normal saline. The albuterol group had a significant decrease in potassium level compared with the normal saline group. In one pilot study, albuterol inhalation (400 mcg in 2 mL of saline repeated every 2 h, until serum potassium <5 mEq/L, with a maximum of 12 doses) lowered potassium rapidly in premature neonates. Some institutions use this first in the 500- to 800-g patients to try to decrease potassium. No adverse effects were reported in any of these studies.

B. **Hyperkalemia without ECG changes**

1. **Stop administration of potassium** in IV fluids and consider stopping any potassium-containing medications or medications known to induce hyperkalemia (see Section III, H).

2. **Check the serum potassium level frequently** (ie, every 1–2 h) until stable.

3. **Furosemide (Lasix)** can be given if renal function is adequate; the usual dose is 1 mg/kg IV (*controversial*). (See Chapter 132.)

4. **Sodium polystyrene sulfonate (Kayexalate)**, or calcium polystyrene sulfonate, a potassium-exchange resin, can be given. One gram of resin removes ~1 mEq of potassium. The usual dose is 1g/kg/dose orally every 6 h or rectally every 2–6 h. (See Chapter 132.) **This therapy should not be used in extremely low birthweight infants because of risk of irritation, concretions, and NEC.** This treatment can cause an increase in sodium and calcium. Repetitive rectal use can cause local bleeding.

5. **Insulin and glucose** can be used (see Section V, A, 2b).

6. **Inhaled albuterol** (*controversial*) (see Section V, A, 2d).

C. **Refractory hyperkalemia.** If all of these measures fail to lower the potassium level, other measures, such as exchange transfusion with freshly washed packed red blood cells reconstituted with plasma, peritoneal dialysis, or hemofiltration and hemodialysis, must be considered. These methods work immediately and are very effective but are limited by the time and complexity involved.

D. **Prevention of nonoliguric hyperkalemia of extremely low birthweight infants.** Potassium should not be administered in the first days of life until good urinary output is established and serum potassium is normal and not rising. Potassium levels should be monitored every 6 h in the first few days of life. Early administration of amino acids (first day of life) may stimulate endogenous insulin secretions and prevent the need for insulin infusion.

54 Hypertension

I. **Problem.** An infant has a systolic blood pressure (BP) >90 mm Hg. **Hypertension is defined as a BP >2 standard deviations above normal** values for age and weight, but the definition can vary widely (see Appendix C.). Others define neonatal hypertension as a systolic BP >95th percentile for age and sex on three separate occasions. It can also be defined as a systolic BP >90 mm Hg and a diastolic BP >60 mm Hg in full-term infants; for premature infants, the values are systolic >80 mm Hg and diastolic >50 mm Hg. The values for normal BP are given in Appendix C (infants [C-1], premature infants[C-2] and infants weighing 401–1000 g [C-3]).

II. **Immediate questions**

A. **How was the BP taken?** Make sure the BP reading is correct and the hypertension is real. **Doppler flow ultrasonography is the most reliable noninvasive method of measurement.** The size of the cuff is important; it should encircle two thirds of the length of the upper extremity. **If the cuff is too narrow, the BP will be falsely elevated.** If measurements are taken by means of an umbilical artery catheter, be certain that the catheter is free of bubbles or clots and the transducer is calibrated; otherwise, erroneous results will occur. **BP reading from an indwelling catheter is the most accurate of all methods. BP rises when the infant is feeding, sucking, or in an upright position.**

B. **Is an umbilical artery catheter in place, or has one been in place in the past?** Umbilical artery catheters are associated with an increased incidence of renovascular hypertension. There is no relation between the duration of catheter placement and the development of hypertension. The hypertension is probably related to the thrombus formation, which leads to disruption of the vascular endothelium of the artery. The following conditions are risk factors to thrombus formation in the aorta: bronchopulmonary dysplasia (BPD), patent ductus arteriosus, hypervolemia, and certain CNS disorders. Improved catheters and the use of heparin have helped decrease the incidence of thrombus formation.

C. **Are symptoms of hypertension present?** Infants with hypertension may be asymptomatic or may have the following symptoms: tachypnea, cyanosis, seizures, lethargy, increased tone, apnea, abdominal distention, fever, and mottling. They may also have congestive heart failure (CHF) and respiratory distress.

D. **What is the BP in the extremities?** The BP in a healthy infant should be higher in the legs than in the arms. If the pressure is lower in the legs, coarctation of the aorta may be the cause of the hypertension.

E. **What is the birthweight and postnatal age of the infant?** Normal BP values increase with increasing birthweight and age. Values rise ~1–2 mm Hg/day during the first week of life and then ~1–2 mm Hg/week over the next 6 weeks.

F. **Is the infant in pain or agitated?** Pain from an invasive procedure, crying, agitation, or suctioning can cause a transient rise in BP. The systolic pressure can be 5 mm Hg lower in sleeping infants.

G. **Does the infant have BPD, patent ductus arteriosus (PDA), or an intraventricular hemorrhage?** Infants with BPD have a significant problem with hypertension (up to 40%). It often occurs after discharge from the nursery. Infants with PDA and intraventricular hemorrhage have a higher incidence of hypertension.

III. **Differential diagnosis.** Hypertension is rare in the healthy term newborn infant. The incidence is anywhere from 0.2% (healthy newborn) to 40% (in infants with chronic lung disease). Hypertension in newborns is primarily of renal origin. Cardiac, endocrine, and pulmonary causes are also described. Approximately 9% of infants who had an umbilical arterial catheter have hypertension.

A. **Common causes of hypertension**
   1. **Renal causes**
      a. **Renal artery stenosis.** The infant is hypertensive from birth. This accounts for 20% of the cases of hypertension in infants. It can be secondary to fibromuscular dysplasia where there is significant renal vessel disease. Congenital rubella infection can cause arterial calcification and renal artery stenosis.
      b. **Renal artery thrombosis.** Most commonly related to umbilical artery catheterization. This is a relatively common cause of hypertension.
      c. **Obstructive uropathy.**
      d. **Renal failure.**
      e. **Infantile polycystic kidneys.**
   2. **Aortic thrombosis.**
   3. **Medications** such as theophylline, caffeine, prolonged use of pancuronium, doxapram, corticosteroids, ocular phenylephrine, dopamine, vitamin D intoxication, and epinephrine.
   4. **Fluid overload.**
   5. **Pain or agitation.**
   6. **BPD.** This is the most common cause of nonrenal hypertension in the neonate. Approximately 40% of patients with BPD have hypertension. The origin is unclear but probably multifactorial (increased renin activity and catecholamine secretion, and hypoxemia may be associated with chronic lung disease). **The majority of these infants develop hypertension after being discharged from the hospital.**
   7. **Coarctation of the aorta,** with an increased incidence of coarctation in Turner syndrome.
   8. **Drug withdrawal.** Especially heroin and cocaine.
   9. **Birth asphyxia.**
B. **Less common causes**
   1. **Renal**
      a. **Renal vein thrombosis.**
      b. **Hypoplasia or dysplasia of the kidneys.**
      c. **Pyelonephritis.**
      d. **Unilateral multicystic dysplastic kidneys.**
   2. **Endocrine/Metabolic**
      a. **Primary hyperaldosteronism.**
      b. **Hyperthyroidism.**
      c. **Adrenogenital syndrome.**
      d. **Congenital adrenal hyperplasia.** Blood gas studies reveal a metabolic alkalosis.
      e. **Cushing disease.**
      f. **Hypercalcemia.**
   3. **Neoplasms.** Neuroblastoma, pheochromocytoma, mesoblastic nephroma, Wilms tumor, others.
   4. **CNS related**
      a. **Increased intracranial pressure secondary to intracranial hemorrhage, hydrocephalus, meningitis, or subdural hemorrhage.**
      b. **Seizures.**
      c. **Subdural hematoma.**
   5. **Closure of abdominal wall defects** (eg, omphalocele or gastroschisis).
   6. **Extracorporeal membrane oxygenation (ECMO).** Hypertension is common in infants undergoing ECMO.
   7. **Prolonged total parenteral nutrition.**
   8. **Pneumothorax.**
   9. **Adrenal hemorrhage.**

IV. Database
  A. Physical examination. In most infants, hypertension is discovered on vital signs with no overt symptoms. Infants can present with CHF with shock. Some infants present with apnea, seizures, irritability, lethargy, tachypnea, or feeding issues.
    1. Check the femoral pulse in both legs, which are absent or decreased in coarctation of the aorta.
    2. Examine the abdomen for masses and to determine the size of the kidneys. An enlarged kidney may indicate tumor, polycystic kidneys, obstruction, or renal vein thrombosis.
  B. Laboratory studies. Figure 54–1 is an overview of a complete evaluation.
    1. Assessment of renal function. To assess renal function, perform the following tests:
      a. Serum creatinine and blood urea nitrogen. If elevated may indicate renal insufficiency, which may be associated with hypertension.
      b. Urinalysis. Red blood cells in the urine suggest obstruction, infection, or renal vein thrombosis.
      c. Urine culture. To rule out pyelonephritis.
      d. Serum electrolytes and carbon dioxide. A low serum potassium level and a high carbon dioxide level suggests primary hyperaldosteronism.
    2. Plasma renin levels (plasma renin activity [PRA]) may be elevated in patients with renovascular disease. Levels will be low in primary hyperaldosteronism. Rarely elevated in normal infants, PRA can be falsely elevated because of medications such as aminophylline. Direct renin assay has been used but normal neonatal values are not readily available.
  C. Radiologic and other studies
    1. Chest radiograph may help rule out CHF.
    2. Renal/Abdominal ultrasonography is the preferred screening test in neonates and should be done in all hypertensive infants to detect abdominal masses as well as kidney obstruction. Color Doppler flow ultrasonography can be used to screen for arterial or venous problems. Infants who had an umbilical artery catheter should have their aorta and renal arteries studied for thrombi.
    3. Cranial ultrasonography to rule out intraventricular hemorrhage.
    4. Echocardiography if a disease such as coarctation is suspected or to evaluate end-organ damage caused by hypertension (eg, left ventricular hypertrophy or decreased contractility).
    5. Intravenous pyelography is usually of limited value in the newborn because of poor renal concentrating ability.
    6. Further studies. The following invasive procedures and laboratory studies are sometimes necessary to further evaluate the infant with hypertension:
      a. Arteriography/Angiography to evaluate renovascular disease or venacavography to evaluate renal vein thrombosis.
      b. Abdominal computed tomography scan in cases of abdominal mass.
      c. Renal scan helps quantitate the function of each kidney. A DMSA renal scan can rule out arterial infarctions.
      d. Renal vein renin level to further evaluate renovascular disease.
      e. Renal biopsy to rule out any intrinsic renal disease.
      f. Twenty-four-hour urinary catecholamines to evaluate for pheochromocytoma.
      g. Urinary 17-hydroxysteroid and 17-ketosteroid levels to evaluate for Cushing syndrome and congenital adrenal hyperplasia.
V. Plan
  A. General. First treat any obvious underlying condition. Stop medications if they are causing hypertension. Correct fluid overload by decreasing fluids and administering diuretics. Always check volume status and restrict sodium and fluid intake. Administer pain medications if necessary. Remove umbilical catheter if possible.

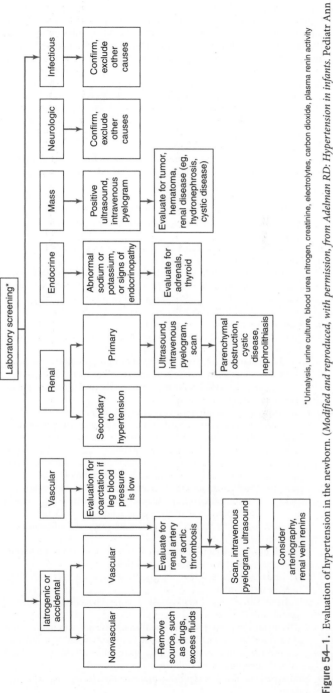

Figure 54–1. Evaluation of hypertension in the newborn. (*Modified and reproduced, with permission, from Adelman RD: Hypertension in infants. Pediatr Ann 1989;18:568.*)

*Urinalysis, urine culture, blood urea nitrogen, creatinine, electrolytes, carbon dioxide, plasma renin activity

B. Drug therapy (see Chapter 132). To guide drug therapy, determine whether the hypertension is **mild, moderate, or life threatening**. **Note that treatment thresholds are unclear, and many of the recommendations are** *controversial.* More studies are necessary to establish guidelines in preterm infants. Some experts believe that any asymptomatic infant with hypertension with no end-organ involvement should not be treated but observed.

1. **Life-threatening hypertension** (BP extremely high with or without symptoms). Avoid too rapid of a decrease in the BP because this may cause cerebral ischemia and hemorrhage. Monitor the BP every 10 min. These medications can be titrated and the BP will begin to fall within 1 h. Choice depends on your institution. (Some advocate nicardipine, others labetalol or hydralazine as first choice.) Five drugs for continuous IV infusion are available:

   a. **Nicardipine.** A calcium channel blocker, one reference stated it was the drug of choice because of its advantages and few side effects (reflex tachycardia). Dose is 1–5 mcg/kg/min constant infusion IV.

   b. **Labetalol** is an α- and β-blocker. Side effects include heart failure and contraindication with BPD. Dose is 0.25–3 mg/kg/h IV infusion.

   c. **Esmolol** is a β-blocker that is short acting. Dose is 100–300 mcg/kg/min IV constant infusion.

   d. **Hydralazine** is a vasodilator. Dose is 0.75–5.0 mcg/kg/min IV constant infusion. Side effects include tachycardia.

   e. **Sodium nitroprusside** is a vasodilator (rarely used). It is difficult to use but has a very short half-life so its effect can be quickly reversed if the pressure drops too far. Dose is 0.5–10 mcg/kg/min IV constant infusion. Use for >72 h or in infants with renal failure can cause thiocyanate toxicity.

2. **Moderate hypertension**

   a. **Begin diuretics** first such as furosemide, hydrochlorothiazide, or chlorothiazide.

   b. **Add a second-line drug (eg, hydralazine or propranolol) if necessary.** Begin with a low dose and increase as necessary. Choice of drug depends on your institution; propranolol is the most extensively used β-blocker and has a low risk of side effects.

   c. **If a third drug is needed with propranolol,** hydralazine can be added.

   d. **Give captopril alone or with a diuretic.** This drug is contraindicated in infants with bilateral renovascular disease. Angiotensin-converting enzyme (ACE) inhibitors also may result in hypotensive events at initiation of therapy and after long-term use. Oliguria and some neurologic complications have been reported after captopril use; therefore, it should be used cautiously.

3. **Patients with mild to moderate hypertension who cannot tolerate oral therapy because of gastrointestinal (GI) problems.** The hypertension is not severe enough to use constant IV infusion so they are good candidates for IV bolus or intermittently administered IV agents. They cannot tolerate oral medications because of issues with their GI tract.

   a. **Begin diuretics first.** Chlorothiazide may be used. Furosemide can also be used, but electrolytes must be followed closely.

   b. **Hydralazine** dose is 0.15–0.6 mg/kg/dose IV bolus every 4 h. Side effects include tachycardia.

   c. **Labetalol** dose is 0.2–1 mg/kg/dose IV bolus. Side effects cause heart failure. Avoid in BPD patients.

   d. **Diazoxide (Hyperstat) (rarely used)** (*controversial* **with many side effects).** As a vasodilator it may cause a rapid and significant drop in BP, which may cause cerebral underperfusion. It also increases blood glucose levels. The dose is 2–5 mg/kg/dose rapid IV bolus.

4. **Mild hypertension** can be controlled by observation (recommended) or oral medications.

    a. Simple observation is best for asymptomatic patients with no readily identifiable cause and is supported in recent reviews.

    b. Diuretics if nonpharmacologic measures fail. Chlorothiazide or hydrochlorothiazide is preferred over furosemide because there are fewer electrolyte disturbances. They work well in cases of volume overload but may cause hypotension when used with other agents. Spironolactone is a potassium-sparing diuretic.

  5. Oral antihypertensive medications. These can be used for infants with mild to moderate hypertension and for those infants with more severe hypertension that are ready to go on long-term oral therapy. More information can be found in Chapter 132. Medication choice depends on your institution's preference.

    a. Propranolol. This should not be used in infants with BPD.

    b. Hydralazine.

    c. Clonidine.

    d. Amlodipine.

    e. Labetalol. Avoid in infants with BPD.

    f. Spironolactone.

    g. Minoxidil.

    h. Isradipine.

    i. Captopril. Captopril may cause renal development problems.

    j. Nifedipine. May cause tachycardia and is not used long term because of side effects.

    k. Hydrochlorothiazide.

    l. Chlorothiazide.

C. Neonatal renovascular hypertension. Enalaprilat (IV ACE inhibitor) has been used with some success but has to be used with extreme caution. Side effects are oliguric acute renal failure and prolonged hypotension. Surgery may be required.

D. Surgical intervention is used for ureteral obstruction, certain tumors, unilateral renal vein thrombosis, renal arterial stenosis, rare cases of polycystic kidney disease, and coarctation of the aorta.

55 Hypoglycemia

I. Problem. An infant has a "low blood glucose level" on Dextrostix or Chemstrip-bG testing. **The exact definition of neonatal hypoglycemia is not agreed on. If symptomatic, no matter what the level, the infant should be treated.** It is not possible to define a single blood glucose level that requires intervention in every newborn. Older definitions used glucose < 30mg/dL in the first 24 h of life and <45mg/dL after 24 h in a newborn (*controversial*). Later, hypoglycemia was defined as a serum glucose <40–45mg/dL in a term or premature infant (*controversial*). Today many institutions have defined it as a serum glucose <45–50 mg/dL (some use <60 mg/dL) in the first 24 h and <50–60 mg/dL thereafter. **It is best to follow your institution's guidelines.** In infants with documented hyperinsulinemic states, a value of <60 mg/dL is considered hypoglycemic (*controversial*).

II. Immediate questions

  A. Has the value been repeated, and has a plasma blood sugar sample been sent to the laboratory? Dextrostix or Chemstrip-bG strips can give incorrect values if the test is not done properly or if the strips used are too old. There can be a wide variation when these results are compared with laboratory-determined plasma levels. Glucose oxidase strips are also quite inaccurate in the low range (<40–50 mg/dL). **Note:** The glucose concentration in whole blood is 10–15% lower than in the plasma. **Never diagnose or treat hypoglycemia based on these screening strips alone.** Always send a serum sample to the laboratory before starting treatment.

B. **Is the infant symptomatic?** Symptoms of hypoglycemia include apnea, hypotonia, inadequate sucking reflex, irritability, irregular respirations, poor sucking or feeding, exaggerated Moro reflex, cyanosis, tremors, pallor, eye rolling, seizures, lethargy, changes in levels of consciousness, temperature instability, and coma. Some infants can have documented hypoglycemia but no symptoms. Rarely, bradycardia, tachycardia, abnormal cry (high pitched), tachypnea, and vomiting present as manifestations of hypoglycemia.

C. **Is the mother a diabetic?** Approximately 40% of infants of diabetic mothers have hypoglycemia. Throughout pregnancy, diabetic mothers have fluctuating hyperglycemia, resulting in fetal hyperglycemia. This fetal hyperglycemia induces pancreatic beta cell hyperplasia, which in turn results in hyperinsulinism. After delivery, hyperinsulinism persists and hypoglycemia results.

D. **How much glucose is the infant receiving?** The normal initial glucose requirement is 5–7 mg/kg/min. If the glucose order was written arbitrarily and not calculated on the basis of body weight, the infant may not be getting enough glucose. (For glucose calculations, see Chapter 8.)

III. **Differential diagnosis**
   A. **Causes of transient hypoglycemia**
      1. **Perinatal stress.**
      2. **Sepsis,** especially Gram negative.
      3. **Asphyxia** or hypoxic-ischemic encephalopathy.
      4. **Hypothermia.**
      5. **Polycythemia.**
      6. **Shock.**
      7. **Infant of a gestational or insulin-dependent diabetic mother.**
      8. **Insufficient glucose administration** (see Section II, D).
      9. **Maternal drugs** such as terbutaline, ritodrine, chlorothiazide, chlorpropamide, labetalol, or propranolol.
     10. **Exchange transfusion.**
     11. **Large for gestational age (LGA) infants.**
   B. **Decreased glycogen stores**
      1. **Intrauterine growth restriction (IUGR)** or small for gestational age.
      2. **Premature/postmature infants.**
      3. **Caloric intake is insufficient.**
   C. **Causes of recurrent or persistent hypoglycemia**
      1. **Hormone excess hyperinsulinism**
         a. **Beckwith-Wiedemann syndrome** (visceromegaly, macroglossia, and hypoglycemia).
         b. **Islet cell adenoma.**
         c. **Adenomatosis.**
         d. **Beta cell hyperplasia or dysplasia.**
         e. **Nesidioblastosis.**
      2. **Hormone deficiencies**
         a. **Growth hormone deficiency.**
         b. **Corticotropin (adrenocorticotropic hormone) unresponsiveness.**
         c. **Thyroid deficiency.**
         d. **Epinephrine deficiency.**
         e. **Glucagon deficiency.**
         f. **Cortisol deficiency,** either from hemorrhage or adrenogenital syndrome.
         g. **Pituitary disorders** (hypoplasia or aplasia of the anterior pituitary).
         h. **Congenital optic nerve hypoplasia.**

    i. Hypothalamic hormone deficiencies.
    j. Midline central nervous system malformations.
  3. Hereditary defects in carbohydrate metabolism
    a. Glycogen storage disease type I.
    b. Fructose intolerance.
    c. Galactosemia.
    d. Glycogen synthase deficiency.
    e. Fructose-1,6-diphosphatase deficiency.
  4. Hereditary defects in amino acid metabolism
    a. Maple syrup urine disease.
    b. Propionic acidemia.
    c. Methylmalonic acidemia.
    d. Tyrosinosis.
    e. 3-Hydroxy-3-methylglutaryl-CoA lyase deficiency.
  5. Hereditary defects in fatty acid metabolism. Medium- and long-chain deficiency.
IV. Database
  A. **History and physical examination.** Evaluate the infant for symptoms of hypoglycemia (see Section II, B). Are there signs of sepsis, shock, or dysmorphism suggesting a syndrome? Is the infant plethoric suggesting polycythemia? Is the growth normal? Intrauterine growth restriction and LGA both cause hypoglycemia. Is there a large liver? Infants with Beckwith Wiedemann syndrome and glycogen storage disease both can have a large liver.
  B. **Laboratory studies**
    1. **Initial studies for transient hypoglycemia**
      a. **Serum glucose level** should be obtained to confirm the bedside paper-strip determination.
      b. **Complete blood count with differential** should be obtained to evaluate for sepsis and to rule out polycythemia.
    2. **Studies for persistent hypoglycemia**
      a. **Initial studies.** One study recommends obtaining only serum glucose, insulin, and ketones. The ratio of insulin to glucose (I/G) is obtained. A level >0.30 indicates a nonhyperinsulinemic cause of hypoglycemia. Serum ketones are low to absent in the presence of hyperinsulinemia.
      b. **Follow-up studies.** If further evaluation is needed, the following tests can be done to help differentiate a metabolic defect, hypopituitarism, and hyperinsulinism:
        i. Insulin.
        ii. Glucose.
        iii. I/G ratio (see Section IV, B, 2a).
        iv. Growth hormone.
        v. Cortisol.
        vi. Free fatty acids.
        vii. Thyroxine (T_4), triiodothyronine (T_3), and thyroid-stimulating hormone (TSH).
        viii. Glucagon.
        ix. Uric acid.
        x. Lactate.
        xi. Alanine.
        xii. Ketones.
        xiii. Amino acids.
        xiv. Somatomedins (insulin-like growth factor [IGF] type I, IGF-II, and IGF-binding proteins).
      c. **Electrospray ionization tandem mass spectrometry** can identify inborn errors of metabolism more rapidly.
  C. **Radiologic and other studies.** An ultrasonogram or computed tomography scan of the pancreas is usually done.

V. Plan

A. Overall plan. Attempt to maintain normoglycemia. Infants at risk for hypoglycemia and those with established hypoglycemia should have glucose screening every 1–2 h until glucose levels are stable and then every 4 h. Once the glucose level is stable, the next step is to determine why the patient is hypoglycemic. Sometimes the cause is obvious, as in the case of an infant of a diabetic mother or one with IUGR. If the cause is not obvious, further workup is necessary.

1. **Asymptomatic hypoglycemia.** The treatment of asymptomatic hypoglycemia is **controversial.** One method of treatment is presented next. Some clinicians treat with early feeding if the infant is term, in the first 6–12 h of life, and not high-risk. Others go by a blood level (usually <25 mg/dL), and treat all such infants with parenteral glucose. Follow your own institution's guidelines.

   a. **Draw a blood sample,** and send it to the laboratory for a STAT baseline plasma glucose level.

   b. **For infants with Dextrostix values of <25 mg/dL or Chemstrip-bG values of <20 mg/dL (confirmed by stat central serum level), insert an intravenous catheter and start a glucose infusion** of ~6 mg/kg/min (calculation in Chapter 8), even if the infant is asymptomatic. (*controversial*) Early feeding is used by some if the infant is term, in the first 6–12 h of life, and not high risk. They recheck the glucose in 30–60 min and start intravenous (IV) treatment only if the repeat blood sugar is still low. Initially, glucose levels should be checked every 30 min until stable. The infusion should be increased until normoglycemia is achieved. A bolus of glucose in the asymptomatic infant is contraindicated because it is thought to result in rebound hypoglycemia (*controversial*).

   c. **For infants with Dextrostix values of 25–45 mg/dL or Chemstrip-bG values of 20–40 mg/dL,** if there are no risk factors for hypoglycemia and the infant is clinically stable, an **early feeding of 5% dextrose in water** or formula can be given. The glucose levels are monitored every 30–60 min until stable and then every 4 h. If the glucose remains low, an IV line should be started with a glucose infusion of 6 mg/kg/min.

2. **Symptomatic hypoglycemia (transient).** Always treat symptomatic hypoglycemia with parenteral glucose.

   a. **Draw a sample for a STAT baseline plasma glucose level.**

   b. **Insert an IV catheter, and start a glucose infusion.** Infuse a mini-bolus (usually not associated with rebound hypoglycemia) of 2 mL/kg of a 10% glucose solution at a rate of 1.0 mL/min. Then give a continuous infusion of glucose at a rate of 6–8 mg/kg/min, and increase the rate as needed to maintain a normal blood glucose (>40–50 mg/dL). The level should be monitored every 30–60 min until stable. **The highest concentration of glucose that can be infused through a peripheral catheter is 12.5%. One study found that 12.5% dextrose in water (DW) was preferred over 10% DW in sick preterm infants weighing 1500–2500 g. If a more concentrated solution is required, a central catheter is needed.** Higher concentrations are hypertonic and may damage the veins. Also, if there is difficulty starting an IV catheter, an umbilical venous catheter can be placed emergently.

   c. **If an IV catheter cannot be inserted, glucagon (see Chapter 132) can be given to infants with adequate glycogen stores** and may be particularly effective in infants of diabetic mothers. It may be less effective in infants who have growth retardation or who are small for gestational age because of poor muscle mass and glycogen stores. The dose is 300 mcg/kg, not to exceed 1.0 mg total dose, and it may be given subcutaneously or intramuscularly while vascular access is being attempted.

3. **Persistent hypoglycemia.** This usually means hypoglycemia persisting or recurring over a period >7 days. **Endocrinologic consultation should be obtained.**

a. **Continue administration of IV glucose.** Continue to increase the rate of IV glucose to 16–20 mg/kg/min. Rates higher than 20 mg/kg/min are usually not helpful. If it is evident at this point that the infant still has problems with hypoglycemia, further workup should be initiated as outlined next.

b. **Perform a definitive workup.** First, obtain blood samples to determine the I/G ratio and serum ketone level. If the diagnosis is still unclear, the definitive workup of an infant with persistent hypoglycemia consists of obtaining a set of laboratory determinations before and 15 min after the parenteral administration of glucagon (0.3 mg/kg/dose). These include serum glucose, ketones, free fatty acids, lactate, alanine, uric acid, insulin, growth hormone, cortisol, glucagon, T_4, and TSH. The results are interpreted as shown in Table 55–1. Urine collections for catecholamines, organic acids, and specific reducing sugars should be sent to the laboratory. The following methods of treatment can be initiated while waiting for results of the glucagon test:

   i. **Consider a trial of corticosteroids,** either hydrocortisone sodium succinate (Solu-Cortef), 5 mg/kg/day, IV or orally every 12 h, or prednisone, 2 mg/kg/day, orally daily.

   ii. **If hypoglycemia persists,** the following medications can be tried. It is not necessary to stop the previous agent when trying a new medication. Choice of treatment is variable and depends on the institution. If dosages are not given, see Chapter 132.

   (a) **Human growth hormone (somatrem [Protropin]),** 0.1 unit/day IM in infants with growth hormone deficiency.

   (b) **Diazoxide.** Chlorothiazide is often used with this for its synergistic effect.

   (c) **Octreotide,** a long-acting analog of somatostatin, is preferred over somatostatin because the latter has a very short half-life. The starting dose is 2–10 mcg/kg/day, subcutaneously divided every 6–8 h, or by continuous IV infusion. Doses up to 40 mcg/kg/day are used.

   (d) **Glucagon.**

   (e) **Nifedipine.** Case reports have shown some success and few side effects.

   (f) **Sus-Phrine (used rarely).** The dose is 0.005–0.01 mL/kg/dose subcutaneously, given every 6 h.

Table 55–1. **DIAGNOSIS OF PERSISTENT HYPOGLYCEMIA BEFORE AND AFTER PARENTERAL GLUCAGON ADMINISTRATION**

Variable	Hyperinsulinism Before	Hyperinsulinism After	Hypopituitarism Before	Hypopituitarism After	Metabolic Defect Before	Metabolic Defect After
Glucose	↓	↑↑↑	↓	↑/N	↓	↓/N
Ketones	↓	↓	N/↓	N	↑	↑
Free fatty acids	↓	↑	N/↓	N	↑	↑
Lactate	N	N	N	N	↑	↑↑
Alanine	N	?	N	N	↑	↑↑
Uric acid	N	N	N	N	↑	↑↑
Insulin	↑↑	↑↑↑	N/↑	↑	N	↑
Growth hormone	↑	↓	↓	↓	↑	↑
Cortisol	↑	↓	↓[a]	↓[a]	↑	↑
TSH and T_4	N	N	↓[a]	↓[a]	N	N

N, normal or no change; ↑, elevated; ↓, lowered; ?, unknown; TSH, thyroid-stimulating hormone; T_4, thyroxine.
[a]Response may vary depending on the degree of hypopituitarism.
Courtesy of Marvin Cornblath, MD, Baltimore, Maryland.

(g) **Rarely used.** Epinephrine, diphenylhydantoin.

(h) **Surgery** to remove most of the pancreas is the treatment of choice in patients with beta cell hyperplasia or nesidioblastosis.

iii. **Medications for persistent hyperinsulinemic hypoglycemia.** Diazoxide (with chlorothiazide), octreotide, and nifedipine are the primary medications used for the long-term treatment of this disorder.

B. **Specific treatment plans**

1. **Neonatal hyperinsulinism.** Pancreatectomy, removing at least 95% of the organ, is usually necessary. Partial pancreatectomy can be done when hypersecretion is shown to be confined to a small area of the pancreas. Some studies have shown that **familial hyperinsulinemic hypoglycemic syndromes of infancy** have been managed effectively with diazoxide and long-acting somatostatin preparations.

2. **Congenital hypopituitarism** usually responds to administration of cortisone and intravenous glucose. Administration of human growth hormone may be necessary. (For dosages, see Chapter 132.)

3. **Metabolic defects**

a. **Type I glycogen storage disease.** Frequent small feedings, avoiding fructose or galactose, may be beneficial.

b. **Hereditary fructose intolerance.** The infant should begin a fructose-free diet.

c. **Galactosemia.** The infant should be placed on a galactose-free diet immediately on suspicion of the diagnosis.

56 Hypokalemia

I. **Problem.** A serum potassium value is 2.8 mEq/L. Normal serum potassium values vary with technique used by the laboratory but are usually between 3.5 and 5 mEq/L. Moderate hypokalemia is 2.5–3.0 mEq/L; severe hypokalemia is <2.5 mEq/L.

II. **Immediate questions**

A. **What is the central serum potassium?** If a low value is obtained by heelstick, central values should be obtained because they may actually be lower than values obtained by heelstick because of the hemolysis of red blood cells.

B. **Are potassium-wasting medications or digitalis being given?** Diuretics may cause hypokalemia. Hypokalemia may cause arrhythmias if digitalis is being administered.

C. **How much potassium is the infant receiving?** Normal maintenance doses are 1–2 mEq/kg/day.

D. **Is diarrhea occurring, or is a nasogastric tube in place?** Loss of large amounts of gastrointestinal (GI) fluids can cause hypokalemia.

III. **Differential diagnosis**

A. **Inadequate maintenance infusion of potassium** (Inadequate intake). For a further discussion, see Chapter 8.

B. **Abnormal potassium losses (GI and renal)**

1. **Medications (most common cause of hypokalemia in the newborn).** Diuretic use, especially long-term therapy, is the most common cause. Any thiazide diuretic may cause hypokalemia. High and continuous doses of spironolactone with hydrochlorothiazide (Aldactazide) have also resulted in hypokalemia. **Amphotericin B** can cause direct renal tubular damage with resulting hypokalemia.

Gentamicin, carbenicillin, and corticosteroids are associated with potassium losses. β-Adrenergic agonists can cause hypokalemia with a case report of epinephrine overdose causing newborn hypokalemia and rhabdomyolysis.

2. **Gastrointestinal tract losses.** Diarrhea, loss of fluid via nasogastric tube, and vomiting may cause hypokalemia. Pyloric stenosis with vomiting and ileostomy can cause hypokalemia.

3. **Primary or secondary hypermineralocorticoidism.** Renal artery stenosis is a cause. In certain forms of congenital adrenal hyperplasia, hypokalemia may occur.

4. **Renal loss of potassium** (other than induced by medications).
   a. **Any cause of polyuria** can be associated with hypokalemia.
   b. **Excessive base administration.**
   c. **Bartter syndrome,** a rare form of potassium wasting, secondary to chloride channels abnormality, is characterized by polyuria, hypokalemia, hyponatremia, and hypercalciuria with risk of nephrocalcinosis with elevated levels of aldosterone and renin.
   d. **Hyperaldosteronism.** Hypertension, hypokalemia, and suppressed renin activity are the three laboratory hallmarks of this disease, an increased potassium secretion from a primary defect of the adrenal gland.
   e. **Cushing syndrome,** hyperfunction of the adrenal cortex, in infants is usually caused by a functioning adrenocortical tumor.
   f. **Proximal renal tubular acidosis type 2.**
   g. **Distal renal tubular acidosis type 1.**

C. **Redistribution of potassium by an increase in intracellular uptake (movement of potassium from serum into the cells)**
   1. **Alkalosis (metabolic or respiratory).** An increase in pH by 0.1 unit causes a decrease in the potassium level by 0.3–1.3 mEq/L. The decrease is less in respiratory than in metabolic alkalosis.
   2. **Insulin.** An increase in insulin causes intracellular uptake in potassium with hypokalemia.
   3. **Medications** cause an increase in intracellular uptake of potassium. These include terbutaline, albuterol, isoproterenol, and catecholamines.

IV. **Database**
A. **Physical examination.** Mild hypokalemia may not cause any symptoms. Symptoms of clinically significant hypokalemia include muscle weakness and decreased tendon reflexes, but these are difficult to evaluate in an infant. In severe hypokalemia, the infant can have lethargy, an ileus, and cardiac arrhythmias. In pyloric stenosis, a **"pyloric olive"** is palpable in 90% of patients.

B. **Laboratory studies**
   1. **Repeat the serum potassium level.**
   2. **Spot checks of urinary electrolytes.** Perform periodic spot checks of urinary potassium levels to determine whether urinary losses are high. Not accurate if diuretics have been administered.
   3. **Serum electrolytes and creatinine** to evaluate renal status.
   4. **Blood gas levels.** An alkalosis may cause or aggravate hypokalemia (ie, as hydrogen ions leave the cells, potassium ions enter the cells, causing decreased serum potassium levels).
   5. **Digoxin level if the patient is on a digitalis preparation.** Remember, hypokalemia can potentiate digitalis-induced arrhythmias.

C. **Radiologic and other studies**
   1. **Abdominal radiograph.** If ileus is suspected, an abdominal radiograph should be obtained. Also, in those infants in whom pyloric stenosis is suspected and an olive cannot be palpated, the diagnostic procedure of choice is abdominal ultrasonography.
   2. **Electrocardiography (ECG).** If hypokalemia is present and the infant is unstable, an ECG may show a prominent U wave with prolonged Q-T interval, flattening of

the T wave, and a depressed ST segment. Ventricular and atrial arrhythmias may also develop. Note that these ECG findings are also seen in hypomagnesemia.

V. **Plan**

A. **General measures.** Hypokalemia is increasing in neonatal intensive care units because of the widespread use of diuretics. The goal of treatment is to increase the potassium intake so that normal blood levels are maintained. Short-term intravenous (IV) potassium administration may cause damage to the veins, and sometimes hyperkalemia, because the potassium does not rapidly equilibrate. **Rapid treatment is not recommended because it can cause hyperkalemia with resultant cardiac complications.** Therefore, corrections are given slowly, often over 24 h. If too large a bolus is given, cardiac arrest may result. Serum potassium levels should be monitored every 4–6 h until correction is achieved. Once levels reach high normal, decrease the amount of potassium given.

B. **Specific measures.** Any specific defects (ie, renal defects, adrenal disorders, and certain metabolic problems) require specific evaluation and therapy.

1. **Inadequate maintenance infusion of potassium.** Calculate the normal maintenance infusion of potassium that should be given and increase the amount accordingly (normal maintenance infusion is 1–2 mEq/kg/day, usually only necessary after the first day of life).

2. **Abnormal potassium losses**

a. **Medications.** If the infant is receiving potassium-wasting medications, increase the maintenance dose of potassium (eg, patients with bronchopulmonary dysplasia on long-term furosemide therapy). Oral supplementation with potassium chloride may be given, 1–2 mEq/kg/day in three to four divided doses (with feedings), adjusted depending on serum potassium levels. It was once thought that a potassium-sparing diuretic decreased the amount of potassium supplementation; however, a randomized study showed that serum electrolytes sodium and potassium were not affected by the addition of spironolactone.

b. **Gastrointestinal losses**

i. **Severe diarrhea** leading to potassium losses can be corrected by treating the cause of the diarrhea, withholding oral feedings to allow the gut to rest, and giving IV potassium (initial dose of potassium chloride, 1–2 mEq/kg/day). Serum potassium levels are monitored, and the IV dose is adjusted.

ii. **Nasogastric drainage.** This amount should be measured each shift and replaced milliliter for milliliter with 1/2 normal saline with 20 mEq of potassium chloride.

iii. **Pyloric stenosis.** Correct dehydration if present and if surgery is indicated.

C. **Renal loss of potassium (other than induced by medications)**

1. **Bartter syndrome.** Potassium supplementation is given orally, starting dosage of 2–3 mEq/kg/day, which is increased as necessary to maintain a normal serum potassium level. Certain forms respond to indomethacin.

2. **Hyperaldosteronism.** Surgery and dexamethasone therapy may be indicated.

3. **Cushing syndrome.** Surgery is usually indicated.

4. **Renal tubular acidosis type 2 and 1.** Alkaline therapy and potassium supplementation if needed.

D. **Redistribution of potassium**

1. **Alkalosis.** Determine the cause of metabolic or respiratory alkalosis and treat the underlying disorder.

2. **Medications.** The medications should be discontinued if possible.

57 Hyponatremia

I. **Problem.** A 7-day-old infant with an intraventricular bleed has a serum sodium level of 127 mEq/L, below the normal accepted value of 135 mEq/L.

II. **Immediate questions**

A. **Is there any seizure activity?** Seizure activity is often seen in patients with extremely low serum sodium levels (usually <120 mEq/L). **This is a medical emergency, and urgent sodium correction is needed.**

B. **How much sodium and free water is the patient receiving? Is weight gain or loss occurring?** Be certain that an adequate amount of sodium is being given and that free water intake is not excessive. The normal amount of sodium intake is 2–4 mEq/kg/day. Weight gain with low serum sodium levels is most likely a result of volume overload, especially in the first day or two of life when weight loss is expected.

C. **What is the urine output?** With syndrome of inappropriate secretion of anti-diuretic hormone (SIADH), urine output is decreased. If the urine output is increased (>4 mL/kg/h), perform a spot check of urine sodium to determine whether sodium losses are high.

D. **Are renal salt-wasting medications being given?** Diuretics such as furosemide may cause hyponatremia.

III. **Differential diagnosis.** When considering the differential, determine if the value is real. Certain conditions can cause pseudohyponatremia. Is the amount of sodium given adequate? Then you need to decide if the hyponatremia is caused by deficit of total body sodium or an excess of free water. Have medications caused the hyponatremia? Deciding the cause dictates the form of treatment. **The most frequent cause of hyponatremia in the neonate is hypotonic hyponatremia caused by excessive fluid administration or retention of free water.**

A. **Exclude pseudohyponatremia.** Laboratory tests reveal a decreased sodium, but serum osmolality is normal. Caused by hyperproteinemia, hyperglycemia, or hyperlipidemia.

B. **Inadequate sodium intake.** Maintenance is usually 2–4 mEq/kg/day.

C. **Hyponatremia with hypervolemia.** This occurs with excess of extracellular fluid. There is a positive water balance. The infants have signs of edema and weight gain. Causes include the following:

1. **Congestive heart failure.**
2. **Sepsis with decreasing cardiac output.**
3. **Neuromuscular paralysis with fluid retention (with pancuronium).**
4. **Renal failure.**
5. **Liver failure.**
6. **Nephrotic syndrome.**

D. **Hyponatremia with hypovolemia.** This occurs with a deficit of extracellular fluid and can be caused by either renal losses or extrarenal losses.

1. **Renal losses (urinary Na >20mEq/L)**
   a. **Diuretics.**
   b. **Mineralocorticoid deficiency.**
      i. **Addison disease.**
      ii. **Hypoaldosteronism.**
      iii. **Congenital adrenal hyperplasia.**
      iv. **Pseudohypoaldosteronism.**
   c. **Osmotic diuresis.** One case report presented this secondary to renovascular hypertension caused by a thrombotic occlusion.
   d. **Obstructive uropathy.**
   e. **Bartter and Fanconi syndrome.**

      f. Renal immaturity. Often very low birthweight infants show increased renal tubular sodium and water loss, causing hyponatremia. (See Chapter 16.)

      g. Renal tubular acidosis.

    2. Extrarenal losses (urinary Na <20mEq/L)

      a. Gastrointestinal (GI) losses such as vomiting, diarrhea, nasogastric tubes.

      b. Third spacing of fluids due to ascites, pleural effusion, ileus, necrotizing enterocolitis, sloughing of skin.

      c. Radiant warmer skin loss.

  E. Hyponatremia with normal extracellular fluid.

    1. Excessive IV fluids, free water or using diluted (hypotonic) formulas is a common cause of the hyponatremia in a neonate. Maternal water intoxication is also a cause of hyponatremia in a newborn. Associated with low urine specific gravity and high urine output.

    2. SIADH occurs more commonly in central nervous system disorders such as intraventricular hemorrhage, hydrocephalus, birth asphyxia, and meningitis but may also be seen with lung disease (pneumothorax and positive pressure ventilation). SIADH is often seen in critically ill premature and term neonates.

    3. Hypothyroidism.

    4. Hypoadrenalism.

  F. Drug-induced hyponatremia. Diuretics (used frequently with bronchopulmonary dysplasia [BPD]) can lead to sodium losses. Indomethacin causes water retention, which causes dilutional hyponatremia. Opiates, carbamazepine, and barbiturates can cause SIADH. Infusion of mannitol or hypertonic glucose can cause hyperosmolality with salt wasting. Infusion of recommended and excessive doses of oxytocin and glucose can both cause transplacental hyponatremia. One study revealed that maternal fluid overload (with glucose-only sodium-free solutions) caused hyponatremia in the infant.

IV. Database

  A. Evaluate the bedside chart

    1. Check for weight loss or gain. Weight gain is more likely to be associated with dilutional hyponatremia.

    2. Check fluid intake and output over a 24-h period. Normally, infants retain two thirds of the fluid administered, and the rest is lost in the urine or by insensible loss. If the input is much greater than the output, the patient may be retaining fluid, and dilutional hyponatremia should be considered.

    3. Assess the urine output and specific gravity. A low urine output with a high specific gravity is more commonly seen with SIADH. In excessive fluid, one sees a low urine specific gravity and a high urine output.

  B. Physical examination. Perform a complete examination and note signs of seizure activity (eg, abnormal eye movements, jerking of the extremities, and tongue thrusting). Check for edema, a sign of volume overload. Look for decreased skin turgor and dry mucous membranes, which are seen in dehydration.

  C. Laboratory studies

    1. Specific tests

      a. Serum sodium and osmolality.

      b. Urine spot sodium, osmolality, and specific gravity.

      c. Serum electrolytes, creatinine, and total protein to assess renal function.

    2. Laboratory results of specific diagnoses

      a. Volume overload (dilutional hyponatremia)

        i. Excess intravenous fluids: Increased urine output and decreased urine osmolality and low specific gravity.

        ii. Other (congestive heart failure or paralysis with fluid retention): Decreased urine output and increased urine specific gravity.

      b. Increased sodium losses

        i. In renal losses, with diuretics and adrenal insufficiency: Increased urine output and urine Na^+ and decreased urine osmolality and specific gravity.

      ii. **In skin and GI losses and with third spacing:** Decreased urine output and sodium and increased urine osmolality and specific gravity.

    c. **SIADH.** The diagnosis is made by documenting the following on simultaneous laboratory studies: low urine output, urine osmolality greater than serum osmolality, low serum sodium level and low serum osmolality, and high urinary sodium level and high specific gravity. A plasma antidiuretic hormone (ADH) concentration and a plasma concentration of atrial natriuretic peptide can be obtained. If they show a high ADH concentration in the presence of low serum osmolality and elevated urinary osmolality, the diagnosis is confirmed.

  D. Radiologic and other studies. None usually needed. Ultrasound of the head may reveal intraventricular hemorrhage as a cause of hyponatremia secondary to SIADH.

V. Plan. Treatment is essential because hyponatremia can cause future problems and is a risk factor for hearing loss.

  A. Emergency measures. If the infant is having **hyponatremia-induced seizures as a result of low sodium** (usually sodium <120 mEq/dL), hypertonic saline solution (3% sodium chloride) should be given. There is *controversy* over the rate and how it should be given. Some give a IV push over 15 min until seizures stop and then a 24-h correction. Others give an infusion hourly until the sodium is >120 mmol/L. Follow institutional guidelines. Rapid corrections, especially in chronic hyponatremia, can cause brain damage (central pontine myelinolysis). **Once symptoms resolve,** and the serum sodium is >120 mEq/dL, a slow correction can be given over 24 h.

    1. **IV push over 15 min** (1–3 mL/kg of 3% NaCl). This method should be reserved for those patients who have seizures, those with repeated apnea requiring intubation, or refractory status epilepticus from hyponatremia (*controversial*).

    2. **Hourly correction:** 2 mL/kg/h of 3% NaCl can be given (should raise the sodium concentration by 2 mmol/L/h).

    3. **24-h correction.** The total body deficit can be calculated (see Section V, C, 2c) and half of that is given over 12–24 h.

  B. General rules (always treat the underlying disorder)

    1. **Hyponatremia with hypervolemia.** Sodium and water restriction.

    2. **Hyponatremia with hypovolemia.** Volume expansion. Give sodium and water to replace what has been lost.

    3. **Hyponatremia with normal extracellular fluid.** Water restriction.

  C. Specific rules

    1. **Volume overload (dilutional hyponatremia)** is treated with fluid restriction. The total maintenance fluids can be decreased by 20 mL/kg/day, and serum sodium levels should be monitored every 6–8 h. The underlying cause must be investigated and treated.

    2. **Inadequate sodium intake**

      a. **The maintenance sodium requirement for term infants is 2–4 mEq/kg/day; it is higher in premature infants.** Calculate the amount of sodium the patient is receiving, using the equations in Chapter 8. Readjust the intravenous sodium intake if it is the cause of hyponatremia.

      b. **If the infant is receiving oral formula only, check the formula being used.** Low-sodium formulas such as Similac PM 60/40 may be used. Use of supplemental sodium chloride or a formula with a higher sodium content may be necessary.

      c. **Calculate the total sodium deficit** using the following equation:

$$\text{(Sodium value desired [130–135 mEq/L] – infants sodium value)} \times \text{[Weight(kg)} \times 0.6] = \text{Total sodium deficit.}$$

The result will be the amount of sodium needed to correct the hyponatremia. Usually, **only half of this amount** is given over 12–24 h.

3. **Increased sodium losses.** Try to treat the underlying cause and increase the sodium administered to replace the losses.

4. **Drug-induced hyponatremia.** If a renal salt-wasting medication such as furosemide is being given, serum sodium levels will be low even though an adequate amount of sodium is being given in the diet. An increase in sodium intake may be required, often the case in infants with BPD who are receiving diuretics. Most are also receiving oral feedings, so an oral sodium chloride supplement can be used. Start with 1 mEq three times/day with feedings and adjust as needed. Some infants may require 12–15 mEq/day. Sodium levels should be kept in the low 130s because higher levels may result in fluid retention when diuretics are used. Indomethacin-induced hyponatremia is treated with fluid restriction.

5. **SIADH. The cause of SIADH is usually obvious; if it is not, further investigation is needed** (eg, ultrasonography of the head) or chest radiograph to rule out lung disease). During treatment, monitor the serum sodium, osmolality, and urine output to determine whether the patient is responding.

   a. **Seizures present or serum sodium is <120 mEq/L.**
      i. **Hypertonic saline** solution (3% sodium chloride). See Section V, A.
      ii. **Lasix,** 1 mg/kg IV, every 6 h.
      iii. **Anticonvulsant therapy.** One study showed that routine anticonvulsant therapy was ineffective and associated with apnea. A case report revealed that phenytoin (suppressive against SIADH) was effective for a neonate with SIADH and seizures.
      iv. **Fluid restriction,** usually 40–60 mL/kg/day free water.

   b. **Seizures not present and serum sodium is >120 mEq/L.**
      i. **Fluid restriction,** usually 40–60 mL/kg/day. (This regimen does not allow for fluid loss that accompanies the use of a radiant warmer or phototherapy.)
      ii. **Lasix** can also be used.

58 Hypotension and Shock

I. **Problem.** The blood pressure (BP) is >2 standard deviations below normal for age. (For normal BP values, see Appendix C.) It is difficult to state a specific blood pressure for every gestational, postnatal age, and weight of an infant that needs treatment. There is debate over normal blood pressures for extremely premature infants. It is best to treat the patient and not the specific number. **Hypotension (diminished BP) is distinct from shock, which is a clinical syndrome of inadequate tissue perfusion with the clinical signs noted below. Hypovolemic shock is the most common cause of shock in a newborn.**

II. **Immediate questions**

A. **What method of measurement was used?** If a cuff was used, be certain that it was the correct width (ie, covering two thirds of the upper arm). A cuff that is too large gives falsely low readings. If measurements were obtained from an indwelling arterial catheter, a "dampened" waveform suggests there is air in the transducer or tubing or a clot in the system, and the readings thus may be inaccurate.

B. **Are symptoms of shock present?** Symptoms of shock include tachycardia, poor perfusion, cold extremities with a normal core temperature, lethargy, narrow pulse pressure, apnea and bradycardia, tachypnea, metabolic acidosis, and weak pulse.

C. **Is the urine output acceptable?** Normal urine output is ~1–2 mL/kg/h. Urine output is decreased in shock because of decreased renal perfusion. If the BP is low but the urine output is adequate, aggressive treatment may not be necessary, because the renal perfusion is adequate. (*Note:* An exception involves the infant with septic shock and hyperglycemia who has osmotic diuresis.)

D. **Is there a history of birth asphyxia?** Birth asphyxia may be associated with hypotension.

E. **At the time of delivery, was there maternal bleeding (eg, abruptio placentae or placenta previa) or was clamping of the cord delayed?** These factors may be associated with loss of blood volume in the infant.

III. **Differential diagnosis.** If a blood pressure is felt to be low, evaluate the infant. If the infant is oxygenating, not acidotic, has normal urine output, and good perfusion, treatment is usually not necessary, regardless of the BP. If the infant is symptomatic (acidotic, not oxygenating, poor or decreased urine output, and poor peripheral perfusion) then the infant is probably not perfusing and has a BP that needs to be treated.

A. **Hypovolemic shock** may be secondary to antepartum or postpartum blood loss or fluid and electrolyte losses.
   1. **Antepartum blood loss (often associated with asphyxia)**
      a. **Abruptio placentae.**
      b. **Placenta previa.**
      c. **Twin-twin transfusion.**
      d. **Fetomaternal hemorrhage.**
   2. **Postpartum blood loss**
      a. **Coagulation disorders (DIC, coagulopathies).**
      b. **Vitamin K deficiency.**
      c. **Iatrogenic causes** (eg, loss of an arterial catheter).
      d. **Birth trauma** (eg, liver injury, adrenal hemorrhage, intracranial hemorrhage, intraperitoneal hemorrhage).
      e. **Pulmonary hemorrhage.**
   3. **Fluid and electrolyte losses.** Volume depletion is common in premature infants.

B. **Septic shock.** Endotoxemia occurs, with release of vasodilator substances and resulting hypotension. It usually involves Gram-negative organisms such as *Escherichia coli* and *Klebsiella* spp but can also occur with Gram-positive organisms such as in group B streptococcal and staphylococcal infections. Hypovolemia can occur with septic shock secondary to loss of plasma.

C. **Cardiogenic shock**
   1. **Birth asphyxia.**
   2. **Metabolic problems** (eg, hypoglycemia [infant of diabetic mother]), hyponatremia, hypocalcemia, acidemia) can cause decreased cardiac output with a decrease in BP.
   3. **Congenital heart disease** (eg, hypoplastic left heart, aortic stenosis, coarctation of the aorta, pulmonary stenosis, tricuspid or mitral atresia, or total anomalous pulmonary venous return).
   4. **Arrhythmias** can cause a decrease in cardiac output.
   5. **Infectious agents** (bacterial or viral) can cause myocardial dysfunction.
   6. **Any obstruction of venous return** (eg, tension pneumothorax, pneumomediastinum, pneumopericardium).

D. **Neurogenic shock.** Birth asphyxia and intracranial hemorrhage can both cause hypotension.

E. **Drug-induced hypotension.** Certain drugs (eg, tolazoline, tubocurarine, nitroprusside, sedatives, magnesium sulfate, digitalis, and barbiturates) cause vasodilation and a drop in BP. Transient hypotension has been seen after exogenous surfactant administration.

F. **Endocrine disorders.** Complete 21-hydroxylase deficiency and adrenal hemorrhage are the most notable endocrine disorders that can cause hypotension and shock. If there is a low serum sodium, high serum potassium, and hypotension, it is important to rule out adrenogenital syndrome.

G. **Extreme prematurity.** Hypotension is very common in extremely low birthweight (ELBW) infants (40% between 27 and 29 weeks, 60–100% between 24 and 26 weeks). Hypotension in this group is rarely secondary to hypovolemia and more likely due to adrenocortical insufficiency, poor vascular tone, and immature catecholamine responses. Hypotension with evidence of end-organ dysfunction in ELBW infants is associated with intraventricular hemorrhage/periventricular leukomalacia (IVH/PVL) and needs to be corrected.

IV. **Database**

A. **Physical examination.** Particular attention is given to signs of blood loss (eg, intracranial or intra-abdominal bleeding), sepsis, or clinical signs of shock (cool extremities, mottling of the skin, tachycardia, decreased urine output).

B. **Laboratory studies**

1. **Complete blood count (CBC) with differential.** Decreased hematocrit (Hct) identifies blood loss; however, the Hct can be normal in patients with acute blood loss. Elevated/decreased white blood cell count and differential may help identify sepsis as the cause.

2. **Coagulation studies (prothrombin time and partial thromboplastin time) and platelet count,** if DIC is suspected.

3. **Serum glucose, electrolytes, and calcium levels** may reveal a metabolic disorder.

4. **Cultures.** Obtain blood and urine for culture and antibiotic sensitivity testing.

5. **Kleihauer-Betke test** should be performed if fetomaternal transfusion is suspected. The test detects the presence of fetal erythrocytes in the mother's blood by a slide elution technique. A smear of maternal blood is fixed and incubated in an acidic buffer. It causes adult hemoglobin to be eluted from erythrocytes; fetal hemoglobin resists elution. After the slide is stained, fetal hemoglobin cells, if present, appear dark, whereas maternal erythrocytes appear clear. Ask the mother's obstetrician to order this test on the mother.

6. **Arterial blood gases** to assess for hypoxia or acidosis.

7. **Plasma lactate.** An increase in plasma lactate can signify anaerobic metabolism and sepsis.

C. **Radiologic and other studies**

1. **Chest radiograph.** An anteroposterior chest radiograph assesses the heart and lungs and rules out any mechanical cause of shock (eg, pneumothorax).

2. **Ultrasonography of the head** in infants in whom intracranial hemorrhage is suspected.

3. **Electrocardiography** if an arrhythmia is suspected.

4. **Echocardiography** in birth-asphyxiated infants to assess myocardial function and left ventricular output. If there is myocardial failure, drug therapy is needed to improve cardiac output. Echocardiography is also useful to rule out a congenital heart lesion. Left ventricular output is important to measure in evaluating mean arterial blood pressure and guiding the management of hypotension. This helps determine if fluids or vasopressors are needed. See Section V, A, 1e.

5. **Central venous pressure (CVP) measurement.** A venous umbilical catheter can be placed above the diaphragm (at the right atrium) to obtain central venous pressure readings. Normal values are 4–6 (very low birthweight) and 5–8 (newborn) mm Hg. Readings are higher in ventilated infants. If the readings are low, hypovolemia is present and transfusion is usually necessary. Recent studies indicate that CVP values in sick ventilated infants are limited but can be used to guide when used serially. The normal range of CVP in VLBW infants may be wider than previously reported at 2.8–13.9 mm with a mean of 4.4–6.1 mm Hg.

V. **Plan**

A. **General measures**

1. **Rapidly assess the infant to determine what is causing the hypotension** in order to direct therapy. The basic decision is whether the infant requires volume replacement or administration of inotropic agents. The decision is not difficult in the majority of patients. Five parameters are useful in making this decision:

    a. **History** to rule out birth asphyxia, blood loss (antepartum or postpartum), drug infusion, and birth trauma (adrenal hemorrhage or liver injury).

    b. **Physical examination** often reveals which organ systems are involved.

    c. **Chest radiograph.** A small heart is seen in volume depletion; a large heart is seen in cardiac disease. Evaluate for pneumothorax. **Transillumination** of the chest may help detect pneumothorax.

    d. **Central venous pressure.** If it is low (<4 mm Hg in VLBW or 5 in newborn), the infant is volume depleted. If it is high (eg, >6 mm Hg in VLBW or >8 in newborn), the infant probably has cardiogenic shock.

    e. **Left ventricular output (LVO) assessed by echocardiogram.**

        i. If **LVO is normal or high with no patent ductus arteriosus (PDA)**, a vasopressor is indicated. If a PDA is present, it should be treated.

        ii. If **LVO is low and the left ventricle shows underfilling,** volume expansion is indicated.

        iii. If **LVO is normal but the left ventricle shows impaired contractility,** dobutamine is indicated.

2. **If cause is uncertain,** start empirical volume expansion with crystalloid (eg, normal saline) (10–20 mL/kg intravenously over 30 min).

    a. **If there is a response,** continue volume expansion.

    b. **If there is no response,** an inotropic agent (eg, dopamine) should be started (see Section V, B, 3).

3. **Provide respiratory support as needed.** Blood gas determinations and clinical examinations will dictate whether supplemental oxygen will suffice or whether intubation and mechanical ventilation are necessary.

4. **Correct any metabolic acidosis with sodium bicarbonate.**

5. **Correct any hypoglycemia or hypocalcemia.**

B. **Specific measures**

1. **Hypovolemic shock**

    a. **Volume expansion using intravenous crystalloid** should be given (for dosage, see Section V, A, 2). Colloids such as albumin or plasma protein fraction (Plasmanate) are to be used with caution. Use of colloids is associated with an increased risk of mortality in critically ill infants. Crystalloids are also preferred over albumin because of no risk of infection, availability, and less cost. No benefit of use of colloids versus crystalloids (normal saline) has been found in preterm infants. If blood loss has occurred and the patient is severely hypovolemic, immediate volume expansion with a crystalloid is essential. Volume expansion should be continued until adequate tissue perfusion is attained as indicated by good urinary output and central nervous system function. Meanwhile, a blood sample should be sent to the laboratory for an Hct value, which is used to determine the specific blood products that should be used in blood replacement therapy.

    b. **Blood replacement therapy**

        i. **Hct <40%.** Packed red blood cells should be given, 5–10 mL/kg over 30–40 min. The following formula may also be used to calculate the volume of packed red blood cells needed. This formula assumes that the total blood volume is 80 mL/kg and the Hct of the packed red blood cells is 70%.

$$\text{Volume required} = \frac{(\text{Weight [kg]} \times \text{Total blood volume}) \times (\text{Desired Hct} - \text{Patient's Hct})}{\text{Hct of transfusion product}}$$

        ii. **Hct >50%.** Normal saline, or fresh-frozen plasma (FFP) should be used. FFP is used only if clotting studies are also abnormal.

        iii. **Hct of 40–50%.** Alternating transfusions of packed red blood cells and normal saline should be given.

2. **Septic shock**
   a. **Obtain cultures** (blood and urine [unless in the first 24 h of life, in which case obtain only blood], lumbar puncture for cerebrospinal fluid culture, and other culture studies as clinically indicated).
   b. **Initiate empirical antibiotic therapy** after culture specimens have been obtained. **Intravenous ampicillin and gentamicin** are recommended. **Vancomycin** may be substituted for ampicillin if staphylococcal infection is suspected (usually seen in infants >3 days old who have invasive monitoring catheters or chest tubes in place). Some institutions are advocating the use of **cefotaxime (especially if there is a concern for central nervous system [CNS] infection)** with vancomycin instead of gentamicin to avoid the nephrotoxicity. (For dosages, see Chapter 132.) Consider using more specific Gram-negative coverage if there are known resistant organisms in your unit.
   c. **Use volume expansion and inotropic agents as needed** to maintain adequate tissue and renal perfusion (see Sections V, B, 1a and V, B, 3e).Usually early on volume expansion is indicated, inotropic agents later.
   d. **Use of corticosteroids.** If volume expansion and inotropic agents have not worked, corticosteroids have been effective. IV corticosteroid therapy for sepsis is *controversial.* Agents such as dexamethasone have been used, however. Studies have shown a single dose may be useful in refractory hypotension or a short course of steroids may be beneficial with no associated adverse effects in neonates. Recent reviews state there is insufficient evidence to support the routine use of steroids in neonatal hypotension.
   e. **Naloxone** has been used in patients with septic shock and persistent hypotension, but its use is *controversial* (for dosage, see Chapter 132). Studies have shown that the effects of naloxone and methylprednisolone may be synergistic in improving the hemodynamics of these patients. Naloxone is rarely helpful in hypoxic ischemic shock. A recent review of naloxone in shock (sepsis, cardiogenic, and hemorrhagic) found it did improve arterial blood pressure, but the review was unclear if this was clinically useful.
   f. **Methylene blue (*controversial*)** has been used in septic shock unresponsive to colloid, inotropic agents, and corticosteroids. One study showed that three of five patients had an increase in BP after given a dose of 1 mg/kg over 1 h IV. Some required a second infusion. Three of five of these patients were weaned off inotropic agents within 72 h. The mechanism by which this works is that methylene blue is a soluble guanylate cyclase inhibitor. Excess nitric oxide is a mediator of hypotension by dilating vascular smooth muscle through activation of soluble guanylate cyclase.
   g. **Double-volume exchange transfusion (*controversial*).** Exchange transfusion with fresh whole blood is beneficial in sepsis. Because of significant risk and few studies, many institutions have not advocated its use.
   h. **Intravenous immune globulin (IVIG) (*controversial*).** In a recent review, IVIG was found to reduce mortality (3% reduction with sepsis). Their conclusion did not support the routine use in sepsis. Some institutions give a single dose in infants with overwhelming sepsis. Veronate (a specific anti-staph IVIG) was recently shown to be ineffective.
   i. **Fresh frozen plasma** is only indicated in DIC and has no benefit in septic infants.
   j. **Granulocyte transfusions.** Many benefits have been documented, but a recent review said insufficient evidence supports routine use.
   k. **Neutrophil transfusions.** A small number of studies have shown a beneficial effect in septic newborns. The ultimate role needs to be evaluated.
   l. **Cytokines.** The two cytokines that have been studied are granulocyte colony-stimulating factor(G-CSF) and granulocyte-macrophage colony-stimulating activity (GM-CSA). A benefit in decreasing the mortality rate has been shown

in some small trials. A recent review states there is insufficient evidence to support its use.

m. Recombinant human activated protein C (rhAPC). It has been shown to reduce mortality in adult sepsis. Insufficient data support its use in neonates, and there is also a high risk of bleeding.

n. Pentoxifylline. Current evidence shows that as an adjunct to antibiotics it may reduce mortality, but the studies have been small.

o. Nitric oxide inhibitors (*controversial*).

p. Extracorporeal membrane oxygenation (ECMO) is sometimes used in newborns with refractory shock.

3. **Cardiogenic shock.** First, treat any obvious cause.

   a. Air leak. If a tension pneumothorax is causing hypotension by obstructing venous return, immediate evacuation of the air is necessary (see Chapter 26).

   b. Arrhythmia. Recognize the arrhythmia and treat it.

   c. Metabolic cause. Metabolic problems need to be corrected.

   d. Asphyxia. The hypotension usually responds to inotropic agents. See following discussion.

   e. In cardiogenic shock, the goal is to improve cardiac output. Inotropic agents should be used IV (for dosages and other pharmacologic information, see Chapter 132). Use of volume expansion is not warranted and may be harmful.

   i. **Dopamine** is the drug of first choice and is superior to dobutamine.(especially in the short-term treatment of hypotension) Previous studies have suggested that higher than traditionally used dosages (≥ 30–50 mcg/kg/min) may be used without causing α-adrenergic side effects such as decreased renal perfusion and decreased urine output. A recent review stated that infants with suspected perinatal asphyxia who were treated with low-dose dopamine (2.5 mcg/kg/min) did not show any improvement in mortality or long-term neurodevelopmental outcome.

   ii. **Dobutamine.** If dopamine fails to improve BP, dobutamine is recommended as a second-line drug. In neonates, it is usually given together with dopamine infusion. *Note:* Dobutamine causes peripheral vasodilation.

   iii. **Other agents (if dopamine or dobutamine do not work).** Dopexamine, epinephrine, hydralazine, isoproterenol, nitroprusside, norepinephrine, phentolamine, amrinone, and milrinone are sometimes used. Choice depends on institutional protocols.

4. **Neurogenic shock.** Neurogenic shock is treated with volume expansion (see Section V, B, 1a) and inotropic agents (see Section V, B, 3e).

5. **Drug-induced hypotension.** Volume expansion (see Section V, B, 1a) usually maintains the BP in cases of drug-induced vasodilation. If the BP cannot be maintained, the drug causing hypotension may need to be discontinued.

6. **Endocrine disorders**

   a. Adrenal hemorrhage is treated with volume expansion and blood replacement and corticosteroids (see Chapter 132).

   b. Congenital adrenal hyperplasia is treated with corticosteroids (see Chapter 132).

7. **Hypotension in ELBW infants.** (Recent studies have revealed that cerebral blood flow autoregulation is lost when blood pressure reaches the fifth percentile in very low birthweight infants.)

   a. The use of antenatal steroids decreases the risk of hypotension in ELBW infants.

   b. Dopamine is more effective than normal saline (as long as there is no evidence of myocardial dysfunction) in increasing BP in preterm infants. It raised BP in 90% of infants, whereas volume supplementation only was 40% effective. If there is evidence of myocardial dysfunction, then dobutamine should be used.

   c. Physiologic doses of hydrocortisone have been used in refractory hypotension (vasopressor resistant) with uncertainty of long-term side effects. Low-dose dexamethasone increases the blood pressure and also decreases pressor requirements in ELBW infants with volume and pressor-resistant hypotension (see part e in this section about echo recommendations prior to hydrocortisone treatment).

   d. **More studies** are needed to evaluate safety of use of crystalloids/dopamine/dobutamine to treat low BP in preterm infants.

   e. **Consider the possibility and role of the left to right PDA shunt** in hypotension in ELBW infants. Studies have revealed that hypotension not responding to vasopressors was significantly associated with a hemodynamically significant PDA. Echocardiography is recommended early to detect shunting before hydrocortisone is used.

   f. **Indomethacin with hydrocortisone** is not recommended because there is an increase in gastric perforations.

59 Is the Infant Ready for Discharge?

  I. **Problem.** The infant in the neonatal intensive care unit (NICU) or newborn nursery is ready to be discharged home. How can we ensure that this discharge is smooth, safe, and complete? The three essential factors for discharge are maintaining a normal body temperature in an open crib; ability to grow at a normal rate; and ability to eat, without respiratory compromise while taking an appropriate volume of feeding.

 II. **Immediate questions**

   A. **What is the corrected age of the infant?** Most preterm infants are discharged 2–4 weeks before their "due date," but there are variations among hospitals. Infants staying beyond their due date are usually on prolonged assisted ventilation, have severe malformations, or are status post–major surgery. The postconceptual age of 36 weeks is a prime time for consideration for discharge.

   B. **Is the infant showing consistent weight gain?** At discharge, the infant should be gaining weight steadily on breast- or bottle-feeds. Most healthy preterm or term infants with no ongoing problems show an average weight gain of 15–30 g/day. If possible, multiple-gestation infants should be discharged home together, which may necessitate extra allowance on weight criteria. A specific weight requirement at discharge is **controversial.** Recent recommendations state that a sustained weight gain is more important than a specific weight. Some institutions require that an infant must weigh at least 1800–2000 g at discharge. Others base discharge more on maturity: ability to feed, gain weight, and keep warm.

   C. **Is the infant maintaining body temperature in an open crib?** The ability to maintain thermal homeostasis without an external source of heat in an open crib with comfortable clothing is a key determinant of fitness for discharge.

   D. **Is the infant feeding satisfactorily? Are any special feeding techniques necessary?** The ability of the infant to breast- or bottle-feed satisfactorily, taking in an adequate number of calories (120 cal/kg/day) in reasonable frequency (every 3–4 h), with each feed not taking >30–40 min, is important. If clinical grounds indicate the need for prolonged tube feeding or gastrostomy tube feeding, the parents must be trained to carry out the feedings at home.

   E. **Are the vital signs stable? Is there a need for home monitoring? Have arrangements been made for parental training in monitor use and in cardiopulmonary resuscitation?** Episodes of apnea of prematurity along with associated bradycardia and desaturation resolve at about the postconceptional age of 36 weeks. If such episodes persist at 36 weeks of age or at discharge, the infants are usually sent home on varying combinations of cardiopulmonary event monitoring, respiratory stimulants (eg, theophylline or caffeine), and supplemental oxygen. Infant cardiopulmonary resuscitation training is arranged for the parents. If theophylline is still being used, then serum levels should be checked before discharge and monitored during follow-up visits; this is not usually necessary with caffeine. If home oxygen therapy is needed, pulse oximetry saturations in room air and in oxygen (supine and in a car seat) are recorded before discharge and checked during each follow-up visit.

F. **Are there medications that need to be continued after discharge?** Infants discharged on medications usually have the first prescription filled in the hospital pharmacy. Before the patient's discharge, the parents should be trained in safely administering the medications. Parents are briefed on the duration of administration, importance of the medication, and probable duration of treatment as well as side effects and risks of discontinuing too soon.

G. **Is the audiology screen completed?** A newborn hearing screen (either an otoacoustic emissions [OAE], measuring the sound waves in the inner ear or an auditory brainstem response [ABR], measuring how the brain responds to sound) **is now recommended before discharge.** Results are recorded in the patient's record and the discharge summary and are also mailed to each state's Newborn Hearing Screening Program. Any "fail" is usually tested again after clinical inspection of the ear and cleaning of the external auditory meatus, if necessary. Brainstem auditory evoked response assessment is essential in other clinical conditions in which there is an increased risk for hearing loss and which progressive losses are possible. Risk factors for hearing loss: family history of hearing loss, in utero TORCH infection, ear and craniofacial anomalies, high bilirubin requiring exchange transfusion, birthweight <1500 g, bacterial meningitis, low Apgar scores 0–3 at 5 min, 0–6 at 10 min, respiratory distress, mechanical ventilation >10 days, ototoxic medication given >5 days, physical features of a syndrome that includes hearing loss (eg, Down syndrome).

H. **Is the newborn metabolic screen completed? If so, is it valid and is a repeat test needed?** (See Chapter 14.) The content of the newborn metabolic screen varies among states. Screening at birth for phenylketonuria, hypothyroidism, and galactosemia is almost universal. Other tests, such as sickle cell screen and cystic fibrosis screen, vary regionally based on prevalence. All initial newborn screens should be done per state protocol but essentially at 48 h after birth and preferably after 24 h of protein feeding. The thyroid screen is invalid if done before 48 h because of the surge of thyroid-stimulating hormone (TSH) at birth. The galactosemia test is valid at birth and invalid after blood transfusion for at least 60 days. Any borderline values or abnormal initial metabolic screen results are repeated with more definitive tests (eg, serum thyroxine, TSH, free thyroxine, and thyroxine-binding immunoglobulin).

I. **Are any immunizations due before discharge?** Preterm infants should be immunized at the normal chronologic age with the same vaccine doses as term infants (**Note:** Birthweight does not matter). If the infant is discharged at ≥2 months of age, give DPT (diphtheria-pertussis-tetanus), Hib vaccine (*Haemophilus influenzae* vaccine), and IPV (polio vaccine inactivated) at the appropriate time. All of these, DPT, Hib, and IPV, can be given as early as 6 weeks of age. **All newborns should be vaccinated with hepatitis B before discharge from the hospital.** Preterm infants (<2000 g) born to HBsAg-negative women usually receive the first hepatitis B vaccine at 1 month of age, regardless of gestational age or birthweight. Infants whose mothers are positive for hepatitis B virus surface antigen or core or "e" antigen (HBsAg, HBcAg, or HBeAg, respectively) need to be given both hepatitis B immunoglobulin and hepatitis B vaccine (high dose) in the first 12 h of life. Preterm infants with chronic lung disease should be considered for respiratory syncytial virus immunoglobulin administration throughout the winter months and influenza vaccination at 6 months of age.

III. **Discharge diagnosis.** A concise list of all the diagnoses for a patient, listed in chronologic order of occurrence, should be generated.

IV. **Database.** Review the initial history, NICU hospital course, and physical examination at discharge. Compose an organized discharge summary by systems or by problems.

A. **History**

1. **Maternal-fetal conditions** (including prenatal diagnostic tests and medications). Maternal diagnoses need to be reviewed (ie, does the mother have idiopathic thrombocytopenic purpura, systemic lupus erythematosus, and so on?).

2. **Labor and delivery.** Premature rupture of membranes, anesthesia, delivery type, and resuscitation.

3. **Birth history.** Apgar scores, head circumference, length, and weight.

B. **Physical examination.** List any significant abnormal findings noted at birth. Perform a complete physical examination, paying careful attention to the following aspects at discharge:

1. **General.** General disposition, spontaneous activity, phenotypic features of note (if any), weight for gestational or chronologic age, and symmetry. Plot the growth chart and record the percentiles for weight, length, and head circumference.

2. **Skin.** Look for hemangiomas, neurocutaneous markers (eg, café au lait), and scars (eg, surgical, deep-line insertion sites, and chest tube or gastrostomy tube sites). Specifically look for erythema, discharge, and unremoved suture threads at incision sites.

3. **Head.** Check for size (occipitofrontal head circumference), shape (dolichocephalic in premature infants), rate of growth, state of the fontanelles (including size, if open), sutures, and presence of cephalhematoma or caput. Watch for intravenous infiltrates and necrotic patches in the scalp.

4. **Eyes.** Look specifically for strabismus, red reflex, nystagmus, nasolacrimal duct obstruction, and abnormalities of the sclera and conjunctiva. Elicit the pupillary reflex, and examine the size, color, shape, and symmetry of the pupils.

5. **Ears, nose, and mouth.** Examine the ears at the time of discharge, paying particular attention to patency and any abnormality (eg, preauricular, postauricular sinuses, skin tags, or abnormalities of pinnae), patency of both nostrils (already confirmed with nasogastric tube passage), and examination of the throat to rule out cleft of the soft palate and submucous clefts. Look for natal teeth or prematurely erupted teeth, thrush (Candida), and other lesions in the mouth.

6. **Face.** Look for characteristic facies, facial asymmetry (eg, facial nerve paresis or paralysis or torticollis), and hemangiomas in the trigeminal area.

7. **Neck.** The neck should be supple and free of lymphadenopathy and sinuses (eg, branchial). Look for anterior midline masses (eg, ectopic thyroid, thyromegaly, or thyroglossal cyst). Examine the site of deep-line insertions in the neck and upper thorax (eg, extracorporeal membrane oxygenation, cannulation, or indwelling catheter).

8. **Cardiovascular (eg, murmur or femoral pulse).** Listen for the presence of both normal heart sounds as well as any extraneous clicks or murmurs over the precordium. Assess for murmurs in the neck and interscapular region (eg, peripheral pulmonic stenosis) and axilla. Feel for peripheral pulses on each limb, including femoral pulses. Note the presence of systolic flow murmur secondary to anemia in premature infants.

9. **Chest.** Note the shape and symmetry of the chest, abnormalities of the sternum, prominence of the costochondral junctions, significant intercostal and subcostal retractions, abnormalities in the breathing pattern, air entry, and accessory breathing sounds (eg, wheeze or rales). Look specifically at the indwelling catheter site, chest tube insertion site (for infection), and sutures.

10. **Abdomen.** Look for distention, dilated veins, and visible gastric or intestinal peristalsis, and auscultate for bowel sounds. Palpate for visceromegaly or abnormal masses. Check the renal angle for fullness, dullness, or bruit (eg, renal artery stenosis). Note the presence of surgical scars, gastrostomy tube, ventriculoperitoneal catheters, and so on.

11. **Genitalia. In males,** look for the position of the urethral meatus (eg, normal, epispadias, or hypospadias), the stream of urine, and circumcision and for the presence of both testes in the scrotum. **In females,** note the vaginal-to-anal distance to screen for ano-rectal anomalies. Examine for hernia (umbilical, inguinal, and femoral).

12. **Spine.** Specifically look for kyphosis and scoliosis, and record any abnormality already radiologically confirmed (eg, hemivertebrae). Record the presence of cutaneous stigmata such as pigmentation, lipoma, or tuft of hair along the vertebral region.

13. **Presacral area.** Examine the lumbosacral region in detail for spina bifida occulta, any sinus tracts, and cutaneous markers (eg, lipoma or pigmentation). Always perform ultrasound examination of deep pilonidal pits and sinuses to look for cord tethering.

14. **Limbs.** Look for symmetry, palpable peripheral pulses in all four limbs, areas of intravenous infiltrates, erythema or induration in areas of cutdowns, and arterial cannulation. Look for normal passive mobility in all joints and assess muscle tone (eg, hypotonia, hypertonia, and contracture).

15. **Joints.** Look for abnormal shape, limitation of movement and stability, especially in the hip joint. Assess the hips for congenital hip dysplasia with the Barlow or Ortolani procedure.

16. **Gross neurologic.** Examine for general body tone, posture, spontaneous activity, symmetry of movements, deep tendon reflexes, presence of or abnormal persistence of neonatal reflexes, and involuntary movements.

C. **Laboratory studies (at discharge)**

1. **Hematocrit and reticulocyte count.** Hematocrit at the time of discharge should be >22% (***controversial***), and the reticulocyte count should be >5% (***controversial***) with adequate supplementation of iron and multivitamins added to the normal dietary intake. Folic acid, B_{12}, and fat-soluble vitamin supplementation may be necessary in infants with short-gut syndrome or loss of distal ileum, including ileocecal valve during surgery. Anemia of prematurity must be noted and followed.

2. **Serum calcium, phosphorus, and alkaline phosphatase.** Extremely premature infants and low birthweight infants must have these parameters checked during inpatient stay and at discharge along with radiographs of the bones to rule out rickets of prematurity. Vitamin D_3 (1,25-dihydroxycholecalciferol) supplementation may be considered in these infants, often as part of a multivitamin (***controversial***).

3. **Repeat newborn metabolic screen.** This is done if necessary for validity, for checking a previously positive screening test, or for a more extensive screen based on clinical suspicion.

4. **Drug levels.** Infants being discharged home on medications such as phenobarbital, theophylline, or caffeine should have levels tested before discharge, and the results should be recorded and the dosage adjusted as necessary.

5. **Bilirubin levels.** Measure the total serum bilirubin and plot on the nomogram, see Figure 92–1 and Chapter 51, Section V, F.

D. **Radiologic and other studies**

1. **Chest radiograph.** A copy of the most recent radiograph should be sent with the parents to the primary physician for follow-up care of chronic lung disease (eg, bronchopulmonary dysplasia [BPD]).

2. **Head ultrasound scan.** Clearly record the findings of the scans in chronologic order, with emphasis on hemorrhage, ventricular size, and areas of echogenicity suggestive of periventricular leukomalacia and porencephalic cysts.

3. **Electroencephalogram.** Record the results, if done more than once, in chronologic order, indicating assessment of cerebral function in infants with seizures.

4. **Electrocardiogram.** Documentation is useful in cases of congenital heart defect, supraventricular tachycardias, or metabolic problems.

5. **Computed tomography scan.** If performed to evaluate any area in the infant's body, comment on the findings and interpretation.

6. **Other tests.** Record the findings and recommendations on pneumograms, barium contrast studies, and so on.

V. Plan. Once a decision has been made for discharge, compile a checklist of active problems and appointments at discharge. Levels of follow up depend on the infant. Recent American Academy of Pediatrics (AAP) recommendations state that level 1 could consist of a telephone call. Different screening assessments could be done on the phone. Level 2 could involve a clinic visit with a neurodevelopmental screening test. Level 3 would involve comprehensive testing done at a clinic visit.

  A. Ophthalmic check. An eye examination for evaluation of retinopathy of prematurity (ROP) is recommended for all infants weighing <1500 g or gestational age of ≤32 weeks and selected infants with a birthweight between 1500 and 2000g or gestational age > 32 weeks who have had an unstable clinical course. Any infant who are believed to have a high risk should also have an examination. Parents need to be told the importance of follow-up examinations and the possible consequences of serious ROP. The examination schedule is as follows:

  1. **Follow-up ≤1 week:** Stage 1 or 2 ROP, zone 1; stage 3 ROP, zone II.
  2. **Follow-up in 1–2 weeks:** Immature vascularization zone I, no ROP; stage 2, ROP zone II; regressing ROP, zone I.
  3. **Follow-up in 2 weeks:** Stage 1 ROP, zone II; regressing ROP: zone II.
  4. **Follow-up in 2–3 weeks:** Immature vascularization zone II, no ROP; stage 1 or 2 ROP, zone III; regressing ROP, zone III.

  B. Audiologic follow-up
  1. **If the infant has a normal ABR and no risk,** a follow-up questionnaire is sent at 6 months.
  2. **If the infant fails the ABR,** rescreen in 2 weeks.
  3. **If the infant passes** but has high risk (one risk factor) (see Section II, G), reevaluate in 3 months for ABR/OAE.

  C. Developmental assessment, including occupational therapy and physiotherapy. The initial examination and evaluation is done in the NICU before discharge to assess the need for early interventional services.

  D. Bilirubin assessment. Before discharge, every infant should be assessed for the risk of developing severe hyperbilirubinemia. The AAP recommends either doing a predischarge bilirubin using TSB or TcB and/or do a clinical assessment of risk factors (See Chapter 51, Section V, F, 1b) or both. Use the predischarge TSB and plot the results on the nomogram to assess the risk of subsequent hyperbilirubinemia. (See Figure 92–1.) **Clinical judgment should be used.** If there are many risk factors, it is best to see those infants earlier and more frequent. If follow-up cannot be done and there is significant risk, it may be best not to discharge the infant. Follow-up recommendations are as follows:

  1. **Infant discharged <24 h** should be seen by age 72 h.
  2. **Infant discharged between 24 and 47.9 h** should be seen by age 96 h.
  3. **Infant discharged between 48 and 72 h** should be seen by age 120 h.

  E. Immunizations (except hepatitis B, which should be given before discharge unless the mother is HBsAg positive) need to be given at 2 months of age.

  F. Circumcision is performed at parental request and with their consent before discharge. The procedure is elective, requires analgesia, and should not be done on small infants, on infants with BPD on oxygen, or on those with ongoing apnea or bradycardia problems or anomalies of the external genitalia (eg, hypospadias, ambiguous genitalia where reconstruction may be needed at a later date). Older infants require formal anesthesia and analgesia.

  G. Social services input. Determine whether this service has been required, including the family's need for housing, financial stability, or other assistance.

  H. Follow-up with the primary care physician. Information on the name, location, and choice of follow-up physician should be available at the time of discharge. In any given case, the specialty physician should personally contact the primary care physician by telephone to discuss the patient or to make arrangements for a preliminary discharge summary to be faxed to the primary physician.

I. **Follow-up clinical assessment.** Parents should be briefed on subspecialty appointments (eg, ophthalmology, pediatric surgery, or neurosurgery) and their importance. Appointments at a neonatal follow-up clinic for monitoring growth and development, with input from a dietitian, social worker, physiotherapist, and developmentalist, are mandatory for very high-risk infants. At the request of the physician, follow-up house visits by a home health nurse to check clinical status, to repeat tests, and to ensure weight gain should be arranged for finite periods, depending on the needs of the individual infant and family. Infants with special needs who require specialized follow-up health surveillance include those with the following conditions:

1. **Lung diseases** (BPD, chronic lung disease).
2. **Central nervous system disorders/Neurologic abnormalities** (seizures, posthemorrhagic hydrocephalus, postmeningitis hydrocephalus and periventricular leukomalacia.
3. **Gastrointestinal diseases** such as gastroesophageal reflux, short gut, and the presence of ostomies.
5. **Congenital heart disease.**
6. **Genetic problems.**
7. **Hearing problems** (hearing loss).
8. **Eye problems** (ROP, other).
9. **Apnea and bradycardia.**
10. **Anemia of prematurity.**

J. **Car seat.** Use infant-only car safety seats with three-point harness systems or convertible car safety seats with five-point harness systems. Blanket rolls may be placed on both sides of the infant and a rolled diaper or blanket can be used between the crotch strap and the infant to reduce slouching. Parents need to bring the car seat before discharge for training on seating the infant, proper positioning, and support. While the infant is in the car seat, check for oxygen saturation in supine and car seat positions, especially for premature infants sent home on oxygen and monitoring for apnea (per the AAP's "Safe Transport of the Preemie" policy statement).

K. **Brief parents on common issues after discharge.** Discuss home temperature and dressing the infant, intercurrent illness and taking temperature, vomiting, bowel movement, diaper rash, sleeping, bathing, stuffy nose and its management, hiccups, crying, breathing pattern, interacting with the infant, going out, visitors and relatives, and a "no smoking" policy inside the house. Review medications, nutrition (type, amount, frequency, and special precautions), and use of supplemental oxygen and the cardiopulmonary monitor as needed.

60 No Stool in 48 Hours

I. **Problem.** No stool has been passed in over 48 h. Ninety-nine percent of term infants and 76% of premature infants pass a stool in the first 24 h of life. Ninety-nine percent of premature infants pass a stool by 48 h.

II. **Immediate questions**

A. **Has a stool been passed since birth?** If a stool has been passed since birth but not in the last 48 h, constipation may be the cause. If a stool has never been passed, imperforate anus or some degree of intestinal obstruction may be present. Table 60–1 shows the time after birth at which the first stool is typically passed.

Table 60–1. **TIME OF FIRST STOOL BASED ON A STUDY OF 500 TERM AND PRETERM INFANTS**

Hours	Full-Term Infants (%)[a]	Preterm Infants (%)[a]
Delivery room (0)	16.7	5.0
1–8	59.5	32.5
9–16	91.1	63.8
17–24	98.5	76.3
24–48	100.0	98.8
>48	—	100.0

[a]Percentages are cumulative.
Based on data from Clark DA: Times of first void and stool in 500 newborns. *Pediatrics* 1977;60:457.

    B. **What is the gestational age?** Prematurity is associated with a delayed passage of stool because of immaturity of the colon and lack of triggering effect of enteral feeds on gut hormones when the patient is maintained on NPO.

    C. **Were maternal drugs used that could cause a paralytic ileus with delayed passage of stool?** Magnesium sulfate, which is used to slow the premature onset of labor, may cause paralytic ileus. Narcotics for pain control or use of heroin by the mother may also cause delayed passage of stool in the neonate.

III. **Differential diagnosis**

    A. **Constipation.**

    B. **Anorectal abnormalities** such as imperforate anus. Imperforate anus may pass meconium if a fistula exists.

    C. **Bowel obstruction**

        1. **Meconium plug** is an obstruction in the lower colon and rectum caused by meconium. It is more common in infants of diabetic mothers (as seen in neonatal small left colon syndrome, in which the plug extends to the splenic flexure) and in premature infants. (**Note:** A rectal biopsy should be considered in all these patients because they have an increased incidence [10–15%] of Hirschsprung disease.)

        2. **Meconium ileus** occurs when meconium becomes obstructed in the terminal ileum. Ninety percent of patients with meconium ileum have cystic fibrosis (CF) and thus should be tested for CF. It is the most common presentation of CF in the neonatal period.

        3. **Hirschsprung disease** accounts for ~15% of infants who have delayed passage of stool. A functional obstruction is caused by aganglionosis of cells in Meissner and Auerbach plexus in the rectum and variable amounts of the distal colon. The affected segment of colon and rectum are aperistaltic.

        4. **Jejunal/Ileal atresia** can occur secondary to meconium ileus, Hirschsprung disease, incarcerated hernia, or intussusception. Signs include abdominal distention, bilious vomiting, and failure to pass meconium.

        5. **Adhesions.** Postoperatively, such as after surgery for necrotizing enterocolitis (NEC), there is a 30% chance of having adhesions.

        6. **Incarcerated hernia** when hernia contents cannot be reduced and the bowel is obstructed. Signs include irritability, cramps, bilious vomiting, and abdominal distention. The risk of incarceration for an inguinal hernia in infancy is 20–30%; the risk of bowel obstruction secondary to an inguinal hernia is 9%.

        7. **Malrotation** is the failure of the gastrointestinal tract to properly rotate and adhere. Volvulus is a specific malrotation of the gut and is a **surgical emergency** because it can cause ischemia of the gut, with resulting shock, bowel necrosis, and possibly death. Malrotation without volvulus formation may present with intermittent episodes of vomiting and abdominal distention. The stooling pattern can be normal.

        8. **Intussusception.** Very rare in newborns.

   9. Duodenal atresia. May pass meconium in the first 24 h, then no stool.
   10. Small left colon syndrome. Approximately 50% have a history of maternal diabetes, and all don't pass meconium in the first 24 h of life.
   D. Other causes
   1. Ileus can be secondary to the following conditions:
      a. Sepsis.
      b. Necrotizing enterocolitis.
      c. Hypokalemia.
      d. Pneumonia.
      e. Maternal use of magnesium sulfate.
      f. Hypothyroidism.
      g. Narcotic analgesic therapy.
   2. Prematurity (see Section II, B).
IV. Database
   A. Physical examination. First, document the patency of the anus (eg, rectal thermometer or feeding tube). Check for abdominal distention or rigidity, bowel sounds, and evidence of a mass. A rectal examination will determine whether muscle tone is adequate, and it may reveal hardened stool in the rectum.
   B. Laboratory findings
      1. Complete blood count with differential and blood culture to rule out sepsis. A urine culture under sterile conditions should also be done.
      2. Urinary drug screening on both mother and infant to detect maternal use of narcotics.
      3. Serum magnesium level to detect hypermagnesemia.
      4. Serum electrolytes, especially to rule out hypokalemia.
      5. Serum thyroxine (T_4) and thyroid-stimulating hormone (TSH) levels to detect hypothyroidism.
   C. Radiologic and other studies
      1. Plain film abdominal radiographs. A flat plate and upright film of the abdomen should be obtained to look for ileus or bowel obstruction in any infant who has not passed stool within 48 h of birth. With Hirschsprung disease or meconium plug, distention of the colon with multiple air-fluid levels is seen. With duodenal atresia, one sees air in the stomach and upper part of the abdomen (the double bubble) with no air in the small or large bowel.
      2. Abdominal radiographs with barium enema should be obtained in all cases of delayed passage of stool if the patient is symptomatic. These will help define the disease process and may be therapeutic. Specific findings for each disease are described in Section V.
V. Plan
   A. Constipation
      1. Digital rectal stimulation can be tried first.
      2. Glycerin suppositories can be used if digital rectal stimulation is unsuccessful.
   B. Anorectal abnormality: Imperforate anus.
      1. Obtain pediatric surgical consultation immediately.
      2. Insert a nasogastric tube for decompression.
      3. Look for other congenital anomalies. Genitourinary tract abnormalities are frequently seen with imperforate anus.
   C. Bowel obstruction
      1. Meconium plug
         a. Barium enema is performed to verify meconium plug. In infants with this problem, the study usually reveals a normal-sized colon with filling defects.
         b. If meconium plug is verified by barium enema, repeated water-soluble enemas are usually given every 4–6 h.
         c. Acetylcysteine (Mucomyst) enema. If water-soluble enemas are ineffective, a dilute 4% solution of acetylcysteine and water can be used as an enema to break down the meconium so the plug can be passed.

   d. **If normal stooling occurs,** monitor closely.
   e. **If an abnormal pattern of stooling recurs,** further workup (eg, rectal biopsy) is necessary to rule out Hirschsprung disease, which may be diagnosed in half of these patients.
2. **Meconium ileus**
   a. **Barium enema** may reveal microcolon. Evidence of perforation, volvulus, or atresia may also be seen.
   b. **Mild obstruction** can be treated with Mucomyst enemas (see Section V, C, 1c).
   c. **Complete obstruction** may be relieved by an hyperosmolar Gastrografin enema. Adequate fluid and electrolyte replacement must be given.
   d. **Operative management** may be necessary in patients not relieved by enemas with passage of meconium within several hours.
3. **Hirschsprung disease**
   a. **Barium enema** usually shows a distal narrowed, aganglionic segment leading to a dilated proximal segment.
   b. **Rectal biopsy,** the definitive diagnosis, is performed to confirm aganglionosis.
   c. **Colostomy** is usually indicated once the diagnosis is confirmed.
4. **Adhesions.** Surgery is usually necessary to lyse the adhesions if a trial of nasogastric decompression fails.
5. **Incarcerated hernia** is a surgical emergency.
6. **Malrotation**
   a. **Barium enema** reveals an abnormally placed cecum.
   b. **Surgical correction** is necessary.
7. **Volvulus**
   a. **Barium enema** reveals obstruction at the midtransverse colon.
   b. **Surgery** should be an immediate intervention.
8. **Intussusception.** Hydrostatic reduction is attempted. If unsuccessful, surgery with operative reduction or resection is done.
9. **Duodenal atresia.** Decompression with nasogastric suction and surgery.
10. **Small left colon syndrome.** Contrast enema is done and is usually diagnostic and therapeutic. Surgery is indicated if the obstruction is recurrent or if there is a perforation.
D. **Ileus**
1. **Ileus caused by sepsis**
   a. **Broad-spectrum antibiotics** are initiated after a sepsis workup (see Chapter 117) is performed. Intravenous ampicillin and gentamicin are recommended. Vancomycin may be substituted for ampicillin if staphylococcal infection is suspected (for dosages, see Chapter 132).
   b. **A nasogastric tube** should be placed to decompress the bowel. The infant should not be fed enterally.
2. **Ileus caused by NEC.** See Chapter 104.
3. **Ileus caused by hypokalemia**
   a. **Treat underlying metabolic abnormalities.** Correct potassium levels (see Chapter 56).
   b. **Place a nasogastric tube** to rest the bowel.
E. **Prematurity.** Conservative treatment is usually recommended in infants who are not vomiting but have progressive abdominal distention, even if microcolon is seen. Treatment consists of a hyperosmolar contrast enema for passage of the stool. (*Note:* Some institutions advocate the use of low-osmolality, water-soluble, iodine-containing contrast enemas because of fewer side effects. Consult a pediatric radiologist for appropriate contrast enema to be used.)
F. **Hypothyroidism.** If the serum T_4 and TSH levels confirm the presence of hypothyroidism, thyroid replacement therapy is indicated. Consultation with an endocrinologist should be obtained before starting this therapy.

61 No Urine Output in 24 Hours

I. **Problem.** Urine output has been scant or absent for 24 h. Oliguria is defined as urine output <0.5–1 mL/kg/h. One hundred percent of healthy premature, full-term, and post-term infants void by 24 h of age. Oliguria is one of the clinical hallmarks of renal failure.

II. **Immediate questions**
A. **Is the bladder palpable?** If a distended bladder is present, it is usually palpable. A palpable bladder suggests there is urine in the bladder. **Credé maneuver** (manual compression of the bladder) may initiate voiding, especially in infants receiving medications causing muscle paralysis.
B. **Has bladder catheterization been performed?** Catheterization determines whether urine is present in the bladder. It is commonly done in more mature infants.
C. **What is the blood pressure?** Hypotension can cause decreased renal perfusion and urine output.
D. **Has the infant ever voided?** If the infant has never voided, consider bilateral renal agenesis, renovascular accident, or obstruction. Table 61–1 shows the time after birth at which the first voiding occurs.
E. **Did the mother have oligohydramnios?** One of the etiologies of oligohydramnios, a decrease in amniotic fluid, can be caused by a decrease in fetal urine production. This can be caused by fetal renal problems such as decreased renal perfusion, obstructive uropathy, and congenital absence of renal tissue (renal agenesis, cystic dysplasia, and ureteral atresia).

III. **Differential diagnosis.** For a complete discussion of acute renal failure, see Chapter 113.
A. **Prerenal causes** (normal kidneys with inadequate renal perfusion)
1. **Sepsis/Shock.** Renal failure occurs in 26% of neonates with sepsis.
2. **Dehydration.**
3. **Hemorrhage.**
4. **Hypotension.**
5. **Asphyxia.** Sixty-one percent of infants with asphyxia have renal failure, 25% of cases are oliguric, and 15% are anuric.
6. **Hypokalemia.**
7. **Heart failure.**
8. **Medications.** Certain medications (eg, indomethacin, captopril, and β-agonists), if given to the mother before delivery, can result in renal insufficiency.
9. **Respiratory distress syndrome.**
10. **Polycythemia.**
B. **Intrinsic renal failure** (structural renal damage)
1. **Renal agenesis.**
2. **Hypoplastic, dysplastic, or polycystic kidneys.**

Table 61–1. **TIME OF FIRST VOID BASED ON A STUDY OF 500 TERM AND PRETERM INFANTS**

Hours	Full-Term Infants (%)[a]	Preterm Infants (%)[a]
Delivery room (0)	12.9	21.2
1–8	51.1	83.7
9–16	91.1	98.7
17–24	100.0	100.0

[a]Percentages are cumulative.
Based on data from Clark DA: Times of first void and stool in 500 newborns. *Pediatrics* 1977;60:457.

3. **Pyelonephritis.**
4. **Vascular accident** (renal artery and vein thrombosis).
5. **Nephritis.**
6. **Infections** such as congenital syphilis, cytomegalovirus, toxoplasmosis, and Gram-negative infections.
7. **Acute tubular necrosis** secondary to shock, dehydration, drugs, toxins, and asphyxia.
8. **Medications.** Some nephrotoxic medications include tolazoline, aminoglycosides, indomethacin, amphotericin, α-adrenergic agents, nonsteroidal anti-inflammatory drugs, diuretics, and acyclovir.

C. **Postrenal causes** (urine is formed but not passed)
1. **Neurogenic bladder** (from myelomeningocele or medications such as pancuronium or heavy sedation).
2. **Urethral stricture.**
3. **Posterior urethral valves** (males only).
4. **Extrinsic compression** (eg, sacrococcygeal teratoma).
5. **Drugs.** Certain medications (eg, acyclovir and sulfonamides) can precipitate within the tubules and cause obstruction.
6. **Systemic candidiasis** with bilateral uteropelvic fungal bezoar formation.

IV. **Database**
A. **Physical examination** may reveal bladder distention, abdominal masses, or ascites. Signs of renal disorders (eg, Potter facies [low-set ears, inner canthal crease, etc.]) should be noted. Urinary ascites may be seen with posterior urethral valves. Oligohydramnios in the mother suggests possible renal problems.
1. **Prerenal.** Signs of volume depletion (tachycardia and hypotension).
2. **Intrinsic renal.** Edema, signs of congestive heart failure, hypertension. Palpable kidneys may mean polycystic kidney, hydronephrosis, or tumors.
3. **Postrenal.** Poor urinary stream, enlarged bladder, and dribbling of urine; urinary ascites with rupture.
B. **Laboratory studies.** The following laboratory tests can be obtained to help establish the diagnosis. Interpret the results as outlined in Table 113–1.
1. **Serum creatinine.**
2. **Serum electrolytes and blood urea nitrogen** also help to evaluate renal function.
3. **Complete blood count (CBC) and platelet count.** An abnormal CBC can be seen in sepsis. Thrombocytopenia can be seen in renal vein thrombosis.
4. **Urinalysis** may reveal white blood cells, suggesting a urinary tract infection.
5. **Arterial blood pH.** A metabolic acidosis can be seen in anything that causes hypovolemia, hypoperfusion, or hypotension, such as sepsis.
6. **Urine osmolality.**
7. **Urine sodium (mEq/L).**
8. **Urine-to-plasma creatinine ratio.**
9. **Fractional excretion of sodium.** See Chapter 113.
10. **Renal failure index.** See Chapter 113.
C. **Radiologic and other studies**
1. **Ultrasonography with Doppler flow studies** of the abdomen and kidneys will rule out urinary tract obstruction and help evaluate for other renal or vascular abnormalities.
2. **Abdominal radiograph studies** may reveal ascites, masses, spina bifida, or an absent sacrum, suggesting a neurogenic bladder.
3. **Voiding cystourethrography** if bladder outlet obstruction is suspected.
4. **Radionuclide renal scanning** may be helpful in obstruction.

V. **Plan.** For management of renal failure, see Chapter 113.
A. **Prerenal**
1. **Treat the specific cause** (eg, sepsis).
2. **A fluid challenge** can be given (10–20 mL/kg of normal saline intravenously).

3. **Treatment may involve volume therapy or inotropic agents.**
4. **Recent reviews found** that low-dose dopamine does not prevent renal dysfunction in indomethacin-treated premature infants.
B. **Renal**
   1. **Pediatric nephrologist consultation**
      a. Supportive measures.
      b. Treat the specific cause.
      c. Restrict fluid intake, and replace insensible losses.
C. **Postrenal**
   1. **Urologic/Pediatric surgical consultation**
      a. **If obstruction is distal to the bladder,** perform initial catheterization. Surgical vesicostomy may be indicated.
      b. **If obstruction is proximal to the bladder,** urologic surgical intervention should be considered (eg, nephrostomy tubes or cutaneous ureterostomy).
      c. **Neurogenic bladder** is initially managed with catheterization.
      d. **Medications resulting in bladder dysfunction** may be stopped, and bladder function is usually restored.

62 Pneumoperitoneum

I. **Problem.** A pneumoperitoneum (an abnormal collection of air in the peritoneal cavity) is seen on an abdominal radiograph. The air can be secondary to perforation of the gastrointestinal (GI) tract (most common), from the respiratory tract, or secondary to iatrogenic causes (uncommon).

II. **Immediate questions**
   A. **Are signs or symptoms of pneumoperitoneum present?** These findings can include abdominal distention, respiratory distress, deteriorating blood gas levels, and a decrease in blood pressure.
   B. **Were signs or symptoms of necrotizing enterocolitis (NEC) present before?** If so, the pneumoperitoneum is most likely to be associated with GI tract perforation.
   C. **Are any signs of air leak present?** If a pneumomediastinum, pulmonary interstitial emphysema, or pneumothorax is present, the peritoneal air collection is more likely to be of respiratory tract origin.
   D. **Is mechanical ventilation being given?** High peak inspiratory pressures (PIPs) > a mean of 34 cm H_2O can be associated with a pneumoperitoneum.
   E. **Did the infant recently undergo abdominal surgery or an invasive procedure such as paracentesis?** Intra-abdominal air is normal in the immediate postoperative period and usually resolves without treatment. Paracentesis can perforate a hollow organ.

III. **Differential diagnosis.** Pneumoperitoneum develops secondary to perforation of the GI tract, from an air leak from the chest, or postoperatively. In a neonate, unless the infant is on high ventilator settings and has air leak syndrome, **the cause is GI perforation until proven otherwise.** Identification of the cause directs treatment.
   A. **Pneumoperitoneum associated with GI perforation**
      1. **Spontaneous perforation (no underlying disease process or cause is present)** occurs most commonly in the stomach of a full-term neonate. In a preterm infant, the most common site is the jejunoileal area. However, isolated perforation can also occur elsewhere in the intestine of a term infant including the appendix and Meckel diverticulum. Isolated rupture at any level of the GI tract is associated with

oral or intravenous indomethacin. A meta-analysis of the effect of early treatment (<96 h) with high doses of steroids for chronic lung disease showed an increased risk of spontaneous GI perforation. An embolic phenomenon secondary to an umbilical artery catheter can also contribute to perforation. Ischemic necrosis secondary to asphyxia or shock may be another cause in the perinatal period.

2. **Secondary perforations (underlying disease process is present).** This group consists of GI perforations caused by an underlying disease process.

   a. **NEC is the most common cause of secondary perforation.** Data show varying results as to whether indomethacin for intraventricular hemorrhage prophylaxis increases spontaneous perforation and perforation with NEC.

   b. **Other causes.** Malrotation with volvulus (rare), meconium ileus, Hirschsprung disease, bowel atresia, omphalocele, ruptured appendix, mesenteric thrombosis, imperforate anus, strangulated hernia, malrotation with midgut volvulus, gastric and duodenal ulcer perforation, peptic ulcer disease complication, Meckel diverticulum, idiopathic gastric necrosis, and pneumatosis cystoides intestinalis.

3. **Traumatic perforations.** An iatrogenic pneumoperitoneum caused by an intervention by a health-care professional.

   a. **Neonatal rectal perforations.** These can be caused by a rectal thermometer or rectal tubes. Because of the shape of the neonatal rectum, when a rectal thermometer is placed to a depth of 2 cm, it impinges on the anterior wall. Any attempt to push it any further may result in perforation. Use of axillary thermometers eliminates this risk totally.

   b. **Nasogastric tube trauma during placement** can cause perforation and pneumoperitoneum.

   c. **Intubation trauma.** During an intubation attempt, the endotracheal tube can be inadvertently placed in the esophagus and then through the posterior wall of the stomach.

   d. **Improperly performed suprapubic bladder aspiration or paracentesis** perforating a hollow organ.

   e. **Normal transient finding following laparotomy or laparoscopy** is the most commonly identified cause of a pneumoperitoneum.

B. **Pneumoperitoneum associated with a respiratory disorder (eg, pneumomediastinum or pneumothorax).** A pulmonary air leak, with or without mechanical ventilation, can extend below the diaphragm resulting in a pneumoperitoneum.

C. **Benign neonatal pneumoperitoneum with no known cause.** There is no clear evidence of GI or respiratory pathology.

D. **"Mimicked" pneumoperitoneum.** A case report of transplacental passage of a nonionic contrast agent ioversol (Optiray) resulted in opacification of the fetal bowel that mimicked a pneumoperitoneum in the infant.

IV. **Database**

A. **Physical examination.** Perform a complete physical examination. Clinical evaluation may not help differentiate if the pneumoperitoneum is of respiratory or GI tract origin. The examination should focus on the pulmonary and abdominal aspects. Abdominal distention and elevation of the diaphragm with increasing respiratory difficulty is a hallmark of pneumoperitoneum. Feeding intolerance and poor activity can also be present.

B. **Laboratory studies**

   1. **Complete blood count and serum electrolyte levels.** Elevation of the white blood cell count or a left shift may signify a GI tract perforation. Hyponatremia can be seen with NEC secondary to third spacing of fluid. Thrombocytopenia also can be seen. These can also serve as preoperative laboratory levels if surgery is planned.

   2. **Arterial blood gas levels** may reveal hypoxemia and increasing PCO_2 levels. Metabolic acidosis can be seen with peritonitis.

C. **Radiologic and other studies.** Some findings can help confirm the diagnosis of free air ("football," "saddle bag," or "arcade sign") on an anterior-posterior supine radiograph of the abdomen, air over the liver on a lateral decubitus view or air below the diaphragm on an upright view. Simple observation of free air is often sufficient particularly if the air leak is large (see Figure 10–21).

1. **Anterior-posterior radiograph of the chest and abdomen.** The chest may show signs of air leak syndrome (pneumomediastinum or pneumothorax) if it is suspected that the intraperitoneal air is from the respiratory tract. The abdomen may show signs of NEC or ileus. Air-fluid levels in the peritoneal cavity usually indicate ileus. The following signs may be seen on a radiograph of a pneumoperitoneum:

   a. **Football sign** is a large oval radiolucency in the shape of an American football on a supine abdominal anteroposterior (AP) radiographic study. The **football sign** can also include when the falciform ligament is seen in the center as a vertical strip surrounded by gas.

   b. **Saddle bag sign** is when the spleen and liver are displaced downward toward the midline.

   c. **Arcade sign** is when air is seen between bowel loops and creates triangular shaped areas of gas.

2. **Lateral decubitus radiographic study of the abdomen** with the right side up is the best examination for the detection of free abdominal air; air (seen as a lucency) is seen over the liver if a perforation has occurred. This is also done to show smaller leaks not appreciated on the AP abdominal film. A lateral decubitus radiograph should be serially taken when NEC is suspected. Lateral decubitus studies showed to be more sensitive in detecting a pneumoperitoneum than upright view studies.

3. **Upright view of the chest abdomen will show air below the diaphragm.** Uprights are rarely done and are difficult to do in sick infants.

4. **Paracentesis.** Air obtained by paracentesis (see Chapter 33) may be tested for its oxygen level. If the oxygen level is high, the air is probably from a respiratory tract leak. If the oxygen if similar to room air or lower, the air is probably from the GI tract. Fluid may be obtained by paracentesis if the diagnosis is still undetermined. If green or brownish fluid is obtained, especially if bacterial are present on the Gram stain, the air is probably of GI tract origin. A microscopic smear of the fluid for white blood cells, which suggests peritonitis.

V. **Plan**

A. **Emergency measures.** Massive accumulation of air in the abdomen may causes respiratory compromise from an immobile diaphragm. In these cases, an emergency paracentesis must be done to reduce the pressure and allow the diaphragm to be mobile.(For the procedure see Chapter 33.)

B. **General measures.** Place a nasogastric tube with low suction.

C. **Specific measures**

   1. **Pneumoperitoneum of GI tract origin.** Unless the pneumoperitoneum is of a known iatrogenic origin (postoperative), **immediate surgical evaluation** is necessary. Exploratory laparotomy is often the treatment of choice, although in some stable patients only a drain is placed.

      a. **Preoperative laboratory values** should be available.

      b. **The infant should be stabilized** as much as possible before being taken to the operating room.

      c. **The surgical team may request a study with a water-soluble contrast medium given through the nasogastric tube** to try to localize the perforation (see Section V, C, 4).

   2. **Pneumoperitoneum of respiratory tract origin.** The pulmonary air leak should be treated.

      a. **For asymptomatic patients,** observation is often the treatment of choice, with follow-up radiographic studies usually performed every 8–12 h but more frequently if the patient's clinical course changes.

   b. For symptomatic patients, emergency paracentesis can be performed. Treatment of coexisting pneumothorax is required if present. Review the ventilator settings to avoid high pressures that will contribute to the problems.
   3. **Traumatic pneumoperitoneum**
      a. Pneumoperitoneum caused by rectal thermometers, suprapubic bladder aspiration, attempted intubation, or paracentesis may require surgical exploration.
      b. Post laparotomy or laparoscopy pneumoperitoneum associated with an uncomplicated surgical procedure will resolve spontaneously.
   4. **If the cause of the pneumoperitoneum is in doubt, a low-osmolality, water-soluble contrast medium (eg, metrizamide) can be given through a nasogastric tube.** If there is a pneumoperitoneum secondary to a GI perforation, contrast material will pass into the peritoneal cavity and confirm the diagnosis. **Barium should never be used because of the morbidity of barium peritonitis.**

63 Pneumothorax

 I. **Problem.** An infant may have a pneumothorax (an accumulation of air in the pleural space). An infant can develop a pneumothorax spontaneously or due to ventilator associated barotrauma.
 II. **Immediate questions**
    A. **Are symptoms of tension pneumothorax present? Tension pneumothorax presents as a medical emergency, and the patient's status will deteriorate acutely.** The following signs and symptoms may be seen with tension pneumothorax: cyanosis, hypoxia, tachypnea, a sudden decrease in heart rate with bradycardia, a sudden increase in systolic blood pressure followed by narrowing pulse pressure and hypotension, an asymmetric chest (bulging on the affected side), distention of the abdomen (secondary to downward displacement of the diaphragm), decreased breath sounds on the affected side, and shift of the cardiac apical impulse (most consistent finding) away from the affected side. A cyanotic upper half of the body with a pale lower half can be seen.
    B. **Is the patient asymptomatic?** A spontaneous pneumothorax occurs in 0.7% of newborns. An asymptomatic pneumothorax is present in 1–2% of neonates. Most of these cases are discovered on chest radiograph at admission. Up to 15% of these infants were meconium stained at birth.
    C. **Is mechanical ventilation being used?** The incidence of pneumothorax in patients receiving positive-pressure ventilation is 15–30%. A life-threatening tension pneumothorax may result from mechanical ventilation.
 III. **Differential diagnosis.** The incidence is higher in those with respiratory distress syndrome (up to 40%). The rates of pneumothorax are declining due to the use of surfactant and improved ventilator management.
    A. **Pneumothorax**
       1. **Symptomatic** pneumothorax (includes tension pneumothorax).
       2. **Asymptomatic** pneumothorax.
       3. **Persistent** pneumothorax.
    B. **Pneumomediastinum.** Air in the mediastinal space that may be confused with a true pneumothorax.
    C. **Congenital lobar emphysema.** Overdistention of one lobe secondary to air trapping occurs most commonly (47%) in the left upper lobe. Other lobe involvement is right

upper lobe (20%), right middle lobe (28%), and lower lobes (rare). The causes of congenital lobar emphysema are probably multifactorial.
  D. **Atelectasis with compensatory hyperinflation.** Compensatory hyperinflation may appear as a pneumothorax on a chest radiograph.
  E. **Pneumopericardium.** In neonates, **pneumopericardium** and **tension pneumothorax** can **both present as sudden and rapid clinical deterioration.** In pneumopericardium, the blood pressure drops, heart sounds are distant or absent, and pulses are muffled or absent. Massive abdominal distention can also be seen. In tension pneumothorax, the blood pressure may initially increase, but then hypotension follows. The chest radiograph easily differentiates the two. A pneumopericardium has a halo of air around the heart (see Figure 10–17). **The more common event is a tension pneumothorax.** If one is unsure and time does not permit radiographic verification, it is better to insert a needle in the chest on the suspected side. If no response, then a needle should be inserted on the other side. If there is still no response, then the diagnosis of pneumopericardium should be considered.
  F. **Congenital cystic adenomatoid malformation.** This rare abnormality results from abnormal embryogenesis. An overgrowth of bronchioles occurs with a decrease in alveolar growth. The infants present with respiratory distress ranging from minor to severe. Tachypnea and cyanosis can be presenting signs that are similar to a pneumothorax. Many of these are detected on ultrasound prenatally. A chest radiograph usually identifies the mass containing air-filled cysts. Rarely a computed tomography scan is needed. (See Chapter 121.)
IV. **Clinical findings**
  A. **Physical examination.** Perform a thorough examination of the chest. Specific findings are discussed in Section II, A. Transillumination is a useful rapid bedside technique in neonates (see Section IV, C).
  B. **Laboratory studies.** Blood gas levels may show decreased PaO_2 and increased PCO_2, with resultant respiratory acidosis.
  C. **Radiologic and other studies**
    1. **Transillumination** of the chest is a rapid bedside method to define the pneumothorax. The room lights are lowered, and a fiberoptic transilluminator is placed along the posterior axillary line on the side on which pneumothorax is suspected. If a pneumothorax is present, the chest "lights up" on that side. The transilluminator may be moved up and down along the posterior axillary line and may also be placed above the nipple. Transilluminate both sides of the chest, and then compare the results. If severe subcutaneous edema is present, transillumination may be falsely positive. Premature infants with pulmonary interstitial emphysema may also have a false-positive transillumination. Large infants with thick chest walls do not transilluminate well. **Always verify the diagnosis of pneumothorax by a chest radiograph if time permits.**
    2. **Chest radiographs** are the method of choice for diagnosing pneumothorax. Early pneumothoraces are difficult to diagnose. Early on, one can see separation of lung from the chest wall with no lung markings in that space The following films will help in making the diagnosis:
      a. **Anteroposterior (AP) view** (see Figure 10–19) of the chest will show the following:
        i. **A shift of the mediastinum** away from the side of pneumothorax (with tension pneumothorax).
        ii. **Depression of the diaphragm** on the side of the pneumothorax (with tension pneumothorax).
        iii. **Displacement of the lung** on the affected side away from the chest wall by a radiolucent band of air.
      b. **Cross-table lateral view** will show a rim of air around the lung ("pancaking"). It will *not* help to identify the affected side. **You must have an AP film to identify what side the pneumothorax is on.** This film must be considered together with the AP view to identify the involved side.

        c. **Lateral decubitus view (shot through the AP position)** will detect even a small pneumothorax not seen on a routine chest radiograph. The infant should be positioned so the side of the suspected pneumothorax is up (eg, if pneumothorax is suspected on the left side, the film is taken with the left side up).

V. Plan

  A. Symptomatic (tension) pneumothorax is an emergency! A 1- to 2-min delay could be fatal. If a tension pneumothorax is suspected, act immediately. It is better to treat in this setting, even if it turns out that there is no pneumothorax. There is no time for x-ray confirmation. If the patient's status is deteriorating rapidly, a needle or catheter over needle can be placed for aspiration, followed by formal chest tube placement. There is no specific sign that distinguishes a tension from a nontension pneumothorax. Signs of a tension pneumothorax from above can also occur in a nontension pneumothorax. Just remember that in a tension pneumothorax there is an ongoing cardiopulmonary deterioration as a result of the progressive increase in intrathoracic pressure.

    1. **Needle aspiration.** A needle aspiration can be done as an emergency. Often times this is all that is necessary if the infant is not being ventilated. This can also be done before placing a chest tube.

      a. **The site of puncture** should be at the second or third intercostal space along the midclavicular line. Cleanse this area with antibacterial solution.

      b. **Connect a 21-, 23- or 25-gauge scalp vein needle** or a 22- or 24-gauge catheter over needle to a 20-mL syringe with a stopcock attached. Have an assistant hold the syringe and withdraw the air.

      c. **Palpate the third rib at the midclavicular line.** Insert the needle above the rib, and advance it until air is withdrawn from the syringe. The needle may be removed before the chest tube is placed if the infant is relatively stable, or it may be left in place for continuous aspiration while the chest tube is being placed. If an Angiocath is used, the needle can be removed and the catheter left in place.

    2. **Chest tube placement** is discussed in Chapter 26. This is necessary in infants on mechanical ventilation.

  B. Asymptomatic pneumothorax

    1. **If positive-pressure mechanical ventilation is the cause of asymptomatic pneumothorax,** a chest tube will probably need to be inserted because the ventilator pressure will prevent resolution of the pneumothorax, and tension pneumothorax may develop. Sometimes needle aspiration is all that is needed. If a pneumothorax develops in a patient who is ready to be extubated, clinical judgment must be used in deciding whether a chest tube should be placed.

    2. **If positive-pressure mechanical ventilation is not being administered,** one of two treatments may be used.

      a. **Close observation with follow-up chest radiographs** every 8–12 h or sooner if the infant becomes symptomatic. The pneumothorax will probably resolve within 24–48 h.

      b. **For more rapid resolution of the pneumothorax** in the asymptomatic patient, give the infant 100% oxygen for 8–12 h, a procedure known as ***nitrogen washout therapy.*** Less nitrogen is able to enter the lungs, and at the same time absorption of nitrogen from the extrapleural space is increased and then exhaled. The total gas tension is decreased, which also facilitates absorption of nitrogen by the blood. The method should be used only in full-term infants in whom retinopathy of prematurity will not be a problem. Some institutions do not routinely give 100% FIO_2.

  C. Persistent pneumothorax (generally defined as a pneumothorax that persists >7 days in the absence of mechanical problems). Sometimes infants who have chest tubes still have air leaks that persist for greater than a week. The majority of these infants have episodes of instability when they reaccumulate air, requiring a new or replacement chest tube and an increase in their ventilator settings. The reason to treat these is to decrease the risk associated with air leaks (air embolus, hypotension, intracranial hemorrhage). There have been reports of treating these with fibrin glue (such as CryoSeal C; ThermoGenesis Corp., Rancho Cordova, CA) in neonates. It was injected in the chest tube with a marked reduction in the air leak. One report used fibrin glue in a 790-g premature infant with no complications. In another study, eight newborns were treated. Six had complete resolution or reduction within 24 h, and two received a second course. Seven of them were <1500 g. Risks include hypercalcemia, localized tissue necrosis, bradycardia, diaphragmatic paralysis, and pneumothorax on the contralateral side. More studies are needed before this treatment can be routinely recommended. This technique is used in adults.

D. **Pneumomediastinum** may progress to a pneumothorax or pneumopericardium. Close observation is required.

E. **Congenital lobar emphysema**
   1. **Asymptomatic.** Conservative management with observation is advocated.
   2. **Symptomatic.** If respiratory failure is occurring, the treatment is usually surgical excision of the affected lobe.

F. **Atelectasis with compensatory hyperinflation**
   1. Chest physiotherapy and postural drainage should be initiated. Chest physiotherapy should be used with caution in premature infants. A study showed an association with intraventricular hemorrhage and porencephaly in extreme premature infants.
   2. Treatment with bronchodilators is indicated. See Chapter 7.
   3. Positioning the infant with the affected (hyperinflated) side down may speed resolution.

G. **Pneumopericardium** should be treated emergently by pericardiocentesis (see Chapter 34).

H. **Cystic adenomatoid malformation.** Surgery is the treatment of choice. Fetal surgery is reported prenatally, and resection of the cyst can be done postnatally.

64 Polycythemia

I. **Problem.** The hematocrit (Hct) is 68% in a newborn. The upper limit of a normal Hct for a newborn peripheral venous sample is 65%. Polycythemia occurs in 0.4–12% of newborn infants and is rare in premature infants <34 weeks' gestation.

II. **Immediate questions**
   A. **What is the central hematocrit (Hct)?** In blood obtained by heelstick, the Hct may be falsely elevated by 5–15%. Treatment should **never** be initiated based on heelstick Hct values alone; a central (peripheral venous phlebotomy) Hct is needed. If the sample is from the umbilical vein or radial artery, the upper limit of normal is 63%.
   B. **Does the infant have symptoms of polycythemia?** Many infants with polycythemia are asymptomatic. One study found that feeding problems and lethargy were the most common symptoms. There are many symptoms and signs of polycythemia, which can include the following:
      1. **Central nervous system.** Lethargy, hypotonia, irritability, jitteriness, weak sucking reflex, vomiting, seizures, tremulousness, apnea, sleepiness, exaggerated startle, cerebrovascular accidents.

2. **Cardiovascular.** Heart murmurs, congestive heart failure, cyanosis, plethora, tachycardia, cardiomegaly.

3. **Respiratory.** Respiratory distress, tachypnea, cyanosis.

4. **Gastrointestinal.** Poor feeding, poor suck, vomiting, necrotizing enterocolitis (NEC).

5. **Renal.** Proteinuria, oliguria, hematuria, renal vein thrombosis.

6. **Hematologic.** Thrombocytopenia, hepatosplenomegaly, thrombosis, disseminated intravascular coagulation (rare), elevated reticulocyte count.

7. **Metabolic.** Hypoglycemia (12–40%), hypocalcemia (1–11%), increased jaundice (hyperbilirubinemia).

8. **Skin.** Plethora or ruddiness.

9. **Miscellaneous.** Testicular infarcts, priapism.

C. **Is the mother diabetic?** Poor maternal control of diabetes during pregnancy leads to chronic fetal hypoxia, which may result in increased neonatal erythropoiesis. Infants of diabetic mothers have a 25–40% incidence of polycythemia. Infants of mothers with gestational diabetes also have an increased incidence (30%) of polycythemia.

D. **What is the infant's age?** The Hct normally rises after birth and reaches a peak at 2 h of age and then slowly decreases. After 48 h of age, hemoconcentration as a result of dehydration may be present.

E. **Is the infant dehydrated?** Dehydration may cause hemoconcentration, resulting in a high Hct. It usually occurs in infants >48 h old.

F. **Does the mother live at a high altitude?** Infants born to mothers at high altitudes have a higher incidence of polycythemia.

G. **Is the infant small or large for gestational age?** Polycythemia is more common in these infants.

III. **Differential diagnosis.** See also Chapter 112.

A. **Falsely elevated Hct.** This finding occurs most often when blood is obtained by heelstick.

B. **Dehydration.** Weight loss and decreased urine output are sensitive indicators of dehydration. Hemoconcentration secondary to dehydration is suspected if >8–10% of the birthweight has been lost. It usually occurs on the second or third day of life.

C. **True polycythemia**

1. **Placental transfusion (hypertransfusion)** occurs with delayed cord clamping (defined as clamping the cord >3 min after delivery of the infant), twin-twin transfusion, maternal–fetal blood transfusion, stripping the cord, and holding the infant below the mother at delivery. Intrapartum asphyxia can cause blood volume to shift from the placenta to the fetus and cause polycythemia.

2. **Iatrogenic polycythemia** is caused by overtransfusion.

3. **Intrauterine hypoxia** may be caused by placental insufficiency. It may be seen in postmature, intrauterine growth restricted, or small for gestational age infants, preeclampsia/eclampsia, and infants with perinatal asphyxia. Maternal smoking, chronic or recurrent abruptio placentae, maternal hypertension, and severe maternal heart, pulmonary or primary renovascular disease may also cause intrauterine hypoxia. Severe maternal diabetes can cause reduced placental blood flow. A pregnancy at a high altitude can also cause this.

4. **Other causes**

   a. **Chromosomal abnormalities** such as Down syndrome and trisomies 13 and 18.

   b. **Beckwith-Wiedemann syndrome.**

   c. **Thyroid disorders.** Neonatal thyrotoxicosis and congenital hypothyroidism.

   d. **Congenital adrenal hyperplasia.**

   e. **Infant of a diabetic mother** has a 22–29% incidence of polycythemia. This occurs with gestational and insulin-dependent diabetes and is due to increased erythropoiesis.

   f. **Maternal use of propranolol.**

5. **Idiopathic.** No specific cause found.

IV. **Database**
   A. **Physical examination.** Evaluate for possible dehydration. The mucous membranes will be dry. Increased skin turgor is usually not seen. True polycythemia is often, but not always, associated with visible skin changes. Ruddiness, plethora, or "pink-on-blue" or "blue-on-pink" coloration may be evident. In males, priapism may be seen secondary to sludging of red blood cells. Clinical signs are listed in Section II, B.
   B. **Laboratory studies**
     1. **Central Hct is essential.**
     2. **Serum glucose.** Hypoglycemia is commonly seen with polycythemia.
     3. **Serum bilirubin.** Infants with polycythemia can have problems with hyperbilirubinemia because of the increased turnover of red blood cells.
     4. **Sodium and blood urea nitrogen** should be obtained if dehydration is being considered. They are usually high, or higher than baseline values, if dehydration is present.
     5. **Urine specific gravity** >1.015 is usually seen with dehydration.
     6. **Blood gas** should be obtained to rule out inadequate oxygenation.
     7. **Platelet count.** Thrombocytopenia can accompany polycythemia.
     8. **Calcium.** Hypocalcemia can also be seen (less common).
   C. **Radiologic and other studies.** These studies are usually not indicated. Cardiomegaly, increased pulmonary vascular markings, and pleural effusions may be seen on a chest radiography. An abnormal electrocardiogram (ECG) and electroencephalogram can be seen, but these tests are not routinely indicated. An ECG can show right ventricular hypertrophy and right and left atrial hypertrophy. Echocardiogram can show increased pulmonary resistance and decreased cardiac output.
V. **Plan.** See also Chapter 112.
   A. **Preventive measures.** One study found that with early cord clamping (clamping within 10 s vs clamping within 11–120 s) of high-risk infants, these infants had fewer manifestations of polycythemia. This may be an effective way to prevent polycythemia in at-risk infants. Another study found that delayed cord clamping at 30–45 s (when compared with immediate cord clamping at 5–10 s) of infants <1500 g did not increase polycythemia rates, but the infants did have higher bilirubin levels. Holding the infant at the level of the introitus at the time of delivery may help minimize the maternal-to-fetal transfusion.
   B. **Falsely elevated Hct (>65%).** If the confirmatory central Hct is normal, no further evaluation is needed. If the central Hct is high, either dehydration or true polycythemia is present (for treatment, see Sections V, C and D).
   C. **Hemoconcentration secondary to dehydration.** If the infant is dehydrated but does not have symptoms or signs of polycythemia, a trial of rehydration over 6–8 h can be attempted. The type of fluid used depends on the infant's age and serum electrolyte status and is discussed in Chapter 8. Usually, 130–150 mL/kg/day is given. The Hct is checked every 6 h and usually decreases with adequate rehydration.
   D. **True polycythemia.** Treatment is usually based on whether or not the infant is symptomatic.
     1. **Asymptomatic infants**
       a. **Central Hct of 65–70%.** If the central Hct is 65–70% and the infant is asymptomatic, only observation may be needed. Many of these patients respond to increased fluid therapy; increases of 20–40 mL/kg/day can be attempted. The central Hct must be checked every 6 h. The Hct normally reaches a peak at 2–4 h of age. If the Hct is 70% at birth, it may be 5–10% higher at 2–4 h of age.
       b. **Central Hct of 70–75%.** If the Hct is 70–75% and the infant is asymptomatic, *controversy* exists as to whether an exchange transfusion should be done. Hydration can be considered. It is best to follow your institutional guidelines.
       c. **Central Hct >75%.** Most neonatologists agree that a partial exchange transfusion should be given, although some *controversy* exists. Institutional guidelines should be followed.

2. **Symptomatic infants**
    a. **Central Hct >65%** in the symptomatic infant. Partial exchange transfusion should be performed (*controversial*). To calculate the volume that must be exchanged, use the following formula (blood volume = 80 mL/kg):

    $$\text{Volume exchanged (mL)} = \frac{(\text{Weight [kg]} \_ \text{Blood volume}) \_ (\text{Hct of patient} - \text{Desired Hct})}{\text{Hct of patient}}$$

    Desired Hct is usually <60, with a goal of bringing it down to 50–55. Partial exchange transfusion may be administered via an umbilical venous catheter. **Care must be taken not to place the catheter in the liver** (see Chapter 38). A low umbilical artery catheter or a peripheral intravenous catheter can also be used. The fluid that can be used for a partial exchange transfusion is Plasmanate, 5% albumin, normal saline, or fresh-frozen plasma (FFP). FFP is usually not recommended because of the risk of HIV transmission, and there is also a risk of infection with Plasmanate and 5% albumin. The decision about which fluid to use depends on a particular institutional preference. Most often, **normal saline is preferred in most institutions.** One study noted that both normal saline and albumin can be used and are effective, but normal saline should be the replacement fluid of choice because it is less costly and infection free. Serial Hct levels should be obtained after transfusion. The partial exchange transfusion procedure is discussed in detail in Chapter 29. **Use these guidelines when performing a partial exchange transfusion:**
        i. Aliquots should not exceed 5 mL/kg and should be removed or delivered over 2–3 min.
        ii. If there is both an umbilical artery catheter (UAC) and umbilical venous catheter (UVC), withdraw blood from the UAC while giving the replacement fluid through the UVC.
        iii. If only a UVC is in place, use the push-pull method: pull out the blood, and then push in the replacement fluid. **Never remove >5 mL/kg.**
        iv. If you have a UVC, UAC, and peripheral venous catheter in, you can use either the UVC or UAC for blood withdrawal and then use the peripheral line for replacement fluid.
3. **Symptoms with a central Hct of 60–65%.** If all other disease entities are ruled out, these infants may indeed be polycythemic and hyperviscous. In these cases, management is *controversial.* Use clinical judgment and institutional guidelines to decide whether or not this infant should have a partial exchange transfusion.
E. **Observe for complications of polycythemia** and disorders that are more common in polycythemic infants.
    1. **Hyperbilirubinemia.**
    2. **Seizures.**
    3. **Necrotizing enterocolitis (NEC)** risk is increased in neonates with hyperviscosity who received a partial exchange transfusion via an UVC with colloid (FFP, albumin, Plasmanate). Recent data suggest that the development of NEC in these infants may be related to partial exchange transfusion with colloid, not the polycythemia.
    4. **Ileus.**
    5. **Renal failure.**
    6. **Peripheral gangrene.**
    7. **Hypocalcemia.**
    8. **Renal vein/Cerebral vein thrombosis.**
    9. **Congestive heart failure.**
    10. **Testicular infarcts/priapism.**

11. **Spontaneous intestinal perforations and intestinal atresia** were also found to be increased in infants with polycythemia.
12. **Stroke.**
13. **Vasospasms.**
F. **Long term follow-up data** (*controversial*)
1. **Note that a partial exchange transfusion decreases viscosity** and ameliorates most symptoms but does not significantly affect or improve long-term neurologic outcomes.
2. **Decreased IQ scores and lower achievement** were reported in infants with hyperviscosity syndrome who had been treated and had not been treated with partial exchange transfusion.
3. **In a study that compared** partial exchange–treated infants with symptomatic polycythemia versus asymptomatic infants who were grouped to either be observed or treated, outcome of the groups was no different. What did affect long-term outcome was perinatal risk factors and race, not polycythemia or partial plasma exchange transfusion.
4. **Recent reviews of short- and long-term outcomes** following partial exchange transfusion in the polycythemic infant found:
   a. **There is no evidence of improvement** in long-term neurologic outcome following partial exchange transfusion in symptomatic or asymptomatic infants.
   b. **There is no evidence of improvement** in early neurobehavioral assessment scores.
   c. **Partial exchange transfusion may be associated** with an earlier improvement in symptoms.
   d. **Partial exchange transfusion increases** the risk of gastrointestinal tract disorders and NEC.
5. **Polycythemic infants are at risk** for speech abnormalities and for fine and gross motor delays.
6. **Umbilical partial exchange transfusion with colloid** increases the risk of NEC.
7. **Recent data suggest** that the cause of impaired long-term outcome is also the cause of polycythemia, both being related with intrauterine fetal hypoxia.

65 Poor Perfusion

I. **Problem.** You receive a report that an infant "doesn't look good" or looks "mottled." Other descriptions may include "a washed-out appearance" or "poor perfusion."
II. **Immediate questions**
   A. **What is the age of the infant?** Hypoplastic left heart syndrome may cause poor perfusion and a mottled appearance. It may be seen at days 1–21 of life (more commonly at day 2 or 3). In an infant <3 days old, sepsis may be a cause. Associated risk factors for sepsis are premature rupture of membranes, maternal infection, and fever.
   B. **What are the vital signs?** If the temperature is lower than normal, cold stress or hypothermia associated with sepsis may be present. Hypotension may cause poor perfusion (see normal blood pressure values in Appendix C). Decreased urine output (<2 mL/kg/h) may indicate depleted intravascular volume or shock.
   C. **Is the liver enlarged? Is there metabolic acidosis, poor peripheral pulse rate, and a gallop present?** These problems are signs of failure of the left side of the heart (eg, hypoplastic left heart syndrome). Poor perfusion occurs because of reduced blood flow to the skin.

D. **If mechanical ventilation is being used, are chest movements adequate and are blood gas levels improving?** Inadequate ventilation can result in poor perfusion. Pneumothorax may also be a cause.

E. **Are congenital anomalies present?** Persistent cutis marmorata (see definition later) may be seen in Cornelia de Lange syndrome and in trisomies 18 and 21. **Chromosome 22q11 deletion syndrome** can present with abnormal vascular tone with hypotension; 75% of these infants have congenital heart defects. **Cornelia de Lange syndrome** consists of multiple congenital anomalies: a distinctive facial appearance, pre- and postnatal growth deficiency, feeding problems, psychomotor delay, behavioral problems, and malformations that mainly involve the upper extremities.

III. **Differential diagnosis**

A. **More common causes**

1. **Sepsis.**
2. **Cold stress,** in general, a skin temperature <36.5°C.
3. **Hypotension,** usually with shock.
4. **Hypoventilation.**
5. **Pneumothorax.**
6. **Necrotizing enterocolitis (NEC).**
7. **Left-sided heart lesions** such as hypoplastic left heart syndrome, coarctation of the aorta, and aortic stenosis.
8. **Cutis marmorata,** a marbling pattern of the skin (the infant appears poorly perfused). May occur in a healthy infant, especially when exposed to cold stress and with other congenital syndromes (Cornelia de Lange syndrome, trisomies 18 [Edwards syndrome] and 21 [Down syndrome]). Persistent mottling can also be seen in hypothyroidism and (CNS) dysfunction.

B. **Less common causes**

1. **Enteroviral infection** presents as overwhelming sepsis.
2. **Periventricular hemorrhage-intraventricular hemorrhage (PVH-IVH).** Presentation varies but can present with extreme signs including sudden onset of poor perfusion, pallor, and hypotonia.
3. **Subgaleal hemorrhage.** Case report of an infant presenting with poor perfusion.
4. **Inborn errors of metabolism.**
5. **Seizures.**
6. **Hematologic.** Bleeding disorders, polycythemia.
7. **Adrenal problems.** Congenital adrenal hyperplasia, Addison disease, adrenal hemorrhage.
8. **Renovascular hypertension.**
9. **Intestinal problems.**

IV. **Database**

A. **Physical examination.** Note the temperature and vital signs. Look for signs of sepsis. The cardiovascular and pulmonary examinations are important because they may suggest cardiac problems or pneumothorax. Signs of trisomy 18 include micrognathia and overlapping digits. Signs of trisomy 21 include a single palmar transverse crease and epicanthal folds.

B. **Laboratory studies**

1. **Complete blood count with differential** to evaluate for sepsis or decreased hematocrit.
2. **Blood gas levels.** These studies reveal inadequate ventilation or the presence of acidosis, which may be seen in sepsis or NEC.
3. **Cultures.** If sepsis is suspected, a complete workup should be considered, especially if antibiotics are to be started. This workup includes cultures of blood, urine, and spinal fluid (if indicated). If enteroviral infection is suspected, send for viral cultures.
4. **Polymerase chain reaction (PCR)** studies of stool, cerebrospinal fluid, nasopharyngeal or throat swab for enterovirus.

C. **Radiologic and other studies**
   1. **Transillumination of the chest** (see Chapter 26, Section III, A) can be performed quickly to help determine whether or not a pneumothorax is present.
   2. **Chest radiograph** if pneumonia, pneumothorax, congenital heart lesion, or hypoventilation is suspected. In left-sided heart lesions, the radiograph shows cardiomegaly with pulmonary venous congestion (except in hypoplastic left heart syndrome, in which the size of the heart may be normal). If a view taken during lung expansion shows that the lungs are down only to the sixth rib or less, hypoventilation should be considered. With hyperventilation, lung expansion is down to the ninth or tenth rib. See Figure 10–14 for radiograph of pneumonia. See Figure 10–19 for radiograph showing a pneumothorax.
   3. **Abdominal radiograph** if NEC is suspected. See Figure 10–22 for a radiograph showing pneumatosis intestinalis seen in NEC.
   4. **Echocardiography** should be performed if a congenital heart lesion is suspected. In hypoplastic left heart syndrome, a large right ventricle and a small left ventricle are seen on the echocardiogram, and there is failure to visualize the mitral or aortic valve. In aortic stenosis, the echocardiogram reveals a deformed aortic valve. In coarctation of the aorta, it reveals decreased aortic diameter.
   5. **Karyotyping or molecular genetic testing** if trisomy 18 or 21 or a deletion is suspected. Cornelia de Lange syndrome has mutations in the NIPBL and SMC3 genes.
V. **Plan**
   A. **General plan.** An initial quick workup should be performed. While checking vital signs and quickly examining the patient, order a STAT blood gas and a chest radiograph. Initiate oxygen supplementation and transilluminate the chest if a pneumothorax is suspected.
   B. **Specific plans**
      1. **Sepsis.** Full cultures and empirical antibiotic therapy may be started at the discretion of the physician.
      2. **Cold stress.** Gradual rewarming is necessary, usually at a rate of $\leq 1°C/h$. It can be accomplished by means of a radiant warmer or incubator or a heating pad. (See Chapter 6.)
      3. **Hypotension or shock.** If the blood pressure is low because of depleted intravascular volume, give crystalloid (normal saline), 10 mL/kg intravenously for 5–10 min. (See Chapter 58.)
      4. **Hypoventilation.** If hypoventilation is suspected, it may be necessary to increase the pressure being given by the ventilator. The amount of pressure must be decided on an individual basis. One method is to increase the pressure by 2–4 cm H_2O and then obtain blood gas levels in 20 min. Another method is to use bag-and-mask ventilation, observing the manometer to determine the amount of pressure needed to move the chest.
      5. **Pneumothorax.** See Chapter 63.
      6. **Necrotizing enterocolitis (NEC).** See Chapter 104.
      7. **Left-sided heart lesions.** Treat with oxygen, possibly diuretics and digoxin if congestive heart failure is present, and infusion of prostaglandin E_1. Surgery is usually indicated in all these patients. Options for hypoplastic left heart syndrome include supportive therapy, a three-staged reconstruction, or cardiac transplantation. For a full discussion of cardiac abnormalities, see Chapter 81.
      8. **Cutis marmorata.** If this condition is secondary to cold stress, treat the patient as described in Section V, B, 2. If the condition persists, consider formal genetic testing for various syndromes noted. Thyroid studies will be necessary if hypothyroidism is suspected. If CNS dysfunction is suspected, this should be evaluated further.
      9. **Periventricular hemorrhage-intraventricular hemorrhage (PVH-IVH).** Initial supportive care (maintain blood pressure, stabilize blood gases, transfuse if necessary, treat for seizures, etc.). After stabilization, close follow up is required. Serial LPs may be necessary. See also Chapter 96.

10. **Subgaleal hemorrhage.** Early recognition, appropriate resuscitation, supportive care as in volume replacement, blood transfusion, and coagulation factors if necessary. Wrapping of the head is *controversial.*

11. **Inborn errors of metabolism.** See Chapter 93.

12. **Seizures.** See Chapter 116.

13. **Hematologic problems.** Blood transfusions and diagnosing and treating the specific bleeding disorder are necessary.

14. **Adrenal insufficiency.** Blood volume replacement and steroid therapy are usually necessary.

15. **Renovascular hypertension.** Usually treated with aggressive medical management as outlined in Chapter 54.

16. **Intestinal problems.** See Chapter 120.

17. **Enteroviral infections.** Supportive management. (See Chapter 83.)

66 Postdelivery Antibiotics

I. **Problem.** Two infants are born within the last hour. One infant's mother had premature rupture of membranes (ROM) but no antibiotics. The other infant's mother was pretreated with antibiotics for a positive group B streptococcus (GBS) culture taken at 36 weeks. Should a sepsis workup be done, and should antibiotics be started in either of these newborns? The incidence of sepsis is 1 in 10 in 1000 live births and 1 in 250 live premature births. **This section focuses on postdelivery antibiotics for early-onset sepsis** because late infections of premature infants with prolonged hospital stays may require a different workup and antibiotic choice.

II. **Immediate questions**

A. **Are there any maternal risk factors for sepsis in the infant?** Risk factors include African race, malnutrition in the mother, maternal colonization with GBS organism, recently acquired sexually transmitted diseases, and maternal age <20 years. Low socioeconomic status and asymptomatic bacteriuria in the mother are associated with increased prematurity and sepsis. Maternal history of a previous infant with GBS infection also increases the risk of sepsis for the unborn infant.

B. **Are there intrapartum risk factors for sepsis in the infant?** These include ROM >18 h, chorioamnionitis (defined as sustained fetal tachycardia, uterine tenderness, purulent amniotic fluid, unexplained maternal temperature ≥38.0°C (>100.4°F), any untreated or incompletely treated infection of the mother, and maternal fever without identifiable cause. The use of fetal scalp electrodes in the intrapartum period increases the risk of infection in the infant. Perinatal asphyxia (defined as a 5-min Apgar score <6) with prolonged ROM also increases the risk of infection in the neonate.

C. **Are there any neonatal risk factors involved?** Neonatal risk factors include male sex, twin birth, prematurity (<37 weeks), low birthweight (<2500 g), and presence of the metabolic disorder galactosemia that increases risk of Gram-negative sepsis.

D. **How long before delivery did the membranes rupture?** ROM that occurs >18 h before birth is associated with an increased incidence of infection in the neonate.

E. **Was the infant monitored during labor?** Fetal tachycardia (>160 beats/min), especially sustained, and decelerations (usually late) can be associated with neonatal infection. Prolonged duration of intrauterine monitoring is a risk factor for early-onset group B streptococcal disease.

F. **Did the mother have a cerclage for cervical incompetence?** Cerclage increases the risk of infection in the infant.

G. **Are signs of sepsis present in the infant?** Signs of sepsis include apnea and bradycardia, temperature instability (hypothermia or hyperthermia), feeding intolerance, tachypnea, jaundice, cyanosis, poor peripheral perfusion, hypoglycemia, lethargy, poor sucking reflex, increased gastric aspirates, and irritability. Other signs include tachycardia, shock, vomiting, seizures, abnormal rash, abdominal distention, and hepatomegaly.

H. **Did the mother have epidural analgesia?** Studies have shown an increase in maternal intrapartum fever with the use of epidural analgesia. Because of this fever, an increase in sepsis evaluations and antibiotic treatment was found. However, the study did not find that epidurals caused infections or even increased the risk of infections.

I. **Was the mother tested for GBS, and did she receive antibiotics if she tested positive?** There are now specific guidelines to follow after delivery if the mother was treated for GBS.

III. **Differential diagnosis**

A. **Infant at increased risk for sepsis.** The factors noted previously can increase the risk of sepsis.

B. **Infant at low risk for sepsis.** Newborns without risk factors noted previously are at low risk of sepsis.

IV. **Database**

A. **Complete maternal, perinatal, and birth history** should be obtained and reviewed in an attempt to identify risk factors. Maternal history is just as important as the birth history.

B. **Physical examination.** Perform a complete physical examination, observing for signs of sepsis (see Section II, G). ***Note:* Clinical observation is important.** One study found that affect, peripheral perfusion, and respiratory status were key predictors in sepsis compared with feeding patterns, level of activity, and level of alertness. The maternal clinical examination should be reviewed with the OB/GYN service.

C. **Laboratory studies**

1. **Complete blood count (CBC) with differential.** An abnormally low or high white blood cell (WBC) count is worrisome. Values <6000 cells/mm^3 or >30,000 cells/mm^3 in the first 24 h of life are abnormal. A band neutrophil count >20% is abnormal. The total leukocyte count is a very unreliable indicator of neonatal infection. ***Note:* A normal WBC count does not rule out sepsis.** Normal WBC counts may be seen in as many as 50% of culture-proven sepsis cases. Only half of infants with WBC <5000 cells/mm^3 or WBC >20,000 cells/mm^3 have positive blood cultures (BCs). The total neutrophil count can be calculated, and normal reference ranges can be found in Tables 66–1 and 66–2. **A single WBC count is not very helpful.** A normal WBC is a better negative predictor for sepsis. **Repeat the WBC count** in 4–6 h. Repeating the WBC count helps increase the utility of the test when it is used to screen for sepsis.

2. **Peripheral blood cultures.** Antibiotic removal device bottles should be used if the mother has received any antibiotics.

3. **Suprapubic aspiration of urine for urinalysis and culture (*controversial*).** Many institutions do not perform this procedure in newborn infants with possible sepsis on day 1 of life because newborns rarely present with a urinary tract infection the first day.

4. **Lumbar puncture for cerebrospinal fluid (CSF) examination.** This procedure is ***controversial;*** some institutions perform a lumbar puncture only if the infant has a positive blood culture, is symptomatic, and will be treated with antibiotics or has signs of central nervous system infection.

5. **Maternal laboratory tests**

   a. **Maternal endocervical culture for GBS, chlamydia, and gonorrhea.**

   b. **Urine analysis and culture.**

   c. **Any other pertinent laboratory studies.**

Table 66–1. **NEONATAL NEUTROPHIL INDICES REFERENCE RANGES (per mm^3)**

Variable	Birth	12 h	24 h	48 h	72 h	>120 h
Absolute total neutrophil count[a]	1800–5400	7800–14,400	7200–12,600	4200–9000	1800–7000	1800–5400
Total immature neutrophil count[b]	<1120	<1440	<1280	<800	<500	<500
I:T ratio[c]	<0.16	<0.16	<0.13	<0.13	<0.13	<0.12

[a]Total count includes mature and immature forms.
[b]Includes all neutrophils except segmented ones.
[c]Ratio of total absolute neutrophil count divided by total immature neutrophil count.
Based on data from Manroe BL et al: The neonatal blood count in health and disease: I. Reference values for neutrophilic cells. *J Pediatr* 1979;95:89.

6. Baseline serum glucose.
7. Arterial blood gas.
8. **Antigen detection assays,** which include the latex agglutination test for GBS, counterimmunoelectrophoresis, and bacterial antigens (GBS, *Streptococcus pneumoniae,* and *Escherichia coli* are available). These tests can be performed on serum, urine, and CSF. Some laboratories do not offer these tests because of poor predictive value.
9. **Other laboratory tests used in the diagnose of sepsis.** None of the following tests should be used alone to diagnose sepsis. If used together, or **repeated values** become more abnormal, they may help in deciding which infant should receive antibiotics.
   a. **Absolute total neutrophil count** is more sensitive than the total leukocyte count but too often is normal in case of infection). See Tables 66–1 and 66–2.
   b. **Total immature neutrophil count** has poor sensitivity; could have a better positive predictive value. See Table 66–1.
   c. **Ratio of immature to total neutrophils (I:T).** The greatest value relies on good negative predictive value; likelihood of infection is minimal if I:T ratio is normal. See Table 66–1.
   d. **C-reactive protein (CRP).** This is a quantitative test with normal values ≤1 mg/dL. An increasing CRP is worrisome and is elevated in 50–90% of infants with sepsis. The main interest in CRP is its negative predictive value if repeated over 1–3 days.

Table 66–2. **REFERENCE RANGES FOR NEUTROPHIL COUNTS IN VERY LOW BIRTHWEIGHT INFANTS (<1500 g)**

Age	Absolute Total Neutrophil Count (mm^3) (min to max)
Birth	500–6000
18 h	2200–14,000
60 h	1100–8800
120 h	1100–5600

Based on data from Mouzinho A et al: Revised reference ranges for circulating neutrophils in very-low-birth-weight neonates. *Pediatrics* 1994;94:76.

  e. **Erythrocyte sedimentation rates** are increased with infection but have a very limited value in diagnosing or monitoring infection.

  f. **Gastric aspirate stain and culture** are of limited value in predicting sepsis. A recent review found no statistical correlation between gastric aspirate examinations and early onset of sepsis.

 10. **Laboratory tests that could be helpful in screening for sepsis but are not routinely used** because of their lack of availability, lack of studies, and wide variations in results:

  a. **Cytokines** regulate the inflammatory response. Many have been identified with sepsis: interleukin (IL-1, IL-6, IL-8), soluble IL-2 receptor, soluble intercellular adhesion molecule-1(ICAM-1), soluble tumor necrosis factor alpha (TNF-α) receptor, E-selectin, IL-1 receptor antagonist, granulocyte CSF (GCSF) and granulocyte macrophage colony-stimulating factor (GM-CSF). IL-6 has been studied the most. These tests are promising but not used routinely.

  b. **Acute phase reactants** have been used to identify infants with sepsis, with the most common being CRP (see Section IV, C, 9d). Other reactants include fibrinogen, fibronectin, ceruloplasmin, prealbumin, haptoglobin, orosomucoids, α-1 antitrypsin, and α-1 antichymotrypsin.

  c. **Procalcitonin, CRP IL-6, IL-8, TNF-α.** Using serial and multiple markers showed the best reliability for predicting sepsis. One study found PCT and TNF-α as the best markers in the diagnosis of sepsis. These can also be used to follow the effectiveness of treatment.

  d. **Cellular antigens.** CD11b and neutrophil CD64 are increased in sepsis.

  e. **Serum procalcitonin** levels are elevated in neonatal sepsis and a negative result is helpful in ruling out sepsis.

 D. **Radiologic studies.** With signs of respiratory infection, obtain a chest radiograph to rule out pneumonia.

V. **Plan**

 A. **General measures.** For the majority of cases, a decision about whether an infant requires a sepsis workup and antibiotics is usually straightforward. These infants either are clinically sick or have a positive history of an increased risk for sepsis and some clinical signs, thereby making the antibiotic decision easy. However, if an infant does not have a clear-cut history and clinical presentation, the decision is difficult. It is important to remember that one single test is often not helpful and to "repeat, repeat, and repeat" the test. Once the decision is made to treat the infant, treatment usually involves 48 h of antibiotics after obtaining cultures. The following guidelines can be used to help make the decision to treat:

  1. **Septic scoring systems.** Some institutions have devised their own septic scoring systems to help decide which infants should be treated. Many studies of scoring systems (using a combination of the laboratory tests mentioned previously) have shown that they all have limited value in screening for sepsis, with a negative panel being a better predictor than a positive panel.

  2. **Centers for Disease Control and Prevention (CDC) recommendations should be followed if possible.** (Prevention of Perinatal Group B Streptococcal Disease. *MMWR*;, 2002(51):RR-11. Available at http://www.cdc.gov/mmwr/PDF/rr/rr5111.pdf. Accessed February 1, 2009). If not possible, other guidelines can be recommended but are not based on sufficient data. In these situations, it is best to follow your institutions recommendations. The CDC now requires universal prenatal screening for vaginal and rectal GBS of all pregnant women at 35–37 weeks. **The following are CDC recommendations for management of a newborn whose mother received intrapartum antimicrobial agents.** (See Figure 117–1.)

   a. **Management of a newborn whose mother received intrapartum antimicrobial agents:**

i. **If the mother received antibiotics for suspected chorioamniotic.** The infant should receive a full diagnostic evaluation (CBC, BCs, chest radiograph, and if clinical sepsis present, lumbar puncture) and receive antibiotics. Duration of treatment depends on results of the septic evaluation and the clinical course. If cultures are negative and there are no signs of infection, antibiotics could be stopped as early as 48 h.

ii. **If the mother received intrapartum antimicrobial agents for a positive GBS:**

(a) **Are there signs of sepsis?** If there are signs of neonatal sepsis, the infant should have a full diagnostic evaluation and antibiotic therapy.

(b) **If there are no signs of neonatal sepsis.**

i. **Gestational age (GA) <35 weeks.** Limited evaluation (CBC and BC). Observe for 48 h. If sepsis is suspected, full diagnostic evaluation and antibiotic therapy.

ii. **GA >35 weeks and duration of intrapartum antimicrobial agents before delivery <4 h.** Limited evaluation. Observe for >48 h. If sepsis suspected, full diagnostic evaluation and antibiotic therapy.

iii. **GA >35 weeks and duration of intrapartum antimicrobial agents before delivery >4 h.** No evaluation is needed and no therapy is needed. Observe for 48 h, unless the infant who was >38weeks' gestation at delivery may be discharged after 24 h if other discharge criteria have been met and a person able to do home observation is present. If this is not possible, the infant should be observed in the hospital at least 48 h.

3. **Infants that do not follow the CDC guidelines.** The CDC states that if maternal prophylaxis for GBS is indicated but was not given, recommendations cannot be made based on insufficient data. The following are general guidelines that can be followed if the infant does not follow CDC guidelines (*controversial*).

a. **If the infant is symptomatic** regardless of history and laboratory values, send culture specimens and initiate empirical antibiotic therapy.

b. **In the presence of chorioamnionitis,** the infant should be treated whether or not the mother received antibiotics before delivery.

c. **In the presence of risk factors** (eg, infant with GBS disease, GBS bacteriuria during pregnancy, delivery <37 weeks, and rupture of membranes >18 h or if the GBS was positive and no antibiotics were given or if the GBS was unknown):

i. **Mother treated with more than two doses of antibiotics.** No treatment is recommended if infant is asymptomatic, but the infant should be observed for at least 48 h.

ii. **Mother inadequately or not treated:**

(a) Some centers would observe the infant for at least 48 h. It is debated whether BCs and CBC should be obtained because the CBC is poorly sensitive and the majority of infections occur before the results of BCs are available.

(b) Another option is to treat the infant after the BC and CBC are obtained. Some centers use selective neonatal chemoprophylaxis (SNC): penicillin G, 50,000 units intramuscularly if >2 kg and 25,000 units for <2 kg given within 1 h of birth. Send culture specimens to the laboratory, and initiate empirical antibiotic therapy.

(c) There is insufficient data from trials to guide clinical practice on giving prophylactic antibiotics to asymptomatic infants born to mothers with risk factors.

iii. **GBS screen is negative.** No treatment is recommended, but it is preferable to observe the infant for 48 h.

d. **In the presence of no risk factors, and the GBS is unknown, or positive.**

i. **If the mother was treated with more than two doses of antibiotics,** one option is to observe the infant for at least 48 h.

      ii. If the mother was treated with less than two doses of antibiotics, one option is to observe the infant for at least 48 h (± BCs and CBC). The second option is to treat (possibly with SNC) after obtaining a BC and a CBC.

B. Antibiotic therapy

  1. If the decision is to treat:

    a. Obtain cultures of the blood, urine, and spinal fluid (cultures of urine and spinal fluid are *controversial*). Any other cultures that seem appropriate should be sent to the laboratory (eg, if there is eye discharge, send a Gram stain and culture).

    b. Ampicillin and gentamicin are the antibiotics most commonly used for empirical initial therapy in a newborn. (For dosing, see Chapter 132.) Recent reviews have documented that in infants (>32 weeks' gestation), once a day gentamicin is superior to multiple doses a day because it achieves higher peak levels and avoids toxic trough levels. Some institutions are adding a third-generation cephalosporin (usually cefotaxime or ceftazidime), especially if there is concern for ampicillin-resistant Gram-negative organisms. Most Gram-negative organisms are now ampicillin resistant.

  2. Discontinuing antibiotics is another *controversial* topic. The following guidelines may be used:

    a. If the cultures are negative and the patient is doing well, antibiotics may be stopped after 48–72 h. A normal I:T ratio and serial negative CRP might help determine whether antibiotics can be stopped because of their high negative predictive value.

    b. If the cultures are negative but the infant had signs of sepsis, some clinicians treat the infant for 7–10 days.

    c. If the cultures are positive, treat accordingly.

C. Beyond antibiotic therapy

  1. Immunoglobulin therapy (*controversial*). Studies show a reduction in mortality in proven infection but less reduction in suspected infection. In a recent review, intravenous immune globulin administration resulted in a 3% reduction in sepsis but was not found to not have any significant effect on mortality. The data do not support the routine use in sepsis. Some institutions give a single dose in infants with overwhelming sepsis.

  2. Fresh-frozen plasma. Its use is only indicated in disseminated intravascular coagulation, and no benefit has been shown in septic infants.

  3. Granulocyte transfusions. Although benefits of granulocyte transfusions have been documented, one review concluded there is insufficient evidence to support the routine use of granulocyte transfusion.

  4. Neutrophil transfusions. A small amount of studies have shown a beneficial effect of neutrophil transfusions in septic newborns. Additional studies are needed.

  5. Cytokines. GCSF and GM-CSF have been tried mostly in studies with small trials showing variable results in reducing mortality. At present insufficient evidence supports the use of cytokines in neonatal sepsis.

  6. Double volume exchange transfusion. Exchange transfusion with fresh whole blood is beneficial in neonatal sepsis. Because of significant risks and few prospective studies on the subject, many institutions have not advocated its use.

  7. Recombinant human activated protein C (rhAPC) reduces mortality in sepsis in adults. Insufficient data support the routine use of rhAPC for the management of sepsis in infants. Bleeding is a side effect.

  8. Pentoxifylline. Current evidence shows that pentoxifylline as an adjunct to antibiotics reduces mortality in neonatal sepsis. The studies have been small, and the results need to be interpreted with caution.

67 Pulmonary Hemorrhage

I. **Problem.** Grossly bloody secretions are seen in the endotracheal tube (ETT). The incidence of pulmonary hemorrhage varies from 0.8–12 per 1000 live births. It has been reported in >11% of infants with a birthweight <1500 g who were treated with surfactant and in 5–7% low birthweight infants with respiratory distress syndrome (RDS). It occurs most commonly in acutely ill infants on mechanical ventilation between 2 and 4 days of age. The mortality rate is higher immediately after pulmonary hemorrhage and can be as high as 50%.

II. **Immediate questions**

A. **Are any other signs or symptoms abnormal?** Typically, an infant with pulmonary hemorrhage is a ventilated low birthweight infant, often from a multiple birth, and 2–4 days old (usually in the first week of life). Late gestation infants with pulmonary hemorrhage usually have low 1 and 5 min APGAR scores. The infant has a sudden deterioration in respiratory status. The infant becomes hypoxic, has severe retractions, and may experience associated pallor, shock, apnea, bradycardia, and cyanosis.

B. **Is the infant hypoxic? Has a blood transfusion recently been given?** Hypoxia or hypervolemia (usually caused by overtransfusion) may cause an acute rise in the pulmonary capillary pressure and lead to pulmonary hemorrhage.

C. **Is bleeding occurring from other sites?** If there is bleeding from multiple sites, coagulopathy may be present, and coagulation studies should be obtained. Volume replacement with colloid or blood products may be needed.

D. **What is the hematocrit (Hct) of the tracheal blood?** If the Hct is close to the venous Hct, it represents a true hemorrhage, and the blood is usually from trauma, aspiration of maternal blood, or bleeding diathesis. If the Hct is 15–20 percentage points lower than the venous Hct, the bleeding is likely hemorrhagic edema fluid. This is seen with the majority of cases of pulmonary hemorrhage (such as those secondary to patent ductus arteriosus [PDA], surfactant therapy, and left-sided heart failure; others discussed later).

III. **Differential diagnosis**

A. **Direct trauma.** Trauma to the airway may be a result of nasotracheal or endotracheal intubation. Vigorous suctioning can also cause tissue trauma. Lung trauma during chest tube insertion can cause hemorrhage.

B. **Aspiration of gastric or maternal blood** is often seen after cesarean delivery. The majority of blood is usually obtained from the nasogastric tube, but blood may be seen in the ETT.

C. **Coagulopathy** may be due to sepsis or due to congenital factors. The role of coagulation abnormalities is unclear as a cause of pulmonary hemorrhage or if it just exacerbates it.

D. **Other disorders associated with pulmonary hemorrhage**

1. **Hypoxia/Asphyxia.** Acute left ventricular failure due to asphyxia is a very important factor in pulmonary hemorrhage.

2. **Hypervolemia** as the result of overtransfusion or fluid overload.

3. **Congenital heart disease/Congestive heart failure** (especially in pulmonary edema caused by PDA).

4. **Pulmonary related.** Respiratory distress syndrome, pulmonary interstitial emphysema, pneumothorax, meconium aspiration, and pneumonia (caused by Gram-negative organisms).

5. **Surfactant administration.** Pulmonary hemorrhage occurred within hours of surfactant therapy and may be related to a rapid increase in pulmonary blood flow

(PBF) because of improved lung function. The increased PBF may cause hemorrhagic pulmonary edema. Reports show a significant relationship between pulmonary hemorrhage and a clinical PDA in surfactant-treated infants. Recent data indicates rescue surfactant therapy did not increase the risk of pulmonary hemorrhage, but prophylactic surfactant did.

6. **Mechanical ventilation or oxygen therapy/toxicity.**
7. **Hematologic disorders.** Severe Rh incompatibility, thrombocytopenia, hemorrhagic disease of the newborn (from failure to administer vitamin K).
8. **Prematurity, intrauterine growth restriction and/or multiple births.**
9. **Severe hypothermia.**
10. **Infection/Sepsis.** Sepsis is an important cause of hemorrhage and is most likely from disseminated intravascular coagulation.
11. **Urea cycle defects with hyperammonemia.**
12. **Rare causes.** Case reports have included pulmonary hemorrhage after RhDNase treatment in a premature infant with chronic lung disease, in a 32-week infant gestational age from microscopic polyangiitis secondary to transfer of maternal MPO-ANCA, and in a premature infant in association with multidrug-resistant *Enterobacter cloacae*. There is also a case report involving an infant with chromosome 22q11 deletion who had multiple dissecting pulmonary arterial aneurysms that were believed to cause the pulmonary hemorrhage.

IV. **Database**
   A. **Physical examination.** Typically, the infant has a sudden deterioration and bloody secretions from the airway. The infant can be pale, limp, and unresponsive, can be fighting the ventilator, or can look well. Note the presence of other bleeding sites, signs of pneumonia, infection, or congestive heart failure. Look for peripheral edema, hepatosplenomegaly, murmur. Listen to the chest for decreased breath sounds.
   B. **Laboratory studies**
      1. **Complete blood count with differential and platelet count.** With pneumonia, sepsis, or other infection, results of these studies may be abnormal. Thrombocytopenia may be seen. The Hct should be checked to determine whether excessive blood loss has occurred.
      2. **Coagulation profile (prothrombin time, partial thromboplastin time, thrombin time, and fibrinogen level)** may reveal coagulation disorders.
      3. **Arterial blood gas levels** detect hypoxia and metabolic acidosis.
      4. **Apt test,** if aspiration of maternal blood is suspected (rarely needed). (See Chapter 49.)
   C. **Radiologic and other studies**
      1. **Chest radiograph** helps rule out pneumonia, RDS, and congestive heart failure. With pulmonary hemorrhage, radiographic findings depend on whether the hemorrhage is focal (patchy, linear, or nodular densities) or massive (the film shows a complete whiteout). The chest radiograph can also be clear.
      2. **Echocardiogram** to evaluate for a PDA.
V. **Plan**
   A. **Emergency measures.** These methods are acceptable modes of treatment.
      1. **Suction the airway** initially (sometimes as often as every 15 min) until bleeding subsides. This is very critical because there is always a risk of secretions blocking the airway. **Percussion should be used with caution and has no primary role in pulmonary hemorrhage.**
      2. **Increase the inspired oxygen concentration.**
      3. **If mechanical ventilation is not being used,** consider initiating its use.
      4. **Increase the positive end-expiratory pressure** to 6–8 cm H_2O; it may cause tamponade of the capillaries. Sometimes higher levels are required to stop the bleeding.

5. **Consider increasing the peak inspiratory pressure** if bleeding does not subside to improve ventilation and raise the mean airway pressure.

B. **General measures**

1. **Support and correct the blood pressure** with volume expansion and colloids (see Chapter 58).

2. **Blood volume and Hct** should be restored with packed red blood cell transfusions. However, in many cases the infant has not had a large volume loss; thus administering excessive fluid volume may only worsen the situation (increasing the left arterial pressure may increase the pulmonary edema).

3. **Correct acidosis.** Bicarbonate infusion may be necessary if the ventilation is adequate.

4. **Treat any underlying disorder.**

C. **Other measures to consider if the preceding methods do not work (*controversial*)**

1. **Consider giving epinephrine** (0.1 mL/kg of 1:10,000) through the ETT *(controversial)*. This may cause constriction of the pulmonary capillaries. One study stated epinephrine and/or 4% cocaine (4 mg/kg) were useful adjuncts to increases in MAP in the management of pulmonary hemorrhage.

2. **Consider high-frequency ventilation.** It is not known if it has any benefits over conventional ventilation, but three studies suggest that high-frequency ventilation improved survival.

3. **Consider using a single dose of surfactant** because it has been reported to improve respiratory status based on the oxygenation index. Case reports have also shown benefit in term infants. Reviews note promising results, but a lack of randomized trials prevents this form being universally recommended.

4. **Steroids.** Because chronic inflammation was found on lung biopsies of infants with pulmonary hemorrhage, and more infants survived with pulmonary hemorrhage who had been on steroids, steroid use can be considered. Methylprednisolone, 1 mg/kg every 6 h, during hospital stay and 1 mg/kg daily thereafter and discontinued after a 4-week period has been reported to be beneficial.

5. **Activated recombinant factor VII (rFVIIa).** A study of two very low birthweight infants who did not respond to conventional treatment were successfully treated with activated rFVIIa (50 mcg/kg per dose twice daily 3 h apart intravenously for 2–3 days). It is a low-volume alternative to blood products and effective as a panhemostatic agent. It is usually used in severe hemorrhages in individuals with hemophilia A and B. **The optimal dose of rFVIIa in low birthweight infants has not been established.**

6. **Hemocoagulase plus mechanical ventilation.** A study was done on 41 infants treated with hemocoagulase (0.25 KU [Klobusitzky unit] through the ETT every 4–6 h) plus mechanical ventilation for pulmonary hemorrhage. Results were promising: the duration of ventilation, pulmonary hemorrhage, and mortality were all decreased compared with controls. Prophylactic use of hemocoagulase in mechanically ventilated neonates has decreased the incidence and duration of pulmonary hemorrhage in some reports.

7. **Diuretics.** Some advocate diuretic therapy (Furosemide, 1 mg/kg) to treat fluid overload.

D. **Specific therapy**

1. **Direct nasotracheal or endotracheal trauma.** If there is significant bleeding immediately after an endotracheal or nasotracheal intubation, trauma is the most likely cause; surgical consultation is indicated.

2. **Aspiration of maternal blood.** If the infant is stable, no treatment is needed because the condition is typically self-limited.

3. **Coagulopathy**

a. **Hemorrhagic disease of the newborn.** Vitamin K, 1 mg intravenously, should be given.

b. **Other coagulopathies.** Fresh-frozen plasma, 10 mL/kg every 12–24 h, may be given. If the platelet count is low, transfuse 1 unit and monitor closely. Monitor the prothrombin time/partial thromboplastin time, platelet count, and fibrinogen level.

4. **PDA,** if hemodynamically significant, treat medically or surgically (Chapter 109).

5. **Sepsis.** Appropriate antibiotics should be started immediately (see Chapters 66 and 117).

68 Rash and Dermatologic Problems

I. **Problem.** A nurse calls you to tell you that an infant has a rash and wants you to evaluate it. A rash is any change of skin that affects its color, appearance, or texture. **Although the majority of rashes in newborns are benign and require no treatment, certain rashes require a workup and intervention.**

II. **Immediate questions**

A. **What are the characteristics of the rash?** Morphology of the lesion aids differential diagnosis. **Is it macular** (flat lesion <1 cm), **papular** (raised up to 1 cm), **nodular** (raised up to 2 cm), **vesicular** (raised, <1 cm, filled with clear fluid), **bullous** (raised, >1 cm, with clear fluid), or **pustular** (raised with purulent fluid)?

B. **Are there petechiae (tiny pinpoint red dots from broken blood vessels), purpura (large flat area of blood under tissue), or ecchymosis (very large bruised area)?** All can result from intradermal bleeding and need to be differentiated from **erythema** (redness of the skin). With erythema, the redness is cleared when pressed and returns when you release. With pressure, petechiae, purpura, and ecchymosis do not blanch. Petechiae on the lower body after a breech delivery or upper body with a vertex presentation can be normal. If widespread, petechiae are considered abnormal. **Petechiae and purpura can signify thrombocytopenia and require a workup.**

C. **Is there a history of a congenital infection?** Obtain a thorough maternal history. TORCH infections are known to cause rashes. The **"blueberry muffin baby"** has widespread purpura and papules and can be seen in rubella (most known), CMV, and syphilis.

D. **Is the infant ill appearing?** A well infant with a rash suggests a benign rash. A febrile or ill-appearing infant with a rash requires a thorough workup searching for an infectious cause.

E. **What medications did the mother receive during pregnancy and delivery? Is the mother breastfeeding and taking any medications?** A rare cause of rash in the infant.

F. **Does the skin lesion make you think of a genetic disorder? Skin lesions can be associated with genetic syndromes.**

1. **Blisters:** Epidermolysis bullosa.

2. **Brown flat patches:** Neurofibromatosis.

3. **Cutis marmorata:** Cornelia de Lange syndrome and in trisomies 18 (Edward syndrome) and 21 (Down syndrome).

4. **Deficient hair and nails:** Ectodermal dysplasias.

5. **Scaly, thick skin:** Ichthyoses.

6. **Thin, fragile skin:** Collagen disorders and hypoplasia of the dermis.

7. **Unformed skin:** Aplasia cutis.

8. **White skin and hair:** Piebaldism, tuberous sclerosis.

III. **Differential diagnosis**
   A. **Benign skin disorders/rashes that usually require no workup or intervention.**
     These rashes are common.
      1. **Erythema toxicum,** the most common newborn rash, consists of erythematous macules with a central papule or pustule. Can be present at birth, typically appear within the first 48 h, and may appear up to 2 weeks of age. More common in full-term infants and more common on the trunk, extremities, and perineum. New lesions can appear after the initial onset and usually disappear after a week.
      2. **Transient neonatal pustular melanosis.** These 2- to 5-mm pustules are usually present at birth on various sites, typically the face and sacrum. Pustules evolve and disappear within 48 h but can leave hyperpigmented scarring that eventually resolves but may persist for months.
      3. **Sebaceous gland hyperplasia** are tiny yellow papules occurring usually on the cheeks and nose. Smaller and more yellow than milia.
      4. **Milia** are tiny (1-mm) white-yellow papules frequently present on face, chin, and forehead. Caused by sebaceous retention cysts.
      5. **Miliaria crystalline.** May appear on scalp or face as vesicular or papular lesions with or without erythema. Exacerbated by heat and humidity, they resolve quickly when the infant is cooled.
      6. **Miliaria rubra ("prickly heat").** Similar fluid-filled vesicles but are surrounded by small red areas.
      7. **Miliaria pustulosis.** Nonerythematous pustules.
      8. **Infantile acropustulosis.** Recurrent areas of pruritic vesicopustules develop on the palmar surface of the hand and plantar surface of the feet. Usually last 7–14 days.
      9. **Seborrheic dermatitis.** Patchy redness and scales on the scalp (**"cradle cap"**), face, skin folds, and behind the ears.
      10. **Neonatal acne.** Erythematous comedones, papules, and pustules. May be present at birth or develop during early infancy; may take several weeks for complete resolution.
      11. **Sucking blister.** Vesicular or bullous lesions present at birth on finger, lips, or hands; no associated erythema that distinguishes these from herpetic lesions.
      12. **Subcutaneous fat necrosis.** Erythematous nodules and plaques occurring during the first few weeks of life and resolving by 2 months of age. Usually on areas of trauma (face, back, arms, legs, and buttocks). Hypercalcemia can occur if these lesions calcify.
      13. **Stork bite ("salmon patch," "angel's kiss").** Pink macules that are dilated superficial capillaries, seen at the nape of the neck, midforehead, and upper eyelids that usually fade within a year. The most common vascular malformation.
      14. **Mongolian blue spot.** A blue black macular discoloration at the base of the spine and on the buttocks. More common in blacks (>90%) and Asians (81%); usually fades over several years.
      15. **Harlequin sign (color change, not Harlequin fetus).** Secondary to vasomotor instability, there is a sharp demarcation of blanching (one side of the body is red and the other is pale) that usually only lasts a few minutes.
      16 **Strawberry hemangioma** is the most common vascular tumor.
      17. **Benign petechiae** are nonblanching erythematous macules present on the lower body after a breech delivery or upper body with a vertex presentation.
   B. **Rashes caused by infections.** These typically require intervention.
      1. **Bacterial infections causing rashes**
        a. *Staphylococcus aureus*
          i. **Impetigo (nonbullous and bullous).** Usually present with intact vesicles, then intact pustules rupture, erode, and dry out to form crusts often secondary to an infected umbilical wound.

ii. **Staphylococcal scalded skin syndrome (SSSS).** Usually presents during the first week of life, starts with marked erythema of the face, then spreads caudally and tends to be most severe in flexural areas. Lesions progress to bullae that are denuded easily.

b. **Cutaneous streptococcus infections.** Uncommon, group A streptococcal infections can have an erysipelas-like eruption. Skin infections caused by group B are very rare. Vesiculopustular lesions, abscesses, and cellulitis have been reported.

c. **Syphilis.** Usually macular or maculopapular eruptions (in congenital syphilis, infants present with vesicles, bullae, and erosions). Hemorrhagic bullae on the palms and soles are characteristic of syphilis.

d. **Listeria monocytogenes.** Small (2- to 3-mm) cutaneous pinkish gray granulomas are characteristic.

2. **Viral infections causing rashes**
   a. **Herpes simplex virus (HSV)**
      i. **Neonatal HSV** is transmitted perinatally and occurs in three forms. Erythematous papules or vesicles progress into pustular clusters with intense erythema.
      ii. **Congenital HSV** is acquired in utero and presents with vesicles apparent the first day of life. Typically associated with low birthweight, chorioretinitis, and microcephaly.
   b. **Varicella**
      i. **Neonatal varicella.** Widespread vesicular or pustular lesions appearing at 3–10 days of life. Mother should have a history of varicella within weeks of birth or symptoms within 2 days after birth.
      ii. **Congenital varicella.** Acquired in utero and marked by erosions or stellate scarring present at birth.
   c. **CMV is the most common congenital infection.** The majority of cases are asymptomatic. If symptomatic, they can have multiorgan disease with petechiae and purpura and jaundice.
   d. **Rubella.** Can have petechiae, but if severe, may have bluish red papules ("blueberry muffin") that appear on the head and trunk and extremities.

3. **Fungal infections causing rashes**
   a. **Candida albicans,** the most common fungal infection that causes problems in neonates, is discussed here. Other species (*Candida parapsilosis, Candida lusitaniae, Candida glabrata,* etc.) are less common.
      i. **Candida diaper dermatitis/oral candidiasis (thrush).** Most common presentation of Candida infections in a normal infant. The diaper rash is usually erythematous with satellite pustules. Oral candidiasis can present with fussiness and refusal to take oral feedings and is characterized by white patches in the oral cavity.
      ii. **Congenital candidiasis.** Acquired in utero, presents with diffuse papules and pustules that may involve the palm and soles. There can be desquamation of these lesions, which may mimic SSSS. Premature infants may present without skin lesions.
      iii. **Neonatal candidiasis.** Contracted through an infected birth canal, there may be many different presentations. Very low birthweight infants can have a burn-like dermatitis with peeling.
   b. **Aspergillus** has been reported to cause cutaneous fungal infections but is rare.
      i. **Primary cutaneous aspergillosis (PCA)** is characterized by lack of involvement of organs except the skin at the time of diagnosis. Preterm infants are at risk for PCA because of vulnerability of their skin and immature host defenses. Risk factors include prematurity, neutropenia, prior use of antibiotics, and glucocorticoid administration. A plaque with an eschar is characteristic

of PCA. Disruption of the skin occurs due to contaminated hand splints, skin maceration caused by oximeter sensor, or adhesive tape.

   ii. **Secondary aspergillosis.** is characterized by involvement of organs, and a maculopapular eruption caused by thrombosis of small vessels.

4. **Parasitic infections that can cause a rash**

   a. **Scabies,** an infestation with the mite *Sarcoptes scabei*, has been reported in infants as young as 2 weeks. Infants tend to have widespread lesions often on the face and scalp (usually not seen in older patients who present with intertriginous locations). They can have papules, nodules, vesicles, and pustules.

   b. ***Toxoplasma gondii* infections** have generalized maculopapular rash.

C. **Rashes that cause scaling** are usually benign and self-limited. Infectious and dietary etiologies need to be ruled out because they need immediate treatment. Genetic and immune etiologies can be considered later in the differential.

1. **Postmaturity.** The majority of term and postmature infants normally shed their skin. The skin appears like parchment paper and peels off. This is a normal physiologic finding that requires no medical treatment.

2. **Seborrheic dermatitis** is usually seen on the scalp and flexure areas. It is a red erythematous rash with yellow scaling. Can be seen in the diaper area and is self-limiting.

3. **Fatty acid deficiency.** Superficial scaling and desquamation can occur. Can be seen in fatty acid deficiency syndrome (where infants have decreased fat stores) or in fat malabsorption. Fatty acid replacement is necessary.

4. **Ichthyoses (also called "Harlequin fetus," "collodion baby").** Several types of ichthyoses are present. These are genetic disorders that cause severe thick scaly skin with restricted movement. The infant can have a shiny tight membrane covering that can peel off. Prone to cracking and secondary infection.

5. **Infantile eczema.** Scaling is present, but eczema is rarely seen in the newborn.

6. **Atopic dermatitis.** Red scaly and itchy rash; rarely seen in the newborn.

7. **Staphylococcal scalded skin syndrome** (see Section III, B, 1a, ii).

8. **Psoriasis.** Can be seen as a diaper rash with dissemination (scaly patches beyond the diaper rash) or can present as erythroderma progressing to pustular psoriasis.

9. **Candida infections** can also cause redness and scaling (see earlier).

10. **Syphilis infections.** See Section III, B, 1c.

11. **Ectodermal dysplasias.** Most common form is X-linked recessive hypohidrotic ectodermal dysplasia with excessive desquamation.

12. **Immunodeficiencies.** Infants with immunodeficiencies can have a red scaly rash (neonatal lupus, AIDS, severe combined immunodeficiency, diffuse cutaneous mastocytosis, Wiskott- Aldrich syndrome, Langerhans cell histiocytosis).

D. **Rashes that cause blisters and bullae.** Infectious and dietary causes need to be ruled out because they require immediate treatment. Then less common causes can be evaluated.

1. **Epidermolysis bullosa.** A group of inherited diseases that cause blistering. Trauma induces the blisters.

2. **Zinc deficiency dermatosis.** Can present as a blistering rash, an eczematous rash on the angle of the mouth, chin, cheeks, and diaper area. It can be red, scaly, and have a dark color at the periphery.

3. **Congenital herpes infection.**

4. **Staphylococcal scalded skin syndrome.**

5. **Less common causes.** Genetic disorders, epidermolytic hyperkeratosis, incontinentia pigmenti, toxic epidermal necrolysis, and bullous mastocytosis.

E. **Rashes that are birthmarks.** The majority of birthmarks are benign and require no treatment. However, if there are many present, they may signify an associated syndrome, or if very large they can be at risk for melanoma and have to be closely followed. Vascular lesions need to be evaluated to see if they interfere with vital organs.

1. **Pigmented lesions: hyperpigmentation**
   a. **Café-au-lait spots (macule).** Benign lesions that are oval or irregular with a light brown color. If they are >4 cm and there are more than six, need to suspect an associated syndrome (think neurofibromatosis, Albright syndrome, Turner and Noonan syndrome, tuberous sclerosis, ataxia-telangiectasis, etc.).
   b. **Mongolian blue spot.** See Section III, A, 14.
   c. **Congenital nevocellular (melanocytic) nevus.** Usually small lesions that are common with a small risk of malignant melanoma.
   d. **Nevus of Ota.** A blue or grayish area involving the orbital and zygomatic area common in Asians and carries the risk of glaucoma.
   e. **Giant hairy nevus (>20 cm).** A large pigmented hairy area that has a high risk of malignant melanoma (5-15% risk).
2. **Diffuse hyperpigmentation** is not normal and can be secondary to Addison disease, biliary atresia, hepatic atresia, sprue, melanism, lentiginosis, porphyria, Hartnup disease, or idiopathic.
3. **Pigmented lesions: hypopigmentation**
   a. **Diffuse or localized loss of pigment** can be secondary to phenylketonuria, Addison disease, traumatic, postinflammation, or genetic.
   b. **Ash-leaf macules.** Small area of hypopigmentation, oval shaped and similar to the leaf of an ash tree; a marker for tuberous sclerosis.
   c. **Hypomelanosis of Ito.** Syndrome (primarily neurologic) with hypopigmented macule or linear/whorled pattern of hypopigmentation.
   d. **Partial albinism (piebaldism).** An autosomal dominant disorder of off-white macules on forehead, scalp, trunk, and extremities. Can be secondary to Addison disease, tuberous sclerosis, vitiligo, and Klein Waardenburg syndrome.
   e. **Albinism.** Genetic disorders that cause abnormal melanin synthesis.
4. **Vascular lesions**
   a. **Port wine stain (nevus flammeus).** This usually presents at birth on the face. It is a permanent capillary angioma. Rarely it is associated with Sturge Weber syndrome or Klippel-Trenaunay syndrome.
   b. **Salmon patch.** See Section III, A, 13.
   c. **Hemangiomas.** Most common benign tumor of vascular endothelium of infancy; more frequent in premature infants.
      i. **Strawberry hemangioma.** A bright red tumor (of dilated mass of capillaries) that protrudes above the skin and can appear anywhere on the body. Usually does not require treatment unless it interferes with vital functions.
      ii. **Cavernous hemangioma.** More deep into the skin and bluish red; usually benign unless it interferes with vital organs.
F. **Rashes that cause petechiae /purpura.** These may relate to birth trauma (considered "normal") or if generalized and recurring can signify a serious infection or hematologic etiology that needs immediate evaluation and treatment.
   1. **Birth trauma.**
   2. **Autoimmune disorders.** Maternal lupus.
   3. **Thrombocytopenia,** usually scattered petechiae.
   4. **Neonatal alloimmune thrombocytopenia (NAIT).** An isoimmune reaction that can cause thrombocytopenia and severe bleeding, including intracranial bleeding.
   5. **Maternal idiopathic thrombocytopenic purpura.** Approximately 80% of cases of thrombocytopenia are caused by autoimmune form.
   6. **Coagulation factor deficiencies.**
   7. **Sepsis/Infectious related.** Usually caused by Gram-negative bacterial sepsis (*Escherichia coli, Pseudomonas*). Listeriosis and Aspergillosis also involved. TORCH infections can all cause these. Rubella, CMV, and syphilis can all cause blueberry muffin lesions (widespread papules and purpura).
   8. **Disseminated intravascular coagulation.**

9. **Purpura fulminans.** Symmetrical and well-defined lakes of confluent ecchymosis without petechiae, with sudden onset and development of hemorrhagic bullae and sudden death. Characteristic of meningococcal sepsis or other life-threatening infection.

10. **TORCH infections.** Rubella, CMV, and syphilis can all cause "blueberry muffin" lesions (widespread papules and purpura).

11. **Maternal drugs.** Salicylates, steroids.

IV. Database

A. **History.** Obtain thorough history from the mother and family and a detailed history from the obstetric department. Is there a family history of skin disorders? Many skin disorders are genetic (ichthyoses, immunodeficiency, albinism). Asking about recent infections (varicella), early infections during the pregnancy (congenital infections), sexual history (syphilis), unusual travel destinations (scabies), and pet history (*Toxoplasma gondii*) may provide some clues to the diagnosis. Does the mother have herpes? Did she have any unusual food products or undercooked food (*Listeria*)? Medications taken by the mother?

B. **Physical examination.** Check vital signs. Is the infant febrile or appear sick, suggesting an infection? Do not just examine the presenting rash, but check the entire body to see if there are signs of the rash anywhere else. The distribution of the rash may be characteristic. Frequent follow-up examinations may document any progression or resolution of the lesions. Examine the eye to check for chorioretinitis (TORCH infections). Hepatosplenomegaly may be seen in congenital TORCH infections.

C. **Laboratory studies**

1. **Sepsis evaluation** labs if infection suspected. Aspirate- appropriate fluid for bacterial, viral, and fungal cultures.

2. **If active bleeding suspected,** send complete blood count with differential, platelet and reticulocyte count, TORCH titers, and sepsis workup.

3. **Potassium hydroxide prep** if Candida suspected (reveals pseudohyphae).

4. **Wright stain** can show polymorphonuclear neutrophils with bullous impetigo, eosinophils with erythema toxicum.

5. **Mineral oil prep** can show mites and ova with scabies.

6. **Tzanck smear** if herpes suspected.

7. **Skin biopsy** is sometimes indicated.

D. **Radiologic and other studies (rarely needed)**

1. Computed tomography (CT) scan or contrast-enhanced magnetic resonance imaging of the head to rule out calcifications if Sturge-Weber syndrome is suspected.

2. Ultrasound, echocardiography, and/or CT scans may be needed to manage hemangiomas.

V. **Plan.** The majority of rashes that occur in the neonate do not require treatment.

A. **Benign skin disorders.** No treatment is necessary.

B. **Rashes that are caused by infections.** See specific infectious disease chapter for more details where appropriate.

1. *Staphylococcus aureus.* Systemic antibiotics.

2. **Streptococcus.** Cutaneous is usually Group-A, treated by penicillin.

3. **Syphilis.** Usually penicillin for 10 days.

4. *Listeria monocytogenes.* Ampicillin and an aminoglycoside such as gentamicin (cephalosporins not active).

5. **Herpes simplex.** Acyclovir 60 mg/kg/day IV divided twice daily only if there is no CNS or disseminated disease.

6. **Varicella.** Acyclovir and varicella zoster immune globulin may decrease the severity of the course and improve outcome. Treatment must begin early in the course of the illness.

7. **Cytomegalovirus.** Ganciclovir (Cytovene) in adults, limited data in pediatrics.

8. **Rubella.** Supportive management.
9. *Candida albicans.* Systemic antifungal medications such as amphotericin B to treat disseminated infection. Topical antifungals are used to treat isolated skin lesions. Thrush is treated by oral nystatin, 0.5 mL inside each cheek twice daily, for 10 days.
10. **Aspergillus.** Voriconazole (VFEND) or amphotericin B if invasive (limited data in infants).
11. **Scabies.** Apply 5% permethrin cream topically; may not be safe in very low birth-weight infants.
12. **Toxoplasmosis.** Most do not require therapy, if needed pyrimethamine and sulfadiazine and folinic acid (leucovorin).

C. **Rashes that cause scaling**
   1. **Postmaturity.** No treatment is necessary.
   2. **Seborrheic dermatitis.** Usually resolves by 1 year; supportive care.
   3. **Fatty acid deficiency.** Replacement of fatty acids through intravenous lipid solutions or diet is necessary.
   4. **Ichthyoses.** Aggressive supportive care, close monitoring of fluid and electrolytes, and meticulous skin care with the goal of preventing infections. Collodion babies frequently have temperature instability and excessive fluid loss.
   5. **Infantile eczema.** Avoid any irritants; use protective creams such as zinc oxide in the diaper area. Short-term topical steroids may be needed.
   6. **Atopic dermatitis.** Emollients and mild topical steroids are used.
   7. **Staphylococcal scalded skin syndrome.** Antibiotics (intravenous penicillinase-resistant, antistaphylococcal [eg, Cloxacillin]), supportive care, and attention to fluid and electrolyte management.
   8. **Psoriasis.** Mild topical steroids and wet dressings are used.
   9. **Candida.** See Section V, B, 9.
   10. **Syphilis.** See Section V, B, 3.
   11. **Ectodermal dysplasias.** Supportive care involving artificial tears.
   12. **Immunodeficiencies.**

D. **Rashes that cause blisters and bullae**
   1. **Epidermolysis bullosa.** Meticulous skin care, infection prevention, and special attention to nutrition and feedings because of the problems with dysphagia from scarring.
   2. **Zinc deficiency dermatosis.** Zinc supplementation.
   3. **Congenital herpes.** See Chapter 127.
   4. **Staphylococcal scalded skin syndrome.** See Section V, C, 7.

E. **Rashes that are birthmarks**
   1. **Hyperpigmented lesions.** Most of these lesions require no treatment. If the lesions are large (>3 cm), removal is recommended. Giant hairy nevi are removed to prevent cancer development.
   2. **Hypopigmented lesions.** Piebaldism is treated with cosmetic camouflage. Albinism should follow sun restriction guidelines and sunblock.
   3. **Vascular lesions.** Many hemangiomas can be closely watched and left to regress. If treatment is necessary, steroid therapy, embolization, excision, occlusion, laser therapy, alpha interferon, and radiotherapy are options. Port wine stains can be treated with laser therapy.

F. **Rashes that cause petechiae and purpura.** These rashes usually require a thorough workup and treatment if there is a bleeding disorder. Infections are treated with antibiotics or antiviral agents. Platelet transfusion and replacement of coagulation factors may be necessary.
   1. **Birth trauma.** No treatment is necessary.
   2. **Autoimmune disorders** such as maternal or neonatal lupus.
   3. **Thrombocytopenia.** See Chapter 125.

  4. **Neonatal isoimmune thrombocytopenia (NAIT).** See Chapter 125.
  5. **Maternal idiopathic thrombocytopenic purpura (ITTP).** See Chapter 125.
  6. **Coagulation factor deficiencies.** See Chapter 125.
  7. **Sepsis/TORCH infections.** See Chapter 127.
  8. **Disseminated intravascular coagulation (DIC).** See Chapter 125.
  9. **Purpura fulminans.** Treat the underlying infection.

69 Sedation and Analgesia in a Neonate

I. **Problem.** An infant with pulmonary hypertension with extreme lability needs sedation. Should the infant be sedated, and which agent is available to use? An infant is having a procedure. Should I use a local anesthetic?

II. **Immediate questions**

  A. **What is the indication for the sedation?** Agitation and movement by the infant during procedures such as extracorporeal membrane oxygenation (ECMO) can risk injury. Certain procedures (eg, magnetic resonance imaging [MRI]) mandate that the infant be immobilized, so sedation is required. Infants with extreme lability on mechanical ventilation may benefit from sedation.

  B. **Why does the infant need analgesia?** If the newborn is to undergo procedures such as elective circumcision, local analgesia is usually administered. For emergency procedures such as chest tube placement, the need for analgesia must be weighed against the delay of administering the analgesic agent.

  C. **If treating for agitation while an infant is on mechanical ventilation, is the infant adequately ventilated?** Hypoxia and inadequate ventilation can result in agitation, and sedation is dangerous in these situations.

  D. **Is sedation needed for a short period (ie, for a diagnostic procedure) or long term?** Certain medications are indicated for short-term sedation (ie, chloral hydrate) and should not be used long term.

III. **Differential diagnosis and indications**

  A. **Indications for analgesia.** Whether a newborn can experience pain remains in the philosophical realm, but they undeniably react to painful stimuli (nociception). Such stimuli elicit both clinical symptoms (eg, tachycardia, hypertension, and decreased oxygenation) and complex behavioral responses in term and preterm infants. By 23 weeks' gestation, the nervous system has developed sufficiently to enable the conduction of nociceptive stimuli from peripheral skin receptors to the brain. The development of the descending inhibiting pathways occurs at a later stage; therefore the more immature infant may have an even lower threshold for noxious stimulus than at a later age. Neonates possibly have an increased sensitivity to pain compared with older age groups. During surgical interventions, the neonate, like the adult, mounts a hormonal response that consists of the release of catecholamines, β-endorphins, corticotropin, growth hormone, and glucagon as well as the suppression of insulin secretion. This response is reduced by prior administration of analgesia or anesthesia. Although we do not know whether or not the neonate experiences psychological distress and lasting psychological sequelae, there are enough reasons to attempt to control exposure to pain as well as other unpleasant experiences.

    1. **Major surgical procedures** such as ligation of the ductus arteriosus, laparotomy, and placement of a central venous catheter require anesthesia. General anesthesia

should be provided by inhalation of anesthetic gases or intravenous (IV) administration of narcotic agents. In all these conditions, **the use of paralytic agents without analgesia is absolutely contraindicated.**

2. Postoperative management

   a. Narcotic agents should always be included in the immediate postoperative period. Supplementary sedation is often provided by benzodiazepines or chloral hydrate, which are useful to combat agitation and potentiate the effect of opiates. It is important to remember that these sedative agents do not have any analgesic effect and, therefore, cannot be given alone to relieve pain.

   b. Other pain-relieving agents have, in general, little role in postoperative management. Acetaminophen has only a weak analgesic effect and should be indicated at this age mostly for its antipyretic action. Aspirin should not be given in neonates because of the risk of bleeding.

3. Minor surgical procedures. Analgesia for so-called minor procedures is mostly provided by local anesthesia, at times supplemented by small doses of opiates or sedative agents.

   a. Unless the child's condition requires extreme urgent action, provide analgesia for procedures such as chest tube insertion and vascular cutdown.

   b. The need for analgesia for circumcision is becoming less controversial and is now widely accepted.

   c. The effectiveness and need for analgesia for more minor procedures such as lumbar puncture have not been demonstrated.

4. "Stressful" conditions. There is wide controversy with regard to providing analgesia or sedation in "stressful" conditions, akin to "anxiolysis" in the adult and pediatric population. The period during which mechanical ventilation and its related routine procedures are provided has been identified as the most frequent time when infants are being "stressed."

   a. The arguments to favor analgesia or sedation for these situations are as follows:

      i. It reduces the level of various biochemical markers of stress such as blood levels of catecholamines, cortisol, and β-endorphin.

      ii. It lessens the duration of hypoxemia associated with endotracheal suctioning.

      iii. Additional argument for its use involves the difficulty in diagnosing discomfort and pain when the infant is under muscle paralysis.

   b. The arguments against such routine use of analgesia or sedation are as follows:

      i. The pharmacokinetic characteristics of narcotic agents in the preterm infant are variable and not always predictable.

      ii. The same assumed "safe" dose for some infants can, for others, result in severe toxicity (eg, hemodynamic and respiratory depression, toxic accumulation, leading to a transient comatose state).

      iii. The prolonged use (sometimes as little as 4 days) of narcotic and sedative agents is associated with the rapid development of tolerance, withdrawal, and encephalopathy and the requirement for higher ventilatory support in the early phase of respiratory distress syndrome. Furthermore, it often delays weaning from mechanical ventilation.

      iv. Treating for "agitation" by sedation can be dangerous when the former is the result of inadequate ventilation or hypoxemia. Therefore, before treating agitation, one must always ensure, by careful physical examination, that the endotracheal tube is not obstructed or misplaced and that adequate ventilating pressures are being used.

B. Indications for sedation

   1. Extreme respiratory lability. Infants who have demonstrated extreme respiratory lability develop hypoxemia rapidly with minimal handling. Infants with severe

pulmonary hypertension and pulmonary vascular hyperreactivity are often candidates for sedation.

2. **Therapeutic procedures.** When it is necessary to prevent the child from moving vigorously (eg, during ECMO), sedation may be needed to prevent accidental dislodgment of the vascular cannulas.

3. **Diagnostic procedures.** Procedures that require the child to be immobilized include imaging procedures such as MRI, cardiac catheterization, and occasionally computed tomography (CT) scan.

IV. **Database**

A. **Physical examination.** Before instituting any type of sedation or analgesia, there must be a clear diagnosis. The physical examination is directed at the underlying condition.

B. **Laboratory studies.** These are usually not needed, except in the context of the underlying disease.

C. **Radiologic and other studies.** Such studies are usually not needed, except in the context of the underlying disease.

V. **Plan**

A. **General management.** Prevention of distress and pain should be a priority in the neonatal unit and in newborn nurseries. Measures to prevent or minimize stress in the neonate should include the following:

1. **Reduce noise (eg, close the incubator door gently).**
2. **Protect the infant from intense light.**
3. **Cluster blood drawings as much as possible.**
4. **Use a spring-loaded lancet for heelstick phlebotomy.**
5. **Replace tape with a self-adhesive bandage.**
6. **Perform intratracheal suctioning only if indicated.**
7. **Use adequate medication before invasive procedures.**

B. **Specific agent.** See also Chapter 132 for additional information.

1. **Pharmacologic management provided by systemic analgesia**

a. **Opiates.** All opiates may lead to respiratory depression and hypotension. Muscular rigidity is seen mostly with the synthetic opiates with rapid IV administration, such as fentanyl (>2 mcg/kg), sufentanil, or especially alfentanil. Muscular rigidity can be counteracted by use of a muscle-relaxing agent (eg, pancuronium) and acutely reversed by naloxone (0.1 mg/kg).

i. **Morphine sulfate** is the most commonly used opioid for sedation during mechanical ventilation. A loading IV dose of 50–200 mcg/kg is followed by IV infusion of 10–40 mcg/kg/h. The peak action occurs in 20 min and lasts for 2–4 h in full-term infants and 6–8 h in preterm infants. The use of morphine infusions reduces pain and stress in mechanically ventilated preterm infants at the expense of increasing the duration of mechanical ventilation.

ii. **Fentanyl (Sublimaze)** is frequently used in neonates for its ability to provide rapid analgesia. It has a faster onset (3–4 min) and shorter duration (30 min) of action and is 13–20 times more potent than morphine. Fentanyl blocks endocrine stress responses and prevents pain-induced increases in pulmonary vascular resistance while hemodynamic stability is better preserved than with morphine because it causes less histamine release. For anesthesia, use IV bolus 10–50 mcg/kg, and for analgesia 1–4 mcg/kg. A continuous IV infusion of 1–3 mcg/kg/h is may be used for ongoing sedation. Tolerance to opioid-induced analgesia and sedation occurs more rapidly than with morphine. A cumulative fentanyl dose of >2.5 mg/kg or a duration of infusion >9 days is predictive of opioid withdrawal syndrome.

iii. **Alfentanil.** Give 20 mcg/kg or by continuous IV, 3–5 mcg/kg/h. (**Note:** Alfentanil has a higher incidence of chest wall rigidity and hypotension than fentanyl; use is discouraged.)

iv. **Sufentanil.** Give 0.2 mcg/kg over 20 min, then continuous IV, 0.05 mcg/kg/h.

b. **Ketamine** is unique; it produces sedation, analgesia, and amnesia. It has a mild effect on the respiratory drive, increases blood pressure, produces bronchodilation, and can be used IV, IM, or enterally. It can provide anesthesia for a short duration at 0.5–2 mcg/kg per dose (IV). Use in the NICU has been limited. It may be of value, possibly in combination with atropine sulfate, for sedation before endotracheal intubation. Infants with severe bronchopulmonary dysplasia and refractory bronchospasm may also benefit from the use of ketamine for its additional bronchodilatory effect.

c. **Thiopental,** a short-acting oxybarbiturate, is used at a dose of 6 mg/kg for anesthetic induction in neonates.

2. **Pharmacologic management provided by local analgesia**

a. **Subcutaneous (SQ) infiltration with lidocaine,** 0.5–1% concentration. Always use solution without epinephrine. **Maximum dose (SQ infiltration): 5 mg/kg or 1 mL/kg of 0.5% or 0.5 mL/kg of 1%.**

b. **Buffered lidocaine** is 1 part sodium bicarbonate with 10 parts 1% lidocaine and is typically prepared in the hospital pharmacy. The pain associated with anesthetic infiltration is reduced by buffering the pH from 7.0 to 7.4.

c. **Topical local anesthetics**

i. **Lidocaine 2.5% and prilocaine 2.5% (EMLA cream).** This is a eutectic anesthetic mixture (ie, liquid at room temperature). A single dose of 0.5–1.25 g of EMLA cream applied under an occlusive dressing provides adequate local anesthesia 60–80 min later. In the term infant, it is an alternative to penile dorsal block for anesthesia during circumcision. The risk of methemoglobinemia (from prilocaine) may restrict its use to the full-term infant, and repeated doses should be avoided.

ii. **Tetracaine 4% gel (Ametop).** Apply 1.5 g 30–60 min prior to the procedure. It has no risk of methemoglobinemia, but its repeated use may lead to contact dermatitis.

iii. **4% Liposomal lidocaine cream (L.M.X.4 or Ela-Max).** Increasingly used in pediatrics for its rapid onset of action (20–30 min) and can be applied with (preferred) or without an occlusive dressing.

3. **Pharmacologic management provided by sedative-hypnotics**

a. **Benzodiazepines** activate gamma-aminobutyric acid (GABA) receptors and produce sedation, anxiolysis, muscle relaxation, amnesia, and anticonvulsant effects. They may improve synchrony with assisted ventilation but offer little pain relief. Side effects include respiratory depression, hypotension, dependence, and occasional neuroexcitability or clonic activity resembling seizures.

i. **Midazolam (Versed)** has a rapid onset of action (1–2 min) and can produce apnea if given too rapidly. Its very short half-life (30–60 min) makes it a good choice for brief rapid sedation. Midazolam is given as a single dose, 50–100 mcg/kg, or by continuous infusion at a rate of 0.4–0.6 mcg/kg/min. Withdrawal may occur when given continuously for >48 h. Combining midazolam with opioids increase the incidence of adverse effects of both agents.

ii. **Lorazepam (Ativan)** has a longer duration of action (8–12 h) and may require less frequent dosing (50–100 mcg/kg every 8 h).

b. **Chloral hydrate** is a sedative-hypnotic used primarily for short-term sedation. It is especially useful during diagnostic procedures such as CT scan and MRI. The onset of action is usually within 10–15 min. Administer 20–50 mg/kg every 6–8 h rectally or orally for sedation. It should not be used long term.

c. **Oral pentobarbital (Nembutal)** may produce less adverse effects than chloral hydrate when used for sedation for MRI or CT scan. The initial dose is 4 mg, which may be supplemented at aliquots of 2 mg/kg every 30 min to a maximum of 8 mg/kg.

   d. **Acetaminophen.** The usual dose is 10–15 mg/kg every 6–8 h by mouth.
      Bioavailability is lower by the rectal route requiring administration at a higher
      dose (30–45 mg/kg).
   4. **Oral sucrose** is a disaccharide composed of fructose and glucose shown to pro-
      mote calming behaviors and reduce distress associated with acute painful events. Gus-
      tatory inputs from the taste buds lead to cholecystokinin release in the brainstem that
      activates descending inhibitory opioid. It is effective for the management of proce-
      dural pain in the neonate. Analgesic effects are present with doses as low as 0.1 mL
      of 24 % sucrose. The usual dose is 0.5–1.5 mL of a 24% sucrose solution given by
      syringe or pacifier 2 min before procedures such as heelstick or venipuncture. The
      potential risk for fluid overload, hyperglycemia, and necrotizing enterocolitis should
      limit this method to infants >34 weeks' gestation. Other sweet-tasting liquids such as
      glucose, mother's milk, and saccharin are reported to be equally effective.
   5. **Nonpharmacologic management.** Physical measures such as the use of swad-
      dling, containment, or facilitated tucking as well as skin-to-skin contact with the
      mother ("kangaroo care") are likely to be efficacious in decreasing the noxious
      effect of the "routine procedures" (such as heelstick) needed for the management
      of the sick infant.

70 Seizure Activity

I. **Problem.** The nurse reports that an infant is having abnormal movements of the extremities consistent with seizure activity. **Neonatal seizures are rarely idiopathic and are a
   common manifestation of a serious central nervous system (CNS) disease.** This is why
   quick intervention is necessary. Common causes include cerebral hypoxia ischemia
   (~30–50%), intracranial hemorrhage (10–17%), metabolic abnormalities (hypocalcemia
   [6–15%] hypoglycemia [6–10%]), CNS infections (5–14%), infarction (7%), inborn errors
   of metabolism (3%), CNS malformations (5%), and unknown (10%).
II. **Immediate questions**
   A. **Is the infant really seizing?** This question is very important and is often initially dif-
      ficult to answer. **"Jitteriness"** is sometimes confused with seizures. In a jittery infant,
      eye movements are normal, hands stop moving if they are grasped, and movements
      are of a fine nature. In an infant who is seizing, eye movements can be abnormal (eg,
      staring, blinking, nystagmoid jerks, or tonic horizontal eye deviation). The hands
      continue to move if grasped, and movements are of a coarser nature. The electroen-
      cephalogram (EEG) is normal with jitteriness and abnormal with seizure activity.
      Most seizures in the neonate are focal.
   B. **Is there a history of birth asphyxia or risk factors for sepsis?** Asphyxia and sepsis
      with meningitis may cause neonatal seizures.
   C. **What is the blood glucose level?** Hypoglycemia is an easily treatable cause of seizures
      in the neonatal period.
   D. **How old is the infant?** The age of the infant is often the best clue to the cause of the
      seizures. Common seizure causes for specific ages are as follows:
      1. **At birth.** Maternal anesthetic agents can cause severe tonic seizures typically in
         the first few hours of life.
      2. **Seizure onset 30 min to 3 days after birth.** Pyridoxine deficiency (B_6-dependent
         seizures).

3. **Day 1.** Metabolic abnormalities such as hypoglycemia, hypocalcemia, hypoxic-ischemic encephalopathy (presenting at 6–18 h after birth and becoming more severe in the next 24–48 h).
4. **Days 2–3.** Drug withdrawal or meningitis.
5. **Day 5 or greater.** Hypocalcemia, TORCH infections , or developmental defects.
6. **More than 1–2 weeks.** Methadone withdrawal, De Vivo syndrome (glucose-transport protein 1 [GLUT 1] deficiency syndrome); earliest seizures observed at 2 weeks of age.

III. **Differential diagnosis.** See also Chapter 116.
  A. **Seizure activity may be secondary to:**
    1. **Hypoxic-ischemic cerebral injury.**
    2. **Intracranial hemorrhage,** including subarachnoid, periventricular-intraventricular, or subdural.
    3. **Neonatal cerebral infarction** is a common cause of seizures in **full-term** infants. Its origin remains unclear, but it is found in ~1 in 4000 infants.
    4. **Metabolic/Electrolyte abnormalities**
      a. **Hypoglycemia.**
      b. **Hypocalcemia.** Neonates exposed to topiramate in utero can have hypocalcemic seizures.
      c. **Hypomagnesemia.**
      d. **Hyponatremia or hypernatremia.**
      e. **Pyridoxine dependence.**
    5. **Infection**
      a. **Meningitis.**
      b. **Sepsis.**
      c. **TORCH infections.**
    6. **Neonatal drug withdrawal** (see Chapter 95). Seizures are an uncommon manifestation of withdrawal. One can see abnormalities on the EEG or seizures in infants exposed to maternal cocaine abuse in utero. Maternal antidepressant exposure is associated with an increased risk for infant convulsions of unknown etiology. Specifically, mothers who were on a selective serotonin reuptake inhibitor had infants with a higher incidence of drug-induced convulsions and convulsions of unknown etiology.
    7. **Inborn errors of metabolism** (see Chapter 93)
      a. **Maple syrup urine disease.**
      b. **Methylmalonic acidemia.**
      c. **Nonketotic hyperglycinemia.**
    8. **Folinic acid responsive seizures** occur when there is an abnormality in the cerebrospinal fluid (CSF) neurotransmitter studies. Very rare disorder; <10 cases have been reported.
    9. **De Vivo syndrome (GLUT-1 deficiency syndrome).** This is a rare condition that is caused by inadequate transport of glucose across the blood-brain barrier.
    10. **Maternal anesthetic agents (rare cause).** If a local anesthetic (eg, mepivacaine) is accidentally injected into the infant's scalp during a pudendal, paracervical, or epidural block, seizures can occur at birth.
    11. **Drug toxicity** from agents such as theophylline or caffeine.
    12. **Developmental abnormalities.** Cerebral malformations can cause seizures. Often, the infant has obvious anomalies of the face or head if developmental abnormalities are present.
    13. **CNS trauma.** Usually, there is a history of a difficult delivery.
    14. **Hydrocephalus.** Twenty percent of infants with periventricular or intraventricular hemorrhage develop posthemorrhagic hydrocephalus.
    15. **Polycythemia with hyperviscosity.**
    16. **Four epileptic syndromes that can present in the newborn period:**

   a. Benign familial neonatal convulsions. Presents usually on the third day of life. They run in families and can have 10–20 seizures a day. Usually outgrow after 1–6 months with no recurring problems.

   b. Benign idiopathic nonfamilial neonatal convulsions, otherwise known as "fifth day fits." Usually start on day 4 to 6 and tend to be over in 24 h. They are benign. Chance of having seizures later on is the same as in the general population.

   c. Early myoclonic encephalopathy presents within hours of birth. Infants usually die within the first 2 years of life.

   d. Early infantile epileptic encephalopathy (Ohtahara syndrome) is a severe epileptic syndrome.

 B. Jitteriness. This benign condition is differentiated from seizures as described in Section II, A.

 C. Benign myoclonic activity is isolated jerky, nonrepetitive movements of an extremity or other part of the body that occurs mainly during sleep and are benign.

IV. Database

 A. History. A detailed history helps diagnose seizure activity. The nurse or physician observing the activity should record a complete description of the event on the chart.

 B. Physical examination, with close attention to the neurologic status. Look at the scalp for evidence of injection during delivery.

 C. Laboratory studies

  1. Metabolic workup

   a. Serum glucose. If the glucose level on paper-strip testing is <40 mg/dL, obtain a central value.

   b. Serum sodium to evaluate for hyponatremia.

   c. Serum ionized and total calcium levels. Only an ionized calcium level is usually necessary, but if this test cannot be done, a total calcium study should be ordered. Ionized calcium is the most accurate measurement of calcium.

   d. Serum magnesium.

  2. Infection workup

   a. Complete blood count with differential. A hematocrit also rules out polycythemia.

   b. Blood, urine, and CSF cultures (for bacteria and viruses). CSF polymerase chain reaction for herpes simplex virus if suspected.

   c. Serum immunoglobulin M (IgM) and IgM-specific TORCH titers. The serum IgM titer may be elevated in TORCH infections.

  3. Urine drug screening, if drug withdrawal is suspected.

  4. Theophylline or caffeine level, if the infant is on this medication and toxicity is suspected.

  5. Blood gas levels to rule out hypoxia or acidosis.

  6. Coagulation studies if there is evidence of hemorrhage.

  7. Studies for inborn errors of metabolism include serum ammonia, lactate, CSF lactate, urine organic acids/serum amino acids.

  8. Lumbar puncture. If blood is in the CSF it may suggest an intraventricular hemorrhage (IVH). Cultures and rapid testing of the fluid should be done to diagnose infection (see Chapters 32 and 101). Check glucose for De Vivo syndrome and CSF neurotransmitters for folinic acid responsive seizures.

 D. Radiologic and other studies

  1. Ultrasound examination of the head. This confirms periventricular-intraventricular hemorrhage (PV-IVH). *Note:* The coexistence of IVH and seizures does not necessarily mean the two are related.

  2. Computed tomography scan of the head to diagnose subarachnoid or subdural hemorrhage. It may also reveal a congenital malformation or cerebral infarction if suspected.

  3. Cranial magnetic resonance imaging is a very sensitive test used to help determine the etiology of the seizures. Its disadvantage is that it is difficult to obtain in an unstable infant. **Magnetic resonance angiography** is helpful in making the diagnosis of cerebral infarction.

4. **Electroencephalography (EEG).** It is usually not possible to perform an EEG during the episode of seizure activity. The EEG is rarely helpful in making a specific diagnosis. This study should be done at some time after seizure activity has been documented; it may confirm seizure activity and may also be used as a baseline study and may show changes consistent with the localization of the lesion in cerebral infarction. The interictal pattern is also helpful in predicting future seizure activity. Focal clonic seizures have a consistent EEG correlation, subtle seizures do not.

V. **Plan**

A. **General measures.** Once it is determined that the infant is having seizures **immediate management is necessary.** The other two diagnoses (jitteriness and benign myoclonic activity) are benign conditions. The following immediate measures should be taken.

1. **Rule out hypoxia** by measurement of blood gases, and start oxygen therapy. Assess the infant's airway and breathing. Intubation and mechanical ventilation may be necessary to maintain ventilation and oxygenation. Correct any metabolic acidosis.

2. **Check the glucose level.** A Dextrostix or Chemstrip-bG paper-strip test should be immediately done to rule out hypoglycemia while a STAT sample is sent to the laboratory for confirmation. If the paper-strip test shows low blood glucose, it is acceptable to give 10% glucose, 2–4 mL/kg IV push, before obtaining results from the laboratory.

3. **Obtain STAT serum calcium, sodium, and magnesium levels.** If these levels were low on earlier values and a metabolic disorder is strongly suspected as the cause of the seizures, it is acceptable to treat the infant before new laboratory values are available.

4. **Anticonvulsant therapy.** If hypoxia and all metabolic abnormalities have been treated or if blood gas and metabolic workup values are normal, start anticonvulsant therapy. For detailed pharmacologic information, see Chapter 132.

a. **Phenobarbital is the first-line drug.** Initially, 20 mg/kg is given as the loading dose, but additional doses of 5 mg/kg up to 40 mg/kg can be given if the seizures have not stopped. Usually is only successful in <50% of patients.

b. **If seizures persist,** give **phenytoin (Dilantin),** 20 mg/kg/dose, at a rate of 1 mg/kg/min or less. **Fosphenytoin may be preferred** at some centers (see dosage in Chapter 132) because it has been associated with fewer side effects than phenytoin (less hypotension, fewer cardiac abnormalities, and less soft tissue injury).

c. **If seizures still persist,** the **third medication** to give is a **benzodiazepine.** Respiratory depression can occur with these medications, but is usually not a problem because most infants are already on mechanical ventilation. Most institutions use lorazepam.

i. **Lorazepam,** given IV, can be repeated four to six times in a 24-h period. It is advantageous to use over diazepam because it causes less sedation and respiratory depression. Dose is 0.05–0.1 mg/kg every 8–12 h.

ii. **Diazepam** is effective if given by a continuous infusion of 0.3 mg/kg/h. Another dose listed was 0.25 mg/kg every 6–8 h.

d. **If seizures persist and other causes have been ruled out, three disorders need to be considered because they are treatable:**

i. **Pyridoxine (B_6)-dependent seizures.** A trial of pyridoxine (vitamin B_6), 50–100 mg given IV with EEG monitoring, is now recommended. With pyridoxine dependency, the seizures stop quickly after the medication is given. Some institutions wait to give this after three medications have been given and failed; some try this after two medications have been given.

   ii. **Folinic acid responsive seizures (rare).** Obtain CSF neurotransmitter studies. Then folinic acid is given at 2.5 mg twice daily (up to 4 mg/kg/day initially) in two doses. After 24 h of treatment, seizures may stop. Folinic acid can be given for 48 h as a trial.
   iii. **De Vivo syndrome (glucose transporter deficiency).** Treatment is a ketogenic diet.
   e. **If seizures still persist,** the following drugs may be used depending on institutional preference:
      i. High-dose phenobarbital (>30 mg/kg to achieve serum level >60 mcg/mL) was effective in one review.
      ii. Midazolam, IV and has also been given intranasally. IV dose is 0.2 mg/kg, then 0.1–0.4 mg/kg/h.
      iii. Pentobarbital, 10 mg/kg IV, then 1 mg/kg/h.
      iv. Thiopental, 10 mg/kg IV, then 2–4 mg/kg/h.
      v. Clonazepam, 0.1 mg/kg orally.
      vi. Valproic acid, 10–25 mg/kg, then 20 mg/kg/day in three doses.
      vii. Chlormethiazole (not available in United States). Initial infusion rate of 0.08 mg/kg/min.
      viii. Paraldehyde. Given rectally (IV preparation no longer available in United States); used as a last effort.
      ix. Lidocaine, 2 mg/kg IV, then 6 mg/kg/h with cardiac monitoring. New infusion doses have been used to decrease cardiac arrhythmias. Not recommended in infants who have been treated with phenytoin or who have congenital heart disease.
   f. **Newer medications.** Lamotrigine, vigabatrin, zonisamide, topiramate, and levetiracetam.
B. **Specific measures**
   1. **Hypoxic-ischemic injury.** Seizures secondary to birth asphyxia usually present at anywhere from 6–18 h of age.
      a. **Careful observation** by the physician and nursing staff is required to detect seizure activity.
      b. **Prophylactic phenobarbital** is used at some institutions (*controversial*). One study stated that the use of phenobarbital within 6 h of birth in infants with hypoxic ischemic encephalopathy decreased the incidence of neonatal seizures. However, anticonvulsant therapy soon after birth to birth-asphyxiated infants cannot be recommended unless larger and more studies are done.
      c. **Restrict fluids to ~60 mL/kg/day.** Monitor serum electrolytes and urine output.
      d. **If seizures begin,** follow the guidelines given in Section V, A, 4.
   2. **Hypoglycemia.** Treat and determine the cause, as outlined in Chapter 55.
   3. **Hypocalcemia.** Give 100–200 mg/kg calcium gluconate slow IV. Make certain that the infant is receiving maintenance calcium therapy (usually 50 mg/kg every 6 h). Monitor the heart rate continuously, and make sure that the IV line is correctly positioned.(See also Chapter 78.)
   4. **Hypomagnesemia.** Give 0.2 mEq/kg magnesium sulfate IV every 6 h until magnesium levels are normal or symptoms resolve. (See Chapter 99.)
   5. **Hyponatremia.** See Chapter 57.
   6. **Hypernatremia.** Treat the seizure activity as described in Section V, A, 4. If hypernatremia is secondary to decreased fluid intake, increase the rate of free water. The amount of sodium needs to be decreased; it should be reduced over 48 h to decrease the possibility of cerebral edema.
   7. **Hypercalcemia.** Usual treatment plans include the following:
      a. **Increase IV fluids by 20 mL/kg/day.**
      b. **Administer a diuretic** (eg, furosemide [Lasix], 1–2 mg/kg/dose every 12 h).
      c. **Administer phosphate,** 30–40 mg/kg/day orally or IV.

8. **Infection.** If sepsis is suspected, a complete workup should be performed and empirical broad-spectrum antibiotic therapy initiated. Remember aminoglycosides have poor CSF penetration. Antiviral therapy (acyclovir) should be considered in infants >1 week of age or sooner if premature rupture of membranes for treatment of herpes simplex virus. Some institutions treat all infants with seizures empirically with acyclovir when there is a high index of suspicion of herpes infection. A complete septic workup includes white blood cell count with differential, blood culture, urine and serum antigen test, lumbar puncture, culture for bacteria and viruses (if indicated), and urinalysis and urine culture (if indicated). CSF polymerase chain reaction and surface cultures should be done if herpes is suspected.

9. **Drug withdrawal syndrome.** Supportive therapy and anticonvulsants are used. See Chapter 95.

10. **Subarachnoid hemorrhage.** Only supportive therapy is necessary. (See Chapter 96.)

11. **Subdural hemorrhage.** Only supportive therapy is necessary, unless the infant has lacerations of the falx and tentorium for which rapid surgical correction is necessary. Hemorrhage over cerebral convexities is treated by subdural taps. (See Chapter 96.)

12. **CNS trauma.** In cases of depressed skull fracture, elevation of the bone may be necessary.

13. **Hydrocephalus.** Repeated lumbar taps may be necessary, or a shunt may be placed. (See Chapter 90.)

14. **Polycythemia.** Partial plasma exchange is necessary. See Chapters 64 and 112.

15. **Cerebral infarction**
    a. **Supportive therapy.**
    b. **Treat the seizures.** Some resolve and others progress to epilepsy.
    c. **Close follow-up** is necessary because of possible neurologic sequelae (eg, hemiplegia, cognitive difficulties, delays in language acquisition, and developmental delay).
    d. **Most of the cases** have a normal outcome.

16. **Accidental injection.** Vigorous support and removal of the drug by diuresis or dialysis is recommended.

71 Traumatic Delivery

I. **Problem.** An infant is noted to have severe bruises after birth, and a nurse observes that the infant is not using his right arm. The birth was traumatic, and the nurse calls you to evaluate the infant. Birth injuries are injuries that occur during the birth process. The incidence is ~2–7 per 1000 live births.

II. **Immediate questions**
   A. **Is there any reason the infant would have a birth injury?** Certain factors predispose the infant to birth injuries. These include fetal macrosomia, dystocia, prolonged or very rapid labor, abnormal presentation (especially breech), cephalopelvic disproportion, small maternal stature, maternal pelvic abnormalities, oligohydramnios, very low birthweight infant, fetal anomalies, use of forceps or vacuum extraction, and prematurity.

B. **Is the injury so serious that it requires immediate attention?** The majority of birth injuries are not serious and do not require immediate treatment. Significant injuries requiring immediate intervention, such as abdominal organ injuries that present as shock and require surgery, need to be identified early. It is important to distinguish and recognize the different injuries so that appropriate treatment can be given.

C. **Was forceps or vacuum extraction used during the delivery?** Studies suggest that the use of midforceps and vacuum extraction may increase the infant's risk of fractures and paralysis.

III. **Differential diagnosis**

A. **Skin**

1. **Petechiae.** In birth trauma, petechiae are usually localized (eg, on the head, neck, upper chest area, and lower back). There is no associated bleeding, and no new lesions appear. If petechiae are diffuse, suspect systemic disease. If there is associated bleeding, suspect disseminated intravascular coagulation.

2. **Forceps injury.** Frequently, linear marks are seen across both sides of the face. The area is usually red.

3. **Subcutaneous fat necrosis** typically involves the shoulders and the buttocks with a well-circumscribed lesion of the skin and underlying tissue. It usually appears between 6 and 10 days of age. Lesion size is 1–10 cm, it can be irregular and hard, and the overlying skin can be purple or colorless.

4. **Ecchymoses.** Bruising can occur after a traumatic delivery, especially when labor is rapid or the infant is premature.

5. **Lacerations** can occur secondary to the use of a scalpel during a cesarean delivery. They usually occur on the buttocks, scalp, or thigh.

6. **Scalp electrode injury.** The site of insertion of the scalp electrode can sometimes become infected (1% of cases) and rarely in premature infants can cause severe bleeding.

B. **Head**

1. **Caput succedaneum.** This is an area of edema over the presenting part of the scalp during a vertex delivery. The area of edema is usually associated with bruising and petechiae. It crosses the midline of the skull and suture lines. The bleeding is external to the periosteum (see Figure 5–1). Hyperbilirubinemia rarely develops.

2. **Cephalhematoma.** Incidence is 1.5–2.5% of all deliveries. This is caused by bleeding that occurs below the periosteum overlying one cranial bone (usually the parietal bone). (See Figure 5–1.) **There is no crossing of the suture lines.** The overlying scalp is not discolored, and the swelling sometimes takes days to become apparent. The incidence of an associated skull fracture is 5% in unilateral lesions and 18% in bilateral lesions and is most often a linear fracture. Hyperbilirubinemia (sometimes significant if the lesion is extensive) may develop.

3. **Subgaleal hemorrhage** is a collection of blood in the soft tissue space under the aponeurosis but above the periosteum of the skull. (See Figure 5–1.) Diffuse swelling of the soft tissue, often spreading toward the neck and behind the ears, can be seen. Periorbital swelling is also evident. Associated symptoms include severe blood loss, shock, anemia, hypotonia, seizures, and pallor.

4. **Intracranial hemorrhage.** See also Chapter 96.

a. **Subarachnoid.** This is usually asymptomatic, but seizures and other complications are rare.

b. **Epidural.** This is very rare and also very difficult to diagnose. Clinical symptoms are usually delayed.

c. **Subdural.** These infants present shortly after birth with stupor, seizures, a full fontanelle, unresponsive pupils, and coma.

5. **Skull fracture.** These are uncommon in neonates; most are linear and are associated with a cephalhematoma. Depressed fractures are often visible and can result in seizures. Fractures at the base of the skull may result in shock.

C. Face
  1. **Fractures.** Fractures of the nose, mandible, maxilla, and septal cartilage can occur. These can often present as respiratory distress or feeding problems.
  2. **Dislocations of the facial bones.** Nasal septal dislocation (the most common facial injury) can occur and present as stridor and cyanosis.
  3. **Facial nerve palsy.** This is the most common cranial nerve injury secondary to birth trauma. It is not increased in deliveries involving forceps, as previously believed. The nerve is injured at the point where it emerges from the stylomastoid foramen.
     a. **Central paralysis** involves the lower half or two thirds of the contralateral side of the face. On the paralyzed side, the nasolabial fold is obliterated, the corner of the mouth droops, and the skin is smooth and full. When the infant cries, the wrinkles are deeper on the normal side and the mouth is drawn to the normal side.
     b. **Peripheral paralysis** involves the entire side of the face. At rest, the infant has an open eye on the affected side. When the infant cries, the findings are similar to those with central paralysis.
D. Eye
  1. **Eyelids.** Edema and bruising can occur. Swollen eyelids should be forced open to examine the eyeball. Laceration of the eyelid can also occur.
  2. **Orbit fracture** can occur rarely. Immediate ophthalmologic evaluation is necessary if disturbances of the extraocular muscle movements and exophthalmos are evident. Severe injuries may result in death.
  3. **Horner syndrome** (miosis, partial ptosis, enophthalmos, and anhidrosis of the ipsilateral side of the face). Delayed pigmentation of the ipsilateral iris can be seen.
  4. **Subconjunctival hemorrhage** is a common finding.
  5. **Cornea.** Haziness can occur secondary to edema. With persistent haziness, suspect rupture of Descemet membrane.
  6. **Intraocular hemorrhage**
     a. **Retinal hemorrhage** can occur most commonly as a flame-shaped or streak hemorrhage found near the optic disk. A subdural hemorrhage can cause preretinal and intraretinal hemorrhages.
     b. **Hyphemas.** Gross blood is seen in the anterior chamber.
     c. **Vitreous hemorrhage.** Indicated by floaters, absent red reflex, and blood pigment seen on slit-lamp examination by the ophthalmologist.
E. **Ear.** Ear injuries can occur because of forceps placed near the ears.
  1. **Abrasions and bruising.**
  2. **Hematomas.**
  3. **Avulsion of the auricle.**
  4. **Laceration of the auricle.**
F. **Vocal cord injuries.** Although these are rare, they can occur as a result of excessive traction on the head during delivery.
  1. **Unilateral paralysis** involves the recurrent laryngeal branch of one of the vagus nerves in the neck. Clinically, hoarseness and mild to moderate stridor with inspiration are seen.
  2. **Bilateral paralysis** is caused by trauma to both recurrent laryngeal nerves. Symptoms at birth include respiratory distress, stridor, and cyanosis.
G. **Neck and shoulder injuries**
  1. **Clavicular fracture is the most common bone fracture during delivery.** If the fracture is complete, symptoms involve decreased or absent movement of the arm, gross deformity of the clavicle, tenderness on palpation, localized crepitus, and an absent or asymmetric Moro reflex. Green-stick fracture usually presents with no symptoms, and the diagnosis is made because of callus formation at 7–10 days.
  2. **Brachial palsy.** This is usually secondary from a prolonged delivery of a macrosomic infant. Trauma to the spinal roots of the fifth cervical through the first thoracic spinal

nerves (brachial plexus) during birth. There are three different presentations. This is usually unilateral and occurs twice as often on the right as the left.

    a. **Duchenne-Erb palsy.** This involves the upper arm and is the most common type (~90% of cases). The fifth and sixth cervical roots are affected, and the arm is adducted and internally rotated. Moro reflex is absent (sometimes it can be asymmetric or weakened), but the grasp reflex is intact.

    b. **Klumpke palsy.** This involves the lower arm because the seventh and eighth cervical and first thoracic roots are injured; it is rare (2.5% of cases). The hand is paralyzed, the wrist does not move, and the grasp reflex is absent (ie, dropped hand). Cyanosis and edema of the hand can also occur. An ipsilateral Horner syndrome (ptosis, miosis, and enophthalmos) can be seen because of injury involving the cervical sympathetic fibers of the first thoracic root. Phrenic nerve paralysis with Klumpke palsy is evident.

    c. **Entire arm (global or total brachial plexus) paralysis.** The entire brachial plexus is damaged. The patient has a flaccid arm, hanging limply with no reflexes.

    3. **Phrenic nerve paralysis.** Difficult breech delivery can rarely cause diaphragmatic paralysis and usually occurs along with upper brachial nerve palsy (75% of cases). It is associated with cyanosis, tachypnea, irregular respirations, and thoracic breathing with no bulging of the abdomen.

    4. **Sternocleidomastoid muscle (SCM) injury** (muscular or congenital torticollis). A well-circumscribed, immobile mass in the midportion of the SCM that enlarges, regresses, and disappears. This results in a transient torticollis after birth. The head tilts toward the involved side, the chin is elevated and rotated, and the patient cannot move the head into normal position.

  H. **Spinal cord injuries** are rare and caused by lateral or longitudinal stretching force of the neck. It can also be caused by torsion of the neck. Symptoms vary, depending on the location of the injury. It occurs with breech deliveries. The higher the injury, the greater is the risk of respiratory problems.

    1. **Infants with a high cervical lesion** usually have severe respiratory depression with paralysis at birth. There is a high rate of mortality.

    2. **Upper or midcervical lesions** usually present without symptoms but can have hypotonia. The mortality rate is high.

    3. **Lesions in the seventh cervical to first thoracic roots** present with paraplegia and urinary and respiratory problems.

    4. **Partial spinal cord injuries.** On neurologic examination, these infants have signs of spasticity.

  I. **Abdominal organ injuries** (uncommon). These injuries should be suspected with shock, increasing abdomen, anemia, and irritability. These infants can be asymptomatic for hours and then crash. Risk factors for these include macrosomia and breech presentation.

    1. **Liver rupture.** The liver is the most common organ affected. Subcapsular hematomas are usually not symptomatic and can present with subtle signs of blood loss such as onset of jaundice, tachypnea, and poor feeding. Rupture of the hematoma presents with sudden circulatory collapse (a hematoma ruptures through the capsule).

    2. **Splenic rupture.** Signs are similar to rupture of the liver; blood loss and hemoperitoneum may be seen.

    3. **Adrenal hemorrhage.** Usually right sided and unilateral. Symptoms include fever, tachypnea, flank mass, pallor, cyanosis, poor feeding, shock, vomiting, and diarrhea.

    4. **Kidney trauma.** Is similar to the other organ injuries with ascites, flank mass, and gross hematuria.

  J. **Extremity injuries**

    1. **Fractured humerus** is the second most common fracture during birth trauma. The arm is immobile, with tenderness and crepitation on palpation. Moro reflex is absent on the affected side.

2. **Fractured femur** may occur secondary to breech delivery. Infants with congenital hypotonia are at risk. Deformity is usually obvious; the affected leg does not move, and there is pain with assisted movement.

3. **Dislocation.** Rare; this usually involves the radial head. Examination reveals adduction, internal rotation of the affected arm, and poor Moro reflex. Palpate lateral and posterior displacement of the radial head.

K. **Genital injuries**

1. **Edema, bruising, and hematoma of the scrotum and penis** can occur, especially in large infants and breech deliveries. Injury does not affect micturition.

2. **Testicular and epididymal injury.** Findings are scrotal swelling, with the infant experiencing vomiting and irritability. A **hematocele** can form if the tunica vaginalis testis is injured; the scrotum will not transilluminate.

IV. **Database**

A. **Physical examination**

1. **Skin.** Look for petechiae, bruising, and any lacerations. Check the side of the face for forceps marks. Look for and palpate any area that looks like fat necrosis.

2. **Head.** Carefully examine the head for any evidence of a caput succedaneum, cephalhematoma, subgaleal hemorrhage, or fracture. Check to see whether the suture lines are crossed; this helps differentiate between the caput succedaneum and cephalhematoma. Depressed skull fractures are obvious; others may require radiologic studies.

3. **Face.** Examine the face at rest and during crying to look for any facial nerve palsy. Check for any signs of respiratory distress (eg, stridor or cyanosis).

4. **Eyes.** Examine the eyeball and the eyelid. Make sure that extraocular muscle movements are normal. Check for the red reflex.

5. **Ears.** Examine the front and back of the ear, looking for lacerations, swelling, and hematomas.

6. **Vocal cords.** If injury is suspected, examine the vocal cords by direct laryngoscopy or use a flexible fiberoptic laryngoscope.

7. **Neck and shoulder injuries.** Carefully examine the neck and the shoulder. Check Moro and grasp reflexes. Examine the arm to see whether movement is normal. Check respirations, and note any thoracic breathing. Make sure the head rests in a normal position and is not tilted.

8. **Spinal cord.** A careful and thorough neurologic examination should be done.

9. **Abdomen.** Examine the abdomen, and check for ascites, masses, and increase in size.

10. **Extremities.** Observe for movement and deformity.

11. **Genitalia.** Examine the testes and the penis; transilluminate the scrotum.

B. **Laboratory studies based on site of trauma**

1. **Skin**

a. **Platelet count.** A normal platelet count excludes neonatal thrombocytopenia.

b. **Serum bilirubin test.** Hyperbilirubinemia may result from reabsorption of blood from extensive ecchymoses.

c. **Serum hematocrit.** Anemia may result from severe ecchymoses.

2. **Head**

a. **Hematocrit.** Blood loss can occur, requiring transfusions, especially in subgaleal hemorrhage.

b. **Serum bilirubin.** Significant hyperbilirubinemia may result from cephalohematoma.

3. **Face.** Arterial blood gas may be indicated in those infants with respiratory distress. Nerve excitability or conduction tests are recommended if there is no improvement in the facial nerve palsy after 3–4 days.

4. **Eyes, ears, or vocal cords.** No laboratory tests are usually required.

5. **Neck and shoulder.** Arterial blood gas helps diagnose hypoxia associated with phrenic nerve paralysis.

6. **Spinal cord.** The usual laboratory tests required for respiratory depression and shock, if indicated.

7. **Abdomen.** Obtain hematocrit, to rule out anemia and blood loss; urine dipstick, to check for hematuria. Consider abdominal paracentesis with fluid sent to the laboratory for cell count with differential.

8. **Extremities and genitalia.** No laboratory tests are usually needed.

C. **Radiologic and other studies**

1. **Head.** Skull radiographs should be obtained to rule out the possibility of skull fractures. A computed tomography (CT) scan can also be obtained and can be useful in the diagnosis of an intracranial hemorrhage.

2. **Face.** Radiographs and a cranial CT scan help diagnose facial fractures.

3. **Eyes.** Radiographs, to rule out orbit fracture, may be indicated.

4. **Neck and shoulder**
   a. **A radiograph of the clavicle** is necessary for confirmation of the diagnosis.
   b. **A radiograph of the chest** for phrenic nerve paralysis shows an elevated diaphragm.
   c. **Fluoroscopy** reveals elevation of the affected side and descent of the normal side on inspiration. Opposite movements occur with expiration.
   d. **Ultrasonogram of the diaphragm** shows abnormal motion on the affected side.
   e. **Magnetic resonance imaging (MRI)** can be used to show nerve root avulsion.
   f. **An electroencephalogram** can reveal the extent of the denervation weeks after the injury.

5. **Spinal cord**
   a. **Cervical and thoracic spine radiographs** should be obtained.
   b. **MRI** is the most reliable method for diagnosing spinal cord injuries.

6. **Abdomen.** Ultrasonogram diagnoses liver and splenic rupture, adrenal hemorrhage, and kidney damage. An abdominal radiograph may reveal a stomach bubble displaced medially in splenic rupture.

7. **Extremities.** A radiography of the extremities confirms the diagnosis.

8. **Genitalia.** Ultrasonography may be diagnostic.

V. **Plan**

A. **Skin**

1. **Petechiae.** No specific treatment is necessary. Traumatic petechiae usually fade in 2–3 days.

2. **Subcutaneous fat necrosis.** The lesions require minimal pressure at the affected site and observation only. They disappear within a couple of months. Closely monitor the first 6 weeks for symptomatic hypercalcemia (vomiting, fever, and weight loss with high serum calcium), which can occur in these infants. This can usually be treated with intravenous hydration, furosemide, and hydrocortisone therapy.

3. **Ecchymoses.** No specific treatment is necessary because they usually resolve within 1 week. Watch for hyperbilirubinemia (reabsorption of blood from a bruised area), anemia (blood loss from bruising), and hyperkalemia.

4. **Lacerations.** If superficial, the edges may be held together with butterfly adhesive strips. If deeper, they should be sutured with 7–0 nylon. Healing is usually rapid. Observe for infections, especially a scalp lesion and caput succedaneum.

B. **Head**

1. **Caput succedaneum.** No specific treatment is necessary. It resolves within several days.

2. **Cephalhematoma.** Usually no treatment is necessary, and it resolves anywhere between 2 weeks and 3 months. In some cases, blood loss and hyperbilirubinemia can occur.

3. **Subgaleal hemorrhage.** If hypovolemic shock develops, it requires immediate treatment. Surgery is done if the bleeding does not subside. Death may occur. Look for coagulopathies and treat as needed.

4. **Intracranial hemorrhage.** Circulatory and ventilatory support are indicated in deteriorating conditions. (See also Chapter 96.)
   a. **Subarachnoid.** Resolution usually occurs without treatment.
   b. **Epidural.** Prompt surgical evacuation for large bleeds. Prognosis is good with early treatment.
   c. **Subdural.** Subdural taps are indicated to drain a large hematoma.
5. **Skull fracture.** Linear fractures do not require treatment. Depressed skull fractures usually require surgery because of seizure risk.

C. **Face**
1. **Facial nerve injury.** No specific therapy is necessary. Full resolution usually occurs within a few months. Neurology consult should be obtained if no improvement in 2–3 weeks.
   a. **Complete peripheral paralysis.** Cover the exposed eye with an eye patch and instill synthetic tears (1% methylcellulose drops) every 4 h. This will prevent irritation from the dryness.
   b. **Electrodiagnostic testing** may be beneficial in predicting recovery.
   c. **In severe cases,** surgery may be necessary.
2. **Fractures. Maxilla, lacrimal, mandible and nose fractures** require immediate evaluation. An oral airway is required, and surgical consultation is needed. The fractures must be reduced and fixated.

D. **Eyes**
1. **Eyelids.** Edema and bruising usually resolve within 1 week. Laceration of the eyelid may require microsurgery.
2. **Orbit fracture.** Immediate ophthalmologic consultation is required.
3. **Horner syndrome.** No treatment is necessary, and resolution usually occurs.
4. **Subconjunctival hemorrhage.** No treatment is necessary because the blood is usually absorbed within 1–2 weeks.
5. **Cornea.** Haziness disappears usually within 2 weeks. If persistent and if rupture of Descemet membrane has occurred, then a white opacity of the cornea will occur. This is usually permanent. Ophthalmologic input is essential.
6. **Intraocular hemorrhage**
   a. **Retinal hemorrhage** usually disappears within 1 week. No treatment is necessary.
   b. **Hyphema.** This usually resolves without treatment within 1 week.
   c. **Vitreous hemorrhage.** If resolution does not occur within 1 year, surgery must be considered.

E. **Ears**
1. **Abrasions and ecchymoses.** These injuries are usually mild and require no treatment, except for keeping the area clean. They resolve spontaneously.
2. **Hematomas.** Incision and evacuation may be indicated.
3. **Avulsion of the auricle.** Surgical consultation is required if cartilage is involved.
4. **Laceration of the ear.** Most of these can be sutured with 7–0 nylon sutures.

F. **Vocal cords**
1. **Unilateral paralysis.** Observe these infants closely. Keeping them quiet and giving small, frequent feedings decreases their risk of aspiration. This condition usually resolves within 4–6 weeks.
2. **Bilateral paralysis.** Intubation is required if there is airway obstruction. ENT consultation and tracheostomy are usually required. The prognosis is variable.

G. **Neck and shoulder**
1. **Clavicular fracture.** Immobilization, and the prognosis is excellent. Pain medication can be given.
2. **Brachial palsy.** Immobilization and physical therapy to prevent contractures, until recovery of the brachial plexus. Recovery depends on the extent of the lesions and is usually good but may take many months. In Erb-Duchenne paralysis, one can see improvement in 2 weeks and recovery is usually complete by 18 months. In Klumpke

paralysis, prognosis is poorer and sometimes never complete. Muscle atrophy and contractures can occur. Orthopedic consultation is recommended early on.

3. **Phrenic nerve paralysis.** Treatment is usually supportive and nonspecific, and the prognosis is usually good. Some infants may require continuous positive airway pressure or mechanical ventilation. Most infants recover in 1–3 months.

4. **Sternocleidomastoid muscle (SCM) injury.** Most recover spontaneously. Passive exercise may be indicated and appropriate positioning of the infant is recommended. If it is not resolved within 1 year, surgery should be considered.

H. **Spinal cord.** Prognosis depends on the level and severity of the injury. Most infants with a severe spinal cord injury do not survive. Treatment is supportive, and some require intubation for respiratory problems. Specific therapy needs to be directed at the bladder, bowel, and skin because these present as ongoing problems.

I. **Abdomen.** Surgical consultation with the prognosis for all of these dependent on early recognition and treatment. Early management strategies that increase survival include volume replacement and identifying and correcting coagulation disorders.

1. **Liver rupture.** Transfusion, laparotomy with evacuation of hematomas, and repair of any laceration.

2. **Splenic rupture.** Transfusion of whole blood and exploratory laparotomy, with preservation of the spleen if possible.

3. **Adrenal hemorrhage.** Management is supportive with packed red blood cells and intravenous steroids usually the only treatment.

4. **Kidney damage.** Use supportive measures. Surgery may be necessary if severe.

J. **Extremities**

1. **Fractured humerus.** Obtain an orthopedic consultation. Immobilize the arm for usually 2 weeks. Displaced fractures may require closed reduction and casting. The prognosis is excellent.

2. **Fractured femur.** Treatment is traction and casting, with an orthopedic consultation. The prognosis is excellent.

3. **Dislocation.** Treatment is immediate reduction with immobilization of the arm.

K. **Genitalia**

1. **Edema and bruising.** These usually resolve within 4–5 days, and no treatment is necessary.

2. **Testicular injury.** Urologic or pediatric surgical consultation is necessary.

3. **Hematocele.** Elevate the scrotum with cold packs. Resolution occurs without other treatment, unless there is a severe underlying testicular injury.

72 Vasospasms and Thromboembolism

I. **Problem.** An infant with an indwelling umbilical artery catheter develops a vasospasm in one leg. The nurse notifies you that another infant with an umbilical line has no pulses in the lower legs and has severely decreased perfusion.

II. **Immediate questions**

A. **Can the catheter be removed?** Evaluate the need for the catheter. If the catheter can be removed, this is the treatment of choice. Vasospasm is most commonly related to the use of umbilical artery catheters (UAC), but it can also occur in other catheters such as radial artery catheters. Over 80% of venous thromboembolism in newborns is secondary to central venous lines. Arterial thrombosis is less common than venous thrombosis. The incidence of UAC-related thrombosis is 14–35% by ultrasound, and up to 64% by angiography. In some cases of thrombosis, the catheter should not be removed so thrombolytic medication can be given through it.

B. **Was a medication given recently through the catheter?** Most medications, if given too rapidly, can cause vasospasm.

C. **How severe is the vasospasm?** Deciding on the severity of the vasospasm may dictate treatment choices (see physical examination).

D. **Is there a pulse in the affected extremity?** A loss of pulse with a thrombus is a medical emergency.

E. **What are the risk factors for vasospasm?** Besides the umbilical catheter, the most common risk factor, infection, polycythemia, hypoxia, maternal diabetes, hypotension, dehydration, intrauterine growth restriction, and an increase in blood viscosity can all increase the risk.

III. **Differential diagnosis**

A. **Vasospasm** is a muscular contraction (spasm) of an **arterial** vessel, manifested by acute color change (white or blue) in the perfused extremity (upper or lower extremity, sometimes only on the toes or fingers). Occasionally, the color change extends to the buttocks and the abdomen. The change in color may be transient or persistent. It may be caused by prior injection of medication or a manifestation of thromboembolism/thromboembolic phenomenon. Arterial blood sampling can also be a predisposing factor.

B. **Thromboembolism.** A **thrombus** is a blood clot formation in an artery or vein and can cause partial or complete obstruction. An **embolus** is a clot that is mobile and lodges in a blood vessel and may cause obstruction or vasospasm. Neonates are the most common affected age group with an incidence of ~41 cases in 100,000 per year. The initial sign is usually that the catheter does not work. One can not infuse fluid or withdraw from the line. Less commonly, thromboembolic phenomenon are due to inherited or acquired thrombophilias (heterozygous factor V Leiden; protein C or S deficiency). Congenital CMV is a rare cause of neonatal aortic thrombosis.

IV. **Database**

A. **History.** Obtain a detailed family history of any inherited clotting or other hematologic disorder. Did any one in the family have a thromboembolism?

B. **Physical examination.** The severity of the vasospasm and thrombosis must be assessed because it dictates treatment. The areas of involvement, appearance of the skin over the involved areas, and pulses of the affected extremity are measures of severity. Compare the affected extremity with the other extremity. A handheld Doppler is useful to assess peripheral arterial flow.

1. **Severe vasospasm** involves a large area of one or both legs, the abdomen, or the buttocks. In the upper extremity, a severe vasospasm includes most of the arm and all of the fingers. The skin may be completely white. Decreased perfusion is present and pulses of the affected extremity are weak but detectable.

2. **Less severe vasospasm** involves a small area of one or both legs (usually some of the toes and part of the foot). In the arm, it can involve part of the extremity and some fingers. The skin has a mottled appearance and pulses are present but can be diminished.

3. **Thrombosis.** If pulses are completely absent, an arterial thrombosis, which is a **medical emergency,** is likely. Persistent bacteremia and thrombocytopenia may be associated with thrombosis.

   a. **Venous thrombosis.** Venous thrombosis in the newborn occurs either from indwelling venous catheters or renal vein thrombosis. With a central venous thrombosis, extremities are swollen and discolored with distended superficial veins. A renal vein thrombosis can cause hematuria, hypertension, thrombocytopenia, and a flank mass.

   b. **Aortic thrombosis.** Aortic thrombosis is rare in newborns. Decreased perfusion and color change of the lower extremities, loss of pulses, blood pressure difference in upper and lower extremities, oliguria, hypertension, and hematuria can be observed. Renal arterial thrombosis can cause the similar renal findings.

c. **Peripheral or central arterial thrombosis.** Arterial thrombosis occurs more frequently in the femoral, iliac, and cerebral arteries. Radial, posterior tibial and dorsalis pedis arterial lines are rarely associated with thrombosis. Weak or absent peripheral pulse, pallor of the extremity, coldness, discoloration, and decreased perfusion of the extremity is seen.

C. **Laboratory studies** are not usually needed for vasospasm. However, the following laboratory tests should be obtained if a thrombosis is suspected and clot dissolving medication is to be used.

1. **Thrombin time.**
2. **Activated partial thromboplastin time (aPTT).**
3. **Prothrombin time/INR.**
4. **Hematocrit.**
5. **Platelet count.** The thrombus itself and the use of heparin can cause thrombocytopenia.
6. **Fibrinogen.**
7. **Genetic tests** may be done to rule out congenital thrombophilia.
8. **CMV work up.** See Chapter 127.

D. **Radiologic and other studies**

1. **Real-time ultrasonography,** with or without color Doppler flow imaging, can be used to diagnose thrombosis. It is the most common study used but can be unreliable. One study showed that this method underestimated the number of venous and arterial thromboses and had significant false-positive results. It can also be used to monitor the progress over time.
2. **Contrast angiography (the gold standard)** is performed through the umbilical artery catheter and can be used to diagnose aortoiliac thrombosis. In several studies, this procedure was found to be the most effective diagnostic technique. A contrast study should be considered before administrating a fibrinolytic agent. Remember this test is difficult to perform in sick neonates.
3. **"Linograms."** Injecting radio-opaque dye directly into the line is sometimes done, but this method may also miss thrombosis.
4. **Venography.** Injection of contrast through peripheral vessels can be done if other studies have failed.
5. **A plain radiograph of the abdomen** should be done to determine catheter placement.

V. **Plan.** Management of vasospasms is ***highly controversial.*** Management of thrombosis is largely based on treatment plans for older children and adults. Lack of organized studies in neonates adds to the problem. Current management protocols for thrombophilia can be obtained from the International Children's Thrombophilia Network (# 1-800-NO-CLOTS). The network was established as a free consultative service and to develop collaborate research studies.

A. **Key points**

1. **Monitor for potential signs of vasospasm** or thromboembolic complications in all infants with any intravascular catheter.
2. **Thromboembolism can occur in newborns** and produce little or no clinical symptoms.
3. **Heparin is often added to neonatal infusions (0.25–1.0 unit/mL).** It extends catheter life and may also decrease the incidence of thrombosis. One study found that 0.25 unit/mL decreased the likelihood of the catheter occluding but had no effect on the frequency of thrombosis. For extremely low birthweight infants, use the lowest dose. Randomized trials have showed that heparin use in umbilical arterial catheters prolonged patency and decreased the incidence of thromboembolic occlusions. Patency of peripheral arterial catheters is also preserved by use of

heparin. There are no randomized trials of heparin use in central venous catheters placed peripherally but its use is common in NICUs.

4. **Umbilical lines should be removed as soon as possible.** The CDC recommends that umbilical artery catheters should not be left in place >5 days. They state umbilical venous catheters should be removed as soon as possible, but can be used up to 14 days.

5. **High umbilical arterial catheters** (see Chapter 23) have a lower incidence of thrombotic complications and a longer catheter life. Low umbilical arterial catheters are associated with an increased incidence of vasospasms and cyanosis.

6. **If possible, use a peripheral arterial line** over an umbilical catheter.

7. **If there is difficulty infusing into the line,** consider a thrombotic event.

8. **Heparinization of flush solution** without heparinization of the infusate is not adequate. Use of intermittent heparin flushes has no benefit over normal saline (NS) flushes.

9. **Always use umbilical artery catheters** with a hole at the end and not the side because the side hole may increase aortic thrombosis risk.

10. **The use of multiple lumen umbilical venous catheters** is associated with a decrease in the need for peripheral intravenous lines in the first week of life but an increase in catheter malfunctions.

11. **Heparin-bonded catheters** versus polyvinyl chloride catheters showed no difference in the incidence of aortic thrombosis or duration of patency.

B. **Vasospasm.** Treatment is *highly controversial,* and guidelines vary extensively. Check your institution's guidelines before initiating treatment. Use of heparin and thrombolytics is not uniformly recommended. If the vasospasm does not resolve with treatment and the tissue ischemia persists, rule out a vascular thrombosis.

1. **Severe vasospasm of the leg**

   a. **If possible, remove the catheter.** The vasospasm should then resolve spontaneously.

   b. **Warming the contralateral leg.** Wrap the entire *unaffected* leg in a warm (not hot) washcloth. This measure should cause reflex vasodilatation of the vessels in the affected leg, and the vasospasm may resolve. Treatment should continue for 15–30 min before a beneficial effect is seen.

   c. **Topical nitroglycerin therapy (*controversial*)** (2% ointment, 4 mm/kg, applied as a thin film over the area). Studies applied it usually once, but some repeated it every 8 h for 2–27 days. Improvement was usually seen within 15–45 min. Three cases had improvement at 12 h, 30 h, and 27 days. Observe for hypotension.

   d. **If it is not possible to remove the catheter (as in a tiny infant) and this is the only catheter,** then a papaverine-containing solution (60 mg/500 mL in $^1/_2$ NS with 1.0 unit/mL heparin) through the catheter as a continuous infusion for 24–48 h can be used (*highly controversial*). If the vasospasm resolves, the infusion may be stopped. If the vasospasm does not resolve, remove the catheter. **Exercise caution using this technique** in premature infants in the first few days of life where the incidence of developing an intracranial hemorrhage is high.

2. **Less severe vasospasm of the leg**

   a. **If possible, remove the catheter.** The vasospasm should then resolve spontaneously.

   b. **Warming the contralateral leg.** Wrap the entire *unaffected* leg in a warm (not hot) washcloth. This measure should cause reflex vasodilatation of the vessels in the affected leg, and the vasospasm may resolve. Treatment should continue for 15–30 min before a beneficial effect is seen.

   c. **Papaverine (*controversial*).** If the treatment just described does not work, administer papaverine hydrochloride, 1 mg intramuscularly, in the unaffected leg. Papaverine is a mild vasodilator; if it is going to work, the effect is usually apparent within 30 min.

    d. Topical nitroglycerine therapy (*controversial*). (2% ointment, 4 mm/kg, applied as a thin film over the area). As in Section V, B, 1c earlier.

    e. If it is not possible to remove the catheter (as in a tiny infant) and this is the only catheter, then a papaverine containing solution (60 mg/500 mL in $^1/_2$ NS with 1.0 unit/mL heparin as in Section V, B, 1d earlier.

   3. Vasospasm from peripheral artery catheters. There has been an increase in the use of peripheral arterial catheters, with an associated increase in vasospasms.

    a. If possible, remove the catheter.

    b. Warm the contralateral arm. Wrap the entire unaffected arm in a warm (not hot) washcloth. This measure should cause reflex vasodilatation of the vessels in the affected arm, and the vasospasm may resolve. Treatment should continue for 15–30 min before a beneficial effect is seen.

    c. Topical nitroglycerine therapy (*controversial*). (2% ointment, 4 mm/kg, applied as a thin film over the area) as in Section V, B, 1c noted earlier.

    d. If it is not possible to remove the catheter (as in a tiny infant) and this is the only catheter, then a papaverine-containing solution (60 mg/500 mL in $^1/_2$ NS) through the catheter as a continuous infusion for 24–48 h can be used (***highly controversial***) as in Section V, B, 1d earlier.

C. Problems after vasospasm with peripheral tissue ischemia. Ischemia can sometimes occur after a vasospasm. Topical 2% nitroglycerin ointment (4 mm/kg of body weight) has been applied to the ischemic area with resolution with no adverse effects except mild episodes of decreased blood pressure (***controversial***).

D. Thromboembolism. If thrombosis is suspected and there is loss of pulses in the affected extremity, it is a **medical emergency.** Symptomatic thrombosis can lead to irreversible organ damage or loss of limbs or digits. The most common treatments are observation with supportive care, anticoagulation therapy with heparin or low molecular weight heparin, thrombolytic agents (clot-dissolving drugs streptokinase, urokinase, and tissue plasminogen activator) or surgery. Clot-dissolving drugs can cause severe bleeding and there are no current randomized trials comparing these treatments. Management is ***highly controversial***. Treatment depends on the extent and severity of the thrombus. Management is identical for peripheral arterial thrombosis, venous thrombosis, and aortic thrombosis.

   1. Mild or minor thrombosis. This can present with decreased limb perfusion, hypertension, and hematuria and can usually be treated with removal of the catheter, supportive care, and close ultrasonographic follow-up. Many of these resolve spontaneously.

   2. Moderate thrombosis has all the findings of mild plus oliguria and congestive heart failure. Can be treated with heparin therapy and with management of systemic hypertension.

   3. Major thrombosis presents with all of the above plus major multiorgan failure. Should be treated aggressively with heparin therapy, antithrombolytic agents, and supportive care. **May require further evaluation for underlying hypercoagulative disorder.**

E. General guidelines for thrombosis treatment. Treatment involves supportive care, heparin therapy, use of thrombolytic medications, or surgery.

   1. Supportive care

    a. Prompt removal of the catheter is indicated unless it is needed to facilitate arteriography or thrombolytic drug infusion.

    b. Treatment of volume depletion, electrolyte abnormalities, sepsis, thrombocytopenia, and anemia is essential. Control hypertension and any coagulation deficiency or hypofibrinogenemia before initiation of treatment.

    c. Emergency consultation with vascular surgery and pediatric hematology is recommended.

    d. Evaluate patients for intraventricular hemorrhage (IVH) before initiating thrombolytic therapy. During treatment, ultrasounds of the head should be obtained at regular intervals.

e. **If the infant has had major surgery in the last 10 days,** or evidence of major bleeding (gastrointestinal, pulmonary or intracranial), anticoagulant and thrombolytic therapy is contraindicated.

f. **Warfarin therapy** is not recommended in neonates.

2. **Heparin therapy.** Low molecular weight heparins are advocated because of the following advantages: reduced need for laboratory monitoring, subcutaneous dosing, longer half-life, decreased risk of osteopenia and heparin-induced thrombocytopenia, and decreased risk of hemorrhage. Monitor platelet counts if heparin is used. Obtain daily CBC and APTT. General recommendations are:

a. **Unfractionated (standard) heparin** load 75 units/kg IV over 10 min, then 28 units/kg/h maintenance through a dedicated IV line. **Adjust based on aPTT 4 h after initiation of after each dosing change.** The target is an aPTT at 60–85 s. Duration of therapy is generally 5–14 days. Always increase or decrease the infusion amount by 10%, depending on the aPTT. If the aPTT >96 s, hold the heparin for 30–60 minutes and start at a lower infusion rate.

b. **Low molecular weight heparin therapy using enoxaparin (Lovenox)** is most widely used in neonates. Other LMWH preparations include dalteparin and reviparin. For therapeutic treatment: <2 months of age, use enoxaparin 1.5 mg/kg/dose every 12 h SQ; if >2 months, 1.0 mg/kg/dose SQ. Follow antifactor Xa levels 4 h after dose with target levels are 0.5–1 unit/mL and adjust accordingly. Multiple adjustments may have to be made to reach the target levels. Some recent studies have indicated that preterm neonates have required higher mean maintenance doses to achieve target levels (1.7 mg/kg q12 h for term neonates and 2.0 mg/kg q 12 h for preterm infants).

c. **If urgent reversal of unfractionated heparin effect is needed,** IV protamine can be given based on the total amount of heparin administered in the previous 2 h. (See Chapter 132.) Stopping the infusion is usually sufficient for LMW heparin and protamine is only partially effective.

3. **Thrombolytic drugs.** Do not use in milder cases, and few studies have been done in very preterm infants. With extensive thrombosis with the possibility of limb loss or organ damage, one of these drugs may be used. Treatment is **controversial,** and it is best to follow institutional guidelines. When using thrombolytic therapy, maintain a platelet count $>50 \times 10^3$ μL and fibrinogen >100 mg/dL using platelet transfusion and cryoprecipitate and. Monitor PT/INR, PTT, and fibrinogen every 4h. If the catheter is still patent, the medications can be given through it. If the catheter is obstructed and needs to be removed, systemic therapy can be used. Streptokinase and urokinase were more commonly used in the past, now recombinant tissue plasminogen activator (tPA) is most commonly used. There are no randomized trials comparing these three medications.

a. **Recombinant tissue plasminogen activator (tPA) (Alteplase)** has become the drug of choice because when compared with the others, it has the lowest risk of allergies, the shortest half-life, and less manufacturing concerns. See Chapter 132 for dosage.

b. **Infusion of intra-arterial streptokinase** has been successful in some infants. For dosage, see Chapter 132. In one study, lower doses of streptokinase, 500 units/kg/h instead of 1000 units/kg/h, was shown to be effective and was well tolerated. In nine preterm infants who had aortoiliac thrombosis a dose of 50 units/kg/h given directly into the clot was effective . Because of systemic side effects (allergic and toxic reactions), its use has declined.

c. **Urokinase.** Previously concerns with viral contamination have been eliminated (see dose in Chapter 132).

4. **Surgery.** Immediate surgery has been successfully performed in neonates and may be indicated in the presence of an occluding embolism, but guidelines are not well established. Surgical options include thrombectomy, microvascular reconstruction, vascular decompression through the use of a fasciotomy, mechanical disruption of the thrombus, and amputation.

73 ABO Incompatibility

I. **Definition.** Isoimmune hemolytic anemia may result when ABO incompatibility occurs between the mother and the newborn infant. This disorder is **most common with blood type A or B infants born to type O mothers.** The hemolytic process begins in utero and is the result of active placental transport of maternal isoantibody. In type O mothers, isoantibody is predominantly 7S-IgG (immunoglobulin G) and is capable of crossing the placental membranes. Because of its larger size, the mostly 19S-IgM (immunoglobulin M) isoantibody found in type A or type B mothers cannot cross. Symptomatic clinical disease, which usually does not present until after birth, is a compensated mild hemolytic anemia with reticulocytosis, microspherocytosis, and early-onset unconjugated hyperbilirubinemia.

II. **Incidence.** Risk factors for ABO incompatibility are present in 12–15% of pregnancies, but evidence of fetal sensitization (positive direct Coombs test) occurs in only 3–4%. Symptomatic ABO hemolytic disease occurs in <1% of all newborn infants but accounts for approximately two thirds of observed cases of hemolytic disease in the newborn.

III. **Pathophysiology.** Transplacental transport of maternal isoantibody results in an immune reaction with the A or B antigen on fetal erythrocytes, which produces characteristic **microspherocytes.** This process eventually results in complete extravascular hemolysis of the end-stage spherocyte. The ongoing hemolysis is balanced by compensatory reticulocytosis and shortening of the cell cycle time, so that there is overall maintenance of the erythrocyte indices within physiologic limits. A paucity of A or B antigenic sites on the fetal (in contrast to the adult) erythrocytes and competitive binding of isoantibody to myriad other antigenic sites in other tissues may explain the often mild hemolytic process that occurs and the usual absence of progressive disease with subsequent pregnancies.

IV. **Risk factors**

A. **A_1 antigen in the infant.** Of the major blood group antigens, the A_1 antigen has the greatest antigenicity and is associated with a greater risk of symptomatic disease. However the hemolytic activity of anti-B antibodies is higher than those of anti-A and may produce a more severe disease in particular among infants of African American descent.

B. **Elevated isohemagglutinins.** Antepartum intestinal parasitism or third-trimester immunization with tetanus toxoid or pneumococcal vaccine may stimulate isoantibody titer to A or B antigens.

C. **Birth order.** Birth order is not considered a risk factor. Maternal isoantibody exists naturally and is independent of prior exposure to incompatible fetal blood group antigens. First-born infants have a 40–50% risk for symptomatic disease. Progressive severity of the hemolytic process in succeeding pregnancies is a rare phenomenon.

V. **Clinical presentation**

A. **Jaundice.** Icterus is often the sole physical manifestation of ABO incompatibility with a clinically significant level of hemolysis. The onset is usually within the first 24 h of life. The jaundice evolves at a faster rate over the early neonatal period than nonhemolytic physiologic pattern jaundice.

B. **Anemia.** Because of the effectiveness of compensation by reticulocytosis in response to the ongoing mild hemolytic process, erythrocyte indices are maintained within a physiologic range that is normal for asymptomatic infants of the same gestational age. Additional signs of clinical disease (eg, hepatosplenomegaly or hydrops fetalis)

393

are extremely unusual but may be seen with a more progressive hemolytic process (see Rh incompatibility, pages 654–658). Exaggerated physiologic anemia may occur at 8–12 weeks of age, particularly when treatment during the neonatal period required phototherapy or exchange transfusion.

VI. **Diagnosis.** Obligatory screening for infants with unconjugated hyperbilirubinemia includes the following studies:

A. **Blood type and Rh factor in the mother and the infant.** These studies establish risk factors for ABO incompatibility.

B. **Reticulocyte count.** Elevated values after adjustment for gestational age and degree of anemia, if any, support the diagnosis of hemolytic anemia. For term infants, normal values are 4–5%; for preterm infants of 30–36 weeks' gestational age, 6–10%. In ABO hemolytic disease of the newborn, values range from 10–30%.

C. **Direct Coombs test (direct antiglobulin test).** Because there is very little antibody on the red blood cell (RBC), the direct Coombs test is often only weakly positive at birth and may become negative by 2–3 days of age. A strongly positive test is distinctly unusual and would direct attention to other isoimmune or autoimmune hemolytic processes.

D. **Blood smear.** The blood smear typically demonstrates **microspherocytes, polychromasia** proportionate to the reticulocyte response, and **normoblastosis** above the normal values for gestational age. An increased number of nucleated RBCs in the cord blood could be a sign of ABO incompatibility.

E. **Bilirubin levels** (fractionated or total and direct). Indirect hyperbilirubinemia is mainly present and provides an index of the severity of disease. The rate at which unconjugated bilirubin levels are increasing suggests the required frequency of testing, usually every 4–8 h until values plateau.

F. **Additional laboratory studies.** Supportive diagnostic studies may be indicated on an individual basis if the nature of the hemolytic process remains unclear.

1. **Antibody identification (indirect Coombs test).** The indirect Coombs test is more sensitive than the direct Coombs test in detecting the presence of maternal isoantibody and identifies antibody specificity. The test is performed on an eluate of neonatal erythrocytes, which is then tested against a panel of type-specific adult cells.

2. **Maternal IgG titer.** The absence in the mother of elevated IgG titers against the infant's blood group tends to exclude a diagnosis of ABO incompatibility.

VII. **Management**

A. **Antepartum treatment.** Because of the low incidence of moderate to severe ABO hemolytic disease, invasive maneuvers before term is reached (eg, amniocentesis or early delivery) are usually not indicated.

B. **Postpartum treatment**

1. **General measures.** The maintenance of adequate hydration (see Chapter 8) and evaluation for potentially aggravating factors (eg, sepsis, drug exposure, or metabolic disturbance) should be considered.

2. **Phototherapy.** Once a diagnosis of ABO incompatibility is established, phototherapy may be initiated before exchange transfusion is given. Because of the usual mild to moderate hemolysis, phototherapy may entirely obviate the need for exchange transfusion or may reduce the number of transfusions required. For guidelines on phototherapy, see Table 51–1 and Figure 92–2.

3. **Exchange transfusion.** See Table 51–1 and Figure 92–3 for guidelines on exchange transfusion and Chapter 29 for exchange transfusion procedure.

4. **Tin (Sn) porphyrin** can decrease the production of bilirubin and reduce the need for exchange transfusion and duration of phototherapy. It is an inhibitor of heme oxygenase, which is the enzyme that allows the production of bilirubin from heme. The dose of Stannsoporfin is 6 μmol/kg IM as a single dose given within 24 h of birth with severe hemolytic disease, and it is available via compassionate use protocol.

5. **Intravenous immunoglobulin (IVIG).** By blocking neonatal reticuloendothelial Fc receptors, and thus decreasing hemolysis of the antibody-coated RBCs, high-dose IVIG (1 g/kg over 4 h) reduces serum bilirubin levels and the need for blood exchange transfusion with ABO or Rh hemolytic diseases. (See Chapter 132.)
6. **Synthetic blood group trisaccharides.** Their use is investigational; studies have shown a decrease in exchange transfusion rates in severe ABO hemolytic disease when A or B trisaccharides were administered.
VIII. **Prognosis.** For infants with ABO incompatibility, the overall prognosis is excellent. Timely recognition and appropriate management of the rare infant with aggressive ABO hemolytic disease may avoid any potential morbidity or severe hemolytic anemia and secondary hyperbilirubinemia and the inherent risks associated with exchange transfusion with the use of blood products.

Selected References

Miqdad AM et al: Intravenous immunoglobulin G (IVIG) therapy for significant hyperbilirubinemia in ABO hemolytic disease of the newborn. *J Matern Fetal Neonat Med* 2004;16:163.

Murray NA et al: Haemolytic disease of the newborn. *Arch Dis Child* 2007;92:83.

Poole J et al: Blood group antibodies and their significance in transfusion medicine. *Transfus Med Rev* 2007;21:58.

74 Air Leak Syndromes

I. **Definition.** The pulmonary air leak syndromes (pneumomediastinum, pneumothorax, pulmonary interstitial emphysema [PIE], pneumopericardium, pneumoperitoneum, and pneumoretroperitoneum) comprise a spectrum of disease with the same underlying pathophysiology. Overdistention of alveolar sacs or terminal airways leads to disruption of airway integrity, resulting in dissection of air into extra-alveolar spaces.
II. **Incidence.** The exact incidence of the air leak syndromes is difficult to determine. **Pneumothorax is the most common of the air leak syndromes, reported to occur spontaneously in 1–2% of neonates.** The incidence increases in preterm infants to about 6%. The incidence also increases in infants with underlying lung disease (such as respiratory distress syndrome [RDS], meconium aspiration, pneumonia, and pulmonary hypoplasia) who are on ventilatory support and in infants who had vigorous resuscitation at birth.
III. **Pathophysiology.** Overdistention of terminal air spaces or airways—the common denominator in all the pulmonary air leaks—can result from uneven alveolar ventilation, air trapping, or injudicious use of alveolar-distending pressure in infants on ventilatory support. As lung volume exceeds physiologic limits, mechanical stresses occur in all planes of the alveolar or respiratory bronchial wall, with eventual tissue rupture. Air can track through the perivascular adventitia, causing PIE, or dissect along vascular sheaths toward the hilum, causing a pneumomediastinum. Rupture of the mediastinal pleura and into the thoracic cavity results in a pneumothorax. Pneumoretroperitoneum and pneumoperitoneum may occur when mediastinal air tracks downward to the extraperitoneal fascial planes of the abdominal wall, mesentery, and retroperitoneum and eventually ruptures into the peritoneal cavity.

A. **Barotrauma. The common denominator of the air leak syndromes is barotrauma.** Barotrauma results whenever positive pressure is applied to the lung. It cannot be avoided in the ill newborn infant needing ventilatory support, but its effects should be minimized. Peak inspiratory pressure (PIP), positive end-expiratory pressure (PEEP), inspiratory time (IT), respiratory rate, and the inspiratory waveform play important roles in the development of barotrauma. Contributing factors include high PIP, large tidal volume, and long IT. It is difficult to determine which of these parameters is the most damaging and which plays the largest role in the development of the air leaks. However, in a case-controlled study, investigators found no relationship between inadvertent overventilation and pneumothoraces in ventilated newborns.

B. **Other causes of lung overdistention.** Barotrauma is not the only cause of lung overdistention. **Atelectatic alveoli in RDS** may cause uneven ventilation and subject the more distensible areas of the lung to receive high pressures, placing them at risk for rupture. Small mucus plugs in the airway in meconium aspiration may cause gas trapping secondary to a ball-valve effect. Other events, such as inappropriate intubation of the right main stem bronchus, failure to wean after surfactant replacement therapy, and vigorous resuscitation or the development of high opening pressures with the onset of air breathing, can also lead to overdistention, with rupture of airway integrity at birth.

C. **Lung injury**
   1. **Large tidal volume.** It has long been considered that lung injury is primarily a result of high-pressure ventilation (barotrauma). Although reports show variable relationships between airway pressures and lung injury, more recent studies support the concept that lung overdistention resulting from high maximal lung volume ("volutrauma") and transalveolar pressure, rather than high airway pressure, is the harmful factor. In infants with low lung compliance, a high PIP may cause only small alveolar distention that may not be associated with significant injury.
   2. **Atelectasis.** The alveolar units in patients with RDS are subjected to a cycle of recruitment and derecruitment. Strategies to decrease this mechanism of atelectatic trauma, optimizing lung recruitment and decreasing lung injury and severity of lung disease, lessen the risk for pulmonary air leak.

IV. **Risk factors**
A. **Ventilatory support.** The infants on ventilatory support, such as the preterm and infants with underlying pulmonary disease, have an increased risk of developing one of the air leak syndromes. Some investigators report an incidence as high as 30%. Factors that contribute to development of air leak include high inspiratory pressure, large tidal volume, and long inspiratory duration.

B. **Meconium staining.** Other infants at risk include those who are meconium stained at birth. In these infants, meconium may be plugged in the airways, with resultant air trapping. During inspiration, the airway expands, allowing air to enter; however, during exhalation, there is airway collapse with resultant trapping of air behind the meconium plugs.

C. **Failure to wean after surfactant therapy.** Studies have shown that prophylactic use of surfactant therapy in infants at risk for RDS is associated with a decrease in the incidence of pneumothorax and PIE. Similar findings were noted in treating premature newborns with established RDS. With the return of pulmonary compliance after receiving surfactant, appropriate decreases in pressure support and more cautious ventilatory management of these infants is necessary immediately after therapy. The clinician must closely watch for improvement in the infant's arterial blood gas levels and must wean ventilatory support as required.

V. **Clinical presentation. Air leak syndromes are potentially lethal, and a high index of suspicion is necessary for the diagnosis.** On clinical grounds, respiratory distress or a deteriorating clinical course strongly suggests air leak. See Section IX for clinical presentation of specific air leak syndromes.

VI. **Diagnosis.** The **definitive diagnosis** of all of these syndromes is made **radiographically.** An anteroposterior (AP) chest radiograph along with a cross-table lateral film is essential in diagnosing an air leak.

VII. **Management.** The best mode of treatment for all of the air leak syndromes is prevention and judicious use of ventilatory support, with close attention to distending pressure, PEEP, and IT. Barotrauma remains a prominent disadvantage to ventilatory support. The careful use of ventilatory pressures and the adjustment of ventilator settings to provide a minimum of barotrauma are extremely important in the neonatal intensive care unit. The use of surfactant therapy for RDS substantially decreases the incidence of pneumothorax and PIE. Earlier treatment is more beneficial than later treatment. A review of six randomized trials found **early surfactant administration with extubation to nasal continuous positive airway pressure (CPAP) was associated with significant reductions in the need for mechanical ventilation and fewer air leak syndromes compared with later selective surfactant administration and continued mechanical ventilation in infants with RDS.** Controlled studies with high-frequency positive pressure ventilation showed a decreased incidence of pneumothorax. In infants with established PIE, high-frequency jet ventilation (HFJV) facilitates resolution of the air leak. In preterm infants born <35 weeks or with birthweight <2000 g who were treated either with rescue HFJV or conventional mechanical ventilation, a meta-analysis showed no significant increase in new air leaks. There were, however, insufficient data to assess the effectiveness of rescue HFJV in preterm infants, and the study was done before the surfactant era and before widespread use of antenatal steroids. In the HiFO Study Group, authors concluded that high-frequency oscillatory ventilation (HFOV) improves oxygenation and reduced the incidence of air leak in infants with severe RDS. However, in a recent meta-analysis, in the use of elective HFOV versus conventional ventilation for acute pulmonary dysfunction in preterm infants, pulmonary air leaks were found to occur more frequently in the HFOV group.

VIII. **Prognosis.** The prognosis for the infant in whom an air leak develops depends on the underlying condition. **In general, if the air leak is treated rapidly and effectively, the long-term outcome should not change; however, it must be remembered that early-onset PIE (<24 h of age) is associated with a high mortality rate.** Chronic lung disease of the newborn, or bronchopulmonary dysplasia, is also associated with severe pulmonary air leak syndromes. Pneumothorax is also described as a risk factor for intraventricular hemorrhage, cerebral palsy, and delayed mental development.

IX. **Specific air leak syndromes**

   A. **Pneumomediastinum**

      1. **Definition.** Pneumomediastinum is air in the mediastinum from ruptured alveolar air that enters the perivascular sheaths dissecting into the hilum, through the visceral pleura into the loose connective tissue spaces of the mediastinum.

      2. **Incidence.** The actual incidence of pneumomediastinum is uncertain because it is usually asymptomatic and may go undetected. It has been reported to occur spontaneously in 25 of 10,000 live births in symptomatic infants. The exact incidence is related to the degree of ventilatory support.

      3. **Pathophysiology.** Pneumomediastinum is preceded by PIE in almost every instance. After alveolar rupture, air traverses fascial planes and passes into the mediastinum.

      4. **Risk factors.** See Section IV.

      5. **Clinical presentation.** Unless accompanied by a pneumothorax, a pneumomediastinum may be totally asymptomatic. **Spontaneous pneumomediastinum** may develop in term infants not on ventilatory support and may be accompanied by mild respiratory distress. Physical findings in addition to respiratory distress may include an increase in AP diameter of the chest and difficulty in auscultating heart sounds.

6. **Diagnosis.** (See Figure 10–18.) Radiographically, pneumomediastinum may present in several ways. The **classic description** is that of a **"wind-blown spinnaker sail"** (a lobe or lobes of the thymus being elevated off the heart), most likely to be seen on a left lateral oblique view. In other cases, a halo may be seen around the heart in the AP projection. This must be distinguished from a pneumopericardium in which air completely surrounds the heart including the inferior border. The cross-table lateral projection will show an anterior collection of air that may be difficult to distinguish from a pneumothorax.

7. **Management.** In isolated pneumomediastinum, close observation is required because it can progress to a pneumothorax. One should resist the temptation to insert a drain into the mediastinum because it will not be beneficial and may cause more problems than it will solve. An oxygen-rich environment can be used in the term infant to attempt nitrogen washout if the pneumomediastinum is believed to be clinically significant.

8. **Prognosis.** The prognosis is good because recovery is frequently spontaneous without treatment.

B. **Pneumothorax.** See also On-Call Problems, Chapter 63.

1. **Definition.** Pneumothorax is air between the visceral pleura of the lungs and the parietal pleural of the chest wall.

2. **Incidence.** The incidence of pneumothorax varies between units. It occurs more frequently in the neonatal period than in any other time of life with an incidence of 1–2%. With the advent of neonatal ventilator care, however, the incidence has risen dramatically. Although the exact incidence is difficult to determine, it is directly related to the degree of ventilatory support delivered. The incidence increases to 30% in the presence of underlying pulmonary disease, especially in patients who require mechanical ventilation. In infants <1000 g birthweight, an incidence of approximately 11% was reported in this population.

3. **Pathophysiology**

   a. **The term infant not on ventilatory support.** Pneumothorax may develop spontaneously. It usually occurs at delivery, when a large initial opening pressure is necessary to inflate collapsed alveolar sacs. It is thought to result from uneven inflation of alveoli throughout the lung combined with the high negative intrathoracic pressure that occurs during the first breath.

   b. **The infant on ventilatory support** has alveolar overdistention secondary to either injudicious use of distending pressure or failure to wean ventilatory pressure when compliance begins to return. A pneumothorax is usually preceded by rupture of the alveoli, with the interstitial air traversing via fascial planes into the mediastinum. Air breaks through the mediastinal pleura to form a pneumothorax.

4. **Risk factors.** See Section IV.

5. **Clinical presentation.** The clinical presentation of the neonate with a pneumothorax depends on the setting in which it develops.

   a. **Term infants with a spontaneous pneumothorax** may be asymptomatic or only mildly symptomatic. These infants usually have tachypnea and mild oxygen needs early, but they may progress to the classic signs of respiratory distress (grunting, flaring, retractions, and tachypnea).

   b. **The infant on ventilatory support** generally has a sudden, rapid clinical deterioration characterized by cyanosis, hypoxemia, hypercarbia, and respiratory acidosis. The most common time for the development of this complication is either immediately after the initiation of ventilatory support or when the infant begins to improve and compliance returns (eg, after surfactant therapy). In either case, other clinical signs may include decreased breath sounds on the involved side, shifted heart sounds, and asynchrony of the chest. When compression of major veins and decreased cardiac output occur because of downward displacement of the diaphragm, signs of shock may be evident.

6. **Diagnosis.** A high index of suspicion is necessary for the diagnosis of pneumothorax.

a. **Transillumination of the chest.** (See Chapter 26.) With the aid of transillumination, the diagnosis of pneumothorax may be made without a chest radiograph. A fiberoptic light probe placed on the infant's chest wall will illuminate the involved hemithorax. Although this technique is beneficial in an emergency, it should not replace a chest radiograph as the means of diagnosis.

b. **Chest radiograph.** (See Figure 10–19.) Radiographically, a pneumothorax is diagnosed on the basis of the following characteristics:

   i. **Presence of air in the pleural cavity** separating the parietal and visceral pleura. The area appears hyperlucent with absence of pulmonary markings.

   ii. **Collapse of the ipsilateral lobes.**

   iii. **Displacement of the mediastinum** toward the contralateral side.

   iv. **Downward displacement of the diaphragm.** In infants with RDS, the compliance may be so poor that the lung may not collapse, with only minimal shift of the mediastinal structures. The AP radiograph may not demonstrate the classic radiographic appearance if a large amount of the intrapleural air is situated just anterior to the sternum. In these situations, the cross-table lateral radiograph will show a large lucent area immediately below the sternum, or the lateral decubitus radiograph (with the suspected side up) will show free air.

c. **Transcutaneous carbon dioxide (tcPco$_2$).** Reference percentiles for tcPco$_2$ level and slope of the trended tcPco$_2$ over various time intervals have been used to detect the occurrence of pneumothorax preclinically. The area under the curve for 5 consecutive min with a 5-min tcPco$_2$ slope >90th percentile shows good discrimination for a pneumothorax. False-positive results such as presence of a blocked or misplaced endotracheal tube may be encountered. If the problem with tcPco$_2$ persists after appropriately suctioning the endotracheal tube, a confirmatory radiograph should be ordered.

7. **Management.** Treatment of a pneumothorax depends on the clinical status of the infant. In infants without respiratory distress, continuous air leak, or need for assisted ventilation, close monitoring and observation may be all that is needed. The pneumothorax typically resolves in 1–2 days. If the pneumothorax affects <15% of a patient's hemithorax, the pneumothorax can resolve spontaneously; otherwise the air must be removed.

a. **Oxygen supplementation.** In the term infant who is mildly symptomatic, an oxygen-rich environment is often all that is necessary. The inspired oxygen facilitates nitrogen washout of the blood and tissues and thus establishes a difference in the gas tensions between the loculated gases in the chest and those in the blood. A diffusion gradient results in rapid resorption of the loculated gas, with resolution of the pneumothorax. This mode of therapy is not appropriate in the preterm infant because of the high oxygen levels needed for washout and resulting increase in oxygen saturation. This makes it unsuitable for premature infants with risk for retinopathy of prematurity.

b. **Decompression.** In the symptomatic neonate or the neonate on mechanical ventilatory support, immediate evacuation of air is necessary. The technique is described in Chapter 63. Placement of a chest tube of appropriate size will eventually be necessary (see Chapter 26).

8. **Prognosis.** See Section VIII.

C. **Pulmonary interstitial emphysema**

1. **Definition.** PIE is dissection of air into the perivascular tissues of the lung from alveolar overdistention or overdistention of the smaller airways.

2. **Incidence.** This disorder arises almost exclusively in the very low birthweight infant on ventilatory support. It may also emerge in the extremely low birthweight infant without mechanical ventilation but receiving ventilatory support by CPAP. Although localized persistent PIE is rarely reported in infants not receiving ventilatory support, it must be considered in any infant with cystic lung lesions. PIE has been reported to occur in at least a third of infants <1000 g who have RDS on the first day of life.

3. **Pathophysiology.** PIE may be the precursor of all other types of pulmonary air leaks. With overdistention of the alveoli or conducting airways, or both, rupture may occur, and there may be dissection of the air into the perivascular tissue of the lung. The interstitial air moves in the connective tissue planes and around the vascular axis, particularly the venous ones. Once in the interstitial space, the air moves along bronchioles, lymphatics, and vascular sheaths or directly through the lung interstitium to the pleural surface. The extrapulmonary air is trapped in the interstitium (PIE), or it may extend and cause pneumomediastinum, pneumopericardium, or pneumothorax. PIE may exist in two forms, either localized (which involves one or more lobes) or diffuse (bilateral).

4. **Risk factors.** See Section IV.

5. **Clinical presentation.** The patient in whom PIE develops may have sudden deterioration. More commonly, however, the onset of PIE is heralded by slow, progressive deterioration of arterial blood gas levels and the apparent need for increasing ventilatory support. Invariably, a diffusion block develops in these patients, with the alveolar membrane becoming separated from the capillary bed by the interstitial air. The response to increased ventilatory support in the face of poor arterial blood gas levels may lead to worsening of PIE and sudden clinical deterioration; however, some infants with severe PIE may actually improve if it progresses to pneumothorax.

6. **Diagnosis.** In infants with PIE, the chest radiograph generally reveals radiolucencies that are either linear or cyst-like. The linear radiolucencies vary in length and do not branch. They are seen in the periphery of the lung as well as medially and may be mistaken for air bronchograms. The cyst-like lucencies vary from 1.0–4.0 mm in diameter and can be lobulated. (See Figure 10–20.)

7. **Management**
   a. **Lessening lung injury.** In general, once PIE is diagnosed, an attempt should be made to decrease ventilatory support and lessen lung trauma. Decreasing the PIP, decreasing the PEEP, or shortening the IT may be required. When decreasing these settings, some degree of hypercarbia and hypoxia may have to be accepted.
   b. **Positioning of the infant** with the involved side down has also proved beneficial in some cases of unilateral PIE.
   c. **Other treatments.** More invasive measures include selective collapse of the involved lung on the side with the worse involvement, with selective intubation or even the insertion of chest tubes before the development of pneumothorax. In cases of severe PIE, surgical resection of the affected lobe may be considered.
   d. **HFV.** Both HFOV and HFJV are used effectively in the treatment of PIE and other types of air leak syndromes. Although these treatment modalities may improve survival of the infant with PIE, the long-term outcome remains uncertain.

8. **Prognosis.** See Section VIII.

D. **Pneumopericardium**
   1. **Definition.** Pneumopericardium is air in the pericardial sac, which is usually secondary to passage of air along vascular sheaths. It is most often a complication of mechanical ventilation and can result in fatal cardiac tamponade, with mortality of 72–83%.

2. **Incidence.** Pneumopericardium is a rare occurrence and the least common form of pulmonary air leak in the neonatal period. The incidence in a study involving very low birthweight neonates was reported at 2%.

3. **Pathophysiology. Pneumopericardium is usually preceded by pneumomediastinum or other air leaks such as PIE or pneumothorax.** The mechanism by which pneumopericardium develops is probably due to passage of air along vascular sheaths. From the mediastinum, air can travel along the fascial planes in the subcutaneous tissues of the neck, chest wall, and anterior abdominal wall and into the pericardial space, causing pneumopericardium.

4. **Risk factors.** See Section IV.

5. **Clinical presentation.** The clinical signs of pneumopericardium range from asymptomatic to the full picture of cardiac tamponade. **The first sign of pneumopericardium may be a decrease in blood pressure or a decrease in pulse pressure.** There may also be an increase in heart rate with distant heart sounds.

6. **Diagnosis.** Pneumopericardium has the most classic radiographic appearance of all the air leaks. (See Figure 10–17.). **A broad radiolucent halo completely surrounds the heart, including the diaphragmatic surface.** This picture is easily distinguished from all the other air leaks by its extension completely around the heart in all projections.

7. **Management.** Treatment of pneumopericardium is essential and requires the placement of a pericardial drain or repeated pericardial taps. Tube drainage is recommended for all neonates because of high risk for reaccumulation. The procedure is described in Chapter 34.

8. **Prognosis.** See Section VIII.

E. **Pneumoperitoneum.** See On-Call Problems, Chapter 62.

1. **Definition.** Pneumoperitoneum is air in the peritoneal cavity that is usually caused by gastrointestinal perforation, but it can also be caused by air that has ruptured from the mediastinum into the peritoneum.

2. **Incidence.** Pneumoperitoneum from passage of air into the chest is rare. It has been reported to occur in ~1% of mechanically ventilated children in intensive care units.

3. **Pathophysiology.** Pneumoperitoneum in the newborn most commonly arises from a perforated hollow viscus or a preceding abdominal operation. It can also be secondary to ventilator-assisted pulmonary air leakage. Air from the ruptured alveoli can flow transdiaphragmatically along the great vessels and esophagus into the retroperitoneum. When air accumulates in the retroperitoneum, rupture into the peritoneal cavity can occur.

4. **Risk factors.** See Section IV.

5. **Clinical presentation.** Depending on the cause and severity, pneumoperitoneum can present with or without associated abdominal findings. Because pneumoperitoneum can occur as a result of pneumothorax, pneumomediastinum, and pulmonary interstitial air, infants can present with signs of respiratory distress, as mentioned earlier.

6. **Diagnosis.** Pneumoperitoneum can be detected in radiographic films as free air under the diaphragm. (See Figure 10–21.)

7. **Management.** Conservative management may be strongly considered if evidence of pulmonary air leak precedes or simultaneously appears with pneumoperitoneum.

8. **Prognosis.** See Section VIII.

F. **Pneumoretroperitoneum.** A pneumoretroperitoneum is the presence of air in the retroperitoneal space. **An isolated pneumoretroperitoneum is rare in neonates.** It can occur when massive intrathoracic pressure from a pneumothorax or pneumomediastinum that causes free air to dissect into the retroperitoneum from the chest. It may suggest necrotizing enterocolitis. On radiograph, one sees air around the kidneys and in the perinephric space.

Selected References

Agrons GA et al: Lung disease in premature neonates: radiopathologic correlation. *Radiographics* 2005;25:1047-1073.

Arda IS et al: Treatment of pneumothorax in newborns: use of venous catheter versus tube. *Pediatr Int* 2002;44:78-82.

Attar MA, Donn SM: Mechanisms of ventilator-induced lung injury in premature infants. *Semin Neonatol* 2002;7:353-360.

Benjamin PK et al: Complications of mechanical ventilation in a children's hospital multidisciplinary intensive care unit. *Respir Care* 1990;35:873-878.

Berk DR, Varch LJ: Localized persistent pulmonary interstitial emphysema in a preterm infant in the absence of mechanical ventilation. *Pediatr Radiol* 2005;35:1243-1245.

Briassoulis GC et al: Air leaks from the respiratory tract in mechanically ventilated children with severe respiratory distress. *Pediatr Pulmonol* 2000;29:127-134.

Carey BE: Neonatal air leaks: pneumothorax, pneumomediastinum, pulmonary interstitial emphysema, pneumopericardium. *Neonatal Netw* 1999;18(8):81-84.

Chan V et al: Neonatal complications of extreme prematurity in mechanically ventilated infants. *Eur J Pediatr* 1992;151(9):636-639.

Davis C, Stevens G: Value of routine radiographic examination of the newborn, based on study of 702 consecutive babies. *Am J Obstet Gynecol* 1930;20:73.

Fiser DH, Walker WM: Tension pneumopericardium in an infant. *Chest* 1992;102:1888-1891.

Greenough A: Air leaks. In Greenough A, Milner AD (eds): *Neonatal Respiratory Disorders.* London, UK: Oxford University Press, 2003:311-319.

Heckmann M et al: Tension pneumopericardium in a preterm infant without mechanical ventilation: a rare cause of cardiac arrest. *Acta Paediatr* 1998;87: 346-348.

Henderson-Smart DJ et al: Elective high frequency oscillatory ventilation versus conventional ventilation for acute pulmonary dysfunction in preterm infants. *Cochrane Database Syst Rev* 2007;3:CD000104.

Hermansen CL, Lorah KN: Respiratory distress in the newborn. *Am Fam Physician* 2007;76:987-994.

HiFO Study Group: Randomized study of high-frequency oscillatory ventilation in infants with severe respiratory distress syndrome. *J Pediatr* 1993;122:609-619.

Hook B et al: Pneumopericardium in very low birth weight infants. *J Perinatol* 1995;15: 27-31.

Horbar JD et al: Trends in mortality and morbidity for very low birth weight infants, 1991-1999. *Pediatrics* 2002;110:143-151.

Joshi VH, Bhuta A: Rescue high frequency jet ventilation versus conventional ventilation for severe pulmonary dysfunction in preterm infants. *Cochrane Database Syst Rev* 2006;1:CD000437.

Kamli CO, Davis PG: Long versus short inspiratory times in neonates receiving mechanical ventilation. *Cochrane Database Syst Rev* 2004;4:CD004503.

Keszler M: High-frequency ventilation: evidence-based practice and specific clinical indications. *Neoreviews* 2006;7:e234-e249.

Keszler M et al: Multicenter controlled trial comparing high-frequency jet ventilation and conventional mechanical ventilation in newborn infants with pulmonary interstitial emphysema. *J Pediatr* 1991;119:85-93.

Laptook AR et al; the NICHD Neonatal Network: Adverse neurodevelopmental outcomes among extremely low birth weight infants with a normal head ultrasound: prevalence and antecedents. *Pediatrics* 2005;115:673-680.

Linder N et al: Risk factors for intraventricular hemorrhage in very low birth weight premature infants: a retrospective case-control study. *Pediatrics* 2003;111:590-595.

Macklin CC: Transport of air along sheaths of pulmonic blood vessels from alveoli to mediastinum. *Arch Intern Med* 1939;64:913.

Makhoul IR et al: Pneumothorax and nasal continuous positive airway pressure ventilation in premature neonates: a note of caution. *ASAIO J* 2002;48:476-479.

Miller MJ et al: Respiratory disorders in preterm and term infants. In Fanaroff AA, Martin RJ (eds): *Neonatal-Perinatal Medicine: Diseases of the Fetus and Infant*. Philadelphia, PA: Mosby, 2006;1128-1146.

Morrow G et al: Pneumomediastinum: a silent lesion in the newborn. *J Pediatr* 1967;70:554-560.

Octave Study Group: Multicentre randomized trial of high against low frequency positive pressure ventilation. Oxford region controlled trial of artificial ventilation. *Arch Dis Child* 1991;66:770-775.

Singh SA: Familial spontaneous pneumothorax in neonates. *Indian J Pediatr* 2005;72:445-447.

Soll RF: Prophylactic versus selective use of surfactant in preventing morbidity and mortality in preterm infants. *Cochrane Database Syst Rev* 2001;2:CD000510.

Soll RF, Blanco F: Natural surfactant extract versus synthetic surfactant for neonatal respiratory distress syndrome. *Cochrane Database Syst Rev* 2001;2:CD000144.

Stevens TP et al: Early surfactant administration with brief ventilation vs. selective surfactant and continued mechanical ventilation for preterm infants with or at risk for respiratory distress syndrome. *Cochrane Database Syst Rev* 2007;4:CD003063.

Walker WM et al: Clinical process improvement: reduction of pneumothorax and mortality in high-risk preterm infants. J Perinatol 2002;22:641-645.

Watkinson M, Tiron I: Events before the diagnosis of a pneumothorax. *Arch Dis Child Fetal Neonatal Ed* 2001;85(3):F201-F203.

Yu VY et al: Pulmonary interstitial emphysema in infants less than 1000g at birth. *Aust Paediatr J* 1986;22:189-192.

75 Anemia

I. **Definition.** Anemia developing during the neonatal period (0–28 days of life) in infants of >34 weeks' gestational age is indicated by a central venous hemoglobin <13 g/dL or a capillary hemoglobin <14.5 g/dL.

II. **Incidence.** Anemia is the most common hematologic abnormality in the newborn. Specific incidence depends on the cause of the anemia.

III. **Pathophysiology**

    A. **Normal physiology.** At birth, **normal values for the central venous hemoglobin in infants of >34 weeks' gestational age are 14–20 g/dL,** with an average value of 17 g/dL. Reticulocyte count in the cord blood of infants ranges from 3–7%. The average mean corpuscular volume of red blood cells (RBCs) is 107 fL. Premature infants have slightly lower hemoglobin and higher mean corpuscular volume and reticulocyte counts. In healthy term infants, **hemoglobin values remain unchanged until the third week of life and then decline, reaching a nadir of 11 g/dL at 8–12 weeks.** This is known as the **"physiologic anemia of infancy."** In preterm infants, this decline is more profound, reaching a nadir of 7–9 g/dL at 4–8 weeks. This exaggerated physiologic anemia of prematurity is related to a combination of decreased RBC mass at birth, increased iatrogenic losses from laboratory blood sampling, shorter RBC life span, inadequate erythropoietin production, and rapid body growth.

In the absence of clinical complications associated with prematurity, infants remain asymptomatic during this process.

B. **Etiologies of anemia.** Anemia in the newborn infant results from one of three processes: loss of RBCs, or hemorrhagic anemia, the most common cause; increased destruction of RBCs, or hemolytic anemia; or underproduction of RBCs, or hypoplastic anemia.

1. **Hemorrhagic anemia**

    a. **Antepartum period** (1 in 1000 live births)

        i. **Loss of placental integrity.** Abruptio placentae, placenta previa, or traumatic amniocentesis (acute or chronic) may result in loss of placental integrity.

        ii. **Anomalies of the umbilical cord or placental vessels.** Velamentous insertion of the umbilical cord occurs in 10% of twin gestations and almost all gestations with three or more fetuses. Communicating vessels (vasa praevia), umbilical cord hematoma (1 in 5500 deliveries), or entanglement of the cord by the fetus may also cause hemorrhagic anemia.

        iii. **Twin-twin transfusion** is observed only in monozygotic multiple births. In the presence of a monochorial placenta, 13–33% of twin pregnancies are associated with twin-twin transfusion. The difference in hemoglobin concentration between twins is >5 g/dL. The survival rate for twin-twin transfusion diagnosed before 28 weeks' gestation is 21%. The anemic donor twin may develop congestive heart disease, whereas the recipient plethoric twin may manifest signs of the hyperviscosity syndrome.

    b. **Intrapartum period**

        i. **Fetomaternal hemorrhage** occurs in 30–50% of pregnancies. The risk is increased with preeclampsia, with the need for instrumentation and with cesarean delivery. In ~8% of pregnancies, the volume of the hemorrhage is >10 mL.

        ii. **Cesarean delivery.** In elective cesarean deliveries, there is a 3% incidence of anemia. The incidence is increased in emergency cesarean deliveries.

        iii. **Traumatic rupture of the umbilical cord.** Rupture may occur if delivery is uncontrolled or unattended.

        iv. **Failure of placental transfusion.** Failure is usually caused by umbilical cord occlusion (eg, a nuchal cord or an entangled or prolapsed cord) during vaginal delivery. Blood loss may be 25–30 mL in the newborn.

        v. **Obstetric trauma.** During a difficult vaginal delivery, occult visceral or intracranial hemorrhage may occur. It may not be apparent at birth. Difficult deliveries are more common with large for gestational age infants, breech presentation, or difficult extraction.

    c. **Neonatal period**

        i. **Enclosed hemorrhage.** Hemorrhage severe enough to cause neonatal anemia suggests obstetric trauma, severe perinatal distress, or a defect in hemostasis.

            (a) **Caput succedaneum** is relatively common and may result in benign hemorrhage.

            (b) **Cephalhematoma** is found in up to 2.5% of births. It is associated with vacuum extraction and primiparity (5% risk of associated linear nondepressed skull fracture).

            (c) **Subgaleal (subaponeurotic) hemorrhage** is a rare but potentially lethal medical emergency caused by rupture of the emissary veins, which are connections between the dural sinuses and the scalp veins. Blood accumulates between the epicranial aponeurosis of the scalp and the periosteum. This potential space extends forward to the orbital margins, backward to the nuchal ridge, and laterally to the temporal fascia. In term infants, this subaponeurotic space may hold as much as 260 mL of blood. Subgaleal hemorrhage is most often associated with vacuum extraction and forceps delivery, but it may also occur spontaneously from an associated coagulopathy.

   (d) **Intracranial hemorrhage** may occur in the subdural, subarachnoid, or subependymal space.
   (e) **Visceral parenchymal hemorrhage** is uncommon. It is usually the result of obstetric trauma to an internal organ, most commonly the liver but also the spleen, kidneys, or adrenal glands.
ii. **Defects in hemostasis.** Defects in hemostasis may be congenital, but more commonly hemorrhage occurs secondary to consumption coagulopathy, which may be caused by the following:
   (a) **Congenital coagulation factor deficiency**
   (b) **Consumption coagulopathy**
      (i) Disseminated congenital or viral infection.
      (ii) Bacterial sepsis.
      (iii) Intravascular embolism of thromboplastin (as a result of a dead twin, maternal toxemia, necrotizing enterocolitis, or others).
   (c) **Deficiency of vitamin K–dependent coagulation factors** (factors II, VII, IX, and X)
      (i) Failure to administer vitamin K at birth usually results in a bleeding diathesis at 3–4 days of age.
      (ii) Use of antibiotics may interfere with the production of vitamin K by normal gastrointestinal flora.
      (iii) Maternal anticonvulsant treatment (phenobarbital, pheytoin).
   (d) **Thrombocytopenia**
      (i) Immune thrombocytopenia may be isoimmune or autoimmune.
      (ii) Congenital thrombocytopenia with absent radii is a syndrome frequently associated with hemorrhagic anemia in the newborn.
iii. **Iatrogenic blood loss.** Anemia may occur if blood loss resulting from repeated venipuncture is not replaced routinely. Symptoms may develop if a loss of >20% occurs within a 48-h period.
2. **Hemolytic anemia**
   a. **Immune hemolysis**
      i. **Isoimmune hemolytic anemia** is caused mostly by Rh incompatibility.
      ii. **Autoimmune hemolytic anemia.**
   b. **Nonimmune hemolysis**
      i. **Bacterial sepsis** may cause primary microangiopathic hemolysis.
      ii. **Congenital TORCH** (*t*oxoplasmosis, *o*ther, *r*ubella, *c*ytomegalovirus, and *h*erpes simplex virus) infections (see Chapter 127).
   c. **Congenital erythrocyte defect**
      i. **Metabolic enzyme deficiency**
         (a) Glucose-6-phosphate dehydrogenase (G6PD) deficiency.
         (b) Pyruvate kinase deficiency.
      ii. **Thalassemia.** Hemolytic anemia secondary to thalassemia is invariably associated with homozygous α-thalassemia and presents at birth. The disorders in β-thalassemia become apparent only after 2–3 months of age.
      iii. **Hemoglobinopathy** may be characterized as unstable hemoglobins or congenital Heinz body anemias.
      iv. **Membrane defects** are usually autosomal dominant.
         (a) **Hereditary spherocytosis** (1 in 5000 neonates) commonly presents with jaundice and less often with anemia.
         (b) **Hereditary elliptocytosis** (1 in 2500 neonates) rarely presents in the newborn infant.
   d. **Systemic diseases**
      i. Galactosemia.
      ii. Osteopetrosis.

e. **Nutritional deficiency.** Vitamin E deficiency occurs with chronic malabsorption but usually does not present until after the neonatal period.
3. **Hypoplastic anemia**
  a. **Congenital disease**
    i. Diamond-Blackfan syndrome (congenital hypoplastic anemia).
    ii. Atransferrinemia.
    iii. Congenital leukemia.
    iv. Sideroblastic anemia.
  b. **Acquired disease**
    i. Infection. Rubella and syphilis are the most common causes.
    ii. Aplastic crisis.
    iii. Aplastic anemia.
IV. **Risk factors.** Prematurity, certain race and ethnic groups, and hereditary blood disorders (see Section III).
V. **Clinical presentation**
  A. **Symptoms and signs.** The four major forms of neonatal anemia may be demonstrated by determination of the following factors: age at presentation of anemia, associated clinical features at presentation, hemodynamic status of the infant, and presence or absence of compensatory reticulocytosis.
  1. **Hemorrhagic anemia** is often dramatic in clinical presentation when acute but may be more subtle when chronic. Both forms have significant rates of perinatal morbidity and mortality if they remain unrecognized. Neither form has significant elevation of bilirubin levels or hepatosplenomegaly.
    a. **Acute hemorrhagic anemia** presents at birth or with internal hemorrhage after 24 h. There is pallor not associated with jaundice and often without cyanosis (<5 g of deoxyhemoglobin) and unrelieved by supplemental oxygen. Tachypnea or gasping respirations are present. Vascular instability ranges from decreased peripheral perfusion (a 10% loss of blood volume) to hypovolemic shock (20–25% loss of blood volume). There is also decreased central venous pressure and poor capillary refill. Normocytic or normochromic RBC indices are present, with reticulocytosis developing within 2–3 days of the hemorrhagic event.
    b. **Chronic hemorrhagic anemia** presents at birth with unexplained pallor, often without cyanosis (<5 g of deoxyhemoglobin), and unrelieved by supplemental oxygen. Minimal signs of respiratory distress are present. The central venous pressure is normal or increased. Microcytic or hypochromic RBC indices are present, with compensatory reticulocytosis. The liver is often enlarged because of compensatory extramedullary erythropoiesis. Hydrops fetalis or stillbirth may occur with failure of compensatory reticulocytosis or intravascular volume maintenance.
    c. **Asphyxia pallida** (severe neonatal asphyxia) is not associated with hemorrhagic anemia at presentation. This disorder must be distinguished clinically from acute hemorrhage because specific immediate therapy is needed for each disorder. Asphyxia pallida presents at birth with pallor and cyanosis, which improves with supplemental oxygen delivery, respiratory failure, bradycardia, and normal central venous pressure.
  2. **Hemolytic anemia.** Jaundice is often seen before diagnostic levels of hemoglobin are obtained, in part because of the compensatory reticulocytosis that is invariably present. The infant usually presents with pallor after 48 h of age. However, severe Rh isoimmune disease or homozygous α-thalassemia presents at birth with severe anemia and, in many cases, hydrops fetalis. Unconjugated hyperbilirubinemia of >10–12 mg/dL, tachypnea, and hepatosplenomegaly may be seen with hemolytic anemia.
  3. **Hypoplastic anemia** is uncommon. It is characterized by presentation after 48 h of age, absence of jaundice, and reticulocytopenia.

4. Other forms of anemia
   a. **Anemia associated with twin-twin transfusion.** If chronic hemorrhage is occurring, there is often a >20% difference in the birthweights of the two infants, the donor being the smaller twin.
   b. **Occult (internal) hemorrhage**
      i. **Intracranial hemorrhage.** Signs include a bulging anterior fontanelle and neurologic signs (eg, a change in consciousness, apnea, or seizures).
      ii. **Visceral hemorrhage.** Most commonly, the liver has been injured. An abdominal mass or distention is seen.
      iii. **Pulmonary hemorrhage.** Partial or total radiographic opacification of a hemithorax and bloody tracheal secretions are seen.

B. History
   1. **Anemia at birth**
      a. **Hemorrhagic anemia.** There may be a history of third-trimester vaginal bleeding or amniocentesis. Hemorrhagic anemia may be associated with multiple gestation, maternal chills or fever postpartum, and nonelective cesarean delivery.
      b. **Hemolytic anemia** may be associated with intrauterine growth retardation (IUGR) and Rh-negative mothers.
   2. **Anemia presenting after 24 h of age** is often associated with obstetric trauma, unattended delivery, precipitous delivery, perinatal fetal distress, or a low Apgar score.
   3. **Anemia presenting with jaundice** suggests hemolytic anemia. There may be evidence of drug ingestion late in the third trimester; IUGR; a family member with splenectomy, anemia, jaundice, or cholelithiasis; maternal autoimmune disease; or Mediterranean or Asian ethnic background.

VI. Diagnosis
   A. **Obligatory initial studies**
      1. Hemoglobin.
      2. RBC indices.
         a. **Microcytic or hypochromic RBC indices** suggest fetomaternal or twin-twin hemorrhage or α-thalassemia (mean corpuscular volume <90 fL).
         b. **Normocytic or normochromic RBC indices** are suggestive of acute hemorrhage, systemic disease, intrinsic RBC defect, or hypoplastic anemia.
      3. **Reticulocyte count (corrected).** An elevated reticulocyte count is associated with antecedent hemorrhage or hemolytic anemia. A low count is seen with hypoplastic anemia. The following formula is used:

Corrected reticulocyte count =

$$\frac{\text{Observed reticulocyte count} \times \text{Observed hematocrit}}{\text{Normal hematocrit for age}}$$

      4. **Blood smear**
         a. **Spherocytes** are associated with ABO isoimmune hemolysis or hereditary spherocytosis.
         b. **Elliptocytes** are seen in hereditary elliptocytosis.
         c. **Pyknocytes** may be seen in G6PD deficiency.
         d. **Schistocytes or helmet cells** are most often seen with consumption coagulopathy.
      5. **Direct antiglobulin test (direct Coombs test).** This test is positive in isoimmune or autoimmune hemolysis.
   B. **Other selected laboratory studies**
      1. **Isoimmune hemolysis.** The blood type and Rh type should be determined and an eluate of neonatal cells prepared.
      2. **Fetomaternal hemorrhage.** The **Kleihauer-Betke test** should be performed. Using an acid elution technique, a maternal blood smear is stained with eosin.

Fetal RBCs containing hemoglobin F resistant to acid elution stain darkly. Adult RBCs voided of their acid-sensitive hemoglobin A do not stain and appear as "ghost cells." A 50-mL loss of fetal blood into the maternal circulation shows up as 1% fetal cells in the maternal circulation. **ABO incompatibility between mother and infant results in an increased clearance rate of fetal cells from the maternal circulation, giving a falsely low result.** Because various conditions may lead to a false-negative result, new and more accurate flow cytometry techniques can be used when the index of suspicion for fetomaternal transfusions is elevated.

3. **Congenital hypoplastic or aplastic anemia.** Bone marrow aspiration is usually indicated.
4. **TORCH infection**
   a. Skull and long-bone films.
   b. IgM levels.
   c. Acute or convalescent serology.
   d. Urine culture for cytomegalovirus.
5. **Consumption coagulopathy**
   a. Prothrombin time (PT) and partial thromboplastin time (PTT).
   b. Platelet count.
   c. Thrombin time or fibrinogen assay.
   d. Factor V and factor VIII levels.
   e. Fibrin split products (D-dimers).
6. **Occult hemorrhage**
   a. Pathologic examination of the placenta.
   b. Cranial or abdominal ultrasonography will help identify the site of bleeding.
7. **Intrinsic RBC defect**
   a. RBC enzyme studies.
   b. Analysis of the globin chain ratio.
   c. Studies of RBC membrane.

VII. **Management.** Treatment of neonatal anemia may involve, individually or in combination, simple replacement transfusion, exchange transfusion, nutritional supplementation, or treatment of the underlying primary disorder.
   A. **Simple replacement transfusion**
      1. **Indications**
         a. **Acute hemorrhagic anemia.**
         b. **Ongoing deficit replacement.**
         c. **Maintenance of effective oxygen-carrying capacity.** There are no universally accepted guidelines; however, those presented next are fairly representative of most common practice.
            i. **Hematocrit <35%** with severe cardiopulmonary disease (eg, intermittent positive-pressure ventilation with mean airway pressure >6 cm H_2O).
            ii. **Hematocrit <30%**
               (a) With mild to moderate cardiopulmonary disease (FIO_2 >35%, continuous positive airway pressure).
               (b) Significant apnea (>9–12 h, or requiring bag-and-mask ventilation).
               (c) "Symptomatic anemia": weight gain <10 g/kg/day at full caloric intake and heart rate >180 beats/min persisting for 24 h.
               (d) If undergoing major surgery.
            iii. **Hematocrit <21%.** Asymptomatic but with low reticulocyte count (<2%).
      2. **Emergency transfusion at birth only**
         a. **Use type O, Rh-negative packed RBCs.**
            i. Adjust the hematocrit to 50%.
            ii. If a medical emergency exists, blood that has not been cross-matched may be given; if time permits, blood may be cross-matched to the mother's blood.

    b. Alternative replacement fluids include normal saline, fresh-frozen plasma, and 5% albumin in saline. Timely infusion of packed RBCs or partial exchange transfusion should follow.

    c. Perform umbilical vein catheterization to a depth of 4–5 cm or until free blood flow is established (see Chapter 38).

    d. Draw initial blood samples for diagnostic studies. Obtain a hemogram and differential, blood type and Rh type, direct Coombs test, and, if indicated, total bilirubin levels. In a medical emergency, transfusion may be started before the results of laboratory testing are known.

    e. Infuse 10–15 mL/kg of replacement fluid over 10–15 min if emergency measures are needed. Once the infant's status is stable, reassess the diagnostic studies, physical examination, and obstetric history.

    f. Calculate the RBC volume. Under controlled circumstances or if simple transfusion is indicated, calculate the volume of packed RBCs needed to achieve the desired increase in RBC mass (see page 327).

    g. The volume of a single transfusion should not exceed 10–20 mL/kg.

B. Exchange transfusion

  1. Indications

    a. Chronic hemolytic anemia or hemorrhagic anemia with evidence of tissue hypoxia (poor perfusion, metabolic acidosis, oliguria).

    b. Severe isoimmune hemolytic anemia with circulating sensitized RBCs and isoantibody.

    c. Consumption coagulopathy.

  2. Technique. See Chapter 29 for the technique of exchange transfusion in neonates.

C. Nutritional replacement

  1. Iron. Iron replacement is useful in the following situations:

    a. Fetomaternal hemorrhage of significant volume.

    b. Chronic twin-twin transfusion (in the donor twin).

    c. Incremental external blood loss (if unreplaced).

    d. Preterm infant (<36 weeks' gestational age).

  2. Folate (especially with serum levels <0.5 ng/mL).

    a. Premature infants weighing <1500 g or <34 weeks' gestational age.

    b. Chronic hemolytic anemias or conditions involving "stress erythropoiesis."

    c. Infants receiving phenytoin (Dilantin).

  3. Vitamin E. Preterm infants of <34 weeks' gestational age, unless they are being breast-fed.

D. Prophylactic

  1. Recombinant human erythropoietin (r-HuEPO) *(controversial).* High doses of erythropoietin are capable of increasing neonatal erythropoiesis and have very little adverse side effect. It decreases the requirement for "late" transfusions (those required past the age of 2–3 weeks); it will not compensate for the anemia secondary to phlebotomy losses. Its use in the very low birthweight infant continues to be *controversial* because the severity of anemia in this group can be more effectively minimized by a restrictive policy for blood sampling and the use of micromethods in the laboratory. The need for transfusions is also reduced when a consistent "protocolized" approach for transfusions is available in the neonatal intensive care unit. It has been also argued that what needs to be avoided, more than the transfusion itself, is the exposure to multiple donors. The allocation of a single donor for each high-risk infant, for a 42-day period, is the most effective way to reach that former goal. Early and late strategies have been used for erythropoietin treatment. (See also Chapter 132.)

    a. Early. Starting on day 1 or 2, 1200–1400 units/kg/week. r-HuEPO is added to the total parenteral nutrition solution, and 1 mg/kg/day of iron is added.

    b. Late. 500–700 units/kg/week given three to five times per week subcutaneously. Supplemental oral iron needs to be provided at 3 mg/kg/day in three divided doses. The iron dose is increased to 6 mg/kg/day as soon as the infant is tolerating full enteral feeds.

2. Nutritional supplementation
   a. Elemental iron, 1–2 mg/kg/day, beginning at 2 months of age and continuing through 1 year of age.
   b. Folic acid, 1–2 mg/week for preterm infants; 50 mcg/day for term infants.
   c. Vitamin E, 25 IU/day, until a corrected age of 4 months is reached.

E. Treatment of selected disorders
   1. Consumption coagulopathy
      a. Treat the underlying cause (eg, sepsis).
      b. Give blood replacement therapy. Perform exchange transfusion or give fresh-frozen plasma, 10 mL/kg every 12–14 h. Platelet concentrate, 1 unit, may be used as a substitute for plasma transfusion.
      c. Perform coagulation studies. Monitor the PTT, PT, and fibrinogen levels and the platelet count.
   2. Immune thrombocytopenia
      a. Isoimmune thrombocytopenia
         i. Consider performing cesarean delivery if the diagnosis has been confirmed and there is an older sibling with immune thrombocytopenia (75% risk of recurrence).
         ii. Give maternal washed platelets when indicated for bleeding diathesis in an infant with a platelet count <20,000–30,000 μL. Exchange transfusion may be used as an alternative.
         iii. Corticosteroid therapy and intravenous immune globulin are *controversial*. See Chapter 132.
      b. Autoimmune thrombocytopenia
         i. Consider performing cesarean delivery if the maternal platelet count is <100,000 μL or the fetal platelet count is <50,000 μL.
         ii. Use of corticosteroids is *controversial*. Under the conditions just mentioned, consider giving corticosteroids to the mother several weeks before delivery. Transfusion of random donor platelets may be given when indicated.

VIII. **Prognosis** depends on the underlying cause, its severity, and how acutely the anemia develops.

Selected References

Alpay F et al: High-dose intravenous immunoglobulin therapy in neonatal immune haemolytic jaundice. *Acta Paediatr* 1999;88:216.

American Academy of Pediatrics: Commentary: neonatal jaundice and kernicterus. *Pediatrics* 2001;108:763.

Bifano EM, Curran TR: Minimizing donor blood exposure in the neonatal intensive care unit: current trends and future prospects. *Clin Perinatol* 1995;22:657.

Blanchette VS, Rand ML: Platelet disorders in newborn infants: diagnosis and management. *Semin Perinatol* 1997;21:53.

Bowman JM: Rh erythroblastosis fetalis. *Semin Hematol* 1975;12:189.

Bowman JM: Immune hemolytic disease. In Nathan DG, Orkin S (eds): *Hematology of Infancy and Childhood,* 5th ed. Philadelphia, PA: Saunders, 1998.

Davis BH: Detection of fetal red cells in fetomaternal hemorrhage using a fetal hemoglobin monoclonal antibody by flow cytometry. *Transfusion* 1998;38:749.

Dickerman JF: Anemia in the newborn infant. *Pediatr Rev* 1984;6:131.

Glader BE: Erythrocyte disorders in infancy. In Avery ME, Taeusch HW (eds): *Schaffer's Diseases of the Newborn,* 5th ed. Philadelphia, PA: Saunders, 1984.

Kates EH, Kates JS: Anemia and polycythemia in the newborn. *Pediatr Rev* 2007;28(1):33-34.

Lee DA et al: Reducing blood donor exposure in low birth weight infants by use of older, unwashed packed red blood cells. *J Pediatr* 1995;126:280.

Litty CA: Neonatal red cell transfusions. *Immunohematology* 2008;24(1):10-14.

Miller DR: Normal values and examination of the blood: perinatal period, infancy, childhood, and adolescence. In Miller DR et al (eds): *Blood Diseases of Infancy and Childhood,* 5th ed. St. Louis, MO: Mosby, 1984.

Ohls R et al: Effects of early erythropoietin therapy on the transfusion requirements of preterm infants below 1250 gm birth weight: a multicenter, randomized, controlled trial. *Pediatrics* 2001;108:934.

Oski FA: Hematologic problems. In Avery GB (ed): *Neonatology, Pathophysiology, and Management of the Newborn,* 2nd ed. Lippincott, 1981.

Oski FA, Naiman JL (eds): *Hematologic Problems in the Newborn,* 3rd ed. Philadelphia, PA: Saunders, 1982.

Pearson HA: Posthemorrhagic anemia in the newborn. *Pediatr Rev* 1982;4:40.

Roberts D et al: Interventions for twin-twin transfusion syndrome: a Cochrane review. *Ultrasound Obstet Gynecol* 2008;31(6):701-711.

Shannon K: Recombinant human erythropoietin in neonatal anemia. *Clin Perinatol* 1995;22:627.

76 Apnea and Periodic Breathing

I. **Definitions.** Simply defined, apnea is the absence of respiratory shorter gas flow for a period of 20 s or more if associated with bradycardia or significant desaturation.
   A. **Central apnea** is of central nervous system (CNS) origin and characterized by the absence of gas flow with no respiratory effort.
   B. **Obstructive apnea** is continued respiratory effort not resulting in gas flow.
   C. **Mixed apnea** is a combination of the central and obstructive types.
   D. **Periodic breathing,** defined as three or more periods of apnea lasting ≥ 3 s within a 20 s period of otherwise normal respiration, is also common in the newborn period. Currently, it is not known whether an association exists between apnea and periodic breathing.
II. **Incidence.** The incidence of apnea and periodic breathing in the term infant has not been adequately determined. More than 50% of infants weighing <1500 g and 90% of infants weighing <1000 g have apnea. Mixed is the most common type of apnea, followed by central and then obstructive. Another 30% have periodic breathing.
III. **Pathophysiology.** Apnea and periodic breathing probably have a common pathophysiologic origin, apnea being a step further along the continuum than periodic breathing. Although the exact pathophysiology of these events has not yet been elucidated, there are many theories.
   A. **Immaturity of respiratory control.** Because apnea is seen most commonly in the premature infant, some type of immaturity of the respiratory control mechanism is thought to play a role in most cases.

1. **Hypoxic response.** The preterm infant is known to have an abnormal biphasic response to hypoxia: a brief period of tachypnea followed by apnea. This response is unlike that seen in the adult or older child in whom hypoxia produces a state of prolonged tachypnea.

2. **Carbon dioxide response.** The carbon dioxide response curve is shifted in the preterm infant, with higher levels of carbon dioxide required before respiration is stimulated.

B. **Sleep-related response.** Sleep states may also play an important role in the development of apnea in the preterm infant. A shift from one sleep state to another is often characterized by instability of respiratory activity in the adult. The preterm infant is sleeping ~80% of the time and has difficulty making the transition between the sleeping and waking states. This may be associated with an increased risk for the development of apnea in the infants.

C. **Protective reflexes** such as the apneic response to noxious substances in the airway may also play a role in the apneic episodes seen in the newborn infant.

D. **Muscle weakness.** Overall muscle weakness (of both the muscles of respiration and the muscles that maintain airway patency) also plays an important role in pathophysiology.

E. **All of the preceding** point to an immature respiratory control mechanism in the preterm infant. Whether the immaturity is operational at the level of the brainstem, the peripheral chemoreceptors, or the central receptors has yet to be determined. What is likely is that apnea results from a combination of immature afferent impulses to the respiratory control centers along with immature efferent pathways from these receptor sites, giving rise to the poor ventilation control.

F. **Pathologic states** can also lead to apnea in the infant. The following disorders are all associated with apnea in the neonatal period:

1. Hypothermia and hyperthermia.
2. Metabolic disturbances such as hypoglycemia and hyponatremia.
3. Sepsis.
4. Anemia.
5. Hypoxemia.
6. CNS abnormalities such as intraventricular hemorrhage (IVH) or stroke.
7. Necrotizing enterocolitis (NEC).
8. Drug withdrawal and drug effects (eg, maternal antepartum magnesium therapy).
9. Gastroesophageal reflux.

IV. **Risk factors**

A. **Preterm infants are at greatest risk for apnea.** Because it is believed to be secondary to immature or poorly developed respiratory control mechanisms, it is especially noted in extremely low birthweight infants.

B. **Sleep positioning.** The "back to sleep" campaign, which was initiated in 1992, has led to a 40% reduction in the incidence of sudden infant death syndrome (SIDS).

C. **Neurologic disorders.** Because respiration depends on the integration of numerous CNS functions, the child with certain neurologic diseases may be at increased risk for the development of apnea. Examples of central neurologic disorders include CNS infection and structural abnormalities (eg, holoprosencephaly); peripheral disorders include Werdnig-Hoffman disease and myasthenia gravis.

D. **Sibling with SIDS.** The Collaborative Home Infant Monitoring Evaluation (CHIME) study showed that the incidence of apnea was the same in siblings of SIDS and normal term infants. Evidence supports an increased chance of obstructive sleep apnea (OSA) in infants with a family history of OSA, SIDS, and an apparent life-threatening event.

E. **Gastroesophageal reflux.** Its relationship to apnea has been the source of much debate, with recent studies showing no temporal relationship to apnea of prematurity, but it is a cause of apnea in the term infant.

V. **Clinical presentation**

A. **Apnea within 24 h after delivery.** Although apnea may be present at any time during the neonatal period, if it presents within the first 24 h of life, it is usually not simple apnea of prematurity. Apnea during this period may be suspected as being associated with infant or maternal conditions (eg, neonatal sepsis, hypoglycemia, intracranial hemorrhage, maternal antepartum magnesium treatment, or maternal exposure to narcotics).

B. **Apnea after the first 24 h of life.** When apnea occurs after the first 24 h of life and is not associated with any other pathologic condition, it may be classified as apnea of prematurity. Apnea may also occur following weaning from prolonged ventilator support and may be associated with intermittent hypoxia secondary to hypoventilation or atelectasis.

VI. **Diagnosis.** A high index of suspicion is necessary to diagnose apnea. If significant apnea is detected, an extensive workup is required to make an accurate diagnosis and develop a logical treatment plan.

A. **Monitoring of infants at risk.** All preterm infants should be closely monitored for the development of this often life-threatening condition. Close attention should be paid to the type of monitoring given to infants in intensive care units. Preterm infants are commonly on heart rate monitors only, and they are identified as having apnea only if the heart rate drops below the monitor alarm limit (usually set at 80 beats/min). In this case, these infants may suffer profound hypoxia before bradycardia develops, or they may have apnea with significant hypoxemia but without a drop in heart rate. To detect apnea, these infants should have continuous monitoring of respiratory activity or monitoring of oxygenation, or both, using either transcutaneous oximetry or pulse oximetry.

B. **History.** A thorough review of maternal septic risk factors, medications, and birth history are required. Additional history of feeding intolerance along with abdominal distention might suggest NEC.

C. **Physical examination.** Specific attention should be paid to physical findings such as lethargy, hypothermia or hyperthermia, cyanosis, and respiratory effort. A thorough physical examination including neurological examination should also be performed.

D. **Laboratory studies**
   1. **Sepsis screen** should include a complete blood cell count with differential and platelet count. Serial C-reactive protein tests will help rule out sepsis and anemia.
   2. **Pulse oximetry** will screen for hypoxia, with arterial blood gas when indicated.
   3. **Serum glucose, electrolyte, and calcium levels** will aid in the diagnosis of metabolic disturbances.

E. **Radiographic studies**
   1. **Chest radiograph** to detect evidence of pathologic lung changes (eg, atelectasis, pneumonia, or air leak).
   2. **Abdominal radiograph** to detect signs of NEC.
   3. **Ultrasonography** of the head to detect IVH or other CNS abnormality.
   4. **Computed tomography scan or magnetic resonance imaging** of the head may also be appropriate in infants with definite signs of neurologic disease.

F. **Other studies**
   1. **Electroencephalography.** An electroencephalogram (EEG) may be necessary to complete the workup if there is any question about the neurologic status of the infant. Apnea as the sole presentation of seizures is uncommon.
   2. **Pneumography.** A pneumogram is another tool in the diagnosis of apnea. Pneumography is especially useful in the infant whose cause of apnea has not yet been identified. Chest leads provide a tracing that gives a continuous recording of heart rate, chest wall movement, pulse oximetry, and airflow via a nasal thermistor. **With the addition of a thermistor, central apnea can easily be distinguished from obstructive apnea.** The addition of the pulse oximeter helps determine whether there are oxygen desaturations during periods of apnea or heart rate drops. This distinction is important for the treatment of the disorder and should be directed specifically to the type of apnea detected. A pH probe for the detection of gastroesophageal reflux is also important for completion of an overall evaluation for apnea.

3. **Polysomnography.** This is a rarely used test. In research-oriented centers, a polysomnogram (a study that monitors specific EEG leads and muscle movement) can be used for a more thorough workup of apnea. This study not only determines the type of apnea that occurs but can also relate it to the sleep stage of the infant.

VII. **Management.** Treatment for apnea must be individualized.

A. **Specific therapy.** If an identifiable cause of apnea is determined, it should be treated accordingly. See On-Call Problems or disease chapter for specific therapies.

B. **General therapy.** If a cause cannot be identified or if one can be identified but is not amenable to treatment (eg, IVH), there are several approaches to treatment.

1. **Respiratory support**

a. **Supplemental oxygen** can be used to be used to alleviate apneic spells, with the mechanism of action to decrease the number of unidentified hypoxic spells. Concern about worsening retinopathy of prematurity does exist, and oxygenation should be monitored.

b. **Continuous positive airway pressure (CPAP)** is used with some success, probably acting by the same mechanism as supplemental oxygen. This method is an invasive therapeutic modality and should be used only when other methods have failed. Many centers are now using a high-flow nasal cannula (HFNC) in lieu of CPAP. HFNC delivers CPAP when used at flows >1 L/min.

c. **Mechanical ventilation** is required in some infants who continue to have apneic spells despite pharmacologic treatment. If the apnea is severe and associated with hypoxia or significant bradycardia, intubation and mechanical ventilation may be indicated.

2. **Pharmacologic therapy.** If the methods just described fail, the next line of approach is to begin administration of respiratory stimulants. (For dosage and other pharmacologic information, see Chapter 132.)

a. **Caffeine** can be used in the treatment of apnea. Recent evidence has demonstrated that caffeine therapy in infants weighing 500–1250 g is associated with improved survival and neurodevelopmental outcome at 18–21 months. The mechanism of benefit is only partially due to a decrease in apneic episodes, which leads to an earlier discontinuation of positive airway pressure, with caffeine also thought to have some neuroprotective effects. Caffeine has fewer side effects, has a greater therapeutic window, does not alter cerebral blood flow, and has a longer half-life than theophylline, so it is the preferred agent. Caffeine levels are no longer considered absolutely necessary in the management of most infants with apnea.

b. **Theophylline** can also be used in the treatment of apnea. The exact mechanism of action is open to debate, but it probably works through a variety of mechanisms, including an effect on the adenosine tissue receptors, direct stimulation of the respiratory centers, and lowering of the threshold to carbon dioxide. Some clinicians think it may act by direct stimulation of the diaphragm.

c. **Doxapram.** Doxapram, a potent respiratory stimulant, is effective when theophylline and caffeine have failed. The duration of treatment with doxapram is limited to 5 days, but the drug may be used longer if indicated. Benzyl alcohol is the preservative used in doxapram. The duration of therapy depends on the cumulative dose of benzyl alcohol, and there have been concerns about long-term neurodevelopmental outcome.

C. **Discharge planning and follow-up.** A major issue in the management of infants with apnea is deciding when to stop administration of methylxanthines and whether or not the infant needs to be discharged on methylxanthines, a home monitor, or both.

1. **Discontinuing medications.** Consider stopping methylxanthine therapy when the apnea has resolved and the infant weighs between 1800 and 2000 g. A more

aggressive approach is to stop therapy when the infant has been apnea free for a period of 7 days, irrespective of age. If the infant remains asymptomatic following the discontinuation of methylxanthine therapy, the child may be discharged without further therapy.

2. **Reinstituting medications.** If symptomatic apnea recurs after discontinuing therapy, methylxanthine therapy should be reinstituted and a decision should be made to discharge the infant on this medication or to keep the infant hospitalized longer. Earlier discharge with monitoring is acceptable in an attempt to shorten the length of hospital stay. The use of home monitors in addition to methylxanthine therapy is ***controversial.*** Therapeutic methylxanthine levels are maintained until the child reaches 52 weeks of postconceptional age; then methylxanthine therapy is discontinued and the recording is checked. If the recording is normal, therapy can be stopped. If the recording is abnormal, the infant may need to be restarted on methylxanthines and monitoring continued. Another attempt can be made to discontinue methylxanthines in 4 weeks.

3. **Home apnea monitoring.** Use of home apnea monitors continues to be ***controversial.*** The CHIME study showed that after 43 weeks postconceptional age, cardiorespiratory events occurred no more frequently in preterm infants than term infants. No study has shown an improved morbidity and mortality with home infant monitoring for apnea. If home monitoring is used, the most appropriate type of monitor has the ability to store and record waveforms. These monitors allow for continued evaluation and management of the infant at risk. Waveform monitors measure transthoracic impedance and electrocardiograms and document captured waveform data, alarms, and physiologic events, which should give clinicians a better understanding of the patient's symptoms.

At present, no standard of care exists among neonatologists, but reasonable indications for home apnea monitor use include the following:

a. Significant event not associated with feeds.

b. Home methylxanthine therapy for apnea.

c. Presence of a tracheotomy.

d. Home oxygen therapy.

VIII. **Prognosis.** The best indicator of prognosis in apnea is etiology. Apnea of prematurity has an excellent prognosis, whereas apnea associated with IVH has a poorer prognosis. In most infants, apnea resolves without the occurrence of long-term deficiencies.

Selected References

McNamara F, Sullivan CE: Obstructive sleep apnea in infants: relation to family history of sudden infant death syndrome, apparent life-threatening events, and obstructive sleep apnea. *J Pediatr* 2000;136(3):318-323.

Miller MJ et al: Respiratory control and apnea of prematurity. In Martin RJ et al (eds): *Neonatal-Perinatal Medicine: Diseases of the Fetus and Infant,* 8th ed. Philadelphia, PA: Elsevier Mosby, 2006:1135-1141.

Peter CS et al: Gastroesophageal reflux and apnea of prematurity: no temporal relationship. *Pediatrics* 2002;109(1):8-11.

Ramanathan R et al: Cardiorespiratory events recorded on home monitors: Comparison of healthy infants with those at increased risk for SIDS. *JAMA* 2001;285(17):2199-2207.

Schmidt B et al: Long-term effects of caffeine therapy for apnea of prematurity. *N Engl J Med* 2007;357(19):1893-1902.

Sreenan C et al: High-flow nasal cannulae in the management of apnea of prematurity: a comparison with conventional nasal continuous positive airway pressure. *Pediatrics* 2001;107(5):1081-1083.

77 Bronchopulmonary Dysplasia

I. **Definition.** Classic bronchopulmonary dysplasia (BPD) is a neonatal form of chronic pulmonary disorder that follows a primary course of respiratory failure (eg, respiratory distress syndrome [RDS], meconium aspiration syndrome) in the first days of life. A "new" form of BPD has been described in extremely low birthweight infants. This occurs in infants who initially had none or modest initial ventilatory and oxygen needs. **BPD is defined as persistent oxygen dependency up to 28 days of life.** The severity of BPD-related pulmonary dysfunction in early childhood is more accurately predicted by an oxygen dependence at 36 weeks' postconceptional age (PCA) in infants <32 weeks' gestational age (GA) and at 56 days of age in infants with older GA. BPD is thus classified at this later postnatal age and is graded according to the type of respiratory support required to maintain a normal arterial oxygen saturation (>89%).

A. **Mild BPD.** Infants who have been weaned from any supplemental oxygen.

B. **Moderate BPD.** Infants who continue to need up to 30% oxygen.

C. **Severe BPD.** Infants whose requirements exceed 30% and/or include continuous positive airway pressure or mechanical ventilation.

II. **Incidence.** The incidence of BPD is influenced by many risk factors, the most important of which is lung maturity. The incidence of BPD increases with decreasing birthweight and affects ~30% of infants with birthweights <1000 g. There is a large variability in rates reported among centers in part related to differences in clinical practices, such as criteria used for the management of mechanical ventilation.

III. **Pathophysiology.** A primary lung injury is not always evident at birth. The secondary development of a persistent lung injury is associated with an abnormal repair process and leads to structural changes such as arrested alveolarization and pulmonary vascular dysgenesis.

A. **The major factors contributing to BPD are as follows:**

1. **Inflammation** is central to the development of BPD. An exaggerated inflammatory response (alveolar influx of numerous proinflammatory cytokines as well as macrophages and leukocytes) occurs in the first few days of life in infants in whom BPD subsequently develops.

2. **Mechanical ventilation.** Volutrauma/barotrauma is one of the key risk factors for the development of BPD. Minimizing the use of mechanical ventilation by the use of early nasal continuous positive airway pressure (NCPAP) and noninvasive ventilatory support (nasal intermittent positive pressure ventilation) has led to lesser rates of BPD.

3. **Oxygen exposure.** Classic BPD observed prior to the availability of exogenous surfactant treatment was always associated with prolonged exposure (>150 h) to an FIO_2 >60%. Hyperoxia can have major effects on lung tissue such as proliferation of alveolar type II cells and fibroblast, alterations in the surfactant system, increases in inflammatory cells and cytokines, increased collagen deposition, and decreased alveolarization and microvascular density. Today, exposure to prolonged high oxygen is limited. Nevertheless, aiming for arterial oxygen saturation in the range 85–93% rather than >92% has led to a decrease in the need for supplemental oxygen at 36 weeks PCA in this postsurfactant era.

B. **Pathologic changes.** Compared with the presurfactant era, lungs of infants currently dying from BPD have normal-appearing airways, less fibrosis, and more uniform inflation. However, these lungs have deficient septation, leading to fewer and larger alveoli with possible reduced pulmonary capillarization that may lead to pulmonary hypertension.

IV. **Risk factors.** Major risk factors are prematurity, white race, male gender, chorioamnionitis, tracheal colonization with ureaplasma, and the increased survival of the extremely low birthweight infant. Other risk factors are RDS, excessive early intravenous

fluid administration, symptomatic PDA, sepsis, oxygen therapy, vitamin A deficiency, and a family history of atopic disease.
V. **Clinical presentation.** BPD is usually suspected in infants with progressive and idiopathic deterioration of pulmonary function. Infants in whom BPD develops often require oxygen therapy or mechanical ventilation beyond the first week of life. Severe cases of BPD are usually associated with poor growth, pulmonary edema, and a hyperreactive airway.
VI. **Diagnosis**
  A. **Physical examination**
    1. **General signs.** Worsening respiratory status is manifested by an increase in the work of breathing, an increase in oxygen requirement, or an increase in apnea-bradycardia, or a combination of these.
    2. **Pulmonary examination.** Retractions and diffuse rales are common. Wheezing or prolongation of expiration may also be noted.
    3. **Cardiovascular examination.** A right ventricular heave, single S_2, or prominent P_2 may accompany cor pulmonale.
    4. **Abdominal examination.** The liver may be enlarged secondary to right-sided heart failure or may be displaced downward into the abdomen secondary to lung hyperinflation.
  B. **Laboratory and radiologic studies.** These studies are intended to rule out differential diagnosis such as sepsis or patent ductus arteriosus (PDA) during the acute nature of the disease and to detect problems related to chronic lung disease or its therapy.
    1. **Arterial blood gas levels** frequently reveal carbon dioxide retention. However, if the respiratory difficulties are chronic and stable, the pH is usually subnormal (pH ≥7.25).
    2. **Electrolytes.** Abnormalities of electrolytes may result from chronic carbon dioxide retention (elevated serum bicarbonate), diuretic therapy (hyponatremia, hypokalemia, or hypochloremia), or fluid restriction (elevated urea nitrogen and creatinine), or all three.
    3. **Urinalysis.** Microscopic examination may reveal the presence of red blood cells, indicating a possible nephrocalcinosis as a result of prolonged diuretic treatment.
    4. **Chest radiograph.** Radiographic findings may be quite variable. Most frequently, BPD appears as diffuse haziness and lung hypoinflation in infants who were very immature at birth and who have persistent oxygen requirements. In other infants, a different picture is seen reminiscent of that originally described by Northway: **streaky interstitial markings, patchy atelectasis intermingled with cystic area, and severe overall lung hyperinflation.** Because those findings persist for a prolonged period, new changes (such as a secondary infection) are difficult to detect without the benefit of comparison to previous radiographs. (See Figure 10–16 for an example of BPD.)
    5. **Renal ultrasonography.** Radiologic studies of the abdomen should be considered during diuretic therapy to detect the presence of nephrocalcinosis. It should be performed when red blood cells are present in the urine.
    6. **Other studies. Electrocardiography** and **echocardiography** are indicated in nonimproving or worsening BPD. Electrocardiograms and echocardiograms could detect cor pulmonale and/or pulmonary hypertension, manifested by right ventricular hypertrophy and elevation of pulmonary artery pressure with right axis deviation, increased right systolic time intervals, thickening of the right ventricular wall, and abnormal right ventricular geometry.
VII. **Management**
  A. **Prevention of BPD**
    1. **Prevention of prematurity and RDS.** Therapies directed toward decreasing the risk of prematurity and the incidence of RDS include improving prenatal care and antenatal corticosteroids.
    2. **Reducing exposure to risk factors.** Successful measures should include minimizing exposure to oxygen, ventilation strategies that minimize the use of excessive tidal volume (above 4–6 mL/kg), prudent administration of fluids, aggressive

closure of PDA, and adequate nutrition. **Early surfactant replacement therapy may be beneficial, but the avoidance of intubation and mechanical ventilation with the initiation of continuous positive airway pressure (CPAP) shortly after birth may prove to be the most effective preventive strategy.**

3. Vitamin A is known to be important in epithelial cell differentiation and repair, and extremely low birthweight infant have low blood levels. A multicenter randomized trial has shown that vitamin A supplementation, 5000 IU administered intramuscularly three times per week for 4 weeks, significantly reduced the rate of BPD. In this study, one additional infant survived without BPD for every fifteen extremely low birthweight infants treated.

4. **Caffeine.** Methylxanthines decrease the frequency of apnea and allow for shorter duration of mechanical ventilation leading to a reduced rate of BPD.

5. **Inhaled nitric oxide (iNO).** Inhaled nitric oxide has been shown in animal models to reduce pulmonary vascular tone and prevent lung inflammation that ensues mechanical ventilation. Recently, two randomized multicenter trials were performed to assess the efficacy of iNO for BPD prevention. Results have been equivocal with a possible beneficial effect within certain subgroups divided according to birthweight or onset of treatment.

B. **Treatment of BPD.** Once BPD is present, the goal of management is to prevent further injury by minimizing respiratory support, improving pulmonary function, preventing cor pulmonale, and emphasizing growth and nutrition.

1. **Respiratory support**

   a. **Supplemental oxygen.** Maintaining adequate oxygenation is important in the infant with BPD to prevent hypoxia-induced pulmonary hypertension, bronchospasm, cor pulmonale, and growth failure. However, the least required oxygen should be delivered to minimize oxygen toxicity. Arterial oxygen saturation (Sao_2) should be monitored during the infant's various activities, including rest, sleep, and feeding. The optimal oxygen saturation level has not been established, and whether the level should exceed the range between 90% and 94% is **controversial.** Nonfrequent blood gas measurements are important for the assessment of trends in pH, $Paco_2$, and serum bicarbonate, but they are of limited use in monitoring oxygenation because they provide information about only one point in time.

   b. **Positive-pressure ventilation.** Mechanical ventilation should be used only when clearly indicated. Problems with air trapping can be significant; thus a ventilatory strategy using a slower rate with longer inspiration and expiration times than when ventilated for RDS should be implemented. Similarly inspiratory pressure needs to be limited at the expense of tolerating $Paco_2$ in excess of 50–60 mm Hg. Nasal CPAP can be useful as an adjunctive therapy after extubation.

2. **Improving lung function**

   a. **Fluid restriction.** Restricting fluid to 120 mL/kg/day is often required. It can be accomplished by concentrating proprietary formulas to 24 cal/oz. Increasing the caloric density further, to 27–30 cal/oz may require the addition of fat (eg, medium-chain triglyceride oil or corn oil) and carbohydrate (eg, Polycose) to avoid excessive protein intake.

   b. **Diuretic therapy.** See Chapter 132.

      i. **Furosemide** (1–2 mg/kg every 12 h, orally or intravenously) is a potent diuretic that is particularly useful for rapid diuresis. It is associated with side effects such as electrolyte abnormalities, interference with bilirubin-albumin binding capacity, calciuria with bone demineralization and renal stone formation, and ototoxicity. When used as a chronic medication, Na^+ and K^+ supplementation are often required.

      ii. **Bumetanide** (0.015–0.1 mg/kg daily or every other day, orally or intravenously). When administered orally, 1 mg of bumetanide (Bumex) has a diuretic effect similar to that of 40 mg of furosemide. Whereas furosemide's bioavailability is 30–70%, bumetanide's bioavailability is >90%. Bumetanide produces side effects similar to those of furosemide, except that it may produce less ototoxicity and less interference with bilirubin-albumin binding.

iii. **Chlorothiazide and spironolactone.** When used in doses of 20 mg/kg/day (chlorothiazide) and 2 mg/kg/day (spironolactone), a good diuretic response can often be achieved. Although less potent than furosemide, this combination is often better suited for chronic management because it has relatively fewer side effects. It may be the diuretic combination of choice when the calciuric effect of furosemide has led to the development of nephrocalcinosis.

c. **Bronchodilators**

i. β_2-**Agonists.** (See Table 7–5.) Inhaled β_2-agonists produce measurable acute improvements in lung mechanics and gas exchange in infants with BPD exhibiting symptoms of increased airway tone. Their effect is usually time limited. Because of their side effects (eg, tachycardia, hypertension, hyperglycemia, and possible arrhythmia), their use (**albuterol,** 0.2 mg/kg/dose nebulized as needed every 2–8 h) should be limited to the management of acute exacerbations of BPD. **Xopenex** (levalbuterol, 0.1 mg/kg/dose nebulized as needed every 8 h) is a nonracemic form of albuterol recently introduced in pediatric and adult populations. Its experience in newborns is limited. Its potential advantages are better and longer efficacy; hence lower doses have a therapeutic effect, enabling a significant reduction in the adverse effects associated with racemic albuterol. If bronchodilators are being used long term, a frequent reevaluation of their benefit is essential.

ii. **Anticholinergic agents.** (See Table 7–5.) The best studied and most available inhaled quaternary anticholinergic is **ipratropium bromide** (nebulized Atrovent, 175 mcg, diluted in 3 mL of normal saline over 10 min every 8 h). Its bronchodilatory effect is more potent than that of atropine and similar to that of albuterol. Combined albuterol and ipratropium therapy has a larger effect than either agent alone. Unlike atropine, systemic effects do not occur because of its poor systemic absorption.

iii. **Theophylline.** The beneficial actions of theophylline include smooth airway muscle dilation, improved diaphragmatic contractility, central respiratory stimulation, and mild diuretic effects. It appears to improve lung function in BPD when levels are maintained at >10 mcg/mL. Side effects are fairly common and may include central nervous system (CNS) irritability, gastroesophageal reflux, and gastrointestinal irritation. Prevention of apnea rather than bronchodilation is the major reason for infants with BPD to receive a methylxanthine treatment.

d. **Corticosteroids.** Although very efficient, the use of postnatal steroids should be limited to severe cases of BPD with a low chance of survival because of impaired gas exchange. Parents should be informed that the use of postnatal steroids could be associated with impaired brain and somatic growth and increased incidence of cerebral palsy. The initiation of steroid therapy in the first day increases the incidence of gastrointestinal perforation in particular when associated with concomitant indomethacin administration. Other side effects include infection, hypertension, gastric ulcer, hyperglycemia, adrenocortical suppression, lung growth suppression, and hypertrophic cardiomyopathy. Because of the central role of inflammation and relative adrenal insufficiency in the pathogenesis of BPD, steroids can be very effective both for prophylaxis or treatment of severe cases. Various steroid regimens have been proposed.

i. **Dexamethasone (DXM),** 0.25 mg/kg twice daily for 3 days and then gradually tapered by a 10% dose decrease every 3 days for a total course of 42 days, is one of the original regimens that has proven efficacious in the treatment of BPD. Because of the concern about the possible neurologic adverse effects, many other regimens of shorter duration or dosage have been used, and no standards have been accepted.

ii. **Methylprednisolone (Solu-Medrol),** a corticosteroid with much weaker genomic activity than DXM, has almost similar nongenomic activity and thus possibly fewer CNS and somatic side effects. In a pilot study, methylprednisolone, 0.6, 0.4, 0.2 mg/kg/dose every 6 h for 3 days, followed by betamethasone, 0.1 mg/kg orally every other day for a total of 21 days, was found to have similar beneficial effects and fewer side effects (eg, periventricular leukomalacia, hyperglycemia) than DXM. These findings still need to be confirmed by large randomized controlled trials.

iii. **Hydrocortisone,** 5 mg/kg/day divided every 6 h for 1 week, then gradually tapered for the following 2 to 5 weeks. In contrast to infants treated with dexamethasone, when compared with nontreated preterm infants, hydrocortisone-treated infants showed no difference in neurocognitive or motor outcome, or in the incidence of brain abnormalities on magnetic resonance imaging, in long-term follow-up studies at 5–8 years.

iv. **Prednisolone,** 2 mg/kg per day orally divided twice per day for 5 days, then 1 mg/kg per dose orally daily for 3 days, and then 1 mg/kg per dose every other day for three doses has been used to wean from oxygen therapy prior to discharge home.

v. **Nebulized corticosteroids** (beclomethasone, 100–200 mcg 4 times/day) produced fewer side effects than oral or parenteral forms but seems to be much less efficacious in the treatment of BPD.

3. **Growth and nutrition.** Because growth is essential for recovery from BPD, adequate nutritional intake is crucial. Infants with BPD frequently have high caloric needs (120–150 kcal/kg/day or more) because of increased metabolic expenditures. Concentrated formula is often necessary to provide sufficient calories and prevent pulmonary edema. In addition, specific micronutrient supplementation, such as antioxidant therapy, may also enhance pulmonary and nutritional status.

C. **Discharge planning.** Oxygen can often be discontinued before discharge from the neonatal intensive care unit. However, home oxygen therapy can be a safe alternative to long-term hospitalization. The need for home respiratory, heart rate, and oxygen monitoring must be decided on an individual basis but is generally recommended for infants discharged home on oxygen. Synagis (palivizumab, humanized monoclonal antibodies against respiratory syncytial virus [RSV]) should be given monthly (15 mg/kg intramuscularly) throughout the RSV season. All parents should be instructed in cardiopulmonary resuscitation.

D. **General care.** Care plans for older infants with BPD should include adapting their routine for home life and involving the parents in their care. Immunizations should be given at the appropriate chronologic age. Periodic screening for chemical evidence of rickets and echocardiographic evidence of right ventricular hypertrophy is recommended. Assessment by a developmental specialist and occupational or physical therapist, or both, can be useful for prognostic and therapeutic purposes.

VIII. **Prognosis.** The prognosis for infants with BPD depends on the degree of pulmonary dysfunction and the presence of other medical conditions. Most deaths occur in the first year of life as a result of cardiorespiratory failure, sepsis, or respiratory infection or as a sudden, unexplained death.

A. **Pulmonary outcome.** The short-term outcome of infants with BPD, including those requiring oxygen at home, is surprisingly good. Weaning from oxygen is usually possible before their first birthday, and they demonstrate catch-up growth as their pulmonary status improves. However, in the first year of life, rehospitalization is necessary for ~30% of patients for treatment of wheezing, respiratory infections, or both. Although upper respiratory tract infections are probably no more common in infants with BPD than in normal infants, they are more likely to be associated with significant respiratory symptoms. Most adolescents and young adults who had moderate to severe BPD in infancy have some degree of pulmonary dysfunction, consisting of airway obstruction, airway hyperreactivity, and hyperinflation.

B. **Neurodevelopmental outcome.** Children with BPD appear to be at an increased risk for adverse neurodevelopmental outcome compared with comparable infants without BPD. Neuromotor and cognitive dysfunction appears to be more common. In addition, children with BPD may be at higher risk for significant hearing impairment and retinopathy of prematurity. They are also at risk for later problems, including learning disabilities, attention deficits, and behavior problems.

Selected References

Cerny L et al: Prevention and treatment of bronchopulmonary dysplasia: contemporary status and future outlook. *Lung* 2008;186:75.

Ehrenkranz RA et al: Validation of the National Institute of Health consensus definition of bronchopulmonary dysplasia *Pediatrics* 2005;105:1194.

Jobe A et al: Bronchopulmonary dysplasia. *Am J Respir Crit Care Med* 2001;163:1723.

Kinsella JP et al: Bronchopulmonary dysplasia. *Lancet* 2006;367:1421.

Rademaker KJ et al: Postnatal hydrocortisone treatment for chronic lung disease in the preterm newborn and long-term neurodevelopmental follow-up. *Arch Dis Child Fetal Neonatal Ed* 2008;93:58.

Van Marter LJ et al: Do clinical markers of barotrauma and oxygen toxicity explain interhospital variation in rates of chronic lung disease? *Pediatrics* 2000;116:1353.

78 Calcium Disorders (Hypocalcemia, Hypercalcemia)

Abnormalities of calcium (Ca^{+2}) and magnesium (Mg^{+2}) metabolism are not infrequent occurrences among infants admitted for neonatal intensive care. Moreover, the disturbances of calcium may be mirrored by magnesium, or conversely, as in hypocalcemia and hypomagnesemia. Infants of diabetic mothers (IDM) and infants with intrauterine growth restriction (IUGR) may present with low serum levels of either Ca^{+2} or Mg^{+2}, or both. Serum values for Ca^{+2} and Mg^{+2} above or below accepted normal values are of concern in any infant and warrant further clinical studies. Magnesium disorders are discussed in Chapter 99.

HYPOCALCEMIA

I. **Definition.** Hypocalcemia is determined as either total serum calcium (tCa^{+2}) or ionized calcium (iCa^{+2}). Clinical chemistry values for serum levels vary by units (ie, mEq/L, mmol/L, or mg/dL) or by gestational age and by day of age following the immediate newborn period. Reference textbooks reflect considerable variance of normal serum values for Ca^{+2} and Mg^{+2}. Interpretation of serum values for any given patient depends on recognition of your institution's laboratory values and range of acceptable values.

A generally accepted value for hypocalcemia is < 2.0 mmol/L (8.0 mg/dL) (1.0 mmol/L = 4.0 mg/dL) for a symptomatic term infant or < 1.75 mmol/L (7.0 mg/dL) for an asymptomatic term infant. A range of normal values for a term newborn can be 2.25–2.65 mmol/L (9.0–10.6 mg/dL) throughout the first week of life. Preterm infant tCa^{+2} levels closely parallel term infants.

Of greater significance is the ionized fraction of Ca^{+2}. It is the active physiologic component and depends on the interaction of tCa^{+2}, normal acid-base status, and normal serum albumin. **Typical iCa^{+2} values for term infants over the first 72 h of life are 1.22–1.24 mmol/L (4.88–4.96 mg/dL).** Preterm infant mean values are similar for 24 and 72 h: 1.21–1.28 mmol/L (4.84–5.12 mg/dL). Interestingly, preterm infants slightly increase their iCa^{+2} levels, whereas term infants experience a slight decline. **Ionized Ca^{+2} levels of <4 mg/dL are generally considered hypocalcemic.**

II. **Incidence.** Hypocalcemia is likely the most common disorder of either Ca^{+2} or Mg^{+2} in newborn infants and it affects both preterm and term infants. It occurs in up to 30% of infants with birthweight <1500 g. Late-onset hypocalcemia is more common in developing countries where cow's milk or formulas with phosphate concentrations are used.

III. **Pathophysiology.** Ionized Ca^{+2} is the biologically important form of Ca^{+2}. The tCa^{+2} levels have repeatedly been shown not to be predictive of iCa^{+2} levels. Therefore, tCa^{+2} levels are unreliable as criteria for true hypocalcemia. In premature infants, it has been shown that tCa^{+2} levels as low as ≤6 mg/dL correspond to iCa^{+2} levels >3 mg/dL.

A. **Early-onset neonatal hypocalcemia.** During the third trimester of pregnancy, the human fetus receives at least 140 mg/kg/day of elemental Ca^{+2} via the umbilical cord. Most of this Ca^{+2} is readily incorporated into the newly forming bones. After delivery, this massive supply of Ca^{+2} is suddenly stopped, and Ca^{+2} must be given enterally.

1. **A full-term infant** receiving 100–120 mL of normal formula would be receiving 50–60 mg/kg/day of Ca^{+2} orally. Despite this drop in supply, full-term infants tolerate the change well and do not become hypocalcemic.

2. **Premature (especially < 28 weeks) or sick infants** often become hypocalcemic during the first 3 days of life. Total serum Ca^{+2} levels can drop to <7 mg/dL and occasionally fall below 6 mg/dL.

3. **Calcium levels** (both iCa^{+2} and tCa^{+2}) usually return to normal within 48–72 h regardless of whether supplemental Ca^{+2} is given. Immunoreactive parathyroid hormone (iPTH) is often low at birth but rises to higher levels within 24–72 h after delivery. Intravenous Ca^{+2} supplementation suppresses this increase in iPTH.

B. **Perinatal stress** presents with hypocalcemia if infants also have asphyxia and acidosis. Resuscitation and the use of alkali to correct acidosis (bicarbonate therapy) may have multiple effects resulting in hypocalcemia (eg, lower iCa^{+2} levels, decreased Ca^{+2} flux from bones, and relative hyperphosphatemia secondary to increased circulating endogenous phosphorous following postasphyxial renal impairment). Additional factors include meconium aspiration syndrome, compromised placental blood flow, sepsis, and shock. Of special note is alkalosis secondary to hyperventilation and hypocarbia after resuscitation. The combination of bicarbonate infusions and hypocarbia can induce an alkalosis with profound hypocalcemia.

C. **Infant of diabetic mother (IDM).** Onset of hypocalcemia is usually early (1–3 days) and may recur throughout the first week. The mechanism for IDM hypocalcemia is unknown. Related factors that have been identified are increased calcitonin levels, decreased bone Ca^{+2} flux, hypomagnesemia, hypoparathyroidism, and hyperphosphatemia. The occurrence and severity of IDM hypocalcemia follows the severity of maternal diabetes and the prenatal management for euglycemic control.

D. **Intrauterine growth restriction (IUGR).** Sporadic hypocalcemia occurs and may be associated with one or more of the known complications of IUGR (eg, hypoglycemia, asphyxia, meconium aspiration, hypothermia, polycythemia, and placental insufficiency).

E. **Nutritional deprivation.** Infants unable to take enteral feeds by 3 days of age need calcium supplementation. Breast milk or calcium enriched formulas provide adequate calcium intake. Because hypocalcemia is related to hypomagnesemia, both elements require supplementation to prevent secondary suppression of parathormone recurrence of hypocalcemia.

F. **Hypomagnesemia** may be secondary to maternal gestational Mg^{+2} losses or secondary to impaired intestinal uptake. Hypomagnesemia frequently occurs with hypocalcemia and must be looked for in any at-risk infant.

G. **Congenital abnormalities** such as the DiGeorge sequence with absence of parathyroid glands and related craniofacial and cardiac anomalies often presents with hypocalcemia.

H. **Maternal hyperparathyroidism** may cause pseudohyperparathyroidism in the newborn.

I. **Other therapeutic modalities** include furosemide-induced hypercalcuria, citrated blood transfusions that reduce iCa due to a citrate-calcium complex and an alkalosis following metabolism of citrate, and inadequate prenatal vitamin D supplementation of the mother or of the infant during the first 6 months of life.

IV. **Risk factors.** There is an increased incidence of hypocalcemia within the first 3 days of life in premature or sick neonates. The risk of hypocalcemia increases with the degree of prematurity. Common risk factors include the following:

A. Infant of diabetic mother carries a 25–50% risk in the newborn.

B. Poor enteral intake.

C. Stress during the perinatal period.

D. Blood or exchange transfusions.

E. Alkalosis.

F. Diuretics such as furosemide.

G. Excessive phosphate intake.

H. Insufficient magnesium intake.

I. Inadequate prenatal vitamin D supplementation of the mother or of the infant during the first 6 months of life.

J. Congenital hypoparathyroidism (eg, DiGeorge syndrome). (See Chapter 80.)

V. **Clinical presentation**

A. **Early-onset hypocalcemia; first week of life:**
 1. Apnea.
 2. Stridor.
 3. Irritability, jitteriness, tremors, or hyperreflexia.
 4. Clonus, tetany, or seizures.
 5. Arrhythmia secondary to prolonged Q-T interval.

B. **Late-onset hypocalcemia; any time after first week:**
 1. Lethargy, apnea.
 2. Feeding intolerance.
 3. Abdominal distention.
 4. Bone demineralization, increased alkaline phosphatase.
 5. Skeletal fractures.

C. **Paradoxically, neonatal hypocalcemia may be asymptomatic** and only an index of suspicion on the basis of risk factors will lead to a correct diagnosis.

VI. **Diagnosis**

A. **Laboratory studies**
 1. **Total and ionized calcium levels** should be available to the patient in the neonatal intensive care unit. Serum tCa^{+2} of <1.75 mmol/L (7.0 mg/dL) is usually diagnostic of hypocalcemia and further confirmed by iCa^{+2} levels of <1.10 mmol/L (4.4 mg/dL). See definition earlier for range of normal values for both tCa^{+2} and iCa^{+2}.
 2. **Serum magnesium levels** of <1.5 mg/dL is indicative of hypocalcemia because they often follow one another.
 3. **Elevated alkaline phosphatase levels** can be seen in chronic hypocalcemia.
 4. **Urinary calcium.** Calcium-to-creatinine ratios (measured in spot urine specimens) >0.21–0.25 are indicative of hypercalciuria. Also, 24-h urinary Ca^{+2} levels >4 mg/kg/24 h indicate hypercalciuria.

B. **Radiologic studies** for bone demineralization, metaphyseal lucencies, and rib and long bone fractures may be helpful for late-onset hypocalcemia. More acutely, the absence of a thymic shadow on chest radiograph suggests the DiGeorge sequence.

C. **Electrocardiographic studies** identify arrhythmias due to Q-T interval changes.

VII. **Management**

A. **Acute treatment** is reserved for the symptomatic hypocalcemic infants with apneic spells, seizures, or cardiac failure with arrhythmia. Dosage is 100–200 mg/kg of 10% calcium gluconate *slowly* by peripheral intravenous route over 15–20 min with constant cardiac monitoring. (See Chapter 132 for more pharmacologic information.)

B. **Maintenance treatment** for infants with limited enteral intake or dependent on parenteral Ca^{+2} intake: An intravenous dosage of 45 mg/kg/day of elemental Ca^{+2} with a calcium-to-phosphate ratio ranging from 1.3:1.0–2:1 is adequate for promoting both Ca^{+2} and phosphate retention. Parenteral nutrition is usually started by day 2 or 3 of life. Intrauterine Ca^{+2} source is ~140 mg/kg/day of elemental Ca^{+2}. Parenteral fluids cannot approximate the intrauterine level of Ca^{+2} intake without some precipitation in solution. Therefore early and continuous maintenance treatment is essential until milk or formula feeds can be successfully initiated.

C. **Vitamin D supplementation** should be started along with parenteral nutrition at 400 IU/day.

D. **Intravenous calcium administration** is not without some risk for complications. The potential problems include extravasation of Ca^{+2} solution and resulting subcutaneous Ca^{+2} deposition with limited joint movement, sloughing of skin, nephrocalcinosis, cardiac arrhythmias with prolonged Q-T intervals, or bradycardia if Ca^{+2} gluconate is given too quickly. Use of an umbilical artery or vein is *not* recommended for administration of Ca^{+2} solutions.

E. **Hypocalcemia secondary to blood transfusions** may require supplementation with Ca^{+2} gluconate. See Chapters 29 and 132 for recommendations and dosage guidelines.

F. **Hypocalcemia secondary to diuretic therapy.** Infants receiving loop diuretics have an increased urinary loss of Ca^{+2}. This loss can be demonstrated by urine calcium-to-creatinine ratio (>0.21–0.25). If hypercalciuria exists, an attempt should be made to substitute furosemide or bumetanide with chlorothiazide, or use in combination. Thiazide diuretics cause Ca^{+2} retention and tend to offset the calciuric effect of loop diuretics. Caution is needed to guard against excessive potassium losses while compensating for diuretic effects on Ca^{+2}.

VIII. **Prognosis.** No long-term effects of hypocalcemia treated in the neonatal period are seen as attributable to known adverse neurobehavioral or neurologic outcomes of preterm or sick term infants. Decreased bone mineralization (osteopenia) and the development of nephrocalcinosis are seen as long-term complications of Ca^{+2} disorders. See Chapter 107 on osteopenia of prematurity for more information on long-term hypocalcemia outcomes.

HYPERCALCEMIA

I. **Definition.** Hypercalcemia is defined as an iCa^{+2} serum level >1.35 mmol/L (5.4 mg/dL) for any infant, irrespective of a tCa^{+2} serum level of more or less than 2.75 mmol/L (11.0 mg/dL). The iCa^{+2} level is the physiologically active component of serum Ca^{+2} and thus the most important determination. Although tCa^{+2} is indicative of hypercalcemia at levels >2.75 mmol/L, it is not a reliable measure.

II. **Incidence** is uncommon and unknown. It is less common than in adults.

III. **Pathophysiology.** Hypercalcemia may be due to parathyroid-related causes or to mechanisms unrelated to the parathyroid.

IV. **Risk factors**

A. **Congenital hyperparathyroidism**

1. Primary, due to genetic defects as either familial hypocalciuria, hypercalcemia, or severe neonatal hyperparathyroidism.

2. Secondary, due to maternal hypoparathyroidism.

B. Maternal hypocalcemia.

C. Jansen metaphyseal chondrodysplasia.

D. Idiopathic infantile hypercalcemia.

E. Williams syndrome.

F. Hypophosphatasia.

G. Subcutaneous fat necrosis.

H. Hyper- or hypothyroidism.

I. Malignancy (very rare in the newborn).

J. Iatrogenic.

    1. Hypophosphatemia due to inadequate dietary intake of phosphorus, especially in preterm infants.

    2. Excessive vitamin D intake.

    3. Excessive Ca^{+2} intake.

    4. Thiazide diuretics.

    5. Extracorporeal life support.

V. **Clinical presentation**

A. Feeding intolerance, constipation, failure to thrive.

B. Polyuria, dehydration.

C. Hematuria, nephrocalcinosis, nephrolithiasis.

D. Lethargy, hypotonia, seizures (rare; only most severe cases of hypercalcemia).

E. Bradycardia, short Q-T interval, hypertension.

F. Paradoxically, hypercalcemia can be asymptomatic unless severe hypercalcemic levels have been reached.

VI. **Diagnosis**

A. **Laboratory**

    1. Serum Ca^{+2} for levels as given above.

    2. Serum total protein and albumin-to-globulin ratio for hypoproteinemia.

    3. Blood gases for acid-base status.

    4. Serum phosphorus for hypophosphatemia.

    5. Urine Ca^{+2} and phosphorus.

    6. Parathyroid hormone, 25-OH vitamin D, 1,25-OH vitamin D.

    7. Thyroid studies.

    8. Alkaline phosphatase for hypophosphatasia.

    9. Serum creatinine.

B. **Imaging studies**

    1. Renal ultrasound for calcifications.

    2. Long-bone studies for demineralization secondary to hyperparathyroidism or osteosclerotic lesions secondary to hypervitaminosis.

VII. **Management.** Treatment depends on the cause and severity of hypercalcemia. Generally, hypercalcemia is mild and a conservative approach is prudent. Immediate steps are to calculate Ca^{+2} and vitamin D intake, and correct or discontinue excesses. **Severity of hypercalcemia dictates treatment.** After hypercalcemia has been resolved, dietary Ca^{+2}, phosphorus, and vitamin D intakes can be recalculated and administered according to basic daily requirements. An endocrine consult is recommended.

A. **Acute symptomatic hypercalcemia**

    1. Increased fluid intake as intravenous saline.

    2. Augment calciuria using furosemide with intravenous saline intake; exercise caution to monitor urine output and serum electrolytes.

B. **Less acute, but severe hypercalcemia, consider:**

    1. Calcitonin, but of limited newborn or neonatal clinical experience.

    2. Glucocorticoids may be effective short term but are not recommended.

    3. Intravenous bisphosphates are promising but of limited newborn or neonatal clinical experience.

C. **Refractory hypercalcemia.** In extreme situations, parathyroidectomy is the last resort.

VIII. **Prognosis.** Complete resolution of hypercalcemia occurs rapidly if it is treated promptly. If unrecognized and not treated it may result in renal and CNS damage.

Selected References

Borgia F et al: Subcutaneous fat necrosis of the newborn: be aware of hypercalcemia. *Paediatr Child Health* 2006;42:316-318.

Camadoo L et al: Maternal vitamin D deficiency associated with neonatal hypocalcemic convulsions. *Nutr J* 2007;19;23-24.

Fox L et al: Neonatal hyperparathyroidism and pamidronate therapy in an extremely premature infant. *Pediatrics* 2007;120:e1350-e1354.

Fridriksson JH et al: Hypercalcemia associated with extracorporeal life support in neonates. *J Pediatr Surg* 2001;36:493-497.

Gabbett MT et al: Neonatal severe hyperparathyroidism: an important clue to the aetiology. *J Paediatr Child Health* 2006;42:813-816.

Hsu SC, Levine MA: Perinatal calcium metabolism: physiology and pathophysiology. *Semin Neonatol* 2004;9:23-36.

Jatana V et al: Deletion 22q11.2 syndrome—implications for the intensive care physician. *Pediatr Crit Care Med* 2007;8:459-463.

Nock ML, Kousiki P: Tables of normal values. In Martin RJ et al (eds): *Fanaroff and Martin's Neonatal-Perinatal Medicine: Diseases of the Fetus and Infant,* 8th ed. Philadelphia, PA: Elsevier Mosby, 2006:1801-1802.

Poomthavorn P et al: Transient neonatal hypoparathyroidism in two siblings unmasking maternal normocalcemic hyperparathyroidism. *Eur J Pediatr* 2008;167:431-434.

Rigo J, DeCurtis M: Disorders of calcium, phosphorus and magnesium metabolism. In Martin RJ et al (eds): *Fanaroff and Martin's Neonatal-Perinatal Medicine: Diseases of the Fetus and Infant,* 8th ed. Philadelphia, PA: Elsevier Mosby, 2006:1509-1520.

Yu VY, Upadhyay A: Neonatal management of the growth- restricted infant. *Semin Fetal Neonatal Med* 2004;9:403-409.

79 Chlamydial Infection

I. **Definition.** *Chlamydia trachomatis* is an obligate intracellular small Gram-negative bacterium that possesses a cell wall, contains DNA and RNA, and can be inactivated by several antimicrobial agents. It is the most common cause of sexually transmitted genital infections. It may cause urethritis, cervicitis, and salpingitis in the mother. In the infant, it may cause conjunctivitis and pneumonia.

II. **Incidence.** The prevalence of *C. trachomatis* in pregnant women varies from 2–15%. The risk of infection to infants born to infected mothers is high; conjunctivitis occurs in 25–50%, and pneumonia in 5–20%.

III. **Pathophysiology.** *C. trachomatis* subtypes B and D through K cause the sexually transmitted form of the disease and the associated neonatal infection. They frequently cause a benign subclinical infection. The infant acquires infection during vaginal delivery through an infected cervix. Infection after cesarean delivery is rare and usually occurs with early rupture of amniotic membranes; however, infection associated with intact membranes has been reported. A recent population-based study from Washington State suggested that maternal *C. trachomatis* infection is associated with an increased risk of preterm delivery and premature rupture of membranes.

IV. **Risk factors.** Risk is inversely proportional to gestational age. Risk factors include vaginal delivery of an infant with an infected mother and cesarean delivery with early rupture of the amniotic membrane of an infected mother.

V. **Clinical presentation**
  A. **Conjunctivitis.** See Chapter 47.
  B. **Pneumonia.** This is one of the most common forms of pneumonia in the first 3 months of life. The respiratory tract may be directly infected during delivery. Approximately half of infants presenting with pneumonia have concurrent or previous conjunctivitis. Pneumonia usually presents at 3–11 weeks of life. The infants experience a gradual increase in symptoms over several weeks. Initially, there is often 1–2 weeks of mucoid rhinorrhea followed by cough and increasing respiratory rate. More than 95% of cases are afebrile. The cough is characteristic, paroxysmal, and staccato, and it interferes with sleeping and eating. Approximately a third of infants have otitis media. Preterm infants may present with apneic spells. *C. trachomatis* has been isolated from tracheal secretions of preterm infants with pneumonia in the first week after birth.

VI. **Diagnosis**
  A. **Laboratory studies**
    1. **Tissue culture.** Because chlamydiae are obligate intracellular organisms, culture specimens must contain epithelial cells. **Culture of the organism is the gold standard** for diagnosing neonatal conjunctivitis and pneumonia. The specificity and sensitivity of culture is nearly 100% with adequate sampling and transport. Material should be obtained from the tarsal conjunctiva (for conjunctivitis) or from nasopharyngeal aspiration or deep suctioning of the trachea (for suspected pneumonia).
    2. **Nucleic acid amplification (NAA) tests** use methods to amplify *C. trachomatis* DNA or RNA sequences. Currently available tests are polymerase chain reaction (Amplicor), transcription-mediated amplification (Aptima Comb 2), and strand displacement amplification (ProbeTec). These tests are approved by the United States Food and Drug Administration (FDA) to be used in adults, but no sufficient data are available in infants.
    3. **Antigen detection tests** include **direct fluorescent antibody** and **enzyme immunoassay** tests. These tests appear to be sensitive and specific when used with conjunctival specimens, but the sensitivity with nasopharyngeal samples is poor. These tests are used infrequently and have largely been replaced by NAA tests.
    4. **DNA probes** are commercially available but not approved for use in children. Any positive probe test should be confirmed by a culture or NAA test.
    5. **Serum anti-chlamydial antibody (IgM)** concentration is difficult to determine and not widely available. In children with pneumonia, a titer >1:32 is diagnostic of infection.
    6. **Other tests.** In cases of pneumonia, the white blood cell count is normal, but there is **eosinophilia** in 70% of cases. Blood gas measurements show mild to moderate hypoxemia.
  B. **Radiologic studies.** In cases of pneumonia, the chest radiograph may reveal hyperexpansion of the lungs, with bilateral diffuse interstitial or alveolar infiltrates.

VII. **Management.** Isolation precautions for all infectious diseases, including maternal and neonatal precautions, breast-feeding, and visiting issues, can be found in Appendix F.
  A. **Prevention.** In high-risk populations, identification and treatment of infected mothers can prevent disease in the infant. Some experts advocate routine testing of pregnant women at high risk during the first trimester and again during the third trimester. Infants born to mothers known to have untreated chlamydial infection should be monitored clinically. Prophylactic antimicrobial treatment is no longer recommended because the efficacy of such therapy is unknown. Additionally, oral erythromycin, the agent most commonly used, is associated with significant risk for **infantile hypertrophic pyloric stenosis (IHPS)**.

B. **Conjunctivitis** is treated with oral erythromycin base or ethylsuccinate (50 mg/kg per day in four divided doses) for 14 days. Topical therapy is ineffective and unnecessary.

C. **Pneumonia** is also treated with erythromycin, 50 mg/kg/day in four divided doses for 14 days. This not only shortens the clinical course but decreases the duration of nasopharyngeal shedding. **IHPS** may occur when infants are treated with erythromycin in the first 2 weeks of life. Because alternative therapies for *C. trachomatis* in the newborn are not well studied, the American Academy of Pediatrics continues to recommend erythromycin to treat neonatal chlamydia infection. Parents should be informed about the signs and potential risks of developing IHPS. Cases of IHPS after the use of oral erythromycin should be reported to MedWatch, the FDA Safety Information and Adverse Event Reporting Program. No isolation measures are necessary.

VIII. **Prognosis.** Infants who are diagnosed and treated early generally recover.

Selected References

American Academy of Pediatrics: Chlamydial trachomatis. In: Pickering LK et al (eds): *Red Book: 2006 Report of the Committee on Infectious Diseases,* 27th ed. Elk Grove Village, IL: American Academy of Pediatrics, 2006;252-257.

Blas MM et al: Pregnancy outcomes in women infected with *Chlamydia trachomatis*: a population-based cohort study in Washington State. *Sex Transm Infect* 2007;83:314-318.

Johnson RE et al: Screening tests to detect *Chlamydia trachomatis* and *Neisseria gonorrhoeae* infections—2002. *MMWR Recomm Rep* 2002;18;51(RR-15):1-38.

Maheshwai N: Are young infants treated with erythromycin at risk for developing hypertrophic pyloric stenosis? *Arch Dis Child* 2007;92:271-273.

Shariat H et al: An interesting case presentation: a possible new route for perinatal acquisition of Chlamydia. *J Perinatol* 1992;12:300-302.

80 Common Multiple Congenital Anomaly Syndromes

I. **Definition.** A **congenital anomaly** is defined as a structural defect, present at birth and different from the norm. These anomalies can be further divided into major anomalies that require medical and surgical care (eg, congenital heart defect, cleft palate, meningomyelocele) and minor anomalies that do not have medical significance (eg, single palmar crease, epicanthal folds, fifth digit clinodactyly). Anomalies themselves can be classified based on the developmental process involved in their formation. Well-defined types of anomalies include malformations, deformations, disruptions, dysplasias, syndromes, associations, and sequences (see Table 80–1). It is also important to understand that these may not be entirely mutually exclusive. Table 81–1 provides an overview of congenital anomalies that are associated with congenital heart disease and Table 81–2 reviews the teratogens associated with some of these lesions.

II. **Incidence.** Among newborns, ~1–3% have more than one major congenital anomaly recognized at birth. These infants often have longer hospital stays and have increased mortality rates. Malformations can cause >20% of neonatal deaths.

III. **General approach to diagnosis.** In the management of multiple congenital anomaly (MCA) syndromes, the neonatologist must deal with complex clinical issues calling for

Table 80–1. **TYPES OF CONGENITAL ANOMALIES**

- **Malformation:** The morphologic defect of an organ or larger region of the body resulting from an intrinsically abnormal developmental process. A primary defect.
- **Deformation:** An alteration in shape and or structure, caused by biomechanical forces that distort otherwise normally developing structure. A secondary defect.
- **Disruption:** A structural defect resulting from an extrinsic insult to an originally normal developmental process.
- **Dysplasia:** An abnormality in the organization or differentiation of cells within a specific tissue type that results in clinically apparent structural changes.
- **Syndrome:** A recognizable pattern of anomalies considered to have a specific cause.
- **Association:** A nonrandom, statistically significant association of multiple anomalies for which no specific etiology has been described.
- **Sequence:** A pattern of multiple anomalies derived from a single abnormality followed by a cascade of secondary effects.

a wide range of diagnostic skills. Without a correct diagnosis of MCA syndrome, many available forms of therapy go underused and others may be tried, although they will be relatively ineffective. Furthermore, unrealistic counseling may be given about prognosis and recurrence risk. Only a few common MCA syndromes are life threatening in the neonatal period. It is important to note, however, that **malformations are the most common cause of death at this critical point** in the life span. Table 80–2 lists symptoms and signs that should alert the clinician to the possibility of cryptogenic malformations or disorders. Obviously, if overt malformations are present, an MCA syndrome will be immediately recognized and diagnostic efforts will shortly follow. However, if external features of the disorder are subtle or nonspecific and the usual procedures associated with intensive newborn support have been started, findings may go unrecognized early. Each manifestation listed in Table 80–2 is more common in infants with MCA syndromes. Underlying etiologies for MCA syndromes include chromosomal abnormalities, monogenic disorders, multifactorial disorders, and unknown. The diagnostic approach to MCA syndromes in neonates is no different from that in older children. Because so many of these children are intubated with multiple lines and tubes, detailed

Table 80–2. **SYMPTOMS AND SIGNS IN NEONATES THAT MIGHT INDICATE A MULTIPLE CONGENITAL ANOMALY SYNDROME**

Prenatal
Oligohydramnios
Polyhydramnios
Decreased or unusual fetal activity
Abnormal fetal problem/position

Postnatal
Abnormalities of size: small for gestational age or large for gestational age, microcephaly or macrocephaly, large or irregular abdomen, small chest, limb-trunk disproportion, asymmetry
Abnormalities of tone: hypotonia, hypertonia
Abnormalities of position: joint contractures, fixation of joints in extension, hyperextension of joints
Midline aberrations: hemangiomas, hair tufts, dimples or pits
Problems of secretion, excretion, or edema: no urination, no passage of meconium, chronic nasal or oral secretions, edema (nuchal, pedal, generalized, ascites)
Symptoms: unexplained seizures, resistant or unexplained respiratory distress
Metabolic disorders: resistant hypoglycemia, unexplained hypo- or hypercalcemia, polycythemia, hyponatremia, thrombocytopenia

assessment of physical characteristics can be challenging. Clinical photographs are essential, especially when a clinical geneticist is not available locally. If specialists in these fields are not available, a telephone call to a university medical center for expert advice is often useful. If the infant is critically ill and suspicion for a MCA syndrome is present, looking for other major malformations is important (eg, echocardiogram, renal/abdominal ultrasound, brain imaging). **The basis for diagnosis of a MCA syndrome in a neonate involves a combination of defining the physical manifestations and diagnostic genetic testing.** Diagnostic problems can also occur because immediate efforts tend to emphasize therapy. Nevertheless, diagnosis will often facilitate or guide therapy more efficiently.

IV. **Genetic testing**
   A. **High-resolution karyotype.** Perhaps the **most common diagnostic genetic test** performed in an infant with MCAs is the **high-resolution karyotype.** This test typically involves the analysis of chromosomes obtained from white blood cells present in a peripheral blood sample and is unaffected by a red blood cell transfusion. Once obtained, these cells are cultured, stimulated to divide, and then a mitotic inhibitor is used to halt cell division in the prometaphase stage. The chromosomes in prometaphase stage are at their longest length, and the number of observable stained bands can reach 800–900. The analysis of a standard 20 cells is then performed microscopically by a trained specialist. This process can take up to 2 weeks for completion. Differences in chromosomal number, large chromosomal deletions or duplications, and translocations can be detected with this test.
   B. **Fluorescent in situ hybridization (FISH)** is a cytogenetic technique where a probe can be used to detect specific DNA sequences. FISH can be performed on preparations that require the culturing and synchronization of cells to detect small chromosomal or submicroscopic deletions. This process is faster than high-resolution karyotyping, but it still can take several days to weeks to complete. FISH also can be done on an interphase or unsynchronized sample. Typically interphase FISH is done to assess for forms of chromosomal aneuploidy. FISH probes can be used to assess for the copy number of a given chromosome. Most commercial laboratories offer a panel to assess for copies of chromosomes 13, 18, 21, X, and Y. This can be done on an interphase sample and a result given within 48 h from reaching the laboratory. This test can be very important in trying quickly to confirm a diagnosis in a critically ill infant with trisomy 13, 18, or 21 or Turner syndrome. In addition to interphase FISH, a complete high-resolution karyotype must be done to assess for a possible translocation.
   C. **Comparative genomic hybridization (CGH)** or **chromosomal microarray analysis (CMA)** is a new cytogenetic technique that can be used to detect chromosomal deletions or duplications. CGH/CMA is a fluorescent technique that compares a reference standard DNA to the patient's DNA. Depending on the laboratory and specific platform used, comparisons are made at hundreds of regions across the entire genome to assess for copy number differences between the two samples. CGH/CMA assesses for common microdeletion and microduplication regions, subtelomeric regions, and pericentromeric regions. This test is not only capable of diagnosing described chromosomal abnormalities, but it can also detect novel changes.

V. **Genetic counseling.** For MCA syndromes, counseling is complex and requires a great deal of sensitivity. First, it is important to have a secure diagnosis, if one is possible. The next step is to establish the parents' understanding of the entire situation and what they have been told by other professionals. Be sure you know what questions the parents want answers to before the factual counseling begins. Do not give excessive details relative to the facts and try to avoid specific predictions, particularly regarding timing and the presence or absence of certain problems relative to the future. Leave some degree of hope, but be honestly realistic, particularly if the parents clearly demand it. Assume frequent follow-up counseling sessions, and outline a long-term program for the child's care and evaluations. Recurrence risk figures and the availability of prenatal diagnosis for subsequent pregnancies are mandatory areas to cover. Remember: You may well view the child's problems much differently than the parents do. Consequently, work with the family from their perspective.

VI. **Chromosomal syndromes.** The most common MCA syndromes diagnosed in the neonatal period are chromosomal.

A. **Trisomy 21 (Down syndrome)**

1. **Incidence.** Trisomy 21 is by far the most common MCA syndrome, occurring in about 1 in 650 live births.

2. **Neonatal mortality.** Is quite small and mostly due to severe cardiac anomalies or congenital leukemias.

3. **Physical findings.** Findings include hypotonia, a poor or absent Moro reflex, flat facial profile, upslanting palpebral fissures, Brushfield spots, anomalous auricles, joint hyperextensibility, excess nuchal skin, fifth digit brachy clinodactyly, and a single transverse palmar crease.

4. **Associated anomalies.** Include congenital heart defects (~50%), most commonly an atrioventricular canal defect or ventricular septal defect. Major gastrointestinal malformations include Hirschsprung disease, duodenal or esophageal atresia, and imperforate anus.

B. **Trisomy 18 (Edwards syndrome)**

1. **Incidence.** Approximately 1 in 5000–7000 live births. There is a 4:1 female-to-male sex ratio.

2. **Neonatal mortality.** Mean life expectancy is 48 days. More than 90% of infants die in the first 6 months. Survival beyond the first year is rare.

3. **Physical findings.** Consist of prenatal and postnatal growth deficiency, decreased subcutaneous fat, initial hypotonia followed by hypertonia, microcephaly, dolichocephaly with a prominent occiput, micrognathia, malformed auricles, short sternum with widely spaced nipples, overlapping digits with hypoplastic nails, and clubbed or rocker-bottom feet.

4. **Associated anomalies.** Congenital heart disease is typically present (95% incidence) and is usually complex. Less frequent anomalies include cryptorchidism, horseshoe kidney, and umbilical or inguinal hernia.

C. **Trisomy 13 (Patau syndrome)**

1. **Incidence.** Approximately 1 in 12,000 live births.

2. **Neonatal mortality.** Mean life expectancy of 130 days. Forty-five percent of infants die in the first month. Survival beyond the first year is rare.

3. **Physical findings.** Consist of low birthweight, microcephaly with sloping forehead, scalp cutis aplasia, microphthalmia, cleft lip and palate, dysplastic ears, redundant nuchal skin, postaxial polydactyly, and overlapping and flexed fingers with hyperconvex nails.

4. **Associated anomalies.** Congenital heart disease is typically present (95% incidence) and usually complex. Renal abnormalities are common and can include polycystic kidneys, hydronephrosis, hydroureters or horseshoe kidney. Holoprosencephaly, cryptorchidism, a single umbilical artery, and inguinal or umbilical hernias are common.

D. **Monosomy X (Turner syndrome)**

1. **Incidence.** Approximately 1 in 2500 live-born females.

2. **Neonatal mortality.** Turner syndrome is usually compatible with survival if the child reaches term. Approximately 98–99% of Turner syndrome fetuses are spontaneously aborted.

3. **Physical findings.** Consist of epicanthal folds, prominent ears, micrognathia, low posterior hairline, excess nuchal skin, webbed neck, broad chest with wide-spaced nipples, hypoplastic nails, peripheral lymphedema of the hands and feet, and pigmented nevi.

4. **Associated anomalies.** Include congenital heart defects, typically a bicuspid aortic valve or aortic coarctation, horseshoe kidney, and gonadal dysgenesis.

E. **22q11.2 Deletion syndrome (DiGeorge syndrome, velocardiofacial syndrome).**
It is now understood that the phenotypes of DiGeorge syndrome (congenital heart disease, hypocalcemia, and immunodeficiency), velocardiofacial syndrome (velopharyngeal incompetence, congenital heart disease, and characteristic facial features), and conotruncal anomaly facial syndrome are all encompassed by and result from the chromosome 22q11.2 deletion.
  1. **Incidence.** Approximately 1 in 5000 live births.
  2. **Neonatal mortality.** Neonatal deaths occur in <10% of cases and are almost exclusively due to cardiac defects.
  3. **Physical findings** consist of a range of malformations including:
     a. **Congenital heart disease** (~75%). Typically conotruncal malformations including tetralogy of Fallot, interrupted aortic arch, ventricular septal defects, or truncus arteriosus.
     b. **Palatal abnormalities** (~70%). Typically velopharyngeal incompetence, submucosal cleft palate, and cleft palate.
     c. **Immune function** (~75%). Typically immunodeficiency occurs as a result of thymic hypoplasia and secondary T-cell abnormalities.
     d. **Craniofacial features.** Typically include microcephaly, malar flattening, mandibular retrusion, overfolded or squared-off helices, prominent nasal root, bulbous nasal tip, hooded eyelids, and hypertelorism. However, some neonates offer no clues to their underlying diagnosis based on their facial features, especially persons of African American heritage.
  4. **Associated anomalies.** Include hypocalcemia (~50%), significant feeding problems (~30%), renal anomalies (~33%), hearing loss (both conductive and sensorineural), and hyperextensibility of hands and fingers.
F. **Williams syndrome (7p11.23 deletion)**
  1. **Incidence.** Approximately 1 in 7500 live births.
  2. **Neonatal mortality.** Is quite small and mostly due to severe cardiac anomalies.
  3. **Physical findings.** Consist of a flat midface, medial eyebrow flare, short palpebral fissures, epicanthal folds, depressed nasal bridge, anteverted nostrils, long philtrum, thick lips, and blue iridae with a stellate pattern.
  4. **Associated anomalies.** Include congenital heart defects (~80%), inguinal or umbilical hernias, hypercalcemia, and feeding difficulties.
VII. **Common sequences**
  A. **Oligohydramnios sequence (Potter sequence)**
     1. **Incidence.** Approximately 1 in 3000–9000 live births.
     2. **Neonatal mortality.** Almost all of these infants die.
     3. **Pathophysiology.** The initial malformations in this sequence are varied, but all lead to oligohydramnios. Primary malformations can include bilateral renal agenesis, severe polycystic kidneys, or a urinary tract obstruction. The resultant oligohydramnios then results in deformations and disruptions including compression deformities of the face and limbs, pulmonary hypoplasia with pneumothoraces, wrinkled skin, and growth restriction. Absent abdominal musculature (prune belly) and cryptorchidism may also be present.
     4. **Associated anomalies.** Include congenital heart defects, esophageal and duodenal atresia, imperforate anus, sirenomelia, hypoplastic nails, Pierre Robin sequence, large fontanelles, wide sutures, flexion contractures, and club feet.
  B. **Amniotic rupture sequence**
     1. **Incidence.** Approximately 1 in 8000–11,000 live births.
     2. **Neonatal mortality.** Variable based on affected tissues and organs.
     3. **Pathophysiology.** The effects of early amnion rupture with entanglement of body parts in bands or strands of amnion is the primary event. The resulting biomechanical forces can lead to disruptions, deformations, and malformations. Viscera that are normally outside the fetus in early embryonic development may be hindered in their return, giving rise to omphalocele and other anomalies.

4. **Physical findings.** Examination of the placenta and amnionic membranes is diagnostic. Aberrant bands or strands are noted, and remnants of the amnion may be rolled up in the umbilical cord.
   a. **Extremities.** Anomalies of the extremities include congenital amputations, constrictions, and distal swellings.
   b. **Craniofacies.** Craniofacial anomalies include microcephaly, encephaloceles, and facial clefts.
   c. **Viscera.** Visceral anomalies include omphaloceles, ectopia cordis, thoracoschisis, and abdominoschisis.

C. **Arthrogryposis (multiple joint contractures)**
   1. **Incidence.** Approximately 1 in 8000 live births.
   2. **Neonatal mortality.** Variable based on etiology.
   3. **Pathophysiology.** Arthrogryposis can result secondarily from varied abnormalities in the developing fetus. Factors that lead to reduced movement including primary neurologic, muscular, or orthopedic problems can all lead to arthrogryposis. Joint contractures can also be secondary to factors that are extrinsic to the developing fetus, such as fetal crowding and constraint. Neurologic abnormalities include meningomyelocele, prenatal spasticity, anencephaly, and hydranencephaly. Muscle abnormalities include muscle agenesis and fetal myopathies. Orthopedic abnormalities include synostosis, joint laxity with dislocations, and aberrant soft tissue fixations.
   4. **Clinical presentation.** The newborn infant is affected by a combination of joint contractures, joint extensions, and joint dislocations. Those with arthrogryposis of central nervous system origin are at increased risk for aspiration and inadequate respiratory movement.

D. **Pierre Robin sequence.** This sequence can occur in isolation or as part of a larger MCA syndrome. The most common associated syndrome is Stickler syndrome.
   1. **Incidence.** Approximately 1 in 8500 live births.
   2. **Neonatal mortality.** Small and mostly due to severe upper airway obstruction at birth.
   3. **Pathophysiology.** The primary event of this sequence is hypoplasia of the mandible, which results in secondary glossoptosis. The glossoptosis then leads to both upper airway obstruction and the development of a cleft palate.
   4. **Clinical presentation.** Infants have micrognathia or a receding chin with a cleft palate. Respiratory distress can occur as a result of upper airway obstruction. Low-set ears may also be present.
   5. **Management.** In mild cases, prone positioning can prevent airway obstruction. In more severe cases, temporary measures for glossoptosis and prevention of airway obstruction include nasal pharyngeal airway, nasal esophageal intubation, lip-tongue adhesion, mandibular distraction, and tracheostomy. Gastric tube feedings are common due to oral feedings causing respiratory distress.

VIII. **Miscellaneous syndromes**
   A. **VATER/VACTERL association.** These conditions are closely related MCA associations. VATER is an acronym that stands for *v*ertebral defects, *a*nal atresia, *t*racheoesophageal fistula, and *r*adial or *r*enal dysplasia. VACTERL is an acronym that stands for *v*ertebral defects, *a*nal atresia, *c*ardiac malformations, *t*racheoesophageal fistula, *r*enal dysplasia and *l*imb abnormalities.
      1. **Incidence.** Approximately 1 in 5000 live births.
      2. **Neonatal mortality.** Small and mostly due to severe cardiac or renal anomalies.
      3. **Clinical presentation.** Aside from the defects described in the acronyms, other features of these disorders include a single umbilical artery and prenatal growth deficiency.
   B. **CHARGE syndrome.** CHARGE is an acronym that stands for *c*oloboma, *h*eart defects, choanal *a*tresia, *r*etarded growth and development, *g*enital abnormalities,

and ear anomalies. CHARGE is an autosomal dominant disorder that results from mutations in the CDH7 gene.

1. **Incidence.** Approximately 1 in 8500–10,000 live births.
2. **Neonatal mortality.** Variable based on the degree of upper airway obstruction and congenital heart disease. Feeding difficulties are a major cause of morbidity in all age groups.
3. **Physical findings.** The major features of CHARGE syndrome include unilateral or bilateral coloboma of the iris, retina, choroid, and or discs with or without microphthalmos (80–90%); cardiovascular malformations including conotruncal defects (75–85%); unilateral or bilateral choanal atresia or stenosis (50–60%); developmental delay and hypotonia (~100%); growth deficiency is typically postnatal with or without growth hormone deficiency (70–80%). Genital abnormalities include cryptorchidism in males and hypogonadotrophic hypogonadism in both males and females. Ear anomalies are both external with anomalous auricles and internal with ossicular malformations, Mondini defect of the cochlea, and absent or hypoplastic semicircular canals.
4. **Associated anomalies.** Include cranial nerve dysfunction resulting in hyposomia or anosmia, unilateral or bilateral facial palsy (40%) and/or swallowing problems (70–90%), and tracheoesophageal fistula (15–20%).

C. **Beckwith-Wiedemann syndrome (BWS)**
   1. **Incidence.** Approximately 1 in 13,000 live births.
   2. **Neonatal mortality.** Infants have ~20% mortality rate, mainly caused by complications of prematurity.
   3. **Physical findings.** Perinatal findings include polyhydramnios, premature birth, macroglossia, linear ear creases, and macrosomia. Hemihyperplasia may be present at birth but can develop over time. Neonatal hypoglycemia is often present and clinically important. Anterior abdominal wall defects, including omphalocele and umbilical hernia, are common.
   4. **Associated anomalies.** Include renal anomalies and an increased risk of mortality associated with Wilms tumor and hepatoblastoma. The estimated risk for tumor development in children with BWS is 7.5%. This increased risk for neoplasia seems to be concentrated in the first 8 years of life. Tumor development is uncommon in affected individuals >8 years of age.

IX. **Teratogenic malformation syndromes**

A. **Fetal alcohol syndrome (FAS).** The incidence is estimated to be 1–2 per 1000 live births. Features include prenatal and postnatal growth deficiency, irritability in infancy, microcephaly, short palpebral fissures, smooth philtrum with thin and smooth upper lip, joint anomalies, and congenital cardiac defects. Brain development and function are the most serious consequences of prenatal alcohol exposure.

B. **Fetal hydantoin (Dilantin) syndrome.** When taken during pregnancy, a two-to threefold increased risk for congenital malformations. Approximately 5–10% of exposed fetuses manifest the embryopathy. Features include mild to moderate prenatal growth deficiency, microcephaly, wide anterior fontanelle, low-set hairline, hirsutism, hypertelorism, strabismus, broad, depressed nasal bridge, cleft lip and palate, digit and nail hypoplasia, and umbilical and inguinal hernias. Similar craniofacial features are also associated with prenatal exposure to carbamazepine, mysoline, and phenobarbital.

C. **Fetal valproate syndrome** was described when an association was made between maternal ingestion of valproic acid and neural tube defects. Additional anomalies of fetal valproate syndrome include narrow bifrontal diameter, epicanthal folds, telecanthus, midface hypoplasia, broad, low nasal bridge with a short nose, long philtrum, micrognathia, long, thin fingers, congenital heart defects, genitourinary anomalies, and clubfeet.

D. **Fetal Accutane (isotretinoin) syndrome** is caused by the maternal use of isotretinoin, an active metabolite of vitamin A, for severe cystic acne. An estimated 25% of fetuses exposed to isotretinoin have a major malformation. Fetal anomalies include congenital heart defects, hydrocephalus, microcephaly, cranial nerve deficits, microtia, and a cleft palate. Pregnancy should wait until 2 years post-treatment with isotretinoin. Ingestion of large amounts of vitamin A may result in the same adverse effects to the fetus.

E. **Diabetic embryopathy.** Children born to insulin-dependent diabetic mothers have a two- to threefold risk for congenital malformations. The cardiovascular, genitourinary, and CNS are the most frequently affected systems. Cardiovascular anomalies include ventricular septal defect (VSD), transposition of great arteries, single umbilical artery, and situs inversus. Anomalies of the genitourinary system consist of renal agenesis and hypospadias and anomalies of the CNS include spina bifida and anencephaly.

F. **Infants of mothers with myotonic dystrophy** vary in their clinical presentation from mild hypotonia and feeding problems to severe respiratory insufficiency causing death. Other abnormalities include a history of polyhydramnios and decreased fetal movement, multiple joint contractures, clubfeet, and facial weakness. The mutation identified to be the cause of myotonic dystrophy is a trinucleotide containing cytosine-thymidine-guanosine that undergoes expansion in females with each transmission from an affected mother to a child. The severity of symptoms and onset of disease increases with transmission of this disorder to family members in subsequent generations.

G. **Infectious (prenatal) diseases** such as toxoplasmosis, rubella, and, cytomegalovirus can result in anomalies including microcephaly, macrocephaly, hydrocephalus, and congenital heart defects. Toxoplasmosis is the most common cause of congenital infections, with an occurrence rate of 0.5–2.5% of all live births.

Selected References

Aase JM: *Diagnostic Dysmorphology*. New York, NY: Plenum, 1990.

Bishara N, Clericuzio C: Common dysmorphic syndromes in the NICU. *Neoreviews* 2008;9: e29-e38.

Gomella TL (ed): *Neonatology: Management, Procedures, On-Call Problems, Diseases and Drugs*, 5th ed. New York, NY: McGraw-Hill, 2004.

Gorlin RJ et al (eds): *Syndromes of the Head and Neck*, 4th ed. New York, NY: Oxford University Press, 2001.

Harper PS: *Practical Genetic Counseling*. New York, NY: Oxford University Press, 2004.

Jones KL: *Smith's Recognizable Patterns of Human Malformation*. Philadelphia, PA: Elsevier Saunders, 2006.

Lalani SR et al: Gene reviews: CHARGE syndrome. Available at: www.genetests.org, 2008.

McDonald-McGinn DM et al: Gene reviews: 22q11.2 deletion syndrome. Available at: www.genetests.org, 2008.

Morris CA: Gene reviews: Williams syndrome. Available at: www.genetests.org, 2008.

Roizen NJ, Patterson D: Down's syndrome. *Lancet* 2003;361:1281-1289.

Schinzel A: *Catalogue of Unbalanced Chromosome Aberrations in Man*, 2nd ed. New York, NY: Walter de Gruyter, 2001.

Shuman C et al: Gene reviews: Beckwith-Wiedemann syndrome. Available at: www.genetests.org, 2008.

81 Congenital Heart Disease

The diagnostic dilemma of the newborn with congenital heart disease must be resolved quickly because therapy may prove lifesaving for some of these infants. Congenital heart disease occurs in ~1% of live-born infants. Nearly half of all cases of congenital heart disease are diagnosed during the first week of life. In patients with complex congenital heart disease, neonatal hospital mortality can be as high as 7%. These patients have a high frequency of multiple congenital anomalies, syndromes, low birthweight, and prolonged length of stay. The most frequently occurring anomalies seen during this first week are patent ductus arteriosus (PDA), D-transposition of the great arteries, hypoplastic left heart syndrome (HLHS), tetralogy of Fallot, and pulmonary atresia.

I. **Classification.** Symptoms and signs in newborns with heart disease permit grouping according to levels of arterial oxygen saturation. Further classification (based on other physical findings and laboratory tests) facilitates delineation of the exact cardiac lesion present.

  A. **Cyanotic heart disease.** Infants with cyanotic heart disease are usually unable to achieve a PaO_2 of >100 mm Hg after breathing 100% inspired oxygen for 10–20 min.

  B. **Acyanotic heart disease.** Infants with acyanotic heart disease achieve PaO_2 levels of >100 mm Hg under the same conditions as noted in Section I, A.

II. **Cyanotic heart disease.** See Figure 81–1.

  A. **100% oxygen test.** Because of intracardiac right-to-left shunting, the newborn with cyanotic congenital heart disease (in contrast to the infant with pulmonary disease) is unable to raise the arterial saturation, even in the presence of increased ambient oxygen.

    1. **Determine PaO_2** while the infant is on room air.

    2. **Give 100% oxygen for 10–20 min** by mask, hood, or endotracheal tube.

    3. **Obtain an arterial blood gas level** while the infant is breathing 100% oxygen.

  B. **Cyanosis.** Care must be taken in evaluating cyanosis by skin color because polycythemia, jaundice, racial pigmentation, or anemia may make clinical recognition of cyanosis difficult.

  C. **Murmur.** The infant with cyanotic congenital heart disease often does not have a distinctive murmur. In fact, the most serious of these anomalies may not be associated with a murmur at all.

  D. **Other studies.** Cyanotic infants may be further classified on the basis of pulmonary circulation on chest radiograph and electrocardiographic findings.

  E. **Diagnosis and treatment.** Figure 81–1 outlines the diagnosis and treatment of cyanotic heart disease.

  F. **Specific cyanotic heart disease abnormalities**

    1. **D-transposition of the great arteries** is the most common cardiac cause of cyanosis in the first year of life, with a male-to-female ratio of 2:1. The aorta comes from the right ventricle and the pulmonary artery from the left ventricle, with resultant separate systemic and pulmonary circuits. With modern newborn care, the 1-year survival rate approaches 90%.

      a. **Physical examination.** Typical presentation is a large, vigorous infant with cyanosis but little or no respiratory distress. There may be no murmur or a soft, systolic ejection murmur.

      b. **Chest radiograph.** This study may be normal, but typically it reveals a very narrow upper mediastinal shadow ("egg on a stick" appearance).

      c. **Electrocardiography (ECG).** There are no characteristic ECG findings.

      d. **Echocardiography is diagnostic.** Typical findings include branching of the anterior great vessel into the innominate, subclavian, and carotid vessels

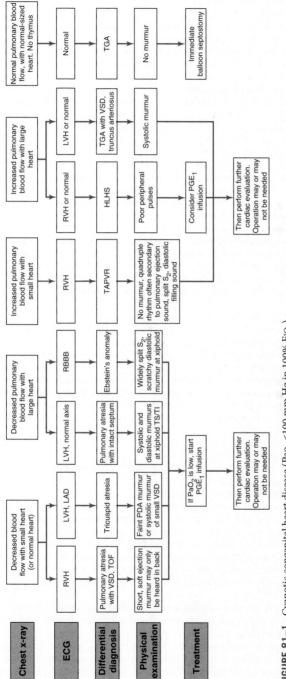

FIGURE 81–1. Cyanotic congenital heart disease (Pao₂ <100 mm Hg in 100% Fio₂).

ECG, electrocardiography; HLHS, hypoplastic left heart syndrome; LAD, left axis deviation; LVH, left ventricular hypertrophy; PDA, patent ductus arteriosus; PGE₁, prostaglandin E1; RBBB, right bundle branch block; RVH, right ventricular hypertrophy; TAPVR, total anomalous pulmonary venous return; TGA, transposition of the great arteries; TI, tricuspid incompetence; TOF, tetralogy of Fallot; TS, tricuspid stenosis; VSD, ventricular septal defect.

and branching of the posterior great vessel into the right and left pulmonary arteries.

e. **Cardiac catheterization.** Like echocardiography, this study is diagnostic and often therapeutic as outlined next.

f. **Treatment.** If severe hypoxia or acidosis occurs, urgent balloon atrial septostomy can be done under echocardiogram guidance in the nursery. Cardiac catheterization with balloon septostomy and subsequent arterial switch operation are methods of treatment.

2. **Tetralogy of Fallot.** Tetralogy of Fallot is characterized by four anomalies: pulmonary stenosis, ventricular septal defect, overriding aorta, and right ventricular hypertrophy (RVH). There is a slight male predominance. Cyanosis usually signifies complete or partial atresia of the right ventricular overflow tract or extremely severe pulmonary stenosis with hypoplastic pulmonary arteries. The degree of right ventricular outflow obstruction is inversely proportional to pulmonary blood flow and directly proportional to the degree of cyanosis. Tetralogy of Fallot with absent pulmonary valve may present with respiratory distress or poor feeding (because of compression of the esophagus or bronchi by the large pulmonary arteries).

a. **Physical examination.** The patient is cyanotic with a systolic ejection murmur along the left sternal border. Loud murmurs are associated with more flow across the right ventricular outflow tract and milder degrees of desaturation. Softer murmurs are associated with less flow and more hypoxia.

b. **Chest radiograph.** The chest radiograph film reveals a small, often "boot-shaped" heart, with decreased pulmonary vascular markings. A right aortic arch is seen in ~20% of these infants.

c. **ECG.** The ECG may be normal or may demonstrate RVH. The only sign of RVH may be an upright T wave in V_4R or V_1 after 72 h of age.

d. **Echocardiography** is usually diagnostic, with the demonstration of an overriding aorta, ventricular septal defect (VSD), and small right ventricular outflow tract.

e. **Treatment.** Pulmonary blood flow may be ductal dependent with severe cyanosis and may respond to ductal dilation using prostaglandin E_1 (see Chapter 132). This measure allows more flexibility for planning cardiac catheterization and surgical correction. Surgery (shunting or total correction) may be considered.

III. **Acyanotic heart disease** (Figure 81–2)

A. **100% oxygen test.** See Section II, A.

B. **Murmur.** The infant who is not cyanotic will have either a heart murmur or symptoms of congestive heart failure.

C. **Diagnosis and treatment.** See Figure 81–2.

D. **Specific acyanotic heart disease abnormalities**

1. **Ventricular septal defect (VSD)** is the most common congenital heart abnormality, with equal sex distribution. Murmurs can be heard at birth but typically appear between 3 days and 3 weeks of age. Congestive heart failure is unusual before 4 weeks of age but may develop earlier in premature infants. Symptoms and physical findings vary with patient age and defect size. Spontaneous closure occurs in half of the patients. Surgical correction is reserved for large, symptomatic VSD's only.

2. **Atrial septal defect (ASD)** is not an important cause of morbidity or mortality in infancy. Occasionally, congestive heart failure can occur in infancy but not usually in the neonatal period.

3. **Endocardial cushion defects** include ostium primum–type ASD with or without a cleft mitral valve and an atrioventricular (AV) canal. These defects are commonly associated with multiple congenital anomalies, especially Down syndrome.

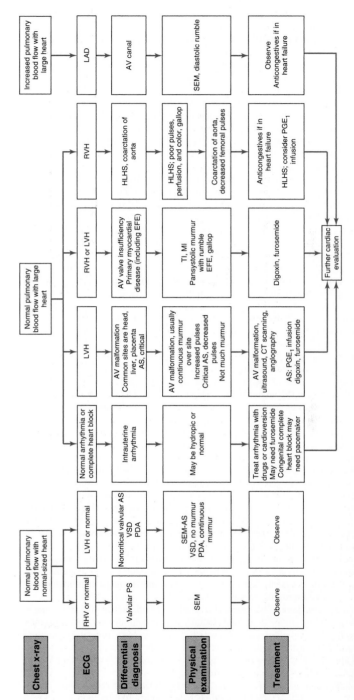

FIGURE 81-2. Acyanotic congenital heart disease (Pao$_2$ >100 mm Hg in 100% Fio$_2$)

AS, aortic stenosis; AV canal, atrioventricular canal; AV malformation, arteriovenous malformation; AV valve, atrioventricular valve; CT, computed tomography; ECG, electrocardiogram; EFE, endocardial fibroelastosis; HLHS, hypoplastic left heart syndrome; LAD, left axis deviation; LVH, left ventricular hypertrophy; MI, myocardial infarction; PDA, patent ductus arteriosus; PGE$_1$, prostaglandin E1; PS, pulmonary stenosis; RVH, right ventricular hypertrophy; SEM, systolic ejection murmur; TI, tricuspid incompetence; VSD, ventricular septal defect.

If marked AV valve insufficiency is present, the patient may have congestive heart failure at birth or in the neonatal period.

a. **Physical examination.** On physical examination, a systolic murmur resulting from AV valve insufficiency may be heard. Cyanosis may be present but is often not severe. Infants with severe pulmonary artery hypertension may have little or no murmur.

b. **Chest radiograph.** Variable findings may include a dilated pulmonary artery or a large heart secondary to atrial dilatation.

c. **ECG.** Left axis deviation (left superior vector) is *always* found; the PR interval may be long, or there may be an RSR′ pattern in V_4R and V_1.

d. **Echocardiography** is usually diagnostic; the echocardiogram usually demonstrates a common AV valve with inlet VSD or a defect in the septum primum with an abnormal mitral valve.

e. **Treatment.** Congestive heart failure is treated with diuretics and digoxin (for dosages, see Chapter 132); early cardiac catheterization with corrective surgery may be needed to prevent pulmonary vascular obstructive disease.

IV. **Hypoplastic left heart syndrome** occurs in both cyanotic and acyanotic forms. In 15% of cases, the foramen ovale is intact and thus prevents mixing at the atrial level, causing cyanosis. Infants with mixing at the atria are acyanotic. HLHS accounts for 25% of all cardiac deaths during the first week of life.

A. **Physical examination.** The infant is typically pale and tachypneic, with poor perfusion and poor to absent peripheral pulses. A loud single S_2 is present, usually with a gallop and no murmur. There is hepatomegaly, and metabolic acidosis is usually present by 48 h of age.

B. **Electrocardiogram** demonstrates small or absent left ventricular forces.

C. **Chest radiograph.** Moderate cardiomegaly is present, often with a large main pulmonary artery shadow.

D. **Echocardiography.** A diagnostic study demonstrates a small or slit-like left ventricle with a hypoplastic ascending aorta.

E. **Treatment.** Systemic blood flow is ductal dependent; therefore, prostaglandin E_1 is of value. Oxygen should not be given, as the resultant dilatation of the pulmonary vessels increases pulmonary blood flow. Respiratory compromise and subsequent dilatation and reduced RV function are undesired effects of oxygen administration. In fact, infants with HLHS and pulmonary overcirculation may require oxygen concentrations <21%. Surgical correction is done in three stages. The first is palliation (the Norwood procedure), redirecting the blood flow so that the right ventricle serves as the "systemic ventricle" and a surgically constructed "shunt" provides pulmonary blood flow. Some surgeons prefer to do a Sano modification of the Norwood, which involves placing a Gore-tex tube from the RV to the MPA. Successful outcome is influenced by gestational age (term infants do much better than preterm infants) and the presence of other major anomalies. The second stage usually consists of a hemi-Fontan or bidirectional Glenn operation or Sano, routing superior vena cava blood to the lungs and closing the systemic-to-pulmonary artery shunt. The third stage (the Fontan procedure) directs remaining systemic venous return directly to the pulmonary circulation. Neonatal cardiac transplantation is a second option, but shortage of organs is a significant deterrent. Compassionate care (keeping the infant comfortable until death) may be appropriate in some instances.

V. **Associated anomalies and syndromes** (Table 81–1). No discussion of heart disease in neonates would be complete without the inclusion of common multiple congenital anomaly (MCA) syndromes associated with heart defects. Many times, recognition of MCA syndromes facilitates identification of the heart defect. Syndromes that tend to present after the newborn period have not been included. See Chapter 80 for a complete discussion of anomalies and syndromes.

VI. **Teratogens and heart disease.** Several teratogens associated with congenital heart disease have been identified (Table 81–2), although there is not a 100% relationship between exposure and heart defects. A history of teratogen exposure may help in the diagnosis.

Table 81–1. **CONGENITAL ANOMALIES ASSOCIATED WITH HEART DEFECTS**

Congenital Anomaly	Heart Defect
Chromosomal anomaly	
Trisomy 21 (Down syndrome)	Atrioventricular canal, ventricular septal defect
Trisomies 13, 15, and 18	Ventricular septal defect, patent ductus arteriosus
Syndrome associated with 4p–	Atrial septal defect, ventricular septal defect
Syndrome associated with 5p–(cri du chat syndrome)	Variable
XO (Turner syndrome)	Coarctation of aorta, aortic stenosis
Syndromes with predominantly skeletal defects[a]	
Ellis-van Creveld syndrome	Atrial septal defect, single atrium
Laurence-Moon-Biedl syndrome	Tetralogy of Fallot, ventricular septal defect
Carpenter syndrome	Patent ductus arteriosus, ventricular septal defect
Holt-Oram syndrome	Atrial septal defect, ventricular septal defect
Fanconi syndrome	Patent ductus arteriosus, ventricular septal defect
Thrombocytopenia–absent radius syndrome	Atrial septal defect, tetralogy of Fallot
Syndromes with characteristic facies[a]	
Noonan syndrome (long arm of chromosome 12)	Pulmonary stenosis
DiGeorge syndrome (chromosome 22 deletion)	Tetralogy of Fallot, aortic arch anomalies
Smith-Lemli-Opitz syndrome	Ventricular septal defect, patent ductus arteriosus
de Lange syndrome	Tetralogy of Fallot, ventricular septal defect
Goldenhar syndrome	Tetralogy of Fallot, variable
Williams syndrome	Supravalvular aortic stenosis, peripheral pulmonary artery stenosis
Asymmetric crying facies	Variable

[a]Not all infants with these syndromes have heart defects.

Table 81–2. **TERATOGENS ASSOCIATED WITH HEART DEFECTS**

Teratogen	Heart Defect
Drugs	
Alcohol	Ventricular septal defect, tetralogy of Fallot, atrial septal defect
Anticonvulsants	Variable, ventricular septal defect, tetralogy of Fallot
Retinoic acid	Aortic arch anomalies
Lithium	Ebstein anomaly of the tricuspid valve
Environmental agents	
Irradiation	Variable
High altitude	PDA; others variable
Maternal factors	
Diabetes	Variable
Maternal lupus	Complete (3rd degree) AV block
Maternal PKU	Ventricular septal defect, coarctation
Infections	
Rubella syndrome	PDA, peripheral pulmonary stenosis
Parvovirus, Coxsackie	Cardiomyopathy
Other viruses	Variable

AV, atrioventricular; PDA, patent ductus arteriosus; PKU, phenylketonuria.

VII. **Abnormal situs syndromes.** Syndromes of abnormal situs relationships are associated with congenital heart disease. For example, an infant with situs inversus totalis and dextrocardia has the same incidence of congenital heart disease as the general population. If, however, there is disparity between thoracic and abdominal situs, the incidence of congenital heart disease is >90%. (Check the chest radiograph to see that the cardiac apex and the stomach bubble are on the same side. Both should be on the left.) Some of these syndromes involve bilateral left-sidedness (two bilobed lungs or multiple spleens) and complex cyanotic congenital heart disease, whereas others have bilateral right-sidedness (two trilobed lungs or an absent spleen) and complex cyanotic congenital heart disease.

VIII. **General principles of management**

A. **Fetal echocardiography**

1. **General considerations.** Fetal echocardiography is now possible in many centers. The optimal gestational age to perform echocardiography is between 18 and 24 weeks when structural abnormalities and arrhythmias can be detected. With early detection of cardiac abnormalities, arrangements can be made for delivery at a center with pediatric cardiac and surgical facilities. If the anomaly is not consistent with life, some families may elect termination of pregnancy.

2. **Indications.** See Table 81–3.

a. **Maternal factors.** Oligohydramnios or polyhydramnios, diabetes, collagen vascular disease, teratogen exposure, or a previous child with congenital heart disease.

b. **Fetal factors.** Suspected cardiac abnormality on obstetric ultrasound examination, pleural fluid, pericardial fluid, heart rate abnormalities, intrauterine growth retardation, or other abnormality on obstetric ultrasound examination.

c. **Genetic factors.** Familial history of chromosomal disorders or congenital heart disease.

B. **Emergency therapy.** Once the specific lesion has been identified as emergent, a decision about therapy must be made. As an example, if confronted with a very cyanotic infant with no murmur, a normal chest radiograph, and a normal ECG and it is believed that the diagnosis of D-transposition of the great arteries is likely, it is necessary to prepare for a **balloon septostomy.**

C. **Prostaglandins.** As a general principle, if an infant is cyanotic and has decreased pulmonary blood flow, the Pao_2 will be improved by promoting flow through the ductus arteriosus via a drip of **prostaglandin E_1** (alprostadil, or Prostin VR Pediatric). Maintaining patency of the ductus will enable stabilization of the infant

Table 81–3. **INDICATIONS FOR FETAL ECHOCARDIOGRAM**

Maternal conditions
Diabetes
Collagen vascular disease
Maternal drug/teratogen exposure

Family conditions
History of congenital heart disease
History of chromosomal or genetic abnormalities

Fetal conditions
Abnormal fetal heart rate
Suspected cardiac malformation on screening ultrasonogram
Presence of other malformations on ultrasonogram
Oligo- or polyhydramnios
Evidence of hydrops fetalis
Intrauterine growth restriction

and subsequent catheterization or surgery to be planned on an urgent rather than emergent basis. Similarly, if poor peripheral pulses and acidosis from poor perfusion are present, infusion of prostaglandin, using the same dose, will open the ductus arteriosus and allow right ventricular blood flow to augment the systemic circulation. This measure is beneficial in critical aortic stenosis, coarctation of the aorta, and HLHS. (For dosage and other pharmacologic information, see Chapter 132.)

   D. **Antiarrhythmic drugs.** Rapid arrhythmias may occur during intrauterine life or after delivery. Arrhythmias are a cause of fetal hydrops and intrauterine death; most often, the rhythm disturbance is a rapid supraventricular tachycardia with a 1:1 ventricular response. Occasionally, atrial flutter with 2:1 block presents before or just after birth. **Digitalis** has been a successful antiarrhythmic agent in this situation, but treatment with adenosine or electrical cardioversion is also sometimes necessary. (See Chapter 42 on Arrhythmias.)

   E. **Pacemaker.** Fetal hydrops can result from congenital complete heart block. If cardiovascular demise is imminent, delivery and **temporary transvenous ventricular pacing may be lifesaving.** It should be followed by urgent surgical placement of a permanent pacemaker. Mothers may have anti-Rho or anti-LA antibodies.

Selected References

Allan LD et al: Prospective diagnosis of 1,006 consecutive cases of congenital heart disease in the fetus. *J Am Coll Cardiol* 1994;23:1452.

Ballard RA, Wernosky G: Cardiovascular system. In Taeusch HW (ed): *Avery's Diseases of the Newborn.* Philadelphia, PA: Elsevier Saunders, 2005:779-901.

Brooks PA, Penny DJ: Management of the sick neonate with suspected heart disease. *Early Hum Dev* 2008;84(3):155-159.

Dallopiccola B et al: A Mendelian basis of congenital heart defects. *Cardiol Young* 1996;6:264.

Dorfman AT et al: Critical heart disease in the neonate: presentation and outcome at a tertiary care center. *Pediatr Crit Care Med* 2008;9(2):193-202.

Jenkins PC et al: A comparison of treatment strategies for hypoplastic left heart syndrome using decision analysis. *J Am Coll Cardiol* 2001;38:1181.

Perry LW et al: Infants with congenital heart disease: the cases. In Ferencz C et al (eds): *Epidemiology of Congenital Heart Disease: The Baltimore-Washington Infant Heart Study 1981-1989.* Mt. Kisco, NY: Futura, 1993.

Rosenthal A: Hypoplastic left heart syndrome. In JH Moller, JIE Hoffman (eds): *Pediatric Cardiovascular Medicine.* New York, NY: Churchill Livingston, 2000.

82 Disorders of Sex Development

   I. **Definition.** Ambiguous genitalia are present when the sex of an infant is not readily apparent after examination of the external genitalia. If the appearance resembles neither a male with a normal phallus and palpable testes nor a female with an unfused vaginal orifice and absence of an enlarged phallic structure, the genitalia are ambiguous and investigation before gender assignment is indicated. Recent trend has been to refer to these disorders as **disorders of sex development** because many of the other terms used are considered pejorative by some patients and professionals. New definitions and classifications are also being proposed in this already very complex area. For the purpose of this on-call manual, the embryology and pathophysiology are reviewed as relevant to the initial evaluation and treatment of patients in the neonatal period.

II. **Incidence.** The quoted incidence of ambiguous genitalia varies according to source and is likely somewhat variable for different ethnic groups; it appears to be approximately 1 in 5000. Congenital adrenal hyperplasia is often considered the most common cause with an incidence quoted from 1 in 14,000 to 1 in 28,000; followed by androgen insensitivity and mixed gonadal dysgenesis. Hypospadias has a frequency of about 1 in 300 births, but only a minority of these patients has a disorder of sex development (usually presenting with hypospadias in combination with cryptorchidism).

III. **Embryology.** The early fetus, regardless of the genetic sex (XX or XY), is bipotential and can undergo either male or female differentiation. The innate tendency of the embryo is to differentiate along female lines.

   A. **Development of the gonads.** Gonadal development occurs during the embryonic period (the third through the seventh to eighth weeks of gestation).

      1. **Testicular differentiation.** Gonadal differentiation is determined by the absence or presence of the Y chromosome. If the **Y chromosome** (more specifically, the sex-determining region of the Y or *SRY* gene) is present, the gonads differentiate as testes. The testes then produce and release testosterone, which is converted to **dihydrotestosterone (DHT)** in the target organ cells by 5a-reductase. DHT induces male differentiation of the external genitalia (see Section III, B, 1). The testes descend behind the peritoneum and normally reach the scrotum by the eighth or ninth month.

      2. **Ovarian differentiation.** In the female fetus, where the Y chromosome/*SRY* gene is absent, the gonads form ovaries (even in 45,X Turner syndrome, histologically normal ovaries are present at birth). As ovaries do not produce testosterone, female differentiation proceeds. Two X chromosomes are needed for differentiation of the primordial follicle. If part or all of the second X chromosome is missing, ovarian development fails, resulting in atrophic, whitish, streaky gonads by 1–2 years of age.

   B. **Development of external genitalia.** This part of sexual differentiation occurs in the fetal period, beginning in the seventh week of gestation and proceeds up to the 14th week (about 16 weeks after the last menstrual period).

      1. **Normal male.** At ~9 weeks postconceptional age, in the presence of systemic androgens (especially DHT), masculinization begins with lengthening of the anogenital distance. The urogenital and labioscrotal folds fuse in the midline (beginning caudally and progressing anteriorly), leading to the formation of the scrotum and the penis.

      2. **Normal female.** In the female fetus, the anogenital distance does not increase. The urogenital and labioscrotal folds do not fuse and instead differentiate into the labia majora and minora. The urogenital sinus divides into the urethra and the vagina.

IV. **Pathophysiology**

   A. **Virilization of female infants (female pseudohermaphroditism).** Many neonates with disorders of sex development belong to this group. They have a 46,XX karyotype, are *SRY* negative, and have exclusively ovarian tissue. The degree of masculinization of the female newborn depends on the potency of the androgenic stimulation to which she is exposed, the stage of development at the time of initial exposure, and the duration of exposure.

      1. The most common cause of excess fetal androgens is an autosomal recessively inherited **enzymatic deficiency in the cortisol pathway,** leading to excessive corticotropin (adrenocorticotropic hormone [ACTH]) stimulation with **congenital adrenal hyperplasia (CAH)** and excessive production of adrenal androgens (dehydroepiandrosterone and androstenedione) and testosterone (Figure 82–1). Most common is **21-hydroxylase deficiency,** which causes inadequate cortisol levels, leading to excessive ACTH stimulation (through feedback to the hypothalamus and

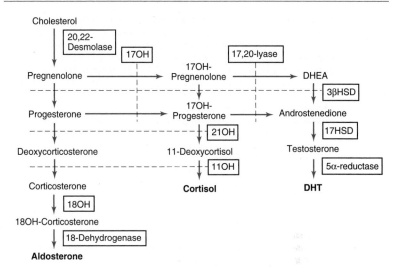

FIGURE 82–1. Adrenal metabolic pathways relevant to normal sex development. 11OH, 11-Hydroxylase; 17OH, 17-hydroxylase; 18OH, 18-hydroxylase; 21OH, 21-hydroxylase; 3βHSD, 3β-hydroxysteroid dehydrogenase; 17HSD, 17-hydroxysteroid dehydrogenase (17-ketosteroid reductase); DHEA, dehydroepiandrosterone; DHT, dihydrotestosterone.

pituitary), adrenal hyperplasia, and excessive production of adrenal androgens (dehydroepiandrosterone and androstenedione) and testosterone, producing virilization. **Two forms** of CAH are seen in neonates, depending on the associated **relative or absolute aldosterone deficiency: a simple virilizing form and a salt-losing form.** In the first form, the salt loss is mild and adrenal insufficiency tends not to occur, except in stressful circumstances. In the second, adrenal insufficiency occurs under basal conditions and tends to manifest in the neonatal period or soon thereafter as an adrenal crisis. The electrolyte status of all infants with 21-hydroxylase deficiency should be monitored because the extent of virilization is not a reliable indicator of the degree of adrenal insufficiency. **11-Hydroxylase enzyme deficiency** is less common and associated with salt retention, volume expansion, and hypertension.

2. **Other, less common causes** are virilizing maternal or fetal tumors or maternal androgen ingestion or topical use.

B. **Inadequate virilization of male infants (male pseudohermaphroditism).** This condition is caused by inadequate androgen production or incomplete end-organ response to androgen. These patients have a 46,XY karyotype and exclusively testicular tissue. These abnormalities are rare, and most require extensive laboratory investigation before a final diagnosis can be confirmed.

1. **Decreased androgen production** can be caused by one of several rare enzyme defects, which are inherited in an autosomal recessive manner. Some of these defects also cause cortisol deficiency and **nonvirilizing adrenal hyperplasia,** and others are specific to the testosterone pathway. Other causes of decreased androgen production include **deficiency of Müllerian-inhibiting substance** (the most common presentation is a male infant with inguinal hernias that contain a uterus or fallopian tubes); **testicular unresponsiveness to human chorionic gonadotropin (hCG) and luteinizing hormone (LH);** and **anorchia** (absent testes caused by loss of vascular supply to the testis during fetal life). The association of

microphallus/micropenis and **hypoglycemia** suggests a **pituitary deficiency** with absence of gonadotropins, ACTH, or growth hormone.

2. **Decreased end-organ response to androgen,** also referred to as **testicular feminization,** can be caused by a defect in the androgen receptor or an unknown defect with normal receptors. It can be total (labial testes with otherwise normal-appearing female genitalia) or, more commonly, partial (incomplete virilization of a male).

3. **5α-Reductase deficiency** results in failure of the external genitalia to undergo male differentiation because of the lack of DHT (see Figure 82–1). The outcome is a neonate with female or a disorder of sex development but with a 46,XY karyotype, normally developed testes, and male internal ducts.

C. **Disorders of gonadal differentiation**

1. **True hermaphroditism.** The presence of both a testis and an ovary (or ovotestes) in the same individual is a rare cause of ambiguous genitalia. Most individuals with true hermaphroditism have a 46,XX karyotype, but mosaics of 46,XX, 45,X, 46,XY, and multiple X/multiple Y have all been reported. The appearance of the genitalia is variable; fertility is poor.

2. **Gonadal dysgenesis**

   a. **Pure gonadal dysgenesis** is characterized by the presence of a streak gonad bilaterally (complete gonadal dysgenesis) or unilaterally (partial gonadal dysgenesis). It is important to distinguish the X-chromosomal from the Y-chromosomal form because the streak gonads in the Y-positive patients carry a significant **risk for tumor development.**

   b. **Mixed gonadal dysgenesis** is characterized by the presence of a unilateral functioning testis and a contralateral streak gonad. All patients have a Y chromosome and some degree of virilization of the external genitalia. Mixed gonadal dysgenesis is associated with a high incidence of **gonadal malignancy** in mid to late childhood.

D. **Chromosome abnormalities, syndromes, and associations.** In general, chromosomal abnormalities do not usually lead to genital abnormalities. However, disruption of normal sex development has been reported occasionally in **trisomies 13 and 18, triploidy, and a number of other chromosomal anomalies.** Single-gene disorders and syndromes such as **Smith-Lemli-Opitz syndrome, Rieger syndrome, CHARGE syndrome** (*c*oloboma, *h*eart defects, choanal *a*tresia, *r*etarded growth and development, *g*enital abnormalities, and *e*ar anomalies), **camptomelic dysplasia,** and others can also be associated with external sexual ambiguity (>90 syndromes with "ambiguous genitalia" were found in a search of a syndrome database). **VACTERL** (*v*ertebral defects, *a*nal atresia, *c*ardiac malformations, *t*racheoesophageal fistula, *r*enal dysplasia and *l*imb abnormalities) association can include abnormally developed genitalia.

V. **Risk factors.** The etiology of disorders of sex development is developmental/genetic. Therefore, there are no definite behavioral risk factors but a history of relatives with genital anomalies, abnormal pubertal development, infertility, or neonatal/infant deaths could be an indicator of increased risk. The question if techniques of assisted reproduction, especially in vitro fertilization with intracytoplasmic sperm injection, may be associated with disorders of sex development and other birth defects remains *controversial* because the abnormalities reported could also be related to the underlying cause of infertility leading to the use of these techniques rather than an association with the process of assisted reproduction.

VI. **Clinical presentation.** Note that the American Academy of Pediatrics issued a policy statement on the evaluation of the newborn with developmental anomalies of the external genitalia in 2000. In 2006, after an International Conference on Intersex, a "Consensus Statement on the Management of Intersex Disorders" was published (see references).

A. **History.** A careful history should be obtained from the parents. **Family history** of early neonatal deaths (a death in early infancy accompanied by vomiting and dehydration may be secondary to CAH), consanguinity of the parents (increased risk for autosomal recessive disorders), and female relatives with amenorrhea and infertility (male pseudohermaphroditism or chromosomal anomalies) are significant, as are a **maternal history** of virilization or CAH and ingestion or topical use of drugs during pregnancy (particularly androgens or progestational agents).

B. Physical examination

1. **A general examination** should address the presence of any of the following: dysmorphic features (syndromes and chromosomal abnormalities), hypertension or hypotension, areolar hyperpigmentation, and signs of dehydration (as signs of CAH).

2. **Genitalia. Gonads:** The number, size, and symmetry of gonads should be evaluated. Palpable gonads below the inguinal canal are usually testes. Ovaries are not found in scrotal folds or in the inguinal region. However, the testes may be intra-abdominal. **Phallus length:** Measured from the pubic ramus to the tip of the glands, a stretched penile length in a full-term infant should be ≥2.0 cm. Reference values for premature infants have been established; ethnic background may influence penile length. **Urethral meatus:** Look for hypospadias (usually accompanied by chordee). **Labioscrotal folds:** Findings can range from unfused labia majora, variable degrees of posterior fusion, and bifid scrotum to fully fused, normal-appearing scrotum. The presence of a vaginal opening or urogenital sinus should be determined. A rectal examination, to determine presence of a uterus, may be considered.

VII. Diagnosis

A. Laboratory studies

1. **Initial evaluation.** An important test in the initial evaluation is the **chromosome analysis.** Most cytogenetic laboratories can now provide preliminary results of a karyotype in a few days. **Fluorescent in situ hybridization techniques (FISH)** allow even faster determination of the sex chromosome status; X- and Y-specific probes are available. Buccal smears are unreliable and therefore obsolete. The remainder of the diagnostic evaluation depends on the sex chromosome status. Blood for **basic biochemical studies** can be obtained at the same time as the karyotype, including 17-hydroxyprogesterone (17-OHP), testosterone, dihydrotestosterone, sodium, and potassium levels. Other tests may be necessary, depending on the results of the karyotype. Biochemical tests are therefore discussed in the context of the different chromosomal constellations.

2. **Normal 46,XX karyotype.** This finding implies virilization of a genetic female and is caused by excessive maternal or fetal androgen. If the mother is not virilized, the infant almost always has **virilizing adrenal hyperplasia.** To confirm the diagnosis, measure the following:

   a. **17-hydroxyprogesterone (17-OHP).** This is the immediate precursor to the enzyme defect in 21-hydroxylase enzyme deficiency and a precursor one step further removed in 11-hydroxylase enzyme deficiency. In infants with either defect, the serum or plasma level of 17-OHP will be 100–1000 times the normal infant level. Note that the 17-OHP level may be somewhat elevated in normal infants within the first 24 h of life; a repeat level several days later may be indicated while fluid and electrolyte balance is monitored. 17-OHP is now measured by many newborn screening programs in the United States and other countries as a screening for CAH.

   b. **Daily serum measurements of sodium and potassium.** Infants with 21-hydroxylase enzyme deficiency usually have relative or absolute aldosterone deficiency and begin to demonstrate hyperkalemia at days 3–5 and hyponatremia 1–2 days later. If hyperkalemia becomes clinically significant before the 17-OHP result is available, empirical treatment with intravenous saline, cortisol, and fludrocortisone may be needed (for dosages, see Section VIII, B, 1a and b).

    c. Serum testosterone. About 3% of infants with ambiguous genitalia are true hermaphrodites, and most have a 46,XX karyotype. If the 17-OHP is not elevated and there is no maternal virilization, a high testosterone level suggests hermaphroditism or fetal testosterone-producing tumor.

3. Normal 46,XY karyotype. The differential diagnosis of an **incompletely virilized genetic male** is extremely complex and includes in utero testicular damage, defects of testosterone synthesis, end-organ resistance, and an enzymatic defect in the conversion of testosterone to dihydrotestosterone. The laboratory evaluation is correspondingly complex and usually proceeds through a number of steps.

    a. Testosterone (T) and dihydrotestosterone (DHT). These hormone levels should be measurable and are higher in newborns than later in childhood. In the male pseudohermaphrodite, testosterone is low in any defect in testosterone production. The T-to-DHT ratio should be between 5:1 and 20:1 when expressed in similar units. A high T-to-DHT ratio suggests 5a-reductase deficiency (see also Section VII A 3c: the hCG stimulation test). **Androstenedione** levels are measured to diagnose **17-ketosteroid reductase deficiency.**

    b. LH and follicle-stimulating hormone (FSH). These hormones are also higher in infancy than they are in childhood. A diagnosis of gonadotropin deficiency is suspected if these values are low in a reliable assay but can be confirmed in infancy only if there are **other pituitary hormone deficits** (see Section VII A, 3d). Note that growth hormone and ACTH deficiency are manifested in the newborn period as **hypoglycemia.** In primary gonadal defects and some androgen-resistant states, LH and FSH are elevated.

    c. hCG stimulation test. hCG is administered to stimulate gonadal steroid production when testosterone values are low (as in gonadotropin deficiency or a defect in testosterone synthesis). Recommendations vary, and the test should be performed under the guidance of a specialist. In general, a dose of 500–1000 units every day or every other day for three doses may be given. Then testosterone and DHT are measured again to evaluate the gonadal response. A rise in the testosterone level confirms the presence of Leydig cells and, by implication, testicular tissue. In patients with 5a-reductase deficiency, the basal T-to-DHT ratio may be normal but elevated after hCG stimulation. It is wise to obtain enough blood after hCG injection to measure other steroid intermediates if the testosterone is low. Considering the complexity of male pseudohermaphroditism, the restrictions in drawing blood from newborns, and the fact that many specific tests can be performed only in special laboratories, involvement of a pediatric endocrinologist in the planning and interpretation of these tests is crucial. In any case, it is always advisable to ask the initial processing laboratory to freeze any remaining serum or plasma.

    d. Assessment of pituitary function. If gonadotropin deficiency due to impairment of pituitary function is suspected (eg, microphallus/micropenis combined with hypoglycemia), thyroid function tests, growth hormone levels, ACTH stimulation test, and imaging studies of the pituitary gland may be indicated.

4. Abnormal karyotype. Mixed gonadal dysgenesis with a dysplastic gonad may be present in infants with abnormal karyotype and abnormal genitalia. **Hormone studies** are unlikely to be revealing in this scenario. Note that a normal karyotype from peripheral white blood cells does not exclude mosaic chromosomal abnormalities and there is a limit in the resolution of conventional karyotypes. **Special genetic testing (FISH analysis, genome microarray analysis, or specific DNA analysis)** may be needed. These techniques may allow detection of *SRY* gene material in 46,XX phenotypic males and be useful in determining whether Y material is present in a 45,X individual, placing the patient at risk for gonadoblastoma.

B. **Radiographic studies**
   1. **Ultrasonography** to evaluate adrenal and pelvic structures. Although a uterus is sometimes palpable on rectal examination shortly after birth (because of enlargement in response to maternal estrogen), ultrasonography seems less invasive. The presence and localization of gonads may also be clarified by ultrasonography. Adrenal ultrasonography is sufficiently sensitive to determine adrenal abnormalities in the majority of patients with untreated adrenal hyperplasia.
   2. **Contrast studies** to outline the internal anatomy (sinography, urethrography, vesicocystoureterography, and intravenous urography) may be indicated in complex cases and before reconstructive surgery.
   3. **Magnetic resonance imaging** has been used to evaluate patients with disorders of sex development but, at least in the neonatal period, sensitivity may only be marginally improved over ultrasound.
VIII. **Management**
   A. **General considerations.** The presence of any disorders of sex differentiation is likely to cause significant emotional and social stresses and anxieties for the family. It is very important to protect the privacy of child and parents while diagnostic studies are in progress. A multidisciplinary team should assist the patient and family throughout the diagnostic process and beyond. Once a diagnosis has been established, gender should be assigned (see Section IX) and a team of specialists should supervise medical treatment (steroid replacement, gonadal removal, reconstructive surgery, etc.) and treatment of psychosocial aspects.
      1. **Early interactions with the parents and general care.** As soon as the abnormality is noted, a physician responsible for the infant should be identified and the parents should be informed. During the initial counseling of the family, gender neutral terms such as "your infant" should be used; gender-specific pronouns should be avoided. A phrase often recommended in this situation is to refer to the genitalia as "incompletely developed." Parents should be informed that it is not possible without further tests to identify the sex of their child. Meet with the parents as soon as possible to discuss the situation in more detail (the delivery room is usually not appropriate for an in-depth discussion). The feelings, impressions, and biases perceived at the time parents first learn about the diagnosis of a sex differentiation disorder often persist. Examining the infant with the parents may be beneficial, but any attempts to identify the sex of the child on the basis of appearance should be resisted, although there is likely to be great pressure to do so from parents, relatives, and hospital personnel. It is important not to complete the birth certificate or make any reference to gender in any of the permanent medical records of the mother or the child. It may be advisable to isolate the child and parents from the inquiries of certain nonessential hospital personnel and the community, but any actions implying that the conditions is shameful or should be "hidden" must be avoided. Parents may want to delay sending out birth announcements and telling anyone outside the immediate family that the infant has been born until a gender assignment has been made. Be aware that many children live the majority of their lives in the community of their birth, and confusion about gender assignment because of premature release of information may have long-term consequences. Parents should be reassured that in most cases the gender will be determined as soon as test results are available, and some specialists discourage the use of unisex/epicene names in the early neonatal period.
      2. **Early referral.** It is advisable to seek consultation from a specialist in the evaluation of children with disorders of sex differentiation (the first specialist involved is often a pediatric endocrinologist) as soon as feasible. It is usually not appropriate to discharge a child from the nursery before a detailed evaluation is done. In most cases, a complete diagnosis, assignment of the sex of rearing, and a plan for future treatment can be accomplished before discharge.

B. **Medical management in the neonatal period and early infancy**
1. **Congenital adrenal hyperplasia.** The most immediate concern in a neonate with abnormal genitalia is whether CAH is present. The onset of adrenal insufficiency occurs between days 3 and 14 in 50% of affected patients. All forms of adrenal hyperplasia have absolute or relative cortisol deficiency and require early diagnosis and replacement therapy to prevent potential life-threatening complications such as vascular collapse.
   a. **Glucocorticoid therapy** should be initiated as soon as possible. Maintenance cortisol replacement therapy is often given orally. **Hydrocortisone** is the oral preparation of choice. (See Chapter 132.) Initial doses usually range from 10–20 mg/m²/day given as three divided doses and often require adjustments for growth and during periods of stress. Alternatively, intramuscular **cortisone acetate** is sometimes used in children <6 months of age out of concern that oral hydrocortisone may be absorbed erratically in these infants. Supervision of replacement therapy and long-term follow-up with a pediatric endocrinologist is advised; institutional practices may vary.
   b. **Mineralocorticoid therapy.** Fludrocortisone acetate at a dose of 0.05–0.1 mg daily (given orally) is often used. Unlike hydrocortisone, the dose of fludrocortisone does not change with increase of body size or during stress. Some endocrinologists also recommend sodium supplementation (1–5 mEq/kg/day).
2. **Incompletely virilized genetic male.** Treatment with **depo-testosterone** might be considered by the team of specialists depending on the results of the diagnostic evaluation.

IX. **Prognosis, gender assignment, long-term care.** Discussion surrounding issues of gender assignment are beyond the scope of this manual. In general, the sex of rearing should be determined only after diagnostic evaluation by a specialist team. In the past, gender assignment had been approached as though individuals are psychosexually neutral at birth and as though healthy psychosexual development is related to the appearance of the external genitals. However, these beliefs have been challenged. It is now believed that prenatal and early exposure of the brain to androgens, if present, influences gender-specific behavioral patterns and sexual identity in addition to the external appearance of the genitalia or their future function. Considering the significance of the decision for the affected patient's emotional, physical, and reproductive health, a highly specialized multidisciplinary team of pediatricians, urologists, endocrinologists, geneticists, psychiatrists, and others is needed, and each case must be approached individually. Specialized treatment centers should provide long-term care to optimize prognosis. The Consortium on Disorders of Sex Development maintains a website with clinical guidelines and information for families (www.dsdguidelines.org) as do many other support groups such as the Intersex Society of North America (www.isna.org), the Congenital Adrenal Hyperplasia Support and Education (CARES) Foundation (www.caresfoundation.org), and others.

Selected References

Al-Alwan I et al: Clinical utility of adrenal ultrasonography in the diagnosis of congenital hyperplasia. *J Pediatr* 1999;135:71.

American Academy of Pediatrics Committee on Genetics: Evaluation of the newborn with developmental anomalies of the external genitalia. *Pediatrics* 2000;106(1):138-141.

American Academy of Pediatrics Section on Urology: Timing of elective surgery on the genitalia of male children with particular reference to the risks, benefits, and psychological effects of surgery and anesthesia. *Pediatrics* 1996;97:590-594.

Cheng PK, Chanoine JP: Should the definition of micropenis vary according to ethnicity? *Horm Res* 2001;55:278-281.

Clayton PE et al: Consensus statement on 21-hydroxylase deficiency from the European Society for paediatric endocrinology and the Lawson Wilkins pediatric endocrine society. *Horm Res* 2002;58:188-195.

Diamond M, Sigmundson HK: Management of intersexuality: guidelines for dealing with persons with ambiguous genitalia. *Arch Pediatr Adolesc Med* 1997;151:1046.

Diamond M, Sigmundson HK: Sex reassignment at birth: long-term review and clinical implications. *Arch Pediatr Adolesc Med* 1997;151:298.

Donahoe PK, Schnitzer JJ: Evaluation of the infant who has ambiguous genitalia, and principles of operative management. *Semin Pediatr Surg* 1996;5:30.

Fletcher MA: The chest, abdomen, genitalia, perineum and back. In Fletcher MA (ed): *Physical Diagnosis in Neonatology*. Philadelphia, PA: Lippincott-Raven, 1998.

Gooren LJ: Androgen-resistance syndromes: considerations of gender assignment. *Curr Ther Endocrinol Metab* 1997;6:380.

Grumbach MM et al: Disorders of sexual differentiation. In Larsen PR et al (eds): *Williams' Textbook of Endocrinology*, 10th ed. Philadelphia, PA: Saunders, 2003.

Hernanz-Schulman M et al: Sonographic findings in infants with congenital adrenal hyperplasia. *Pediatr Radiol* 2002;32:130.

Houk CP et al: Summary of consensus statement on intersex disorders and their management. International Intersex Consensus Conference. *Pediatrics* 2006;118(2):753-757.

Hughes IA: Congenital adrenal hyperplasia: 21-hydroxylase deficiency in the newborn and during infancy. *Semin Reprod Med* 2002;20(3):229-242.

Hughes IA: Disorders of sex development: a new definition and classification. *Best Pract Res Clin Endocrinol Metab* 2008;22(1):119-134.

Hyun G, Kolon TF: A practical approach to intersex in the newborn period. *Urol Clin North Am* 2004;31(3):435-443.

Lee MM, Donahoe PK: The infant with ambiguous genitalia. *Curr Ther Endocrinol Metab* 1997;6:216.

Lee PA: A perspective on the approach to the intersex child born with genital ambiguity. *J Pedatr Endocrinol Metab* 2004;17(2):133-140.

Lee PA et al; International Consensus Conference on Intersex: Consensus statement on management of intersex disorders. *Pediatrics* 2006;118(2):e488-e500.

Low Y, Hutson JM; Murdoch Children's Research Institute Sex Study Group: Rules for clinical diagnosis in babies with ambiguous genitalia. *J Paediatr Child Health* 2003;38(6):406-413.

Diamond DA: Sexual differentiation: normal and abnormal. In Wein A et al (eds): *Campbell-Walsh Urology*, 9th ed. Philadelphia, PA: Saunders, 2007.

Ogilvy-Stewart AL, Brain CE: Early assessment of ambiguous genitalia. *Arch Dis Child* 2004;89(5):401-407.

Rangecroft L; British Association of Paediatric Surgeons Working Party on the Surgical Management of Children Born With Ambiguous Genitalia: Surgical management of ambiguous genitalia. *Arch Dis Child* 2003;88(9):799-801.

Reiner WG: Assignment of sex in neonates with ambiguous genitalia. *Current Opin Pediatr* 1999;11:363.

Schober JM: Quality-of-life studies in patients with ambiguous genitalia. *World J Urol* 1999;17:249.

Tuladhar R et al: Establishment of a normal range of penile length in preterm infants. *J Paediatr Child Health* 1998;34:471-473.

Warne G et al: A long-term outcome study of intersex conditions. *J Pediatr Endocrinol Metab* 2005;18:555-567.

Zaontz MR, Packer MG: Abnormalities of the external genitalia. *Pediatr Clin North Am* 1997;44:1267.

83 Enteroviruses and Parechoviruses

I. **Definition.** Enteroviruses are a large group of viral pathogens represented by two genera of the family Picornaviridae. They are all of a single strand of RNA in a capsid of individually distinct polypeptides. The capsid proteins impart antigenicity and facilitate transfer of RNA into the cells of newly infected hosts.

The genus of **enteroviruses** contains five subgroups of species, each with well-known human infant pathogenicity. They are coxsackieviruses A and B, enteroviruses, echoviruses, and poliovirus. Within each subgroup many numbered subspecies exist, for example, 24 coxsackieviruses A, 6 coxsackieviruses B, 34 echoviruses, 5 enteroviruses, and the polioviruses (types 1, 2, and 3).

The genus of human **parechoviruses** is made up of two species (types 1 and 2). They were formerly thought to be human enteroviruses 22 and 23, but following the discovery of capsid proteins distinctly different from those of the genus enterovirus, they have been relegated to a single genus.

II. **Incidence.** Enteroviruses are of worldwide distribution and produce human illness of varying severity, from mild coryza to life-threatening multisystem disease. The diseases have some seasonal variation such as summer-fall in temperate zones but of little variation in the more tropical regions of the world.

Of special interest to neonatologists is the now well-established enteroviral transplacental passage, enteroviruses detected in breast milk, and vertical passage of enteroviruses within first-degree family members without clinical signs of illness. Enteroviral illnesses are transmitted by the oral to fecal route and, to a lesser extent, respiratory droplets. Incubation periods are typically 3–6 days. All subgroups of enteroviruses are linked to nursery and NICU outbreaks of enteroviral diseases.

Numerous outbreaks of nonpolio neonatal enterovirus have been reported for newborn nurseries, NICUs, and maternity units over the past three decades. Overall incidence for newborn and neonatal infants is variable, but one report gave an incidence of all neonatal nonpolio enteroviral diseases in 666 infants cultured sequentially in the summer and fall 1981 as 12.8%. More specifically, the Centers for Disease Control and Prevention (CDC) have reported from the National Enterovirus Surveillance System (NESS), 1983–2003, that neonatal enteroviral illnesses accounted for 11.4% of all reports. Most common neonatal serotypes were echovirus serotype 11 (14%), and coxsackievirus serotypes B 2, 4, 5 (33.2%). Neonatal deaths were reported as 3.3%. More recently, for the year 2007, the CDC reported, through the resources of NESS, 444 cases of neonatal enterovirus infections of which 25% were identified as coxsackievirus B1.

III. **Pathophysiology.** Human enteroviruses manifest disease in nearly all body systems. Paradoxically, signs of disease can be mild to nearly nonexistent or life threatening within the same serotype. Host susceptibility seems to be the distinguishing factor. For the great majority of children and adults, enterovirus and parechovirus illnesses are mild, but for the neonate, a more susceptible host, enteroviruses and parechovirus can cause serious multiorgan dysfunction and death. Some human enteroviruses are more pathogenic than others. Examples of the more serious infections by nonpolio enterovirus serotypes are echo 11, coxsackie B3, coxsackie A9, enterovirus 71, and parechoviruses 1 and 2.

A. **Echovirus 11** has been particularly associated with neonatal fatalities. Most pathologic findings have been extensive hepatic necrosis with adrenal hemorrhage and acute tubular necrosis as less frequent additional findings.

B. **Coxsackievirus B3 (CVB3)** neonatal infections have been marked by hepatitis, disseminated intravascular infection, fever, thrombocytopenia, and intracranial hemorrhage. CVB3 has also been closely associated with antenatal maternal infection and positive virus cultures from placenta, cord, and infant tissues at death. All circumstances suggested transplacental viral passage.

C. **Coxsackie A9**, although much less common than CVB3, has a more protean spectrum of neonatal morbidity. It may present as aseptic meningitis, a nonspecific sepsis-like illness, myocarditis, pneumonia, or disseminated intravascular coagulation.

D. **Enterovirus 71** has been less frequently reported but has been identified with aseptic meningitis, encephalitis, acute flaccid paralysis, and acute cardiopulmonary disease. Community-wide outbreaks in 2003 and 2005 in Denver, Colorado, revealed involvement of infants 4 weeks of age and upward with most having central nervous system (CNS) disease.

E. **Parechovirus** infections are perhaps the most recently recognized cause of enteroviral-like illness in neonates. Because of its former categorization as an echovirus, its more distinct pathophysiologic elements were obscured. It is now recognized as an agent for nursery outbreaks of diarrhea coupled with respiratory illnesses. It has been associated with small clusters of patients with necrotizing enterocolitis. More specific to parechoviruses are the CNS manifestations, which include seizures and meningoencephalitis. Other conditions have included myocarditis and conjunctivitis.

IV. **Risk factors**

A. **Infants born to mothers** who have symptoms of enterovirus around the time of the delivery have a higher chance of being infected.

B. **Risk of severe infection** is higher if the infant is infected during the first 2 weeks of life.

V. **Clinical presentations.** As previously noted, the clinical presentation of nonpolio enterovirus diseases are varied and overlap with the many subspecies and serotypes. In neonates the signs that suggest an enteroviral outbreak in a nursery might include a cluster of infants with similar findings of coryza, morbilliform rash, low-grade fever, or cough. The latter is a most unusual occurrence in neonates, prompting close observation and investigation. A sepsis-like illness is frequently ascribed to enteroviral illnesses. Sepsis evaluation is often negative, but findings of lethargy, poor feeding, and fever are hallmarks suggesting sepsis.

VI. **Diagnosis.** Because of the myriad of known human enteroviruses, specific diagnostic tests have been difficult to develop. Cell culture has been the standard method for isolation and diagnosis, but specific serotype identification requires expensive neutralization assays or genomic sequencing in laboratories specializing in these test procedures. Of more practical application is polymerase chain reaction (PCR) assays for virus RNA. PCR is readily available in commercial laboratories but lacks specificity for serotyping. Advanced PCR techniques are required to further identify most enterovirus subspecies.

Specimens for cell culture or PCR assays should include cerebrospinal fluid, blood, urine, nasal swabs, throat swabs, and stool specimens.

VII. **Management.** No specific therapy for human enteroviruses exists. Overall care involves supportive measures, close observation for organ-specific disease (eg, meningitis, myocarditis), and diagnostic testing to confirm infection. In cases of severe neonatal disease, high-dose human immune globulin has been suggested, but depending on antibody per lot of immune globulin, efficacy varies. Observation for bacterial colonization and secondary infection is appropriate, especially for staphylococcal disease. If fulminate hepatic disease is present, oral neomycin therapy to minimize gut flora may be beneficial.

VIII. **Prognosis.** The illness is usually mild and recoverable. Mortality is increased with the more severe forms of the infection.

Selected References

American Academy of Pediatrics: Enteroviruses (nonpolio) infections: Group A and B coxsackieviruses, echoviruses, and numbered enteroviruses. In Pickering LK et al (eds): *Red Book: 2006 Report of the Committee on Infectious Diseases*, 27th ed. Elk Grove Village, IL: American Academy of Pediatrics, 2006:284-285.

Centers for Disease Control and Prevention: Increased detections and severe neonatal disease associated with coxsackievirus B1 infection–United States, 2007. *MMWR Morb Mortal Wkly Rep* 2008:57:553-536.

Cheng LL et al: Probable intrafamilial transmission of coxsackievirus B3 with vertical transmission, severe early onset neonatal hepatitis, and prolonged viral RNA shedding. *Pediatrics* 2006;118:e929-e933.

Cherry JD: Enteroviruses and parechoviruses. In Remington JS et al (eds): *Infectious Diseases of the Fetus and Newborn Infant*, 6th ed. Philadelphia, PA: Elsevier Saunders, 2006:783-822.

Khetsuriani N et al: Neonatal enterovirus infections reported to the national enterovirus surveillance system in the United States, 1983–2003. *Pediatr Infect Dis J* 2006; 25:889-893.

Ouellet A et al: Antenatal diagnosis of intrauterine infection with coxsackievirus B3 associated with live birth. *Infect Dis Obstet Gynecol* 2004;12:23-26.

Perez-Velez CM et al: Outbreak of neurologic enterovirus type 71 disease: a diagnostic challenge. *Clin Infect Dis* 2007;45:950-957.

Verboon-Maciolek MA et al: Severe neonatal parechovirus infection and similarity with enterovirus infection. *Pediatr Infect Dis J* 2008;27:241-245.

84 Eye Disorders of the Newborn and Retinopathy of Prematurity

AMBLYOPIA

I. **Definition.** Amblyopia, or "lazy eye," is a reduction in vision when there is a difference in the quality of the images recorded by each eye and sent to the brain. The eyes and the brain must work in conjunction for vision to develop correctly. If the pathways to the visual cortex are not properly stimulated, the visual cortex cannot mature appropriately. Thus, when the brain selectively disregards the eye with the poor visual image, the visual system for that eye develops more slowly than for the eye that sent the good image. Vision loss ranges from mild (worse than 20/25) to severe (legal blindness, 20/200 or worse).

II. **Incidence.** Amblyopia is a major public health problem with the estimated prevalence of 1–4% in the United States. The condition affects approximately 2 to 3 out of every 100 children. Amblyopia was shown in the Visual Acuity Impairment Survey sponsored by the National Eye Institute (2004) to be the leading cause of monocular vision loss in adults 20–70 years of age.

III. **Pathophysiology.** Amblyopia may be caused by any condition that affects normal visual development or use of the eyes. Animal studies and clinical studies in infants and young children support the concept of a critical period during infancy and childhood for developing amblyopia. The developing brain is sensitive, and amblyopia may occur as early as the first few weeks of life. There are three general etiologies for amblyopia in the neonate.

   A. **Strabismus.** Strabismus, the preference of one eye when the visual axes are misaligned, is the most common contributing factor. Small, intermittent deviations commonly seen in many infants are rarely associated with amblyopia. This type of divergence decreases with time, as visual acuity and binocularity develop. Amblyopia develops in a consistently deviating eye whether it is from esotropia, exotropia, or hypertropia. This can be recognized in the first few months of life after the newborn period.

B. **Refractive errors.** Refractive errors, the second most common cause of amblyopia, can be difficult to detect. Amblyopia resulting from refractive errors can be divided into two types: anisometropic and isometropic. Anisometropic amblyopia results from significant inequality of the refractive errors in each eye, blunting the development of the visual pathway in the affected eye. Bilateral hyperopia (farsightedness) is the most common refractive error to cause amblyopia. Severe unilateral hyperopia, myopia (nearsightedness), and astigmatism also may cause profound vision loss. Isometric amblyopia occurs when the refractive errors in the two eyes are equal. Severe refractive errors in both eyes can cause isometropic amblyopia that is bilateral.

C. **Deprivation.** The least common condition, congenital or early-acquired opacity, causes deprivation amblyopia. This can be the most severe and damaging type. Cataracts, corneal lesions, or ptosis block or distort the retinal image formation. This can affect one or both eyes and may develop as early as 2–4 months. It is critical that these be diagnosed and treated as early as possible.

IV. **Risk factors.** These include low birthweight, prematurity, familial factors, and certain congenital anterior lens opacities with significant anisometropia.

V. **Clinical presentation.** Diagnosis is made during the newborn or early infant eye examination or when there is evidence of reduced visual acuity that cannot be explained by physical abnormalities. Opacities, structural eye pathology such as optic nerve lesions, and abnormalities of central visual pathways must be excluded.

VI. **Management.** Treatment is individualized depending on the cause. The treatment for strabismus is patching of the preferred eye or surgical correction. Refractive amblyopia is treated with patching or glasses. Surgical interventions are needed for deprivation amblyopia.

VII. **Prognosis.** Most vision loss from amblyopia is preventable or reversible with the right intervention for the individual etiology. The recovery depends on the maturity of the visual connections, the length of deprivation, and the age at which therapy is begun. Early diagnosis is optimal.

ANOPHTHALMOS/MICROPHTHALMOS

Anophthalmos is an eye that cannot be found on a routine examination. In cases of anophthalmos, a rudimentary eye may be seen on MRI, CT scan, or ultrasound. **Microphthalmos** is described as an eye with a corneal diameter <9 mm in a term birth. Colobomas and persistent fetal vasculature are frequently associated with microphthalmos.

COLOBOMA

Coloboma is a developmental gap generally located inferiorly in the eye. A coloboma can be recognized as an inferior "keyhole" notch in the pupil caused by missing iris tissue, which does not affect vision. A coloboma can also include the optic nerve, macula, and other parts of the retina, which result in legal blindness. Colobomas are also an integral finding in CHARGE (*c*oloboma, *h*eart defects, *a*tresia choanae, *r*etarded growth, *g*enital hypoplasia, and *e*ar anomalies) association.

CONGENITAL CATARACTS

I. **Definition.** A nonspecific reaction to a change in the lens metabolism leading to lens opacification. Cataracts are one of the main treatable causes of visual impairment in infancy.

II. **Incidence.** Estimates are 1.2–6.0 cases per 10,000 in the United States. About 25% of cataracts are hereditary; the most frequent mode of transmission is autosomal dominant. About a third are sporadic.

III. **Pathophysiology.** Any process that alters the glycolytic pathway or epithelial cell mitosis of the avascular lens causes cataracts.

A. **Metabolic causes** include hypoglycemia, mannosidosis, hypoparathyroidism, maternal diabetes, galactosemia, hypocalcemia, and vitamin A or D deficiency.

B. **Cataracts** may be seen with **congenital infections** such as rubella, herpes simplex, and varicella.

C. **Other causes** include *in utero* radiation exposure and associations with specific syndromes (trisomy 21, Stickler, Smith-Lemli-Opitz).

IV. **Risk factors.** See pathophysiology.

V. **Clinical presentation.** The newborn infant presents with a white pupillary reflex or leukocoria. Cataracts lead to varying degrees of visual impairment from blurred vision to blindness depending on the extent of the opacity and the location. Cataracts in neonates may be transient and disappear spontaneously in several weeks. Lens opacities in infants may be isolated or associated with other eye anomalies or systemic conditions. The cataracts seen with congenital rubella are characteristically total or near-total opacities in a smaller than normal lens. Abnormalities of the retinal pigment, "salt and pepper" changes, are typically seen.

VI. **Diagnosis.** The initial workup would consider the many causes and associations. Maternal and infant history would direct laboratory evaluation. An irregular red reflex suggests a congenital cataract might be present. Ophthalmologic slit lamp confirms the presence of a cataract and may be able to identify the time when the insult occurred in utero.

VII. **Management.** If the cataract directly threatens vision, then **prompt** surgical removal is indicated to avoid legal blindness from deprivation amblyopia. Infants will require significant visual rehabilitation.

A. **Optical devices** are used to provide focus after the lost lens. Contact lenses are used early. Parents are taught to insert and remove the lens.

B. **Occlusion therapy** of the better eye to reverse amblyopia may be necessary. The amount of time per day for occlusion remains *controversial*.

VIII. **Prognosis.** There can be a high association of significant genetic anomalies with cataracts especially if they are bilateral. Genetic counseling is suggested. There is the potential for long-term visual loss directly from the glaucoma or secondary to amblyopia or retinal detachment.

CONGENITAL GLAUCOMA

I. **Definition.** Increased ocular pressure in the aqueous humor (anterior fluid of the eye) that eventually causes damage to the optic nerve and permanent loss of vision if not treated.

II. **Incidence.** It is estimated to affect <0.05% of patients.

III. **Pathophysiology.** Primary congenital glaucoma is caused by structural abnormalities of the eye drainage channels, the trabecular meshwork. These are typically autosomal recessive and present at birth. Secondary causes such as retinopathy of prematurity, aniridia, persistent fetal vasculature, homocystinuria, congenital rubella syndrome, and numerous syndromes present after the neonatal period with symptoms similar to those of primary glaucoma.

IV. **Risk factors.** Boys are at greater risk than girls, except in Japan where it is reversed. Up to 10% can have a family history of glaucoma.

V. **Clinical presentation.** Clinically, photophobia, lacrimation, buphthalmos, and eye rubbing are typical.

VI. **Diagnosis.** The diagnosis is made by measuring intraocular pressure.

VII. **Management.** Periodic monitoring of ocular pressure and vision is necessary. Infants usually require surgery to increase drainage.

VIII. **Prognosis.** The sooner the treatment, the better the outcome. If left untreated, there is increased risk for blindness.

CORNEAL OPACITIES

Corneal opacity is a generic description for an opacified lens and associated with a wide variety of etiologies.

I. Congenital glaucoma.
II. Persistent fetal vasculature.
III. Birth trauma (forceps). This usually clears in a few days but may leave corneal scarring in the visual axis or may induce significant refractive error, which leads to poor vision.
IV. Sclerocornea is a nonprogressive, usually bilateral, anomaly where the cornea is replaced by an opaque sclera-like tissue, which is devastating to vision.
V. Dermoid tumors of the cornea may affect vision if located centrally. If the tumors are located peripherally, they can induce a refractive error. These may be isolated or part of Goldenhar syndrome.
VI. Peter anomaly is characterized by central corneal opacity and variable iris-corneal or lens-corneal adhesions. This is uncommon but a frequent cause of corneal transplants in infants. The periphery of the cornea is usually normal. This has an association with fetal alcohol syndrome. Corneal surgery is often reserved for bilateral cases because the prognosis for good vision following even initially successful corneal transplantation is guarded. In unilateral cases, poor vision is expected because of amblyopia in the affected eye.

NASOLACRIMAL DUCT OBSTRUCTION

A congenital obstruction caused by an imperforate membrane at the end of the nasolacrimal duct. This is the most common abnormality of the lacrimal apparatus and is found in 2–6% of all newborns. Symptoms are usually seen within the first few weeks of life. Persistent tearing, crusting or matting of the eyelids, and spilling of tears in absence of conjunctival infection are classic signs of obstruction. There also may be mucopurulent material refluxing from the punctum when pressure is placed over the lacrimal sac. Acute dacryocystitis or orbital or facial cellulitis may be secondary complications.

Initially, conservative management consists of application of warm soaks and daily massage of the nasolacrimal sac in an attempt to rupture the membrane. If mucopurulent discharge is noted, ophthalmic antibiotics may be administered. Conservative management is recommended for the first year of life because the majority of these obstructions resolve spontaneously or with massage. Tear duct probing may surgically treat unresolved obstructions.

RETINOPATHY OF PREMATURITY

I. Definitions
   A. **Retinopathy of prematurity (ROP)** is a disorder of the developing retinal vasculature resulting from interruption of normal progression of newly forming retinal vessels. Vasoconstriction and obliteration of the advancing capillary bed are followed in succession by neovascularization extending into the vitreous, retinal edema, retinal hemorrhages, fibrosis, and traction on, and eventual detachment of, the retina. In most cases, the process is reversed before fibrosis occurs. **Advanced stages may lead to blindness.**
   B. **Retrolental fibroplasia (RLF).** As originally described, the condition was seen only in its most advanced form, after extensive fibrosis and scarring had already occurred behind the lens. It was, therefore, termed *retrolental fibroplasia*. It is now understood that several recognizable changes occur in the developing vasculature before end-stage fibrosis occurs, making this condition a true retinopathy. Because it is found chiefly in premature infants, it is called *retinopathy of prematurity*.
   C. **Cicatricial ROP.** The term *cicatricial ROP* refers to fibrotic disease.
II. **Incidence.** ROP represents ~20% of blindness in preschool children in the United States. Of particular concern are the increasing numbers of survivors weighing <1000 g who have the highest incidence of ROP. The U.S. National Institutes of Health (NIH) sponsored the Cryotherapy for Retinopathy of Prematurity (CRYO-ROP) study in 1986–1987, which showed that 65.8% of infants weighing <1251 g developed ROP of any stage. Two percent of infants weighing 1000–1250 g developed threshold stage

III+ disease eligible for treatment, whereas 15.5% of infants weighing <750 g did so. **Threshold disease occurred at a median postconceptional age of 36–37 weeks, regardless of gestational age at birth or chronologic age.** A study of earlier treatment, the ETROP (Early Treatment for Retinopathy of Prematurity) study, carried out in 2002, showed little difference in the overall incidence of the disorder and time of onset from the earlier CRYO-ROP study. The International NO-ROP Group, however, published data in 2005 suggesting that severe ROP in larger infants is an emerging worldwide issue.

III. Pathophysiology

   A. **Historical perspective.** RLF was first described by Terry in the 1940s and was associated with the use of oxygen in newborn infants by Patz in 1984. The **first epidemic,** estimated to be responsible for 30% of cases of blindness in preschool children by the end of the 1940s, occurred during a period of relatively liberal oxygen administration. After this association was recognized, oxygen use in nurseries was curtailed. Although the incidence of RLF fell, mortality rates in newborn infants increased. In the 1960s, improved oxygen monitoring techniques made possible the cautious reintroduction of oxygen into the nursery. Despite improved oxygen monitoring, however, a **second epidemic** of RLF (ROP) appeared in the late 1970s and is associated with the increased survival of very low birthweight infants.

   B. **Normal embryology of the eye.** In the normally developing retina, there are no retinal vessels until about 16 weeks' gestation. Until then, oxygen diffuses from the underlying choroidal circulation. At 16 weeks, in response to a stimulus (experimental evidence suggests relative hypoxia *stimulating the release of angiogenic factors* as the retina thickens), cells derived from mesenchyme traveling in the nerve fiber layer emanate from the optic nerve head. These cells are the precursors of the retinal vascular system. A fine capillary network advances through the retina to the ora serrata, or retinal edge. More mature vessels form behind this advancing network. Vascularization on the nasal side of the ora serrata is complete at about 8 months gestation, whereas that on the temporal side is ordinarily complete at term. Once it is completely vascularized, the retinal vasculature is no longer susceptible to insults of the type that lead to ROP.

   C. Causes

      1. **There appear to be two phases in the development of ROP:**

         a. **Early vasoconstriction and obliteration of the capillary network** in response to high oxygen concentrations noted experimentally or another vascular insult.

         b. **Vasoproliferation,** which follows the period of high oxygen exposure or insult, perhaps in response to angiogenic factors released by the hypoxic retina. Considerable evidence has been developed to support this hypothesis. Phelps and Rosenbaum studied kittens made hyperoxic and then allowed to recover in room air (21% oxygen) or 13% oxygen. Those recovering in the hypoxic environment had worse retinopathy than those recovering in room air, suggesting that retinal hypoxia may play a role. *In vitro,* an angiogenic factor, vascular endothelial cell growth factor (VEGF), is produced in the hypoxic retina. Evidence suggests that it plays an important role in ROP. Lofqvist and Smith have published data suggesting that insulin-like growth factor 1 and IGF binding protein 3 are important modulators of ROP.

IV. **Risk factors.** The association of ROP with oxygen alone is not so clear. Transient hyperoxemia alone is not considered sufficient. Many other factors, such as extreme prematurity, maternal complications, apnea, sepsis, hyper- and hypocapnia, vitamin E deficiency, intraventricular hemorrhage, anemia, exchange transfusion, hypoxia, lactic acidosis, bright light, and possibly early erythropoietin use have been implicated. The pathophysiology of ROP is still unclear. Experimental studies have focused chiefly on the role of oxygen, and oxygen monitoring is an important part of the care of the premature infant, although **extreme prematurity is known to be the most significant risk factor.**

V. **Clinical presentation.** Several methods of classification of ROP have been used. With development of the **International Classification of ROP,** there is general agreement on the staging of active disease.

- **Stage I:** A thin demarcation line develops between the vascularized region of the retina and the avascular zone.
- **Stage II:** This line develops into a ridge protruding into the vitreous.
- **Stage III:** Extraretinal fibrovascular proliferation occurs with the ridge. Neovascular tufts may be found just posterior to the ridge (Figure 84–1).
- **Stage IV:** Fibrosis and scarring occur as the neovascularization extends into the vitreous. Traction occurs on the retina, resulting in partial retinal detachment.
- **Stage V:** Complete retinal detachment.
- **Plus disease:** (eg, stage III+) may occur when vessels posterior to the ridge become dilated and tortuous.
- **Pre plus disease:** Dilation and tortuosity of posterior pole vessels in zone 1; less severe than plus disease.
- **Aggressive posterior ROP (AP-ROP):** Rapidly progressive ROP primarily zone 1.

VI. **Diagnosis. Ophthalmoscopic examination** by an experienced examiner usually confirms the diagnosis. A 2006 joint statement by the American Academy of Pediatrics, American Association for Pediatric Ophthalmology and Strabismus, and American Academy of Ophthalmology provided updated recommendations for ROP screening examinations in premature infants. These recommendations are evolving and may change as longer-term ROP outcomes are recognized.

A. **Infants weighing ≤1500 g or ≤30 weeks' gestation** and those weighing >1500 g with an unstable clinical course should have dilated eye examinations starting at 4–6 weeks of age or 31–33 weeks postmenstrual age. Examinations should continue every 2–3 weeks until retinal maturity is reached, if no disease is present.

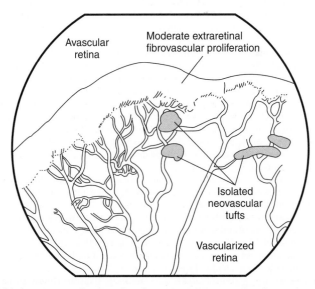

Avascular retina

Moderate extraretinal fibrovascular proliferation

Isolated neovascular tufts

Vascularized retina

FIGURE 84–1. Schematic drawing of moderate stage III retinopathy of prematurity. Optic nerve head is shown at the bottom, and periphery of the retina is at the top. *(Reproduced, with permission, from Garner A: International classification of retinopathy of prematurity.* Pediatrics *1984;74:127.)*

B. Infants with ROP or very immature vessels should be examined every 1–2 weeks until vessels are mature or the risk of threshold disease has passed. Those at greatest risk should be examined every week.

VII. Management

A. **Circumferential cryopexy** has been proven to be an effective treatment for progressive (stage III+) disease in an attempt to prevent further progression by destroying cells that may be releasing angiogenic factors. Results of the large collaborative NIH-sponsored trial indicate that cryopexy carried out at stage III+ can reduce the incidence of severe visual impairment by ~50% if performed within 72 h of detecting threshold disease. Although myopia is a common feature of ROP, 10-year follow-up shows significant improvement in visual acuity of treated versus control eyes. It is imperative that an ophthalmologist skilled in cryopexy perform the procedure.

B. **Laser photocoagulation.** Data suggest that this technique is equally effective yet safer than cryopexy. In 1994, the Laser ROP Study Group was formed to carry out a meta-analysis of four laser-ROP trials. Treatment was based on the same criteria used in the CRYO-ROP trial. Recognizing the limitations of a meta-analysis, the study group concluded that laser therapy is at least as effective as cryotherapy for ROP, despite a small risk of cataract formation. Ten-year follow-up of a small group of patients suggests better outcomes with laser photocoagulation. More recently, the ETROP study (2002) demonstrated improved outcomes with treatment at any stage when plus disease is present.

C. **Oxygen for treatment of ROP.** In an attempt to reduce angiogenic factors from the hypoxic retina and the progression of ROP from prethreshold to threshold (III+) levels, oxygen therapy was attempted in a large collaborative trial, the Supplemental Therapeutic Oxygen for Prethreshold Retinopathy of Prematurity (STOP-ROP) study. Oxygen saturations were targeted at 96–99% in the treatment group and 89–94% in the conventional group once prethreshold ROP was diagnosed. No significant difference was seen in the rate of progression to threshold disease between the two groups, although there was a significant increase in chronic lung disease in the high saturation group. The appropriate saturation ranges remain *controversial* and under study, although most neonatal intensive care units keep infants <1250 g at saturations <95% when in supplemental oxygen.

D. **Vitamin E.** The administration of pharmacologic doses of vitamin E for ROP has been studied with no proof of clear benefit. Reported side effects include sepsis, necrotizing enterocolitis, and intraventricular hemorrhage. Even so, maintenance of normal serum vitamin E levels is a prudent management objective. (See Chapter 132.)

E. **Decreased lighting intensity.** A prospective, randomized, multicenter trial of 409 premature infants weighing <1251 g and 31 weeks gestation concluded that a reduction in ambient light exposure does not alter the incidence of ROP.

F. **Additional experimental therapies** include VEGF receptor blockers. Data are limited. Further work is needed.

G. **Retinal reattachment.** Stage IV disease has been treated by attempts at retinal reattachment without significant success to date. Reattachment of late retinal detachments in childhood has met with more success.

H. **Vitrectomy** has not substantially improved the outcome in cicatricial disease.

I. **Follow-up eye examinations** are advocated every 1–2 years for infants with fully regressed ROP and every 6–12 months for those with cicatricial ROP. Premature infants are at risk for myopia even in the absence of ROP and should have an eye examination by 6 months of age.

VIII. Prognosis.
Ninety percent of cases of stage I and stage II disease regress spontaneously. Current information suggests that ~50% of cases of stage III+ disease regress spontaneously. Of those that do progress to stage III+, the incidence of unfavorable structural outcomes can be reduced by ~50% and unfavorable visual outcomes by ~30% if circumferential cryopexy is carried out by a skilled ophthalmologist. Laser photocoagulation

appears equally and possibly more effective than cryopexy. Sequelae of regressed disease such as myopia, strabismus, amblyopia, glaucoma, and late detachment require regular follow-up.

Selected References

Common Newborn Eye Disorders

Amaya L: The morphology and natural history of congenital cataracts. *Surv Ophthalmol* 2003;48:125.

Berk AT: Ocular and systemic findings associated with optic disc colobomas. *J Pediatr Ophthalmol Strabismus* 2003;40:272.

Donahue R: Pediatric strabismus. *N Engl J Med* 2007;356:1040.

Haddad MA: Causes of visual impairment in children: a study of 3,210 cases. *J Pediatr Ophthalmol Strabismus* 2007;44:232.

Lloyd IC: Advances in the management of congenital and infantile cataract. *Eye* 2007;21:1307.

Muir KW: Central corneal thickness: congenital cataracts and aphakia. *Am J Ophthalmol* 2007;144:502.

National Eye Institute: Amblyopia. Available at: www.nei.nih.gov/health/amblyopia.

Olitsky S: Diagnosis and treatment of lacrimal duct obstruction. *J Pediatr Ophthalmol Strabismus* 2007;44:80.

Powell C et al: Screening for correctable visual acuity deficits in school-age children and adolescents. *Cochrane Database Syst Rev* 2005;1:CD005023.

Roche O et al: Nonpenetrating external trabeculectomy for congenital glaucoma—a retrospective study. *Ophthalmology* 2007;114:1994.

Sanlaville D, Verlies A: CHARGE syndrome: an update. *Eur J Hum Genet* 2007;15:389.

U.S. Preventative Services Task Force: Screening for visual impairment in children younger than age 5 years. Update of the evidence form randomized controlled trials, 1999-2003. Rockville, MD: Agency for Healthcare Research and Quality, 2004. Accessed at: http://www.ahrq.gov/clinic/3rduspstf/visionscr/vischup.htm.

Williams C et al: Amblyopia treatment outcome after screening before or at age 3 years: follow up from randomized trial. *BMJ* 2002;324:1459.

Retinopathy of Prematurity

Adamis AP et al: Inhibition of VEGF prevents ocular neovascularization in a primate. *Arch Ophthalmol* 1996;114:6671.

Aher SM, Ohlsson A: Early versus late erythropoietin for preventing red blood cell transfusion in preterm and/or low birth weight infants. *Cochrane Database Syst Rev* 2006;3:CD004865.

American Academy of Pediatrics, Section on Ophthalmology; American Academy of Ophthalmology; American Association for Pediatric Ophthalmology and Strabismus: Screening examination of premature infants for retinopathy of prematurity. *Pediatrics* 2006;117:572-576 and Erratum, *Pediatrics* 2006;118(3):1324.

American Academy of Pediatrics and American College of Obstetrics and Gynecology: In Lockwood C, Lemons J (eds): *Guidelines for Perinatal Care*, 6th ed. Atlanta, GA: ACOG, 2007:262-264.

Cryotherapy for Retinopathy of Prematurity Cooperative Group: Multicenter trial of cryotherapy for retinopathy of prematurity: three-month outcome. *Arch Ophthalmol* 1990;108:195.

Cryotherapy for Retinopathy of Prematurity Cooperative Group: Multicenter trial of cryotherapy for retinopathy of prematurity: ophthalmological outcomes at 10 years. *Arch Ophthalmol* 2001;119:1110.

Early Treatment for Retinopathy of Prematurity Cooperative Group: The incidence and course of retinopathy of prematurity: findings from the Early Treatment for Retinopathy of Prematurity study. *Pediatrics* 2005;116 (1):15-23.

Flynn JT: Retinopathy of prematurity. *Pediatr Clin North Am* 1987;34:1847.

Garner A: International classification of retinopathy of prematurity. *Pediatrics* 1984;74:127.

Gilbert C et al: Characteristics of infants with severe retinopathy of prematurity in countries with low, moderate, and high levels of development: implications for screening programs. *Pediatrics* 2005;115:e518-e525.

Good WV for the Early Treatment for Retinopathy of Prematurity Cooperative Group: Final Results of the Early Treatment for Retinopathy of Prematurity (ETROP) Randomized Trial. *Trans Am Opthalmol Soc* 2004;102:233-250.

International Committee for the Classification of Retinopathy of Prematurity. The international classification of retinopathy of prematurity revisited. *Arch Ophthalmol.* 2005;123:991-999.

Laser ROP Study Group: Laser therapy for retinopathy of prematurity. *Arch Ophthalmol* 1994;112:154.

Lofqvist C et al: IGFBP3 suppresses retinopathy through suppression of oxygen-induced vessel loss and promotion of vascular regrowth. *PNAS* 2007;104(25):10589-10594.

Lutty GA et al: Proceedings of the Third International Symposium on Retinopathy of Prematurity: an update on ROP from the lab to the nursery (November 2003, Anaheim, California. *Molecular Vision* 2006;12:532-580.

Ng E et al: A comparison of laser photocoagulation with cryotherapy for threshold retinopathy of prematurity at 10 years: Part 1. Visual function and structural outcome. *Ophthalmology* 2002;109:928.

Palmer EA et al: Incidence and early course of retinopathy of prematurity. *Ophthalmology* 1991;98:1628.

Phelps DL: Role of vitamin E therapy in high-risk neonates. *Clin Perinatol* 1988;15:955.

Phelps DL, Rosenbaum AL: Effects of marginal hypoxemia on recovery from oxygen-induced retinopathy in the kitten model. *Pediatrics* 1984;73:1.

Reynolds JD et al: Lack of efficacy of light reduction in preventing retinopathy of prematurity. *N Engl J Med* 1998;338:1572.

Shweiki D et al: Vascular endothelial growth factor induced by hypoxia may mediate hypoxia-initiated angiogenesis. *Nature* 1992:359:843.

STOP-ROP Multicenter Study Group: Supplemental therapeutic oxygen for prethreshold retinopathy of prematurity (STOP-ROP), a randomized, controlled trial: I. Primary outcomes. *Pediatrics* 2000;105:295.

85 Gonorrhea

I. **Definition.** Infection with ***Neisseria gonorrhoeae* (a Gram-negative diplococcus)** is a reproductive tract infection that is an important infection in pregnancy because of transmission to the fetus or neonate.

II. **Incidence.** The prevalence of gonococcus infection among pregnant women is ~1–8 in 1000. If routine ophthalmic prophylaxis was not used, it is estimated that a third of newborn infants born to infected mothers would become infected.

III. **Pathophysiology.** *N. gonorrhoeae* primarily affects the endocervical canal of the mother. The infant may become infected during passage through an infected cervical canal or by contact with contaminated amniotic fluid if rupture of membranes has occurred.

IV. **Clinical presentations**

A. **Ophthalmia neonatorum.** The most common clinical manifestation is gonococcal ophthalmia neonatorum. This occurs in 1–2% of cases of positive maternal gonococcal infection despite appropriate eye prophylaxis. For a description of this disease, see Chapter 47.

B. **Gonococcal arthritis.** The onset of gonococcal arthritis can be at any time from 1–4 weeks after delivery. It is secondary to gonococcemia. The source of bacteremia has been attributed to infection of the mouth, nares, and umbilicus. The most common sites are the knees and ankles, but any joint may be affected. The infant may present with mild or moderate symptoms. Drainage of affected joint and antibiotics are necessary.

C. **Amniotic infection syndrome** occurs when there is premature rupture of membranes, with inflammation of the placenta and umbilical cord. The infant may have clinical evidence of sepsis. This infection is associated with a high infant mortality rate.

D. **Sepsis and meningitis.**

E. **Scalp abscess** is usually secondary to intrauterine fetal monitoring.

F. **Stomatitis.**

V. **Diagnosis**

A. **Mother.** Endocervical scrapings should be obtained for culture.

B. **Infant.**

1. **Gram stain** of any exudate, if present, should be obtained.

2. **Culture.** Material may be obtained by swabbing the eye or nasopharynx or the orogastric or anorectal areas. Blood should be obtained for culture. Cultures for concomitant infection with *Chlamydia trachomatis* should also be done. Gonococcal cultures from nonsterile sites (eg, the pharynx, rectum, and vagina) should be done using selective media.

3. **Spinal fluid studies.** Cell count, protein, culture, Gram stain, and others should be ordered.

VI. **Management.** Isolation precautions for all infectious diseases, including maternal and neonatal precautions, breast-feeding, and visiting issues, can be found in Appendix F.

A. **Hospitalization.** Infants with clinical evidence of ophthalmia neonatorum, scalp abscess, or disseminated infection should be hospitalized. Complete sepsis evaluation including lumbar puncture should be performed. Tests for concomitant *C. trachomatis*, congenital syphilis, and HIV infection should be performed. Results of the maternal tests for hepatitis B surface antigen should be confirmed.

B. **Antibiotic therapy**

1. **Maternal infection.** Most infants born to mothers with gonococcal infection do not experience infection; however, because there have been some reported cases, it is recommended that full-term infants receive a single injection of ceftriaxone (125 mg intravenously [IV] or intramuscularly [IM]) and that premature infants receive 25–50 mg/kg (maximum, 125 mg).

2. **Nondisseminated infection,** including ophthalmia neonatorum, treatment is ceftriaxone (25–50 mg/kg/day IV or IM, not to exceed 125 mg) given once. Alternative treatment for ophthalmia is cefotaxime (100 mg/kg IV or IM) as a single dose. Infants with ophthalmia should have their eyes irrigated with saline immediately and at frequent intervals until the discharge is eliminated. Topical antibiotics are inadequate and unnecessary with systemic therapy. Infants with conjunctivitis should be hospitalized and evaluated for disseminated infections (sepsis, arthritis, meningitis).

3. **Disseminated infection** treatment is ceftriaxone (25–50 mg/kg IV or IM once a day for 7 days) or cefotaxime (50–100 mg/kg/day IV or IM in two divided doses for 7 days). For **meningitis,** continue treatment for 10–14 days.

C. **Isolation.** All infants with gonococcal infection should be placed in contact isolation until effective parenteral antimicrobial therapy has been given for 24 h.

VII. **Prognosis** is excellent if treatment is started early.

References

American Academy of Pediatrics: Gonococcal infections. In Pickering LK et al (eds): *Red Book: 2006 Report of the Committee on Infectious Diseases,* 27th ed. Elk Grove Village, IL: American Academy of Pediatrics, 2006:301-309.

Embree JE: Gonococcal infections. In Remington JS et al (eds): *Infectious Diseases of the Fetus and Newborn Infant.* Philadelphia, PA: Elsevier Saunders, 2006:393-401.

86 Hematuria

I. **Definition.** Hematuria is the presence of gross or microscopic blood in the urine. More than 5-10 red blood cells per high-power field (HPF) are usually considered significant. Some authors recommend two of three urinalyses show microhematuria before evaluation is undertaken. A red-stained diaper usually signifies hematuria but may be due to bile pigments, porphyrins, or urates.

II. **Incidence.** Hematuria is not a common problem in newborns. Transient hematuria is common in critically ill neonates. Normal newborns do not have hematuria.

III. **Pathophysiology.** Hematuria may originate from the glomeruli, renal tubules and interstitium, or urothelium. Common causes include:

  A. **Trauma.** Birth or iatrogenic, such as bladder aspiration or catheterization.

  B. **Vascular.** Renal vein or renal artery thrombosis, hyperosmolar infusions into umbilical catheters.

  C. **Renal.** Renal cortical or medullary necrosis, neonatal glomerulonephritis (most commonly caused by syphilis).

  D. **Infection.**

  E. **Neoplasms.** Rhabdomyosarcoma, Wilms tumor, neuroblastoma, or nephroblastoma, urinary tract obstruction (urolithiasis after Lasix administration), autosomal recessive polycystic kidney disease or infection.

  F. **Hematologic.** Coagulopathy, hemorrhagic disease of the newborn.

  G. **Perinatal asphyxia.**

IV. **Risk factors** include coagulopathy, urinary tract infection, obstruction, maternal diabetes (renal vein thrombosis), indwelling urinary catheters, umbilical artery catheter, and traumatic delivery.

V. **Clinical presentation**

  A. **History.** A maternal history of diabetes may arouse suspicion of renal vein thrombosis. The birth history and Apgar scores may suggest perinatal asphyxia. Has Vitamin K been given? (hemorrhagic disease of the newborn).The presence of an umbilical artery catheter with hematuria should immediately raise the possibility of aortic or renal artery thrombosis.

  B. **Physical examination** may reveal the presence of an abdominal mass (obstruction, neoplasm, or renal vein thrombosis). Note if an umbilical artery catheter is in place.

VI. **Diagnosis**

  A. **Laboratory studies**

    1. **Urinalysis.** Microscopic examination and dipstick testing confirm the presence of blood or other causes of "red urine." **Red blood cell casts** are seen with intrinsic renal disease such as glomerulonephritis. **Bacteria or white blood cells** suggest urinary tract infection.

2. **Urine culture.** Collection of urine by bladder aspiration or catheterization is preferred and outlined in Chapters 24 and 25.
3. **Serum urea nitrogen and creatinine levels** may reveal renal insufficiency.
4. **Coagulation studies.** Prothrombin time, partial thromboplastin time, and thrombin time may provide clues to disseminated intravascular coagulation (DIC) or hemorrhagic disease of the newborn. Thrombocytopenia suggests renal vein thrombosis.

B. **Radiologic studies**
1. **Ultrasonography** shows neoplasms, renal vein thrombosis, or obstruction in the urinary tract.
2. **Ancillary testing** such as intravenous urography, arteriography, and nuclear scans may be indicated.

VII. **Management.** Treatment is directed at the underlying cause.

VIII. **Prognosis** depends on the etiology.

Selected References

Ballard RA, Wernosky G: Clinical evaluation of renal and urinary tract disease. In Taeusch HW et al (eds): *Avery's Diseases of the Newborn*. Philadelphia, PA: Elsevier Saunders, 2005.

Meyers KE: Evaluation of hematuria in children. *Urol Clin N Am* 2004;31:559-573.

87 Hepatitis

Hepatitis may be produced by many infectious and noninfectious agents. Typically, viral hepatitis refers to several clinically similar diseases that differ in cause and epidemiology. These include hepatitis A, B, C, D (delta), E, and G. Chronic, lifelong infection has only been documented with hepatitis B virus (HBV) and hepatitis C (HCV) virus.

The differential diagnosis of a newborn liver disease includes idiopathic neonatal hepatitis (giant cell), biliary atresia, metabolic disorders, antitrypsin deficiency, cystic fibrosis, iron storage disease, and other infectious agents that cause hepatocellular injury (eg, cytomegalovirus [CMV], rubella, varicella, toxoplasmosis, *Listeria,* syphilis, and tuberculosis, as well as bacterial sepsis, which can cause nonspecific hepatic dysfunction). Table 87–1 outlines various hepatitis panel tests useful in the management of this disease. Isolation precautions for all infectious diseases, including maternal and neonatal precautions, breast-feeding, and visiting issues, can be found in Appendix F.

HEPATITIS A

I. **Definition.** Hepatitis A virus (**HAV; infectious hepatitis**) is caused by a RNA virus transmitted by the fecal-oral route. A high concentration of virus is found in stools of infected persons, especially during the late incubation and early symptomatic phases. Children, especially neonates, may excrete HAV for a more prolonged period than has been noted in adults. HAV RNA was detected in neonatal stool samples for 4–5 months in 23% of infants diagnosed with HAV infection. Incubation period is 15–50 days. There is no chronic carrier state.

II. **Incidence.** The true incidence of HAV infection in neonates is unknown. The overall incidence of HAV infection in the U.S. population decreased significantly after the introduction of HAV (26,150 cases/year from 1980–1999 to 5683 cases/year in 2004).

Table 87–1. HEPATITIS TESTING

Specific Test	Description
HAV	Etiologic agent of "infectious" hepatitis
Anti-HAV	Detectable at onset of symptoms; lifetime persistence
Anti-HAV-IgM	Indicates recent infection with HAV; positive up to 4–6 months postinfection
Anti-HAV-IgG	Signifies previous HAV infection; confers immunity
HBV	Etiologic agent of "serum" hepatitis
HBsAg	Detectable in serum; earliest indicator of acute infection or indicative of chronic infection if present >6 months
Anti-HBs	Indicates past infection with and immunity to HBV, passive antibody from HBIG, or immune response from HBV vaccine
HBeAg	Correlates with HBV replication; high-titer HBV in serum signifies high infectivity; persistence for 6–8 weeks suggests a chronic carrier state
Anti-HBe	Presence in carrier of HBsAg suggests a lower titer of HBV and resolution of infection
HBcAg	No commercial test available; found only in liver tissue
Anti-HBc	High titer indicates active HBV infection; low titer presents in chronic infection
Anti-HBc-IgM	Recent infection with HBV positive for 4–6 months after infection; detectable in "window" period after surface antigen disappears
Anti-HBc-IgG	Appears later and may persist for years if viral replication continues
HVC	Etiologic agent of hepatitis C
Anti-HCV	Serologic determinant of hepatitis C infection

IgM and IgG, immunoglobulins M and G; HAV, hepatitis A virus; anti-HAV, antibody to HAV (IgM and IgG sub-classes); anti-HAV-IgM, IgM class antibody to HAV; anti-HAV-IgG, IgG class antibody to HAV; HBV, hepatitis B virus; HBsAg, hepatitis B surface antigen; anti-HBs, antibody to HBsAg; HBeAg, hepatitis B e antigen; anti-HBe, antibody to HBeAg; HBcAg, hepatitis B core antigen; anti-HBc, antibody to HBcAg; anti-HBc-IgM, IGM class antibody to HBcAg; anti-HBc-IgG, IgG class antibody to HBcAg; HVC, hepatitis C virus; anti-HCV, antibody to hepatitis C.

III. **Pathophysiology.** In addition to fecal-oral transmission, parenteral transmission is possible via blood transfusion. Maternal-infant transmission appears to be a very rare; however, both intrauterine and perinatal transmission have been documented in case reports. The risk of transmission is limited because the period of viremia is short, and fecal contamination does not occur at the time of delivery.

IV. **Risk factors.** The newborn infant born to an infected mother whose symptoms began between 2 weeks before and 1 week after delivery is at risk. Risk factors for postnatal acquisition of HAV include poor hygiene, poor sanitation, contact with infected individual (which can be nosocomial), and recent travel to a developing country where the disease is endemic.

V. **Clinical presentation.** Most infants (>80%) are asymptomatic, with mild abnormalities of liver function.

VI. **Diagnosis**

A. **IgM (immunoglobulin M) antibody to hepatitis A virus (anti-HAV-IgM)** is present during the acute or early convalescent phase of disease. In most cases it becomes detectable 5–10 days after exposure and can persist for up to 6 months after infection. **Anti-HAV-IgG** appears in the convalescent phase, remains detectable, and confers immunity. Research laboratories also can detect virus in blood or stool by means of reverse transcriptase polymerase chain reaction (RT-PCR).

B. **Liver function tests (LFTs).** Characteristically, the transaminases (alanine transaminase [ALT] and aspartate transaminase [AST]) and serum bilirubin levels (total and direct) are elevated, whereas the alkaline phosphatase level is normal.

VII. **Management**

A. **Immune serum globulin (ISG),** 0.02 mL/kg intramuscularly (IM), should be given to the newborn whose mother's symptoms began between 2 weeks before and

1 week after delivery. If an outbreak of hepatitis A is documented in the nursery, postexposure prophylaxis with ISG should be given to susceptible health-care workers as well as exposed neonates who may have close contact with infectious secretions. HAV vaccines are now available and routinely recommended for all children (12–23 months old). The effectiveness of HAV vaccines in postexposure prophylaxis is unknown; therefore, they are currently not recommended.
- B. **Isolation.** The infant should be isolated with enteric precautions.
- C. **Breast-feeding** is not contraindicated.

VIII. **Prognosis** for HAV-infected infants is favorable. Less than 20% are clinically symptomatic after infection. Chronic carrier state does not exist.

HEPATITIS B

I. **Definition.** Hepatitis B virus (HBV; serum hepatitis) is caused by a DNA-containing, 42-nM-diameter hepadnavirus. It has a long incubation period (45–160 days) after exposure.

II. **Incidence.** Each year in the United States, ~20,000 infants are born to HBV-infected pregnant women, and without immunoprophylaxis ~5500 would become chronically infected.

III. **Pathophysiology.** In the fetus and neonate, transmission has been suggested by the following mechanisms:
- A. **Transplacental transmission** either during pregnancy or at the time of delivery secondary to placental leaks. This is rare and accounts for <5% of neonatal infection.
- B. **Natal transmission** by exposure to HBV in amniotic fluid, vaginal secretions, or maternal blood accounts for 90% of neonatal infections. The role of the mode of delivery in the transmission of HBV from mother to infant has not been fully determined.
- C. **Postnatal transmission** by fecal-oral spread, blood transfusion, or other mechanisms.

IV. **Risk factors**
- A. **Factors associated with higher rates of HBV transmission** to neonates include the following:
  1. The presence of HBeAg and absence of anti-HBe in maternal serum: attack rates of 70–90%, with up to 90% of these infants being chronic carriers, compared with 15% of infants of anti-HBe-positive mothers. In HBeAg negative and HBsAg positive mothers, the transmission rate is <10%, however, those infants are at risk for acute hepatitis and acute fulminant hepatitis.
  2. Asian racial origin, particularly Chinese, with attack rates of 40–70%.
  3. Maternal acute hepatitis in the third trimester or immediately postpartum (70% attack rate).
  4. Higher-titer HBsAg in maternal serum (attack rates parallel the titer).
  5. Antigenemia present in older siblings.
- B. **Factors not related to transmission** include the following:
  1. The particular HBV subtype in the mother.
  2. The presence or absence of HBsAg in amniotic fluid.
  3. The presence or titer of anti-HBc in cord blood.

V. **Clinical presentation.** Maternal hepatitis B infection has not been associated with abortion, stillbirth, or congenital malformations. Prematurity has occurred, especially with acute hepatitis during pregnancy. Fetuses or newborns exposed to HBV present a wide spectrum of disease. Because of the long incubation period, the infants do not present in the neonatal period. Even after the neonatal period, they are rarely ill; jaundice appears <3% of the time. Various clinical presentations include the following:
- A. **Mild transient acute infection.**
- B. **Chronic active hepatitis with or without cirrhosis.**
- C. **Chronic persistent hepatitis.**
- D. **Chronic asymptomatic HBsAg carriage.**
- E. **Fulminant fatal hepatitis B (rare).**
- F. **Hepatocellular carcinoma in older children and young adults.**

VI. **Diagnosis**
   A. **Differential diagnosis.** Major diseases to consider include biliary atresia and acute hepatitis secondary to other viruses (eg, hepatitis A, CMV, rubella, and herpes simplex virus).
   B. **Liver function tests (LFTs).** ALT and AST levels may be markedly increased before the rise in bilirubin levels.
   C. **Hepatitis panel testing** (see Table 87–1)
      1. **Mother.** Test for HBsAg, HBeAg, anti-HBe, and anti-HBc.
      2. **Infant.** Test for HBsAg and anti-HBc-IgM. Most infants demonstrate antigenemia by 6 months of age, with peak acquisition at 3–4 months. Cord blood is not a reliable indicator of neonatal infection because contamination could have occurred with antigen-positive maternal blood or vaginal secretions and possible noninfectious antigenemia from the mother.

VII. **Management**
   A. **HBsAg-positive mother.** If the mother is HBsAg positive, regardless of the status of her HBe antigen or antibody, the infant should be given hepatitis B immune globulin (HBIG), 0.5 mL IM, within 12 h after delivery. Additionally, hepatitis (HB) vaccine is given at birth, at 1 month and at 6 months of age. If the first dose is given simultaneously with HBIG, it should be administered at a separate site, preferably in the opposite leg. For preterm infants weighing <2 kg, this initial dose of vaccine should not be counted in the required three-dose schedule, and the subsequent three doses should be initiated when the infant is 30 days old. HBIG and HB vaccinations do not interfere with routine childhood immunizations.
   B. **Infant born to mother whose HBsAg status is unknown.** Test the mother as soon as possible. While awaiting the results, give the infant HB vaccine within 12 h of birth. If the mother is found to be HBsAg positive, the infant should receive HBIG (0.5 mL) within 7 days of birth. If the infant is preterm and the maternal HBsAg status cannot be determined within the initial 12 h after birth, HBIG should be given as well as HB vaccine.
   C. **Isolation.** Precautions are needed in handling blood and secretions.
   D. **Breast-feeding.** HBsAg has been detected in breast milk of HBsAg-positive mothers but only with special concentrating techniques. Studies have shown that, with appropriate immunoprophylaxis (HBIG and HB vaccine), breast-feeding of infants of chronic HBV carrier mothers pose no additional risk for the transmission of the hepatitis B virus. Therefore, breast-feeding should be encouraged.
   E. **Vaccine efficacy.** The overall protective efficiency rate in neonates given HB vaccine and HBIG exceeds 90%. The World Health Organization recommends that all countries add HB vaccine to their routine childhood immunization programs. Such programs (in Taiwan) have been shown to lower the incidence of chronic HBsAg carrier state, fulminant hepatic failure, and hepatocellular carcinoma.
   F. **Prevention of HB vaccine failure.** Failure of immunoprophylaxis (HBIG and HB vaccine) does occasionally occur in mothers with a high viral load at time of delivery. The use of maternal antiviral agents like lamivudine in the last trimester of pregnancy is being studied.

VIII. **Prognosis.** The majority of perinatally infected infants remain clinically healthy. Approximately 30–50% develop persistently elevated values on liver function tests. About 5% have moderately severe histopathologic changes on liver biopsy. Late complications including cirrhosis and hepatocellular carcinoma are rare.

HEPATITIS C

   I. **Definition.** Hepatitis C virus (HCV) is a single-stranded RNA virus that accounts for 20% of all cases of acute hepatitis.
   II. **Incidence.** Estimates of HCV seroprevalence in children have ranged from 0.2–0.4%. The true incidence of neonatal HCV is unknown.

III. **Pathophysiology.** Hepatitis C is transmitted primarily by parenteral means. Historically, exposure to blood and blood products was the most common source of infection; however, because of screening tests to exclude infectious donors, the risk of HCV is <0.01% per unit transfused. Vertical perinatal transmission of HCV is ~5%. Intrauterine infection accounts for 30–50% of the cases; the rest is presumably acquired intrapartum.

IV. **Risk factors**

   A. **Maternal HIV coinfection** is associated with a two to threefold increase in risk of transmission.

   B. **Maternal HCV viremia** correlates with transmission. However, viremia levels fluctuate considerably over time and no "safe level" can be defined below which transmission may never occur.

   C. **Gender.** Girls are twice as likely to be infected as boys.

   D. **Mode of delivery.** Cesarean delivery does not seem to offer any protection except if the mother is coinfected with HIV.

V. **Clinical presentation.** The average incubation period is generally 6–7 weeks, with a range of 2–26 weeks. Infants with acute hepatitis C typically are asymptomatic or have a mild clinical illness. Approximately 65–70% of patients experience chronic hepatitis, 20% cirrhosis, and 1–5% hepatocellular carcinoma.

VI. **Diagnosis** of HCV infection in infants can be made by detecting **anti-HCV IgG** in serum after 12–18 months of age. Testing for anti-HCV IgG earlier may detect maternal transplacentally acquired antibodies. For earlier diagnosis, **HCV RNA by PCR** can be performed as early as 2 months of age. PCR carries a low sensitivity if used at birth. All children born to HCV-infected women need to be tested with PCR at 2–3 months of age and again at 6 months of age. Two positive tests are highly suggestive of infection. Regardless of PCR testing, anti-HCV IgG needs to be done at 12–18 months. LFTs may be elevated and fluctuate widely over time. The interval between exposure to HCV or onset of illness and detection of anti-HCV IgG may be 5–6 weeks. Assays for anti-HCV IgM are not available.

VII. **Management**

   A. **If the mother was infected during the last trimester,** the risk of transmission to the infant is highest. Immune globulin prophylaxis is not recommended. It does not appear that a vaccine against hepatitis C will be available for at least another several years.

   B. **Breast-feeding.** Advise mothers that transmission of virus is theoretically possible; but no cases have been confirmed to result from breast-feeding. Currently, HCV infection is not believed to be a contraindication to breast-feeding.

   C. **Treatment.** The Food and Drug Administration has approved use of interferon-alfa-2b in combination with ribavirin for the treatment of HCV in children 3–17 years of age. Children seem to have a higher sustained virologic response compared with adults with fewer adverse events.

VIII. **Prognosis.** A recent study from Italy looking at 10-year follow-up after putative exposure to HCV in untreated patients showed undetectable viremia in 7.5%, persistent viremia in 92%, and decompensated cirrhosis in 1.8%. The few children with chronic HCV infection who cleared viremia spontaneously were more likely to have genotype 3. Of infants treated, 27.9% achieved a sustained virologic response. Risk factors for end-stage liver disease included perinatal exposure, maternal drug use, and infection with HCV genotype 1a. Children with such features should be considered for early treatment.

HEPATITIS D

Hepatitis D virus (HDV), also known as *delta hepatitis,* is a defective RNA virus that cannot survive independently and requires the helper function of DNA virus hepatitis B. Therefore, it occurs either as coinfection with hepatitis B or as superinfection of a hepatitis B carrier. Transmission form mother to newborn infant is uncommon. Prevention of hepatitis B infection prevents hepatitis D. There are, however, no available treatments to prevent HDV in HBsAg carriers before or after exposure. Management should be similar to that for hepatitis B infection (see prior discussion). Diagnosis of HDV is based on the detection of antibody to HDV (anti-HDV) by radioimmunoassay or enzyme immunoassay. HDV testing should be assessed in known carriers of hepatitis B because coinfection may lead to acute or fulminate hepatitis or a more rapid progression of chronic hepatitis.

HEPATITIS E

Hepatitis E virus (HEV) is a nonenveloped, positive sense, single-stranded RNA virus. Transmission is by fecal-oral route. HEV is not transmitted readily from person to person so, unlike HAV, familial clusters of disease are unusual. Unlike other viral hepatitis, HEV is found in wild and domestic animals, especially in swine. HEV particularly common in the Indian subcontinent, where some studies have shown HEV to be the most common etiology for acute viral hepatitis. In the United States, HEV infection is uncommon and generally occurs in travelers returning from endemic areas or swine workers. However, seroprevalence is higher than expected based on clinical disease, possibly because of exposure to infected animals. HEV commonly causes an acute illness with jaundice, malaise, fever, and arthralgia. Hepatitis E is clinically indistinguishable from hepatitis A. It is rarely symptomatic in children <15 years old. There is a very high maternal mortality when HEV is acquired during pregnancy, especially during the third trimester. Mother to infant transmission is high (50–100%). Fetal loss or early neonatal mortality is also significant. Commercial kits are now available to detect anti-HEV IgG and IgM. Definitive diagnosis may be made by demonstrating viral RNA in serum or stool by RT-PCR. The only treatment is supportive. A recombinant HEV phase III clinical trial in adults was recently completed and demonstrated the vaccine to be safe and highly effective.

HEPATITIS G

Hepatitis G virus (HGV), or GBV-C, is a positive, single-strand RNA virus that has been classified in the family Flaviviridae. Despite extensive study, HGV has not been identified as a causative agent of any type of liver disease or any other known clinical condition. The virus is transmitted by parenteral exposure to blood and blood products from HGV-infected persons. The prevalence of HGV RNA in blood donors ranges from 1–4%. Coinfection with HCV and HIV is common, and HGV may be protective against HIV progression in adults. Vertical transmission has been documented, with transmission rates of ≥60%. No biochemical or clinical signs of hepatitis are observed in HGV-infected infants.

Selected References

American Academy of Pediatrics: Hepatitis A-E. In Pickering LK et al (eds): *Red Book: 2006 Report of the Committee on Infectious Diseases*, 27th ed. Elk Grove Village, IL: American Academy of Pediatrics, 2006:326-361.

Bradley SJ: Hepatitis. In Remington JS et al (eds): *Infectious Diseases of the Fetus and Newborn Infant*. Philadelphia, PA: Elsevier Saunders, 2006:823-843.

Chang MH: Hepatitis B virus infection. *Semin Fetal Neonatal Med* 2007;12:160-167.

Davison SM et al: Perinatal hepatitis C virus infection: diagnosis and management. *Arch Dis Child* 2006;91:781-785

Emerson SU, Purcell RH: Hepatitis E. *Pediatr Infect Dis J* 2007;26:1147-1148.

European Paediatric Hepatitis C Virus Network: A significant sex—but not elective Cesarean section—effect on mother-to-child transmission of hepatitis C infection. *J Infect Dis* 2005;192:1872-1879.

Fagan EA et al: Symptomatic neonatal hepatitis A disease from a virus variant acquired in utero. *Pediatr Infect Dis J* 1999;18:389-391.

Fischler B: Hepatitis C virus infection. *Semin Fetal Neonatal Med* 2007;12:168-173.

Hill JB et al: Risk of hepatitis B transmission in breast-fed infants of chronic hepatitis B carriers. *Obstet Gynecol* 2002;99:1049-1052.

Lin HH et al: Transplacental leakage of HBeAg-positive maternal blood as the most likely route in causing intrauterine infection with hepatitis B virus. *J Pediatr* 1987;111:877-881.

Patra S et al: Maternal and fetal outcomes in pregnant women with acute hepatitis E virus infection. *Ann Intern Med* 2007;147:28-33.

Rosenblum LS et al: Hepatitis A outbreak in a neonatal intensive care unit: risk factors for transmission and evidence of prolonged viral excretion among preterm infants. *J Infect Dis* 1991;164:476-482.

Shrestha MP et al: Safety and efficacy of a recombinant hepatitis E vaccine. *N Engl J Med* 2007;356:895-903.

Stapleton JT: GB virus type C/Hepatitis G virus. *Semin Liver Dis* 2003;23:137-148.

Thomas SL et al: A review of hepatitis C virus (HCV) vertical transmission: risks of transmission to infants born to mothers with and without HCV viraemia or human immunodeficiency virus infection. *Int J Epidemiol* 1998;27:108-117.

Towers CV et al: The presence of hepatitis B surface antigen and deoxyribonucleic acid in amniotic fluid and cord blood. *Am J Obstet Gynecol* 2001;184:1514-1518.

van Zonneveld M et al: Lamivudine treatment during pregnancy to prevent perinatal transmission of hepatitis B virus infection. *J Viral Hepat* 2003;10:294-297.

Wirth S et al: Peginterferon alfa-2b plus ribavirin treatment in children and adolescents with chronic hepatitis C. *Hepatology* 2005;41:1013-1018.

Withers MR et al: Antibody levels to hepatitis E virus in North Carolina swine workers, non-swine workers, swine, and murids. *Am J Trop Med Hyg* 2002;66:384-388.

Zanetti AR et al: Multicenter trial on mother-to-infant transmission of GBV-C virus. The Lombardy Study Group on Vertical/Perinatal Hepatitis Viruses Transmission. *J Med Virol* 1998;54:107-112.

88 Human Immunodeficiency Virus (HIV)

I. **Definition.** HIV is an enveloped RNA virus that is a member of the lentivirus subfamily of retroviruses. Infection is most commonly secondary to HIV-1. HIV-2 is rare in the United States but more common in West Africa. HIV results in a broad spectrum of disease, with **AIDS** representing the most severe end of the clinical spectrum.

II. **Incidence.** The Joint United Nations Program on HIV/AIDS approximated that 33.2 million people worldwide were infected with HIV-1 at the end of 2007. More than 95% of the total cases reside in developing countries. Every day, > 6800 persons become infected with HIV and >5700 persons die from AIDS, mostly because of inadequate access to HIV prevention and treatment services. An estimated 1200 children become infected with HIV every day, mostly acquiring infection vertically from their mothers. The mother-to-child transmission (MTCT) of HIV-1 has been reduced significantly over the past 10–15 years in developed countries; however, transmission rate in developing countries is still high at ~26%.

III. **Pathophysiology.** HIV-1 is particularly tropic for CD4$^+$ T cells and cells of monocyte or macrophage lineage. After infection of the cell, viral RNA is uncoated and a double-strand DNA transcript is made. This DNA is transported to the nucleus and integrated into the host genome DNA. There is eventual destruction of both the cellular and humoral arms of the immune system. As well, HIV-1 gene products or cytokines elaborated by infected cells may affect macrophage, B-lymphocyte, and T-lymphocyte function. Hypergammaglobulinemia caused by HIV-induced polyclonal B-cell activation is often detected in early infancy. Disruption of B-cell function results in poor secondary antibody synthesis and response to vaccination. As well, profound defects in cell-mediated immunity occur, allowing a predisposition to opportunistic infections such as fungus, *Pneumocystis jiroveci* pneumonia (PCP), and chronic diarrhea. The virus can also invade the central nervous system and produce psychosis and brain atrophy.

IV. **Risk factors**

A. **High-risk mother.** Any infant born to a high-risk mother is at risk. High-risk mothers include intravenous (IV) drug users, hemophiliacs, spouses of bisexual males, women from areas where the disease is more prevalent in heterosexuals, and spouses of hemophiliacs. Several mechanisms for viral transmission exist, including maternal disease state, fetal exposure to infected maternal body fluids, depressed maternal immune response, and breast-feeding. Maternal plasma HIV RNA level is the best single predictor of MTCT risk. Other risk factors include mode of delivery, duration of rupture of membranes, prematurity and low birthweight, cervicovaginal viral load, low CD4+ cell count, maternal symptomatic HIV disease/AIDS, viral subtype and host genetic factors. MTCT may occur in utero, intrapartum, or postpartum through breast-feeding. Transplacental infection has been proven by evidence of infection in aborted first-trimester fetal tissues as well as isolation of HIV-1 in blood samples obtained with 48 h of birth. Potential routes of infection include mixture of maternal and fetal blood and infection across the placenta when its integrity is compromised (eg, placentitis [syphilitic] and chorioamnionitis).

B. **Blood transfusion.** Screening of blood donors has reduced but has not totally eliminated the risk because some newly infected persons are viremic but seronegative for 2–4 months and because some infected persons (5–15%) are seronegative. The current risk of transmission of HIV per unit transfused is 1 in 2 million. (See also Chapter 12.)

C. **Breast milk.** Breast-feeding is the predominant means of postnatal HIV transmission to infants and accounts for an estimated third to half of all MTCT events in breast-feeding populations. HIV-1 RNA and proviral DNA have been detected in both the cell-free and cellular portions of breast milk. Colostrum viral load appears to be particularly high. Risk from breast milk is highest when maternal primary infection occurs within the first few months after delivery. In areas where infant formula is accessible, affordable, safe, and sustainable, avoidance of breast-feeding has represented one of the main components of prevention efforts of MTCT of HIV-1 for many years. Complete avoidance of breast-feeding by HIV-1-infected women has been recommended by the American Academy of Pediatrics (AAP) and the Centers for Disease Control and Prevention (CDC) and remains the only means by which prevention of breast-feeding transmission of HIV-1 can be absolutely ensured. In developing countries where local sanitary conditions are poor and access to infant formulas is limited, the avoidance of breast-feeding may not be practical.

V. **Clinical presentation.** Disease progression after vertical HIV-1 infection is highly variable.

A. **Incubation period.** The median age of onset of symptoms is approximately 12–18 months for untreated and perinatally infected infants. Most children have delayed onset of mild symptoms and survive beyond 5 years of age. In a small group of untreated children (15–20%), the disease progresses rapidly with subsequent mortality before 4 years of age.

B. **Signs and symptoms.** The newborn is usually asymptomatic or may have low birthweight, weight loss, or failure to thrive (if infected in utero). The frequency of different opportunistic pathogens among HIV-infected children decreased significantly with the application and widespread use of highly active antiretroviral therapy (**HAART**). In the pre-HAART era, serious bacterial infection, herpes zoster, disseminated *Mycobacterium avium* complex (MAC), PCP, and candidiasis were common. History of a previous AIDS-defining opportunistic infection was a predictor of developing a new infection. In the HAART era, descriptions of opportunistic infections among HIV infected children have been limited because of the substantial decreases in morbidity and mortality among children receiving HAART. Nonspecific features of infection include hepatosplenomegaly, lymphadenopathy, and fever. Neurologic disease may be either static (delayed attainment of milestones) or progressive, with impaired brain growth, failure to reach milestones, and progressive motor deficits. Common CT scan findings include basal ganglia calcification and cortical atrophy. Cardiac abnormalities including pericardial disease, myocardial dysfunction, dysrhythmias, and cardiomyopathies are common, particularly in advanced disease. Development of opportunistic infections, particularly PCP; progressive neurologic disease; and severe wasting are associated with poor prognosis.

VI. **Diagnosis.** Diagnosis is based on suspicion of infection based on epidemiological risk or clinical presentation, and confirmation by different virologic assays in infants <18 months old or serologic tests if the infant is >18 months old.

A. **All other causes of immunodeficiency must be excluded.** These include both primary and secondary immunodeficiency states. Primary immunodeficiency diseases include DiGeorge syndrome, Wiskott-Aldrich syndrome, ataxia-telangiectasia, agammaglobulinemia, severe combined immunodeficiency, and neutrophil function abnormality. Secondary immunodeficiency states include those caused by immunosuppressive therapy, starvation, and lymphoreticular cancer.

B. **Laboratory studies**

1. **HIV serology.** Antibodies against HIV-1 are found in all infants born to mother with HIV infection because of transplacental passage of immunoglobulin G. HIV serology (enzyme-linked immunoabsorbent assay [ELISA] or Western blot) should not be used to diagnose HIV infection in infants <18 months of age. The routine serologic testing of these infants is informative only if the test result is negative. If the mother's HIV-1 serostatus is unknown, rapid HIV-1 antibody testing (ELISA) of the newborn infant may identify HIV-1 exposure so that antiretroviral prophylaxis can be initiated within the first 12 h of life if test results are positive.

2. **Virologic assays** (HIV-1 DNA and RNA polymerase chain reaction [PCR]) are considered the **gold standard** for diagnosis of HIV in infants and children <18 months. With the use of these tests, HIV infection may be diagnosed as early as the first day after birth in some infants and by 1 month of age in most infected infants. **The HIV-1 DNA PCR** assay is the preferred diagnostic tool. Amplification of proviral DNA allows detection of cells that harbor quiescent provirus as well as cells with actively replicating virus. Approximately 30% of infants with HIV infection have a positive DNA PCR in samples obtained by 48 h of age. A positive result identifies infants who were infected in utero. The test routinely can detect 1–10 DNA copies. The test will be positive in 93% and 99% of all infected infants by 2 weeks and 1 month of age, respectively. **HIV-1 RNA PCR** assays detect plasma (cell-free) viral RNA by PCR amplification. These assays are available as either "standard" or "ultrasensitive," and the lower limit of detection when using the ultrasensitive assays is in the range of 50–75 HIV-1 copies per mL of plasma. The reported sensitivity for RNA assays range from 25–50% within the first few days of life to 100% by 6–12 weeks of age. HIV-1 RNA assays are commonly used for quantifying the amount of virus present as one predictor of disease progression. They are used in follow-up testing of patients during treatment for HIV-1 infection. When HIV-1 RNA quantitative assays are used for diagnosis of infants and young children, a plasma viral load of 10,000 copies/mL is generally required before the assay result is interpreted as positive. Zidovudine (ZDV) prophylaxis does not appear to alter the diagnostic sensitivity of either HIV DNA PCR or RNA assays. The effect of combination antiretroviral maternal and infant treatment on sensitivity of viral diagnostic testing is unknown.

A perinatally HIV-exposed infant is determined to be infected with the presence of two positive results of HIV virologic assays performed on the infant's blood obtained at two different occasions, one of them obtained after 8 weeks of age. Cord blood should not be used because of the possibility of contamination with maternal blood. Virologic assays should be performed: within the first 48 h after birth, at 14 days, between 1 and 2 months, and at 3–6 months of age. A positive test confirmed at 2 weeks of age warrants a change in the recommended

ZDV prophylactic monotherapy. Infection with HIV can be reasonably excluded with two or more negative virologic assays, at least one of which is performed after 1 month and another performed after 4 months in the absence of breast-feeding. In the absence of hypogammaglobulinemia, two or more negative HIV-specific antibody tests performed beyond 6 months of age in a child without clinical evidence of HIV disease can reasonably exclude HIV infection. Follow-up tests should include either two negative ELISA tests between 6 and 18 months or one negative ELISA at 18–24 months. The p_{24} antigen assay is less sensitive than DNA or RNA PCR and is generally not recommended. Viral HIV-1 culture is labor intensive and poses a significant biohazard risk. It is largely supplanted by DNA and RNA PCR virologic assays.

3. **Rapid tests.** A number of rapid serologic tests for detection of IgG antibodies against HIV-1 are now available (www.fda.gov/cber/products/testkits.htm). Rapid HIV-1 antibody tests are comparable with ELISAs in both sensitivity (99.3–100%) and specificity (98.6–100%). As with routine ELISAs, confirmation of positive results is necessary, but confirmation of a negative result is not. These tests are valuable as a screening tool for pregnant women with no or limited prenatal care or for infants with unknown maternal HIV status. These tests have the potential to reduce MTCT risk, with immediate provision of antiretroviral prophylaxis and formula feeding to prevent postnatal transmission.

4. **Surrogate markers for disease.** Immunologic abnormalities found in HIV-infected infants include hypergammaglobulinemia, a low $CD4^+$ T-lymphocyte count, or a decreased $CD4^+$ percentage.

C. **Presence of a "marker" disease** that indicates cellular immunodeficiency. Marker diseases include candidiasis, cryptococcosis, *Mycobacterium avium* infection, Epstein-Barr virus infection, PCP, strongyloidiasis, and Kaposi sarcoma. Cytomegalovirus (CMV) infection and toxoplasmosis are included if toxoplasmosis occurs >1 month after birth and CMV infection presents >6 months after birth.

VII. **Management.** Isolation precautions for all infectious diseases, including maternal and neonatal precautions, breast-feeding, and visiting issues, can be found in Appendix F.

A. **Prevention.** MTCT can take place in utero, during labor, at delivery and postnatally through breast-feeding. Before the widespread use of MTCT interventions (described later), transmission rates in the United States ranged from 16–30%. More recently, MTCT has dropped below 1–2%.

1. **Identification of HIV infection in pregnant women.** A prerequisite for the application of successful MTCT interventions is identifying mothers who are HIV positive. The CDC issued revised guidelines in 2006 regarding the HIV testing in pregnant women. The guidelines recommended that HIV screening be included in the routine panel of prenatal screening tests for all pregnant women. HIV screening is recommended after the patient is notified that testing will be performed unless the patient declines (opt-out screening). Separate written consent for HIV testing should not be required, and a general consent for medical care should be considered sufficient to encompass consent for HIV testing. Repeat screening in the third trimester is recommended in certain jurisdictions with elevated rates of HIV infection among pregnant women. The AAP and American College of Obstetricians and Gynecologists issued a recommendation similar to the CDC with all organizations supporting routine testing and the opt-out strategy. Most guidelines now state that health-care providers have a responsibility not only to offer, but to recommend, antenatal HIV testing. The benefits of antenatal HIV testing extend beyond the potential to reduce vertical transmission risk and include the opportunity to evaluate the infected woman's health status, to initiate HAART if required, and to allow the woman to reduce the risk of transmitting HIV to her sexual partner.

2. **Antiretroviral prophylaxis and treatment.** Antiretroviral drugs are prescribed to HIV-infected pregnant women to treat their own disease and to decrease

MTCT of HIV. Antiretroviral drugs reduce perinatal transmission by several mechanisms, including lowering maternal antepartum viral load, and pre- and postexposure prophylaxis of the fetus and newborn infant. For optimum prevention of perinatal HIV transmission, combined antepartum, intrapartum, and infant antiretroviral prophylaxis are recommended. Use of HAART is associated with substantial improvements in AIDS-free survival in pregnant women. The ACTG 076 trial published in 1994 showed that an intensive regimen of oral ZDV given prenatally, intrapartum, and postpartum decreased perinatal transmission risk by two thirds when compared with placebo. Widespread implementation of trial regimen led to sharp decreases in perinatal HIV transmission. Furthermore, since the late 1990s, most HIV-infected women in the United States have been prescribed combination regimens, which further reduced the risk. Widespread use of HAART, which is usually composed of three antiretrovirals from two drug classes, has substantially reduced MTCT rates to below 1–2%. Antiretroviral therapy or prophylaxis should be recommended to all pregnant HIV-infected women regardless of plasma HIV RNA copy number or $CD4^+$ cell count. According to the 2007 Public Health Service Task Force recommendations, HAART should be considered the standard of care for all pregnant women with HIV infection even those who do not require treatment for their own health. Regimens for prophylaxis against perinatal HIV transmission should include a three-drug combination from two classes of antiretroviral drugs. The use of ZDV alone is *controversial* but may be considered for those women initiating prophylaxis with plasma HIV RNA levels <1000 copies/mL on no therapy. ZDV should be included in the antenatal antiretroviral regimen unless there is severe toxicity or documented resistance. Other drugs used include nevirapine (NVP), lamivudine (3TC), and didanosine (ddI). The CDC provides periodic updates of new drugs and new treatment recommendations on the web at www.aidsinfo.nih.gov.

3. **Safety of antiretroviral drugs (ARVDs) during pregnancy.** There are limited human safety data on the antenatal use of ARVDs. Efavirenz is a category D drug and thus contraindicated in pregnancy. Women are at increased risk of Nevirapine (NVP) related hepatotoxicity. Lactic acidosis is a relatively uncommon side effect of nucleoside reverse transcriptase inhibitor (NRTI) drugs. HAART in pregnancy may increase the risk of gestational diabetes, preeclampsia, and premature delivery. Although animal studies suggest an increased risk of malformations associated with the use of certain ARVDs, to date there appears to be no increased risk of congenital malformations associated with HAART exposure in pregnancy according to a registry data (www.apregistry.com). ZDV treatment in infants is associated with a transient anemia. In utero exposure to HAART was shown to result in mild but statistically significant hematologic abnormalities like neutropenia and thrombocytopenia.

4. **Mode of delivery.** Data from individual patient meta-analysis and a randomized control trial confirmed that cesarean section (CS) performed before labor and rupture of membranes reduces MTCT by 50–80%, independent of the use of antiretroviral therapy or ZDV prophylaxis. Elective CS is associated with a higher rate of postpartum complications among HIV-infected women than is vaginal delivery. The added benefit of elective CS on reducing risk of MTCT in women with low-plasma HIV RNA loads (<1000 copies/mL) is uncertain, and some experts now recommend that women in this category can be offered a vaginal delivery. The use of invasive procedures in labor (eg, amniocentesis, fetal scalp electrodes, operative vaginal delivery, and episiotomy) should be avoided because of the potential risk for enhanced transmission.

5. **Postdelivery.** Thoroughly clean off amniotic fluid and blood. Isolate the infant with the same precautions as for hepatitis B (blood and secretion precautions). Initiate ZDV at 2 mg/kg, four times per day for 6 weeks. Obtain serial laboratory

evaluation as discussed. Breast-feeding must be discouraged. Ensure that the infant has the best possible follow-up care.

B. **General supportive care.**

1. **Intravenous immune globulin (IVIG).** HIV-infected infants are appropriate candidates for routine IVIG prophylaxis (400 mg/kg/dose every 28 days). See Chapter 132.

2. **Vaccines.** Routine immunization schedules should be followed for DaTP (diphtheria-tetanus-acellular pertussis), IPV (inactivated polio), HBV (hepatitis B vaccine), Hib (*Haemophilus influenzae* type b), hepatitis A vaccine, and PCV (pneumococcal conjugate vaccine, Prevnar). Influenza vaccine is given annually. MMR (measles-mumps-rubella) should be administered to HIV-infected children at 12 months of age unless they are severely immunocompromised. The second dose of MMR may be given as early as 4 weeks after the first dose rather than waiting until school entry. HIV-infected children may be at an increased risk for morbidity from varicella zoster infection. Varicella vaccine should be administered to HIV-infected children ≥12 months of age if they have no or mild symptoms of HIV (CDC categories N1 and A1), and a second dose should be given 3 months later.

3. **Nutrition.** Close nutritional monitoring should be part of the routine care of these children.

4. **Pneumocystis jiroveci prophylaxis.** CDC guidelines state that all infants born to HIV-infected women receive prophylaxis for 1 year beginning at 4–6 weeks regardless of CD4+ lymphocyte count. If HIV infection is excluded, then prophylaxis can be stopped. The drug of choice for this is trimethoprim-sulfamethoxazole. The need for prophylaxis after 1 year can be determined by the degree of immunosuppression as determined by CD4+ T-lymphocyte count.

5. **Other aspects of supportive care.** Neurodevelopmental supportive services include preschool early intervention programs and school-based developmental disability programs. Aggressive management and protocols for pharmacologic and nonpharmacologic pain management should be used.

VIII. **Prognosis.** In developed countries, perinatally acquired HIV infection follows a bimodal course; about a third of the children die or become symptomatic within the first 2 years of life and the remainder in the next several years. Only a minority of patients remain asymptomatic by 8 years. Clinical and laboratory factors associated with poor prognosis include being born to mothers with low CD4+ counts or high viral load, high virus copy number in the cord blood, and early manifestation of symptoms (opportunistic infections, encephalopathy, and hepatosplenomegaly). Use of HAART has substantially reduced both mortality and morbidity and improved quality of life in HIV-infected children. Children with HIV infection acquired through blood transfusion tend to have prolonged asymptomatic period. In developing countries, the prognosis is worse, with one study showing 89% of the infected children have died by 3 years of age, 10% were in HIV disease category B or C, and only ~1% remained without HIV symptoms.

Selected References

American Academy of Pediatrics: Human immunodeficiency virus infection. In Pickering et al (eds): *Red Book: 2006 Report of the Committee on Infectious Diseases,* 27th ed. Elk Grove Village, IL: American Academy of Pediatrics, 2006:378-401.

Branson BM et al; Centers for Disease Control and Prevention (CDC): Revised recommendations for HIV testing of adults, adolescents, and pregnant women in health-care settings. *MMWR Recomm Rep* 2006;55(RR-14):1-17.

Fowler MG et al: Reducing the risk of mother-to-child human immunodeficiency virus transmission: past successes, current progress and challenges, and future directions. *Am J Obstet Gynecol* 2007;197:S3-S9.

Joint United Nations Program on HIV/AIDS (UNAIDS): *2007 AIDS epidemic Update.* Geneva, Switzerland: UNAIDS, 2007. Available at: http://www.unaids.org/en/KnowledgeCentre/HIVData/EpiUpdate/EpiUpdArchive/2007default.asp.

Magder LS et al: Risk factors for in utero and intrapartum transmission of HIV. *J Acquir Immune Defic Syndr* 2005;38:87-95.

Read JS; Committee on Pediatric AIDS, American Academy of Pediatrics: Human milk, breast-feeding, and transmission of human immunodeficiency virus type 1 in the United States. *Pediatrics* 2003;112:1196-1205.

Read JS; Committee on Pediatric AIDS, American Academy of Pediatrics: Diagnosis of HIV-1 infection in children younger than 18 months in the United States. *Pediatrics* 2007;120:e1547-e1562.

The European Mode of Delivery Collaboration: Elective caesarean section versus vaginal delivery in preventing vertical HIV-1 transmission: a randomized clinical trial. *Lancet* 1999;353:1035-1039.

Thorne C, Newell ML: HIV. *Semin Fetal Neonatal Med* 2007;12:174-181.

U.S. Public Health Service: *Public Health Service Task Force Recommendations for Use of Antiretroviral Drugs in Pregnant HIV-1-Infected Women for Maternal Health and Interventions to Reduce Perinatal HIV-1 Transmission in the United States,* November 2, 2007. Available at: http://aidsinfo.nih.gov/contentfiles/PerinatalGL.pdf.

89 Hyaline Membrane Disease (Respiratory Distress Syndrome)

I. **Definition.** Hyaline membrane disease (HMD) is another name for respiratory distress syndrome (RDS). This clinical diagnosis is warranted in a preterm newborn with respiratory difficulty, including tachypnea (>60 breaths/min), chest retractions, and cyanosis in room air that persists or progresses over the first 48–96 h of life, and a characteristic chest radiographic appearance (uniform reticulogranular pattern and peripheral air bronchograms). The clinical course of the disease varies with the size of the infant, severity of disease, use of surfactant replacement therapy, presence of infection, degree of shunting of blood through the patent ductus arteriosus (PDA), and whether or not assisted ventilation was initiated.

II. **Incidence.** HMD occurs in 44% of infants with birthweight between 501 and 1500 g. The incidence is inversely proportional to the gestational age and birthweight. The incidence and severity of HMD are expected to decrease after the increase in use of antenatal steroids in recent years. Survival has improved significantly, especially after the introduction of exogenous surfactant, and is now at >90%. During the surfactant era, HMD accounts for <6% of all neonatal deaths, but declines in HMD mortality have been greater for white than for black infants.

III. **Pathophysiology.** Surfactant deficiency is the primary cause of HMD, often complicated by an overly compliant chest wall. Both factors lead to progressive atelectasis and failure to develop an effective functional residual capacity (FRC). Surfactant is a surface-active material produced by airway epithelial cells called type II pneumocytes. This cell line differentiates, and surfactant synthesis begins at 24–28 weeks' gestation. Type II cells are sensitive to and decreased by asphyxial insults in the perinatal period. The maturation of this cell line is delayed in the presence of fetal hyperinsulinemia. The maturity of type II cells is enhanced by the administration of antenatal corticosteroids and by chronic intrauterine stress such as pregnancy-induced hypertension, intrauterine growth restriction, and twin gestation. Surfactant, composed chiefly of phospholipid (75%) and protein (10%), is produced and stored in the characteristic lamellar bodies of type II pneumocytes. This lipoprotein is released into the airways, where it functions to decrease surface tension and maintain alveolar expansion at physiologic pressures.

A. **Lack of surfactant.** In the absence of surfactant, the small airspaces collapse; each expiration results in progressive atelectasis. Exudative proteinaceous material and epithelial debris, resulting from progressive cellular damage, collect in the airway and directly decrease total lung capacity. In pathologic specimens, this material stains typically as eosinophilic hyaline membranes lining the alveolar spaces and extending into small airways.

B. **Presence of an overly compliant chest wall.** In the presence of a chest wall with weak structural support secondary to prematurity, the large negative pressures generated to open the collapsed airways cause retraction and deformation of the chest wall instead of inflation of the poorly compliant lungs.

C. **Decreased intrathoracic pressure.** The infant with HMD who is <30 weeks' gestational age often has immediate respiratory failure because of an inability to generate the intrathoracic pressure necessary to inflate the lungs without surfactant.

D. **Shunting.** The presence or absence of a cardiovascular shunt through a PDA or foramen ovale, or both, may change the presentation or course of the disease process. Shortly after birth, the predominant shunting is right to left across the foramen ovale into the left atrium, which may result in venous admixture and worsening hypoxemia. After 18–24 h, left-to-right shunting through the PDA may become predominant as a result of falling pulmonary vascular resistance, leading to pulmonary edema and impaired alveolar gas exchange. Unfortunately, this usually occurs when the infant is starting to recover from HMD and can be aggravated by surfactant replacement therapy.

IV. **Risk factors.** Table 89–1 lists factors that increase or decrease the risk of HMD.

V. **Clinical presentation**

A. **History.** The infant is often preterm, either by dates or by gestational examination, or has a history of asphyxia in the perinatal period. Infants have some respiratory difficulty at birth, which becomes progressively more severe. The classic worsening of the atelectasis seen on chest radiograph and increasing oxygen requirement for these infants have been greatly modified by the availability of exogenous surfactant therapy and our increased ability to provide effective mechanical ventilatory support.

Table 89–1. RISK FACTORS THAT INCREASE OR DECREASE THE RISK OF HYALINE MEMBRANE DISEASE

Increased Risk	Decreased Risk
Prematurity	Chronic intrauterine stress
Male sex	Prolonged rupture of membranes
Familial predisposition	Maternal hypertension
Cesarean delivery without labor	Narcotic/cocaine use
Perinatal asphyxia	IUGR or SGA
Chorioamnionitis	Corticosteroids
Multiple gestation	Thyroid hormone
Maternal diabetes	Tocolytic agents

IUGR, intrauterine growth retardation; SGA, small for gestational age.

B. **Physical examination.** The infant with HMD exhibits tachypnea, grunting, nasal flaring, and retractions of the chest wall. The infant may have cyanosis in room air. Grunting occurs when the infant partially closes the vocal cords to prolong expiration and develop or maintain some FRC. This mechanism actually improves alveolar ventilation. The retractions occur and increase as the infant is forced to develop high transpulmonary pressure to reinflate atelectatic air spaces.

VI. **Diagnosis**

A. **Chest radiograph.** An anteroposterior chest radiograph should be obtained for all infants with respiratory distress of any duration. The typical radiographic finding of HMD is a uniform reticulogranular pattern, referred to as a ground-glass appearance, accompanied by peripheral air bronchograms. (See Figure 10–12.) During the clinical course, sequential radiographs may reveal air leaks secondary to mechanical ventilatory intervention as well as the onset of changes compatible with bronchopulmonary dysplasia (BPD) (see Figure 10–16).

B. **Laboratory studies**

1. **Blood gas sampling** is essential in the management of HMD. Usually, intermittent arterial sampling is performed. Although there is no consensus, most neonatologists agree that arterial oxygen tensions of 50–70 mm Hg and arterial carbon dioxide tensions of 45–60 mm Hg are acceptable. Most would maintain the pH at or above 7.25 and the arterial oxygen saturation at 88–95%. In addition, continuous transcutaneous oxygen and carbon dioxide monitors or oxygen saturation monitors, or both, are proving invaluable in the minute-to-minute monitoring of these infants.

2. **Sepsis workup.** A partial sepsis workup, including complete blood cell count and blood culture, should be considered for each infant with a diagnosis of HMD because early-onset sepsis (eg, infection with group B streptococcus or *Haemophilus influenzae*) can be indistinguishable from HMD on clinical grounds alone.

3. **Serum glucose levels** may be high or low initially and must be monitored closely to assess the adequacy of dextrose infusion. Hypoglycemia alone can lead to tachypnea and respiratory distress.

4. **Serum electrolyte levels including calcium** should be monitored every 12–24 h for management of parenteral fluids. Hypocalcemia can contribute to more respiratory symptoms and is common in sick, nonfed, preterm, or asphyxiated infants.

C. **Echocardiography** is a valuable diagnostic tool in the evaluation of an infant with hypoxemia and respiratory distress. It is used to confirm the diagnosis of PDA as well as to document response to therapy. Significant congenital heart disease can be excluded by this technique as well.

VII. **Management**

A. **Prevention**

1. **Antenatal corticosteroids.** According to the systematic review of 21 studies (3885 women and 4269 infants), treatment with antenatal corticosteroids is associated with an overall reduction in neonatal death, RDS, IVH, NEC, respiratory support, intensive care admissions, and systemic infections in the first 48 h of life. Use of antenatal betamethasone to enhance fetal pulmonary maturity is now established and generally considered to be standard of care. The recommended glucocorticoid regimen consists of the administration to the mother of two 12-mg doses of betamethasone given intramuscularly 24 h apart. Dexamethasone is no longer recommended because of increased risk for cystic periventricular leukomalacia among very premature infants exposed to the drug prenatally.

2. **Several preventive measures** may improve the survival of infants at risk for HMD and include **antenatal ultrasonography** for more accurate assessment of gestational age and fetal well-being, **continuous fetal monitoring** to document fetal well-being during labor or to signal the need for intervention when fetal distress is discovered,

tocolytic agents that prevent and treat preterm labor, and **assessment of fetal lung maturity** before delivery (lecithin-to-sphingomyelin [L-S] ratio and phosphatidyl-glycerol; see Chapter 1) to prevent iatrogenic prematurity.

B. **Surfactant replacement** (see also Chapter 7) is now considered a standard of care in the treatment of intubated infants with HMD. Since the late 1980s, >30 randomized clinical trials involving >6000 infants have been conducted. Systematic reviews of these trials demonstrate that surfactant, whether used prophylactically in the delivery room or in the treatment of the established disease, leads to a significant decrease in the risk of pneumothorax and the risk of death. These benefits were observed in both the trials of natural surfactant extracts and synthetic surfactants. Prophylactic surfactant replacement to prevent HMD in infants born at <30 weeks' gestation has reduced the risk of death or BPD but may result in some infants being intubated and receiving treatment unnecessarily. A recent consensus statement recommends surfactant prophylaxis (within 15 min of birth) to almost all infants <27 weeks' gestation. Prophylaxis should be considered for infants >26 weeks but <30 weeks' gestation, if intubation is needed at the delivery room resuscitation, or if the mother has not received prenatal corticosteroids. Currently, long-term follow-up studies have not shown significant differences between surfactant-treated patients and nontreated control groups with regard to PDA, IVH, ROP, NEC, and BPD. Evidence exists that the length of stay on mechanical ventilation and total ventilator days have been reduced with the use of surfactant at all gestational age levels, even with the increase of extremely low birthweight infants. A dramatic fall in deaths from HMD began in 1991. This probably reflected the introduction across the nation of surfactant replacement therapy. In long-term follow-up studies, no adverse effects attributable to surfactant therapy have been identified.

C. **Respiratory support**

1. **Endotracheal intubation and mechanical ventilation** are the mainstays of therapy for infants with HMD in whom apnea or hypoxemia with respiratory acidosis develops. Mechanical ventilation usually begins with rates of 30–60 breaths/min and inspiratory-expiratory ratios of 1:2. An initial positive inspiratory pressure of 18–30 cm H_2O is used, depending on the size of the infant and the severity of the disease. A positive end-expiratory pressure of 4–5 cm H_2O results in improved oxygenation, presumably because it assists in the maintenance of an effective FRC. The lowest possible pressures and inspired oxygen concentrations are maintained in an attempt to minimize damage to parenchymal tissue. Ventilators with the capacity to synchronize respiratory effort may generate less inadvertent airway pressure and lessen barotrauma. The early use of high-frequency oscillatory ventilation (HFOV) has become a popular and frequently used ventilator mode for low birthweight infants. Review of the evidence from 15 randomized controlled trials showed variable results between studies and no clear overall benefit or harm resulting from HFOV. Insufficient evidence exists to recommend the routine use of HFOV instead of conventional ventilation for preterm infants with lung disease.

2. **Continuous positive airway pressure (CPAP) and nasal synchronized intermittent mandatory ventilation (SIMV).** Nasal CPAP (NCPAP) or nasopharyngeal CPAP (NPCPAP) may be used early to delay or prevent the need for endotracheal intubation. To minimize lung injury associated with intubation and mechanical ventilation, there has been a recent interest in using CPAP as an initial treatment strategy to treat HMD even in very low and extremely low birthweight infants. In some centers, this practice has been used successfully and resulted in decreased incidence of BPD. In addition, according to a systematic review of six randomized controlled clinical trials, early surfactant replacement therapy with extubation to NCPAP is associated with less need of treatment in ventilator, lower incidence of BPD, and fewer air leak syndromes compared with later selective surfactant replacement and continued mechanical ventilation, with

extubation from low ventilator support. A low treatment threshold ($FiO_2 \leq 0.45$) is preferable to later, selective surfactant therapy by transient intubation using a higher threshold ($FiO_2 > 0.45$) at the time of respiratory failure and initiation of mechanical ventilation. NCPAP and NPCPAP may be used on extubation and may decrease the chance of reintubation. **Nasal SIMV is a potentially useful way of augmenting NCPAP.** The relatively recent ability to synchronize the ventilator breaths with the infant's own respiratory cycle has made this mode of ventilation feasible. In three trials, nasal SIMV has reduced the incidence of symptoms of extubation failure when compared with NCPAP.

3. **Complications.** Pulmonary air leaks, such as pneumothorax, pneumomediastinum, pneumopericardium, and pulmonary interstitial emphysema, may occur (see Chapter 74).Chronic complications include respiratory problems such as BPD (see Chapter 77) and tracheal stenosis.

D. **Fluid and nutritional support.** In the very ill infant, it is now possible to maintain nutritional support with parenteral nutrition for an extended period. The specific needs of preterm and term infants are becoming better understood, and the nutrient preparations available reflect this understanding (see Chapter 8 and 9).

E. **Antibiotic therapy.** Antibiotics that cover the most common neonatal infections are usually begun initially. Aminoglycoside dosing intervals are increased for the premature infant.

F. **Sedation** is commonly used to control ventilation in these sick infants. **Phenobarbital** has been used to decrease the infant's activity level. **Morphine, fentanyl,** or **lorazepam** may be used for analgesia as well as sedation, but there is significant controversy surrounding such treatment. Reported advantages of treatment include improved ventilator synchrony and pulmonary function. Decreased adverse long-term neurological sequelae have been suggested. Neuroendocrine responses to mechanical ventilation are alleviated by opioid treatment, which may be beneficial in the long term. However, clinicians should consider adverse effects of medication, especially opioids, including hypotension with morphine and chest wall rigidity with fentanyl. Tolerance, dependence, and withdrawal occur with all the opioids and benzodiazepines. In addition, pharmacologic treatment does not decrease adverse sequelae, at least in the short term. The most significant gaps in knowledge include the inability to assess chronic pain in this population and the long-term effects of treatment. Minimal handling to avoid pain is an important means to decrease need for pain management in ventilated infants. Muscle paralysis with **pancuronium** for infants with HMD remains ***controversial.*** Sedation might be indicated for infants who "fight" the ventilator and exhale during the inspiratory cycle of mechanical ventilation. This respiratory pattern may increase the likelihood of complication such as air leak and, therefore, should be avoided. Sedation of infants with fluctuating cerebral blood flow velocity theoretically decreases the risk of IVH.

VIII. **Prognosis.** Although the survival of infants with HMD has improved greatly, the prognosis for survival with or without respiratory and neurologic sequelae is highly dependent on birthweight and gestational age. Major morbidity (BPD, NEC, and severe IVH) and poor postnatal growth remain high for the smallest infants.

Selected References

Aly H: Nasal prongs continuous positive airway pressure: a simple yet powerful tool. *Pediatrics* 2001;108:759.

Bhakoo ON et al: Spectrum of respiratory distress in very low birthweight neonates. *Ind J Pediatr* 2000;67:803.

Bhuta T, Henderson-Smart DJ: Rescue high-frequency oscillatory ventilation versus conventional ventilation for pulmonary dysfunction in preterm infants. *Cochrane Database Syst Rev* 2000;2:CD000438.

Cotton R: Hyaline membrane disease: from tragedy to triumph. *Perspect Neonatol* 1999;1:4.

Davis P et al: Nasal intermittent positive pressure ventilation (NIPPV) versus nasal continuous positive airway pressure (NCPAP) for preterm neonates after extubation. *Cochrane Database Syst Rev* 2001;3:CD002272.

De Klerk A, De Klerk R: Nasal continuous positive airway pressure and outcomes of preterm infants. *J Paediatr Child Health* 2001;37:161.

Fanaroff AA, Martin RJ (eds): *Neonatal-Perinatal Medicine—Diseases of the Fetus and Infant,* 6th ed. St. Louis, MO: Mosby, 2002.

Fanaroff AA et al: Trends in neonatal morbidity and mortality for very low birthweight infants. *Am J Obstet Gynecol* 2007;196:147.e1-8.

Frisbie WP et al: The increasing racial disparity in infant mortality: respiratory distress syndrome and other causes. *Demography* 2002;41:773.

Greenough A et al: Synchronized mechanical ventilation for respiratory support in newborn infants. *Cochrane Database Syst Rev* 2001;1:CD000456.

Hall RW et al: Do ventilated neonates require pain management? *Semin Perinatol* 2007;31:289.

Henderson-Smart DJ et al: Elective high frequency oscillatory ventilation versus conventional ventilation for acute pulmonary dysfunction in preterm infants. *Cochrane Database Syst Rev* 2007;(3):CD000104.

Ho JJ et al: Continuous distending pressure for respiratory distress syndrome in preterm infants. *Cochrane Database Syst Rev* 2000;2:CD002975.

Jobe AH: Glucocorticoids in perinatal medicine: misguided rockets? *J Pediatr* 2000;137:1.

Kuo CY et al: Study of plasma endothelin-1 concentrations in Taiwanese neonates with respiratory distress. *Chang Gung Med J* 2001;24:239.

Levine EM et al: Mode of delivery and risk of respiratory diseases in newborns. *Obstet Gynecol* 2001;97:439.

Lotze A et al: Multicenter study of surfactant (beractant) use in the treatment of term infants with severe respiratory failure. *J Pediatr* 1998;132:40.

Malloy MH, Freeman DH: Respiratory distress syndrome mortality in the United States, 1987 to 1995. *J Perinatol* 2000;20:414.

Merritt TA et al: Immunologic consequences of exogenous surfactant administration. *Semin Perinatol* 1988;12:221.

Miller MJ et al: Respiratory disorders in preterm and term infants. In Fanaroff AA, Martin RJ (eds): *Neonatal-Perinatal Medicine: Diseases of the Fetus and Infant,* 7th ed. St. Louis, MO: Mosby, 2002.

Moriette G et al: Prospective randomized multicenter comparison of high-frequency oscillatory ventilation and conventional ventilation in preterm infants of less than 30 weeks with respiratory distress syndrome. *Pediatrics* 2001;107:363.

National Institutes of Health: NIH Consensus Development Panel on the effect of corticosteroids for fetal maturation on perinatal outcomes. *JAMA* 1995;273:413.

Northway WH Jr et al: Pulmonary disease following respirator therapy of hyaline-membrane disease. *N Engl J Med* 1967;76:357.

O'Shea et al: Randomized placebo-controlled trial of a 42-day tapering course of dexamethasone to reduce the duration of ventilator dependency in very low birth weight infants: outcome of study participants at 1-year adjusted age. *Pediatrics* 1999;104:15.

Plavka R et al: A prospective randomized comparison of conventional mechanical ventilation and very early high frequency oscillatory ventilation in extremely premature newborns with respiratory distress syndrome. *Intensive Care Med* 1999;25:68.

Rimensberger PC et al: First intention high-frequency oscillation with early lung volume optimization improves pulmonary outcome in very low birth weight infants with respiratory distress. *Pediatrics* 2000;105:1202.

Roberts D, Dalziel S: Antenatal corticosteroids for accelerating fetal lung maturation for women at risk of preterm birth. *Cochrane Database Syst Rev* 2006;3:CD004454.

Soll RF: Prophylactic natural surfactant extract for preventing morbidity and mortality in preterm infants. *Cochrane Database Syst Rev* 2000;2:CD000511.

Soll RF, Morley CJ: Prophylactic versus selective use of surfactant for preventing morbidity and mortality in preterm infants. *Cochrane Database Syst Rev* 2001;2:CD000510.

Stevens TP et al: Early surfactant administration with brief ventilation vs. selective surfactant and continued mechanical ventilation for preterm infants with or at risk for respiratory distress syndrome. *Cochrane Database Syst Rev* 2007;4:CD003063.

Sweet D et al: European consensus guidelines on the management of neonatal respiratory distress syndrome. *J Perinat Med* 2007;35:175.

Yu V et al: Pulmonary interstitial emphysema in infants less than 1000g at birth. *Aust Paediatr J* 1986;22:189.

90 Hydrocephalus and Ventriculomegaly

I. **Definition. Hydrocephalus** is dilation of the cerebral ventricular system secondary to an accumulation of cerebral spinal fluid (CSF) and a disturbance in CSF circulation. It is usually associated with increased intracranial pressure (ICP) and an enlarging head. The measurable occipital-frontal head circumference (OFC) may exceed the growth percentiles for gestational age or chronological age. Typically, an OFC of >2 standard deviations of normal is consistent with macrocephaly due to hydrocephalus. Occasionally hydrocephalus may be present with normal head size but with marked ventricular dilation.

CSF is produced largely from the choroid plexus of each ventricle throughout the cerebral ventricular system. Approximately 80% is choroid plexus in origin, and the remainder is contributed from the substance of the brain and spinal cord. CSF flows posterior from the lateral ventricles through the third ventricle into the aqueduct of Sylvius and through to the fourth ventricle. It ultimately reaches the subarachnoid space by way of the foramina of Magendie and Luschka. CSF enters the venous circulation by way of the absorptive arachnoid villi that line the superior sagittal sinus. Any disturbance of the flow or absorption of CSF leads to accumulation and hydrocephalus. Two mechanisms exist to explain pathologic CSF accumulation:

A. **Noncommunicating hydrocephalus** is the result of obstruction anywhere along the ventricular CSF pathway from the third ventricle to the subarachnoid cisterna (ie, cisterna magna). Also known as obstructive hydrocephalus, noncommunicating hydrocephalus is an obstruction to the progressive flow of CSF. It is any blockage of CSF that keeps it from reaching the subarachnoid space and the normal resorptive function of the arachnoid villi (eg, blockage may be aqueductal stenosis, ventriculitis, or a clot following an extensive intraventricular hemorrhage).

B. **Communicating hydrocephalus** results when CSF is able to pass through all the foramina, including the foramina at the base of the brain (cisterna magna), but is not absorbed into the venous drainage of the cerebral circulation because of obliteration of the arachnoid villi. Various disease processes can result in obliteration of the arachnoid villi causing CSF accumulation throughout the cerebral ventricular system (ie, following bacterial meningitis or an extensive subarachnoid hemorrhage).

II. **Incidence.** The incidence of neonatal hydrocephalus alone is unknown. When included in the diagnosis of spina bifida it occurs in 2–5 births in 1000.

III. **Pathophysiology**
   A. **Congenital hydrocephalus (CH)** refers to progressive ventricular enlargement, starting prior to birth and readily apparent on the first day of life. All typical forms of CH are noncommunicating or obstructive in presentation. CH results from developmental malformations of the brain that disturb CSF pathways. Most malformations occur between 6 and 17 weeks of gestation. Fetal hydrocephalus is usually severe and accompanied by other serious anomalies of the brain, namely holoprosencephaly or encephalocele. Fifty percent of CH cases presenting as fetal hydrocephalus are associated with myelomeningocele, Arnold Chiari malformation, aqueduct stenosis, or the Dandy-Walker malformation.
   B. **Postinfectious hydrocephalus** may be either communicating or noncommunicating. Bacterial inflammation of the meninges and subsequent arachnoiditis sets the stage for loss of the CSF absorptive sites and communicating hydrocephalus (eg, group B streptococcus, *Escherichia coli,* and *Listeria* monocytogenes). Conversely, a ventriculitis leads to obstruction within the ventricular system, usually the floor of the third ventricle and within the aqueduct of Sylvius. Examples of ventriculitis-related hydrocephalus are tuberculosis and toxoplasmosis. Indirectly related to the CSF circulatory disturbance can be the formation of a postinfectious subdural effusion with ICP and subsequent hydrocephalus.
   C. **Posthemorrhagic ventricular dilatation (PVD) and posthemorrhagic hydrocephalus (PHH).** It is important to distinguish between PVD and PHH. The distinction is one of timing, progression of ventricular enlargement, and whether or not there is evidence for ICP. PVD follows germinal matrix/intraventricular hemorrhage (GM/IVH) in nearly a third of all cases. It follows the more severe hemorrhages and can present as asymmetric or symmetric dilation of the lateral ventricles. PVD may present early within the first week posthemorrhage as an acute ventricular dilation or slowly become progressive over ≥2 weeks. By definition, hydrocephalus must present with some sign of increased ICP. An important clinical differential is that PVD does not present with signs of increasing pressure. Moreover, recognizing PVD and following it closely will reveal if it is self-limiting and possibly self-resolving without intervention. It may simply represent ventriculomegaly due to disturbed CSF flow following hemorrhage. Hemorrhagic blood and clots may dissipate and allow resumption of CSF circulation.

   PHH may acutely complicate a massive IVH, but more typically evolves posthemorrhage and presents as either communicating or obstructive noncommunicating hydrocephalus with ICP. A helpful overview by Goddard-Feingold et al suggests the following outcomes of ventriculomegaly post GM/IVH as:
   1. PVD that resolves leaving normal ventricles.
   2. Transient PHH that resolves (ie, "arrested") leaving some residual but static ventriculomegaly.
   3. PHH that is progressive and requires intervention to maintain a stable ICP.
   4. Ventriculomegaly with cerebral atrophy and no ICP.
   D. **Other ventriculomegalies.** Ventriculomegaly that reflects cortical atrophy has been called hydrocephalus *ex vacuo;* the term is no longer used because the condition is not a true hydrocephalus. Ventriculomegaly with loss of periventricular white matter is a complication of periventricular hemorrhagic infarction (PVHI). It is almost always unilateral, or if bilateral, decidedly asymmetric. PVHI with loss of periventricular white matter may present as a large extended porencephalic cyst. Increasing ICP is not a factor in either ventriculomegaly with cortical atrophy or periventricular white matter loss.
IV. **Risk factors.** Congenital malformations (eg, aqueductal stenosis), intracranial neoplasms, CNS bleeds, and infections are some risk factors for the development of hydrocephalus.
V. **Clinical presentation**
   A. **Head circumference.** Foremost in clinical assessment is regular and frequent OFC measurements of at-risk infants. Rapidly increasing head size of ≥2 cm per week remains the hallmark clinical finding. Additionally, findings on examination of the

head may reveal distended scalp veins, separating sutures, a full or bulging fontanel, or a cerebral bruit. All are signs pointing to significant increasing ICP and PHH.

B. **Apnea with bradycardia.** Apnea with bradycardia in association with post GM/IVH monitoring is a strong clinical sign of increasing ICP.

C. **Gastrointestinal.** Feeding intolerance with or without vomiting are suspect associations with PHH.

D. **Eye findings.** Increased appearance of sclera above the iris is suggestive of increased ICP. Although inconsistent in preterm and term infants, if seen it is an important observation and sometimes referred to as the "setting-sun sign."

E. **Behavioral state changes.** Irritability or lethargy, not previously attributed to the infants' day-to-day behavior, are noteworthy when seen with any of the signs noted above.

VI. **Diagnosis**

A. **Antenatal diagnosis.** Fetal hydrocephalus may be detected by fetal ultrasound as early as 15–18 weeks' gestation. Amniocentesis is advisable to evaluate chromosomal abnormalities associated with hydrocephalus (trisomies 13 and 18), fetal gender (X-linked aqueductal stenosis), and α-fetoprotein levels. Maternal serology may establish an unsuspected intrauterine infection (eg, toxoplasmosis, syphilis, or cytomegalovirus).

B. **Newborn physical examination.** The OFC must be carefully measured regularly and consistently. A rate of head growth >2 cm/week usually signals the rapid progression of ventricular dilation.

1. Make note of the parents' head sizes. Some parents might have a constitutionally large head size and so might their infant. Normal for adult women is 54 ±3 cm, and for men 55 ±3 cm. No further evaluation of the infant would be required unless there are risk factors for an enlarging head or signs of increased ICP.

2. Fifty percent of infants with X-linked aqueductal stenosis have a characteristic flexion deformity of the thumb.

3. Infants with Dandy-Walker malformation have occipital cranial prominence.

4. Funduscopic examination may reveal chorioretinitis indicative of an intrauterine infection.

5. A cerebral bruit may signal the presence of an arteriovenous malformation of the vein of Galen or increased ICP secondary to hydrocephalus or subdural effusion.

C. **Cranial ultrasonography (cUS)** is the most important screening tool for premature infants at risk for ventriculomegaly or hydrocephalus (see Figure 10–4). Of singular importance is the fact that ventricular dilation may precede clinical signs of hydrocephalus by days or weeks. Clearly, signs of increasing OFC dictate a screening cUS. Likewise, infants of difficult labor and delivery and those who may have needed resuscitation measures are candidates for screening cUS. In our institution a decision is made to screen by the seventh day of life or earlier, depending on the severity of disease and the stability of the patient. Subsequent cUS studies are carried out at 5- to 10-day intervals as clinically needed or by earlier findings. Screening by 2 weeks of age detects 98% of cases of PHH.

D. **Computed tomography cranial scanning** remains useful for image studies in selected patients. It provides the following useful information:

1. Ventricular dilation identification.

2. Determination of the size of the cerebral mantle.

3. Detection of associated CNS anomalies.

4. Detection of parenchymal destruction (eg, calcification or cysts).

5. Determination of a likely site of disturbance of CSF dynamics.

E. **Magnetic resonance imaging (MRI)** has become the most effective means of detailing brain injury, hypoxic ischemic events, hemorrhage, malformations, and ventriculomegaly. Fetal brain imaging with new ultrafast MRI studies negates the motion artifact of the fetus that has previously limited fetal MRI studies. Ultrafast MRI now lends itself to in utero imaging for congenital anomalies of the brain and fetal hydrocephalus. For the infant with GM/IVH and at risk for PVHI, studies by MRI are more accurate at documenting parenchymal loss and the formation of porencephalic cysts.

VII. Management
   A. In the presence of significant fetal hydrocephalus:
      1. Pulmonary maturity and prompt cesarean delivery.
      2. If the lungs are immature, there are three options:
         a. Immediate delivery with the risks of prematurity.
         b. Delayed delivery (with the risks of persistently increasing ICP) until the lungs are mature. Administer antenatal steroids for induction of lung maturity, and deliver the infant as soon as lung maturity is established.
         c. Fetal surgery options of in utero ventricular drainage with a ventriculoamniotic shunt or transabdominal external drainage.
      3. Consultation. Ideal management calls for a team approach with the obstetrician, neonatologist, neurosurgeon, ultrasonographer, geneticist, ethicist, and family members.
   B. Hydrocephalus associated with congenital aqueductal stenosis or neural tube defects. Decompress by prompt placement of a ventricular bypass shunt into an intracranial or extracranial compartment.
   C. Post hemorrhagic hydrocephalus
      1. Mild hydrocephalus usually arrests within 4 weeks of progressive ventricular dilation or returns to normal within the first few months of life.
      2. Temporizing measures
         a. Serial lumbar punctures (LPs) may be instituted if there is communicating hydrocephalus. Removal of 10–15 mL/kg CSF is frequently necessary. Approximately two thirds of this group of infants undergo arrest with partial or total resolution, and one third still require extracranial shunting of CSF.
         b. Drugs to decrease CSF production. Acetazolamide may be administered with or without furosemide (see Chapter 132) with limited clinical improvement. Complications include significant metabolic acidosis, hypercalciuria, and nephrocalcinosis.
         c. Ventricular drainage can be done by direct or tunneled external ventricular drain or by a subcutaneous ventricular catheter that drains to a reservoir or to subgaleal or supraclavicular spaces. This is indicated for infants who have not responded adequately to LPs and who are not good candidates for placement of an extracranial shunt. The incidence of infection with these devices is ~5%. Of more recent development has been the success of a third ventriculostomy. It is an endoscopic procedure that creates a communication from the floor of the third ventricle directly into the subarachnoid space at the level of the foramina of the cisterna magna. It has been particularly promising for obstructive PHH with occlusion of the aqueduct of Sylvius.
      3. Permanent management. The method of choice is placement of ventriculoperitoneal (VP) shunts. The outcome is better with "early" shunting. It remains *controversial* whether an elevated CSF protein level increases the risk of shunt complications and whether shunting should be delayed in patients with a high CSF protein content. VP shunt placement is indicated in nearly all cases to facilitate control of OFC, improved head control, skin care, general nursing care, and patient comfort. VP shunt function depends on shunt valve integrity. The Holter valve was a standard device for almost 50 years, but its limitations included overdrainage of CSF causing symptoms of headache and dizziness and renewed obstruction because of collapse of the ventricles (the slit ventricle syndrome). Newer valves combine programmable magnetic valves with added antisiphon controls for protection against overdrainage when the patient is in the upright position.
            Long-term complications of shunts include scalp ulceration, infection (usually staphylococcal), arachnoiditis, occlusion, development or clinical worsening of an inguinal hernia or hydrocele, organ perforation (secondary to intraperitoneal contact of a catheter with a hollow viscus), slit ventricle syndrome (symptoms of raised ICP in the presence of slit ventricles), blindness, endocarditis, and renal and heart failure. Age of <6 months appears to be a major risk factor for shunt infection in infants.

VIII. **Prognosis**
    A. **Outcomes have significantly improved** with modern neurosurgical techniques for PHH. Long-term survival now approaches 90% with functioning shunts in place.
    B. **Predictors of unfavorable outcome**
        1. Cerebral mantle width <1 cm before shunt placement.
        2. As to the cause of hydrocephalus, prognosis decreases in the following order: communicating hydrocephalus and myelomeningocele > aqueduct stenosis > Dandy-Walker malformation.
        3. Reduced size of the corpus callosum is associated with decreased nonverbal cognitive skills and motor abilities.
        4. In preterm infants with PHH, poor long-term outcome is directly correlated with the severity of IVH, the presence of PVHI or cystic PVL, the need for VP shunt, shunt infections, and a high number of shunt revisions.

Selected References

Baldauf J et al: Endoscopic third ventriculostomy in children younger than 2 years of age. *Childs Nerv Syst* 2007;23:623-626.

Cohen AR: Disorders in head shape and size. In Martin RJ et al (eds): *Fanaroff's and Martin's Neonatal-Perinatal Medicine: Diseases of the Fetus and Newborn*, 8th ed. Philadelphia, PA: Elsevier Mosby, 2006:998-1003.

Goddard-Feingold J et al: The newborn nervous system. In Taeusch W, Ballard R (eds): *Avery's Diseases of the Newborn*, 7th ed. Philadelphia, PA: Saunders, 1998:863.

Khalid HK, Magram G: Siphon regulatory devices: their role in the treatment of hydrocephalus. *Neurosurg Focus* 2007;22: E5-E14.

Koch D, Wagner W: Endoscopic third ventriculostomy in infants of less than 1 year of age: which factors influence the outcome? *Childs Nerv Syst* 2004;20:405-411.

Kondageski C et al: Experience with the Strata valve in the management of shunt overdrainage. *J Neurosurg* 2007;106:95-102.

Volpe JJ: *Neurology of the Newborn*, 4th ed. Philadelphia, PA: Saunders, 2001.

Whitby E et al: Ultrafast magnetic resonance imaging of central nervous system abnormalities in utero in the third trimester of pregnancy: comparison with ultrasound. *Br J Obstet Gynaecol* 2001;108:519-526.

Zimmerman RA, Bilaniuk LT: Neuroimaging evaluation of cerebral palsy. *Clin Perinatol* 2006;33:517-544.

91 Hyperbilirubinemia, Direct (Conjugated Hyperbilirubinemia)

HYPERBILIRUBINEMIA

Jaundice is the most common transitional finding, occurring in 60–70% of term newborns and ~80% of infants born prematurely. An elevation of serum bilirubin concentration >2 mg/dL is found in virtually all newborns in the first several days of life. Jaundice becomes clinically apparent at serum bilirubin concentration of >5 mg/dL.

Bilirubin is the end product of the catabolism of heme derived primarily from the breakdown of red blood cell hemoglobin. The rate-limiting step in this production is the oxidation of heme to form a green pigment called biliverdin, a process controlled by the enzyme **heme oxygenase.** Each molecule of heme catabolized results in equimolar quantities of bilirubin and carbon monoxide. Other sources of heme include heme-containing proteins such as myoglobin, cytochromes, and nitric oxide synthase. Bilirubin exists in several forms in the blood but is predominantly bound to serum albumin; other compounds, such as drugs and metal ions, may compete with bilirubin for albumin binding sites. Elevated concentration of free unconjugated bilirubin, and possibly other forms, can enter the central nervous system (CNS) and become toxic to cells. The precise mechanism is unknown.

Inside liver cells, unconjugated bilirubin is bound immediately to intracellular proteins, the most important one being ligandin. It is then converted into an excretable and soluble form through the process of conjugation that consist of the transfer of one or two glucuronic acid residues from uridine diphosphoglucuronic acid (UDPGA) to form a monoglucuronide or diglucuronide conjugate. Uridine diphosphoglucuronyl transferase (UDPGT) is the major enzyme involved in this process. Conjugation is impaired in newborns due to reduced UDPGT activity and a relatively low level of uridine diphosphoglucuronic acid. Conjugated bilirubin is water soluble and can be excreted in the urine, but most of it is rapidly excreted as bile into the intestine. Conjugated bilirubin is further metabolized by bacteria in the intestine and excreted in the feces.

Hyperbilirubinemia presents as either unconjugated hyperbilirubinemia or conjugated hyperbilirubinemia. The two forms involve different pathophysiologic causes with distinct potential complications. In contrast to unconjugated hyperbilirubinemia, which can be transient and physiologic in the newborn period, conjugated hyperbilirubinemia is always pathologic. See Chapter 92 for a discussion of unconjugated hyperbilirubinemia.

HYPERBILIRUBINEMIA, CONJUGATED (DIRECT)

I. **Definition.** Conjugated hyperbilirubinemia is defined as a conjugated bilirubin concentration of >1.5–2 mg/dL or more than 10–20% of total serum bilirubin (TSB). It is the biochemical marker of **cholestasis** and a sign of hepatobiliary dysfunction. Unlike physiologic unconjugated hyperbilirubinemia, typically known as "physiologic jaundice of the newborn," it is important to emphasize that there is no physiologic conjugated hyperbilirubinemia. Chapter 50 provides information on the rapid "on-call" assessment and management.

II. **Incidence.** Conjugated hyperbilirubinemia affects approximately 1 in every 2500 infants and is less common than unconjugated hyperbilirubinemia.

III. **Pathophysiology.** Normal bile production involves two main processes: bile acid uptake by the hepatocytes from the blood, and bile excretion into the biliary canaliculus. Bile uptake from the blood is an active process facilitated by two main receptors at the basolateral membranes called Na taurocholate cotransporting polypeptide and organic anion transporting proteins. Bile secretion at the canalicular membrane is mediated by the bile salt export pump, and some other important canalicular transporters, called MRP2 and MDR3, which transport conjugated bilirubin and phospholipids into bile. In healthy newborns, the cellular processes that regulates bile flow are immature and do not function at the normal adult level, making them more susceptible to cholestasis.

IV. **Risk factors** include infections, sepsis, neonatal hepatitis, ABO incompatibility, trisomy 21, and the use of total parenteral nutrition (TPN).

V. **Clinical presentation.** Prolonged clinical jaundice is the main presenting complaint of conjugated hyperbilirubinemia, along with pale (acholic) stools and dark urine. The Cholestasis Guideline Committee recommends that any infant noted to be jaundiced at 2 weeks of age be evaluated for cholestasis. Breast-fed infants who have a **normal history and physical examination and can reliably be monitored** may be evaluated for cholestasis at 3 weeks of age if jaundice is persistent. No single screening test can predict which infant will develop cholestasis, so it is critical that care providers are able to recognize clinical signs and gather history relevant to detection of cholestasis, such as persistent jaundice, pale/clay-colored stools, and dark urine. The **differential diagnosis of conjugated hyperbilirubinemia** (ie, cholestasis) is extensive. It can be classified based on the anatomic location of the pathologic process (extrahepatic vs intrahepatic causes) or it can be categorized into broad etiologic causes, such as infectious, familial, metabolic, toxic, chromosomal, vascular, and bile duct anomalies. Recent understanding in molecular genetics has pointed to new directions of investigations that resulted in identification of the molecular mechanisms of a subset of hepatobiliary diseases that often can lead to ongoing liver dysfunction. The most common differential diagnoses of neonatal cholestasis are as follows: extrahepatic biliary atresia (25%), genetic intrahepatic cholestasis (25%—includes progressive familial intrahepatic cholestasis [PFIC], Alagille syndrome, bile acid synthetic defect), metabolic diseases (20%), idiopathic neonatal hepatitis (15%), α-1-antitrypsin deficiency (10%), and viral (5%). See Table 91–1 for a list of differential diagnoses.

Table 91–1. CAUSES OF CONJUGATED HYPERBILIRUBINEMIA

Extrahepatic biliary disease
Biliary atresia
Choledochal cyst
Bile duct stenosis
Spontaneous perforation of the bile duct
Cholelithiasis
Neoplasms

Intrahepatic biliary disease
Intrahepatic bile duct paucity (syndromic or nonsyndromic)
Progressive intrahepatic cholestasis
Inspissated bile

Hepatocellular disease
Metabolic and genetic defects
α_1-antitrypsin deficiency, cystic fibrosis, Zellweger syndrome, Dubin-Johnson syndrome, Rotor syndrome, and galactosemia
Infections
Total parenteral nutrition
Idiopathic neonatal hepatitis
Neonatal hemochromatosis

Miscellaneous
Shock, extracorporeal membrane oxygenation (ECMO)

INTRAHEPATIC CHOLESTASIS WITH NORMAL BILE DUCTS
Infection
Viral: hepatitis B virus; non-A, non-B hepatitis virus; cytomegalovirus; herpes simplex virus; coxsackievirus; Epstein-Barr virus; adenovirus
Bacterial: *Treponema pallidum, Escherichia coli,* group B streptococcus, *Staphylococcus aureus, Listeria monocytogenes;* urinary tract infection caused by *E. coli* and other Gram-negative organisms
Other: *Toxoplasma gondii*

Genetic disorders and inborn errors of metabolism: Progressive familial intrahepatic cholestasis, Dubin-Johnson syndrome, Rotor syndrome, galactosemia, hereditary fructose intolerance, tyrosinemia, α_1-antitrypsin deficiency, Byler disease, recurrent cholestasis with lymphedema, cerebrohepatorenal syndrome, congenital erythropoietic porphyria, Niemann-Pick disease, Menkes' kinky hair syndrome

Idiopathic neonatal hepatitis

Total parenteral nutrition–induced cholestasis

A. **Specific diseases**
   1. **Biliary atresia** is the single most common cause of liver transplantation in children. It is a progressive idiopathic inflammatory process that leads to chronic cholestasis and fibrosis of both the intrahepatic and extrahepatic bile ducts and subsequent biliary cirrhosis. It has a worldwide estimated incidence of 1 in 15,000 live births, with the highest incidence in Taiwan and French Polynesia (1 in 3000 live births). There are two distinct phenotypes identified: the embryonic or fetal form is less common, associated with an earlier onset of cholestasis and multiple congenital anomalies, and the perinatal or acquired form, occurring in 80% of cases, without associated congenital anomalies. In the perinatal or acquired form, infants are presumed to have a normal and patent biliary system at birth that subsequently undergoes progressive inflammation and fibroobliteration due to a perinatal insult. One theory as to the etiology is the potential role of viral infection as the initiator of bile duct injury with a secondary immune-mediated progression of the disease. It is critical to confirm or exclude the diagnosis of biliary atresia as the cause of conjugated hyperbilirubinemia by 45–60 days of age. Evidence suggests that early surgical intervention leads to a better outcome and prognosis.
   2. **Genetic intrahepatic cholestasis.** There are multiple forms of genetic intrahepatic cholestasis, each with different clinical features and variable clinical presentation and prognosis. Some progressive familial forms (formerly called PFIC) are potentially fatal; the syndromic paucity of intrahepatic bile ducts (Alagille syndrome) tends to have a more favorable prognosis. The pathogenetic mechanisms of this group of disorders have been defined only partially, and the techniques of molecular genetics have only been recently applied. These disorders, although individually rare, are collectively common.
      a. **Alagille syndrome** is a syndromic condition characterized by paucity of bile ducts thought to be due to altered embryogenesis, and it is also known as arteriohepatic dysplasia. It is a genetic disorder, transmitted as autosomal dominant inheritance with variable expression. Genetic basis has been identified to be mutations in *JAG1* on chromosome 20p. Its major clinical features include a paucity of the intrahepatic bile ducts (chronic cholestasis), cardiovascular anomalies (peripheral pulmonic stenosis), skeletal abnormalities (butterfly vertebrae), ophthalmologic finding (posterior embryotoxon), and "typical facies" (facial shape of an inverted triangle, with broad forehead, deep-set eyes, mild hypertelorism, straight nose with flattened tip, prominent chin, and small low-set malformed ears). The abnormality of bile ducts is considered to be the most consistent finding in Alagille syndrome; however, the paucity of bile ducts may not be present in 20–40% of young infants. Therefore repeated liver biopsies may be needed in patients with clinically suspected diagnosis but not confirmed on initial histologic diagnosis. Long-term prognosis depends on severity and duration of cholestasis, severity of cardiovascular defect, and liver status as it relates to need for liver transplantation.
      b. **Progressive familial intrahepatic cholestasis** (PFIC) is a group of genetic disorders, with autosomal recessive inheritance and characterized by progressive intrahepatic cholestasis. The predominant mechanism for the intrahepatic cholestasis is altered canalicular transport. Currently, three types of PFIC are recognized.
         i. **PFIC-1 was originally called Byler disease.** It presents with conjugated hyperbilirubinemia early in life, typically within the first 3 months. Diarrhea, pancreatitis, and deficiency of fat-soluble vitamins are seen. Cirrhosis is seen by the first decade of life, and liver transplantation is usually needed by the second decade of life.

ii. **PFIC-2 is caused by bile salt export pump (BSEP) deficiency,** resulting in altered bile acid transport. It has a presentation similar to PFIC-1 with no evidence of pancreatitis. Serum gamma glutamyl transpeptidase (γ-GTP) is not elevated despite cholestasis.

iii. **PFIC-3 is due to multidrug resistance protein 3 (MDR3) deficiency,** resulting in altered phospholipid transport into the canaliculus. It is clinically similar to PFIC-1 and PFIC-2, except that PFIC-3 has an elevated level of γ-GTP.

3. **Metabolic disorders.** (See Chapter 93.) In the neonatal period, several inborn metabolic disorders can result in hepatocellular injury that can give rise to a clinical syndrome of neonatal hepatitis. The most common metabolic disease that presents as cholestasis is α-1-antitrypsin deficiency. Metabolic diseases that can present with rather fulminant liver dysfunction include galactosemia, tyrosinemia, and hereditary fructose intolerance. Hereditary fructose intolerance does not present in the neonatal period unless the infant was exposed to a fructose-containing diet.

a. **Galactosemia.** The most well-known metabolic disorder that presents with prolonged jaundice is galactosemia. It has an estimated incidence of 1 in 23,000 to 1 in 50,000. It is caused by deficiency of the enzyme galactose-1-phosphate uridyltransferase (GALT) resulting in accumulation of galactose-1-phosphate and other metabolites that are thought to be toxic to the liver and other organ systems. The gold standard of diagnosis is measurement of GALT activity in the erythrocytes. Clinical presentation is variable and nonspecific in the neonatal period (occurs after ingestion of galactose-containing formula) and includes vomiting, loose stools, prolonged jaundice, irritability, and poor weight gain. Continued ingestion of galactose results in multiorgan toxicity with hepatomegaly, worsening liver dysfunction, splenomegaly, renal dysfunction, and CNS involvement. These infants while on lactose-containing formula have galactose in the urine, resulting in a positive reducing substance in the urine (Clinitest) but negative urine test for glucose (glucose oxidase). A cataract may be detected on examination. "Oil-drop" cataracts are highly typical of galactosemia and may resolve with treatment if diagnosed early. The incidence of neonatal sepsis, specifically due to *Escherichia coli* and other Gram-negative organisms is more frequent in galactosemic infants. The reason for this unique predisposition for newborns with GALT deficiency remains unclear. Treatment for galactosemia consists of immediate removal of galactose in the diet as soon as diagnosis is suspected. Liver disease usually improves, but long-term neurodevelopmental complications may develop later despite good dietary control.

b. **Tyrosinemia.** Biochemical basis for this disorder is a defect in tyrosine metabolism due to lack of fumarylacetoacetate hydrolase. It is inherited as autosomal recessive disorder that clinically presents with hepatocellular damage, renal tubular dysfunction, and neuropathy. One characteristic pattern of tyrosinemia is a very high α-fetoprotein. For those patients who survived infancy, they are at high risk of developing hepatocellular carcinoma.

c. **Zellweger or cerebrohepatorenal syndrome.** This is a peroxisomal disorder characterized by the absence of peroxisomes and deranged mitochondria. It is inherited as an autosomal recessive trait and presents in the neonatal period with cholestasis, hepatomegaly, profound hypotonia, and dysmorphic features. Diagnosis is confirmed by the presence of abnormal levels of very-long-chain fatty acid in the serum. Most infants die within 1 year. Survivors beyond 1 year of age have severe mental retardation and seizures.

d. **α-1-Antitrypsin deficiency.** The most common inherited cause of neonatal hepatitis syndrome, with an incidence of 1 in 1600 to 1 in 2000 live births in

North American and European population, α-1-antitrypsin is the most abundant proteinase inhibitor, and it acts by inhibiting destructive proteases. Clinical diagnosis is made by documenting low serum concentration of α-1-antitrypsin and identifying the phenotypic variant based on differences in isoelectric point (Pi), with M normal and Z most deficient. There are several phenotypes; however, the homozygous Pi (protease inhibitor) ZZ is the most likely associated with neonatal liver disease and adult emphysema. Despite carrying the same mutation only 10–15% of newborns present clinically. Treatment is mostly supportive or liver transplantation if cirrhosis is progressive. Outcome is related to severity of neonatal liver disease; 50% of children are clinically normal by 10 years of age, 5–10% require liver transplantation, and in 20–30% of patients, cholestasis resolves with residual evidence of cirrhosis that may eventually require liver transplantation.

4. **Idiopathic neonatal hepatitis** is a diagnosis given to neonatal hepatitis with liver histology showing giant cell multinucleated hepatocytes where no known infectious or metabolic has been found. Diagnosis is one of exclusion. Management is mostly supportive. Overall prognosis is difficult to estimate but generally good for infants whose liver disease resolves in the first year.

5. **Infection**
   a. **Congenital infections (TORCH [*t*oxoplasmosis, *o*ther infections, *r*ubella, *c*ytomegalovirus, and *h*erpes simplex virus).** Congenitally acquired infections have a spectrum of manifestations but are usually asymptomatic. They share clinical similarities such as hepatosplenomegaly, jaundice, petechial rash, and intrauterine growth restriction. Liver dysfunction is a possible presentation with any of these viral agents, but it is most common with herpes simplex infection. Vertical transmission of hepatitis viruses (B and C) is generally asymptomatic, but clinical hepatitis, including hepatic failure, may develop later.
   b. **Bacterial infections.** Cholestatic jaundice has been linked predominantly with Gram-negative infections (particularly *E. coli*). Recent studies point to endotoxinemia and the subsequent release of cytokines during infections as the major factors in sepsis-associated cholestasis. The development of a disproportionate elevation of serum bilirubin in comparison with serum alkaline phosphatase and serum aminotransferases should be considered an early warning sign of an underlying infection. Sepsis-related cholestasis should be part of the differential diagnosis of new-onset or worsening jaundice in a hospitalized patient.

6. **Total parenteral nutrition (TPN)-related cholestasis.** The frequency, not necessarily the severity, of cholestasis is partly a function of the degree of prematurity. Cholestasis develops in >50% of infants with birthweight of <1000 g and <10% of term infants after prolonged hyperalimentation. Of infants who require long-term TPN for intestinal failure, 40–60% develop TPN-related liver disease. Pathogenesis is unknown but thought to be multifactorial and directly related to prematurity, low birthweight, episodes of sepsis, and duration of TPN use. One of the most important contributing factors is lack of enteral feeding leading to decreased gut hormone secretion, reduction of bile flow, and biliary stasis. Even small oral feedings (continuous or bolus) during hyperalimentation may prevent TPN-related liver disease. The resumption of normal enteral feeds is associated with improvement of cholestasis in 1–3 months, with minimal or no residual fibrosis and normal hepatic function. Hepatic complications are potentially reversible if TPN is discontinued before significant liver damage has ensued.

7. **Inspissated bile.** The "inspissated bile syndrome" is the term traditionally used for conjugated hyperbilirubinemia resulting from severe jaundice associated with hemolysis due to Rh or ABO incompatibility, although a multifactorial cause

cannot be entirely excluded. Intrahepatic cholestasis is found on liver biopsy, and cholestasis is probably related to direct hepatocellular damage produced by unconjugated hyperbilirubinemia. Prognosis is generally good.

VI. **Diagnosis.** Evaluation of cholestasis can be extensive; therefore, it should be individualized to establish a diagnosis efficiently and promptly. Figure 91–1 provides a concise algorithm for an infant with conjugated hyperbilirubinemia.

A. **Laboratory studies**

1. **Bilirubin levels (total and direct).** The most important initial investigation in a persistently jaundiced infant is determining the fractionated serum bilirubin levels. Conjugated hyperbilirubinemia is defined as conjugated or direct reacting bilirubin >20% of total bilirubin level.

2. **Liver enzymes.** Serum aspartate transaminase (AST) and serum alanine transaminase (ALT) are sensitive indicators of hepatocellular inflammation but are neither specific nor of any prognostic value. They may be helpful in monitoring the course of the disease. Alkaline phosphatase is nonspecific because it is found in the liver, kidney, and bone.

3. **Prothrombin time and partial thromboplastin time** may be more reliable indicators of liver synthetic function.

4. **γ-Glutamyl transpeptidase (GGT)** is an enzyme in the biliary epithelium. Elevated levels are a very sensitive marker of biliary obstruction or inflammation. A normal level makes biliary atresia an unlikely diagnosis. Normal levels of GGT in presence of cholestasis indicate failure of bile excretion at the canalicular level and can be seen in progressive familial hepatic cholestasis.

5. **Complete blood count, C-reactive protein, blood and urine cultures** should be considered to screen for any clinical evidence of infection.

6. **Serum cholesterol, triglycerides, and albumin levels.** Triglyceride and cholesterol levels may aid in nutritional management and assessment of liver failure. Albumin is a long-term indicator of hepatic function.

7. **Ammonia levels** should be checked if liver failure is suspected.

8. **Serum glucose levels** should be checked if the infant appears ill. Metabolic disorders may present with hypoglycemia along with conjugated hyperbilirubinemia.

9. **Urine testing for reducing substances** is a simple screening test that should always be performed to screen for metabolic disease especially for galactosemia. Galactose in the urine results in a positive reducing substance in the urine on a Clinitest but has a negative urine test for glucose (glucose oxidase).

10. **TORCH titers and urine cultures for CMV.** The use of TORCH titers is less preferable; direct identification of viral infection or measurement of specific IgM antibodies should be done for rapid diagnosis. PCR-based diagnostic studies are extremely helpful and specific.

11. **Other tests.** More specific tests are indicated in the investigation of the specific causes of conjugated hyperbilirubinemia.

   a. **Urine organic acid and plasma amino acid** are screens for inborn errors of metabolism as a cause of neonatal liver dysfunction. High concentrations of tyrosine and methionine, and their metabolic derivatives, are seen in the urine in case of tyrosinemia.

   b. **α-1 Antitrypsin serum level.** Decreased serum α-1 antitrypsin concentration and liver biopsy showing periodic acid-Schiff-positive cytoplasmic granules will reveal variable degrees of hepatic necrosis and fibrosis.

   c. **Sweat test.** For diagnosis of cystic fibrosis.

B. **Radiologic studies**

1. **Chest radiograph.** Presence of cardiovascular or situs anomalies may be suggestive of biliary atresia. Skeletal abnormalities, such as butterfly vertebrae, may be consistent with a diagnosis of Alagille syndrome.

2. **Ultrasonography.** A simple and noninvasive test that should be done in all infants presenting with cholestasis. This procedure should be done after a 4-h fast; a small

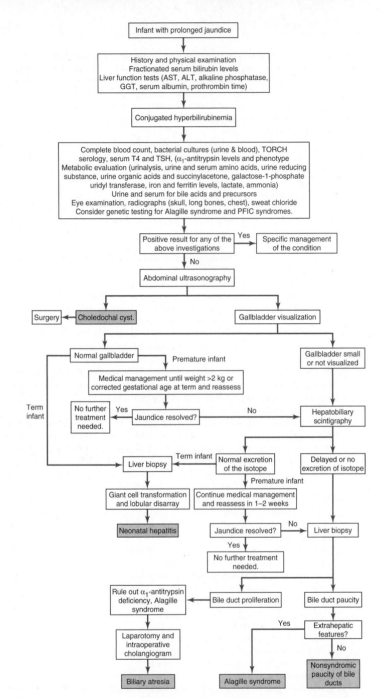

FIGURE 91–1. An approach to a full-term or premature infant with cholestasis. (*Reproduced, with permission, from Venigalla S, Gourley GR: Neonatal cholestasis. Semin Perinatol 2004;28:348-355.*) ALT, alanine transaminase; AST, aspartate transaminase; PFIC, progressive familial intrahepatic cholestasis; TORCH, *t*oxoplasmosis, *o*ther infections, *r*ubella, *c*ytomegalovirus, and *h*erpes simplex virus.

or absent gallbladder is suggestive of biliary atresia, whereas the presence of a normal-looking gallbladder makes this diagnosis unlikely. Ultrasound is a sensitive method for recognizing other surgical causes of neonatal cholestasis, such as a choledochal cyst or structural abnormalities of the biliary tree.

3. **Hepatobiliary scanning.** Contrast agents are taken up by the liver and excreted into the bile. HIDA (hepatobiliary iminodiacetic acid), EHIDA (ethyl hepatobiliary iminodiacetic acid), and PIPIDA (*p*-isopropylacetanilideiminodiacetic acid) are technetium labeled and provide a clear image of the biliary tree after intravenous injection. Serial images are taken for up to 24 h or until gut activity is visualized. Nonvisualization of contrast material within the intestine in 24 h is considered an abnormal finding indicative of biliary obstruction or hepatocellular dysfunction. Sensitivity of this test for biliary atresia is high, but specificity is low because many patients without anatomic obstruction may not excrete the tracer. **Neonatal hepatitis, hyperalimentation,** and **septo-optic dysplasia** are reported causes of absent gastrointestinal contrast excretion and must be considered in the diagnosis of biliary atresia. It is thought that administration of phenobarbital for several days prior to the study may improve precision of the test.

4. **Endoscopic retrograde cholangiopancreatography.** Sensitivity and specificity are excellent. This procedure can be both diagnostic and therapeutic in cases of cholestasis caused by bile duct stones. It is technically demanding and currently has a limited role in the evaluation of cholestasis in neonates. A more recent study has reported an improved success rate and low complications in the hands of an expert endoscopist.

C. **Other studies**

1. **Percutaneous liver biopsy** is the single most definitive procedure in the evaluation of neonatal cholestasis; however biopsy interpretation requires a pathologist with expertise in pediatric liver disease. If a liver biopsy is obtained early in the course of biliary atresia, findings may be indistinguishable from hepatitis. Evidence supports that liver biopsy can be performed safely in young infants; it is therefore recommended that liver biopsy be performed in infants with undiagnosed cholestasis.

2. **Magnetic resonance cholangiopancreatography (MRCP).** The few reports available to date regarding the use of MRCP in children are encouraging, but firm conclusions are not possible. The procedure requires deep sedation or general anesthesia. Based on current available data, this modality is not routinely recommended in the evaluation of cholestasis in neonates.

VII. **Management.** Rapid "on-call" assessment and management is discussed in Chapter 50.

A. **Medical management.** Few conditions causing neonatal cholestasis are treatable, and these conditions (ie, biliary atresia and choledochal cyst) need timely diagnosis and management. Medical treatment is mostly supportive and should be directed toward promoting growth and development and in treating the other complications of chronic cholestasis, such as pruritus, malabsorption, nutritional deficiencies, and portal hypertension. Generally, management involves dietary manipulation and fat-soluble vitamin support. There is no evidence that any medical management alters the natural history of cholestasis.

1. **Special formula.** Elemental formula containing medium-chain triglycerides is preferable because it can be better absorbed regardless of luminal concentration of bile acids.

2. **Medium-chain triglycerides (MCTs).** Long-chain triglycerides are poorly absorbed in the absence of sufficient bile salts. Therefore, infants with cholestasis often require a diet that includes MCTs, which can be absorbed without the action of bile salts. Formulas containing MCTs include Portagen and Pregestimil. Breast-fed cholestatic infants should be given supplemental MCT.

3. **Vitamin supplementation.** Fat malabsorption also interferes with maintenance of adequate levels of fat-soluble vitamins in these infants. Supplementation of vitamins A, D, E, and K is needed. Extra vitamin K supplementation may be necessary if a bleeding tendency develops.

4. **Dietary restrictions.** Removal of galactose and fructose from the diet may prevent the development of cirrhosis and other manifestations of galactosemia and hereditary fructose intolerance, respectively. Dietary restrictions may also be used to treat tyrosinemia but usually are less successful. Most other metabolic causes of cholestatic jaundice have no specific therapy.

B. **Pharmacologic management.** See Chapter 132.

1. **Ursodeoxycholic acid (UDCA, Actigall)** is a naturally occurring dihydroxy bile acid that appears to help cholestasis two ways: substitution in the bile acid pool for more hydrophobic bile acids, and stimulation of bile flow. It was found to lower levels of aminotransferases in patients with viral hepatitis, and to lower biochemical markers and slow the progression of hepatic fibrosis in PFIC. Recommended dose is 20 mg/kg/day in divided doses. The only common side effect is diarrhea, which usually responds to dose reduction.

2. **Phenobarbital.** Mode of action is to enhance bile acid synthesis, increase bile flow, and induce hepatic microsomal enzymes. Recommended dose is 3–5 mg/kg/day. Use is limited by its behavioral and sedative side effects.

3. **Cholestyramine** binds bile acids in the intestinal lumen thereby decreasing enterohepatic circulation of bile acids, which leads to increased fecal excretion and increased hepatic synthesis of bile acids from cholesterol, which may lower serum cholesterol levels. Side effects include binding of fat-soluble vitamins, metabolic acidosis, and constipation.

4. **Rifampin** is effective in the management of pruritus due to cholestasis, but experience is very limited in neonates. Patients should be monitored for hepatotoxicity and idiosyncratic hypersensitivity reaction, such as renal failure, hemolytic anemia, and thrombocytopenia.

C. **Surgical management**

1. **Kasai procedure.** Surgical procedure such as Kasai portoenterostomy should be done to establish biliary drainage in patients diagnosed with biliary atresia. Optimal results are obtained if the procedure is done before 8 weeks of age. The most significant predictor of long-term outcome is resolution of jaundice. The procedure is used as a bridge to transplantation.

2. **Liver transplantation.** When end-stage liver disease is inevitable, liver transplantation is the last resort. Biliary atresia remains the most common indication for liver transplantation in the United States. Overall, the success of liver transplantation has improved significantly. A review of a single center 9-year experience reports patient survival of 94% and 92% at 1 and 5 years, respectively. Long-term complications include immunosuppression, infection, renal failure, and growth retardation.

VIII. **Prognosis.** Based on individual etiologies (see Section V).

Selected References

American Academy of Pediatrics: Subcommittee on hyperbilirubinemia. Management of hyperbilirubinemia in the newborn infant 35 or more weeks of gestation. *Pediatrics* 2004;114:297-316.

Balistreri WF: Neonatal cholestasis. *J Pediatr* 1985;106:171-184.

Balistreri WF, Bezerra JA: Intrahepatic cholestasis: summary of an American Association for the Study of Liver Diseases single-topic conference. *Hepatology* 2005;42:222-235.

Balistreri WF, Bezerra JA: Whatever happened to "neonatal hepatitis"? *Clin Liver Dis* 2006;10:27-53.

Bernstein J et al: Bile-plug syndrome: a correctable cause of obstructive jaundice in infants. *Pediatrics* 1969;43:273-276.

Berry GT: Inborn errors of carbohydrate, ammonia, amino acid and organic acid metabolism. In Taeusch HW et al (eds): *Avery's Diseases of the Newborn*, 8th ed. Philadelphia, PA: Elsevier Saunders, 2005:227-257.

Bosch AM: Classical galactosemia revisited. *J Inherit Metab Dis* 2006;29:516-525.

Cies JJ, Giamalis JN: Treatment of cholestatic pruritus in children. *Am J Health Syst Pharm* 2007;64:1157-1162.

Darwish AA et al: Pediatric liver transplantation using left hepatic segments from living related donors: surgical experience in 100 recipients at Saint-Luc University Clinics. *Pediatr Transplant* 2006;10:345-353.

Dennery PA, Seidman DS: Neonatal hyperbilirubinemia. *N Engl J Med* 2001;344:581-590.

Halamek LP, Stevenson DK: Neonatal jaundice and liver disease. In: Fanaroff AA, Martin RJ (eds): *Neonatal—Perinatal Medicine: Diseases of the Fetus and Infant*, 7th ed. St. Louis, MO: Mosby, 2002:1309-1350.

Harb R, Thomas DW: Conjugated hyperbilirubinemia: screening and treatment in older infants and children. *Pediatr Rev* 2007;28:83-91.

Kamath BM, Piccoli DA: Heritable disorders of the bile ducts. *Gastroenterol Clin North Am* 2003;32:857-875.

Kelly DA: Liver complications of pediatric parenteral nutrition—epidemiology. *Nutrition* 1998;14:153-537.

Landing BH et al: Time course of the intrahepatic lesion of extrahepatic biliary atresia: a morphometric study. *Pediatr Pathol* 1985;4:309-319.

Mack CL: The pathogenesis of biliary atresia: evidence of a virus-induced autoimmune disease. *Semin Liver Dis* 2007;27: 233-242.

Madan A et al: Neonatal hyperbilirubinemia. In: Tauesch HW et al (eds): *Avery's Diseases of the Newborn*, 8th ed. Philadelphia, PA: Elsevier Saunders, 2005:1226-1256.

Maisels MJ: Neonatal jaundice. *Pediatr Rev* 2006;27:443-454.

McKiernan PJ: Neonatal cholestasis. *Semin Neonatol* 2002;7:153-165.

Moseley RH: Sepsis and cholestasis. *Clin Liver Dis* 2004;8:83-94.

Moyer V et al: Guideline for the evaluation of cholestatic jaundice in infants: recommendations of the North American Society for Pediatric Gastroenterology, Hepatology and Nutrition. *J Pediatr Gastroenterol Nutr* 2004;39:115-128.

Pashankar D, Schreiber RA: Neonatal cholestasis: a red alert for the jaundiced newborn. *Can J Gastroenterol* 2000;14: 67D-72D.

Roberts EA: Neonatal hepatitis syndrome. *Semin Neonatol* 2003;8:357-374.

Sinha J et al: Bile duct paucity in infancy. *Semin Liver Dis* 2007;27: 319-323.

Sokol RJ, Mack C: Etiopathogenesis of biliary atresia. *Semin Liver Dis* 2001;2:517-524.

Suchy F: Neonatal cholestasis. *Pediatr Rev* 2004;25:388-396.

Tomar BS: Hepatobiliary abnormalities and parenteral nutrition. *Indian J Pediatr* 2000;67: 695-701.

Vanderhoof JA et al: Gastrointestinal disease. In MacDonald MG et al (eds): *Avery's Neonatology: Pathophysiology and Management of the Newborn*, 6th ed. Philadelphia, PA: Lippincott Williams & Wilkins, 2005:940-964.

Varadarajulu S et al: Technical outcomes and complications of ERCP in children. *Gastrointest Endosc* 2004;60:367-371.

Venigalla S, Gourley GR: Neonatal cholestasis. *Semin Perinatol* 2004;28:348-355.

Zinn AB: Inborn errors of metabolism. In Martin RJ et al (eds): *Neonatal-Perinatal Medicine: Diseases of the Fetus and Infant*, 8th ed. Philadelphia, PA: Mosby Elsevier, 2006:1597-1658.

92 Hyperbilirubinemia, Indirect (Unconjugated Hyperbilirubinemia)

I. **Definition.** When the rate of bilirubin production exceeds the rate of elimination, the end result is an increase in the total serum bilirubin (TSB), a clinical condition called hyperbilirubinemia. The accumulation of bilirubin (the yellow-orange pigment) in the skin, the sclera, and the mucosa is called jaundice. See Chapter 91 for a basic overview of bilirubin metabolism and hyperbilirubinemia. Chapter 51 provides information on rapid "on-call" assessment and management.

II. **Incidence.** Neonatal hyperbilirubinemia is a common problem. Approximately 60–70% of term infants and ~80% of preterm infants develop jaundice in the first week of life. Incidence is higher in populations living at higher altitudes. Incidence also varies with ethnicity. It is lower in African Americans and higher in East Asians, Greeks living in Greece, and American Indians.

III. **Pathophysiology**

A. **Physiologic jaundice.** In full-term newborns, a physiologic progressive elevation of serum unconjugated bilirubin develops to a mean peak of 5–6 mg/dL between 60 and 72 h of age. Premature neonates may experience higher mean peak concentrations as much as 10–12 mg/dL by the fifth day of life. Physiologic ranges of TSB remain *controversial* because levels are affected by several factors, such as gestational age, birthweight, disease state, degree of hydration, nutritional status, and ethnic background. Data from recent studies suggest that the upper limits of TSB levels (95th percentile) found in diverse populations of normal newborn maybe as high as 17–18 mg/dL. Studies published on predominantly breast-fed infants suggest that a typical peak for TSB is approximately 8–9 mg/dL.

1. **Exclusion criteria for diagnosis of physiologic jaundice:**
   a. Jaundice appearing within the first 24 h of life.
   b. TSB level >95th percentile for age in hours based on a nomogram for hour-specific serum bilirubin concentration. (See Figure 1–1.)
   c. Bilirubin level increasing at a rate >0.2 mg/dL/h or >5 mg/dL/day.
   d. Direct serum bilirubin level >1.5–2.0 mg/dL or >10–20% of the TSB.
   e. Jaundice persisting for >2 weeks in full-term infants.

2. **Physiology.** Benign neonatal bilirubinemia, better known as physiologic jaundice, is a nonpathologic condition that develops in virtually all newborns due to distinctive aspects of normal newborn physiology that predisposes them to increased bilirubin production and limited elimination. Because recent data suggest that the upper limit of "physiologic jaundice" in diverse populations is a TSB level of 17–18 mg/dL, a stable 4- to 5-day-old breast-fed infant with bilirubin levels of 15–16 mg/dL may not need an elaborate workup for hyperbilirubinemia but will require close follow-up to ensure that bilirubin levels do not continue to rise to critical levels.

3. **Mechanisms that predispose newborn infants to hyperbilirubinemia:**
   a. **Increased bilirubin synthesis** due to larger red blood cell (RBC) mass, increased hemoglobin breakdown up to two to three times the adult rate (due to shorter life span of neonatal RBCs), and increased rate of RBC degradation in the bone marrow before release to the circulation.
   b. **Decreased binding and transport.** Decreased hepatic uptake of bilirubin from plasma due to decreased plasma albumin and liver transfer protein, ligandin.
   c. **Impaired conjugation and excretion.** Relatively reduced transferase (uridine diphosphate glucuronyltransferase [UDPGT]) activity in the newborn liver resulting in decreased mono- and diglucuronide bilirubin conjugates that can be excreted in the bile.

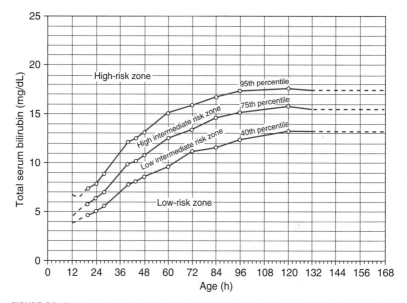

FIGURE 92–1. Nomogram for designation of risk in well newborns at ≥36 weeks gestation with birthweight ≥2000 g or ≥35 weeks' gestational age with birthweight ≥2500 g based on the hour-specific serum bilirubin values. (*Reproduced, with permission, from Bhutani VK et al: Predictive ability of a pre-discharge hour-specific serum bilirubin for subsequent significant hyperbilirubinemia in healthy term and near-term newborns.* Pediatrics 1999;103:6-14.)

      d. **Enhanced enterohepatic circulation.** Conjugated bilirubin is unstable and can be hydrolyzed by the intestinal enzyme β-glucuronidase to its unconjugated form, which can be readily absorbed through the intestinal mucosa. Sterility of intestinal mucosa prevents further formation of the more excretable products urobilin and stercobilin.

   B. **Breast-feeding (BF) and jaundice.** Most studies indicate that breast-feeding is a significant risk factor for hyperbilirubinemia. Jaundice associated with breast-feeding is divided into two types based on the age of onset: **Early-onset breast-feeding-associated jaundice** occurs within the first week of life, with an incidence of (12.9% in infants having a bilirubin level >12 mg/dL; **Late-onset breast milk jaundice** occurs after the first week of life, with 2–4% of infants having a bilirubin level of >10 mg/dL at 3 weeks.

     1. **Breast-feeding-associated jaundice.** Caloric deprivation (ie, starvation and increased enterohepatic circulation) had been implicated as the cause of BF jaundice. The mechanism for so-called starvation jaundice is unclear but may involve shifts in bilirubin pools, less efficient conjugation, and enhanced bilirubin absorption in the intestines. Meconium contains a significant amount of bilirubin that can be reabsorbed. Breast-fed infants pass fewer stools in the first few days of life, which may result in delayed clearance of meconium, thereby increasing bilirubin absorption.

     2. **Breast milk (BM) jaundice.** Prolonged indirect hyperbilirubinemia, beyond the second to third week of life, has been reported to occur in as much as 10–30% of breast-fed infants and may persist up to 3 months of age. Different theories had been considered as the cause for BM jaundice, but no single and exclusive cause has been identified. Some infants with prolonged BM jaundice have been found to have Gilbert syndrome. Although BM jaundice was considered by some

experts as an extension of physiologic jaundice, kernicterus has been reported in apparently healthy term and late preterm infants, and therefore it cannot be considered totally benign. A study of 736 jaundiced newborns showed that among the infants with jaundice appearing between day 4 and day 7 of life, BM jaundice was the more common cause, occurring in almost 50% of cases.

C. **Pathologic unconjugated hyperbilirubinemia**
1. **Disorders of production**
   a. **Hemolytic disease** results in the destruction of the RBCs and is the most common cause of pathologic hyperbilirubinemia in the newborn period. The process may begin in fetal life or immediately after birth depending on the etiology.
   b. **Blood group incompatibilities**
      i. **Rh (D-antigen) incompatibility** as well as other antigens in the Rh blood-group system (c, C, e, E, cc, and Ce) can cause immune-mediated hemolytic disease. Alloimmunization occurs when as little as 0.1 mL of RBC from an Rh (D)-positive fetus cross the placenta into the circulation of an Rh (D)-negative mother. The initial response in the maternal circulation is the production of immunoglobulin (Ig) M that does not cross the placenta and then later followed by Ig G, which in subsequent pregnancies crosses the placenta and causes a hemolytic process that can begin in utero. The severe form of this process can result in erythroblastosis fetalis with hydrops. (See Chapter 115.)
      ii. **ABO incompatibility** occurs in 3% of all infants. Antigens present on the surface of RBCs react with antibodies in the plasma of opposing blood types, resulting in ABO incompatibility with sensitization. Hemolytic disease related to blood groups is generally limited to group A or B infants born to group O mothers. Risk of recurrence of ABO hemolytic disease is reported to be as high as 88% in those infants with the same blood type as their index sibling. ABO incompatibility is somewhat protective of Rh sensitization because the fetal ABO-incompatible RBCs are rapidly destroyed in the maternal circulation, thereby decreasing the opportunity of Rh antigen to mount an immune response. (See Chapter 73.)
   c. **Red cell enzyme deficiencies**
      i. **Glucose-6-phosphate dehydrogenase deficiency (G6PD)** is the most common enzyme deficiency known to affect millions of people. The major function of G6PD is in preventing oxidative damage of cells. The G6PD gene is located on the X chromosome. Prevalence of hyperbilirubinemia is twice that of general population in males who carry the defective gene and in homozygous females. Although it is more common in the African, Middle Eastern, southern European, and Asian populations, the ease of migration and intermarriage has transformed G6PD deficiency into a more global problem. This enzyme deficiency has recently been listed among the 10 most important factors contributory to nonhemolytic neonatal jaundice.
      ii. **Pyruvate kinase deficiency** is inherited in an autosomal recessive manner and most common in northern European descendants. It presents in the newborn period with jaundice, anemia, and reticulocytosis. Kernicterus has been reported. This condition has to be considered in a newborn with a nonspherocytic, direct antiglobulin test (DAT) negative hemolytic anemia.
   d. **Hemoglobinopathies,** as developmental differences in globin chain synthesis, are responsible for the different clinical manifestations of α-chain and β-chain defects in the perinatal period. Although these conditions generally do not present in the newborn period, patients with deletion of three α-globin genes (Hemoglobin H) are often born with hypochromic hemolytic anemia and are at risk for developing severe hyperbilirubinemia.
   e. **Infection,** as sepsis, causes hyperbilirubinemia by increasing bilirubin concentrations via hemolysis, and it may impair conjugation leading to decreased

excretion of bilirubin. Both early- and late-onset jaundice are reported to be one of the more common clinical manifestations of urinary tract infection.

f. Increased erythrocyte load

   i. Blood sequestration. Extravascular blood can result in increased bilirubin production due to breakdown of red blood cells. The catabolism of 1 g of hemoglobin yields 35 mg of bilirubin. Traumatic birth may result in obvious and occult hemorrhages, such as bruising cephalhematomas and intracranial bleeding followed by moderate to severe hyperbilirubinemia.

   ii. Polycythemia. Increased RBC mass is a known risk factor for hyperbilirubinemia due to an increase in the bilirubin load presented to the liver for conjugation and excretion.

   iii. Infants of diabetic mothers have high erythropoietin levels causing ineffective erythropoiesis and polycythemia that contributes to hyperbilirubinemia.

2. Disorders of bilirubin clearance

a. Crigler-Najjar syndrome (CNS) type I, a rare autosomal recessive disease characterized by almost complete absence of hepatic uridine diphosphate glycosyltransferase (UGT) activity. TSB is commonly >20 mg/dL. The diagnosis of CNS-I can usually be made by microassay of UGT activity or by measurement of menthol glucuronide in urine after oral menthol. Treatment consists of exchange transfusion soon after birth, followed by daily phototherapy for 12–24 h and liver transplantation later on. The use of tin-protoporphyrin may help decrease the bilirubin level temporarily and may shorten the need for daily phototherapy. Oral calcium supplementation makes phototherapy more efficient. TSB is unresponsive to phenobarbital therapy.

b. Crigler-Najjar syndrome type II, also known as Arias disease, is more common than CNS-I and typically benign. CNS-II can occur as an autosomal recessive and dominant inheritance. It is caused by a single base pair mutation leading to decrease but not totally absent enzyme activity. TSB rarely exceeds 20 mg/dL and is lowered by phenobarbital administration. A definitive diagnosis is made by identifying the genetic defect.

   For routine clinical practice, CNS-I and CNS-II can be differentiated by their response to phenobarbital therapy and bile analysis. In CNS-I, bile is totally devoid of bilirubin conjugates, whereas bilirubin monoconjugates are present in CNS-II and some diconjugates may be detectable after phenobarbital treatment.

c. Gilbert syndrome is characterized by mild, lifelong, unconjugated hyperbilirubinemia in the absence of hemolysis or evidence of liver disease. Autosomal dominant and recessive patterns of inheritance have been suggested. Hepatic glucuronidating activity is 30% of normal, resulting in an increased proportion of monoglucuronide. Although it is most commonly diagnosed in young adulthood, studies have shown that neonates who carry the genetic marker for Gilbert syndrome have a more rapid rise and duration of neonatal jaundice. It is important to remember that Gilbert syndrome is a condition with no consequences for adults, but it can put a neonate at significant risk for hyperbilirubinemia and the potential for complications of bilirubin encephalopathy.

d. Lucey-Driscoll syndrome, also known as transient familial neonatal hyperbilirubinemia, has TSB concentrations that usually reach ≥20 mg/dL. The sera of affected neonates and their mothers are found to contain a high concentration of an unidentified UGT inhibitor when tested in vitro.

3. Metabolic and endocrine disorders

a. Galactosemia. Jaundice maybe one of the presenting signs; however, infants with significant hyperbilirubinemia due to galactosemia typically have other presenting signs and symptoms such as poor feeding, vomiting, and lethargy. Hyperbilirubinemia during the first week of life is almost always unconjugated, and then it becomes mostly conjugated during the second week, reflective of developing liver disease.

b. **Hypothyroidism.** Prolonged jaundice is found in up to 10% of newborns diagnosed with hypothyroidism. It is due to deficient activity of UGT. Early-onset hyperbilirubinemia has been reported as the only presenting sign of congenital hypothyroidism. Treatment with thyroid hormone improves hyperbilirubinemia.

4. **Increased enterohepatic circulation**

a. Conditions that cause gastrointestinal obstruction (eg, pyloric stenosis, duodenal atresia, annular pancreas) or a decrease in gastrointestinal motility may result in exaggerated jaundice due to increased shunting of bilirubin. Blood swallowed during delivery and decreased caloric intake may also be contributing factors.

b. **Breast-feeding jaundice**

i. **Breast-feeding-associated jaundice** is thought to be primarily due to poor breast-feeding practices and poor enteral intake leading to a state of relative starvation and delayed meconium passage with increased enterohepatic circulation of bilirubin.

ii. **Breast milk jaundice.** Increased intestinal absorption of bilirubin facilitated by enzyme β-glucuronidase appears to be the explanation for increased jaundice in breast-fed infants.

5. **Substances affecting binding of bilirubin to albumin.** Certain drugs occupy bilirubin-binding sites on albumin and increase the amount of free unconjugated bilirubin that can cross the blood-brain barrier. Drugs in which this effect may be significant include aspirin and sulfonamides. Chloral hydrate competes for hepatic glucuronidation with bilirubin and thus increases serum unconjugated bilirubin. Common drugs used in the neonates such as penicillin and gentamicin also compete with bilirubin for albumin-binding sites.

IV. **Risk factors.** Sepsis, acidosis, lethargy, asphyxia, temperature instability, G6PD deficiency, hemolytic disease (ABO or G6PD deficiency), borderline prematurity (35–38 weeks), exclusive breast-feeding, East Asian ethnicity, cephalohematoma or significant bruising, male sex, American Indian infants, maternal diabetes, family history of neonatal jaundice, and use of oxytocin in labor.

V. **Clinical presentation**

A. **Clinical assessment**

1. **Monitor for jaundice.** All newborn infants should be monitored routinely for development of jaundice. Each nursery should have an established guideline for the routine assessment of jaundice. Jaundice is visible when the serum bilirubin level approaches 5–7 mg/dL. It is detected in some infants by pressing lightly on the skin with a finger. The yellow color is seen more easily in the "fingerprint" area than in the surrounding skin. Progression of jaundice is cephalocaudal, so that for a given bilirubin level, the face appears more yellow than the rest of the body. The ability of clinicians to evaluate jaundice varies widely, but newborns with TSB levels >12 mg/dL almost always appear "jaundiced."

2. **History.** Family history of jaundice, anemia, splenectomy, or metabolic disorder is significant and may suggest underlying etiology for jaundice. Maternal history of infection or diabetes may increase the newborn's risk for jaundice. Breast-feeding and factors affecting normal gastrointestinal function in the newborn period increase the tendency for more severe jaundice.

3. **Physical examination.** Physical examination may also be helpful in determining the cause of jaundice. Areas of bleeding such as cephalhematoma, petechiae, or ecchymoses indicate blood extravasations. Hepatosplenomegaly may signify hemolytic disease, liver disease, or infection. Physical signs of prematurity, plethora with polycythemia, pallor with hemolytic disease, and large infants with maternal diabetes all can be associated with jaundice. Omphalitis, chorioretinitis, microcephaly, petechiae, and purpuric lesions suggest infectious causes of increased serum bilirubin.

4. **Neurologic examination.** The appearance of subtle abnormal neurologic signs heralds the onset of early bilirubin encephalopathy. See discussion under Section

VIII, B. Clinical signs may include lethargy, poor feeding, vomiting, and hypotonia. The persistently hyperbilirubinemic infant may go on to experience seizures. The progression of neurologic changes parallels the stages of bilirubin encephalopathy from acute to chronic and irreversible changes.

VI. Diagnosis

A. Basic laboratory studies

1. Total serum bilirubin

   a. TSB level determination is indicated in all infants who develop jaundice in the first 24 h of life. Jaundice appearing that early is almost always associated with a pathologic process.

   b. Total bilirubin level and the direct fraction have to be obtained. Indirect bilirubin (also called the unconjugated fraction) is derived by subtracting the direct fraction from the TSB.

   c. Indicated for all infants with progressive jaundice and/or prolonged jaundice.

   d. All bilirubin levels should be interpreted based on the infant's age in hours.

2. Blood type and Rh status in both mother and infant

   a. ABO and Rh incompatibility can be easily diagnosed by comparing infant and maternal blood types.

   b. Cord blood can be sent for routine blood typing of the newborn infant.

3. Direct antibody test (also known as Coombs test)

   a. Detects antibodies bound to the surface of red blood cells.

   b. Usually positive in hemolytic disease as a result of isoimmunization.

   c. Does not correlate with severity of jaundice.

   d. Can be obtained from the cord blood.

4. Complete blood count and differential

   a. Presence of anemia may be suggestive of a hemolytic process; polycythemia increases risk for exaggerated jaundice.

   b. Evaluate RBC morphology; spherocytes suggest ABO incompatibility or hereditary spherocytosis.

   c. Evaluate for indices suggestive of infection (ie, leukopenia, neutropenia, and thrombocytopenia).

5. Reticulocytes

   a. Elevation suggests hemolytic disease.

   b. Can also be elevated in cases of occult or overt hemorrhage.

6. Other laboratory tests

   a. Urine should be tested for reducing substances (to rule out galactosemia if the infant is receiving a galactose-containing formula) and for infectious agents.

   b. If hemolysis is present, in the absence of ABO or Rh incompatibility, further testing by hemoglobin electrophoresis, G6PD screening, or osmotic fragility testing may be required to diagnose RBC defects.

   c. Prolonged jaundice (>2 weeks of life) may require additional tests for thyroid and liver function, blood and urine cultures, and metabolic screening workup, such as plasma amino acid and urine organic acid measurements.

7. Measurement of serum albumin because bilirubin-albumin binding weakens the correlation between TSB level and bilirubin encephalopathy. **Measurement of serum albumin** may help assess the total albumin bilirubin binding sites available and thereby suggest an albumin infusion. It may be useful in the determination of exchange transfusion. (See Figure 92–3.)

B. **Transcutaneous bilirubinometry (TcB)** is a portable lightweight instrument that uses reflectance measurements on the skin to determine the amount of yellow color present in the skin. A multicenter evaluation of TcB measurement correlates well with laboratory TSB measurement. Accuracy is independent of race, birthweight, and gestational age (>30 weeks), and postnatal age of the newborn. A TcB value of >13 mg/dL should be correlated with TSB.

C. **Expired carbon monoxide (CO) breath analyzer.** An equimolar amount of CO is produced for every molecule of bilirubin formed from the degradation of heme. Measurement of CO in end-tidal breath is an index of total bilirubin production (End-tidal CO corrected for ambient CO). This method can alert the attending physician to the presence of hemolysis irrespective of the timing of jaundice.

VII. **Management.** Three methods of treatment are commonly used to decrease the level of unconjugated bilirubin: exchange transfusion, phototherapy, and pharmacologic therapy. As previously noted, controversy persists as to what levels of serum bilirubin warrant therapy, especially in otherwise healthy full-term infants. Low birthweight infants are excluded from the following guidelines. The authors suggest that each institution and its practicing physicians establish their criteria for phototherapy and exchange transfusion by gestational age, weight groups, postnatal age, and the infant's condition consistent with current standard of pediatric practice.

A. **Practice guidelines.** In 2004, the American Academy of Pediatrics (AAP) promulgated evidence-based recommendations to reduce the incidence of severe hyperbilirubinemia and acute encephalopathy in infants ≥35 weeks' gestation (*Pediatrics* 2004;114(1):297-316). The guidelines include: to promote and support successful breast-feeding, to perform a systematic risk assessment for severe hyperbilirubinemia prior to discharge, to provide early and focused follow-up for the high-risk patient, and to initiate immediate therapeutic intervention when indicated (ie, start phototherapy or exchange transfusion to prevent development of severe hyperbilirubinemia or bilirubin encephalopathy).

B. **Phototherapy**
   1. **Indication.** Most infants with increasing jaundice are treated with phototherapy when it is believed that bilirubin levels could enter the toxic range. (See Figure 92–2.)
   2. **Factors influencing effective phototherapy**
      a. **Spectrum of light delivered.** The blue-green region of the visible spectrum is the most effective.
      b. **Energy output.** More effective reduction in TSB with high-intensity phototherapy. Conventional phototherapy has an irradiance of 6–12 $\mu W/cm^2/nm$. High-intensity phototherapy provides an irradiance of >25 $\mu W/cm^2/nm$. Light intensity is a function of the distance from the light source; therefore, light source should be as close to the infant as possible (12–16 in).
      c. **Surface area exposed.** Maximize the skin exposure to the light source. Systems that provide light source under the infant and standard lighting above are recommended. To maximize exposure, infants should be naked in servo-controlled incubators.
   3. **Side effects.** Phototherapy is relatively safe and easy to use. Minor side effects include rashes, dehydration, and ultraviolet light irradiation. No changes in growth, development, and infant behavior have been reported.
      a. **Bronze baby syndrome.** With conjugated hyperbilirubinemia, phototherapy causes photodestruction of copper porphyrins, causing urine and skin to become bronze.
      b. **Congenital erythropoietic porphyria** is a rare disease in which phototherapy is contraindicated. Exposure to visible light of moderate to high intensity produces severe bullous lesions on exposed skin and may lead to death.
      c. **The retinal effects** of phototherapy to the exposed infant's eyes are unknown; however, animal studies suggest that retinal degeneration may occur. Eye shields must be used. The infant's eyes should be covered with opaque patches for overhead lamp phototherapy.

C. **Exchange transfusion** (see also Chapter 29). Exchange transfusion is used when the risk of kernicterus for a particular infant is significant. A double-volume exchange replaces 85% of the circulating red blood cells and decreases the bilirubin level to about half of the pre-exchange value. It appears that no specific level of bilirubin can be considered safe or dangerous for all infants because patient-to-patient variations

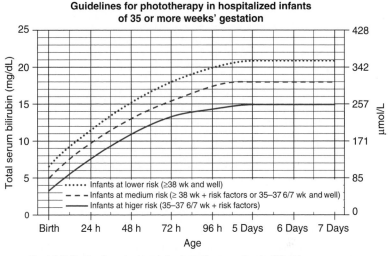

FIGURE 92–2. Guidelines for phototherapy in hospitalized infants of ≥35 weeks' gestation. (*Reproduced, with permission, from the American Academy of Pediatrics, Subcommittee on Hyperbilirubinemia: Management of hyperbilirubinemia in the newborn infant 35 or more weeks of gestation.* Pediatrics *2004;114:297-316.*) TSB, total serum bilirubin.

exist for the permeability of the blood-brain barrier. Clinical practice parameters published by the AAP in July 2004 provide guidelines for exchange transfusions in healthy newborns 35 or more weeks of gestation. (See Figure 92–3.)

1. **Exchange transfusion should be considered in the following circumstances:**
   a. There is evidence of an ongoing hemolytic process and TSB level failed to decline by 1–2 mg/dL with 4–6 h of intensive phototherapy.
   b. Rate of rise indicates that the level will reach 25 mg/dL within 48 h.
   c. High concentration of TSB and early signs of bilirubin encephalopathy.
   d. Hemolysis causing anemia and hydrops fetalis.
      Note: Direct or conjugated fraction should not be subtracted from the TSB when considering exchange transfusion.
2. **General guidelines**
   a. Generally, type O Rh-negative blood is used for ABO or Rh incompatibility. If the infant is type A or B and the mother is of the same blood type, type-specific, Rh-negative donor blood can be use.
   b. Donor blood must always be crossmatched with maternal serum.
   c. Donor blood should be warmed to about 37°C.
   d. Use fresh blood that is no more than 4 days old.
   e. Consider calcium gluconate infusion during the course of the exchange transfusion because citrate (blood preservative) chelates calcium.
   f. Obtain parental consent.

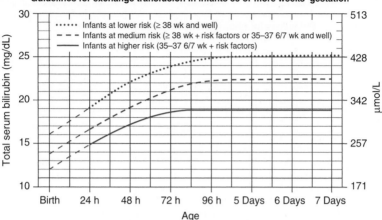

Guidelines for exchange transfusion in infants 35 or more weeks' gestation

- The dashed lines for the first 24 h indicate uncertainty due to a wide range of clinical circumstances and a range of responses to phototherapy.
- Immediate exchange transfusion is recommended if infant shows signs of acute bilirubin encephalopathy (hypertonia, arching, retrocollis, opisthotonos, fever, high-pitched cry) or if TSB is ≥5 mg/dL (85 μmol/L) above these lines.
- Risk factors: isoimmune hemolytic disease, G6PD deficiency, asphyxia, significant lethargy, temperature instability, sepsis, acidosis.
- Measure serum albumin and calculate B/A ratio (see legend).
- Use total bilirubin. Do not subtract direct reacting or conjugated bilirubin.

Note that these suggested levels represent a consensus of most of the committee but are based on limited evidence, and the levels shown are approximations. During birth hospitalization, exchange transfusion is recommended if the TSB rises to these levels despite intensive phototherapy.

The following B/A ratios can be used together with but in not in lieu of the TSB level as an additional factor in determining the need for exchange transfusion:

	B/A Ratio at Which Exchange Transfusion Should be Considered	
	Risk Category	TSB μmol/L/Alb, μmol/L
Infants ≥38 0/7 wk	8.0	0.94
Infants 35 0/7–36 6/7 wk and well or ≥38 0/7 wk if higher risk or isoimmune hemolytic disease or G6PD deficiency	7.2	0.84
Infants 35 0/7–37 6/7 wk if higher risk or isoimmune hemolytic disease or G6PD deficiency	6.8	0.80

If the TSB is at or approaching the exchange level, send blood for immediate type and crossmatch. Blood for exchange transfusion is modified whole blood (red cells and plasma) crossmatched against the mother and compatible with the infant.

FIGURE 92–3. Guidelines for exchange transfusion in infants ≥35 weeks' gestation. (*Reproduced, with permission, from the American Academy of Pediatrics, Subcommittee on Hyperbilirubinemia: Management of hyperbilirubinemia in the newborn infant 35 or more weeks of gestation. Pediatrics 2004;114:297-316.*) B/A, bilirubin/albumin ratio; G6PD, glucose-6-phosphate dehydrogenase deficiency; TSB, total serum bilirubin

3. **Bilirubin levels.** TSB can be decreased by 50% of the pre-exchange level. Rebound increase in TSB is expected after an exchange transfusion as bilirubin in tissues "migrates" back into circulation.

4. **Adverse events.** Observational studies have reported a high rate of adverse events; however, the majority of these events are asymptomatic, transient, and treatable laboratory abnormalities such as thrombocytopenia, hypocalcemia, and metabolic acidosis. More recent studies have reported mortality rates of 0.5–2%. Exchange transfusion is not risk free; therefore the procedure should only be done after intensive phototherapy has failed and the risk of bilirubin encephalopathy outweighs the risk of the procedure.

D. **Pharmacologic therapy**

1. **Phenobarbital**

   a. **Action.** Phenobarbital (dose: 2.5 mg/kg/day) affects the metabolism of bilirubin by increasing the concentration of ligandin in liver cells, inducing production of glucuronyl transferase and enhancing bilirubin excretion.

   b. **Indications.** Used to treat CNS-II and Gilbert syndrome. It can also be used as an adjunct therapy in cases of exaggerated neonatal jaundice, but it takes 3–7 days to become effective. Phenobarbital is not helpful in immediate treatment of unconjugated hyperbilirubinemia in the newborn period.

2. **Metalloporphyrins.** A synthetic heme analog, metalloporphyrin inhibits heme oxygenase (HO), the rate-limiting enzyme in the catabolism of heme. By acting as a competitive inhibitor, the metalloporphyrin decreases the production of bilirubin. Tin-mesoporphyrin (SnMP) is a potent HO inhibitor that has been extensively studied. Strong evidence suggests that a single dose of SnMP reduces the need for phototherapy and exchange transfusion. It is as effective as a single intramuscular injection (6 mmol/kg) in patients with hemolytic disease, resulting in a significant drop in TSB concentration and avoiding the need for exchange transfusion. The only immediate untoward effect noted was a non-dose-dependent, mild, transient erythema when used in conjunction with phototherapy in a preterm infant. SnMP is available only for investigational or "compassionate" use in certain carefully prescribed circumstances. It remains an unlicensed drug at this time.

3. **Albumin.** Administration of intravenous albumin may be helpful because an increased reserve of albumin provides more binding sites for free bilirubin and therefore reduces the unbound fraction that maybe protective against bilirubin toxicity. An albumin level <3.0 g/dL can be considered as one risk factor for lowering the threshold for phototherapy (dose: 1 g/kg over 2 h). (See Chapter 132.)

4. **Intravenous γ-globulin** decreases the need for exchange transfusions in Rh and ABO immunization. It is recommended if the TSB is rising despite intensive phototherapy or a TSB level is within 2–3 mg/dL of the exchange level. Dose: 0.5–1 g/kg over 2 h. (See Chapter 132.)

VIII. **Prognosis**

A. **General.** Unconjugated bilirubin in high concentration can cross the blood-brain barrier and can penetrate the brain cells, which may lead to neuronal dysfunction and death. The exact mechanism of bilirubin-induced neuronal cell injury is not completely understood; however, high concentrations of unconjugated bilirubin can have neurotoxic effects on cellular membranes and intracellular calcium homeostasis resulting in neuronal excitotoxicity and mitochondrial energy failure. The factors that determine toxicity of bilirubin in neurons of neonates is complex and not completely understood. Specific bilirubin concentrations that put a preterm infant at risk for kernicterus have not been identified. The incidence of kernicterus in this group is unknown, and the relationship of serum bilirubin and neurodevelopmental outcome in the very low birthweight infant remains unclear.

B. **Encephalopathy**

1. **Transient.** Early bilirubin-induced neurologic dysfunction is transient and reversible. The auditory system serves as an objective window for looking at the central nervous system in cases of severe hyperbilirubinemia, and it can be

used as an early predictor of bilirubin encephalopathy. **Auditory brainstem responses (ABRs)** show significant prolongation of latency of specific wavelengths. These changes may be reversed with either exchange transfusions or with spontaneous decrease in bilirubin levels. More recent data suggest that with marked hyperbilirubinemia, complete recovery of the ABR may be delayed.

2. **Acute bilirubin encephalopathy** is a preventable neurologic sequela of untreated severe hyperbilirubinemia. It is an evolving encephalopathy that can progress in three clinical phases over several days. The major clinical features involve disturbances in level of consciousness, tone and movement, and brainstem function, especially relating to feeding and cry. The severity of abnormalities appears to correlate with both the severity and duration of hyperbilirubinemia.

   a. **Initial phase** is noted by lethargy, hypotonia, decreased movement, and poor suck. Clinical findings are nonspecific. A high index of suspicion is needed to recognize these signs as a signal of impending acute bilirubin encephalopathy. Prompt therapeutic intervention is critical to prevent deterioration and poor prognosis.

   b. **Intermediate phase** has cardinal signs of moderate stupor, irritability, and increased tone. Infant may exhibit backward arching of the neck (retrocollis) or of the back (opisthotonos). Fever has been reported to occur during this phase of the syndrome.

   c. **Advanced phase** is characterized by deep stupor or coma, increased tone, inability to feed, and a shrill cry. Seizures may occur. This is an ominous stage of acute bilirubin encephalopathy suggesting irreversible central nervous system injury, and the later development of chronic bilirubin encephalopathy occurs in most infants.

3. **Chronic bilirubin encephalopathy** is a devastating and disabling neurologic disorder, also called **kernicterus,** and is characterized by a clinical tetrad:

   a. Choreoathetoid cerebral palsy.
   b. High-frequency sensorineural hearing loss.
   c. Palsy of vertical gaze.
   d. Dental enamel hypoplasia.

   Cognitive deficits are unusual but can be severe. **Mortality rate can be as high as 10%. Kernicterus** is a pathologic diagnosis, describing the yellow discoloration of the deep nuclei of the brain. Clinically the correct terminology is **bilirubin encephalopathy.** Severity varies from mild to severe in children and adults. Mildly affected individuals remain highly functional; moderately affected individuals have more prominent dystonia and are likely to have athetoid movements. Severely affected individuals have speech difficulty and a more disabling dystonia to the point of not being ambulatory. This is a form of static encephalopathy, in which the degree of disability may change slightly overtime but only within limits and is never dramatic. Brainstem regions that are typically affected by bilirubin encephalopathy are the following: globus pallidus, subthalamic nucleus, metabolic sector of the hippocampus, oculomotor nuclei, ventral cochlear nuclei, and the Purkinje cells of the cerebellar cortex. The pattern of involvement is similar across different ages of affected individuals. Bilirubin encephalopathy is not a reportable condition in the United States; therefore, its prevalence is not known.

Selected References

Ahlfors CE, Wennberg RP: Bilirubin-albumin binding and neonatal jaundice. *Semin Perinatol* 2004;28:334-339.

American Academy of Pediatrics; the American College of Obstetricians and Gynecologists: Neonatal complications. In *Guidelines for Perinatal Care*, 6th ed. Atlanta GA: ACOG; 2007:251-259.

American Academy of Pediatrics. Clinical practice guideline: management of hyperbilirubinemia in the newborn infant 35 weeks or more weeks of gestation. *Pediatrics* 2004;114:297-316.

Basu K et al: A new look on neonatal jaundice. *J Indian Med Assoc* 2002;100:556-560.

Dennery PA: Metalloporphyrins for the treatment of neonatal jaundice. *Curr Opin Pediatr* 2005;17:167-169.

Dinesh D: Review of positive direct antiglobulin tests found on cord blood sampling. *J Paediatr Child Health* 2005;41:504-507.

Frank JE: Diagnosis and management of G6PD deficiency. *Am Fam Physician* 2005;72:1277-1282.

Funato M et al: Follow-up study of auditory brainstem responses in hyperbilirubinemic newborns treated with exchange transfusion. *Acta Paediatr Jpn* 1996;38:17-21.

Garcia FJ, Nager AL: Jaundice as an early diagnostic sign of urinary tract infection in infancy. *Pediatrics* 2002;109:846-851.

Ghaemi S et al: Late onset jaundice and urinary tract infection in neonates. *Indian J Pediatr* 2007;74: 47-49.

Gottstein R, Cooke RW: Systematic review of intravenous immunoglobulin in haemolytic disease of the newborn. *Arch Dis Child Fetal Neonatal Ed* 2003;88:F6-F10.

Gourley GR: Breastfeeding, neonatal jaundice and kernicterus. *Semin Neonatol* 2002;7:135-141.

Halamek LP, Stevenson DK: Neonatal jaundice and liver disease. In Fanaroff AA, Martin RJ (eds): *Neonatal—Perinatal Medicine: Diseases of the Fetus and Infant*, 7th ed. St. Louis, MO: Mosby, 2002:1309-1350.

Hosono S et al: Effects of albumin infusion therapy on total and unbound bilirubin values in term infants with intensive phototherapy. *Pediatr Int* 2001;43:8-11.

Jackson JC: Adverse events associated with exchange transfusion in healthy and ill newborns. *Pediatrics* 1997;99:E7.

Jansen PLM: Diagnosis and management of Crigler-Najjar syndrome. *Eur J Pediatr* 1999;158:S89-S94.

Kappas A et al: Sn-Mesoporphyrin interdiction of severe hyperbilirubinemia in Jehovah witness newborns as an alternative to exchange transfusion. *Pediatrics* 2001;108:1374-1377.

Katz MA et al: Recurrence rate of ABO hemolytic disease of the newborn. *Obstet Gynecol* 1982;59:611-614.

Keenan WJ et al: Morbidity and mortality associated with exchange transfusion. *Pediatrics* 1985;75:417-441.

Koenig JM: Evaluation and treatment of erythroblastosis fetalis in the neonate. In Christensen RD (ed): *Hematologic Problems of the Neonate*. Philadelphia, PA: Saunders, 2000:185-207.

Madlon-Kay DJ: Recognition of the presence and severity of newborn jaundice by parents, nurses, physicians, and icterometer. *Pediatrics* 1997;100:E3.

Maisels MJ: Jaundice. In MacDonald MG et al (eds): *Avery's Neonatology: Pathophysiology & Management of the Newborn*, 6th ed. Philadelphia, PA: Lippincott Williams & Wilkins, 2005:768-846.

Murray NA, Roberts IA: Haemolytic disease of the newborn. *Arch Dis Child Fetal Neonatal Ed* 2007;92:F83-F88.

Patra K et al: Adverse events associated with neonatal exchange transfusion in the 1990s. *J Pediatr* 2004;144:626-631.

Phibbs R: Advances in the theory and practice of exchange transfusions. *Calif Med* 1966;105:442-453.

Reiser DJ: Neontal jaundice: physiologic variation or pathologic process. *Crit Care Nurs Clin North Am* 2004;16:257-269.

Rogers PA, Stevenson DK: Developmental biology of heme oxygenase. *Clin Perinatol* 1990;17:275-291.

Roy-Chowdhury N et al: Presence of the genetic marker for Gilbert syndrome is associated with increased level and duration of neonatal jaundice. *Acta Paediatr* 2002;91:100-101.

Rubaltelli FF et al: Transcutaneous bilirubin measurement: a multicenter evaluation of a new device. *Pediatrics* 2001;107:1264-1271.

Shapiro SM et al: Hyperbilirubinemia and kernicterus. *Clin Perinatol* 2006;33:387-410.

Sharma P et al: Brainstem evoked response audiometry (BAER) in neonates with hyper-bilirubinemia. *Indian J Pediatr* 2006;73:413-416.

Smitherman H et al: Early recognition of hyperbilirubinemia and its emergent management. *Semin Fetal Neonatal Med* 2006;11:214-224.

Steiner LA, Gallagher PG: Erythrocyte disorder in the perinatal period. *Semin Perinatol* 2007;31:254-261.

Ticker F et al: Congenital hypothyroidism and early severe hyperbilirubinemia. *Clin Pediatr* 2003;42:365-366.

Valaes T et al: Control of jaundice in preterm newborns by an inhibitor of bilirubin produc-tion: Studies with Tin-Mesoporphyrin. *Pediatrics* 1994;93:1-11.

Volpe JJ: Bilirubin and brain injury. In Volpe JJ (ed): *Neurology of the Newborn*, 4th ed. Philadel-phia, PA: Saunders, 2001:521-546.

Vogt BA, Avner ED: The kidney and urinary tract. In Fanaroff AA, Martin RJ, eds. *Neonatal-Perinatal Medicine: Diseases of the Fetus and Infant*. 7th ed. Philadelphia, PA: Mosby, 2002:1521-1522.

Watchko JF: Hyperbilirubinemia and bilirubin toxicity in the late preterm infant. *Clin Perinatol* 2006;33:839-852.

Watchko JF: Kernicterus and the molecular mechanisms of bilirubin-induced CNS injury in newborns. *Neuromolecular Med* 2006;8:513-529.

Wong RJ et al: Neonatal jaundice and liver disease. In Martin RJ et al (eds): *Neonatal Perina-tal Medicine: Diseases of the Fetus and Infant*, 8th ed. Philadelphia, PA: Mosby Elsevier, 2006:1419-1465.

93 Inborn Errors of Metabolism with Acute Neonatal Onset

Inborn errors of metabolism (IEMs) are a group of disorders that are of great importance to physicians treating newborns. The immediate diagnosis and appropriate treatment of these conditions are often directly linked to the patient's outcome to the extremes of avoiding death or irreversible brain damage. Pediatricians may feel overwhelmed by the number and com-plexity of these disorders (Table 93–1) and the interpretation of laboratory tests needed to establish the diagnosis. This chapter, therefore, concentrates on the symptom patterns, labo-ratory tests and their interpretation, as well as the initial stabilization of the patient rather than discussing details of the specific biochemical and genetic defects or special treatment meas-ures of IEMs. Usually, the patient's ongoing treatment is supervised by a geneticist specially trained in biochemical genetics.

    I. **Classification**

        A. **Classification by time of onset.** Because of the nature of this manual, we con-centrate here on metabolic disorders with onset in the neonatal period and early infancy. Be aware, however, that onset of a disease in later infancy or even in ado-lescence and adulthood does not exclude the diagnosis of an IEM. It is also impor-tant to realize that, even with comprehensive and well-organized neonatal screening programs, a number of IEMs present clinically before they are detected by screening tests or before the test result is available to the treating physicians.

Table 93–1. INBORN ERRORS OF METABOLISM PRESENTING IN THE NEONATAL PERIOD AND INFANCY

Disorders of carbohydrate metabolism
Galactosemia
Fructose-1,6-bisphosphatase deficiency
Glycogen storage disease (types IA, IB, II, III, and IV)
Hereditary fructose intolerance

Disorders of amino acid metabolism
Maple syrup urine disease
Nonketotic hyperglycinemia
Hereditary tyrosinemia
Pyroglutamic acidemia (5-oxoprolinuria)
Hyperornithinemia-hyperammonemia-homo citrullinemia syndrome
Lysinuric protein intolerance
Methylene tetrahydrofolate reductase deficiency
Sulfite oxidase deficiency

Disorders of organic acid metabolism
Methylmalonic acidemia
Propionic acidemia
Isovaleric acidemia
Multiple carboxylase deficiency
Glutaric acidemia type II (multiple acyl-CoA dehydrogenase deficiencies)
HMG-CoA lyase deficiency
3-Methylcrotonoyl-CoA carboxylase deficiency
3-Hydroxyisobutyric aciduria

Disorders of pyruvate metabolism and the electron transport chain
Pyruvate carboxylase deficiency
Pyruvate dehydrogenase deficiency
Electron transport chain defects

Disorders of the urea cycle
Ornithine-transcarbamylase deficiency
Carbamyl phosphate synthetase deficiency
Transient hyperammonemia of the neonate
Argininosuccinate synthetase deficiency (citrullinemia)
Argininosuccinate lyase deficiency
Arginase deficiency
N-Acetylglutamate synthetase deficiency

Lysosomal storage disorders
GM_1 gangliosidosis type I (β-galactosidase deficiency)
Gaucher disease (glucocerebrosidase deficiency)
Niemann-Pick disease types A and B (sphingomyelinase deficiency)
Wolman disease (acid lipase deficiency)
Mucopolysaccharidosis type VII (β-glucuronidase deficiency)
I-cell disease (mucolipidosis type II)
Sialidosis type II (neuraminidase deficiency)
Fucosidosis

Peroxisomal disorders
Zellweger syndrome
Neonatal adrenoleukodystrophy
Single enzyme defects of the peroxisomal β-oxidation
Rhizomelic chondrodysplasia punctata
Infantile Refsum disease

(*Continued*)

Table 93–1. INBORN ERRORS OF METABOLISM PRESENTING IN THE NEONATAL PERIOD AND INFANCY *(CONTINUED)*

Miscellaneous disorders
Adrenogenital syndrome (21-hydroxylase and other deficiencies)
Disorders of bilirubin metabolism (Crigler-Najjar syndrome and others)
Pyridoxine-dependent seizures
α_1-Antitrypsin deficiency
Fatty acid oxidation disorders (short, medium, and long chain)
Cholesterol biosynthesis defects (Smith-Lemli-Opitz syndrome)
Congenital disorders of protein glycosylation (carbohydrate-deficient glycoprotein syndromes)
Neonatal hemochromatosis

HMG, 3-hydroxy-3-methylglutaryl; CoA, coenzyme A.

The use of **tandem mass spectrometry** in newborn screening is now widespread. Due to the large amount of biochemical information obtained through tandem mass spectrometry analysis, physicians involved in newborn care now often encounter new issues regarding the follow-up evaluations and referrals of patients with a positive screening test.

B. **Classification by clinical presentation.** Subdividing IEMs by clinical presentation may be the most useful approach to aid in establishing the correct diagnosis. Note that some **syndromes with dysmorphic features** are now known to be IEMs (eg, Smith-Lemli-Opitz syndrome or Zellweger syndrome [see Section IX, A and B]). Other classic examples of IEMs are discussed only briefly because they are clinically asymptomatic in the neonatal period (eg, phenylketonuria [PKU]). Note that some **skeletal dysplasias** and disorders affecting bone and cartilage formation (not discussed here) are, strictly speaking, also IEMs (eg, rhizomelic chondrodysplasia punctata and hypophosphatasia). The following classification system serves as the basis for the more detailed sections of this chapter. IEMs may present with the following:

1. **Encephalopathy with or without metabolic acidosis.**
2. **Impairment of liver function.**
3. **Impairment of cardiac function.**
4. **Dysmorphic syndromes.**
5. **Less commonly, nonimmune hydrops fetalis.**

C. **Classification according to the biochemical basis of the disease.** A concept that divides IEMs according to their biochemical characteristics helps in understanding the pathogenesis of symptoms and different approaches to treatment but seems to be of less utility for those providing patient care.

II. **Incidence.** By some estimates, IEMs may account for as much as 20% of disease among full-term infants not known to have been born at risk. Cumulatively, an IEM may be present in >1 in 500 live births.

III. **Pathophysiology.** Metabolic processes are catalyzed by genetically encoded enzyme proteins. The classical mechanism of a metabolic defect is lack or deficiency of an enzyme resulting in **substrate accumulation** and conversion of intermediary metabolites to products not usually present. In addition, end products of the normal pathway will be deficient. Symptoms may result from an increased level of the normal substrate (eg, in urea cycle disorders, the substrate ammonia is toxic and leads to cerebral edema, central nervous system [CNS] dysfunction, and eventually death). Additionally, a **lack of normal end products** of metabolism can lead to symptoms (eg, lack of cortisol in 21-hydroxylase deficiency [see Chapter 82]). The **alternative products may interfere with normal metabolic processes** (eg, accumulated propionyl-CoA may participate in reactions normally using acetyl-CoA in propionic acidemia).

Finally, an **inability to degrade end products** of a metabolic pathway may lead to symptoms (eg, myocardial dysfunction in **glycogen storage disease** type II or hepatomegaly in glycogen storage disease type I). The time of clinical presentation often relates to the question of whether the symptoms are caused by metabolites that are able to prenatally transport across the placenta. These are usually of low molecular weight and, therefore, prenatally removed from the fetus and cleared by the maternal metabolism.

IV. **Risk factors.** Inborn errors of metabolism are genetic disorders. Therefore, there are no definite behavioral or environmental risk factors for the presence of an inborn metabolic defect (although environment and especially nutrition may affect presentation). A history of relatives with mental retardation, protein avoidance, and, for many disorders, neonatal or childhood deaths or severe illness (liver disease, abnormal heart function, mental and physical decline, episodic illness) could be an indicator of increased risk. A history of protein avoidance, liver dysfunction/failure, or mental changes in pregnancy and labor may be seen in female carriers of x-linked inherited urea cycle defects. Presence of consanguinity and, for a number of inborn errors, ethnic background are also risk factors.

V. **Clinical presentation.** Although there are several specific situations, listed next, in which an IEM must be considered, the safest guideline for clinical practice is that **an IEM should be considered in any sick newborn.** The newborn has a "limited repertoire" of symptoms that are often nonspecific. The differential diagnosis of symptoms such as **poor feeding, lethargy, hypotonia, vomiting, hypothermia, seizures, and disturbances of breathing** is extensive. Although the diagnosis of sepsis is often at the top of the differential diagnosis list, it is important for a timely diagnosis and in the best interest of the patient to evaluate for other causes, including IEMs, at the same time that laboratory investigations are initiated to rule out sepsis. This can be accomplished with a relatively small number of laboratory tests readily available in most hospitals, as discussed in the following sections.

A. **An IEM must be strongly considered under the following circumstances:**

1. **History of unexplained neonatal deaths in the family** (prior siblings or male infants on the mother's side of the family).

2. **Infants who are the offspring of consanguineous matings** (because of the higher incidence of autosomal recessive conditions; autosomal recessive inheritance is common among IEMs).

3. **Onset of signs and symptoms after a period of good health** that may be as short as a few hours.

4. **The infant may have had an uneventful perinatal and early newborn course.** It is not uncommon for infant with an IEM to have no significant perinatal history.

5. **The introduction and progression of enteral feedings may be related to the symptoms.**

6. **Failure of usual therapies to alleviate the symptoms or inability to prove a suggested diagnosis** such as sepsis, CNS hemorrhage, or other congenital or acquired conditions.

7. **Progression of symptoms.**

8. **Although patients with an IEM might be born prematurely, they are typically full-term infants.** An exception is the diagnosis of transient hyperammonemia of the neonate, a condition that typically affects preterm infants. Although this condition is briefly discussed in this chapter, the exact cause of the hyperammonemia in these patients remains unclear and may well be related to prematurity rather than being a typical IEM.

B. **Signs and symptoms** seen in different IEMs are summarized in Table 93–2. Table 93–3 lists some of the conditions with which infants with IEM have been misdiagnosed. Keep in mind that **symptoms may overlap** with frequent neonatal conditions; for example, a child with an IEM may have transient tachypnea of the newborn

Table 93–2. SIGNS AND SYMPTOMS AND ASSOCIATED METABOLIC DISORDERS

Neurologic (hypotonia, lethargy, poor sucking, seizures, coma)
Glycogen storage disease, galactosemia, organic acidemias, hereditary fructose intolerance, maple syrup urine disease, urea cycle disorders, hyperglycinemia, pyridoxine dependency, peroxisomal disorders, congenital disorders of glycosylation, fatty acid oxidation disorders, and respiratory chain defects

Hepatomegaly/Liver dysfunction
Lysosomal storage diseases, galactosemia, hereditary fructose intolerance, glycogen storage disease, tyrosinemia, α_1-antitrypsin deficiency, Gaucher disease, Niemann-Pick disease, Wolman disease, fatty acid oxidation defects, and respiratory chain defects

Hyperbilirubinemia
Galactosemia, hereditary fructose intolerance, tyrosinemia, α_1-antitrypsin deficiency, Crigler-Najjar syndrome, and other disorders of bilirubin metabolism

Nonimmune hydrops
Gaucher disease, Niemann-Pick disease, GM_1 gangliosidosis, congenital disorders of glycosylation

Cardiomegaly/Cardiomyopathy
Glycogen storage disease type II, fatty acid oxidation defects, and respiratory chain defects

Macroglossia
GM_1 gangliosidosis, glycogen storage disease type II

Abnormal odor
Maple syrup urine disease (odor of maple syrup or burnt sugar)
Isovaleric acidemia, glutaric acidemia (odor of sweaty feet)
HMG-CoA lyase deficiency (odor of cat urine)

Abnormal hair
Argininosuccinic acidemia, lysinuric protein intolerance, Menkes kinky hair syndrome

Hypoglycemia
Galactosemia, hereditary fructose intolerance, tyrosinemia, maple syrup urine disease, glycogen storage disease, methylmalonic acidemia, propionic acidemia, fatty acid oxidation defects, and respiratory chain defects

Ketosis
Organic acidemias, tyrosinemia, methylmalonic acidemia, maple syrup urine disease

Metabolic acidosis
Galactosemia, hereditary fructose intolerance, maple syrup urine disease, glycogen storage disease, organic acidemias

Hyperammonemia
Urea cycle defects, transient hyperammonemia of the neonate, organic acidurias, HMG-CoA lyase deficiency, fatty acid oxidation disorders

Neutropenia
Organic acidemias, especially methylmalonic acidemia and propionic acidemia; nonketotic hyperglycinemia, carbamyl phosphate synthetase deficiency

Thrombocytopenia
Organic acidemias, lysinuric protein intolerance

Dysmorphic features
Glutaric aciduria type II, 3-hydroxyisobutyric aciduria, Smith-Lemli-Opitz syndrome, peroxisomal disorders, congenital disorders of glycosylation

Renal cysts
Glutaric aciduria type II, peroxisomal disorders

Abnormalities of the eye (eg, glaucoma, retinopathy)
Galactosemia, lysosomal storage disorders, peroxisomal disorders

Abnormal fat distribution/inverted nipples
Congenital disorders of glycosylation

Epiphyseal stippling in radiograph
Peroxisomal disorders (Zellweger syndrome, neonatal adrenoleukodystrophy, rhizomelic chondrodysplasia punctata)

HMG, 3-hydroxy-3-methylglutaryl; CoA, coenzyme A.

Table 93–3. **MISDIAGNOSES OF METABOLIC DISEASE IN THE NEWBORN INFANT**

Bacterial sepsis
Acute viral infection
Asphyxia
Gastrointestinal tract obstruction
Hepatic failure, hepatitis
Central nervous system catastrophe
Persistent pulmonary hypertension
Cardiomyopathy
Neuromuscular disorder

or be at risk for sepsis for unrelated reasons. Occasionally, two conditions may be present with a causative relationship. A typical example is the frequently quoted but still unexplained increased incidence of *Escherichia coli* sepsis in infants with galactosemia.

C. **Asymptomatic IEMs in the newborn.** Untreated PKU does not cause any symptoms in the newborn. It causes irreversible brain damage while the patient appears clinically well. Verify that newborn screening tests have been done and check results as soon as available. Early detection of PKU in the newborn allows a well established treatment plan that prevents extreme mental retardation. (See Section XI)

D. To guide the clinician in the diagnostic workup, **signs and symptoms** are discussed **further for five different major clinical presentations**: IEM presenting with encephalopathy, IEM presenting with liver disease, IEM presenting with impairment of cardiac function, IEM presenting as dysmorphic syndromes, and IEM presenting as nonimmune hydrops (Sections VI to X). Flow diagrams in Figures 93–1 and 93–2 are designed to assist in the diagnostic workup. Details regarding the different **laboratory tests** are outlined in Section XII.

VI. **Major clinical presentation. Inborn errors of metabolism presenting with encephalopathy.** Encephalopathies associated with IEMs are clinically often indistinguishable from those caused by a hypoxic-ischemic insult or other CNS insult (hemorrhage or infectious disease). **Abnormal tone** (hypotonia as well as hypertonia may be of central origin) and **abnormal movements and seizures** clearly indicate CNS involvement. Clinically, seizures may present as lip smacking, tongue thrusting, bicycling movements of the lower extremities, opisthotonos, tremors, or generalized tonic-clonic movements. In severe encephalopathy, burst suppression pattern may be seen on **electroencephalography (EEG) using conventional multilead EEG or bedside monitoring with amplitude integrated encephalography (aEEG).** Discontinuous patterns detected by aEEG may be seen with less severe encephalopathy.

A. Laboratory evaluation

1. **Acute evaluation. In any patient with encephalopathy of any degree,** careful **evaluation of the acid-base status** is advisable. Some IEMs present with quite pronounced metabolic acidosis In addition to an arterial or venous blood gas, the following tests (for details, see Section XII) should be performed as part of the **acute evaluation** of patients with encephalopathy:

a. **Arterial or venous blood gas**

i. When interpreting the venous or arterial blood gas of a newborn, the **alterations in respiratory status** that are so frequent in this patient group must be taken into careful consideration. An isolated respiratory acidosis is likely pulmonary, and a metabolic or mixed acidosis, especially shortly after delivery, may be related to perinatal events.

ii. In case of a **severe and prolonged metabolic acidosis** without presence of an underlying condition (such as septic or hypovolemic shock and

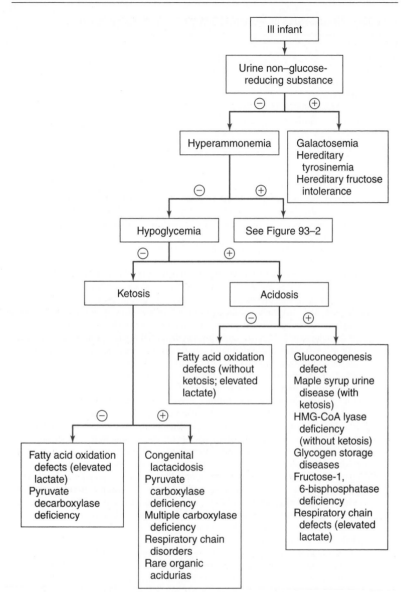

FIGURE 93–1. Algorithm for the diagnosis of metabolic disorders of acute onset (guideline only; for details, see text and references).

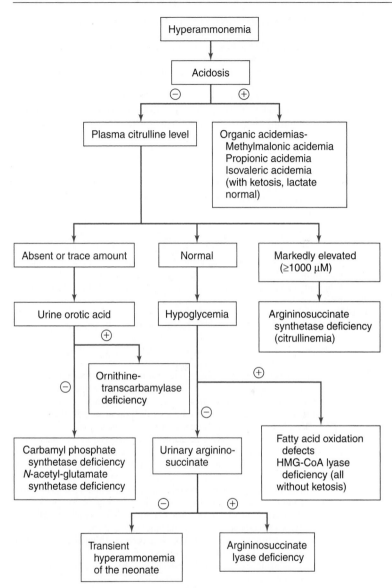

FIGURE 93–2. Algorithm for the differential diagnosis of hyperammonemia (guideline only; for details, see text and references).

malperfusion) explaining the finding, it is mandatory to evaluate whether **acidic metabolites** (eg, the excessive production of lactic acid) could be the cause of the imbalance. When considering compensatory mechanisms (eg, respiratory correction of a metabolic acidosis), remember that the resulting blood gas should reflect a mixed acid-base status.

  iii. Presence of an **isolated respiratory alkalosis** is suspicious for central disturbance of the respiratory pattern (hyperpnea), and **hyperammonemia** should be ruled out in this situation. Ammonia directly stimulates the respiratory center resulting in primary hyperventilation, which in turn leads to respiratory alkalosis.

  b. **Serum electrolytes** with calculation of the anion gap.
  c. **Ammonia level.**
  d. **Lactate and pyruvate levels and ratio.**
  e. **Urine collection** should be initiated and collected urine refrigerated or, ideally, frozen.

 2. **Other causes of encephalopathy should be assessed by appropriate studies** (eg, imaging studies, sepsis workup, lumbar puncture) as indicated and outlined in other sections of this manual. If cerebrospinal fluid (CSF) is obtained, it is advisable to freeze a sample for possible future testing (eg, ~1–2 mL for tests such as CSF amino acid analysis to rule out nonketotic hyperglycinemia [NKH]). If an IEM remains a diagnostic possibility after the initial evaluation, the analysis of plasma amino acids and urine organic acids should be arranged.

B. **Differential diagnosis.** Although the **differential diagnosis** of IEMs associated with encephalopathy is extensive, the following conditions are discussed in more detail because of either their frequency or clinical significance. (Items 1-4 below are typically without severe metabolic acidosis at presentation; items 5 and 6 are typically associated with a severe metabolic acidosis.)

 1. **Urea cycle defects (and transient hyperammonemia of the neonate).**
   a. **Clinical presentation.** Presentation with hyperammonemia (not caused by liver dysfunction) with three major diagnostic possibilities:
     i. A primary defect of one of the enzymes of the urea cycle (that degrades ammonia produced in the metabolism of amino acids). The most common urea cycle defect is **ornithine-transcarbamylase deficiency (OTC),** which is transmitted in an X-linked recessive fashion. Newborn patients, therefore, are usually male. **Female heterozygotes** can be symptomatic, depending on the X-chromosome inactivation pattern in the liver, but females usually present later in life. It is important to note that a mother heterozygous for OTC deficiency may develop symptoms (hyperammonemia) at the time of delivery because of the metabolic stresses of labor and delivery. The other urea cycle defects are inherited in an autosomal recessive fashion, with **carbamyl phosphate synthetase deficiency** the second most common.
     ii. **An organic acidemia as an underlying cause** with secondary impairment of the urea cycle (see Section VI, B, 5).
     iii. **Transient hyperammonemia of the neonate (THAN),** a condition usually seen in premature infants. By anecdotal report, the frequency of THAN seems to have declined over the last few years.
   b. **Diagnosis.** Information regarding the diagnostic workup of patients with hyperammonemia is outlined in Figure 93–2. Quantitative measurement of plasma amino acids and orotic acid is necessary to establish the exact diagnosis. Urine organic acids should also be examined.
   c. **Treatment.** Initial treatment is similar, independent of the final diagnosis (see Section XIII, A). Immediate transfer to a facility able to perform hemodialysis is strongly advised when hyperammonemia is detected. The use of medication

such as sodium phenylacetate and butyrate should be supervised by a biochemical geneticist. In some defects (eg, argininosuccinate lyase deficiency), substitution of arginine (intravenous arginine hydrochloride) may alleviate symptoms; arginine becomes secondarily deficient as a metabolite of the cycle located after the deficient reaction. Long-term **protein restriction** is necessary (see Section XIII, B, 1). Acute treatment of THAN is similar to that of inborn errors of the urea cycle, but deficiency of the metabolic pathway is temporary and normal protein intake is tolerated later in life.

    d. Outcome (especially in regard to CNS damage) is much more favorable for THAN compared with the inherited urea cycle defects.

2. **Maple syrup urine disease (MSUD).** Accumulation of **branched-chain amino acids (leucine, isoleucine, and valine)** is secondary to a defect in the decarboxylase involved in the catabolism of these amino acids. 2-Keto metabolites of the three amino acids also accumulate. Leucine is the amino acid that has been implied to be the most neurotoxic.

    a. **Clinical presentation.** Presentation is commonly after the second week of life but may be as early as at 24 h of age and, therefore, may precede the report of the **neonatal screening** test result. Typical symptoms are feeding intolerance, lethargy, signs of encephalopathy such as hypotonia or posturing, abnormal movements, or frank seizures (late in the course). **Typical odor** (maple syrup or "burnt sugar") may not be prominent, and metabolic acidosis is a late presentation of untreated MSUD.

    b. **Diagnosis.** Diagnosis is by quantitative amino acid analysis (elevated leucine, isoleucine, valine, and glycine) and detection of 2-keto metabolites in urine organic acid analysis. The 2,4-dinitrophenylhydrazine (DNPH) test detects 2-keto acids and may be available at certain specialized laboratories.

    c. **Treatment.** Restrict all protein acutely while providing high amounts of glucose and fluid (see Section XIII, A). Later, provide formula low in leucine, valine, and isoleucine with restriction of natural protein. **Dialysis** may be needed as acute therapy if severe encephalopathy has developed. Some patients may show response to thiamine (see Section XIII, B, 3).

3. **Nonketotic hyperglycinemia (NKH) (glycine encephalopathy)**

    a. **Clinical presentation.** A **typical presentation** for NKH is a patient suffering from a severe encephalopathy that is rapidly progressing and eventually results in respiratory arrest, but standard evaluation for IEMs and other causes of this presentation does not reveal any abnormalities (no acidosis, hypoglycemia, or hyperammonemia and no other organ system affected). **Pronounced and sustained "hiccoughs"** in an encephalopathic infant have been described as a typical observation in NKH.

    b. **Diagnosis.** Hyperglycinemia in plasma is typical but may not be pronounced in young infants because of decreased renal reabsorption of this amino acid. In addition, other IEMs also result in increased blood glycine levels, such as MSUD (which is sometimes referred to as ketotic hyperglycinemia). This diagnostic situation is one of the few indications for **urine amino acids** to detect the high renal glycine excretion.

        A more specific diagnostic test is to determine the **CSF-to-plasma glycine ratio** because an elevation of glycine in the CSF is specific for NKH. A CSF-to-blood glycine ratio of >0.08 is considered abnormal (0.02–0.08 is uncertain; <0.02 is normal).

    c. Treatment options remain limited at this point. Restoration of normal glycine levels in blood can be achieved (through hydration or the use of sodium benzoate (see Section XIII, A, 5), but the glycine accumulation in CSF remains unaffected. Several medications (dextromethorphan, diazepam, and even strychnine) have been used to try to affect the CNS symptomatology but have achieved only limited success.

    d. Outcome. Patients may survive because the respiratory depression has the potential to improve, but severe brain damage is the rule. A few patients with a transient form of NKH have been reported.

4. **Peroxisomal disorders**

    a. Clinical presentation. Defects of peroxisome biogenesis (eg, Zellweger syndrome and neonatal adrenoleukodystrophy) and some of the peroxisomal single enzyme defects (eg, multifunctional enzyme deficiency) present with encephalopathy in the neonatal period. Patients are **extremely floppy** as a result of severe central hypotonia and develop **seizures** (usually within the first week of life). Hepatomegaly, renal and hepatic cysts, and skeletal or retinal abnormalities may also be found.

    b. Diagnosis. Most peroxisomal defects can be detected by analysis of **very long chain fatty acids** (VLCFAs) (with carbon chains of 24 and more) in plasma. To fully exclude a peroxisomal defect, additional studies such as plasmalogen levels in red blood cells, phytanic acid, and others (see Section XII, C, 8) are necessary.

5. **Organic aciduria/acidemias (OAs).** This group of IEMs is complex, and many clinicians feel overwhelmed by the biochemical details regarding these conditions. Relevant clinical information is as follows:

    a. Clinical presentations. Many OAs present later in infancy. Three conditions commonly present in the neonatal period and are clinically nearly indistinguishable: **methylmalonic acidemia, propionic acidemia,** and **isovaleric acidemia.** Diagnostic landmarks are encephalopathy with severe acidosis, hyperammonemia, and seizures; an unusual **odor** (most noticeable in urine [see Table 93–2]) may be noted; **neutropenia** and **thrombocytopenia** may occur. More OAs are listed in Table 93–1.

    b. Diagnosis. Analysis of plasma amino acids and urine organic acids is the appropriate **diagnostic evaluation** for OAs. Interpretation of these tests by an experienced biochemical geneticist familiar with the clinical presentation of the patient is strongly recommended.

    c. Treatment. If this diagnosis is suspected, the following **treatment** should be initiated: hydration and glucose infusion (both at least 1.5 times the maintenance level), treatment of hyperammonemia (see Section XIII A and especially XIII, A, 5), and careful correction of metabolic acidosis with bicarbonate while ensuring appropriate ventilation. Involvement of a geneticist in the diagnostic workup and treatment is strongly recommended. Some OAs may partially respond to vitamins (see Section XIII, B, 3).

6. **Congenital lactic acidosis (LA).** Some possible causes of LA in a neonate are **pyruvate dehydrogenase (PDH) defect, pyruvate carboxylase defect,** and **mitochondrial respiratory chain defects** (most common are defects of complex I and/or IV).

    a. Clinical presentation. Lactic Acidosis may be difficult to differentiate clinically from hypoxic-ischemic encephalopathy, sepsis, and other conditions that result in metabolic acidosis, poor perfusion, and shock. Clinical scenarios that make acidosis due to congenital LA more likely are very severe LA (especially if LA is unexpected or more severe than clinical history explains), **growth retardation** resulting in birth of a small for gestational age infant, some mild **dysmorphic features,** and anatomic abnormalities of the brain. **Multiorgan disease** unexplained by other causes (eg, hypertrophic cardiomyopathy or cataracts) may occur. Hypoglycemia with LA may be a presentation of a glycogen storage disease (see Section VII, F).

    b. Diagnosis. Once an increase of lactic acid is found, determination of the **lactate–pyruvate ratio** further guides the diagnostic process (see Section XII, C, 1). The common biochemical concept of metabolic disorders leading to LA is a deficiency to provide energy through aerobic metabolism, which depends on conversion of pyruvate to metabolites of the citrate cycle and an intact mitochondrial respiratory chain. In some patients with LA, muscle biopsies (Section XII, C, 10) or sequencing of mitochondrial DNA (Section XII, C, 11) may be needed to establish diagnosis.

   c. **Treatment.** Be aware that PDH deficiency is one of the rare exceptions to the treatment approach to provide high levels of glucose to the patient; the LA may worsen.

C. Other rare but significant IEMs with encephalopathy include the following:

   1. **Fatty acid oxidation disorders with dicarboxylic aciduria.** Although the most common fatty acid oxidation defect (medium-chain acyl-CoA dehydrogenase deficiency [MCAD]) does rarely causes illness in a neonate, SCAD, LCAD (short- and long-chain acyl-CoA dehydrogenase deficiencies, respectively), or other fatty acid oxidation disorders may present in the neonatal period (see Section VIII, A).

   2. **Multiple carboxylase deficiency.**

   3. **Holocarboxylase synthetase deficiency.**

   4. **Glutaric acidemia type II** (a defect of the electron transport flavoprotein or its dehydrogenase).

   5. **Pyroglutamic acidemia** (5-oxoprolinuria, a defect in glutathione synthetase).

   6. **Molybdenum cofactor deficiency** (xanthine oxidase deficiency or sulfite oxidase deficiency). One diagnostic clue to xanthine oxidase deficiency may be a significantly **low plasma uric acid level.** A commercial test is available to determine urine sulfite excretion in urine.

   7. **HMG-CoA lyase deficiency.**

   8. **Pyridoxine-dependent seizures** are a rare condition for which treatment is available. Patients present with seizures in the neonatal period or in early infancy that are refractory to treatment with anticonvulsants but show dramatic improvement with administration of vitamin B_6 (100 mg of pyridoxine intravenously).

   9. **Congenital disorders of glycosylation (CDG)** typically present during infancy but may also present in neonates with acute encephalopathy, seizures, and stroke-like episodes. Many types of CDGs have been described in recent years. With a neonatal presentation of the more common types of CDG (type Ia is the most common), patients are usually hypotonic. **Cerebellar atrophy** may be noted on pre- or postnatal imaging studies. Psychomotor development is delayed later in life, and ataxia, dyskinesia, and muscle weakness become prominent. **Severe feeding problems and failure to thrive** are typical; intractable diarrhea in a neonate has been reported. **Unusual fat pads in the buttock area and inverted nipples** are believed to be quite characteristic findings.

   These autosomal recessive conditions are characterized by **defects in the glycosylation of proteins** (see Section XII, C, 9 for diagnostic testing). They are multisystem disorders. Other than neurologic involvement, hepatic dysfunction with abnormal liver enzymes, pericardial effusions, nephrotic syndrome, nonimmune hydrops, and facial dysmorphic features (broad nasal bridge, prominent jaw and forehead, large ears, strabismus) have been described in infants.

VII. **Major clinical presentation. Inborn errors of metabolism presenting with liver disease.** Several IEMs result in liver disease that may present in the neonatal period with the following: **liver enlargement, jaundice, hepatocellular dysfunction, and hypoglycemia.** The initial evaluation in these patients consists of routine tests (eg, bilirubin levels, glucose measurement, liver function tests, and imaging studies). Considering that the liver is the main organ of amino acid metabolism, analysis of plasma amino acid patterns helps in the assessment of liver function; this is a more elaborate and expensive test, however. Many synthetic functions of the liver can be partially evaluated by routine tests such as glucose, cholesterol, total protein, and albumin levels. The following conditions are discussed in more detail because of either their frequency or clinical significance.

A. **Galactosemia** does not present in an affected newborn until the patient is receiving galactose. Breast milk and most formulas contain **lactose** (a disaccharide of glucose and galactose); most soy formulas do not. Typical symptoms are **hyperbilirubinemia** (which may be unconjugated initially but later becomes mainly conjugated); then signs of **liver dysfunction** (which may include **coagulopathy, hypoglycemia, hypoalbuminemia,** and **ascites**) and **hepatomegaly** develop. **Cataracts** may be diagnosed as early because the disease manifests in the neonatal period. If untreated, symptoms may worsen to encephalopathy with cerebral edema, metabolic acidosis (hyperchloremia and hypophosphatemia), and renal dysfunction. Patients with galactosemia have an increased risk for *E. coli* **sepsis** (reasons remain unclear). **Testing urine** for reducing substances is an initial screening test (see Section XII, B, 7). If galactose has been discontinued, reducing substance testing may be falsely negative and blood tests are essential to make a diagnosis. Galactosemia is due to a defect in either **galactose-1-phosphate uridyltransferase (GALT)** (classic galactosemia) or UDP galactose 4-epimerase (rare variant); red blood cells are used to measure GALT activity, or accumulation of galactose-1-phosphate is measured. Treatment consists of galactose restriction in the diet; the diet is relatively strict and difficult to follow. Even if compliance with the diet is good, many patients show **developmental delays,** and females suffer **ovarian failure** later in life.

B. **Hepatorenal tyrosinemia.** Tyrosinemia type I, or hepatorenal tyrosinemia, usually presents in infancy but has been described in neonates who developed **severe liver dysfunction,** including hyperbilirubinemia, hypoglycemia, hyperammonemia, coagulopathy, hypoalbuminemia with ascites, and anasarca. This IEM also causes renal disease with mainly tubular dysfunction (amino aciduria or glucosuria) and results in hypophosphatemia and hyperchloremic metabolic acidosis. **Cardiomyopathy** can also develop, so that the clinical presentation may overlap with disorders of fatty acid metabolism and respiratory chain defects. Although altered tyrosine levels are also found with liver dysfunction as a result of other causes, the presence of **succinylacetone** in urine is a finding specific for tyrosinemia (see Section XII, C, 4). Plasma cysteine might be low; plasma α-fetoprotein may be markedly increased. The only long-term treatment option is liver transplantation.

C. α_1-**Antitrypsin deficiency (AATD).** This IEM may present in neonates and infants as **hyperbilirubinemia,** which is usually prolonged and conjugated (with signs of cholestasis) but may resolve spontaneously within the first 6 months of life. These children may then not present again clinically until **liver cirrhosis** with portal hypertension has developed. An adult manifestation of AATD is the development of **emphysema** as early as in the third or fourth decade of life, a disease process much accelerated by smoking. The cause of AATD is a mutation in the *AATD* gene (designated as **Z mutation**), which, in homozygous carriers, results in deficiency of AAT, which is an inhibitor of an elastase, a degrading enzyme of neutrophils. The defect in this enzyme inhibition results in destruction of pulmonary or hepatic tissue. Diagnosis is confirmed by **genotyping** and routinely available in most hospitals because of the frequency with which the test is performed in the workup of adults with emphysema. Although the symptoms during early life may resolve spontaneously and not all patients develop liver and lung manifestations, the neonatologist or pediatrician has the opportunity to ensure a diagnosis early in life, possibly enabling the patient to prevent serious disease later through early behavior modification.

D. **Inborn errors of bilirubin metabolism.** Inherited defects in the metabolism of bilirubin include defects in conjugation (**Crigler-Najjar syndrome**) and uptake and excretion of bilirubin (**Dubin-Johnson and Rotor syndromes**). These conditions result in either indirect or direct hyperbilirubinemia. Dubin-Johnson and Rotor syndromes are rarely diagnosed in the newborn period.

E. **Fatty acid oxidation (FAO) disorders** may present with a combination of encephalopathy and cardiac and liver dysfunction. These conditions are discussed in more detail in Section VIII, A. The **liver dysfunction** may be mild with less severe hypoalbuminemia and coagulopathy than in other IEMs; **hyperammonemia** may be present if more significant liver dysfunction develops. The clinical presentation is dominated by severe and generalized hypotonia and cardiomyopathy. Succinylacetone will be negative, whereas tyrosine metabolites may be present in urine organic acids. Analysis of an **acyl carnitine profile** is helpful in making the diagnosis (see Section XII, C, 5).

F. **Glycogen storage disease type I (von Gierke disease).** The clinical presentation of glycogen storage disorders in the newborn period may be limited to **hypoglycemia,** which is usually severe and may be accompanied by LA. In von Gierke disease, the hypoglycemia is unresponsive to glucagon injection. **Liver enlargement and dysfunction** usually develop shortly thereafter (as soon as within 1–2 weeks). **Hyperlipidemia** may be present. Glycogen storage disorders are diagnosed by liver biopsy with enzyme analysis (see Section XII, C, 10).

G. **Peroxisomal disorders.** Patients with disorders of peroxisomal biogenesis such as Zellweger syndrome and neonatal adrenoleukodystrophy develop **hepatomegaly** early in life that usually progresses to fibrosis and cirrhosis. The clinical presentation is usually dominated by **central hypotonia and seizures** (see Section VI, B, 4a). **Dysmorphic features** are present (Section IX, B). See Section XII, C, 8 for specific diagnostic tests.

H. **Others.** Other inherited conditions that may present with hepatocellular dysfunction, sometimes as early as in the neonatal period, are as follows:

1. **Neonatal hemochromatosis.**
2. **Hereditary fructose intolerance.**
3. **Defects in carnitine metabolism.**
4. **Other glycogen storage diseases.**
5. **Lysosomal storage disorders** (Niemann-Pick disease may present with neonatal hepatitis).
6. **Congenital disorders of glycosylation.** See Section VI, C, 9.

VIII. **Major clinical presentation.** Inborn errors of metabolism presenting with impairment of cardiac function:

A. **Fatty acid oxidation disorders** are to be suspected in any neonate with impairment of cardiac function; cardiac arrhythmias occur in some. Additional symptoms such as encephalopathy (Section VI, C, 1) or impaired liver function (Section VII, E), rhabdomyolysis and muscle weakness, and/or retinopathy may be present. FAO disorders affecting the dehydrogenase steps of the beta-oxidation are subdivided according to the length of the carbon chain of the fatty acids that accumulate: short chain acyl-CoA dehydrogenase (SCAD), medium chain acyl-CoA dehydrogenase (MCAD), and long chain acyl-CoA dehydrogenase (LCAD) deficiency. In addition, deficiency of long chain 3-hydroxyl acyl CoA dehydrogenase (LCHAD), other enzymes of the trifunctional enzyme complex, and defects resulting in an inability to metabolize fatty acids properly due to defects of the plasma membrane carnitine transporter or carnitine palmitoyl transferase I or II have been described. Many of these IEMs are associated with severe **cardiomyopathy** usually resulting in cardiac failure. In addition to cardiomyopathy, patients may also suffer from **encephalopathy** and **myopathy; hepatomegaly** also occurs, and with low glucose intake or intercurrent illnesses, patients characteristically develop **hypoketotic hypoglycemia.** Maternal fatty liver of pregnancy and HELLP (hemolysis, elevated liver enzymes, and low platelets) syndrome have been associated with FAO defects, especially LCHAD and SCAD.

Acyl carnitine profile analysis by mass spectrometry (Sections XII, C, 5 and 6) helps to establish the diagnosis, which is then confirmed by enzyme assays in cultured fibroblasts. Newborn screening using the tandem mass spectrometry technique, now the predominant means for routine newborn screening, will detect FAO defects. Total and free **carnitine levels** should be determined (Section XII, C, 5). Treatment of FAO disorders consists of avoidance of prolonged periods without carbohydrate intake. Intravenous or oral carnitine may be indicated. Although medium-chain triglycerides are contraindicated in MCAD, they may be a good source of energy in the other conditions and can be given as commercially available medium-chain triglyceride (MCT) oil or through formulas with high levels of MCT oil as the predominant fat source.

B. Pompe disease. The cardiomyopathy of Pompe disease may (although not typically) present as early as in the neonatal period. Of diagnostic help are **electrocardiographic changes,** some of which are fairly characteristic: shortening of the PR interval, marked left-axis deviation, T-wave inversion, and enlarged QRS complexes. The diagnosis is confirmed by measurement of the deficient enzyme (α-glucosidase or acid maltase) in leukocytes or cultured fibroblasts (Section XII, C, 10).

C. Hepatorenal tyrosinemia. Type I tyrosinemia may present with cardiomyopathy in addition to liver and renal tubular dysfunction (see Section VII, B).

D. Congenital disorders of glycosylation (see Section VI, C, 9). Pericardial effusions have been observed in affected patients.

IX. Major clinical presentation. Inborn errors of metabolism presenting as dysmorphic syndromes. Several dysmorphic syndromes are now known to be due to an underlying metabolic defect. With the ongoing progress in molecular, cell, and developmental biology and human genetics, it is likely that more and more conditions initially described as syndromes will eventually be found to be IEMs or genetic conditions secondary to other molecular mechanisms. Examples of disorders in this category include the following:

A. Smith-Lemli-Opitz syndrome. The metabolic basis of Smith-Lemli-Opitz syndrome is a defect in 7-dehydrocholesterol dehydrogenase, resulting in an **accumulation of 7-dehydrocholesterol** and typically low cholesterol levels in plasma. Dietary cholesterol supplementation is now routinely given to patients, and other therapies such as treatment with simvastatin are being investigated. The main clinical signs of this relatively common syndrome, with an estimated frequency of 1 in 20,000, are as follows:

1. **Growth deficiency** (usually postnatal) and microcephaly.
2. **Dysmorphic features,** including a high forehead, ptosis, epicanthal folds, strabismus, rotated and low-set ears, a nose with a wide tip, and micrognathia.
3. **Hypospadias** in males.
4. **Syndactyly** of the second and third toes.
5. **Other common findings** include cataracts, hypotonia and significant psychomotor retardation.

B. Zellweger syndrome and other peroxisomal disorders. Although Zellweger syndrome and **neonatal adrenoleukodystrophy** were initially described based on clinical characteristics, they are now known to be disorders of peroxisome biogenesis, as is **infantile Refsum disease.** These three conditions are all clinical phenotypes of defects in peroxisomal biogenesis and function (hence the term *Zellweger spectrum*). The diagnosis is established by measurement of VLCFAs and other biochemical parameters affected by peroxisomal dysfunction (see Section XII, C, 8). Typical findings are as follows:

1. **Dysmorphic features,** including a high forehead, a wide and flat nasal bridge, epicanthal folds, and dysplastic ears; the fontanelles are wide open.
2. **Severe hypotonia, seizures,** and lack of psychomotor development.
3. **Hepatomegaly** with fibrosis.
4. **Ocular abnormalities** (corneal clouding, cataract, and retinal changes).
5. **Punctate calcifications** of the skeleton.
6. **Small renal cortical cysts.**

C. Pyruvate dehydrogenase (PDH) deficiency. Patients with congenital lactic acidosis (LA) (see Section VI, B,6) resulting from PDH deficiency often display dysmorphic features, including a high and prominent forehead, a widened nasal bridge, a small anteverted nose, and dysmorphic and enlarged ears.

D. **Congenital defects of glycosylation** (see Section VI, C, 9). Dysmorphic features include broad nasal bridge, prominent jaw and forehead, large ears, and strabismus. **Unusual fat pads in the buttock area and inverted nipples** are believed to be characteristic findings.

X. **Major clinical presentation. Inborn errors of metabolism presenting as nonimmune hydrops.** Although the differential diagnosis of nonimmune hydrops is extensive and this condition is discussed in other sections of this manual, **two groups** of **inherited disorders that can present with hydrops** are briefly mentioned here. *Note:* Congenital disorders of glycosylation rarely presents with nonimmune hydrops fetalis (based on a small number of case reports).

A. **Inherited hematologic conditions** (eg, glucose-6-phosphate dehydrogenase deficiency and pyruvate kinase deficiency), the hydrops is due to anemia and heart failure.

B. **Genetic conditions with disturbed lysosomal function.** Cases of hydrops have been reported in **GM$_1$ gangliosidosis, Gaucher disease, Niemann-Pick disease,** and other genetic conditions with disturbed lysosomal function. Although the occurrence of hydrops in lysosomal disorders is well established, little has been published about the possible mechanism. The presence of **hepatomegaly, dysostosis multiplex,** and abnormal **vacuolated mononuclear cells** in the peripheral blood smear are diagnostic clues. Presence of a lysosomal storage disorder should be considered in any hydropic patient without established etiology, and involvement of a geneticist and consequent specific enzymatic essays using white blood cells or fibroblasts are both warranted.

XI. **Phenylketonuria.** Although PKU is an IEM of foremost interest because of its frequency and well-established treatment that prevents the extreme mental retardation characteristic of untreated PKU, it is not discussed in detail here because **untreated PKU does not cause symptoms in the neonate.** Even though the patient is clinically well, **irreversible brain damage** occurs as a result of accumulating phenylalanine and its metabolites. Therefore patients benefit enormously from detection by neonatal screening for PKU.

A. If an **abnormal neonatal screening** for PKU is reported, formula or breast milk must be discontinued and hydration provided (short-term enteral feedings with electrolyte solutions are feasible; intravenous therapy is usually not mandated). The patient should immediately (within hours) be referred to a geneticist for further evaluation (including differentiation between classic PKU and hyperphenylalaninemia), initiation of diet, and family education, training, and counseling.

B. Occasionally, the clinician takes care of a **child of a mother with PKU;** considering that this child is an obligate heterozygote for PKU combined with the high frequency of the PKU allele in the general population (1 in 20), this child has a 1 in 80 risk of being affected, and measurement of phenylalanine levels after enteral feedings are established is mandatory. Although institutional practices vary, many geneticists recommend early quantitative amino acid analysis rather than routine newborn screening in this scenario. Newborns of affected mothers with insufficient treatment manifest with **microcephaly, congenital heart disease,** and **mental deficiencies** (even if the infant is not homozygous for PKU).

XII. **Diagnosis**

A. **Prenatal.** The ability to diagnose IEMs prenatally has increased in recent years. Biochemical methods (eg, detection of metabolites in amniotic fluid and enzyme assays using cultured cells) as well as DNA analysis (mutation detection) are used. Diagnostic procedures routinely available are **chorionic villus sampling** and **amniocentesis.** In some centers, analysis of **fetal cells in maternal circulation** or **preimplantation testing of the embryo with in vitro fertilization** may also be offered. In some cases, in utero treatment can be achieved (eg, dietary control in maternal PKU or experimental therapies such as fetal stem cell treatment). Otherwise, appropriate therapies may be instituted immediately after delivery of the infant. Prenatal counseling is essential so that parents are well educated and able to make an informed decision regarding continuation of the pregnancy.

B. Postnatal. These postnatal tests are usually the initial tests done to evaluate for the possibility of a metabolic disorder while obtaining quick results and limiting the number of secondary tests that may be needed; considering that the limitation of the blood volume drawn is often a significant concern in neonates. Although some of these laboratory tests and their significance in aiding the diagnostic process have already been discussed, details regarding the specifics of these tests and their interpretations are briefly outlined here. Refer also to Table 93–4.

1. **Blood cell count with differential, hemoglobin, and platelets.** Be aware that neutropenia (especially when accompanied by metabolic acidosis) not only is typically found in sepsis and poor perfusion but may be present in a patient with organic acidopathy (most common are propionic acidemia, methylmalonic acidemia, and isovaleric acidemia). Thrombocytopenia may be present. These IEMs are also accompanied by hyperammonemia; measurement of an ammonia level is mandatory in a newborn with acidosis, leukopenia, or thrombocytopenia with no established diagnosis.

2. **Blood gas.** Interpretation of the acid-base status is important in the differential diagnosis and has already been discussed (see Section VI, A, 1a). IEMs must be especially considered in the scenario of a **severe metabolic acidosis** or **respiratory alkalosis** (note that although hyperventilation may be induced by the painful stimulus with a blood draw, a pure respiratory alkalosis should not easily be dismissed as artifact). Ammonia measurement is indicated in this situation to rule out an organic aciduria with secondary hyperammonemia or a urea cycle defect causing a respiratory alkalosis as a result of the direct stimulation of the respiratory center by ammonia with hyperventilation. Be aware that excess heparin in a blood gas specimen may mimic a metabolic acidosis. Those specimens that are not instantly processed should be stored in ice water.

3. **Electrolyte determination.** In addition to the interpretation of the different electrolyte components, the **anion gap** should be calculated. The concentration of negatively and positively charged electrolytes is compared: Add the sodium and potassium levels (in mEq/L), and subtract the sum of the chloride and bicarbonate concentrations. An excess of negatively charged ions (eg, lactate or metabolites found in an organic acidopathy) is suggested if the anion gap is >17 mEq/L (consult with you local laboratory because cutoffs may vary some depending on essays and methods used). Be aware that in a hemolyzed specimen, potassium is released from cells that will distort the anion gap calculation (artificially increased).

   Disturbance of electrolytes is also found in other inherited conditions (eg, adrenogenital syndrome [see Chapter 82]).

4. **Ammonia level.** Although the measurement of ammonia levels can be of foremost importance in making the diagnosis of an IEM, this test is unfortunately very susceptible to artifacts, resulting in a false elevation of ammonia levels. Several precautions must be strictly followed to avoid incorrect test results.

   a. **The specimen must be placed on ice** at the bedside.

   b. **Timely transfer to the laboratory** with instant preparation of the sample for analysis. If samples have to be stored, the blood must be centrifuged and the plasma maintained at –20°C. Without strict adherence to these precautionary measures, false elevation by as much as 60–100 mcg/dL may occur. Normal neonatal levels are up to 80 mcg/dL. IEMs typically result in levels in the hundreds and thousands. If a result is equivocal, a repeat measurement must be done quickly since the hyperammonemia in IEM most likely will be progressive.

5. **Liver function tests.** Transaminases (aspartate aminotransferase [**SGOT**] and alanine aminotransferase [**SGPT**]) are released from hepatocytes with cell damage. Gamma glutamyl transferase (**GGT**) is produced in the liver cell but also present in bile ducts. It is a very sensitive indicator of liver dysfunction and/or cholestasis; it may be elevated even with fairly minor exposures to medications/toxins. **Conjugated bilirubin** and **alkaline phosphatase** are elevated with cholestasis.

Table 93–4. **LABORATORY FINDINGS SUGGESTIVE OF METABOLIC DISEASE**

Variable	Galactosemia	Glycogen Storage Disease	Maple Syrup Urine Disease	Nonketotic Hyperglycinemia	Glutaric Acidemia Type II	Organic Acidemia	Disorders of Pyruvate Metabolism	Disorders of the Urea Cycle	Transient Hyperammonemia of the Newborn
Hypoglycemia	+	+	±	−	±	±	±	−	−
Metabolic acidosis with or without elevated anion gap	+	±	+	−	±	+	+	±	±
Respiratory alkalosis	−	−	−	−	−	−	−	+	+
Hyperammonemia	−	−	−	−	−	+	−	+	+
Urine ketones	−	±	+	−	−	+	±	−	−
Urine abnormal odor or color	−	−	+	−	+	+	−	−	−
Neutropenia or thrombocytopenia	−	−	−	−	−	+	−	−	−

Guidelines only; for details, see text and references.

Cholesterol, albumin, and coagulation factor levels reflect the **synthetic function** of the liver. The **plasma amino acid pattern** is affected by liver dysfunction. **Ammonia** levels are increased in liver failure.

6. **Urine testing for ketones.** The presence of ketones in the urine of a neonate should always be considered abnormal. One of the IEMs that typically results in strongly positive testing is MSUD.

7. **Urine testing for reducing substances.** The main indication in the neonate is suspected galactosemia. It is important that a nonenzymatic essay is done. A negative test does not rule out the diagnosis. Even a few hours of galactose restriction may result in a negative test. Consider which enteral nutrition the patient is receiving. For example, soy formulas are often galactose free, whereas breast milk is not (lactose ["milk sugar"] is a disaccharide of glucose and galactose).

8. **Lipid levels and profile.** Low cholesterol may be noted in patients with Smith Lemli Opitz syndrome. Hyperlipidemia may be present in some glycogen storage disorders.

C. **Laboratory testing more specific for IEMs.** Although some of the following tests might still be available through laboratories at many larger hospitals or through reference laboratories, we consider them to be a second line of more specific tests. The following tests are usually performed to further evaluate a specific diagnosis or abnormalities found on previous testing or to confirm a diagnosis that is clinically suspected.

1. **Lactic acid level and lactate-to-pyruvate ratio.** Determination of lactate and pyruvate levels may be indicated in the evaluation of patients with severe metabolic acidosis. When excess lactate is present, the anion gap (see Section XII, B, 3) is elevated. Lactic acid is best obtained from a central line or arterial specimen because even short stasis of blood (venous sampling using a tourniquet) may result in a significant increase in lactate. The lactate-to-pyruvate ratio is normal (15–20) in PDH deficiency and defects of gluconeogenesis (glycogen storage diseases) and elevated to >25 in pyruvate decarboxylase deficiency and mitochondrial defects of the respiratory/electron transport chain.

2. **Amino acid analysis.** Amino acid analysis must be quantitative to aid in the diagnosis of IEMs. Amino acid analysis of urine is usually not indicated in the evaluation of newborns. There are only a few indications for this test: to rule out cystinuria with renal calculi or to demonstrate a high renal glycine when NKH is suspected (see Section VI, B, 3). **Plasma amino acid results** are best evaluated (in a sample obtained after a 4-h fast) by concentrating on certain patterns of abnormalities rather than on single abnormal values that may be nutritional or artifacts (eg, taurine is often increased with delayed analysis of the sample). Discussion of the many diagnostic patterns of plasma amino acids abnormalities is beyond the scope of this manual. Interpretation of results by an experienced biochemical geneticist who is aware of the clinical presentation and nutritional status of the patient is strongly recommended.

   Plasma amino acid analysis not only is indicated in classic IEMs of amino acid metabolism (eg, MSUD or PKU) but also helps evaluate urea cycle defects because several metabolites of the urea cycle are chemically amino acids (eg, citrulline, arginine, and ornithine; see Figure 93–2). Conditions resulting in hyperammonemia often show elevated glutamine levels (glutamine synthesis incorporates ammonia).

   At least 1–2 mL of blood should be obtained. Laboratories usually request heparinized blood or samples without additives. Samples should be sent on ice. If analysis is to be deferred to a later time, serum or plasma should be separated and frozen.

3. **Urine organic acid analysis.** This complex analytic test is usually performed by laboratories specializing in biochemical genetics. In expert hands, this test can provide an enormous amount of information. Urine organic acid analysis helps establish the diagnosis of organic acidemias. The most common of this large

group of disorders are methylmalonic acidemia, propionic acidemia, and isovaleric acidemia (see Section VI, B, 5). Most laboratories request at least 5–10 mL of "fresh" urine. As soon as the specimen is collected, it should either be transported to the laboratory on ice or frozen at –20°C.

4. **Succinylacetone in urine.** This test is specific for hepatorenal tyrosinemia. A sample is collected and used to wet a filter paper (as used for the routine neonatal screening tests). After air drying, the sample can be forwarded to the testing laboratory by mail or courier services.

5. **Acyl carnitine profile.** Fatty acids that are metabolized in the mitochondria are conjugated with carnitine to facilitate their transport into the mitochondrion. The acyl carnitine profile determines the levels of fatty acid metabolites of different carbon length allowing for the recognition of diagnostic patterns for different fatty acid oxidation defects (note that VLCFAs with carbon chains of 24 or longer are metabolized in the peroxisome; Section XII, C, 8). Acylcarnitine profiles are now often evaluated as part of the newborn screening by tandem mass spectrometry; alternatively the test is performed by specialized biochemical genetics laboratories. Dried whole blood spot samples placed on filter paper cards are used. An additional test useful in patients with suspected fatty acid oxidation defect is the determination of **total and free carnitine plasma levels** (measured in heparinized blood).

6. **Tandem mass spectrometry ms/ms.** TMS detects a large number of disorders of amino and organic acid metabolism as well as fatty acid oxidation defects. This makes it a valuable tool for newborn screening, and TMS is **now used routinely by many neonatal metabolic screening programs**; many laboratories also accept samples obtained beyond the neonatal period from infants presenting with symptoms suggestive of an inborn error of metabolism. Testing is easily done (blood spot samples mailed to laboratories) and usually quite cost effective.

7. **Galactosemia testing.** To measure galactose-1-phosphate levels and GALT activity, whole blood is usually requested by the laboratory because the metabolites and enzyme are localized in the erythrocytes. Blood must therefore be obtained before blood transfusions. An alternative in already transfused patients is to evaluate the heterozygous parents of the patient because heterozygote detection is possible with the enzymatic assay.

8. **Peroxisomal function tests.** Measurement of VLCFAs is done by gas chromatography. Normally, only trace amounts of fatty acids with carbon chains of 24 carbons or more are detectable. Measurement of VLCFAs, therefore, detects all peroxisomal disorders that affect the degradation of these compounds. Note that VLCFAs will be normal in a small subgroup of patients with peroxisomal defects (eg, rhizomelic chondrodysplasia punctata). Tests assessing other aspects of peroxisomal function (eg, plasmalogens, phytanic acid, or pipecolic acid measurements) may be necessary. Most of these analyses are done on plasma obtained from EDTA blood. The red blood cell pellet of the sample should also be sent to the laboratory (separated) because plasmalogen levels are evaluated in red blood cells. Samples do not need to be frozen.

9. **Transferrin electrophoresis analysis.** A suspected diagnosis of carbohydrate-deficient glycoprotein syndromes (see Section VI, C, 9) is first evaluated by electrophoresis analysis of a glycoprotein, usually transferrin. The measurement of transferrin levels is inappropriate as a diagnostic test for these conditions (levels usually normal). Involvement of a geneticist is essential as electrophoresis patterns are not abnormal in all patients and further specialized testing may be indicated.

10. **Muscle, liver, and skin biopsies.** In patients with lactic acidosis, **skeletal muscle biopsies** may be needed to establish diagnosis of a mitochondrial respiratory chain defect. Examination by electron microscopy, special stains, and enzyme essays may also be needed. Certain IEM may require determination of enzyme activities in

cultured skin fibroblasts. Glycogen storage disorders may require **liver biopsies** to establish the exact diagnosis.

11. **DNA analysis and sequencing.** Molecular defects are now known for many genetic conditions, including IEMs. Although diagnoses can usually be established through biochemical testing, analysis of **genomic or mitochondrial DNA** may be indicated in certain scenarios. Considering the complexity of these tests and the associated cost, DNA testing should usually be initiated and supervised by a geneticist. The discussion of specifics is beyond the scope of this manual.

D. **Postmortem evaluation when an IEM is suspected.** If an IEM is suspected as a possible cause of death in a newborn or young infant, we recommend obtaining the following samples postmortem:

1. **Blood.** Blood should be collected. If no central access was established, a postmortem cardiac puncture may be necessary to obtain a sufficient volume of blood. Serum as well as plasma should be frozen. Also, keep the red blood cell pellets (not frozen). EDTA blood (nonseparated) and blood spots on filter paper should be kept to allow for later isolation of DNA.

2. **Urine.** Collect urine, if possible, and freeze it at –20°C. If no urine could be obtained but urine organic acid analysis is indicated, swabs of the bladder surface can be obtained on autopsy to attempt urine organic acid analysis.

3. **Skin.** A full-thickness sterile skin biopsy should be obtained (skin to be cleansed with alcohol, not iodine). Store in a sterile culture medium (if not available, serum from the patient may be used). Do not freeze the specimen, and transport it immediately to a tissue culture laboratory for fibroblast culture and storage.

4. **CSF.** If a lumbar puncture was not performed before death, a lumbar or ventricular puncture can be obtained postmortem. This procedure may be indicated to rule out infection or an IEM. In addition to obtaining cultures, we recommend freezing a 1- to 2-mL CSF specimen at –20°C.

5. **A percutaneous liver biopsy** may be performed to obtain a specimen soon after death (freeze for enzyme analysis) or if the family did not consent to a full autopsy.

6. **A full autopsy and consultation with a geneticist** (even postmortem) may be helpful if an IEM is suspected. The geneticist may give special recommendations for postmortem specimens to be obtained on autopsy (eg, frozen or specially prepared samples rather than standard formalin processing). Genetic counseling may be indicated.

XIII. **Management.** For most IEMs, therapy is currently restricted to dietary measures and in some cases special medications and vitamin supplementation. In some metabolic disorders, **liver, bone marrow, or stem cell transplantation** may be an option.

A. **Acute care while awaiting results of diagnostic studies**

1. **Supportive care** following the standards of neonatal and intensive care includes securing an **airway,** supporting **respiration** and **circulation,** and establishing **intravenous access.** General measures may also include correction of the acid-base balance, electrolyte abnormalities, and **hydration** status. Assisted ventilation may be required in severely affected neonates, and aggressive **antibiotic therapy** is frequently indicated because of the overlap in symptomatology with bacterial disease.

2. **Nutritional measures.** An acutely ill newborn will receive nothing by mouth. For almost all IEMs, a **supply of sufficient glucose** to avoid a catabolic state is strongly indicated. Try to achieve a caloric intake of 80–100 kcal/kg/day. **Eliminate protein** acutely (24–48 h) but not over prolonged periods because breakdown of endogenous protein may otherwise occur and may worsen the patient's clinical status. **Intravenous lipids may be contraindicated** in certain FAO defects.

3. **Hemodialysis or peritoneal dialysis** may be needed to remove toxic metabolites and in cases in which acidosis is intractable. Exchange transfusions are not effective, and early transfer to a facility where hemodialysis is possible is mandatory in these situations (eg, hyperammonemia).

4. **Vitamin treatment.** Several IEMs have vitamin-responsive forms. Often, a combination of vitamin cofactors (vitamin B_{12}, biotin, riboflavin, thiamine, pyridoxine, and folate) is considered while specific test results are still outstanding. Give vitamins only after appropriate specimens have been obtained for full metabolic investigation and after consultation with a geneticist. **Carnitine substitution** may be indicated in some patients (eg, FAO defects or OAs). Carnitine (L-carnitine) may be given intravenously (IV) (30–50 mg/kg/day, some recommend to give a loading dose followed by divided doses; some patients may need higher doses) or carnitine orally (usually at higher doses than IV).

5. **Medications to treat hyperammonemia.** In patients with hyperammonemia, several medications can be used to provide an alternative pathway for ammonia excretion. These include **sodium phenylacetate, sodium phenylbutyrate,** and **sodium benzoate.** A sodium phenylacetate/sodium benzoate 10%/10% preparation is commercially available in the United States. Because of the intrinsic side effects, different indications, coordination with nutritional interventions, and frequent dosage adjustments necessary, the use of these medications should be initiated and supervised by an experienced biochemical geneticist.

6. **Other medications.** In tyrosinemia, NTBC (2-[2-nitro-4-trifluoromethylbenzoyl]-1,3-cyclohexanedione) may be used to prevent tyrosine degradation and production of succinylacetone.

B. **Long-term therapy**

1. **Diet.** One of the classic principles for the treatment of IEMs is the restriction of the substance leading to the accumulation of a toxic metabolite (eg, phenylalanine in PKU). In some disorders (eg, urea cycle defects), the overall protein intake is restricted. Careful monitoring is necessary to avoid essential amino acid deficiencies.

2. **Provision of a deficient substance.** This is effective when the deficient product is readily available and can reach the appropriate tissue (eg, cortisol and mineralocorticoid in 21-hydroxylase deficiency). Carnitine replacement may be needed in organic acidurias because carnitine is lost through renal excretion of metabolites bound to carnitine. Patients with urea cycle defects (with the exception of arginase deficiency) require arginine (and/or citrulline in some defects) replacement due to decreased synthesis.

3. **Vitamin, cofactor, and other disease-specific therapy.** Large doses of specific cofactors may increase the activity of partially deficient enzymes: vitamin B_6 (homocystinuria), vitamin B_{12} (methylmalonic acidemia), biotin (multiple carboxylase deficiency), thiamine (MSUD), and riboflavin (glutaric acidemia II). A subgroup of patients with **PKU** may respond to commercially available **sapropterin dihydrochloride** with a reduction of phenylalanine levels. For a number of lysosomal storage disorders, **enzyme replacement** therapies are either commercially available or under clinical investigation.

4. **Supportive therapy** may help to reduce the morbidity associated with specific IEMs. **Splinting** may reduce deformities in mucopolysaccharidoses. **Splenectomy** may be indicated for thrombocytopenia associated with Gaucher disease.

5. **Long-term therapy.** Genetic disorders require lifelong nutritional, medical, and laboratory monitoring by a team of specialists in these disorders. Many times, intercurrent illnesses and stress may precipitate the recurrence of symptoms.

6. **Early intervention and special education programs** may be beneficial in those disorders characterized by intellectual impairment. Families may find a forum for their concerns and stresses and resources for valuable information in **family support groups** such as the Genetic Alliance (www.geneticalliance.org), the National Organization for Rare Disorders (NORD; www.rarediseases.org), and numerous other disease- and syndrome-specific support groups.

7. As mentioned, liver, bone marrow, or stem cell transplantation may be a treatment option in some IEMs.

Table 93–5. USEFUL RESOURCES FOR THE CLINICIAN IN THE EVALUATION, DIAGNOSIS, AND TREATMENT OF NEWBORNS WITH INBORN ERRORS OF METABOLISM.

- Genetics Home Reference (ghr.nlm.nih.gov) maintained by the National Library of Medicine of the United States.
- Gene Clinics (www.geneclinics.org), a publicly funded database maintained by the University of Washington in Seattle.
- Multiple databases at the National Center for Biotechnology Information (NCBI) (www.ncbi.nlm.org), which includes Online Mendelian Inheritance of Man (OMIM).
- Laboratory resources:
  1. GeneTests database (http://www.genetests.org), a helpful resource to localize a laboratory for a specific genetic test. This is a publicly funded database maintained through the University of Washington.
  2. The American Association for Clinical Chemistry publishes DORA (The Directory of Rare Analyses).
  3. Published test catalogs or websites of major regional referral laboratories are often also helpful resources.

XIV. **Prognosis.** Due to the great variety of inborn errors of metabolism, prognosis ranges from extremely favorable with normal development and life expectancy to severe physical and/or mental disability and death. In general, early diagnosis and, if available, treatment seem associated with more favorable outcomes.

XV. **Additional resources.** In order to assist the clinician with the care of newborns with inborn errors of metabolism, Table 93–5 provides a listing of useful resources for the clinician.

Selected References

Antoun H et al: Cerebellar atrophy: an important feature of carbohydrate deficient glycoprotein syndrome type 1. *Pediatr Radiol* 1999;29:194.

Baumgartner MR, Saudubray JM: Peroxisomal disorders. *Sem Neonatol* 2002;7:85-94.

Blau N et al: *Physicians Guide to the Treatment and Follow-up of Metabolic Diseases.* Berlin: Springer, 2005.

Bosch AM: Classical galactosemia revisited. *J Inherit Metabol Dis* 2006;29:516-525.

Burin MG et al: Investigation of lysosomal storage diseases in nonimmune hydrops fetalis. *Prenat Diagn* 2004;24:653-657.

Burton BK: Inborn errors of metabolism in infancy: a guide to diagnosis. *Pediatrics* 1998;102:E69.

Carpenter KH, Wiley V: Application of tandem mass spectrometry to biochemical genetics and newborn screening. *Clin Chim Acta* 2002;322:1.

Christodoulou J, Wilcken B: Perimortem laboratory investigation of genetic metabolic disorders. *Semin Neonatol* 2004;9:275-280.

Clarke JTR: *A Clinical Guide to Inherited Metabolic Diseases,* 3rd ed. Cambridge, UK: Cambridge University Press, 2006.

Clayton PT: Inborn errors presenting with liver dysfunction. *Semin Neonatol* 2002;7:49-63.

Clayton PT et al: Hypertrophic obstructive cardiomyopathy in a neonate with the carbohydrate-deficient glycoprotein syndrome. *J Inherit Met Dis* 1992;15:857.

Coman DJ et al: Enzyme replacement therapy for mucopolysaccharidoses: opinions of patients and families. *J Pediatr* 2008;152:723-727.

Cowan TM: Neonatal screening by tandem mass spectrometry. *NeoReviews* 2005;6:e539-e548.

Dagli AI et al: Testing strategies for inborn errors of metabolism in the neonate. *NeoReviews* 2008;9:e291-e298.

de Koning TJ et al: Recurrent nonimmune hydrops fetalis associated with carbohydrate-deficient glycoprotein syndrome. *J Inherit Metab Dis* 1998;21:681.

Enns GM: Inborn errors of metabolism masquerading as hypoxic-ischemic encephalopathy. *NeoReviews* 2005;6:e549-e558.

Enns GM, Packman S: Diagnosing inborn errors of metabolism in the newborn: clinical features. *NeoReviews* 2001;2:183-191.

Enns GM, Packman S: Diagnosing inborn errors of metabolism in the newborn: laboratory investigations. *NeoReviews* 2001;2:192-200.

Fernandes J et al: *Inborn Metabolic Diseases: Diagnosis and Treatment*, 4th ed. Heidelberg, Germany: Springer, 2006.

Garganta CL, Smith WE: Metabolic evaluation of the sick neonate. *Semin Perinatol* 2005:29:164-172.

Gehrmann J et al: Cardiomyopathy in congenital disorders of glycosylation. *Cardiol Young* 2003;13:345-351.

Hellström-Westas L et al: *An Atlas of Amplitude-Integrated EEGs in the Newborn*, 2nd ed. London, UK: Informa Healthcare, 2008.

Hicks JM, Young DS: *DORA 2005–2007. The Directory of Rare Analyses.* American Washington, DC: Association for Clinical Chemists, 2005.

Hoffmann et al: *Inherited Metabolic Diseases.* Philadelphia: Lippincott Williams and Wilkins, 2002.

Hudak ML et al: Differentiation of transient hyperammonemia of the newborn and urea cycle enzyme defects by clinical presentation. *J Pediatr* 1985;107:712.

Jaeken J, Matthijs G: Congenital disorders of glycosylation: a rapidly expanding disease family. *Annu Rev Genomics Hum Genet* 2007;8:261-287.

Kahler SG: Metabolic disorders associated with neonatal hypoglycemia. *NeoReviews* 2004; 5:e377-e381.

Kaye C; Committee on Genetics: Introduction to the newborn screening fact sheets. *Pediatrics* 2006;118:1304-1312.

Kooper AJA et al: Lysosomal storage diseases in non-immune hydrops fetalis pregnancies. *Clinica Chimica Acta* 2006;371:176-182.

Leonard JV, Morris AAM: Urea cycle disorders. *Semin Neonatol* 2002;7:27-35.

Leonard JV, Morris AAM: Diagnosis and early management of inborn errors of metabolism presenting around the time of birth. *Acta Paediatrica* 2006;95:6-14.

Malklova E, Albahari ZA: Screening and diagnosis of congenital disorders of glycosylation. *Clin Chim Acta* 2007;385:6-20.

Marsden D et al: Newborn screening for metabolic disorders. *J Pediatr* 2006;148:577-584.

National Organization for Rare Disorders (NORD): *NORD Resource Guide,* 5th ed. Danbury, CT: NORD, 2005.

Nyhan WL et al: *Atlas of Metabolic Diseases,* 2nd ed. London, UK: Hodder Arnold, 2005.

Ogier de Baulny H: Management and emergency treatment of neonates with suspicion on inborn errors of metabolism. *Semin Neonatol* 2002;7:17-26.

Ogier de Baulny H et al: Methylmalonic and propionic acidemias: management and outcomes. *J Inherit Metal Dis* 2005;28:415-423.

Ogier de Baulny H, Saudubray JM: Branched chain organic acidurias. *Semin Neonatol* 2002;7:65-74.

Pasquali M et al: Biochemical findings in common inborn errors of metabolism. *Am J Med Genet (Part C)* 2006;142C:64-76.

Porter FD: Smith-Lemli-Opitz syndrome: pathogenesis, diagnosis and management. *Eur J Hum Genet* 2008;16(5):535-451.

Prasad VK, Kurtzberg J: Emerging trends in transplantation of inherited diseases. *Bone Marrow Transplantation* 2008;41:99-108.

Raghuveer TS et al: Inborn errors of metabolism in infancy and early childhood: an update. *Am Fam Physician* 2006;73:1981-1990.

Rinaldo P, Matern D: Disorders of fatty acid transport and mitochondrial oxidation: challenges and dilemmas of metabolic evaluation. *Genet Med* 2000;2:338.

Roe CR: Inherited disorders of mitochondrial fatty acid oxidation: a new responsibility for the neonatologist. *Semin Neonatol* 2002;7:37-47.

Saudubray JM et al: Clinical approach to inherited metabolic disorders in neonates: an overview. *Semin Neonatol* 2002;7:3-15.

Saudubray JM et al: Clinical approach to treatable inborn metabolic diseases: an introduction. *J Inherit Metab Dis* 2006;29:261-274.

Seashore MR, Seashore CJ: Newborn screening and the pediatric practitioner. *Sem Perinatol* 2005;29:182-188.

Servidei S et al: Hereditary metabolic cardiomyopathies. *Adv Pediatr* 1994;41:1.

Shimozawa N: Molecular and clinical aspects of peroxisomal diseases. *J Inherit Metab Dis* 2007;30:193-197.

Stone DL, Sidransky E: Hydrops fetalis: lysosomal storage disorder in extremis. *Adv Pediatr* 1999;46:409-440.

Valle D et al: The online metabolic and molecular bases of inherited disease. New York, NY: McGraw-Hill. Available at: www.ommbid.com.

van der Knaap WS et al: Congenital nephrotic syndrome: a novel phenotype of type I carbohydrate-deficient glycoprotein syndrome. *J Inherit Met Dis*1996;19:787.

Wilcken CJE, Christodoulou J: Neonatology for the generalist. Clinical approach to inborn errors of metabolism presenting in the newborn period. *J Paediatr Child Health* 2002;38:511-517.

Wraith JE: Lysosomal disorders. *Semin Neonatol* 2002;7:75-83.

Yu H, Patel SB: Recent insights into the Smith-Lemli-Opitz syndrome. *Clin Genet* 2005:68:383-391.

94 Infant of a Diabetic Mother

Maternal diabetic control is a key factor in determining fetal outcome. Data indicate that perinatal morbidity and mortality rates in the offspring of women with diabetes mellitus have improved with dietary management and insulin therapy. The use of oral hypoglycemic agents is *controversial*, and there is some concern about worse maternal and neonatal outcomes as compared to treatment with insulin. However, complications may still arise in the infant, including hypoglycemia, hypocalcemia, hypomagnesemia, perinatal asphyxia, respiratory distress syndrome (RDS), other respiratory illnesses, hypertrophic cardiomyopathy, hyperbilirubinemia, polycythemia, renal vein thrombosis, macrosomia, birth injuries, and congenital malformations. Because of a better current understanding of the pathophysiology of diabetic pregnancies, these complications can be recognized and treated.

I. Definition

A. White's classification. White's classification system is based on the age at onset, duration of the disorder, and complications and is predictive of perinatal mortality. It is currently used to group women with diabetes during pregnancy and provide a

Table 94–1. **WHITE'S MODIFIED CLASSIFICATION OF DIABETES IN PREGNANCY**

White's Class	Description
Gestational diabetes A1	Diet-controlled gestational diabetes**(fasting glucose < 105 mg/dL 2 h postprandial glucose < 120 mg/dL)
Gestational diabetes A2	Insulin-treated gestational diabetes** (fasting glucose > 105 mg/dL 2 h postprandial glucose > 120 mg/dL)
A	Abnormal GTT at any age or of any duration; treated only by diet therapy
B	Onset at age ≥ 20 y and duration <10 y
C	Onset at age 10–19 y or duration of 10–19 y
D	Onset before 10 y of age, duration > 20 y, benign retinopathy, or hypertension (not pregnancy induced)
D1	Onset before age 10 y
D2	Duration > 20 y
D3	Calcification of vessels of the leg (macrovascular disease), formerly called Class E
D4	Benign retinopathy (microvascular disease)
D5	Hypertension (not pregnancy induced)
R	Proliferative retinopathy or vitreous hemorrhage
F	Nephropathy with > 500 mg/d proteinuria
RF	Criteria for both classes R and F
G	Many pregnancy failures
H	Evidence of arteriosclerotic heart disease
T	Prior renal transplantation

**Any degree of glucose intolerance with onset or first recognition during pregnancy.
Classes B through T require insulin treatment. Class R,F,RF,H,T have no onset or duration criterion, but usually occur with long standing diabetes.
Modified from Brown FM, Hare JW: *Diabetes Complicating Pregnancy: The Joslin Clinic Method.* 2nd ed. New York:Wiley-Liss, 1995.

method to compare groups of infants. The original table was produced in 1949 and was most recently revised in the 1980's (see Revised White's Classification, Table 94–1). A major change was placing gestational diabetes in its own category. Newer classifications have been suggested but none are widely adopted.

B. **The Expert Committee on the Diagnosis and Classification of Diabetes Mellitus.** Table 94–2 presents the nomenclature of the Expert Committee on the Diagnosis and Classification of Diabetes Mellitus (American Diabetes Association, Alexandria, VA). This classification defines the illness based on the etiology of the disease. It discourages the use of terms such as insulin-dependent diabetes (IDDM) and the use of roman numerals type I and type II. Preferred terms are Type 1 diabetes mellitus, Type 2 diabetes mellitus, other types, and gestational diabetes mellitus. It is important to note that any type of diabetes can progress through clinical phases of being normoglycemic to hyperglycemic, being asymptomatic and symptomatic during their clinical history.

II. **Incidence.** It is estimated that 3–10% of all pregnancies are complicated by diabetes, and 90% of these are women with gestational diabetes. Women with a family history of type 2 diabetes mellitus, Asian, Native American, Middle eastern, African and Hispanic women, or obesity are at higher risk.

III. **Pathophysiology**

A. **Macrosomia.** Macrosomia is the classic presentation of the infant of a poorly controlled diabetic mother (IDM). It is the result of biochemical events along the maternal hyperglycemia-fetal hyperinsulinemia pathway, as described by Pedersen.

Table 94–2. NOMENCLATURE OF THE EXPERT COMMITTEE ON THE DIAGNOSIS AND
CLASSIFICATION OF DIABETES MELLITUS

Class	Description
I. Type 1 diabetes	Beta cell destruction usually leading to absolute insulin deficiency (immune or idopathic).
II. Type 2 diabetes	May range from predominantly insulin resistance with relative insulin deficiency to a predominantly secretory defect with insulin resistance.
III. Other specific types	Genetic defects of beta cell function, genetic defects in insulin action, diseases of exocrine pancreas, endocrinopathies, drug or chemical induced, infections, uncommon forms of immune mediated diabetes, other genetic syndromes sometimes acssociated with diabetes.
IV. Gestational diabetes mellitus	Any degree of glucose intolerance with onset or first recognition during pregnancy. A fasting plasma glucose of > 126 mg/dL (7.0 mmol/L) or a casual glucose > 200 mg/dL (11.1 mmol/L) meets the minimal criteria for the diagnosis of gestational diabetes. If the diagnosis is not clear, repeat on a subsequent day. If hyperglycemia is confirmed, no further testing needed. If the diagnosis is unclear, perform a 1 or 2 step oral glucose tolerance test.

Based on data from Diagnosis and Classification of Diabetes Mellitus. *Diabetes Care* 2002; 229: S43-S48.

Macrosomia occurs in 15–45% of diabetic pregnancies and plays a role in both birth injuries, including shoulder dystocia, brachial plexus injuries, subdural hemorrhage, cephalohematoma, and the increased rate of asphyxia seen in infants of diabetic mothers. Hispanic diabetic women have higher rates of macrosomia than other ethnic groups.

B. **Small for gestational age.** Mothers with renal, retinal, or cardiac diseases are more likely to have small for gestational age or premature infants, poor fetal outcome, fetal distress, or fetal death.

C. **Specific disorders frequently encountered in IDMs**

1. **Metabolic disorders**

a. **Hypoglycemia** is often defined as a blood glucose level <45mg/dL in a preterm or term infant. However this is a very *controversial* issue. Today many institutions have defined it as <45–50 mg/dL (some use <60mg/dL) in the first 24 h and < 50–60mg/dL thereafter. **It is best to follow your institution's guidelines.** Hypoglycemia is present in up to 40% of IDMs, most commonly in macrosomic infants. It usually presents within 1–2 h after delivery. According to Pedersen, at birth the transplacental glucose supply is terminated, and, because of high concentrations of plasma insulin, blood glucose levels fall. Mothers with well-controlled blood glucose levels have fewer infants with hypoglycemia. Hypoglycemia in small for gestational age infants born to mothers with diabetic vascular disease is caused by decreased glycogen stores; it appears 6–12 h after delivery.

b. **Hypocalcemia.** Hypocalcemia has various definitions, but **serum levels <7 mg/dL in an asymptomatic term infant and <8 mg/dL in a symptomatic term infant. Ionized calcium levels of less than 4 mg/dl are considered hypocalcemic.** The incidence is up to 50% of IDMs. The severity of hypocalcemia is related to the severity of maternal diabetes and involves decreased function of the parathyroid glands. Serum calcium levels are lowest at 24–72 h of age.

c. **Hypomagnesemia.** A serum magnesium level <1.6 mg/dL in any infant indicates hypomagnesemia. It is related to maternal hypomagnesemia and the severity of maternal diabetes.

2. **Cardiorespiratory disorders**
   a. **Perinatal asphyxia.** In a prospective study, 27% of infants of diabetic mothers, White class B-R-T, suffered asphyxia. Nephropathy appearing in pregnancy, maternal hyperglycemia before delivery, and prematurity were significant risk factors.
   b. **Hyaline membrane disease or RDS**
      i. **Incidence.** The incidence has decreased to only 3% of IDMs because of better management of diabetes during pregnancy. Most cases are the result of premature delivery, delayed maturation of pulmonary surfactant production, or delivery by elective cesarean.
      ii. **Fetal lung maturity.** Pulmonary surfactant production in the IDM is deficient or delayed principally in class A, B, and C diabetics. Fetal hyperinsulinism may adversely affect the lung maturation process in the IDM by interfering with the incorporation of choline into lecithin.
      iii. **Cesarean delivery.** Infants delivered by elective cesarean are at risk for RDS because of lack of appropriate surfactant production and decreased prostaglandin production and increased pulmonary vascular resistance.
   c. **Other causes of respiratory distress**
      i. **Transient tachypnea of the newborn** occurs especially after elective cesarean delivery. This disorder may or may not require oxygen therapy and usually responds by 72 h of age. (See Chapter 128)
      ii. **Hypertrophic cardiomyopathy** is the result of increased fat and glycogen deposition in the myocardium and may lead to congestive heart failure. Its incidence varies widely and has been reported as high as 43% in IDMs. One study performed routine echocardiographic scan and found hypertropic myopathy is 30% of IDMs. Symptomatic hypertrophic cardiomyopathy occurs in approximately 12% of IDMs.
3. **Hematologic disorders**
   a. **Hyperbilirubinemia.** Bilirubin production is apparently increased in the IDM secondary to prematurity, macrosomia, hypoglycemia, polycythemia, and delayed clearance.
   b. **Polycythemia and hyperviscosity.** The cause of polycythemia is unclear but may be related to increased levels of erythropoietin in the IDM, increased red blood cell production secondary to chronic intrauterine hypoxia in mothers with vascular disease, and intrauterine placental transfusion resulting from acute hypoxia during labor and delivery.
   c. **Renal venous thrombosis** is a rare complication most likely caused by hyperviscosity, hypotension, or disseminated intravascular coagulation. It is usually diagnosed by ultrasonography and may present with hematuria and an abdominal mass.
4. **Congenital malformations** occur more frequently in infants born to diabetic mothers than in the general population. It is suspected that poor diabetic control in the first trimester is associated with a higher percentage of congenital malformations. Congenital malformations account for a significant portion of perinatal deaths and include cardiac defects (eg, transposition of the great vessels, ventricular septal defect, or atrial septal defect), renal defects (eg, agenesis), gastrointestinal tract defects (eg, small left colon syndrome or situs inversus), neurologic defects (eg, anencephaly or meningocele syndrome), skeletal defects (eg, hemivertebrae or caudal regression syndrome), unusual facies, and microphthalmos.
IV. **Risk factors.** The following factors or conditions may be associated with an increased risk for problems in IDMs:
   A. **Maternal class of diabetes.** Historic studies have correlated the degree of glucose control with perinatal mortality. Historical data also correlates White's classification with increased mortality (ie, Class A 5 % mortality vs. Class C and D 18% mortality).

1. **Women with gestational diabetes, class A B, C diabetes (without vascular or renal disease)** are prone to deliver macrosomic infants. Poor feeding occurs in many of these infants (Class B–D and higher in Class F).

2. **Diabetic women with renal, retinal, cardiac, and vascular disease** have the most severe fetal problems.

B. **Hemoglobin A_{1C}.** To decrease perinatal morbidity and mortality rates, the diabetic woman should attempt to achieve good metabolic control before conception. Elevated hemoglobin A_{1C} levels during the first trimester appear to be associated with a higher incidence of congenital malformations.

C. **Diabetic ketoacidosis.** Pregnant women with insulin-dependent diabetes are apt to develop diabetic ketoacidosis. The onset of this complication may be life threatening for the mother and fetus or may lead to preterm delivery.

D. **Preterm labor.** Premature onset of labor in a diabetic woman is a serious problem because of the increased likelihood of RDS in the fetus. Furthermore, sympathomimetic agents used to prevent preterm delivery may be associated with maternal hyperglycemia, hyperinsulinemia, and acidosis.

E. **Immature fetal lung profile.** Diabetic women who present between 36 and 39 weeks' gestation may undergo amniocentesis to evaluate fetal lung maturity. A mature lecithin-to-sphingomyelin ratio may not ensure normal respiratory function in the IDM. However, the presence of phosphatidylglycerol in the amniotic fluid is more apt to be associated with normal neonatal respiratory function (see also Chapter 1).

V. **Clinical presentation**

A. **At birth,** the infant may be large for gestational age or, if the mother has vascular disease, small for gestational age. The size of most infants is appropriate for gestational age; however, if macrosomia is present, birth trauma may occur.

B. **After birth,** hypoglycemia can present as lethargy, poor feeding, apnea, or jitteriness in the first 6–12 h after birth. Jitteriness that occurs after 24 h of age may be the result of hypocalcemia or hypomagnesemia. Signs of respiratory distress secondary to immature lungs can be noted on examination. Cardiac disease may be present as an enlarged cardiothymic shadow on a chest radiograph or by physical evidence of heart failure. Gross congenital anomalies may be noted on physical examination.

VI. **Diagnosis**

A. **Laboratory studies.** The following tests must be closely monitored in the IDM:

1. **Serum glucose levels** should be checked at delivery and at 1/2, 1, 1 and 1/2, 2, 4, 8, 12, 24, 36, and 48 h of age. Glucose levels should be checked with bedside measurement tools. Readings <40 mg/dL at the bedside should be verified by serum glucose measurements.

2. **Serum calcium levels** should be obtained at 6, 24, and 48 h of age. If serum calcium levels are low, serum magnesium levels should be obtained because they may also be low.

3. **The hematocrit** should be checked at birth and at 4 and 24 h of age.

4. **Serum bilirubin levels** should be checked as indicated by physical examination.

5. **Other tests.** Arterial blood gas levels, complete blood cell counts, cultures, and Gram stains should be obtained as clinically indicated.

B. **Radiologic studies** are not necessary unless there is evidence of cardiac, respiratory, or skeletal problems.

C. **Electrocardiography and echocardiography** should be performed if hypertrophic cardiomyopathy or a cardiac malformation is suspected.

VII. **Management**

A. **Initial evaluation.** Upon delivery, the infant should be evaluated in the usual manner. In the transitional nursery, blood glucose levels and the hematocrit should be obtained. The infant should be observed for jitteriness, tremors, convulsions, apnea, weak cry, and poor sucking. A physical examination should be performed, paying particular attention to the heart, kidneys, lungs, and extremities.

B. **Continuing evaluation.** Over the first several hours after delivery, the infant should be assessed for signs of respiratory distress. During the first 48 h, observe for signs of jaundice and for renal, cardiac, neurologic, and gastrointestinal tract abnormalities.

C. **Metabolic management**
   1. **Hypoglycemia.** See Chapter 55.
   2. **Hypocalcemia.** See Chapter 78.
      a. **Calcium therapy.** Symptomatic infants should receive 10% calcium gluconate IV. The infusion should be given slowly to prevent cardiac arrhythmias, and should be monitored for signs of extravasation. After the initial dose, maintenance is by continuous IV infusion. The hypocalcemia should respond in 3–4 days; until then, serum calcium levels should be monitored every 12 h.
      b. **Magnesium maintenance therapy.** Magnesium is usually added to IV fluids or given orally as magnesium sulfate 50%, 0.2 mL/kg/day (4 mEq/mL). (See Chapter 99.)

D. **Management of cardiorespiratory problems**
   1. **Perinatal asphyxia.** Close observation for fetal distress should continue. (See Chapter 110.)
   2. **Hyaline membrane disease.** Obtaining amniotic fluid for a fetal lung maturity profile is still an option and can decrease the incidence of hyaline membrane disease. However, some infants must be delivered even if the lung profile is immature.
   3. **Cardiomyopathy.** The treatment of choice is with propranolol (for dosage information, see Chapter 132). Digoxin is contraindicated because of possible ventricular outflow obstruction.

E. **Hematologic therapy**
   1. **Hyperbilirubinemia.** Frequent monitoring of serum bilirubin levels may be necessary. Phototherapy and exchange transfusion for infants with hyperbilirubinemia are discussed in Chapters 51 and 92.
   2. **Polycythemia.** See Chapters 64 and 112.
   3. **Renal venous thrombosis.** Treatment consists of fluid restriction and close monitoring of electrolytes and renal status. Supportive therapy is indicated to ensure adequate blood circulation. Nephrectomy is usually only a last resort in unilateral disease. (See Chapter 72.)

F. **Management of morphologic and functional problems**
   1. **Macrosomia and birth injury**
      a. **Fractures of the extremities** should be treated with immobilization.
      b. **Erb palsy** can be treated with range-of-motion exercises.
   2. **Congenital malformations.** If a gross malformation is discovered, a specialist should be consulted.

VIII. **Prognosis.** Less morbidity and mortality occur with adequate control during the diabetic pregnancy. Preconceptual counseling is used as an adjunct to preventive health care of the diabetic patient. The known pregnant diabetic is currently receiving better health care than before, but the challenge is early identification of women with biochemical abnormalities of gestational diabetes. The risk of subsequent diabetes in the infants of these women is (risk of type 1 around 1%, type 2 50%, risk of GDM 35%. The risk of cerebral palsy and epilepsy is 3 to 5 times higher in these infants. Evidence suggests an increased incidence of obesity and metabolic syndrome during childhood. If diabetes is poorly controlled during pregnancy, a higher risk of neurodevelopmental deficits is reported as the child grows.

Selected References

Cheng YW, Caughey AB: Gestational diabetes: diagnosis and management. *J Perinatol* 2008;28:657-664.

Chmait R, Moore T: Endocrine disorders in pregnancy. In Taeusch HW et al (eds): *Avery's Diseases of the Newborn.* Philadelphia, PA: Elsevier Saunders, 2005:71-86.

Cowett RM: The infant of the diabetic mother. *NeoReviews* 2002;3(9):173-189.

Csaba IF et al: Relationship of maternal treatment with indomethacin to persistence of fetal circulation syndrome. *J Pediatr* 1978;92(3):484.

Expert Committee on the Diagnosis and Classification of Diabetes Mellitus: Report. *Diabetes Care* 2003;26:S5-S20.

Diagnosis and Classification of Diabetes Mellitus: Report. *Diabetes Care* 2006;29:S43-S48.

Frantz ID, Epstein MF: Fetal lung development in pregnancies complicated by diabetes. *Semin Perinatol* 1978;2(4):347-352.

Key TC et al: Predictive value of early pregnancy glycohemoglobin in the insulin-treated diabetic patient. *Am J Obstet Gynecol* 1987;156(5):1096-1100.

Landon MB et al: Diabetes mellitus complicating pregnancy. In Gabbe SG et al (eds): *Obstetrics: Normal and Problem Pregnancies.* Philadelphia, PA: Churchill Livingstone, 2007.

Mimouni F et al: Perinatal asphyxia in infants of insulin-dependent diabetic mothers. *J Pediatr* 1988;113(2):345-353.

Rosenn B, Tsang RC: The effects of maternal diabetes on the fetus and neonate. *Ann Clin Lab Sci* 1991;21(3):153-170.

Schaefer UM et al: Congenital malformations in offspring of women with hyperglycemia first detected during pregnancy. *Am J Obstet Gynecol* 1997;177(5):1165-1171.

Smith BT et al: Insulin antagonism of cortisol action on lecithin synthesis by cultured fetal lung cells. *J Pediatr* 1975;87(6 Pt 1):953-955.

Stephenson MJ: Screening for gestational diabetes mellitus: a critical review. *J Fam Pract* 1993;37(3):277-283.

Tsang RC et al: Diabetes and calcium disturbances in infants of diabetic mothers. In Merkatz IR, Adam P (eds): *The Diabetic Pregnancy. A Perinatal Perspective.* New York, NY: Grune and Stratton, 1979:207-225.

Way GL et al: The natural history of hypertrophic cardiomyopathy in infants of diabetic mothers. *J Pediatr* 1979;95(6):1020-1025.

White P: Diabetes mellitus in pregnancy. *Clin Perinatol* 1974;1(2):331-347.

95 Infant of a Drug-Abusing Mother

Existing studies on the neonatal effects of drug exposure in utero are subject to many confounding factors. Many studies have relied on the history obtained from the mother, which is notoriously inaccurate. In addition to recall bias, there is a considerable incentive to withhold information. Testing of urine for drugs of abuse does not reflect drug exposure throughout pregnancy and does not provide quantitative information. Many women who abuse drugs are multiple drug abusers and also drink alcohol and smoke cigarettes. It is thus difficult to isolate the effects of any one drug. Social and economic deprivation is common among drug abusers, and this factor not only confounds perinatal data but has a major effect on long-term studies of infant outcome.

I. **Definition.** An infant of a drug-abusing mother (IDAM) is one whose mother has taken drugs that may potentially cause neonatal withdrawal symptoms. The constellation of signs and symptoms associated with withdrawal is called the neonatal withdrawal syndrome. Table 95–1 lists the drugs associated with this syndrome.

Table 95–1. **DRUGS CAUSING NEONATAL WITHDRAWAL SYNDROME**

Opiates	Barbiturates	Miscellaneous
Codeine	Butalbital	Alcohol
Heroin	Phenobarbital	Amphetamine
Meperidine	Secobarbital	Chlordiazepoxide
Methadone		Clomipramine
Morphine		Cocaine
Pentazocine		Desmethylimipramine
Propoxyphene		Diazepam
		Diphenhydramine
		Ethchlorvynol
		Fluphenazine
		Glutethimide
		Hydroxyzine
		Imipramine
		Meprobamate
		Phencyclidine
		Selective serotonin reuptake inhibitors (SSRIs) (especially paroxetine)

II. **Incidence.** Maternal drug abuse has increased over the past decade. It is estimated that ~5–10% of deliveries nationwide are to women who have abused drugs (excluding alcohol) during pregnancy. The incidence is considerably higher in inner-city hospitals.

III. **Pathophysiology.** Drugs of abuse are of low molecular weight and usually water soluble and lipophilic. These features facilitate their transfer across the placenta and accumulation in the fetus and amniotic fluid. The half-life of drugs is usually prolonged in the fetus compared with an adult. Most drugs of abuse either bind to various central nervous system (CNS) receptors or affect the release and reuptake of various neurotransmitters. This may have a long-lasting trophic effect on developing dendritic structures. In addition, some drugs are directly toxic to fetal cells. The developing fetus may also be affected by the direct physiologic effects of a drug. Many of the fetal effects of cocaine, including its putative teratogenic effects, are thought to be due to its potent vasoconstrictive property.

Some drugs appear to have a partially beneficial effect. The incidence of respiratory distress syndrome (RDS) is decreased after maternal use of heroin and possibly also cocaine. These effects are probably a reflection of fetal stress rather than a direct maturational effect of these drugs. Particularly in the case of cocaine, the decreased incidence of RDS is more than offset by the considerable increase in preterm deliveries after its use. The major concern in IDAMs is the long-term outcome. The importance of direct and indirect effects of drugs on the developing CNS predominates, and the risks of drug abuse far outweigh the benefits. Pathophysiology of specific drugs are:

A. **Opiates.** Opiates bind to opiate receptors in the CNS; part of the clinical manifestations of narcotic withdrawal result from α_2-adrenergic super-sensitivity (particularly in the locus ceruleus).

B. **Cocaine.** Cocaine prevents the reuptake of neurotransmitters (epinephrine, norepinephrine, dopamine, and serotonin) at nerve endings and causes a supersensitivity or exaggerated response to neurotransmitters at the effector organs. It also affects the permeability of nerves to sodium ions. Cocaine is a CNS stimulant and a sympathetic activator with potent vasoconstrictive properties. It causes a decrease in uterine and placental blood flow with consequent fetal hypoxemia. It causes hypertension in the mother and the fetus with a reduction in fetal cerebral blood flow.

C. **Alcohol.** Ethanol is an anxiolytic-analgesic with a depressant effect on the CNS. Both ethanol and its metabolite, acetaldehyde, are toxic. Alcohol crosses the placenta and also impairs its function. The risk of affecting the fetus is related to alcohol dose, but there is a continuum of effects and no known safe limit.

IV. **Risk factors.** Associated with an increased incidence of drug abuse are the following:
  A. **Maternal history**
    1. **Poor social and economic circumstances.**
    2. **Poor antenatal care.**
    3. **Teenage or unwed mothers.**
    4. **Poor education.**
    5. **Associated conditions include infectious diseases** (hepatitis B, syphilis, and other sexually transmitted diseases), HIV-positive serology, multiple drug abuse, poor nutritional status, and anemia.
  B. **Obstetric complications**
    1. **Premature delivery.**
    2. **Premature rupture of membranes.**
    3. **Chorioamnionitis.**
    4. **Fetal distress.**
    5. **Intrauterine growth retardation (IUGR).**
    6. **With cocaine use,** the following may be present (in addition to the conditions just mentioned):
      a. **Hypertension.**
      b. **Abruptio placentae.**
      c. **Cardiac.** Arrhythmias, myocardial ischemia, and infarction.
      d. **Cerebrovascular accident.**
      e. **Respiratory arrest.**
      f. **Fetal demise.**

V. **Clinical presentation.** Signs and symptoms of drug withdrawal are listed in Table 95–2. These signs essentially reflect CNS "irritability," altered neurobehavioral organization, and abnormal sympathetic activation. Although each drug may have its own effects, these signs and symptoms must be noted for every IDAM (because of multiple

Table 95–2. SIGNS AND SYMPTOMS OF NEONATAL ABSTINENCE

Hyperirritability
  Increased deep-tendon and primitive reflexes
  Hypertonus, hyperacusis
  Tremors
  High-pitched cry
Seizures
Wakefulness
Increased rooting reflex
Uncoordinated or ineffectual sucking and swallowing
Regurgitation and vomiting
Loose stools and diarrhea
Tachypnea, apnea
Yawning, hiccups
Sneezing, stuffy nose
Mottling
Fever
Failure to gain weight
Lacrimation

drug abuse); conversely, drug abuse should be suspected in infants exhibiting these signs and symptoms. Signs and symptoms for specific drugs are:

A. Opiates. Infants born to opiate-addicted mothers show an increased incidence of IUGR and perinatal distress. Even when these infants are not small for gestational age, they have lower weight and a smaller head circumference compared with drug-free infants.

1. **Signs and symptoms of withdrawal occur in 60–90% of exposed infants.** The onset of symptoms may be minutes after delivery up to 1–2 weeks' of age, but most infants exhibit signs by 2–3 days of life. The onset of withdrawal may be delayed beyond 2 weeks in infants exposed to methadone (parents should be appropriately informed).

2. **The clinical course is variable, ranging from mild symptoms of brief duration to severe symptoms.** The clinical course may be protracted, with exacerbations or recurrence of symptoms after discharge. Restlessness, agitation, tremors, wakefulness, and feeding problems may persist for 3–6 months. A blunted ventilatory response to carbon dioxide has been shown. There is a reduced incidence of both RDS and hyperbilirubinemia.

B. Cocaine

1. **Symptoms seen in neonates exposed to cocaine in utero** are irritability, tremors, hypertonia, a high-pitched cry, hyperreflexia, frantic fist sucking, feeding problems, sneezing, tachypnea, and abnormal sleep patterns. A specific cocaine withdrawal syndrome has not been described. The symptoms just mentioned may be a reflection of cocaine intoxication rather than withdrawal, and after an initial period of irritability and overactivity, a period of lethargy and decreased tone has been described.

2. *Controversial* cocaine associations

   a. **In the neonate, the following have been described:** Necrotizing enterocolitis, transient hypertension, and reduced cardiac output (on the first day of life), intracranial hemorrhages and infarcts, seizures, apneic spells, periodic breathing, abnormal electroencephalogram, abnormal brainstem auditory evoked potentials, abnormal response to hypoxia and carbon dioxide, and ileal perforation. These reports were mostly case reports or insufficiently controlled case series with numerous confounding factors (notably, various other perinatal and gestational risk factors, including multiple drug and alcohol usage). There are large case-control studies that have found no association between cocaine exposure and intraventricular hemorrhage. Despite earlier concerns, there does not appear to be an increased risk of SIDS.

   b. **Cocaine has been suggested as a teratogen.** Its teratogenic potential is presumed to be due to its vascular effects, although direct toxicity on various cell lines may also play a role. Numerous CNS anomalies as well as cardiovascular abnormalities, limb reduction defects, intestinal atresias, and other malformations have been attributed to cocaine. However, most of these associations were derived from case reports, case series, or poorly controlled studies, and a detailed examination of the data does not substantiate most of these teratogenic associations. An exception appears to be an increased risk of genitourinary tract defects associated with cocaine exposure during gestation. Moreover, there does not appear to be a dysmorphism recognizable as a "cocaine syndrome." Cocaine is associated with an increased incidence of spontaneous abortion, stillbirth, abruptio placentae, premature labor, and IUGR.

C. Alcohol is probably the foremost drug of abuse today. **The risk that an alcoholic woman will have a child with fetal alcohol syndrome (FAS) is ~35–40%.** However, even in the absence of FAS, and also with lower alcohol intakes, there is an increased risk of congenital anomalies and impaired intellect. It is estimated that alcohol is the major cause of congenital mental retardation today. **FAS consists of the following:**

1. **Prenatal or postnatal growth retardation, CNS involvement** such as irritability in infancy or hyperactivity in childhood, developmental delay, hypotonia, or intellectual impairment.
2. **Facial dysmorphology.** Microcephaly, microphthalmos, or short palpebral fissures, a poorly developed philtrum, a thin upper lip (vermilion border), and hypoplastic maxilla.

   Numerous congenital anomalies have been described after exposure to alcohol in utero both with and without full-blown FAS. CNS symptoms may appear within 24 h after delivery and include tremors, irritability, hypertonicity, twitching, hyperventilation, hyperacusis, opisthotonos, and seizures. Symptoms may be severe but are usually of short duration. Abdominal distention and vomiting are less frequent than with most other drugs of abuse. In premature infants of women who were heavy alcohol users (>7 drinks/week), there is an increased risk of both intracranial hemorrhage and white matter CNS damage.

D. **Barbiturates.** Symptoms and signs of withdrawal are similar to those observed in narcotic-exposed infants, but symptoms usually appear later. Most infants become symptomatic toward the end of the first week of life, although onset may be delayed up to 2 weeks. The duration of symptoms is usually 2–6 weeks.

E. **Benzodiazepines.** Symptoms are indistinguishable from those of narcotic withdrawal, including seizures. The onset of symptoms may be shortly after birth.

F. **Phencyclidine (PCP).** Symptoms usually begin within 24 h of birth, and the infant may show signs of CNS "hyperirritability" as in narcotic withdrawal. Gastrointestinal symptoms of withdrawal are less common.

G. **Marijuana.** Studies have suggested a slightly shorter duration of gestation and somewhat reduced birthweight, but the extent of these differences was of no clinical importance. The drug may have some mild effect on a variety of newborn neurobehavioral traits.

H. **Selective serotonin reuptake inhibitors (SSRIs).** Symptoms may include irritability, seizures, myoclonus, hyperreflexia, jitteriness, persistent crying, shivering, increased tone, and feeding difficulties. It may be difficult to make a clinical distinction between symptoms of withdrawal and those of a neonatal variant of the serotonin syndrome. Among this group of drugs, the reported incidence of withdrawal appears highest with paroxetine, but it is not clear whether this reflects the epidemiology of the use of this drug or its pharmacokinetic properties.

VI. **Diagnosis**

A. **History.** Many, if not most, drug abusers withhold this information. Details of the extent, quantity, and duration of abuse are unreliable. However, the history is the simplest and most convenient means of diagnosis.

B. **Laboratory tests.** The most commonly used tests to detect drugs of abuse are immunoassays (enzymatic assays or radioimmunoassays). They are, however, subject to a low rate of false-negative and, because of cross-reactivity, false-positive testing. They are thus viewed as screening tests. When it is either medically or legally important, these tests should be supplemented by the more sensitive and specific chromatographic or mass spectrometric tests.

   1. **Urine** is easily obtained and is the most common substance used for drug testing. It reflects intake only in the last few days before delivery. Urine may be obtained from both the mother and the infant (in whom it may persist for a longer time).

      a. **False-negative immunoassays** may be due to dilution (low specific gravity) or high sodium chloride content (detected by high specific gravity). Various adulterants may also affect detection; this is unlikely in the neonate but may occur in maternal urine.

      b. **False-positive immunoassays.** Although these depend on the specific assay used, the following have been reported:

         i. **Detected as morphine.** Codeine (found in many cold and cough medications and in analgesics). About 10% of codeine is metabolized to morphine in the liver. The consumption of baked goods containing poppy seeds (eg, bagels) can result in detectable amounts of morphine in the urine. These are "physiologic" false-positive results, but chromatography or mass spectrometry may determine the source by quantitative assays of other metabolites.

  ii. **Detected as amphetamines.** Ranitidine, chlorpromazine, ritodrine, phenylpropanolamine, ephedrine, pseudoephedrine, phenylephrine, phentermine, and phenmetrazine. Some of these (eg, phenylpropanolamine, pseudoephedrine, and phenylephrine) are found in many over-the-counter preparations.

  iii. **Very high concentrations of nicotine** (probably higher than those obtained in smokers) have shown false-positive in vitro testing for morphine and benzoylecgonine.

2. **Meconium** is easily obtained, and drugs may be found up to 3 days after delivery. It reflects drug use after the first trimester, has a lower rate of false negatives, is a more sensitive test than urine for detecting drug abuse, and reflects usage over a longer period than is detectable by urine testing. Its main disadvantage is that the specimen requires processing before testing and hence places an additional burden on the laboratory. The ability to detect drugs is reduced after formation of fed stools.

3. **Hair.** This is by far the most sensitive test available for detection of drug abuse. Hair grows at 1–2 cm/mo; hence maternal hair can be segmented and each segment analyzed for drugs. Thus details of drug abuse throughout pregnancy may be obtained. There is a quantitative relationship between amounts of drug used and amounts incorporated in growing hair. Hair may be obtained from the mother or the infant (in whom it will reflect usage only during the last trimester). Hair may also be obtained from the infant a long time after delivery should symptoms occur that suggest in utero drug exposure that was previously unsuspected. The test requires processing before assay, is more expensive, and is currently not as widely available as other test methods

4. **Routine laboratory testing.** Routine laboratory tests are usually not required in IDAMs (other than tests to confirm the diagnosis). Laboratory tests are required to rule out other causes of particular signs and symptoms (eg, calcium and glucose for cases of jerky movements) or to follow up and manage some particular complication of drug abuse appropriately.

C. **Other studies.** A **scoring system** has been devised for assessment of withdrawal signs. Commonly called the **Finnegan score,** after its originator, the score was devised for neonates exposed to opiates in utero. Its usefulness for assessing signs after exposure to other drugs or for guiding management in these cases has not been established, but it can be used as a guide. The scoring system is shown in Table 95–3. Other tools for assessing neonatal abstinence are the **Lipsitz tool, the Neonatal Narcotic Withdrawal Index, and the Neonatal Withdrawal Inventory**, but these are less commonly used.

VII. **Management.** Manifestations of drug withdrawal in many infants resolve within a few days, and drug therapy is not required. Supportive care suffices in many, if not most, infants. It is not appropriate to treat prophylactically infants of drug-dependent mothers. The infant's withdrawal score should be assessed to monitor the progression of symptoms and the adequacy of treatment.

A. **Supportive care**

1. **Minimal stimulation.** Attempt to keep the infant in a darkened, quiet environment. Reduce other noxious stimuli.

2. **Swaddling and positioning.** Use gentle swaddling with positioning that encourages flexion rather than extension.

3. **Prevent excessive crying with a pacifier, cuddling, and so on.** Feedings should be on demand if possible, and treatment should be individualized based on the infant's level of tolerance.

Table 95–3. MODIFIED FINNEGAN'S SCORING SYSTEM FOR NEONATAL WITHDRAWAL

Signs and symptoms are scored between feedings.

Cry:	High-pitched	2
	Continuous	3
Sleep hours after feed:	1 h	3
	2 h	2
	3 h	1
Moro reflex:	Hyperactive	2
	Marked	3
Tremors when disturbed:	Mild	2
	Marked	3
Tremors when undisturbed:	Mild	3
	Marked	4
Muscle tone increased:	Mild	3
	Marked	6
Convulsions:		8
Feedings:		
	Frantic sucking of fists	1
	Poor feeding ability	1
	Regurgitation	1
	Projectile vomiting	1
Stools:	Loose	2
	Watery	3
Fever:	100–101°F	2
	> 101°F	2
Respiratory rate:	>60/min	1
	Retractions	2
Excoriations:	Nose	1
	Knees	1
	Toes	1
Frequent yawning:		1
Sneezing:		1
Nasal stuffiness:		1
Sweating:		1

Total scores per day   ( )
Once an objective score has been attained, a dose for treatment can be decided on.

Initiated by Loretta Finnegan, MD, and modified by J. Yoon, MD. Initiated by Finnegan LP et al: A scoring system for evaluation and treatment of neonatal abstinence syndrome: a new clinical and research tool. In Morselli PL et al (eds): *Basic and Therapeutic Aspects of Perinatal Pharmacology.* New York, NY: Raven Press,1975.)

   B. **General drug treatment. Warning: Naloxone (Narcan) may precipitate acute drug withdrawal in infants exposed to narcotics. It should not be used in infants born to mothers suspected of abusing opiates.**
       The general aim of treatment is to allow sleep and feeding patterns to be as close to normal as possible. When supportive care is insufficient to do this, or if symptoms are particularly severe, drugs are used. Indications for drug treatment are progressive irritability, continued feeding difficulty, and significant weight loss. A score >7 on the Finnegan score for three consecutive scorings (done every 2–4 h during the first 2 days) may also be regarded as an indication for treatment. However, the Finnegan score should not be followed slavishly and treated as a definitive laboratory value

(eg, this is not like treating diabetes by monitoring blood and urine sugar levels). Many centers use the Finnegan score only every 12 h and increase the frequency of its application if the infant's scores rapidly escalate. Drugs used for withdrawal are discussed next. Additional treatment may be required for some symptoms (eg, dehydration or convulsions). There have been very few clinical trials in this area, and drug therapy is based largely on anecdotal evidence and hence is variable. Cumulative reports suggest that drugs that act on the relevant receptors are superior to sedatives. When compared with opiates, phenobarbital, at doses required to suppress symptoms of withdrawal, may impair sucking in infants withdrawing from maternal opiates, and may require a more protracted duration of treatment.

1. **Morphine.** A recent randomized trial comparing morphine with tincture of opium showed that infants treated with morphine required a somewhat longer duration of treatment but had better weight gain. An appropriate schedule of treatment would be to start at a morphine dose of 0.04 mg/kg every 4 h. Dosage may be increased every 4 h, at increments of 0.04 mg/kg until symptoms are under control (absent side effects). Once the symptoms are under control (eg, Finnegan score <8), treatment is maintained at that dosage for 72 h and then weaning is commenced. Weaning is done by decreasing the daily dose by 10% every day, as long as symptoms do not relapse. If the infant becomes symptomatic during weaning, the dose is increased back to the last previous dose that had controlled the symptoms. There are no reports of any maximal dose of morphine used for withdrawal, but prudence suggests that infants be closely watched for side effects, and some centers recommend cardiorespiratory monitoring if morphine dosage exceeds 0.8 mg/kg/day. As mentioned, there is a paucity of controlled trials on this topic, and treatment schedules are highly variable between institutions. The schedule just suggested is within the range of common practice but is not carved in stone.

2. **Paregoric (camphorated opium tincture).** This has 0.4 mg/mL morphine equivalent and is thought to be more "physiologic" than nonnarcotic agents. Treated infants have a more physiologic sucking pattern, a higher calorie intake, and better weight gain than those treated with phenobarbital. Paregoric controls seizures related to narcotic withdrawal better than phenobarbital. It controls symptoms in >90% of infants with withdrawal after narcotic exposure. Potential disadvantages are due to other constituents present in the preparation: Camphor is a CNS stimulant, and paregoric also contains alcohol, anise oil, and benzoic acid, a metabolite of benzyl alcohol. **In full-term infants,** start with 0.2 mL every 3–4 h; if no improvement is seen within 4 h, increase the dose by 0.05-mL steps up to a maximum of 0.5 mL every 3–4 h. **In premature infants,** start 0.05 mL/kg every 4 h and increase with increments of 0.02 mL/kg every 4 h until symptoms are controlled, up to a maximum of 0.15 mL/kg every 4 h. Once the withdrawal score is stable for 48 h, the dosage may be tapered by 10% each day.

3. **Opium tincture, also called tincture of opium,** this is similar to paregoric and has the advantage of fewer additives than paregoric. It has a 10 mg/mL morphine equivalent and should be diluted to provide the same (morphine) dosage as paregoric. (See Chapter 132.)

4. **Phenobarbital** is an adequate drug for controlling withdrawal from narcotics, especially those of irritability, fussiness, and hyperexcitability. It is not as effective as paregoric for control of gastrointestinal symptoms or seizures after narcotic exposure. It is not suitable for dose titration because of its long half-life. It is mainly useful for treatment of withdrawal from nonnarcotic agents. The dosage is a 20 mg/kg loading dose, followed by 4 mg/kg/day maintenance. Once symptoms have been controlled for 1 week, decrease the daily dose by 25% every week.

5. **Chlorpromazine** is quite effective in controlling symptoms of withdrawal from both narcotics and nonnarcotics. It has multiple untoward side effects (it reduces

seizure threshold, cerebellar dysfunction, and hematologic problems) that make it **potentially undesirable** for use in neonates when alternatives can be used. The dosage is 3 mg/kg/day, divided into 3–6 doses/day.

6. **Clonidine** has been used for withdrawal from both narcotic and nonnarcotic agents. The dosage is 3–4 mcg/kg/day, divided into four doses per day.

7. **Diazepam** has been used to treat withdrawal from narcotics. One study showed a greater incidence of seizures after methadone withdrawal when infants were treated with diazepam rather than paregoric. When used to treat methadone withdrawal, it also impairs nutritive sucking more than methadone does alone. It may produce apnea when used with phenobarbital. It may be used for treatment of withdrawal from benzodiazepines and possibly also for the hyperexcitable phase after cocaine exposure. The dosage is 0.5–2 mg every 6–8 h.

8. **Combination therapy.** In one study, the combination of diluted tincture of opium (1:25 dilution of opium tincture to water) in combination with phenobarbital was superior to treatment with diluted tincture of opium alone. Patients given this combination spent less time with severe withdrawal and required less diluted tincture of opium, and duration of hospitalization was reduced by 48%.

C. **Long-term management.** If the infant is discharged after 4 days, an early appointment with the pediatrician should be arranged and the parents should be informed as to possible signs of delayed-onset withdrawal. Minor signs and symptoms of drug withdrawal may continue for a few months after discharge. This places a difficult infant in a difficult home situation. There are a few reports of an increased incidence of child abuse in these circumstances. Thus frequent follow-up visits and close involvement of social services may be required.

D. **Breast-feeding.** The various drugs of abuse may be presumed to enter breast milk, and there have been case reports of intoxication in breast-fed infants whose mothers had continued to abuse drugs. Mothers on low-dose methadone have been allowed to breast-feed, but this required close supervision, and there was a constant concern that unsupervised weaning would precipitate withdrawal. A recent study demonstrated that concentration of methadone in breast milk, even at peak maternal plasma levels, was low in the perinatal period. The mothers had been receiving methadone doses of 76 ± 22 mg. The data support recommendations of breast-feeding for women on methadone maintenance. However, methadone-dependent women require special considerations and support and should also be counseled as to the unknown CNS effects of long-term exposure to small amounts of methadone present in breast milk.

VIII. **Prognosis.** During the first few years of life, infants exposed to drugs in utero may have various neurobehavioral problems. Prognosis is largely dependent on the drug used.

A. **Opiates.** There are increased risks of sudden infant death syndrome (SIDS) and strabismus. A substantial proportion of children demonstrate good catch-up growth by 1–2 years of age, although they may still be below the mean. There are limited data on long-term follow-up, but at 5–6 years of age these children appear to function within the normal range of mental and motor development. Some differences have been found in various behavioral, adaptive, and perceptual skills. At 9 years of age, there is a trend, in opiate-exposed children, to score lower than controls in some measures of language processing. Some children require special education classes. A positive and reinforcing environment can improve infant outcome significantly.

B. **Cocaine.** No major deficits in motor development have been found after gestational exposure to cocaine. By 1–6 years of age, there is no significant differences in weight, height, and head circumference between cocaine-exposed and nonexposed children. However, there is an interaction between cocaine exposure and IUGR status. The negative effect of IUGR status at birth, on weight at 6 years of age, was greater in the noncocaine-exposed infants than on those exposed to cocaine. Similarly, the negative effect of IUGR status on height was greater in the IUGR infants without cocaine exposure. Gestational cocaine exposure may, however, be associated with long-term effects on behavior. Cocaine-exposed children exhibited more behavioral problems (both internalizing and externalizing) on follow-up to age 7 years, and these issues were related to degree of cocaine exposure during gestation. A long-term study found a 4.4 point decrease in IQ at 4.5–7 years of age after gestational exposure to cocaine. In addition, cocaine-exposed children are more likely to be referred for special education services at school when compared with unexposed children.

C. **Phencyclidine.** Very few studies have been done, but at 2 years of age these infants appear to have lower scores in fine motor, adaptive, and language areas of development. Although weight, length, and head circumference are somewhat reduced at birth, most children demonstrate adequate catch-up growth.

D. **Marijuana.** There is no definitive evidence of long-term dysfunction. Some scientific studies have found that infants born to women who used marijuana during their pregnancy display altered responses to visual stimulation, increased tremors, and a high-pitched cry, which may indicate problems with nervous system development. During preschool and early school years, marijuana-exposed children have been reported to have more behavioral problems and difficulties with sustained attention and memory than nonexposed children.

Researchers are not certain whether any effects of maternal marijuana use during pregnancy persist as the child grows up; however, because some parts of the brain continue to develop into adolescence, it is also possible that certain kinds of problems will become more evident as the child matures.

Selected References

Jansson LM et al: Concentrations of methadone in breast milk and plasma in the immediate perinatal period. *J Hum Lact* 2007;23:184-190.

Kuschel C: Managing drug withdrawal in the newborn infant. *Sem Fetal Neonatal Med* 2007;12:127-133.

Langenfeld S et al: Therapy of the neonatal abstinence syndrome with tincture of opium or morphine drops. *Drug Alcohol Depend* 2005;77:31-36.

Oei J, Lui K: Management of the newborn infant affected by maternal opiates and other drugs of dependency. *J Paediatr Child Health* 2007;43:9-18.

Rayburn WF: Maternal and fetal effects from substance use. *Clin Perinatol* 2007;34:559-571.

Ruchkin V, Martin A: SSRIs and the developing brain. *Lancet* 2005;365:451-453.

Schempf AH: Illicit drug use and neonatal outcomes: a critical review. *Obstet Gynecol Surv* 2007;62:749-757.

Shankaran S et al: Impact of maternal substance use during pregnancy on childhood outcome. *Sem Fetal Neonatal Med* 2007;12:143-150.

96 Intracranial Hemorrhage

An **Intracranial hemorrhage (ICH)** can occur in term and preterm infants. An ICH occurring in term infants tends to be subdural, subarachnoid, or subtentorial and is most related to birth trauma, hypoxic-ischemic events, coagulopathies (eg, thrombophilias or thrombocytopenia), and of an undetermined cause. An ICH in preterm infants is periventricular or intraventricular in location but originating from vascular rupture within the subependymal germinal matrix. Preterm infants may have periventricular hemorrhagic infarctions of white matter that follow germinal matrix-intraventricular hemorrhages.

SUBDURAL HEMORRHAGE (SDH)

I. **Definition.** SDH involves tears of veins or venous sinuses traversing the subdural space. Vascular structures most affected are superficial cerebral veins, infratentorial posterior fossa venous sinuses, the inferior sagittal sinus, and tentorial sinuses and veins (eg, vein of Galen). Blood may accumulate and cause acute symptoms of intracranial pressure or reside as a hematoma that slowly evolves as a chronic subdural hematoma with increasing fluid accumulation and increasing intracranial pressure.

II. **Incidence.** SDH is uncommon in term and preterm infants. When it occurs, it usually follows a traumatic delivery of a late preterm or term infant. Among 111 asymptomatic term infants studied prospectively by MRI, 9 had SDH (8.0%), 3 after spontaneous vaginal deliveries and 6 after instrumented deliveries. None required treatment, and all were free of hematoma by 4 weeks of age. Moreover, all infants were normal at 2 years. Although SDH is the least common of all ICH and often self-resolving, it can be a serious to catastrophic event clinically.

III. **Pathophysiology.** SDH is typically related to traumatic events surrounding the delivery and birth. Undue pressure on the skull and torsion may produce shear forces resulting in rupture of superficial cerebral bridging veins, or tears in the dura or dural reflections (eg, the falx cerebri or tentorium and associated venous sinuses). These events are usually found over the cerebrum or within the posterior fossa. Occasionally skull fractures accompany these findings. Timing of the onset of SDH and clinical findings may be acute or delayed. As noted, clinical signs may be minimal to none with the SDH self-resolving; however, subtle findings of slight irritability or a seemingly hyperalert state may foretell an underlying accumulating SDH with delayed onset of more serious neuropathic circumstances. Latent SDH can lead to a subdural hematoma and subdural effusion with increasing intracranial pressure.

IV. **Risk factors** include precipitous delivery, instrumented deliveries using midforceps or vacuum assist (extraction), or circumstances involving a large for gestational age infant and cephalopelvic disproportion.

V. **Clinical presentation.** Signs include lethargy alternating with irritability, or asymmetric hypotonia of upper and lower extremities on the contralateral side of the SDH. More specific to SDH is impaired third cranial nerve function ipsilateral to the SDH. Focal seizures may present at any time. Signs of increasing intracranial pressure may include a bulging fontanel, deviations of eye movements, and increasing occipital-frontal head circumference. Other observations are decreased feeding, intermittent vomiting, and failure to thrive, which are more often related to late post-SDH neuropathic events.

VI. **Diagnosis**
   A. **Laboratory**
      1. **Hematocrit.** Unexplained anemia.
      2. **Total serum bilirubin.** Persistent newborn jaundice.
      3. **Cerebral spinal fluid (CSF) studies** are indicative but not diagnostic of SDH. Emphasis on ICH hemorrhage can be taken if a combination of CSF findings is seen: large numbers of red bloods cells (especially if crenated), xanthochromia, elevated protein content, and hypoglycorrhachia.
   B. **Radiologic studies**
      1. **Computed tomographic (CT) scanning** readily identifies most SDH.
      2. **Magnetic Resonance Imaging (MRI)** is best for detailing posterior fossa lesions and accumulations of blood or effusion.
      3. **Ultrasonography (US)** does not readily lend itself to SDH identification, except for possible midline shifts.

VII. **Management.** Documentation of risk factors and appropriate cogent observation are the most important first clinical steps. Careful and repeated neurologic examinations will reveal neurologic signs that should be followed by laboratory and imaging studies.

VIII. **Prognosis.** The outcome of SDH ranges from early death, to minimal or no disabling conditions. Much of the neurologic outcome of SDH depends on accompanying conditions soon after birth (eg, prematurity, birth asphyxia, shock, hypoxic-ischemic encephalopathy, or infection). Massive tentorial tears and hemorrhage dictate death or severe and long-term handicap. Infants with major SDH can have mortality rates upward to 45%. Conversely, as in most cases noted by Whitby et al, SDH can be limited, produce few clinical signs, and have a good outcome. More than 50% of infants with minimal early clinical findings and later good outcomes have been largely found to have had small cerebral convexity SDH hemorrhages.

SUBARACHNOID HEMORRHAGE (SAH)

I. **Definition.** SAH identifies blood that has accumulated between the arachnoid mater and the pia mater (ie, within the subarachnoid space). The arachnoid mater is an avascular membrane situated below the dura mater, and together with the pia mater constitutes what is known as the leptomeninges. Unlike adult SAH, which is arterial, infant SAH is venous in origin coming from bridging veins within the subarachnoid space. Rarely, it may be arterial coming from leptomeningeal arteries of the subarachnoid space. One must specify SAH as primary in origin when coming from the vasculature of the subarachnoid space. Otherwise SAH is secondary to blood that may be an extension of an intraventricular hemorrhage (IVH) or an extravasation of blood from a cerebral or cerebellar hemorrhage or infarction.

II. **Incidence.** A small SAH is not infrequently seen in preterm and term newborn infants. It is of limited significance unless other conditions are present such as prematurity, hypoxic-ischemic encephalopathy, coagulopathies, birth trauma, or asphyxia. Primary bleeding within the subarachnoid space is usually self-limited, and it is the most common ICH seen in newborns.

III. **Pathophysiology.** Rupture of the small arteries, veins, and capillaries of the subarachnoid space can be associated with trauma in term infants or birth asphyxia in preterm infants. But it is most often of undetermined cause and of little consequence.

IV. **Risk factors.** See pathophysiology.

V. **Clinical presentation.** As with SDH, clinical signs may be nonexistent with SAH, especially in the full-term infant. Mild to intermittent irritability or lethargy may herald the onset of seizures on the second to the third day of life. Rarely, SAH with catastrophic consequences befalls an infant, most likely a preterm infant with severe coexisting perinatal asphyxia.

VI. **Diagnosis**
   A. **Laboratory.** CSF findings in SAH mirror those already discussed for SDH.
   B. **Radiologic studies.** CT and MRI studies establish the existence of primary SAH or identify other lesions that may be the source of secondary subarachnoid blood accumulation.

VII. **Management.** Close observation and repeated neurologic examinations suffice for those infants at risk but without signs of SAH. Supportive and expectant care is appropriate. Anticonvulsant medication and intravenous fluid therapy are needed if the infant has lethargy and/or seizure activity. Serum electrolyte and urine output monitoring for possible syndrome of inappropriate antidiuretic secretion is recommended if a significant amount of SAH has been identified. Follow-up is important for serial measurement of head circumference. Some develop posthemorrhagic hydrocephalus due to obliteration of CSF resorption sites within the ventricles and subarachnoid space. (See Chapter 90).

VIII. **Prognosis.** The majority of SAH are mild and uncomplicated with good outcomes. Those infants who have seizures that resolve prior to discharge from the hospital have an expected 90% uncomplicated outcome. Infants who develop long-term complications are largely within the category of having coexisting problems associated with birth trauma or perinatal asphyxia.

INTRACEREBRAL PARENCHYMAL HEMORRHAGE

I. **Definition.** Intracerebral parenchymal hemorrhage is commonly referred to as **periventricular hemorrhagic infarction (PVHI)**. It is a hemorrhage into periventricular white matter following local venous infarction. In preterm infants, it is usually bilateral and results in periventricular leukomalacia, which subsequently may form multiple small cystic lesions. In term infants it tends to be unilateral and forms a large single porencephalic cyst.

II. **Incidence.** The occurrence of PVHI may be as much as 10–15% in an overall population of infants with ICH.

III. **Pathophysiology.** PVHI is most likely venous in origin, either from venous thrombosis followed by infarction or from venous stasis subsequent to germinal matrix hemorrhage and intraventricular hemorrhage. The latter events cause increased intravascular pressure that leads to rupture of parenchymal vessels and loss of tissue perfusion. Neither mechanism is clearly delineated and may simply represent a consequence of subependymal hemorrhage and IVH. Affected preterm infants have hemorrhagic venous infarction of subcortical and periventricular white matter, whereas affected term infants develop subcortical hemorrhage with infarction of overlying cortex.

IV. **Risk factors.** PVHI is often associated with coexisting hypoxic ischemic encephalopathy following a perinatal hypoxic event.

V. **Clinical presentation.** PVHI presents with clinical signs of severe central nervous system disturbance consistent with coexisting disease processes and findings reflective of severe SDH, SAH, or IVH.

VI. **Diagnosis.** Imaging studies are required to delineate the hemorrhagic and infarcted areas of the brain.

   A. **CT scanning** reveals much of the hemorrhagic damage that can be seen.

   B. **MRI** is more specific for hemorrhage and hypodensities suggest evolving areas of damage.

   C. **Cranial US studies** have been particularly useful to identify PVHI. Bassan and coworkers defined PVHI by US imaging as an echodense lesion of periventricular white matter with an associated germinal matrix (GM) and IVH. If the PVHI is unilateral or bilateral, it is always an asymmetric lesion. If the GM/IVH is bilateral, the PVHI is on the side of greatest hemorrhage.

VII. **Management.** PVHI requires observational and supportive care as for severe SDH or SAH. If a midline shift is suggested, neurosurgical consultation is suggested. Subsequent posthemorrhagic hydrocephalus (PHH) is always a threat, and careful follow-up care is warranted with neurosurgical support as needed.

VIII. **Prognosis.** Follow-up care to determine long-term outcome is essential. The outlook will change depending on recovery from initial findings and comorbidities. Documentation of brain injury through imaging studies will assist in foretelling ultimate long-term outcomes. Neurodevelopmental studies of preterm infants with PVHI have indicated that significant cognitive and/or motor delays complicate overall recovery in at least two thirds of survivors.

INTRACEREBELLAR PARENCHYMAL HEMORRHAGE (ICPH)

I. **Definition.** ICPH is most often seen in preterm infants with complications of labor and delivery who require intense respiratory management. ICPH in term infants is almost always associated with birth trauma.

II. **Incidence.** Reports vary by gestational age. In neuropathologic reports, preterm infants <1500 g have an occurrence of 15–25%. A recent report using cranial US has redefined the incidence as 2.8% in a population of <1500 g infants, and an incidence of 8.7% for the smallest infants weighing <750 g.

III. **Risk factors.** Traumatic delivery.

IV. **Pathogenesis.** Four mechanisms for ICPH are possible:

  A. **Primary hemorrhage** into either cerebellar hemisphere or into the vermis.

  B. **Venous infarction.**

  C. **A large IVH or SAH** extending into the posterior fossa or into the cerebellum proper.

  D. **Direct trauma to the posterior fossa** with rupture of cerebellar bridging veins or the occipital sinuses. This is seen primarily in term infants. Most ICPH is unilateral and focal with a predilection to the right cerebellar hemisphere.

V. **Clinical presentation.** Generally ICPH causes overall neurologic signs much as previously discussed with other ICH. **Unique to ICPH** in clinical presentation is profound and early respiratory compromise with apnea or respiratory rate irregularity and bradycardia.

VI. **Diagnosis.** Although the posterior fossa does not lend itself to cranial US studies, newer techniques using the mastoid fontanel have opened the posterior fossa and the cerebellum to imaging and more direct identification of ICPH.

VII. **Management.** All management modalities presented for other ICH patients apply to infants with confirmed or suspected ICPH. The recent findings by Limperopoulos et al have shown that for infants at risk for ICPH the added combination of shock, acidosis, and patent ductus arteriosus are closely related and warrant close attention with support and diagnostic efforts specific for ICPH.

VIII. **Prognosis.** Short-term outcomes reveal that ICPH preterm infants have required extended periods of assisted ventilation and have experienced longer periods of hospitalization when compared with control study infants. Consistent with other ICH, long-term outcomes require regular assessment and monitoring for neuromotor and behavioral difficulties.

GERMINAL MATRIX AND INTRAVENTRICULAR HEMORRHAGE (GM/IVH)

I. **Definition.** GM/IVH is predominantly a lesion of preterm infants; it is perhaps the single most threatening complication of preterm birth and portends lifelong neurologic consequences. GM/IVH is a consequence of early gestational age and the vulnerability of the immature cerebral vasculature. Perinatal stress factors related to GM/IVH are birth asphyxia, hypoxemia, hypotension, and acidosis.

The germinal matrix, located between the caudate nucleus and the ependymal lining of the lateral ventricle, is normally not seen on cranial US. When germinal matrix hemorrhage occurs, it becomes readily identified by US and is seen as subependymal bleeding originating between the groove of the thalamus and the head of the caudate nucleus. Bleeding may be confined to the germinal matrix or it may rupture into either lateral ventricle, and thereby become a unilateral or bilateral GM/IVH.

IVH seldom occurs in term infants, but if it occurs it is largely confined to circumstances of birth injury. By 36 weeks' postconceptional age (PCA), the germinal matrix has involuted in most infants, though some residual may persist. If IVH occurs in term infants, it originates most often in the choroid plexus; however, residual subependymal germinal matrix may also be a point of origin. Following hemorrhage, venous thromboses result in thalamic infarction.

II. **Incidence.** Specific incidence figures are largely unknown, but the occurrence of GM/IVH is approximately 25–40% for all preterm infants. These estimates are based largely on data from 1990–2000; however, for the last decade there has been a reduction to a lower range of occurrence at 2–20%. Rates vary by gestation with the greatest risk of GM/IVH in preterm infants with birthweight <750 g. Because IVH is seldom seen in term infants, their incidence rates are exceptionally low and associated with birth-related injury or asphyxia. Curiously, 2–3% of seemingly normal term infants, when studied prospectively, have been noted to have a 2–3% incidence of "silent" IVH.

III. **Pathophysiology.** The germinal matrix is a weakly supported and highly vascularized area. The blood vessels (not readily distinguishable as arterioles, venules, or capillaries) in this area of immature cerebrum are especially prone to hypoxic-ischemic injury.

The vessels are irregular, with large luminal areas, and readily rupture. The germinal matrix begins to involute after 34 weeks' PCA, and thus the peculiar vulnerability and predilection for GM/IVH for preterm infants lessens but is not totally removed. Late preterm infants (34–37 weeks' gestation) may have IVH that reflect those of early preterm infants. **Fluctuations in cerebral blood flow (CBF)** play an important role in the pathogenesis of GM/IVH because sick premature infants have **pressure-passive cerebral circulation.** A sudden rise or fall in systemic blood pressure can result in an increase in CBF with subsequent rupture of the germinal matrix vessels. Decreases in CBF can result in ischemic injury to the germinal matrix vessels and surrounding tissues, which rupture following reperfusion.

The unique deep venous anatomy at the level of the foramen of Monroe and the open communication between the germinal matrix vessels and the venous circulation contribute to the importance of abrupt or sharp fluctuations in cerebral venous pressure. Given this anatomic proximity, rupture through the germinal matrix subependymal layer results in entrance of blood into the lateral ventricles in nearly 80% of affected infants.

A. Neuropathologic consequences of IVH

1. **Germinal matrix ventricular-subventricular zone contains the migrating cells of origin for the cerebral cortex.** It is the site of production of neurons and glial cells of the cerebral cortex and basal ganglia. Germinal matrix destruction may result in impairment of myelinization, brain growth, and subsequent cortical development.

2. **Periventricular hemorrhagic infarction** is venous in origin, associated with severe and usually asymmetric IVH, and invariably occurs on the side with the larger amount of intraventricular blood. It is a distinct pathologic event following venous stasis; it is often mistakenly described as an "extension" of IVH, of which it is not. Moreover, PVHI is neuropathologically distinct from periventricular leukomalacia (PVL). See preceding discussion under PVHI.

3. PHH is more common in those infants with the highest grade of hemorrhage. It is most frequently attributable to obliterative arachnoiditis either over the convexities of the cerebral hemispheres with occlusion of the arachnoid villi or in the posterior fossa with obstruction of outflow of the fourth ventricle. Rarely, aqueductal stenosis is caused by an acute clot or reactive gliosis.

4. PVL is a frequent accompaniment of IVH but is not directly caused by IVH. PVL is an ischemic brain injury followed by necrosis of periventricular white matter adjacent to the lateral ventricles. It is usually a nonhemorrhagic, **symmetric** lesion, resulting from hypotension, apnea, and other hypoxic-ischemic events known to decrease CBF.

IV. **Risk factors.** Prematurity and respiratory distress have remained as the most closely related clinical circumstances to GM/IVH. As mentioned earlier, the immature cerebral vascular structures of preterm infants are extremely vulnerable to volume and pressure changes and to hypoxic and acidotic changes. Secondarily, respiratory distress, and its attendant limitations for oxygenation, further attenuates the immature vasculature of the preterm brain. Birth asphyxia, pneumothorax, shock/hypotension, acidosis, hypothermia, and therapeutic volume and/or osmolar overloads all serve to multiply the risk for GM/IVH. Even procedures that we perceive as routine in the care of premature infants may also be contributory, such as tracheal suctioning, abdominal examination, and handling to reposition or to instill mydriatics for an eye examination.

Of growing importance for the understanding of preterm GM/IVH is the possible role of fetal and neonatal **inflammatory responses.** Chorioamnionitis and funisitis may be harbingers of postnatal cerebral vascular events leading up to GM/IVH. Fetal inflammatory responses and subsequent neonatal hypotension and sepsis are closely related processes to IVH. Mediators of the inflammatory response are cytokines. Their vasoactive properties may be the source of exaggerated blood pressure changes that overwhelm the pressure passive state of the germinal matrix.

V. **Clinical presentation.** The clinical presentation is diverse, and diagnosis requires neuroimaging confirmation. Signs may mimic those of other ICH or common neonatal disorders, such as metabolic disturbances, asphyxia, sepsis, or meningitis. IVH may be totally asymptomatic, or there may be subtle symptoms (eg, a bulging fontanel, a sudden drop in hematocrit, apnea, bradycardia, acidosis, seizures, and changes in muscle tone or level of consciousness). A catastrophic syndrome is characterized by rapid onset of stupor or coma, respiratory abnormalities, seizures, decerebrate posturing, pupils fixed to light, or a profound flaccid quadriparesis.

VI. **Diagnosis**

  A. **Cranial US** (see Chapter 10 for examples) is the procedure of choice for screening and diagnosis. CT scanning and MRI are acceptable alternatives but are more expensive and require transport to the imaging service. They are valuable for a more definitive diagnosis or documentation of static brain injury prior to discharge from the hospital. Two systems for classifying GM/IVH have been advanced for clinical use. The older and most time honored has been that of Papile, based originally on CT scanning but adapted for interpretation of cranial US imaging. The second is the classification promulgated by Volpe, based also on cranial US imaging. The utility of classification schema resides in the ability of clinicians to communicate degrees of severity and to have a source of information for comparison of lesions as well as having a means to follow progression or regression and recovery of the initial insult of IVH. The GM/IVH classification by Papile gives classes I to IV. Classes I and II are small hemorrhages. Class I is hemorrhage only seen in the germinal matrix. Class II shows hemorrhage from the germinal matrix extending into the lateral ventricles but without ventricular dilation. Classes III and IV are moderate to severe lateral ventricular hemorrhages, the former with acute ventricular dilation, the latter with parenchymal hemorrhages.

  IVH classification by Volpe offers a somewhat different perspective. His class I is confined to the germinal matrix with little or no IVH. Class II is an IVH seen on parasagittal view and extends into >50% of the lateral ventricles. Class III is IVH >50% on parasagittal view with distention of the lateral ventricles. Lastly, Volpe points out that cranial US findings of any periventricular echodensity is an obvious and more serious intracranial vascular insult, such as PVHI or PVL.

  A cranial US is indicated for screening sick preterm infants for IVH from the first day of life and throughout the hospitalization. Typically a cranial US is done between day 1 and day 7, depending on clinical presentation and institutional protocols, keeping in mind that at least 50% of GM/IVH occurs on day 1, 90% by day 4 of life. Of all GM/IVH identified by day 4 of life, 20–40% progress to a more extensive hemorrhage. Most clinicians obtain a final cranial sonogram, CT, or MRI before discharge or at 36 weeks' PCA.

  B. **Laboratory studies.** CSF initially shows elevated red and white blood cells, with elevated protein concentration. The degree of elevation of CSF protein correlates approximately with the severity of the hemorrhage. It is frequently difficult to distinguish IVH from a "traumatic tap." Within a few days after hemorrhage, the CSF becomes xanthochromic, with a decreased glucose concentration as in other forms of ICH. Often, the CSF shows a persistent increase in white blood cells and protein and a decreased glucose level, making it difficult to rule out meningitis except by negative cultures.

VII. **Management**

  A. **Prenatal prevention**

   1. **Avoidance of premature delivery.**

   2. **Transportation in utero.**

   3. **Data suggest that active preterm labor may be a risk factor for early IVH** and there may be a protective role for cesarean delivery. However, Anderson et al showed that cesarean birth before the active phase of labor resulted in a lower frequency of severe IVH and less progression to severe IVH, although it did not affect the overall incidence of IVH.

4. **Antenatal steroid therapy.** Several large multicenter trials have shown a clear efficacy of antenatal steroids in reducing IVH. In one study the incidence of GM hemorrhage or IVH was two- to threefold lower in infants whose mothers received a complete course of antenatal steroids compared with those whose mothers received no steroids or an incomplete course (<48 h). Moreover, this beneficial effect appears to be independent of the improvement in respiratory status. The prevention of IVH may be a composite effect of enhanced vascular integrity, decreased respiratory distress, and possibly altered cytokine production. Blickstein and coworkers have reported that antenatal steroids (given between 24 and 32 weeks' gestation) as a completed course (48 h) resulted in a 2.5 times less incidence of GM/IVH (7.7% vs 19.4%) for singleton and multiple births.

B. **Postnatal prevention**
   1. **Avoid birth asphyxia.**
   2. **Avoid large fluctuations in blood pressure.**
   3. **Avoid rapid infusion of volume expanders or hypertonic solutions.**
   4. **Use prompt but cautious cardiovascular support to prevent hypotension.**
   5. **Correct acid-base abnormalities.**
   6. **Correct abnormalities of coagulation.**
   7. **Avoid poorly synchronized mechanical ventilation;** consider sedation and in difficult situations pharmacologic paralysis.
   8. **Postnatal pharmacologic intervention with indomethacin.** Ment et al reported in 1994 that low-dose prophylactic indomethacin significantly lowered the incidence and severity of IVH but did not appear to be of benefit in the prevention or extension of early IVH. Subsequent reviews and reports over the ensuing years have not confirmed indomethacin prophylaxis for prevention of IVH, and the approach remains *controversial*. There are reports of reduced cerebral blood flow after indomethacin as well as no difference in long-term neurologic outcome for treated versus nontreated infants. More recently, Ment et al have reported on long-term follow-up of school-age preterm infants, indicating improved vocabulary scores with a striking favorable gender response to indomethacin therapy for male subjects. In the same year, Miller et al have reported less white matter injury following three to six doses of low-dose indomethacin therapy for infants of <28 weeks' gestation. Much of the controversy today surrounding low-dose prophylactic indomethacin therapy for the prevention or amelioration of GM/IVH are the continuing concerns for indomethacin-related complications of necrotizing enterocolitis, spontaneous intestinal perforation, decreased renal function (albeit transient in most cases), and the threat of persistent pulmonary hypertension.

C. **Management of acute hemorrhage**
   1. **General supportive care** to maintain a normal blood volume and a stable acid-base status.
   2. **Avoid fluctuations** of arterial and venous blood pressures.
   3. **Follow-up serial imaging** (cranial US or CT scanning) to detect progressive hydrocephalus. See the previous section on hydrocephalus.

VIII. **Prognosis**
   A. **Short-term outcome of GM/IVH is directly related to birthweight, gestational age, and the ensuing severity of the hemorrhagic insult to the immature brain.** For the years 1995–1996 and 1997–2002, very low birthweight infants in the NICHD Neonatal Research Network saw survival steady at 84–85%. Meanwhile the occurrence of severe IVH remained unchanged at 12%. A broader view of the 1997–2002 infants weighing 501–1500 g reveals 15% mortality, 25% survival with short-term complications of bronchopulmonary dysplasia, severe IVH, and necrotizing enterocolitis, and approximately a 60% survival for infants without the short-term complications just described. However, the long-term outcomes remain very much in question.

B. **Long-term major neurologic sequelae of GM/IVH depend primarily on the extent of associated parenchymal injury and any added effects of the short-term complications.** From the NICHD studies just noted, long-term outcomes of seemingly normal extremely low birthweight infants at time of hospital discharge are worrisome. At 8–9 years of age, and in comparison with control term infants, studies now reveal strikingly lower IQ scores, greater learning problems, poor motor skills, markedly increased behavioral problems, and considerable hearing loss. Clearly, despite increased numbers of survivors for very low birthweight infants, with or without demonstrable GM/IVH, they are encountering lifelong disabilities.

Selected References

Anderson G et al: The effect of cesarean section on intraventricular hemorrhage in the preterm infant. *Am J Obstet Gynecol* 1992;166:1091-1099.

Bassan H et al: Neurodevelopmental outcome in survivors of periventricular hemorrhagic infarction. *Pediatrics* 2007;120:785-792.

Blickstein I et al; Israel Neonatal Network: Plurality-dependent risk of severe intraventricular hemorrhage among very low birth weight infants and antepartum corticosteroid treatment. *Am J Obstet Gynecol* 2006:194:1329-1333.

Eichenwald EC, Stark AR: Management and outcomes of very low birth weight. *N Engl J Med* 2008:358:1700-1711.

Hill A, Volpe JJ: Neurologic disorders: intracranial hemorrhage. In Avery GB et al (eds): *Neonatology: Pathophysiology and Management of the Newborn,* 4th ed. Philadelphia, PA: Lippincott, 1994:1127-1134.

Kaukola T et al: Population cohort associating chorioamnionitis, cord, inflammatory cytokines and neurologic outcome in very preterm, extremely low birth weight infants. *Pediatr Res* 2006:59:478-483.

Laughon M et al: Factors associated with treatment for hypotension in extremely low gestational age newborns during the first postnatal week. *Pediatrics* 2007:119:273-280.

Leviton A et al: Antenatal corticosteroids appear to reduce the risk of postnatal germinal matrix hemorrhage in intubated low birth weight newborns. *Pediatrics* 1993;91: 1083-1088.

Limperopoulos C et al: Cerebellar hemorrhage in the preterm infant: ultrasonographic findings and risk factors. *Pediatrics* 2005;116:717-724.

Ment LR et al: Low dose indomethacin and prevention of intraventricular hemorrhage: a multicenter randomized trial. *Pediatrics*1994;93:543-550.

Ment LR et al: A functional magnetic resonance imaging study of the long term influences of early indomethacin exposure on language processing in the brains of prematurely born children. *Pediatrics* 2006;118:961-970.

Miller SP et al: Prolonged indomethacin exposure is associated with decreased white matter injury detected with magnetic resonance imaging in premature newborns at 24 to 28 weeks' gestational birth. *Pediatrics* 2006;117:1626-1631.

Morrison S: Intracranial hemorrhage in the premature infant. In Fanaroff AA, Martin RJ (eds): *Neonatal-Perinatal Medicine: Diseases of the Fetus and Infant*, 7th ed. St. Louis, MO: Mosby, 2002:655-656.

Papile L: Intracranial hemorrhage. In Fanaroff AA, Martin RJ (eds): *Neonatal-Perinatal Medicine: Diseases of the Fetus and Infant*, 7th ed. St. Louis, MO: Mosby, 2002: 879-887.

Perlman JM et al: Bilateral cystic periventricular leukomalacia in the preterm infant: associated risk factors. *Pediatrics* 1996;97:822-827.

Shalak L, Perlman JM: Hemorrhagic-ischemic cerebral injury in the preterm infant: current concepts. *Clin Perinatol* 2002;29:745-763.

Synnes AR: Neonatal intensive care unit characteristics affect the incidence of severe intraventricular hemorrhage. *Med Care* 2006;44:754-759.

Tauscher MK et al: Association of histologic chorioamnionitis, increased levels of cord blood cytokines, and intracerebral hemorrhage in preterm neonates. *Biol Neonate* 2003; 83:166-170.

Vannucci RC, Palmer C: Hypoxia-ischemia: neuropathology, pathogenesis and management. In Fanaroff AA, Martin RJ (eds): *Neonatal-Perinatal Medicine: Diseases of the Fetus and Infant*, 7th ed. St. Louis, MO: Mosby, 2002:848-849.

Vasileiadis GT et al: Uncomplicated intraventricular hemorrhage is followed by reduced cortical volume at near-term age. *Pediatrics* 2004:114:e367-e372.

Volpe JJ: Intracranial hemorrhage: germinal-matrix intraventricular hemorrhage of the premature infant. In Volpe JJ (ed): *Neurology of the Newborn*, 4th ed. Philadelphia, PA: Saunders, 2001.

Volpe JJ: Intracranial hemorrhage: subdural, primary subarachnoid, intracerebellar, intra-ventricular (term infant), and miscellaneous. In Volpe JJ (ed): *Neurology of the Newborn*, 4th ed. Philadelphia, PA: Saunders, 2001:397-492.

Whitby EH et al: Frequency and natural history of subdural haemorrhages in babies and rela-tion to obstetric factors. *Lancet* 2004;363:846-851.

Wright L: Editorial commentary on antenatal corticosteroid treatment. In Fanaroff AA et al (eds): *The Yearbook of Neonatal-Perinatal Medicine*. Philadelphia, PA: Elsevier Mosby, 2007:185-186.

Yager JY, Vannucci RC: Intracranial hemorrhage. In Fanaroff AA, Martin RJ (eds): *Neonatal-Perinatal Medicine: Diseases of the Fetus and Infant*, 7th ed. St. Louis, MO: Mosby, 2002:894-895.

97 Intrauterine Growth Restriction (Small for Gestational Age)

I. **Definition.** In the past, the terms **intrauterine growth restriction (IUGR)** and **small for gestational age (SGA)** were used interchangeably. Although related, they are not synonymous. **IUGR is the failure to attain optimal intrauterine growth, whereas SGA describes an infant whose weight is lower than population norms or lower than a predetermined cutoff weight.** SGA infants are defined as having a birthweight **below the 10th percentile** for gestational age or **>2 standard deviations below the mean** for gestational age.

The **ponderal index,** arrived at by the following formula, can be used to identify infants whose soft tissue mass is below normal for the stage of skeletal development. A ponderal index <10th percentile may be used to identify IUGR infants. Thus all IUGR infants may not be SGA, and all SGA infants may not be small as a result of a growth-restrictive process.

$$\text{Ponderal index} = \frac{\text{Birthweight} \times 100}{\text{crown-heel length}^3}$$

A. **Symmetric IUGR** (HC = Ht = Wt, all <10%). The head circumference (HC), length (Ht), and weight (Wt) are all proportionately reduced for gestational age. Symmetric IUGR is due to either decreased growth potential of the fetus (congenital infection or genetic disorder) or extrinsic conditions that are active early in pregnancy.

B. **Asymmetric IUGR** (HC = Ht < Wt, all <10%). Fetal weight is reduced out of proportion to length and head circumference. The head circumference and length are closer to the expected percentiles for gestational age than is the weight. In these infants, brain growth is usually spared. The usual causes are uteroplacental insufficiency, maternal malnutrition, or extrinsic conditions appearing late in pregnancy.

II. **Incidence.** About 3–10% of all pregnancies are associated with IUGR, and 20% of still-born infants are growth retarded. The perinatal mortality rate is *5–20* times higher for growth-retarded fetuses, and serious short- or long-term morbidity is noted in half of the affected surviving infants. IUGR is estimated to be the predominant cause for low birthweight in developing countries. It is estimated that a third of infants with birth-weights <2500 g are in fact growth retarded and not premature. **Term infants with birth-weights <3rd percentile have a higher morbidity and a 10 times higher mortality than appropriate for gestational age infants.** In the United States, uteroplacental insufficiency is the leading cause of IUGR. An estimated 10% of cases are secondary to congenital infection. Chromosomal and other genetic disorders are reported in 5–15% of IUGR infants. Estimation of IUGR may vary based on neonatal or fetal growth charts used to define IUGR.

III. **Pathophysiology.** Fetal growth is influenced by fetal, maternal, and placental factors.

A. **Fetal factors** (Table 97–1)

1. **Genetic factors.** Approximately 20% of birthweight variability in a given population is determined by fetal genotype. Genetic determinants of fetal growth have their greatest impact in early gestation during the period of rapid cell development. Racial and ethnic backgrounds influence size at birth irrespective of socioeconomic status. Males weigh an average of 150–200 g more than females at birth. This weight increase occurs late in gestation. Birth order affects fetal size; infants born to primiparous women weigh less than subsequent siblings. Genetic disorders such as achondroplasia, Russell-Silver syndrome, and leprechaunism also present with IUGR.

2. **Chromosomal anomalies.** Chromosomal deletions or imbalances result in diminished fetal growth. Nearly 20% of fetal growth restriction is due to chromosomal aberrations. Growth retardation is observed as a major feature of uniparental disomy (eg, Silver Russell syndrome), short-arm deletion of chromosome 4, long-arm deletion of chromosome 13, and trisomies 13, 18, and 21. Additional X chromosomes beyond norm are associated with diminished birthweight (eg, XXY, XXXY). The risk for recurrence of fetal aneuploidy is 1%.

3. **Congenital malformations.** Anencephaly, gastrointestinal atresia, Potter syndrome, and pancreatic agenesis are examples of congenital anomalies associated with IUGR. Frequency of IUGR increases as the number of congenital defects increases.

4. **Fetal cardiovascular anomalies** (with the possible exception of transposition of the great vessels and tetralogy of Fallot). Abnormal hemodynamics are thought to be the basis of IUGR.

Table 97–1. FETAL FACTORS IN INTRAUTERINE GROWTH RESTRICTION

Genetic factors
    Racial, ethnic, and population differences
    Genetic disorders
    Chromosomal disorders
    Female sex
    Congenital anomalies
Congenital infections
Inborn errors of metabolism

5. **Congenital infection.** TORCH infections (*t*oxoplasmosis, *o*ther, *r*ubella, *c*ytomegalovirus, and *h*erpes simplex virus) are often associated with IUGR and account for ~5% of IUGR fetuses (see Chapter 127). Cytomegalovirus and rubella are associated with severe IUGR. The incidence of IUGR is highest when infection occurs in the first trimester. The clinical findings in different congenital infections are nonspecific and overlap considerably. IUGR with rubella causes damage during organogenesis and results in a decreased number of cells, whereas cytomegalovirus infection results in cytolysis and localized necrosis within the fetus.

6. **Inborn errors of metabolism.** Transient neonatal diabetes, galactosemia, and phenylketonuria are other disorders associated with IUGR. Single-gene defects associated with impaired insulin secretion or action are associated with impaired fetal growth (ie, leprechaunism). (See Chapter 93.)

B. **Maternal factors** (Table 97–2)

1. **Reduced uteroplacental blood flow.** Maternal disorders such as preeclampsia-eclampsia, chronic renovascular disease, and chronic hypertensive vascular disease often result in decreased uteroplacental blood flow and associated IUGR. Impaired delivery of oxygen and other essential nutrients is thought to limit organ growth and musculoskeletal maturation. Risk of placental thrombi is increased in conditions of inherited thrombophilias (factor V Leiden mutation, prothrombin G20210A mutation, protein C and S deficiencies, antithrombin III deficiency, anticardiolipin antibody, factor VIII deficiency, methylenetetrahydrofolate reductase mutation).

2. **Maternal malnutrition.** The major risk factors for IUGR include small maternal size (height and prepregnancy weight) and low maternal weight gain. Low body mass index, defined as (weight [kg]/height [m^2])/100, is a major predictor of IUGR. Maternal malnutrition leads to deficient substrate supply to the fetus. Total caloric consumption rather than protein or fat consumption appears to be the principal nutritional influence on birthweight. Famine causes a modest

---

Table 97–2. MATERNAL FACTORS IN INTRAUTERINE GROWTH RESTRICTION (IUGR)

Pregnancy-induced hypertension (>140/90 mm Hg)
Weight gain (<0.9 kg/every 4 weeks)
Fundal lag (<4 cm for gestational age)
Cyanotic heart disease
Heavy smoking
Residing at high altitude
Substance abuse and drugs
Short stature
Low socioeconomic class
Anemia (hematocrit <30%)
Asthma
Prepregnancy weight (<50 kg)
Prior history of IUGR
Chronic hypertension, diabetes mellitus
Collagen vascular disorders such as lupus
Renal disease
Severe maternal malnutrition
Multiple pregnancy
Low maternal age
Preeclampsia
Inherited thrombophilias

decline in birthweight, and in developing countries, severe maternal malnutrition is the leading cause of IUGR. Negative effects on birthweight are most pronounced when starvation occurs in the last trimester.

3. **Multiple pregnancies.** Impaired growth results from failure to provide optimal nutrition for more than one fetus in utero. There is a progressive decrease in weight of singletons, twins, and triplets. In parabiotic twins, the smaller twin has decreased nutrient delivery secondary to abnormal placental blood flow resulting from arteriovenous communication in the chorionic plate.

4. **Maternal drug use.** See also Chapter 95.

   a. **Cigarettes and alcohol.** Chronic abuse of cigarettes or alcohol is demonstrably associated with IUGR. The effects of alcohol and tobacco seem to be dose dependent, with IUGR becoming more serious and predictable with heavy abuse.

   b. **Heroin.** Maternal heroin addiction is also often associated with IUGR.

   c. **Cocaine.** Cocaine use in pregnancy is associated with increased rates of IUGR. The cause of IUGR may be mediated by placental insufficiency or direct toxic effect on the fetus.

   d. **Others.** Other drugs and chemical agents causing IUGR include known teratogens, antimetabolites, and therapeutic agents such as trimethadione, warfarin, and phenytoin. Each of these agents causes characteristic malformation syndromes. Repeated use of antenatal steroids and lithium use are also associated with low birthweight.

5. **Maternal hypoxemia.** Hypoxemia is seen in mothers with hemoglobinopathies, especially sickle cell disease, and they often have IUGR infants. Infants born at high altitudes tend to have lower mean birthweights for gestational age.

6. **Other maternal factors.** Maternal short stature, young maternal age, short interpregnancy interval, uterine anomalies, low socioeconomic class, primiparity, grand multiparity, and low prepregnancy weight are associated with subnormal birthweight.

C. **Placental factors**

1. **Placental insufficiency.** In the first and second trimesters, fetal growth is determined mostly by inherent fetal growth potential. By the third trimester, placental factors (ie, an adequate supply of nutrients) assume major importance for fetal growth. When the duration of pregnancy exceeds the nurturing capacity of the placenta, placental insufficiency results with subsequent impaired fetal growth. This phenomenon occurs mostly in post-term gestations but may occur at any time during gestation.

2. **Anatomic problems.** Various anatomic factors, such as multiple infarcts, aberrant cord insertions, umbilical vascular thrombosis and hemangiomas are described in IUGR placentas. IUGR is twice as common with a two vessel cord pregnancy as compared with three vessel cord pregnancies. Premature placental separation may reduce the surface area exchange, resulting in impaired fetal growth. An adverse intrauterine environment is apt to affect both placental and fetal development; hence IUGR infants usually have small placentas.

3. **Others.** Placental mosaicism where the placental cytogenetics is different from the fetal cytogenetics) may account for ~15% of IUGR. Risk of recurrence is not known. Fibrin deposition in the decidua basalis and intervillous space and mesenchymal dysplasia associated with an increased risk of thrombosis are also associated with IUGR.

D. **Placental pathology in IUGR infants**

1. **Uteroplacental insufficiency** (UPI) is seen in almost 70% of infants with IUGR. Impaired oxygen extraction and nutrient delivery (glucose and amino acids; see later) lead to fetal hypoglycemia and hypoxia. The latter is associated with decrease in cell size and numbers, lighter brain weight, and lower DNA content. Pathologically, inadequate invasion of spiral arteries, trophoblast dysfunction,

increased apoptosis, decrease in the thickness of syncytiotrophoblast, and abnormalities of the villi are seen in the placenta.

2. **IUGR fetuses** have downregulation of placental amino acid and lipoprotein lipase transporters Na^+/K^+ ATPase and Na^+/H^+ exchanger, leading to lower plasma amino acid levels and decreased fatty acid transfer. Genetic imprinting may also play a role (eg, alterations of the placenta-specific gene IGF-2 in knockout mice have IUGR fetuses).

3. **Fetal endocrine responses** include alterations in the hypothalamic- pituitary axis, resulting in elevated corticotropin-releasing hormone, adrenocorticotropic hormone, and cortisol with a decrease in insulin-like growth factor-1 (IGF-1). Thyroid-stimulating hormone is high, but thyroxine and triiodothyronine are low, as are serum vitamin D and osteocalcin. High cortisol levels are associated with decreased postnatal catchup growth and worse neurodevelopmental outcomes.

IV. **Risk factors** are related to fetal, maternal, or placental factors and outlined in Tables 97–1, 97–2, and 97–3.

V. **Clinical presentation.** The patient's history will raise the index of suspicion regarding suboptimal growth. The infant will have a reduced birthweight for gestational age. Using growth charts and the Ballard score can help assess gestational age and intrauterine and postnatal growth. Infants with IUGR have a characteristic physical appearance. They are thin with loose peeling skin (secondary to loss of subcutaneous tissue), a scaphoid abdomen, and a disproportionately large head.

VI. **Diagnosis**

A. **Establishing gestational age.** Determining the correct gestational age is imperative. The last menstrual period, size of the uterus, time of quickening (fluttering movements in the abdomen caused by fetal activity, appreciated by the mother for the first time), and early ultrasound measurements are used to determine gestational age.

B. **Fetal assessment**

1. **Clinical diagnosis.** Manual estimations of weight, serial fundal height measurements, and maternal estimates of fetal activity are simple clinical measures. Imprecision and inconsistency have prevented widespread confidence in these clinical methods.

2. **Ultrasonography.** Because of its reliability to date pregnancy, detect impaired fetal growth by anthropomorphic measurements, and detect fetal anomalies, ultrasonography currently offers the greatest promise for diagnosis. The following anthropomorphic measurements are used in combination to predict growth impairment with a high degree of accuracy.

Table 97–3. PLACENTAL FACTORS IN INTRAUTERINE GROWTH RESTRICTION

Two-vessel cord
Abruptio placentae, placental hematoma, placenta previa
Hemangioma
Single umbilical artery
Infarction
Aberrant cord insertion
Umbilical vessel thrombosis
Circumvallate placentation
Confined placental mosaicism
Massive perivillous fibrin deposition (immune mediated)
Chronic villitis of unknown etiology (VUE)
Placental mesenchymal dysplasia

    a. **Biparietal diameter (BPD).** When serial measurements of BPD are less than optimal, 50–80% of infants have subnormal birthweights.
    b. **Abdominal circumference.** The liver is the first organ to suffer the effects of growth retardation. Reduced growth of the abdominal circumference (<5 mm/week) is the earliest sign of asymmetric growth retardation and diminished glycogen storage. Abdominal circumference <10th percentile for age is suggestive of growth retardation.
    c. **Ratio of head circumference to abdominal circumference.** This ratio normally changes as pregnancy progresses. In the second trimester, the head circumference is greater than the abdominal circumference. At about 32–36 weeks' gestation, the ratio is 1:1, and after 36 weeks the abdominal measurements become larger. Persistence of a head-to-abdomen ratio <1 late in gestation is predictive of **asymmetric IUGR.**
    d. **Femur length.** Femur length appears to correlate well with crown-heel length and provides an early and reproducible measurement of length. Serial measurements of femur length are as effective as head measurements for detecting symmetric IUGR.
    e. **Placental morphology and amniotic fluid assessment** may help in distinguishing a constitutionally small fetus from a growth-retarded fetus. For example, placental aging with oligohydramnios suggests IUGR and fetal jeopardy, whereas normal placental morphology with a normal amount of amniotic fluid suggests a constitutionally small fetus.
    f. **Placental volume measurements** may be helpful in predicting subsequent fetal growth. Placental weight/volume is decreased before fetal growth decreases. IUGR with decreased placental size is more likely to be associated with fetal acidosis.
 3. **Doppler measurements** in both maternal and various fetal vascular beds are increasingly used to detect, monitor, and optimize time of delivery in IUGR infants. Doppler studies are more helpful in diagnosing moderate to severe IUGR than mild IUGR. The various groups of vessels used are as follows:
    a. **Uterine artery.** To predict IUGR as early as 12–14 weeks. Persistent abnormality at 23–24 weeks has nearly 75% sensitivity in predicting IUGR.
    b. **Umbilical artery (UA).** To evaluate placental insufficiency. Normally, the UA resistance declines with pregnancy. Increased pulsatility index (PI), decreased end diastolic velocity (EDV) and absent or reversed EDV (AREDV) occur with worsening fetal compromise. AREDV is associated with 20–68% mortality.
    c. **Fetal cerebral Doppler,** usually the middle cerebral artery pulsatility index (MCA PI) and middle cerebral artery peak systolic velocity (MCA PSV) have been used to assess fetal well-being. With worsening IUGR, MCA PSV increases. Abnormal MCA PI precedes MCA PSV changes. Changes in MCA PI are not as consistent in predicting mortality.
    d. **Venous Doppler** (ductus venosus, vena cava, and umbilical vein [UV]) provides information about fetal cardiovascular and respiratory responses. Decreased venous blood flow in the UV and an abnormal deep or retrograde 'a' wave in ductus venosus is suggestive of ventricular decompensation.
    e. **Aortic isthmus (AoI).** Absolute flow velocities are decreased in growth-restricted fetuses. Retrograde flow in the AoI correlates strongly with adverse perinatal outcome.
 4. **Biophysical profile (BPP)** is used for noninvasive fetal monitoring.
 5. **Cardiotocography (CTG)** is used more commonly in Europe to assess timing of delivery.
 6. **Compensated versus decompensated fetus.** Persistence of UPI results in fetal adaptation to maintain adequate cerebral oxygenation and growth.

    a. **UPI results in increased placental vascular resistance and fetal hypoxemia** by reducing umbilical blood flow. The fetus responds by redistribution of blood to the brain (brain sparing) by cerebral vasodilatation, mesenteric vasoconstriction, preferential shunting through the foramen ovale, increased fractional extraction of oxygen (O_2), polycythemia, and a relative decrease in fetal O_2 consumption. Fetal growth velocity and weight gain are decreased. Nonstress test (NST), BPP, and CTG are normal. Decreased or absent diastolic flow in the umbilical artery, increased diastolic component in the MCA are seen. The fetus is hypoxemic but does not have cerebral hypoxemia at this stage.

    b. **With worsening fetal compromise,** there is cerebral hypoxemia and acidemia associated with no fetal weight gain, oligohydroamnios, and decreased fetal heart rate variability, abnormal NST, CTG, and BPP. Umbilical arteries show absent or reversal of end diastolic flow (AREDV). Deep 'a' wave is seen in the ductus venosus suggestive of ventricular dysfunction. With severe acidosis, MCA PI and MCA PSV decrease, suggesting imminent collapse of the fetus.

C. Neonatal assessment. See also Chapter 4.

  1. **Reduced birthweight** for gestational age is the simplest method of diagnosing IUGR. However, this method tends to misdiagnose constitutionally small infants.

  2. **Physical appearance.** When infants with congenital malformation syndromes and infections are excluded, the remaining groups of IUGR infants have a characteristic physical appearance. These infants in general are thin, with loose, peeling skin because of loss of subcutaneous tissue, a scaphoid abdomen, and a disproportionately large head.

  3. **Appropriate growth charts should be used.** Several growth charts are available to assess intrauterine and postnatal growth.

  4. **A ponderal index** <10th percentile helps identify neonates with IUGR, especially those with birthweight <2500 g.

  5. **Ballard score.** Gestational age can also be assessed by means of the Ballard scoring system. This examination is accurate within 2 weeks of gestation in infants weighing <999 g at birth and is most accurate at 30–42 h of age. Plotting the individual growth parameter alone may not show IUGR. Use the ponderal index as shown in Section I. IUGR infants have a higher rating on this scale than premature infants with similar weights. See Chapter 4 for Ballard examination and scoring.

D. Observe for the following complications:

  1. **Hypoxia**

    a. **Perinatal asphyxia.** IUGR infants frequently have birth asphyxia because they tolerate the stress of labor poorly. IUGR accounts for a large proportion of stillborn infants with hypoxia in utero.

    b. **Persistent pulmonary hypertension (persistent fetal circulation).** Many IUGR infants are subjected to chronic intrauterine hypoxia, which results in abnormal thickening of the smooth muscles of the small pulmonary arterioles. This, in turn, reduces pulmonary blood flow and results in varying degrees of pulmonary artery hypertension. Because of this, IUGR infants are at risk for persistent pulmonary hypertension. Hyaline membrane disease is less frequently seen in IUGR because these infants tend to manifest advanced pulmonary maturity secondary to chronic intrauterine stress.

    c. **Respiratory distress syndrome.** Several reports suggest accelerated fetal pulmonary maturation in association with IUGR secondary to chronic intrauterine stress. McIntire et al suggest that the incidence of respiratory distress syndrome is inversely proportional to the gestational age and birthweight percentile.

    d. **Meconium aspiration.** Postterm IUGR infants are at risk for meconium aspiration.

    e. **Patent ductus arteriosus (PDA).** Conflicting data suggest that hemodynamically significant PDA may be bigger and occur earlier in IUGR infants than in appropriate for gestational age (AGA) infants, but spontaneous closure of PDA is more frequent in IUGR infants <1000 g birthweight. IUGR infants with PDA are at greater risk for pulmonary hemorrhage, intraventricular hemorrhage (IVH), necrotizing enterocolitis (NEC), and renal failure.

2. **Hypothermia.** Thermoregulation is compromised in IUGR infants because of diminished subcutaneous fat insulation. Infants with IUGR secondary to fetal malnutrition late in gestation tend to be thin as a result of loss of subcutaneous fat.

3. **Metabolic**

    a. **Hypoglycemia.** Carbohydrate metabolism is seriously disturbed, and IUGR infants are highly susceptible to hypoglycemia as a consequence of diminished glycogen reserves and decreased capacity for gluconeogenesis. Oxidation of free fatty acids and triglycerides is reduced in IUGR infants, which limits alternate fuel sources. Hyperinsulinism, excess sensitivity to insulin, and deficient catecholamine release during hypoglycemia suggest abnormality of counterregulatory hormone mechanisms during periods of hypoglycemia in IUGR infants. Hypothermia may potentate the problem of hypoglycemia.

    b. **Hyperglycemia.** Very low birthweight infants have low insulin secretion, resulting in hyperglycemia.

    c. **Hypocalcemia.** Hypocalcemia may occur in IUGR infants after asphyxia.

    d. **Liver disease.** IUGR infants are at higher risk for developing cholestasis associated with parenteral nutrition. There is also an increased risk of nonfatty liver disease in children born SGA.

    e. **Other.** Hypertriglyceridemia, increased sympathetic tone, and reduced concentrations of IGF-I are associated with increased aortic intimal thickness in IUGR infants.

4. **Hematologic disorders.** Hyperviscosity and polycythemia may result from increased erythropoietin levels secondary to fetal hypoxia associated with IUGR. Thrombocytopenia, neutropenia, and altered coagulation profile are also seen in IUGR infants. Polycythemia may also contribute to hypoglycemia and lead to cerebral injury. There are an increased number of nucleated red cells secondary to extramedullary hematopoiesis. Persistent elevated nucleated red cell counts are associated with worse prognosis.

5. **Altered immunity.** IUGR infants have decreased immunoglobulin G (IgG) levels. In addition, the thymus is reduced in size by 50% and peripheral blood lymphocytes are decreased. Reduction in total white cell count, neutrophils, monocyte and lymphocyte subpopulations, and thrombocytopenia may occur, and selective suppression of helper and cytotoxic T cells can be seen.

6. **Others.** IUGR infants are at increased risk of developing NEC, particularly when associated with an absent or reversed end diastolic flow on an umbilical artery Doppler. Preterm IUGR infants are at increased risk of pulmonary hemorrhage, chronic lung disease, more severe IVH, NEC, and renal failure.

VII. **Management.** Antenatal diagnosis is the key to proper management of IUGR.

    A. **History of risk factors.** The presence of maternal risk factors should alert the obstetrician to the likelihood of fetal growth retardation. Ultrasonography confirms the diagnosis. Correctable causes of impaired fetal growth warrant immediate attention.

    B. **Delivery and resuscitation.** The optimal timing for delivery of IUGR infants is still debated, but Doppler measurements provide an important tool for monitoring fetal well-being. However, in a large trial no differences in perinatal mortality or neurodevelopmental quotient were noted at 2 years when IUGR infants were delivered early or late. IUGR infants have a two- to threefold increased risk of preterm delivery when fetal growth standards are used for diagnosis. IUGR infants delivered before 28–30 weeks have worse outcomes. Outcomes are more favorable with cesarean delivery. Delivery is usually undertaken when the lungs are mature or when biophysical data obtained by monitoring reveal fetal distress. Labor is particularly stressful to IUGR fetuses. Skilled resuscitation should be available because perinatal depression is common.

C. **Prevention of heat loss.** Meticulous care should be taken to conserve body heat (see Chapter 6).

D. **Hypoglycemia.** Close monitoring of blood glucose levels is essential for all IUGR infants. Hypoglycemia should be treated promptly with parenteral dextrose and early feeding, as outlined in Chapter 55.

E. **Hematologic disorders.** A central hematocrit reading should be obtained to detect polycythemia.

F. **Congenital infection.** IUGR infants should be examined for congenital malformations or signs of congenital infections. Many intrauterine infections are clinically silent, and screening for these should be done routinely in IUGR infants. (See the discussion of TORCH infections in Chapter 127.)

G. **Genetic anomalies.** Screening for genetic anomalies should be done as indicated by the physical examination.

VIII. **Prognosis.** Mortality increases with decreasing gestational age when IUGR is also present. Mortality decreases by 48% for each week that the fetus remains in utero before 30 weeks' gestation. **Neurodevelopmental morbidities are seen 5–10 times more often in IUGR infants compared with AGA infants.** Neurodevelopmental outcome depends not only on the cause of IUGR but also on the adverse events in the neonatal course (eg, perinatal depression or hypoglycemia). Many studies reveal evidence of minimal brain dysfunction, including hyperactivity, short attention span, and learning problems. Preterm IUGR infants also show alterations in early neurobehavioral functions like attention-interaction capacity and cognitive and memory dysfunction that persist. Increased risk of cerebral palsy, a wide spectrum of learning disabilities, mental retardation, pervasive developmental disorders, and neuropsychiatric disorders are seen in later years.

A. **Symmetric versus asymmetric IUGR.** Infants with symmetric IUGR caused by decreased growth potential generally have a poor outcome, whereas those with asymmetric IUGR in which brain growth is spared usually have a good outcome. Neuroimaging studies using MRI and ultrasound show that preterm IUGR infants have a high incidence of white matter loss and reduced myelination in the internal capsule associated with decreased cortical gray matter volume by as much as 28%. The total brain volume is also reduced by 10% compared with AGA infants, particularly in the hippocampal, parietal, and parieto-occipital areas. These alterations may be due both to a decrease in size and number of neurons, neuronal degeneration, and loss of dendritic branches as shown in animal models.

B. **Preterm IUGR** infants have a higher incidence of abnormalities than the general population because they are subjected to the risks of prematurity in addition to the risks of IUGR. Outcomes are significantly poorer for children whose brain growth failure occurred before 26 weeks' gestation.

C. **Chromosomal disorders.** IUGR infants with major chromosomal disorders have a 100% incidence of disability.

D. **Congenital infections.** Infants with congenital rubella or cytomegalovirus infection with microcephaly have a poor outcome, with a disability rate >50%.

E. **Learning ability.** The school performance of IUGR infants is significantly influenced by social class; children from higher social classes score better on achievement tests.

F. **Adult disorders.** Epidemiologic evidence indicates that obesity, insulin-resistant diabetes, hypertension, and cardiovascular diseases are more common among adults who were IUGR at birth. Alterations in coronary vascular bed, increased thickness of the interventricular septum, decreased left ventricular end-diastolic diameter, altered elastin and collagen content, decreased aortic compliance, increased resting heart rate, and elevated blood pressure have been noted in adolescents and young adults.

G. **Risk for recurrence of IUGR** in subsequent pregnancies depends on the underlying condition. The presence of previous fetal growth retardation, preeclampsia, abruption, infarction, and acquired or inherited thrombophilias increase the risk of fetal growth retardation in the subsequent pregnancies. Placental pathologic examination should be attempted in all IUGR infants. Elimination of known risk factors like smoking, drugs, and maternal anemia can help decrease the risk of fetal growth retardation. In selected cases, folic acid, aspirin, and supplementation with L-arginine to improve placental blood flow may improve outcomes. Early antenatal screening and serial Doppler ultrasounds are helpful in management.

Selected References

Barker DJP: Fetal and infant origin of adult disease. *Brit Med J* 1993;301:1111.

Baschat AA: Doppler application in the delivery timing of the preterm growth restricted fetus: another step in the right direction. *Ultrasound Obstet Gynecol* 2004;23:111-118.

Baschat AA: Fetal responses to placental insufficiency: An update. *Brit J Obstet Gynaecol* 2004;111:1031-1041.

Baserga MC, Sola A: Intrauterine growth restriction impacts tolerance to total parenteral nutrition in extremely low birth weight infants. *J Perinatol* 2004;24:476-481.

Battaglia FC, Lubchenco LO: A practical classification of newborn infants by weight and gestational age. *J Pediatr* 1967;17:159.

Botsis D et al: Doppler assessment of the intrauterine growth-restricted fetus. *Ann NY Acad Sci* 2006;1092:297-303.

Brodszki J et al: Impaired vascular growth in late adolescence after intrauterine growth restriction. *Circulation* 2005;111:2623-2628.

Del Rio M et al: Doppler assessment of the aortic isthmus and perinatal outcome in preterm fetuses with severe intrauterine growth restriction. *Ultrasound Obstet Gynecol* 2008; 31:41-47.

Fouron JC, Audibert F: Best timing of birth in placental insufficiency. *NeoReviews* 2006; 4:e195-e202.

Fowden AL et al: Intrauterine programming of physiological systems: causes and consequences. *Physiology* 2006;21:29-37.

Garite TJ et al: Intrauterine growth restriction increases morbidity and mortality among premature neonates. *Am J Obstet Gynecol* 2004;191:481-487.

Hack M, Fanaroff AA: Outcomes of children of extremely low birthweight and gestational age in 1990s. *Semin Neonatol* 2000;5:89-106.

Hay WW et al: Intrauterine growth restriction. *NeoReviews* 2001;2:129-138.

Jones HN et al: Regulation of placental nutrient transport. *Placenta* 2007;28:763-774.

Kamoji VM et al: Extremely growth-retarded infants: is there a viability centile? *Pediatrics* 2006;118;758-763.

Kinzler W, Kaminsky L: Fetal growth restriction and subsequent pregnancy risks. *Semin Perinatol* 2007;31:126-134.

Kleigman RM, Das UG: Intrauterine growth retardation. In Fanaroff AA, Martin RJ (eds): *Neonatal-Perinatal Medicine: Diseases of the Newborn.* St. Louis, MO: Mosby, 2002;13:228-262.

Koch J et al: Prevalence of spontaneous closure of the ductus arteriosus in neonates at a birth weight of 1000 grams or less. *Pediatrics* 2006;117:1113-1121.

Koklu E et al: Increased aortic intima-media thickness is related to lipid profile in newborns with intrauterine growth restriction. *Horm Res* 2006;65:269-275.

Lackman F et al: The risks of spontaneous preterm delivery and perinatal mortality in relation to size at birth according to fetal versus neonatal growth standards. *Am J Obstet Gynecol* 2001;84:946-953.

Mari G et al: Middle cerebral artery peak systolic velocity: a new Doppler parameter in the assessment of growth restricted fetuses. *Ultrasound Obstet Gynecol* 2007;29:310-316.

Mari G et al: Gestational age at delivery and Doppler waveforms in the very preterm intrauterine growth-restricted fetuses as predictors of perinatal mortality. *J Ultrasound Med* 2007;26:555-559.

McIntire DD et al: Birth weight in relation to morbidity and mortality among newborn infants. *N Engl J Med* 1999;340:1234.

Nobili V et al: Intrauterine growth retardation, insulin resistance, and nonalcoholic fatty liver disease in children. *Diabetes Care* 2007;10:2638-2640.

Orro AS, Dixon SD: Perinatal cocaine and methamphetamine exposure. *J Pediatr* 1987;111:571.

Pardi G et al: Placental fetal relationship in IUGR fetuses: a review. *Placenta* 2002;23(suppl A): S136-S141.

Rakza T et al: Early hemodynamic consequences of patent ductus arteriosus in preterm infants with intrauterine growth restriction. *J Pediatr* 2007;151:624-628.

Sherry B et al: Evaluation and recommendations for growth references for very low birth weight (≤1500 grams) infants in the United States. *Pediatrics* 2003;111:750-758.

Sibley CP et al: Placental phenotypes of intrauterine growth. *Pediatr Res* 2005;58:827-832.

Skilton MR et al: Aortic wall thickness in newborns with intrauterine growth restriction. *Lancet* 2005;365:1484-1486.

The GRIT study group: Infant wellbeing at 2 years of age in growth restriction intervention trial. *Lancet* 2004;364:513-520.

Thomas P et al: A new look at intrauterine growth and impact of race, altitude, and gender. *Pediatrics* 2000;106:e21.

Thompson DK et al: Perinatal risk factors altering regional brain structure in the preterm infant. *Brain* 2007;130:667-677.

Tolsa CB et al: Early alterations in structural and functional brain development in premature infants born with intrauterine growth restriction. *Pediatr Res* 2004;56:132-138.

Urban G et al: State of the art: non-invasive ultrasound assessment of the uteroplacental circulation. *Semin Perinatol* 2007;31:232-239.

98 Lyme Disease and Pregnancy

I. **Definition.** Lyme disease was first reported in 1977, following an unusual cluster of adults and children with oligoarticular arthritis in a certain neighborhood of Lyme, Connecticut. Subsequently, a multisystem disease was described and attributed to the spirochete *Borrelia burgdorferi*. Lyme disease manifests as a spectrum of skin, musculoskeletal, cardiac, and neurologic findings. It is a vector-borne disease following the bite of an Ixodes tick—usually the black-legged *Ixodes scapularis*, commonly known as the deer tick.

The species Ixodes includes additional subspecies (eg, *I. pacificus, I. dammini,* and *I. ricinus*) that contribute to a worldwide distribution of the disease and known to be endemic in North and South America, Europe, Asia, Africa, and Australia. **Prenatal exposure to B. burgdorferi and the development of gestational borreliosis can result in maternal Lyme disease with placentitis and transplacental infection of the fetus and newborn.**

II. **Incidence.** In 2006, 19,931 cases of Lyme disease were reported to the Centers for Disease Control and Prevention, an incidence of nearly double that reported in 1991 and 1992. In the United States, 44 continental states reported cases of Lyme disease, with an incidence of 8.2 in 100,000 nationwide. In the 10 northeastern states with greatest disease prevalence, the incidence was 30.2 in 100,000. No specific data for the number of pregnancy related Lyme disease are available; however, for U.S. women in the childbearing age groups 15–19 years to 40–44 years, for the period 1992–2004, the disease incidence was lowest for the 15–19 year old group at 4 in 100,000 and highest for the older group at 8 in 100,000. These data suggest a relatively low exposure to Lyme borreliosis for childbearing women. Estimates for active infection following exposure to a deer-tick bite are only 1–3%. Presumably the number of infected pregnant women in the United States is small.

III. **Pathophysiology**

A. **Transmission.** The Ixodes tick lives a 2-year life cycle consisting of three life stages: larval, nymph, and adult. The preferred murine reservoirs for the larval and nymph tick are the white-footed field mouse, and for the adult tick it is the white-tailed deer. The larval stage emerges from eggs in early summer and feeds on previously infected mice from which they acquire the *Borrelia burgdorferi* spirochete. The infected nymph stage emerges the next spring and is the most likely source of human infection because the activity of the feeding nymph corresponds to the outdoor activity of humans in spring and summer. The adult tick may infect as well before laying eggs in summer and dying soon afterward.

B. **Human spirochetemia.** Following the tick bite, the incubation period of the spirochetes is 1–55 days with a median of 11 days, followed by the first clinical signs of disease. The disease is characterized by "early" and "late" manifestations. Early disease is in two stages. Early stage I is confined to reactions in the skin. Early stage II is dissemination of the spirochetes from the site of the bite through the skin and into the bloodstream and organ tissues. Spirochete dissemination is presumed to be facilitated by the surface of the organism binding to human plasminogen and subsequently binding to integrins, matrix glycosaminoglycans, and extracellular matrix proteins. These complexes may explain the propensity of the spirochetes to localize to collagen fibrils in the extracellular matrices of the heart, nervous system, and bone joints. Late Lyme disease (or stage III) occurs months to a year or more after dissemination.

C. **Placentitis and transplacental disease.** By the end of the 1980s, a number of case reports had confirmed the transplacental passage of *B. burgdorferi* by way of identification of spirochetes in placental tissues, umbilical vessels, and fetal brain, heart, spleen, kidneys, bone marrow, liver, and adrenal glands. Moreover, in 1989, MacDonald reported finding 13 cases of transplacental transmission of *B. burgdorferi* by way of fetal tissue cultures or immunoserology.

D. **Newborn disease secondary to B. burgdorferi remains undefined.** A number of reviews have documented fetal demise, stillbirths, preterm and near-term births, and newborns with hyperbilirubinemia, petechial rashes, respiratory distress, and various birth defects, all thought to be related to gestational borreliosis. The most frequently studied newborn condition has been a variety of congenital heart defects, but none have been confirmed as a clinical syndrome unique to infants of mothers with documented gestational borreliosis. Indeed, a number of infants with evidence for either placental disease or positive serology have been reported as being well at birth and in follow-up.

IV. **Risk factors.** Maternal Lyme disease is a result of exposure to deer ticks in known endemic areas of the United States or other endemic areas of the world. Once the expectant mother presents with a history of outdoor exposure or has dogs or cats in the home, possibly known tick embedment, and cutaneous lesions consistent with early (stage I) disease, prompt antibiotic therapy lessens the risk for transplacental transmission of spirochetes. There are no other known predilections to Lyme disease related to pregnancy.

V. **Clinical presentation**

A. **Maternal**

1. **Early disease (stage I).** The cutaneous stage begins with a papule at the site of the tick bite, becoming an annular erythematous migrating rash (also known as erythema chronicum migrans) with central clearing. Rash may last 3–4 weeks. The early stage is often accompanied by low-grade fever, evanescent arthralgias, myalgia, fatigue, headache, and neck muscle stiffness.

2. **Dissemination (stage II).** Lyme disease progresses over time, usually 30 days and beyond, to present with persistence of the rash with more definition as annular and migratory. This stage is accompanied by worsening fatigue, severe malaise, and migratory musculoskeletal pain. Approaching 6 weeks postexposure in the untreated patient, target organs of systemic disease become more apparent, namely arthritis, nervous system involvement, and cardiac manifestations. The arthritis may be monoarticular or pauciarticular with joint swelling. The central and peripheral nervous systems form a triad of manifestation starting with meningitis, and progressing to cranial nerve palsies and peripheral radiculopathies.

3. **Late Lyme disease (stage III).** Months after exposure to disease, arthralgias and arthritis persist and recur. They may be monoarticular or oligoarticular. The knees are the most often affected joint with marked swelling, but with pain that is less than that of rheumatoid type arthritis. On rare occasions chronic neurologic conditions of encephalopathy, demyelination, or dementia have been reported.

B. **Neonatal**

1. **As already noted, no specific clinical presentation of Lyme disease in the newborn or neonatal period has been described.** Of importance is the maternal history of disease, and whether or not she has been adequately treated. Placental pathology in suspect cases may offer information that would prompt testing and perhaps treatment for at-risk neonates.

2. **Congenital Lyme disease as a clinical entity has been reviewed and found not to be substantive.** In particular, congenital heart defects have been reviewed in large follow-up studies of mothers with positive *B. burgdorferi* serology. Williams et al reported in 1999 a cohort study of > 5000 cord blood serologic surveys within a highly endemic area for Lyme disease (New York State). They did not find any correlation of congenital heart defects or other major or minor malformations attributable to positive maternal or cord blood serology. In 2001, Elliott et al reported a search of the world literature for teratogenic effects of gestational Lyme disease. They concluded that no effect was found, and any otherwise adverse pregnancy outcome was of low risk in the face of adequately treated gestational borreliosis. More recently, Walsh et al searched the worldwide literature for obstetric associations to Lyme disease with these conclusions:

a. **Women who are seropositive at conception** have no increased incidence of adverse pregnancy.

b. **Women who develop a confirmed diagnosis** of Lyme disease in pregnancy should receive appropriate antimicrobial treatment.

c. **Women with Lyme disease in pregnancy** and who have been appropriately treated have shown no association with specific adverse fetal outcomes.

VI. **Diagnosis.** Laboratory testing for Lyme disease should follow, if careful history taking and physical examination strongly suggest active disease.

    A. **Early (stage I) disease.** Diagnosis is made largely on clinical grounds (history of exposure, rash, and symptoms). Antibodies are slow to develop, and false-negative and false-positive test results are frequently encountered.

    B. **Early (stage II) disease.** Dissemination of the disease is diagnosed clinically as described earlier, and the following serologic screening tests should be obtained:

        1. **Enzyme immunoassay (EIA).**

        2. **Immunofluorescent-antibody assay (IFA).**

        3. **If both tests are negative, no further testing is needed,** and clinical reevaluation for other conditions is indicated. Screening tests are known to have high false-positive rates.

        4. **If either or both are positive, they should be followed by:**

            a. **Western immunoblot standardized for antibodies to *B. burgdorferi.*** Subsequently, positive Western blot assays should include specific immunoglobulin G (IgG) and immunoglobulin M (IgM). If the Western blot assays are negative, the false-positive EIA or IFA testing suggests other spirochetal diseases, that is, syphilis, leptospirosis, an intercurrent viral disease (eg, Epstein–Barr), or an autoimmune condition such as lupus erythematosus.

    C. **Late disease.** If late disease is suspected, only a positive IgG immunoblot is needed.

VII. **Management**

    A. **Maternal**

        1. **Early disease (stage I)**

            a. **Amoxicillin,** 500 mg orally three times daily for 14–28 days.

            b. **Cefuroxime axetil (alternative),** 500 mg orally twice daily for 14–28 days. *(**Note:** Doxycycline is the drug of choice for Lyme disease, except in pregnancy or in children <8 years of age.)*

    B. **Newborn**

        1. **Treat if infant is thought to be symptomatic at birth,** especially if mother is confirmed with Lyme disease but has not been adequately or appropriately treated. Consider:

            a. **Ceftriaxone,** 75–100 mg/kg/day intravenously (IV) divided every 12 h for 14–28 days.

            b. **Penicillin (alternative),** 200,000–400,000 units/kg/day, IV divided every 4 h for 14–28 days. Obtain infectious disease consult prior to starting therapy.

            c. **Cefotaxime (alternative),** 150 mg/kg/day, IV divided every 8 h for 14–28 days.

        2. **If the infant is asymptomatic at birth,** given low risk for active disease, current recommendations do not call for empirical treatment, especially if the mother was appropriately treated during pregnancy. Placental pathology may offer information helpful in the decision to treat or not; consultation with an infectious disease specialist is recommended.

        3. **Lyme disease is *not* a contraindication for breast-feeding.** No evidence is known for the passage of *B. burgdorferi* to the infant through breast-feeding.

VIII. **Prognosis.** Prompt diagnosis and antibiotic therapy is essential. One study revealed 25% of infants had adverse outcomes, 15% were sick or had an abnormality, 8% resulted in fetal death, and 2% resulted in neonatal death. Antibiotic therapy resulted in only 15% with adverse outcomes. Long-term follow-up is important for recurrence of the disease.

Selected References

American Academy of Pediatrics. Lyme disease. In Pickering LK et al (eds): *Red Book: 2006 Report of the Committee on Infectious Diseases,* 27th ed. Elk Grove Village, IL: American Academy of Pediatrics, 2006;428-433.

Centers for Disease Control and Prevention: Lyme disease case definition for public health purposes. *Morb Mort Wkly Rep* 1997;46(RR):20-1.

Centers for Disease Control and Prevention: Lyme Disease—United States 2003–2005. *Morb Mortal Wkly Rep* 2007;56(23):573-576.

Elliott DJ et al: Teratogen update: Lyme disease. *Teratology* 2001;64:276-281.

Gibbs RS et al: Maternal and fetal infectious disorders. In Creasy RK et al (eds): *Maternal-Fetal Medicine: Principles and Practice*, 5th ed. Philadelphia, PA: Elsevier Saunders, 2004:758-760.

MacDonald AB: Gestational Lyme borreliosis: implications for the fetus. *Rheum Dis Clin North Am* 1989;15:657-677.

Shapiro ED, Gerber MA: Lyme disease. In Remington JS et al (eds): *Infectious Diseases of the Fetus and Newborn Infant*, 6th ed. Philadelphia, PA: Elsevier Saunders, 2006:485-497.

Walsh CA et al: Lyme disease in pregnancy: case report and review of the literature. *Obstet Gynecol Surv* 2007;62:41-50.

Williams CL et al: Maternal Lyme disease and congenital malformations: a cord blood serosurvey in endemic and control areas. *Paediatr Perinat Epidemiol* 1995;9:320-330.

99 Magnesium Disorders (Hypomagnesemia, Hypermagnesemia)

The disturbances of magnesium (Mg^{+2}) and calcium (Ca^{+2}) are closely interrelated. Calcium disorders are discussed in Chapter 78.

HYPOMAGNESEMIA

I. **Definition.** Normal serum levels for Mg^{+2} are typically given as 0.5–1.0 mmol/L (1.2–2.6 mg/dL). Hypomagnesemia is usually seen as any value <0.66 mmol/L (1.6 mg/dL); however, clinical signs do not manifest until levels have dropped <0.5 mmol/L (1.2 mg/dL).

II. **Incidence.** True incidence in neonates is not well characterized, but neonates appear to be more predisposed than other groups of patients.

III. **Pathophysiology.** Mg^{+2} is a key trace element for maintaining skeletal integrity, and it acts as a catalyst for intracellular enzymes for adenosine triphosphate (ATP) activation in skeletal and myocardial contractility. It is also integral to protein synthesis, vitamin D metabolism, parathyroid function, and calcium homeostasis.

IV. **Risk factors**
   A. **Hypocalcemia.**
   B. **Inadequate intake of Mg^{+2}.**
   C. **Infant of diabetic mother** reflecting maternal Mg^{+2} deficiency secondary to gestational diabetes.
   D. **Intrauterine growth restriction,** especially if the mother had preeclampsia.
   E. **Inherited renal wasting.**
   F. **Hypoparathyroidism.**
   G. **Associated hypocalciuria and nephrocalcinosis.**
   H. **Secondary to furosemide- or gentamicin-induced loss.**
   I. **Citrated blood exchange transfusions.**
V. **Clinical presentation**
   A. Same as in hypocalcemia (Chapter 78, Section V); may also present as seizures.
   B. May be masked as hypocalcemia but with symptoms that persist after adequate calcium gluconate therapy.

VI. **Diagnosis.** Laboratory testing to establish serum levels as noted earlier.
   A. **Serum magnesium levels.**
   B. **Total and ionized calcium levels.**
VII. **Management.** Acute hypomagnesemia should be treated with **intravenous magnesium sulfate.** See Chapter 132 for dosing information. Infusion must be monitored closely for cardiac arrhythmias and hypotension. Maintenance Mg^{+2} can be by parenteral nutrition solutions or by oral feeds with a fivefold dilution of Mg^{+2} salt solution.
VIII. **Prognosis.** Hypomagnesemia generally has a good outcome if diagnosed promptly and treated adequately. The exception is a clinical presentation that includes hypomagnesemia-induced seizures with follow-up studies suggesting ≥20% incidence of neurologic abnormalities.

HYPERMAGNESEMIA

I. **Definition.** Reference levels of serum Mg^{+2} signifying hypermagnesemia vary from >1.15 mmol/L (2.3 mg/dL) to >1.5 mmol/L (3.0 mg/dL). Hypermagnesemia is uncommon in a NICU population of patients, but in certain circumstances it must be recognized.
II. **Incidence.** Occurs rarely except in infants whose mothers were treated with Mg^{+2} sulfate, where it occurs more frequently.
III. **Pathophysiology.** Increased serum Mg^{+2} levels depress the central nervous system and decrease skeletal muscle contractility.
IV. **Risk factors**
   A. Increased maternal serum levels following Mg^{+2} sulfate therapy for pregnancy-related hypertension or preeclampsia (most common cause).
   B. Excessive Mg^{+2} sulfate administration to an infant for hypomagnesemia (iatrogenic medication error) or following administration of Mg^{+2} containing antacid; especially if hydration and urine output are low. Hypermagnesemia can also be caused by magnesium sulfate enemas, which are contraindicated in neonates.
V. **Clinical presentation**
   A. Birth depression, hypotonia, hypotension, hyporeflexia.
   B. Respiratory depression, apnea.
   C. Poor suck, decreased gastrointestinal motility, increased gastric aspirates, abdominal distention, and delayed meconium passage.
   D. Meconium plug syndrome, intestinal perforation.
   E. Urinary retention.
   F. Symptoms may mimic hypercalcemia.
   G. Paradoxically, hypermagnesemia may be asymptomatic despite appreciable Mg^{+2} levels.
VI. **Diagnosis**
   A. **Laboratory studies**
      1. Serum Mg^{+2} determination.
      2. Serum calcium levels. Always determine calcium levels with Mg^{+2} abnormalities.
   B. **Electrocardiogram** may reveal a shortened Q-T interval.
VII. **Management**
   A. Urinary excretion is the only mechanism for decreasing serum Mg^{+2} levels. Hydration is paramount; usually by intravenous route if patient is symptomatic. Monitoring of serum electrolytes, urine output, and acid-base status is needed.
   B. With acute symptomatology, IV calcium gluconate in dosage as for hypocalcemia (Chapter 78) may relieve symptoms.
   C. Furosemide diuresis may facilitate Mg^{+2} excretion, but close monitoring of electrolytes is needed.
   D. Aminoglycosides should not be used because they may potentiate the neuromuscular manifestations of hypermagnesemia.

E. Respiratory support may be needed in severely effected infants (eg, severe apnea).

F. Only rarely has exchange transfusion or peritoneal dialysis been needed.

VIII. **Prognosis.** Typically it is good following treatment, especially if normal renal function has been preserved.

Selected References

Banerjee S et al: Lower whole blood ionized magnesium concentrations in hypocalcemic infants of gestational diabetic mothers. *Magnes Res* 2003;16:127-130.

Ernst JA, Neal PR: Minerals and trace elements. In Polin RA, Fox WW (eds): *Fetal and Neonatal Physiology*, 2nd ed. Philadelphia, PA: Saunders, 1998:332-343.

Hsu SC, Levine MA: Perinatal calcium metabolism: physiology and pathophysiology. *Semin Neonatol* 2004;9:23-36.

Maggioni A et al: Intravenous correction of neonatal hypomagnesemia: effect on ionized magnesium. *J Pediatr* 1998;132:652-655.

Narchi H:Delayed intestinal transit and arrhythmias due to iatrogenic neonatal hypermagnesemia. *Int Pediatr* 2002;17(3):154-155.

100 Meconium Aspiration

I. **Definition.** Meconium is the first intestinal discharge of the newborn infant and is composed of epithelial cells, fetal hair, mucus, and bile. Intrauterine stress may cause in utero passage of meconium into the amniotic fluid. The meconium-stained amniotic fluid may be aspirated by the fetus when fetal gasping or deep breathing movements are stimulated by hypoxia and hypercapnia. The presence of meconium in the trachea may cause airway obstruction as well as an inflammatory response, resulting in severe respiratory distress. The presence of meconium in amniotic fluid can be a **warning sign of fetal distress** but is not a sensitive independent marker of fetal distress. Mothers with meconium-stained amniotic fluid should be carefully monitored during labor.

All infants that are meconium stained do not develop meconium aspiration syndrome (MAS). MAS is defined by Faranoff as respiratory distress in an infant born through meconium-stained amniotic fluid (MSAF) whose symptoms cannot be otherwise explained. Hallmarks include early onset of respiratory distress in a meconium-stained infant with poor lung compliance, hypoxemia, and a characteristic radiograph of the lungs.

II. **Incidence.** The incidence of meconium-stained amniotic fluid (MSAF) varies from 8–20% of all deliveries. Of infants born through a meconium-stained amniotic fluid. 5% go on to develop meconium aspiration syndrome. Meconium aspiration primarily affects **term and postmature infants.** The passage of meconium in an asphyxiated infant <34 weeks' gestation is unusual and may represent bilious reflux secondary to intestinal obstruction.

III. **Pathophysiology**

A. **In utero passage of meconium.** Control of fetal meconium passage depends on hormonal and parasympathetic neural maturation. After 34 weeks' gestation, the incidence of meconium-stained amniotic fluid increases from 1.6% between 34 and 37 weeks' gestation to 30% at ≥42 weeks. The exact mechanisms for in utero passage of meconium remain unclear, but fetal distress and vagal stimulation are two probable factors.

B. **Aspiration of meconium.** After intrauterine passage of meconium, deep irregular respiration or gasping, either in utero or during labor and delivery, can cause aspiration of the meconium-stained amniotic fluid. Before delivery, the progression of the aspirated meconium is, as a rule, impeded by the presence of the viscous liquid that normally fills the fetal lung and airways. Therefore, the distal progression occurs mostly after birth in conjunction with the reabsorption of lung fluid. Early consequences of meconium aspiration include airway obstruction, decreased lung compliance, and increased expiratory large airway resistance.

1. **Airway obstruction.** Thick meconium-stained amniotic fluid can result in acute upper airway obstruction. As the aspirated meconium progresses distally, total or partial airway obstruction may occur. In areas of total obstruction, atelectasis develops, but in areas of partial obstruction a ball-valve phenomenon occurs, resulting in air trapping and alveolar hyperexpansion. Air trapping increases the risk of air leak to 20–50%.

2. **Chemical pneumonitis.** With distal progression of meconium, chemical pneumonitis develops, with resulting bronchiolar edema and narrowing of the small airways. Meconium at the alveolar level may inactivate existing surfactant. Uneven ventilation resulting from areas of partial obstruction, atelectasis, and superimposed pneumonitis causes carbon dioxide retention and hypoxemia.

3. **Pulmonary hypertension.** A third of infants with meconium aspiration develop persistent pulmonary hypertension of newborn (PPHN). Meconium aspirated into the lung stimulates the release of proinflammatory cytokines and vasoactive substances. Pulmonary vascular resistance also increases as a direct result of alveolar hypoxia, acidosis, and hyperinflation of the lungs. The increase in pulmonary vascular resistance may lead to atrial and ductal right-to-left shunting and further hypoxia.

IV. **Risk factors.** The following factors are associated with an increased risk of meconium passage and subsequent tracheal aspiration:
A. **Postterm pregnancy.**
B. **Preeclampsia-eclampsia.**
C. **Maternal hypertension.**
D. **Maternal diabetes mellitus.**
E. **Abnormal fetal heart rate and non reassuring fetal heart rate tracing.**
F. **Intrauterine growth retardation.**
G. **Abnormal biophysical profile.**
H. **Oligohydramnios.**
I. **Heavy smoking, chronic respiratory or cardiovascular disease in the mother.**
J. **Low five minute apgar score.**
K. **Presence of fetal distress.**
L. **Ethnicity.** Black Americans and Africans have an increased risk when compared to other ethnic groups. Pacific Islander and indigenous Australian ethnicity also have increased risk.
M. **Homebirth.** An increased risk of MAS was noted after a planned home birth.

V. **Clinical presentation.** The presentation of an infant who has aspirated meconium-stained amniotic fluid is variable. Symptoms depend on the severity of the hypoxic insult and the amount and viscosity of the meconium aspirated.
A. **General features**
1. **The infant.** Infants with meconium aspiration syndrome often exhibit signs of postmaturity: They are small for gestational age with long nails and peeling yellow- or green-stained skin. These infants may have respiratory distress at birth or in the transition period. If there has been significant perinatal asphyxia, they may have respiratory depression with poor respiratory effort and decreased muscle tone. Meconium staining on the skin is proportional to the length of exposure and meconium concentration. With heavy meconium, staining of the umbilical cord begins within 15 min of exposure and with light meconium after

an hour. Yellow staining of the newborn's nails requires 4–6 h; staining of the vernix caseosa takes ~12 h.

2. **The amniotic fluid.** The meconium present in amniotic fluid varies in appearance and viscosity, ranging from a thin green-stained fluid to a thick "pea soup" consistency. Although meconium aspiration syndrome can occur in the presence of thin stained amniotic fluid, the majority of infants who become ill have a history of thick meconium-stained fluid.

B. **Airway obstruction.** Early meconium aspiration syndrome is characterized by airway obstruction. Large amounts of thick meconium, if not removed, can result in an acute large airway obstruction. These infants may be apneic or have gasping respirations, cyanosis, and poor air exchange. The airway must be rapidly cleared by endotracheal suctioning. Later, as the meconium is driven down to more distal airways, the smaller airways are affected, resulting in air trapping and scattered atelectasis.

C. **Respiratory distress.** The infant who has aspirated meconium into the distal airways but does not have total airway obstruction manifests signs of respiratory distress secondary to increased airway resistance, decreased compliance, and air trapping (**ie, tachypnea, nasal flaring, intercostal retractions, increased anteroposterior (AP) diameter of the chest,** and **cyanosis**). Some infants **may have a delayed presentation,** with only mild initial respiratory distress, which becomes more severe hours after delivery as atelectasis and chemical pneumonitis develop.

Note: Many infants with meconium-stained amniotic fluid appear normal at birth and exhibit no signs of respiratory distress.

D. **Other pulmonary abnormalities.** If air trapping develops, there may be a noticeable increase in AP diameter of the chest. Auscultation often reveals decreased air exchange, rales, rhonchi, or wheezing.

VI. **Diagnosis**

A. **Laboratory studies.** **Arterial blood gas levels** characteristically reveal hypoxemia. Hyperventilation may result in respiratory alkalosis in mild cases, but infants with severe disease usually manifest respiratory acidosis as a result of airway obstruction, atelectasis, and pneumonitis. If the patient has suffered perinatal asphyxia, combined respiratory and metabolic acidosis is present.

B. **Radiologic studies.** A **chest radiograph** typically reveals hyperinflation of the lung fields and flattened diaphragms. There are coarse, irregular patchy infiltrates. A pneumothorax or pneumomediastinum may be present. The severity of radiographic findings may not always correlate with the clinical disease. (See Figure 10–13.)

C. **Cardiac echocardiogram.** Pulmonary hypertension with the resultant hypoxemia from right-to-left atrial and ductal shunt is a frequently associated finding in infants with meconium aspiration pneumonia.

VII. **Management**

A. **Prenatal management.** The key to management of meconium aspiration lies in prevention during the prenatal period.

1. **Identification of high-risk pregnancies.** The approach to prevention begins with recognition of predisposing maternal factors that may cause uteroplacental insufficiency and subsequent fetal hypoxia during labor. In pregnancies that continue past the due date, induction as early as 41 weeks may help prevent meconium aspiration.

2. **Monitoring.** During labor, careful observation and fetal monitoring should be performed. Any signs of fetal distress (eg, appearance of meconium-stained fluid with membrane rupture, loss of beat-to-beat variability, fetal tachycardia, or deceleration patterns) warrant assessment of fetal well-being by scrutiny of fetal heart tracings and fetal scalp pH. If the assessment identifies a compromised fetus, corrective measures should be undertaken or the infant should be delivered in a timely manner.

3. **Amnioinfusion.** In mothers with moderate or thick meconium-stained amniotic fluid, amnioinfusion is effective in reducing the occurrence of variable fetal heart rate decelerations by relieving umbilical cord compression during labor. However, its efficiency in altering the risk or severity of meconium aspiration has not been well demonstrated.

B. **Delivery room management.** Chapter 3 discusses the delivery room management of the meconium-stained infant. The appropriate pediatric intervention in an infant born through meconium-stained fluid depends on whether the infant is "vigorous" as demonstrated by spontaneous respirations, a heart rate >100 beats per min, spontaneous movements, or extremities in a flexion position. For those vigorous infants, routine care only should be provided regardless of the meconium consistency. Those infants who are depressed should be intubated as quickly as feasible and the endotracheal tube connected to a meconium trap aspirator attached to a wall suction at a pressure of 100 mm Hg. Positive pressure ventilation should be avoided, if possible, until tracheal suctioning is accomplished.

C. **Management of the newborn with meconium aspiration.** Infants with meconium below the vocal cords are at risk for pulmonary hypertension, air leak syndromes, and pneumonitis and must be observed closely for signs of respiratory distress.

1. **Respiratory management**
   a. **Pulmonary toilet.** If suctioning the trachea does not result in clearing of secretions, it may be advisable to leave an endotracheal tube in place in symptomatic infants for pulmonary toilet. Chest physiotherapy every 30 min to 1 h, as tolerated, will aid in clearing the airway. Chest physiotherapy is contraindicated in labile infants when associated PPHN is suspected.
   b. **Arterial blood gas levels.** On admission to the neonatal intensive care unit, arterial blood gas measurements to assess ventilatory compromise and supplemental oxygen requirements should be obtained. If the patient requires >0.4 FIO_2 or demonstrates pronounced lability, an arterial catheter for frequent sampling should be inserted.
   c. **Oxygen monitoring.** A pulse oximeter provides important information regarding the severity of the child's respiratory status and also assists in preventing hypoxemia. Comparing oxygen saturation values from a probe placed on the right arm to those from a probe placed on the lower extremities may help identify those infants with right-to-left ductal shunting secondary to pulmonary hypertension.
   d. **Chest radiograph** should be obtained after delivery if the infant is in distress. A chest radiograph may also help determine which patients will experience respiratory distress. However, the radiograph often poorly correlates with the clinical presentation.
   e. **Antibiotic coverage.** Meconium inhibits the normally bacteriostatic quality of amniotic fluid. Because it is difficult to differentiate meconium aspiration from pneumonia radiographically, infants with infiltrates on a chest radiograph should be started on broad-spectrum antibiotics (ampicillin and gentamicin; for dosages, see Chapter 132) after appropriate cultures have been obtained.
   f. **Supplemental oxygen.** A major goal is to prevent episodes of alveolar hypoxia leading to hypoxic pulmonary vasoconstriction and the development of PPHN. For that purpose, supplemental oxygen is provided "generously," such that arterial oxygen tension is maintained at least in the range of 80–90 mm Hg. Some clinicians may elect to maintain PaO_2 at a higher level because the risk of retinopathy should be negligible among full-term infants. The same goal of preventing alveolar hypoxia requires cautious weaning from oxygen therapy. Many of the patients are very labile, and weaning from oxygen should be made slowly, sometimes at a pace of 1% at a time. The prevention of alveolar hypoxia includes a high index of suspicion for the diagnosis of air leak as well as efforts to minimize handling of the child.

    g. Mechanical ventilation. Patients with severe disease who are in impending respiratory failure with hypercapnia and persistent hypoxemia require mechanical ventilation. Those infants who do not respond to conventional ventilation should be given a trial of high-frequency ventilation (HFV).

        i. Rate settings. Ventilation must be tailored to the individual patient. These patients typically require higher inspiratory pressures and faster rates than those with HMD. Modes of ventilation that allow the infant to regulate the frequency of the mechanically aided breath (assist/control or pressure support ventilation) may be preferable. In addition, relatively short inspiratory time allows for adequate expiration in patients prone to air trapping.

        ii. Pulmonary complications. The clinician must maintain a high index of suspicion for air leak. For any unexplained deterioration of clinical status, the possibility of a pneumothorax should be considered and appropriate evaluation undertaken. With the development of atelectasis, air trapping, and decreased lung compliance, high mean airway pressures may be required in a patient who is at risk for air leak. The approach to ventilation must be directed at preventing hypoxemia and providing adequate ventilation at the lowest mean airway pressure possible to reduce the risk of catastrophic air leak.

    h. HFV. Both high-frequency jet ventilation and high-frequency oscillatory ventilation are efficacious in infants in whom adequate ventilation cannot be maintained on conventional ventilation without using excessive ventilatory pressures. It has also been used to maximize the beneficial effects of inhaled nitric oxide.

    i. Surfactant. Infants with severe meconium aspiration syndrome who require mechanical ventilation and have radiologic evidence of parenchymal lung disease are likely to benefit from early surfactant therapy. Because of the frequently associated pulmonary hypertension, close monitoring at the time of surfactant therapy is required to prevent the consequences of transient airway obstruction that may develop during the tracheal instillation of surfactant. (See Chapter 132.)

    j. Inhaled nitric oxide. The frequently associated pulmonary hypertension can be effectively treated by inhaled nitric oxide. It causes selective pulmonary arterioles vasodilatation by acting directly on the vascular smooth muscle where it activates guanylate cyclase, thus increasing cyclic guanosine monophosphate. Given by inhalation it has only a local effect because it is inactivated by hemoglobin once it reaches the intravascular compartment. As such it has minimal effects on other body systems, but methemoglobin levels need to be closely monitored. (See Chapter 132.)

    k. Extracorporeal membrane oxygenation (ECMO). Patients who cannot be ventilated by the therapies just mentioned may be candidates for ECMO. Oxygenation index ($FIO_2 \times$ mean airway pressure $\overline{Paw} \times 100 \div PaO_2$) >40 in association with a $\overline{Paw} \geq 20$ cm H_2O may predict infants who require ECMO. Compared with other population subsets that require ECMO, infants with meconium aspiration have a high survival rate (93–100%). (See Chapter 13.)

  2. General management. Infants who have aspirated meconium and require resuscitation often develop metabolic abnormalities such as hypoxia, acidosis, hypoglycemia, and hypocalcemia. Because these patients may have suffered perinatal asphyxia, surveillance for any end-organ damage is essential (see Chapter 110).

VIII. Prognosis. Complications are common and associated with significant mortality. New modalities of therapy such as administration of exogenous surfactant, HFV, inhaled nitric oxide, and ECMO have reduced the mortality to <5%. In patients surviving severe meconium aspiration, bronchopulmonary dysplasia or chronic lung disease may result from prolonged mechanical ventilation. Those with a significant asphyxial insult may demonstrate neurologic sequelae.

Selected References

Fanaroff AA. Meconium aspiration syndrome: historical aspects. J Perinatol. 2008 Dec;28 Suppl 3:S3-7.

Lacaze-Masmonteil T: Expanded use of surfactant therapy in newborns. *Clin Perinatol* 2007;34:179.

Walsh MC, Faranoff JM: meconium stained fluid: approach to the mother and the baby. *Clin Perinatol* 2007;34:653.

Xu H et al: Intrapartum amnioinfusion for meconium-stained amniotic fluid: a systematic review of randomised controlled trials. *BJOG* 2007;114(4):383-390.

101 Meningitis

I. **Definition.** Neonatal meningitis is an infection of the meninges and central nervous system (CNS) in the first month of life. This is the most common time of life for meningitis to occur.

II. **Incidence.** The incidence is ~ 0.16–0.45 per 1000 live births in developed countries. The incidence may be higher in underdeveloped countries.

III. **Pathophysiology.** In most cases, infection occurs because of hematogenous seeding of the meninges and CNS. In cases of CNS or spinal anomalies (eg, myelomeningocele), there may be direct inoculation by flora on the skin or in the environment. Neonatal meningitis is often accompanied by **ventriculitis,** which makes resolution of infection more difficult. There is also a predilection for vasculitis, which may lead to hemorrhage, thrombosis, and infarction. Subdural effusions and brain abscess may also complicate the course.

  Most organisms implicated in neonatal sepsis also cause neonatal meningitis. Some have a definite predilection for CNS infection. Group B streptococcus (GBS) (especially type III) and the Gram-negative rods (especially *Escherichia coli* with K1 antigen) are the **most common causative agents.** Other causative organisms include *Listeria monocytogenes* (serotype IVb), other streptococci (*enterococci, Streptococcus pneumoniae*), and other Gram-negative enteric bacilli (*Klebsiella, Enterobacter,* and *Serratia* spp). In the very low birthweight infant, coagulase-negative staphylococci need to be considered as a causative organisms in bacterial meningitis.

  With CNS anomalies involving open defects or indwelling devices (eg, ventriculoperitoneal shunts), staphylococcal disease (*Staphylococcus aureus* and *Staphylococcus epidermidis*) is more common, as is disease caused by other skin flora, including streptococci and diphtheroids. Many unusual organisms, including fungi and anaerobes, have been described in case reports of neonatal meningitis.

IV. **Risk factors.** Premature infants with sepsis have a much higher incidence (up to threefold) than term infants of CNS infection. The characteristics of some bacteria make them more virulent, especially for neonates (eg, capsular polysaccharide of GBS type III, *E. coli* K1, and *L. monocytogenes* serotype IVb all contain sialic acid in high concentrations). Infants with CNS defects necessitating ventriculoperitoneal shunt procedures also are at increased risk.

V. **Clinical presentation.** The clinical presentation is usually nonspecific and indistinguishable from those caused by sepsis. Meningitis must be excluded in any infant being evaluated for sepsis or infection. Signs and symptoms of meningitis include lethargy, irritability, temperature instability, respiratory distress, abdominal distension, apnea, or cyanotic episodes. Late manifestations of meningitis are a bulging anterior fontanelle, seizures, and coma. Syndrome of inappropriate antidiuretic hormone may accompany meningitis.

VI. **Diagnosis**
  A. **Laboratory studies.** Cerebrospinal fluid (CSF) examination is critical in the investigation of possible meningitis and the only way to confirm the diagnosis. Approximately 15–50% of all infants with positive CSF cultures for bacteria have negative blood cultures. The technique for obtaining CSF fluid and CSF normal values is discussed in Chapter 32.
    1. **Culture.** CSF culture is the gold standard for the diagnosis of bacterial meningitis. It may be positive in association with a normal or minimally abnormal CSF analysis.
    2. **CSF pleocytosis** is variable. There are usually more cells with Gram-negative rods than with GBS disease. Normal values range from 0–35 white blood cells (WBC), some of which may be polymorphonuclear cells. A recent study suggests that a normal CSF leukocyte profile in the neonate is similar to the normal adult profile, containing up to 5 WBCs/mm^3. Reactive pleocytosis may be seen secondary to CNS hemorrhage.
    3. **A Gram-stained smear** can be helpful in making a more rapid definitive diagnosis and identifying the initial classification of the causative agent.
    4. **Cerebrospinal glucose levels must be compared with serum glucose levels.** Normal CSF values are half to two thirds of serum values.
    5. **CSF protein** is usually elevated, although normal values for infants, especially premature infants, may be much higher than in later life, and the test may be confounded by the presence of blood in the specimen.
  B. **Radiologic studies** are recommended to detect the complications of meningitis, especially when the clinical course is complicated. Infection with certain microorganisms such as *Citrobacter koseri* and *Enterobacter sakazakii* predispose for development of brain abscesses. The most useful and noninvasive method of imaging is ultrasonography, which provides information regarding ventricular size, inflammation (echogenic strands), and the presence of hemorrhage. Computed tomography or magnetic resonance imaging (MRI) are useful in detecting cerebral abscesses and later in the treatment course in identifying areas of encephalomalacia that may dictate prolonged therapy.
VII. **Management.** Isolation precautions for all infectious diseases, including maternal and neonatal precautions, breast-feeding, and visiting issues, can be found in Appendix F.
  A. **Drug therapy.** For drug dosages and other pharmacologic information, see Chapter 132. (*Note:* Dosages for ampicillin, nafcillin, and penicillin G are **doubled** when treating meningitis.)
    1. **Empirical therapy.** Optimal antibiotic selection depends on culture and sensitivity testing of causative organisms. **Ampicillin** and **gentamicin** are usually started as empirical therapy for suspected early sepsis or meningitis.
    2. **Gram-positive meningitis (GBS and *Listeria*).** **Penicillin or ampicillin** is the drug of choice. These infections usually respond well to treatment. Administration for 14 days is indicated.
    3. **Staphylococcal disease.** Because of the increased prevalence of methicillin-resistant staphylococci both in the nosocomial setting and in the community, **vancomycin** should be substituted for penicillin or ampicillin as initial coverage.
    4. **Gram-negative meningitis.** Most clinicians would use **ampicillin plus cefotaxime** as initial therapy especially for infants >1 week of age or for infants being admitted from home after discharge from the hospital. Further therapy is dictated by sensitivity results. Duration of therapy is usually 21 days. Studies have shown no advantage for intrathecal or intraventricular gentamicin.
    5. **Repeat lumbar puncture** 48 h into antibiotic therapy is recommended to document CSF sterilization. Persistence of infection may indicate a focus, such as obstructive ventriculitis, subdural empyema, or multiple small vessel thrombi. Infants with repeat positive CSF cultures after initiation of appropriate antibiotics are at risk for complications as well as a poor outcome. In general, ~3 days are

required to sterilize the CSF in infants with Gram-negative meningitis, whereas in Gram-positive meningitis, sterilization usually occurs within 36–48 h. Follow-up CSF examination is recommended until sterility is documented. External ventricular drainage may be indicated in certain cases complicated by ventriculitis. Treatment should continue until 14 days after cultures are negative or for 21 days, whichever is longer.

6. **Adjunctive therapy.** Contrary to childhood meningitis, dexamethasone does not seem to improve the outcome of neonatal meningitis. Other therapies focusing on enhancing the immune system in the newborn, such as hematopoietic growth factors or intravenous immune globulins, do not seem to help either.

B. **Supportive measures and monitoring for complications.** Head circumference should be measured daily, and neurologic examination should be performed frequently. Imaging studies (especially MRI) may be helpful for prognosis. All neonates with meningitis should undergo long-term neurodevelopmental follow-up.

VIII. **Prognosis.** The **mortality rate** has decreased over the past 15 years to 3–13% compared with 25–30% from earlier decades. There is a higher incidence ($\geq$50%) of neurodevelopmental sequelae in survivors, and this figure has not changed over the years.

Selected References

Daoud AS et al: Lack of effectiveness of dexamethasone in neonatal bacterial meningitis. *Eur J Pediatr* 1999;158:230-233.

Doctor BA et al: Clinical outcomes of neonatal meningitis in very-low birth-weight infants. *Clin Pediatr* 2001;40:473-480.

Heath PT et al: Neonatal meningitis. *Arch Dis Child Fetal Neonatal Ed* 2003;88:F173-F178.

Malbon K et al: Should a neonate with possible late onset infection always have a lumbar puncture? *Arch Dis Child* 2006;91:75-76.

Martin-Ancel A et al: Cerebrospinal fluid leukocyte counts in healthy neonates. *Arch Dis Child Fetal Neonatal Ed* 2006;91:F357-F358.

Philip AG: Neonatal meningitis in the new millennium. *NeoReviews* 2003;4:e73-e80.

Smith PB et al: Comparison of neonatal Gram-negative rod and Gram-positive cocci meningitis. *J Perinatol* 2006;26:111-114.

102 Methicillin-Resistant *Staphylococcal Aureus* (MRSA) Infections

I. **Definition.** Infection with **MRSA (clustered Gram-positive cocci)** causes a variety of localized and invasive suppurative infections and toxin-mediated syndromes like toxic shock syndrome and scalded skin syndrome. MRSA infections used to be limited to health-care facilities (HC-MRSA) and were strictly nosocomial; however, a significant increase in community-acquired MRSA (CA-MRSA) was noted recently.

II. **Incidence.** The methicillin-sensitive *Staphylococcus aureus* normally colonizes the nose, umbilicus, and the groin area by 1 week of age with a colonization rate of 20–90%. Maternal anogenital colonization with MRSA is usually ~3.5%, with little or no risk for early-onset disease in the newborn. There are several documented outbreaks of invasive CA-MRSA that developed in healthy newborn infants discharged from normal newborn nurseries as well as neonatal intensive care units (NICUs). The majority of MRSA infections in the NICU are of late onset. The incidence of disease in the newborn is not known because most literature describes outbreaks of MRSA infection. A recent study showed NICU colonization rate of 10.4%, with a mean time to acquire MRSA of 17 days.

III. **Pathophysiology.** If the newborn infant is exposed to MRSA, whether from the community or the hospital, then he or she will colonize with more virulent strains that are more likely to cause invasive disease. MRSA has specific virulence factors that make it more invasive than methicillin-sensitive *Staphylococcus aureus*. These include staphylococcal chromosome cassette (SCC) *mecA*, Panton-Valentine leukocidin (PVL), and staphylococcal enterotoxins. The SCC *mecA* has the genes that encode antibiotic resistance. PVL genes lead to the production of cytotoxins that form pores in the cellular membrane and cause tissue necrosis and cell lysis.

IV. **Risk factors** for MRSA infection outbreaks include overcrowding, inconsistent handwashing, invasive procedures (eg, central lines, endotracheal intubations, nasogastric tubes), and prolonged hospital stay.

V. **Clinical presentations.** Invasive MRSA disease is likely to be preceded by colonization (skin, umbilicus, and nasopharynx). The source of the bacteria could be a health-care worker, another patient, equipment, or a family member.

   A. **Bloodstream infections** are usually catheter related. Common clinical signs are nonspecific and include apnea or hypoxia, fever, elevated C-reactive protein, and leukocytosis.

   B. **Septic arthritis and osteomyelitis.** *S. aureus* is the primary cause of septic arthritis and osteomyelitis in the neonate. Symptoms are nonspecific, such as poor feeding or increased irritability. Signs include soft tissue swelling and erythema.

   C. **Endocarditis.** Neonates with congenital heart disease and percutaneous central catheters are at a higher risk for endocarditis.

   D. **Skin and soft tissue infections.** *S. aureus* is the most common pathogen causing pustulosis and cellulitis in the neonate. MRSA has virulence factors that contribute to the pathogen's ability to damage the neonatal skin that is already compromised.

   E. **Surgical site infections.**

VI. **Diagnosis.** The gold standard for diagnosing a bloodstream infection is a positive blood culture. Diagnosing arthritis and osteomyelitis can be challenging. In addition to a blood culture, the work-up should include a joint aspirate, bone culture (if surgical debridement is done), radiography, and possibly magnetic resonance imaging. Echocardiography (to diagnose endocarditis) is strongly recommended in infants with more than one positive blood culture. For skin and soft tissue infections, incision and drainage, with subsequent Gram stain and culture of aspirated fluid, is recommended.

VII. **Management**

   A. **Eradication of colonization.** Adult intensive care unit studies demonstrated that eradication of MRSA colonization using a combination of 5 days of intranasal mupirocin and three daily chlorhexidine baths resulted in reducing MRSA infections. There are no similar studies in neonates; however, mupirocin has been used effectively in controlling outbreaks of MRSA in NICU populations. Detailed recommendations for the prevention and control of MRSA colonization and infection in the NICU were published recently.

   B. **Antibiotic therapy.** Vancomycin remains the first-line therapy for MRSA, and many NICUs with endemic MRSA use vancomycin as an empirical therapy for late-onset sepsis while awaiting culture results. In cases of vancomycin intermediate *S. aureus* (VISA) or vancomycin allergy, linezolid has been used effectively. Treatment duration depends on the specific infection. For skin and soft tissue infections and bacteremia, a 7- to 10-day course is generally appropriate. In cases of endocarditis and osteomyelitis, 6–8 weeks of treatment is necessary. In patients with extensive disease with persistently positive blood cultures despite therapeutic doses of vancomycin, both rifampin and gentamicin can be used for synergy.

Table 102–1. GUIDELINES FOR OUTBREAKS OF MRSA IN THE NICU

Recommendation Type, Rating Category*	Consensus Recommendation
Hand hygiene	
IA	A waterless, alcohol-based hand hygiene product should be made available and easily accessible; soap and water should be used if hands are visibly soiled.
IA	Monitoring of hand hygiene is a key component in preventing MRSA transmission in the NICU. Direct observations of hand hygiene practices on a regular basis, or consistent enforcement of proper hand hygiene (eg. use of a unit guard, providing feedback), contribute to increased rates of compliance.
Cohorting and isolation	
IA	MRSA-positive infants should be placed under contact precautions and cohorted (placed in a designated room or area), as should the supplies used in the care of these infants.
IA	Gloves and gowns should be worn when caring for or visiting infants known or suspected to be MRSA positive.
IA	Masks should be worn for aerosol-generating procedures, such as suctioning. The environment in the area of the infant should be kept clean and neat at all times.
NR/UI	Disposal of infant supplies used in the care of the MRSA-positive cohort should be decided by the institution's infection control experts.
IA	Whenever possible, nurses should be cohorted (designated exclusively) for care of MRSA-positive infants. Other HCWs should also be cohorted to the maximum extent allowed by the institution's resources.
II	If cohorting of nurses is not possible, nurses should care for the noncohorted patients before working with the cohorted neonates, when feasible.
II	The number of people (including HCWs and visitors) who enter a room or area designated for MRSA-positive infants should be limited to the minimum possible.
II	Cohorting of infants should be maintained until the last infected or colonized infant has been discharged from the NICU.
Neonatal surveillance cultures	
IB	Infants in the NICU should be screened periodically to detect MRSA colonization. The frequency of screening should increase (eg, To once per week) when clusters of colonization are detected; after evidence suggests a halt in transmission, it may decrease to a lower frequency (eg, to once per month) until the investigation is over.
IA	Although cultures of swab specimens from multiple body sites, including nares, throat, rectum, and umbilicus, have been used to detect MRSA colonization, culture of nasal or nasopharyngeal specimens alone is sufficiently sensitive to detect MRSA colonization in neonates.
Screening of HCWs	
IB	Screening of HCWs in response to a cluster of MRSA colonization or infection in the NICU should be performed only to corroborate or refute epidemiologic data that link an HCW to transmission.
Decolonization	
IB	Mupirocin may be used for decolonization of neonates and/or HCWs if deemed necessary by the affected institution (off-label use).
Environmental cultures	
IA	Environmental cultures should be performed in response to a cluster of MRSA colonization or infection in the NICU only to corroborate or refute epidemiologic data that link an environmental source to transmission.

(*Continued*)

Table 102–1. GUIDELINES FOR OUTBREAKS OF MRSA IN THE NICU *(CONTINUED)*

Recommendation Type, Rating Category*	Consensus Recommendation
Molecular analysis	
IA	When investigating an outbreak, molecular analysis with pulsed-field gel electrophoresis or a comparable molecular epidemiologic tool should be performed to assess the relatedness of strains found in NICU patients, HCWs, and the environment.
IB	If the hospital cannot perform genotyping in-house, then the isolates should be sent to a suitable laboratory for molecular analysis.
Communication	
II	Open communication between regional NICUs is essential to prevent spread between NICUs at different institutions, particularly when an infant is transferred from one NICU to another.
II	In the intake of a transferred patient, the receiving facility should be able to determine whether the infant has been screened previously for MRSA, and if so, the date, specimen source, and result of the culture.
II	In the intake of a transferred patient, the receiving facility should be able to determine whether the transferring institution currently knows of any MRSA-positive infants in its NICU.
IB	The receiving facility should consider isolation and screening of any infant transferred from another NICU, regardless of the transferring institution's MRSA status.
II	Standardized instruction sheets describing methods to prevent transmission of MRSA should be developed as a resource for parents and visitors of infants in NICUs in which MRSA has been detected.
Regulation	
IA	Overcrowding increases the likelihood of MRSA transmission in the NICU; institutions should adhere to all appropriate licensing requirements.
IA	Agency HCWs should be oriented to and monitored periodically for compliance with the institution's infection control and hand hygiene procedures.
II	Logs of shifts worked by agency HCWs should be updated frequently to ensure that, in the case of an epidemiologic investigation, transmission links to these staff may be evaluated.
IC	Hospitals must comply with all local and state regulations regarding the reporting of MRSA in NICUs.
Hospital and public health collaboration	
II	Hospital officials should collaborate with state and local public health officials to conduct surveillance for MRSA in NICUs, facilitate interinstitutional communication and coordination of prevention activities, and provide laboratory support to allow detection of shared MRSA clones among NICUs in multiple institutions.

HCW, health care worker.

Reproduced with permission from Gerber et al: Management of outbreaks of methicillin-resistant *Staphylococcus aureus* infection in the neonatal intensive care unit: a consensus statement. *Infect Control Hosp Epidemiol* 2006;27:139-145.

*Rating categories are defined as follows. **IA:** Strongly recommended for implementation and strongly supported by well-designed experimental, clinical, or epidemiologic studies. **IB:** Strongly recommended for implementation and supported by some experimental, clinical, or epidemiologic studies and a strong theoretical rationale. **IC:** Required by state or federal regulations, rules, or standards. **II:** Suggested for implementation and supported by suggestive clinical or epidemiologic studies or a theoretical rationale. **NR/UI:** No recommendation or unresolved issue for which evidence is insufficient or no consensus regarding efficacy exists. Definitions from Boyce et al.

VIII. **Prevention**

A. **Hand hygiene.** The Centers for Disease Control and Prevention recommend using an alcohol-based hand sanitizer before touching patients, after touching patients, after removing gloves, and after touching the patient care environment and equipment due to the ability of MRSA to survive on inanimate objects. Alcohol-based hand sanitizers improve compliance with hand hygiene policies as well as improve the skin integrity of health-care workers.

B. **Controlling outbreaks.** During an outbreak, many measures are instituted concurrently. In 2006, Gerber et al released a consensus statement from the Chicago Department of Public Health on the management of outbreaks of MRSA in a NICU. Their recommendations included an alcohol-based rub for hand hygiene, isolation and cohorting of MRSA-colonized infants, and regular neonatal surveillance cultures (see Table 102–1). They also emphasized the use of molecular typing as an integral part of control because it can determine the ongoing transmission of a particular clone. They did not make a recommendation for decontamination with mupirocin; this intervention was left to the discretion of the primary clinical care team because the efficacy of this strategy is still uncertain.

Selected References

American Academy of Pediatrics: Staphylococcal infections. In: Pickering LK et al (eds): *Red Book: 2006 Report of the Committee on Infectious Diseases,* 27th ed. Elk Grove Village, IL: American Academy of Pediatrics, 2006:598-610.

Andrews WW et al: Genital tract methicillin-resistant *Staphylococcus aureus*: risk of vertical transmission in pregnant women. *Obstet Gynecol* 2008;111:113-118.

Carey AJ et al: Hospital-acquired infections in the NICU: epidemiology for the new millennium. *Clin Perinatol* 2008;35:223-249.

Centers for Disease Control and Prevention (CDC): Community-associated methicillin-resistant *Staphylococcus aureus* infection among healthy newborns—Chicago and Los Angeles County, 2004. *MMWR Morb Mortal Wkly Rep* 2006;55:329-332.

Cimolai N: Staphylococcus aureus outbreaks among newborns: new frontiers in an old dilemma. *Am J Perinatol* 2003;20:125-136.

Gerber SI et al: Management of outbreaks of methicillin-resistant *Staphylococcus aureus* infection in the neonatal intensive care unit: a consensus statement. *Infect Control Hosp Epidemiol* 2006;27:139-145.

Kim YH et al: Clinical outcomes in methicillin-resistant *Staphylococcus aureus*-colonized neonates in the neonatal intensive care unit. *Neonatology* 2007;91:241-247.

McDonald JR et al: Methicillin-resistant *Staphylococcus aureus* outbreak in an intensive care nursery: potential for interinstitutional spread. *Pediatr Infect Dis J* 2007;26:678-683.

103 Multiple Gestation

I. **Definition.** A multiple gestation occurs when more than one fetus is carried during a pregnancy.

II. **Incidence.** In 2005, the overall rate of twin births was 32.2 in 1000 live births and the rate of triplet births was 1.6 in 10,000 live births. The incidence of multiple gestation pregnancies is probably underestimated. Fewer than half of twin pregnancies diagnosed by ultrasonography during the first trimester are delivered as twins, a phenomenon that has been termed *vanishing twin*. Two gestational sacs can be identified with ultrasonography by 6 weeks' gestation. In addition, routine screening for maternal α-fetoprotein (AFP) may identify pregnancies with multiple gestations at an early gestational age. About a third of twins in the United States are monozygotic. Between 1980 and 1994, there was a 42% increase in the number of twin births in the United States. The rate of triplet births escalated more rapidly, increasing 100% between 1980 and 1989. By 2001, the rate of higher-order multiples had leveled off while the rate of twin births continued to increase. The incidence of monozygotic twinning is remarkably constant at 3–5 per 1000 pregnancies, whereas the rate for dizygotic twinning varies from 4–50 per 1000 pregnancies.

III. **Pathophysiology.** Placental classification and determination of zygosity are important in the pathophysiology of twins.

    A. **Classification.** Placental examination affords a unique opportunity to identify two thirds to three fourths of monozygotic twins at birth.

        1. **Twin placentation is classified according to the placental disk** (single, fused, or separate), number of chorions (monochorionic or dichorionic), and number of amnions (monoamniotic or diamniotic) (Figure 103–1).

        2. **Heterosexual (assuredly dizygotic) twins** always have a dichorionic placenta.

        3. **Monochorionic twins** are always of the same sex. All monochorionic twins are believed to be monozygotic. In 70% of monozygotic twin pregnancies, the placentas are monochorionic, and the possibility exists for commingling of the fetal circulations. Less than 1% of twin pregnancies are monoamniotic.

    B. **Placental complications.** Twin gestations are associated with an increased frequency of anomalies of the placenta and adnexa; for example, a single umbilical artery or velamentous or marginal cord insertion (6–9 times more common with twin gestation). The cord is more susceptible to trauma from twisting. The vessels near the insertion are often unprotected by Wharton jelly and are especially prone to thrombosis when compression or twisting occurs. Intrapartum fetal distress from cord compression and fetal hemorrhage from associated vasa previa are potential problems with velamentous insertion of the cord.

    C. **Determination of zygosity.** The most efficient way to identify zygosity is as follows:

        1. **Gender examination.** Male-female pairs are dizygotic. The dichorionic placenta may be separate or fused.

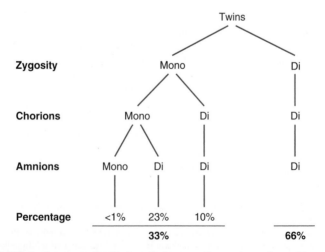

FIGURE 103–1. Percentage distribution of twins according to placental type. Mono, Monoamniotic; Di, diamniotic.

2. **Placental examination.** Twins with a monochorionic placenta (monoamniotic or diamniotic) are monozygotic. Care should be taken not to confuse apposed fused placentas for a single chorion. If doubt exists on a gross inspection of the dividing membranes, a transverse section should be studied. The zygosity of twins of the same sex with dichorionic membranes cannot be immediately known. Genetic studies are needed (eg, blood typing, human leukocyte antigen typing, DNA markers, and chromosome marking) to determine zygosity.

IV. **Risk factors.** Assisted reproductive technology accounted for 1% of all U.S. births in 2004 but 18% of all multiple births. The incidence of dizygotic twinning increases with a family history of twins, maternal age (peak at 35–39 years), previous twin gestation, increasing parity, maternal height, fecundity, social class, frequency of coitus, and exposure to exogenous gonadotropins, clomiphene, or in vitro fertilization. The risk of twinning decreases with undernourishment. Ethnic background (African Americans > Caucasians > Asians) is a preconception risk factor for naturally conceived multiple gestation births.

V. **Clinical presentation.** Twins are more likely to have prematurity, intrauterine growth restriction, congenital anomalies, and twin-twin transfusion.

   A. **Prematurity and uteroplacental insufficiency** are the major contributors to perinatal complications. In 2005, 60% of twins were born prior to 37 weeks, 22% prior to 34 weeks and 64% of triplets were born before 34 weeks' gestation.

   B. **Intrauterine growth restriction.** The incidence of low birthweight in twins is ~50-60%, a figure that is 5-7 times higher than the incidence of low birthweight in singletons. In general, the more fetuses in a gestation, the smaller their weight for gestational age (Figure 103-2). Twins tend to grow at normal rates up to about 30–34 weeks'

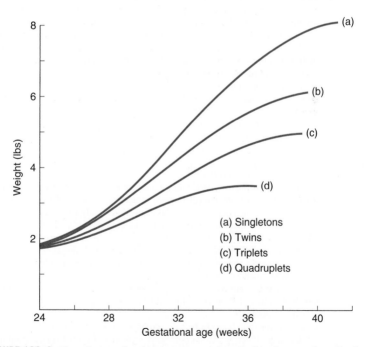

FIGURE 103-2. Growth curve showing the mean weights of infants from single and multiple pregnancies by gestational age. *(From Phelan MC: Twins. In Stevenson RE et al [eds]:* Human Malformations and Related Anomalies. *New York: Oxford University Press, 1993. Modified from McKeown T, Record RG: Observations of foetal growth in multiple pregnancy in man.* J Endocrinol *1952;8:386.)* Reproduced by permission of the Society for Endocrinology.

gestation when they reach a combined weight of 4 kg. Thereafter, they grow more slowly. Two thirds of twins show some signs of growth restriction at birth.

C. **Uteroplacental insufficiency.** The incidence of acute and chronic uteroplacental insufficiency is increased in multiple gestations. Five-minute Apgar scores of 0–3 are reported for 5–10% of twin gestations. These low scores may relate to acute stresses of labor, cord prolapse (1–5%), or trauma during delivery superimposed on chronic uteroplacental insufficiency.

D. **Congenital anomalies.** Birth defects are two to three times more common in monozygotic twins than in singletons or dizygotic twins, who have a 2–3% incidence of major defects diagnosed at birth. Three mechanisms are postulated for the increased frequency of structural defects in monozygotic twins: deformations caused by intrauterine space constraint, disruption of normal blood flow secondary to placental vascular anastomoses, and defects in morphogenesis. Such defects are usually discordant in monozygotic twins; however, in purely genetic conditions (eg, chromosomal abnormalities or single-gene defects), concordance would be the rule. Twins conceived by in vitro fertilization have twice the risk of major congenital anomalies compared with twins conceived naturally.

1. **Anomalies unique to multiple pregnancies.** Certain anomalies, such as conjoined twins and acardia, are unique to multiple pregnancies.

2. **Deformations.** Twins are more likely to suffer from intrauterine crowding and restriction of movement, leading to synostosis, torticollis, facial palsy, positional foot defects, and other defects.

3. **Vascular disruptions.** Disruptions related to monozygotic vascular shunts may result in birth defects. Acardia occurs from an artery-to-artery placental shunt, in which reverse flow leads to the development of an amorphous recipient twin. In utero death of a co-twin may result in a thromboembolic phenomena, including disseminated intravascular coagulation, cutis aplasia, porencephaly or hydranencephaly, limb reduction defects, intestinal atresias, or gastroschisis.

4. **Malformations.** Monozygotic twinning results in an increased frequency of the following specific malformations:
   a. Sacrococcygeal teratoma.
   b. Sirenomelia sequence, including VACTERL association (*v*ertebral abnormalities, imperforate *a*nus, *c*ardiac abnormalities, *t*racheoesophageal fistula, *r*enal dysplasia, and *l*imb deformities).
   c. Cloacal exstrophy sequence.
   d. Holoprosencephaly sequence.
   e. Anencephaly.

E. **Twin-twin transfusion syndrome**

1. **Vascular anastomoses.** Almost all monochorionic placentas demonstrate vascular anastomoses, whereas dichorionic placentas rarely do. Vascular anastomoses may be superficial direct communications easily visible on inspection between arteries (most common) or veins (uncommon), deep connections from arteries to veins via villi, or combinations of superficial and deep connections.

2. **Incidence.** Despite the high frequency of vascular anastomosis in monochorionic placentation, the twin-twin transfusion syndrome is relatively uncommon (~15% of monochorionic gestations).

3. **Clinical manifestations.** Clinically, the twin-twin transfusion syndrome is diagnosed when twins have a hemoglobin difference of >5 g/dL and is due to artery-to-vein anastomoses.
   a. **The donor twin** tends to be pale and have a low birthweight, oligohydramnios, anemia, hypoglycemia, decreased organ mass, hypovolemia, and amnion nodosum. Donor twins often require volume expansion, red blood cell transfusion, or both.
   b. **The recipient twin** is frequently plethoric and has a high birthweight, polyhydramnios, polycythemia or hyperviscosity, increased organ mass, hypervolemia,

and hyperbilirubinemia. Recipient twins often require partial exchange transfusion.

    c. **Infants born with twin-twin transfusion syndrome** have an increased risk of being diagnosed with antenatally acquired severe cerebral lesions and are at an increased risk of neurodevelopmental sequelae even when treatment is initiated antenatally.

    d. **Very low birthweight infants** who are multiple births may have an increased risk of mortality and intraventricular hemorrhage compared with singletons.

VI. Diagnosis. Multiple gestation is usually diagnosed prenatally by ultrasound as early as 5 weeks (can see gestational sacs) and by an increased AFP (in twin pregnancies, the average AFP is double that found in a singleton pregnancy).

VII. Management

  A. Site of delivery. When a complicated twin gestation has been identified, delivery should ideally be conducted at a high-risk perinatal center with experienced pediatric delivery teams in attendance.

  B. Physical examination. Infants should be examined for evidence of intrauterine growth restriction, congenital anomalies, and twin-twin transfusion syndrome. Central hematocrits should be obtained in both infants. When one of the infants has a congenital anomaly, the other twin is at increased risk for complications. In particular, death of one fetus puts the others at risk for fetal disseminated intravascular coagulation.

  C. Complications in newborn period. The second-born twin is more likely to develop respiratory distress syndrome, bronchopulmonary dysplasia, and die.

  D. *Controversial* **issue: Cobedding of multiples.** Coincident with the rise in multiple births has been an interest in cobedding of multiples. Although cobedding multiples has become common practice, the safety or the benefit of this practice has not been definitively established.

  E. Economic considerations. It has been estimated that the perinatal health care costs associated with plural births were 4 times higher for twins and 11 times higher for triplets than those of a singleton birth. The increasing rate of plural births and the concordant decline in mortality has increased the need for medical and social services for these children and their families.

  F. Risks beyond the neonatal period

    1. Catch-up growth. In monozygotic twins, birthweight differences may be as much as 20%, but the lighter twin has a remarkable ability to make up intrauterine growth deficits.

    2. Social problems. Parents of multiple births may have an increased level of stress and may respond differently to their children compared with singletons. Counseling for parents of twins may be invaluable.

VIII. Prognosis. Although perinatal mortality rates for singleton pregnancies have continued to fall during the last decade, there has been little change in mortality rates for multiple pregnancies.

  A. Twins. The perinatal death rate for twins is 9 times the rate for first-born singletons and 11 times the rate for second-born singletons.

    1. Monoamniotic twins. Monoamniotic twins have the highest mortality rate among the different types of twins, largely because of cord entanglement.

    2. Monozygotic twins. Monozygotic twins have a perinatal mortality and morbidity rate that is two to three times that of dizygotic twins. Diamniotic monochorionic twins have a mortality rate of 25%, and dichorionic twins, a mortality rate of 8.9%.

    3. Fetal death in twins. When the cause of death is intrinsic to one dichorionic fetus and does not threaten the other fetus, complications are rare. Hazardous intrauterine environments threaten both twins, whether monochorionic or dichorionic. With monochorionic placentas, the incidence of major complications or death in the surviving twin is ~50%.

  B. Triplets. The neonatal mortality rate for triplets is 18.8%, and the perinatal mortality rate is 25.5%.

Selected References

Bryan E: The impact of multiple preterm births on the family. *BJOG* 2003;110:24-28.

Callahan TL et al: The economic impact of multiple-gestation pregnancies and the contribution of assisted-reproduction techniques to their incidence. *N Engl J Med* 1994;331:244-249.

Hansen M et al: The risk of major birth defects after intracytoplasmic sperm injection and in vitro fertilization. *N Engl J Med* 2002;346:725-730.

Hayes EJ et al: Very-low-birthweight neonates: do outcomes differ in multiple compared with singleton gestations? *Am J Perinatol* 2007;24:373-376.

Linder N et al: Risk factors for intraventricular hemorrhage in very low birth weight premature infants: a retrospective case-control study. *Pediatrics* 2003;111:e590-e595.

Lopriore E et al: Incidence, origin, and character of cerebral injury in twin-to-twin transfusion syndrome treated with fetoscopic laser surgery. *Am J Obstet Gynecol* 2006;194:1215-1220.

Lopriore E et al: Long-term neurodevelopmental outcome in twin-to-twin transfusion syndrome treated with fetoscopic laser surgery. *Am J Obstet Gynecol* 2007;196:231.e1-231.e4.

MacDorman MF et al: Annual summary of vital statistics—2001. *Pediatrics* 2002;110:1037-1052.

Martin JA et al: Births: Final data for 2005. *Natl Vital Stat Rep* 2007;56:1-103.

Shinwell ES et al: Effect of birth order on neonatal morbidity and mortality among very low birthweight twins: a population based study. *Arch Dis Child Fetal Neonatal Ed* 2004;89:F145-F148.

Tomashek KM, Wallman C; Committee on Fetus and Newborn, American Academy of Pediatrics: Cobedding twins and higher-order multiples in a hospital setting. *Pediatrics* 2007;120:1359-1366.

Wright VC et al: Assisted reproductive technology surveillance—United States, 2001. *MMWR Surveill Summ* 2004;53:11-20.

104 Necrotizing Enterocolitis and Spontaneous Intestinal Perforation

NECROTIZING ENTEROCOLITIS

I. **Definition.** Necrotizing enterocolitis (NEC) is an ischemic and inflammatory necrosis of the bowel primarily affecting premature neonates after the initiation of enteral feeding.

II. **Incidence.** NEC is predominantly a disorder of preterm infants, with an incidence of 6–10% in infants weighing <1500g. Although 10% of all cases of NEC occur in term infants, the incidence is highest in premature infants. NEC has an overall mortality of 10–30%.

III. **Pathophysiology.** A multifactorial theory has been suggested in which several risk factors including prematurity, formula feedings, ischemia, and bacterial colonization interact to initiate mucosal damage via a final common pathway involving activation of the inflammatory cascade. Mucosal damage results in an invasion of the bowel wall by gas producing bacteria, resulting in an intramural gas accumulation (pneumatosis intestinalis). This sequence of events may progress to transmural necrosis or gangrene of the bowel and finally to multiple sites of bowel perforation and peritonitis.

IV. **Risk factors**
   A. **Prematurity.** There is an inverse relationship between gestational age and a risk for developing NEC. This may involve immature mucosal barrier, mucosal enzymes, and various gastrointestinal hormones. Premature infants may have an imbalance between pro- and anti-inflammatory factors and thus have an increased activation of inflammatory mediators and a decreased inactivation of specific mediators like platelet-activating factor, which has been linked to NEC. An inability to autoregulate the intestinal microcirculation effectively and differences in bacterial colonization may also make preterm infants more susceptible to NEC.
   B. **Enteral feedings.** NEC is rare in unfed infants, and 90–95% infants with NEC have received at least one enteral feed. Enteral feeding provides necessary substrate for proliferation of enteric pathogens. Hyperosmolar formulas or medications may alter mucosal permeability and cause mucosal damage. Human milk, with the benefit of providing immunoprotective as well as local growth promoting factors, significantly lowers the risk for NEC. Moreover, enteral immunoglobulin A-immunoglobulin G (IgA-IgG) feeds also decreased the risk for NEC in preliminary clinical studies. Use of trophic phase of feeding followed by slow advancements of feeding volume decreases the incidence of NEC.
   C. **Bacterial colonization and viral enteritis.** Bacteria including *Escherichia coli, Klebsiella* species, *Clostridia* species, and *Staphylococcus epidermidis* are implicated in NEC. Blood cultures are positive in only 20–30% of cases. Alternatively, viral enteritis from viruses like enterovirus and rotavirus may compromise the mucosal barrier leading to secondary sepsis from enteric organisms. In some centers, rotavirus may be responsible for as many as 30% of all NEC cases.
   D. **Hypoxic/ischemic events** play a greater role in term and near-term infants, although bowels in preterm infants are also susceptible to ischemic events. During periods of circulatory stress, as in perinatal asphyxia, blood is diverted away from the splanchnic circulation (diving reflex). The resulting intestinal ischemia followed by reperfusion may lead to bowel damage. An imbalance between vasodilating (nitric oxide and others) and vasoconstricting molecules (endothelin 1, and others) in newborns may lead to a defective autoregulation of splanchnic blood flow. For example, infants with NEC have been shown by Doppler flow velocimetry to have a higher flow resistance in the superior mesenteric artery in the first day of life. Similarly, infants with congenital heart disease may have a compromised bowel perfusion, making them susceptible to ischemic injury. Intrauterine growth restricted infants, infants with polycythemia, and infants receiving exchange transfusions are also at risk for bowel ischemia and thus susceptible to NEC.
   E. **Medications.** Maternal venlafaxine therapy and questionable correlation with NEC was recently reported.
V. **Clinical presentation.** In preterm infants, the onset of NEC follows initiation of enteral feeds and is usually diagnosed between 14 and 20 days of age. In contrast, term infants who develop NEC usually do so within the first week of life. Clinical presentation may vary from abdominal distension (the most frequent early sign, noted in 70% of cases), ileus, increased volumes of gastric aspirate, bilious aspirate (two third of cases), or frank signs of shock, bloody stools, perforation, and peritonitis. NEC may also present insidiously with nonspecific signs such as labile temperature, apnea, bradycardia, or other signs of suspected neonatal sepsis. Guaiac-positive stools are quite common in preterm infants being fed by nasogastric tube and are not a useful indicator of NEC.
   Clinical recognition of NEC can be categorized into stages of disease progression and upon systemic, gastrointestinal (GI), and radiographic findings (also known as the **Bell criteria**).
   A. **Stage I: Suspected NEC**
      1. Systemic signs are nonspecific, including apnea, bradycardia, lethargy, and temperature instability.
      2. GI findings include feeding intolerance, recurrent gastric residuals, and abdominal distension.
      3. Radiographic findings may be normal or nonspecific.

B. **Stage II: Proven NEC**
   1. Systemic signs include stage I signs plus abdominal tenderness and thrombocytopenia.
   2. GI findings are prominent abdominal distension, tenderness, bowel wall edema, absent bowel sounds, and gross blood in stools.
   3. Radiographic findings are most often pneumatosis intestinalis, with or without portal venous gas, or ascites.
C. **Stage III: Advanced NEC**
   1. Systemic signs include respiratory and metabolic acidosis, respiratory failure, hypotension, decreased urine output, neutropenia, and disseminated intravascular coagulation.
   2. GI findings include a tense distended abdomen with spreading abdominal wall edema, induration, and discoloration.
   3. Radiographic findings most likely reveal a pneumoperitoneum.

VI. **Diagnosis.** A high index of suspicion must be maintained for any infant with a combination of risk factors enumerated under Section IV.
   A. **Clinical diagnosis.** NEC is a tentative diagnosis in any infant presenting with the triad of feeding intolerance, abdominal distension, and gross blood in stools. Alternatively, the earliest signs may be identical to those of neonatal sepsis.
   B. **Laboratory studies.** The following studies should be performed and repeated as necessary:
      1. **Complete blood cell count (CBC) with differential.** The white blood count may be normal but is frequently either elevated with an increased left shift or low (leukopenia). Thrombocytopenia is often seen. Fifty percent of cases of proven NEC have a platelet count <50,000 μL.
      2. **C-reactive protein** may not be elevated initially or in cases of severe NEC because an infant is unable to produce an effective inflammatory response.
      3. **Cultures.** Blood, urine, stool, and spinal fluid specimens should be sent for cultures for possible bacterial, viral, and fungal pathogens.
      4. **Electrolytes.** Electrolyte imbalances such as hyponatremia and hypernatremia as well as hyperkalemia are common.
      5. **Arterial blood gas measurements.** Metabolic or combined respiratory and metabolic acidosis may be seen.
      6. **Coagulation studies.** If thrombocytopenia or bleeding are found, extended coagulopathy screening should be undertaken. Prolonged prothrombin time, prolonged partial thromboplastin time, decreased fibrinogen, and increased fibrin split products most likely indicate that disseminated intravascular coagulation (DIC) is taking place.
      7. **Biomarkers** are being investigated to diagnose and predict the course of NEC such as breath hydrogen, inflammatory mediators in blood, urine or stool, and genetic markers, but all have drawbacks that limit their use. Further studies of genomic and proteomic markers are ongoing.
   C. **Radiographic studies.** (See Figure 10–22.)
      1. **Flat plate radiograph of the abdomen.** Abnormal bowel gas patterns, ileus, a sentinel loop of dilated bowel, or areas suspicious for pneumatosis intestinalis may be present. If pneumatosis intestinalis and/or intrahepatic portal venous gas (in the absence of umbilical venous catheter) are found, they are confirmatory for NEC.
      2. **Lateral decubitus and cross-table lateral studies of the abdomen.** Presence of free air is indicative of intestinal perforation. Serial radiographic studies of the abdomen should be obtained every 6–8 h in the presence of pneumatosis intestinalis or portal venous gas. They portend the increased risk of pneumoperitoneum. Serial radiographs may be discontinued with clinical improvement after 48–72 h.
      3. **Abdominal sonography.** Sonographs may be useful in the presence of nonspecific clinical and radiologic findings or in infants with NEC not responding to medical management. Free gas and focal fluid collections can be viewed by sonography in infants with perforation when free air cannot be seen radiographically.

4. **Abdominal paracentesis.** (See Chapter 33.) Needle aspiration of the peritoneal cavity may occasionally be performed to obtain fluid for Gram stain and culture in infants with ascites or peritonitis in the absence of clinical improvement, unchanged abdominal radiographic appearance, and an absence of a pneumoperitoneum.

VII. **Management.** The main principle of management for confirmed NEC is to treat it as an acute abdomen with impending septic peritonitis. The goal is to prevent progression of disease, intestinal perforation, and shock. If NEC occurs in epidemic clusters, affected cases should be considered for isolation.

A. **Medical management**

1. **Nothing by mouth** to allow gastrointestinal rest for 7–14 days (shorter course for stage I NEC). Total parenteral nutrition can provide basic nutritional needs.

2. **Gastric decompression** with Replogle orogastric tube at low intermittent or continuous suctioning.

3. **Close monitoring of vital signs and abdominal circumference.**

4. **Monitor for gastrointestinal bleeding.** Check all gastric aspirates and stools for frank blood.

5. **Respiratory support** as needed to maintain acceptable blood gas parameters. Progressive abdominal distension causing loss of lung volume may increase the need for positive-pressure ventilation.

6. **Circulatory support.** Volume replacement may be needed for third-space losses leading to circulatory shock. Ionotropic support may be needed to maintain normal blood pressure.

7. **Strict fluid intake and output monitoring.** Try to maintain urine output of 1–3 mL/kg/h. Remove potassium from intravenous fluids in the presence of hyperkalemia or anuria.

8. **Removal of umbilical arterial and venous catheters** and placement of peripheral venous and arterial catheters depends on severity of illness.

9. **Laboratory monitoring.** Check CBC and electrolyte panel every 12–24 h until stable. Obtain blood and urine cultures prior to starting antibiotics.

10. **Antibiotic therapy.** Treat with parenteral antibiotics for 10–14 days. Start ampicillin and gentamicin (or cefotaxime). Consider vancomycin (in place of ampicillin) in the presence of central lines or if a staphylococcus infection is suspected. Add anaerobic coverage with metronidazole or clindamycin if peritonitis or bowel perforation is suspected. Current evidence does not suggest or refute the use of lactoferrin as an adjunct to antibiotic therapy.

11. **Monitoring for DIC.** Infants in stage II and III may develop DIC and require fresh-frozen plasma and cryoprecipitate. Packed red blood cell transfusions and platelet transfusions may also be needed.

12. **Radiographic studies.** Abdominal flat plate with lateral decubitus of cross-table lateral studies every 6–8 h in the acute stage to detect a bowel perforation.

13. **Surgical consultation in confirmed NEC (stage II and III).**

B. **Surgical management.** A pneumoperitoneum is an absolute indication for surgical intervention. Relative indications for surgery include portal venous gas, abdominal wall cellulitis, fixed dilated intestinal segment by a radiograph (sentinel loop), a tender abdominal mass, and clinical deterioration refractory to medical management.

1. **Exploratory laparotomy.** The bowel is examined and necrotic segments are resected. A portion of viable bowel is used to create an enterostomy and mucous fistula. Reanastomosis takes place after 8–12 weeks. If NEC only involves a short segment of bowel and a limited resection, a primary anastomosis is used by some surgeons to avoid complications associated with ileostomy and the need for a second surgery for reanastomosis.

2. **Primary drain placement** is an option in unstable preterm infants <1500 g. Recent experience has shown this technique to have similar mortality, need for total parenteral nutrition, and length of hospital stay. In situations of widespread

areas of intestinal necrosis, the abdomen may be closed after placement of a drain and re-explored later. A poor prognosis is associated with severe short bowel syndrome, therefore forgoing further treatment may be considered.

C. **Prevention.** Different strategies have been proposed to prevent NEC. These include use of enteral antibiotics, judicious use of parenteral fluids, enteral IgG and IgM, antenatal corticosteroids, delayed or slow feeding advancement, breast milk feeds, and use of enteral probiotics.

1. **Human milk** prevents NEC. Although mother's own milk is ideal, a meta-analysis of four randomized clinical trials of donor human milk versus formula suggest that 100% human milk feeds is protective against NEC.

2. **Feeding protocols.** Slow advancement of feeds decreases the risk of NEC in some studies but remains *controversial*.

3. **Probiotics.** There has been recent work promoting the use of probiotics to decrease the risk for NEC in preterm infants. Although a few trials in preterm infants have shown a decreased incidence of NEC in the treated groups, additional studies regarding the safety of probiotics in this fragile population are awaited before routine treatment with probiotics can be recommended.

VIII. **Prognosis**

A. **Short term.** About 30% infants with pneumatosis intestinalis have mild disease and are managed medically. NEC with perforation is associated with a mortality of 20–40%.

B. **Long-term complications**

1. **Significant growth delay and adverse neurodevelopmental outcomes** can be seen in infants with surgical NEC.

2. **Recurrence of NEC** may occur in ~5% of cases.

3. **Colonic strictures** may occur in 10–20% cases. They present with recurrent abdominal distension and persisting feeding intolerance. A contrast enema is usually diagnostic.

4. **Short bowel syndrome** may develop in infants undergoing extensive resection of bowel. The traditional limits of intestinal length for successful survival are at least 20 cm of viable small bowel remaining with an intact ileocecal valve, or 40 cm of viable small bowel remaining without an ileocecal valve. Short bowel syndrome is further complicated by prolonged total parenteral nutrition, cholestasis, and central line infections. Intestinal transplantation, with variable outcome, remains an option for some of these infants.

SPONTANEOUS INTESTINAL PERFORATION

I. **Definition.** Spontaneous intestinal perforation (SIP) is a distinct entity that differs clinically and histologically from NEC. The perforation typically occurs suddenly, without a defined prodrome, usually within the first 2 weeks of life.

II. **Incidence.** SIP occurs in ~7% of extremely low birthweight infants. It occurs most commonly in infants ≤26 weeks' gestation.

III. **Pathophysiology.** The mucosa is robust with no signs of necrosis or ischemia. The submucosa is thinned and there is a focal absence or nonseptic necrosis of the muscularis. Pneumatosis is absent. Perforation is usually on the antimesenteric surface of the distal ileum. Certain pathogens, Candida and Staphylococcus epidermidis, commonly grow from peritoneal cultures from patients with SIP but it is not known if these play a role in the etiology of the disease.

IV. **Risk factors.** Prematurity, patent ductus arteriosus, outborn status (requiring transport to the neonatal intensive care unit), early postnatal steroid use during the first week of life and hypotension requiring pressors have been linked with occurrence of SIP. Recent studies have shown an association between use of indomethacin in the first 3 days of life and SIP. Combined use of indomethacin and hydrocortisone increase the risk for SIP. Other factors (chorioamnionitis and antenatal indomethacin) have not been proven but are believed to be a risk for SIP.

V. **Clinical presentation.** A sudden deterioration with abdominal distension, bluish discoloration over abdomen, hypotension, and metabolic acidosis is often seen. It usually follows a prolonged period of gasless abdomen radiographs. It usually occurs before starting feeds or during early phases of trophic feeds.

VI. **Diagnosis** can be made by seeing free air on abdominal radiograph (flat plate or left lateral decubitus view). (See Figure 10–21.)

VII. **Management**

    A. **Medical management** is similar to management for NEC as described earlier.

    B. **Surgical management** can be a laparotomy with primary repair or placement of a peritoneal drain.

VIII. **Prognosis.** Morbidity and mortality, as compared with intestinal perforation following NEC, is lower. However, infants who develop SIP do have a higher risk for periventricular leukomalacia and death as compared with infants of similar gestational age.

Selected References

Ahmad I et al: Risk factors for spontaneous intestinal perforation in extremely low birth weight infants. *Open Pediatric Medicine Journal* 2008;2:11-15.

Attridge JT et al: New insights into spontaneous intestinal perforation using a national data set: SIP is associated with early indomethacin exposure. *J Perinatol* 2006;26:93-99.

Berseth CL et al: Prolonged small feeding volumes early in life decreases the incidence of necrotizing enterocolitis in very low birth weight infants. *Pediatrics* 2003;111:529-534.

Caplan M: Neonatal necrotizing enterocolitis. In Martin RJ et al (eds): *Neonatal-Perinatal Medicine*, 8th ed. Philadelphia, PA: Mosby Elsevier, 2005:1403-1410.

Caplan MS, Jilling T: The pathophysiology of necrotizing enterocolitis. *NeoReviews* 2001;2(5):E103-E109.

Clark DA, Munshi UK: Development of the gastrointestinal circulation in the fetus and newborn. In Polin RA et al (eds): *Fetal and Neonatal Physiology*, 3rd ed. Philadelphia, PA: Saunders, 2004:701-705.

Emil S et al: Factors associated with definitive peritoneal drainage for spontaneous intestinal perforation in extremely low birth weight neonates. *Eur J Pediatr Surg* 2008;18(2):80-85.

Foster J, Cole M: Oral immunoglobulin for preventing necrotizing enterocolitis in preterm and low birth-weight neonates [review]. *Cochrane Database Syst Rev* 2004;1:CD001816.

Gordon PV, Attridge JT: Understanding clinical literature relevant to spontaneous intestinal perforations. *Am J Perinatol* 2009;26(4):309-316.

McGuire W, Anthony M: Donor human milk versus formula for preventing necrotizing enterocolitis in preterm infants; systemic review. *Arch Dis Child Fetal Neonatal Ed* 88:F11-F14.

Mohan P, Abrams SA: Oral lactoferrin for the treatment of sepsis and necrotizing enterocolitis in neonates. *Cochrane Database Syst Rev* 2009;(1):CD007138.

Moss RL et al: Laparotomy versus peritoneal drainage for necrotizing enterocolitis and perforation. *N Engl J Med* 2006;354:2225-2234.

Murdoch EM et al: Doppler flow velocimetry in the superior mesenteric artery on the first day of life in preterm infants and the risk of neonatal necrotizing enterocolitis. *Pediatrics* 2006; 118:1999-2003.

Pietz J et al: Prevention of necrotizing enterocolitis in preterm infants: a 20-year experience. *Pediatrics* 2007;119:e164-170.

Schanler RJ: Probiotics and necrotizing enterocolitis in premature infants. *Arch Dis Child Fetal Neonatal Ed* 2006;91:F395-F397.

Schanler RJ et al: Randomized trial of donor human milk vs. preterm formula as substitutes for mother's own milk in the feeding of extremely premature infants. *Pediatrics* 2005;116(2):400-406.

Schulzke SM et al: Neurodevelopmental outcomes of very low-birth-weight infants with necrotizing enterocolitis. *Arch Pediatr Adolesc Med* 2007;161:583-590.

Silva CT et al: Correlation of sonographic findings and outcome in necrotizing enterocolitis. *Pediatr Radiol* 2007;37:274-282.

Sisk PM et al: Early human milk feeding is associated with a lower risk of necrotizing enterocolitis in very low birth weight infants. *J Perinatol* 2007;27:428-433.

Treichel M et al: Is there a correlation between venlafaxine therapy during pregnancy and a higher incidence of necrotizing enterocolitis? *World J Pediatr* 2009;5(1):65-67.

Tyson JE, Kennedy KA: Trophic feedings for parenterally fed infants. *Cochrane Database Syst Rev* 2005;3:CD000504.

Walsh MC, Kliegman RM: Necrotizing enterocolitis: treatment based on staging criteria. *Pediatr Clin North Am* 1986;33(1):179-201.

Watterberg KL et al: Prophylaxis of early adrenal insufficiency to prevent bronchopulmonary dysplasia: a multicenter trial. *Pediatrics* 2004;114:1649-1657.

Young C et al: Biomarkers for infants at risk for necrotizing enterocolitis: Clues to prevention? *Pediatr Res* 2009. [Epub ahead of print]

105 Neural Tube Defects

I. **Definitions.** Neural tube defects (NTDs) are malformations of the developing brain and spinal cord. In normal development, the closure of the neural tube occurs over a 4- to 6-day period with completion around the 29th day postconception, often before a woman has realized that she is pregnant. Most current hypotheses consider NTDs to be defects from failure of a neural tube closure rather than other theories describing the reopening of a previously closed tube. Most likely, the closure starts at several distinct sites rather than being one continuous process. The nomenclature for NTDs is not standardized and is thus often confusing. Frequently used terms are as follows:

A. **Anencephaly** is the defective closure of the upper or rostral end of the anterior neural tube. Hemorrhagic and degenerated neural tissue is exposed through an uncovered cranial opening extending from the lamina terminalis to the foramen magnum. Infants with anencephaly have a typical appearance with prominent eyes when viewed face on. **Craniorachischisis totalis** (a neural platelike structure without skeletal or dermal covering resulting from complete failure of neural tube closure) and **myeloschisis** or **rachischisis** (in which the spinal cord is exposed posteriorly without skeletal or dermal covering because of failure of posterior neural tube closure) are other, less frequent open lesions.

B. **Encephalocele** (herniation of brain tissue outside the cranial cavity resulting from a mesodermal defect occurring at or shortly after anterior neural tube closure) is usually a closed lesion. Approximately 80% of encephaloceles occur in the occipital region.

C. **Myelomeningocele** is often also referred to as **spina bifida** (protrusion of the spinal cord into a sac on the back through a deficient axial skeleton with variable dermal covering). Considering that strictly speaking "spina bifida" only describes the bony defect, the term **spinal dysraphism** is considered more accurate by some. More than 80% of defects in this category occur in the lumbar region, and ~80% are not covered by skin. In contrast to myelomeningoceles, **meningoceles** (closed lesions involving the meninges only) usually do not result in neurologic deficits.

D. **Spina bifida occulta and occult spinal dysraphism** are disorders of the caudal neural tube that are covered by skin (skin dimples or only very small skin lesions are present). These dysraphic disturbances range from cystic dilation of the central canal (**myelocystocele**), over bifid spinal cords with or without a separating bony, cartilaginous, or fibrous septum (**diastematomyelia** or **diplomyelia**), to a **tethered cord with a dermal sinus** or other visible changes such as hair tufts, lipomas, or hemangiomas. The term *spina bifida occulta* is used incorrectly when it is applied to an incomplete ossification of the posterior vertebral arch, a frequent and insignificant finding that is neither clinically nor genetically related to NTDs.

II. **Incidence.** Ninety-five percent of children with NTDs are born to couples with no family history of such defects.

A. Statistics related to NTDs are to be interpreted with caution and in the context of population, location, and time because occurrence of NTDs is affected by many epidemiologic and medical factors (see Sections II, B, D and III, A–F).

B. The overall worldwide incidence has been quoted as ~1 in 1000 live births. More recently, frequency has been given as ~0.2 per 1000 live births.

C. Spina bifida occulta, myelomeningocele, and anencephaly are the more frequently encountered NTDs.

D. At early embryonic stages, the incidence of NTDs is as high as 2.5%; many abort spontaneously.

E. The California Birth Defects Monitoring Program reported the following frequencies of NTDs in live-born infants for 11 California counties for 1990–1992: all NTDs, 0.6 per 1000 live births; anencephaly, 0.2 per 1000 live births. The National Center for Health Statistics (Centers for Disease Control) reports a downward trend for NTDs (data include most of the U.S. states): Spina bifida cases decreased from a level of 0.28 per 1000 live births in 1995 to 0.21 in 2000 and 0.18 in 2005. The frequency of anencephaly was 0.13 per 1000 live births in 1997, 0.10 in 2000, and 0.11 in 2005.

F. In the early 1990s, the annual medical costs of NTDs for the United States were estimated to be $200 million. Highest annual medical expenditures are reported for the first year of life at $41,460 (U.S. privately insured patients, 2001–2003 data); annual costs then decrease throughout childhood and young adulthood to reach $10,134 per year at age 45–64.

G. Countries that have implemented mandatory fortification programs have reported a 30–50% reduction in incidence. For the United States, a 19% reduction in the birth prevalence of NTDs was reported after the introduction of folic acid fortification of the U.S. food supply.

H. **Geographic variation, sex, race, and social class**
   1. The incidence is higher in females versus males.
   2. The risk is approximately doubled for infants born to Hispanic women compared with white women. The risk seems lower in Ashkenazi Jews than in whites of European descent.
   3. Some populations with frequent consanguineous matings have an increased risk.
   4. The risk for African-Americans and Asians is lowest (but the incidence in northern China is higher: 5–6 in 1000 births).
   5. The risk is increased in infants of particularly young or particularly older mothers of lower socioeconomic class. This increase may be related to nutritional factors, considering the observation by the March of Dimes that, among women surveyed in 2001, those least likely to consume a vitamin preparation containing folic acid were women 18–24 years old, those who did not attend college, and those with annual incomes <$25,000.

III. **Pathophysiology.** The causes of NTDs seem to be multifactorial in most cases of anencephaly, encephalocele, myelomeningocele, and meningocele. Interactions between genetic and environmental factors result in disturbance of normal development. Recognized causes or contributing factors include the following:

A. **Nutritional and vitamin deficiencies.** Main concern: folic acid deficiency; other deficiencies linked to NTDs: vitamin B_{12} and zinc.

B. **Chromosome abnormalities,** including trisomies 13 and 18, triploidy, unbalanced translocations, and ring chromosomes.

C. **Genetic syndromes.** NTDs have been observed as part of a variety of syndromes, some with Mendelian inheritance patterns. A typical example is **Meckel-Gruber syndrome** (autosomal recessive), which presents with encephalocele, microcephaly, polydactyly, cystic dysplastic kidneys, and other anomalies of the urogenital system. Genetic references and databases list >50 syndromes associated with NTDs in the differential diagnosis.

D. **Teratogens**
   1. Nitrates (cured meat, blighted potatoes, salicylates, and hard water).
   2. Antifolates (aminopterin, methotrexate, phenytoin, phenobarbital, primidone, carbamazepine, and valproic acid).
   3. Thalidomide.
   4. Hyperglycemia in infants of diabetic mothers.
   5. The question of whether fertility drugs such as clomiphene are associated with NTDs remains ***controversial.*** Lead and glycol ethers have also been suspected to be associated with NTDs.
   6. Potential effect of exposure to hazardous waste in incidence of NTDs remains ***controversial.***

E. **Maternal hyperthermia.** The potential of hyperthermia to result in NTDs remains ***controversial.***

F. **Other causes.** An overall increase in birth defects has been reported in infants of teenage mothers (<20 years old) compared with those mothers in the 25- to 29-year age range. The relative risk of nervous system defects in infants of teen mothers is 3.4 times that for children of 25-to 29-year-old mothers. Although a low body mass index does not increase the risk for NTDs, obesity does. The parents' ages are not related to the occurrence of NTDs per se; the risk for twins seems higher (a two- to fivefold increase).

IV. **Risk factors**
   A. **The occurrence of NTDs appears higher in the following:**
      1. Women with insulin-dependent diabetes mellitus (the risk appears to be influenced by the level of control).
      2. Women with seizure disorders who are being treated with valproic acid or carbamazepine.
      3. Women with a family history of NTDs.
   B. **The recurrence risk is as follows:**
      1. Two to three percent with one affected sibling. Some types of NTDs may be folic acid resistant, and even with folic acid treatment, a residual risk of ~1% remains.
      2. Approximately 4–6% with two affected siblings; higher if other associated findings suggest a syndrome/condition with possible Mendelian inheritance.

V. **Clinical presentation.** Clinical presentations of the most severe NTDs are the obvious cranial defect in anencephaly and open spinal defects of the thoracic and/or lumbar spine with open spinal NTDs, both with exposure of neural tissue. NTDs with an intact skin cover may show an obvious mass (such as an occipital encephalocele) or be more subtle. Subtle findings include: bulging of the skin cover over the occipital or spinal defect, small openings sometimes missed on initial examination, dimples, or hair patches. See Section I for definitions and description of the different NTDs.

VI. **Diagnosis**
   A. **Prenatal screen using maternal serum α-fetoprotein (AFP)** at 14–16 weeks' gestation. Elevated levels (>2.5 multiples of the mean, which are adjusted to gestational age) are indicative of open NTDs at a sensitivity of 90–100%, a specificity of 96%, and a negative predictive value of 99–100% but a low positive predictive value.
   B. **Prenatal diagnosis.** Documentation of an elevated maternal serum AFP is followed by:
      1. **Genetic counseling.** The patient should receive counseling on the risk of NTDs and other conditions with elevated AFP (gastroschisis or other conditions leading

to fetal skin defects) in her fetus. Causes of possible false-positive results (imprecise dates or twin pregnancies) need to be investigated. Options regarding further evaluation (see later) are to be discussed, and nondirective counseling regarding treatment options should be provided.

2. Detailed fetal ultrasonography with anomaly screening. In skilled hands, a detailed ultrasonogram (now often enhanced by three-dimensional images) can be extremely sensitive and specific for detection of NTDs. Sonographic determination of the level of the lesion is useful in predicting the ambulatory potential of fetuses with NTDs. Ultrasonography is also done to rule out other major congenital defects.

3. **Measurement of the amniotic fluid AFP and acetylcholinesterase.** Amniocentesis is usually done between 16 and 18 weeks' gestation, although it can technically be done as early as 14 weeks' gestation. If indicated, a karyotype can also be obtained. The detection rate for anencephaly and open spina bifida is 100% when results of amniotic fluid acetylcholinesterase and AFP are combined, with a false-positive rate of only 0.04%.

VII. Management

A. Prevention of NTDs

1. The **British Medical Research Council (MRC)** demonstrated in 1991 that high-dose folate (4 mg/day), reduced the recurrence risk of NTDs by 72%.

2. Based on results from the MRC, the **U.S. National Institute of Child Health and Human Development (NICHD), Centers for Disease Control and Prevention (CDC),** and **American Academy of Pediatrics (AAP)** published recommendations regarding folic acid intake for women of childbearing age. The **American Academy of Pediatrics Committee on Genetics** gives the following recommendations in their policy statement from 1999 (reaffirmed in 2007):

   a. **All women of childbearing age who are capable of becoming pregnant should consume 0.4 mg of folic acid daily.** The committee encourages food fortification. In the absence of optimal fortification, supplementation is encouraged. Use of a multivitamin with 0.4 mg of folic acid is quoted as the most convenient, inexpensive, and direct way to meet the recommended dosage.

   b. **Women with a previous pregnancy resulting in a fetus affected by an NTD should consume 4 mg of folic acid.** High levels of folic acid intake should not be achieved by use of over-the-counter multivitamin preparations. The higher-level folic aid intake is also recommended for certain other high-risk persons.

   c. **Folic acid should ideally be taken before conception** and at least through the first few months of gestation. See the AAP Policy Statement for further details of the recommendations.

3. Sources of folic acid

   a. **Dietary.** The average diet in the United States used to contain about 0.2 mg of folate, which is less bioavailable than folic acid. Folate intake of 0.4 mg/day can be achieved through careful selection of folate-rich foods (spinach and other leafy green vegetables, dried beans, peas, liver, and citrus fruits). **Since January 1998, enriched grains (including flour, bread, rolls, cornmeal, pasta, and rice) in the United States are fortified with folic acid by order of the U.S. Food and Drug Administration.** Some countries have opted against food fortification due to concerns about adverse effects (masking of vitamin B_{12} deficiency, potential promotion of tumor growth) and issues relating to freedom of choice. Some countries have invested in extensive public heath programs to promote appropriate folate intake in women of childbearing age rather than adopting a measure affecting the entire population.

   b. **Supplementation.** Folic acid is available over the counter and by prescription. Prenatal vitamins typically contain 0.8 or 1 mg of folic acid. A survey by the March of Dimes revealed that only 27% of nonpregnant women 18–45 years of age took a vitamin preparation containing folic acid in 2001. Awareness of the U.S. Public Health Service recommendation regarding folic acid did more than double from 1995–2002 (from 15–32%) for the same group. Multiple sources are available to provide educational material: March of Dimes (www.marchofdimes.com), Centers for Disease Control and Prevention (www.cdc.gov), American Academy of Pediatrics (www.aap.org), American College of Obstetrics and Gynecology (www.acog.org).

4. **Current epidemiologic and biochemical evidence** suggests that NTDs are not primarily due to folate insufficiency but rather arise from changes in the metabolism of folate and possibly vitamin B_{12} in predisposed women. The mechanisms may also involve homocysteine metabolism. Polymorphisms of methylene tetrahydrofolate reductase and other genes encoding proteins involved in folate metabolism may be associated with an increased frequency of NTDs. Due to the homocysteine-lowering effect of folic acid, **supplementation may also reduce the risk for cardiovascular disease.** Some studies suggest that **folate and vitamin supplementation may also reduce the risk for other birth defects** (including congenital heart defects, orofacial clefts, urinary tract and limb defects, or even occurrence of trisomy 21). Other reports suggest an inverse association between folate intake and breast cancer, childhood neuroblastoma, and acute lymphoblastic leukemia. Promotion of tumor growth and the obscuring of vitamin B_{12} deficiency have been discussed as **potential adverse effects** of folate supplementation. A possible increase in twin rates with multivitamin use and folic acid supplementation has been discussed.

5. **Intestinal hydrolysis of dietary folate** is not impaired in mothers who have had infants with NTDs, although the response curve to a folate-enriched meal appears to differ significantly from that of mothers who have not had infants with NTDs.

B. **Specific management**

1. **Anencephaly**

   a. **Approximately 75% of anencephalic infants are stillborn.** Most live-born infants with anencephaly die within the first 2 weeks of birth.

   b. **Considering the 100% lethality of anencephaly,** usually only **supportive care** is given: warmth, comfort, and enteral nutrition. Support services for the family, including social work and genetic and general counseling, are essential. There are some ethically *controversial* issues regarding the extent of care and other issues (eg, organ donation), and it may be advisable to involve other support systems (eg, ethics committees, support groups, or religious guidance—if desired by the family). For family support or other resources, see Section VII, B, 3h.

2. **Encephalocele**

   a. **Physical examination and initial management.** In addition to the general principles of neonatal resuscitation, an especially careful physical examination is indicated. Look for **associated malformations.** As mentioned in Section III, C, some genetic reference texts and databases list in >50 syndromes associated with NTDs. We recommend that the child be given nothing by mouth until the **consultations** by subspecialties such as neurosurgery are obtained and a treatment plan has been formulated. **Imaging studies** (ultrasonography, computed tomography, and magnetic resonance imaging) should be arranged. Genetic evaluation and testing should be initiated early, considering the turnaround time of many tests that may be ordered (eg, karyotype and others).

   b. **Neurosurgical intervention** may be indicated to prevent ulceration and infection, except in those cases with massive lesions and marked microcephaly. The encephalocele and its contents are often excised because the brain tissue within is frequently infarcted and distorted. Surgery may be deferred, depending on the size, skin coverage, and location. **Ventriculoperitoneal (VP) shunt** placement may be required because as many as 50% of cases have secondary hydrocephalus.

   c. **Counseling and long-term outcome.** A multidisciplinary approach is necessary to counsel the family regarding recurrence risk, long-term outcome, and follow-up. For family support and other resources, see Section VII, B, 3h. The degree of **deficits** is determined mainly by the extent of herniation and location; one or both cerebral hemispheres, the cerebellum, and even the brainstem can be involved. **Visual deficits** are common with occipital encephaloceles. **Motor and intellectual deficits** are found in ~50% of patients.

3. **Myelomeningocele.** Although fetal surgery for NTDs remains *controversial,* many maternal-fetal specialists believe that this option should be mentioned to parents if the lesion is detected early in pregnancy. The website of the Meningomyelocele Study (MOMS) provides an overview of the MOMS randomized controlled study on intrauterine surgery (www.spinabifidamoms.com). After birth, a multidisciplinary team approach, including the primary care physician, geneticist, genetic counselor, neonatologist, urologist, neurosurgeon, orthopedic surgeon, and social worker, is necessary.

a. **Physical examination** should include careful evaluation for other malformations (see Section III, C). In addition, special efforts should be made to correlate motor, sensory, and sphincter function and reflexes to the functional level of lesion (Table 105–1). Voluntary muscle movements are difficult to elicit in newborns with myelomeningocele and therefore are not helpful during initial evaluation. Furthermore, motor examination may be distorted initially by reversible spinal cord dysfunction above the level of the actual defect induced by exposure of the open cord.

i. **Extent of neurologic dysfunction** tends to correlate with the level of the spinal cord lesion.

ii. **Paraplegia** typically below the level of the defect.

iii. **The presence of the anal wink and anal sphincter tone** suggests functioning sacral spinal segments and is prognostically important. In one study, 90% of patients with a positive anocutaneous reflex were determined to be "dry" on a regimen of intermittent catheterization as opposed to 50% of those with a negative reflex.

b. **Initial management.** In addition to following the general principles of neonatal resuscitation and newborn care, appropriate management of the spinal lesion is essential.

Table 105–1. **CORRELATION OF THE LEVEL OF MYELOMENINGOCELE WITH LEVELS OF CUTANEOUS SENSATION, SPHINCTER FUNCTION, REFLEXES, AND POTENTIAL FOR AMBULATION**

Level of Lesion	Innervation	Cutaneous Sensation (Pinprick)	Sphincter Function	Reflexes	Ambulation Potential
Thoracolumbar	T12–L2	Groin (L1) Anterior upper thigh (L2)	—	—	Full braces Wheelchair bound
Lumbar	L3–L4	Anterior lower thigh and knee (L3) Medial leg (L4)	—	Knee jerk	May ambulate with braces and crutches
Lumbosacral	L5–S1	Lateral leg and medial foot (L5) Sole of foot (S1)	—	Ankle jerk	May ambulate with or without short leg braces
Sacral	S2–S4	Posterior leg and thigh (S2) Middle of buttock (S3) Medial buttock (S4)	Bladder and rectal function	Anal wink	May ambulate without braces

i. There are institutional differences in the specifics of how to cover the lesion, and provision of a **sterile cover** can be achieved by several means. Some surgeons request that the infant be placed in a sterile plastic bag; others prefer application of plastic wrap to cover the lesion. Many recommend avoiding contact with gauze or other material that could adhere to the tissue and result in mechanical damage when removed. It is advisable to try to keep the defective area moist while avoiding bacterial contamination. If tolerated, the patient should be positioned on the side. Fecal contamination should be avoided, which sometimes is easier with methods covering the site only rather than placement of the infant's complete lower body in a plastic bag.

ii. Be aware that a high rate of **latex allergies** are reported in patients with NTDs. All patients with myelodysplasia should be considered at risk for anaphylaxis and other allergic complications. **Latex avoidance** is practiced as a preventive protocol. One study showed that after 6 years of a latex-free environment, the prevalence of latex sensitization fell from 26.7% to 4.5% of children with spina bifida. A resource regarding issues relating to latex allergy is the website of the American Latex Allergy Association (www.latexallergyresources.org).

iii. In most centers, patients are started on antibiotics and given nothing by mouth.

iv. Arrange for **imaging studies** to evaluate for hydrocephalus or other malformations detected or suspected on physical examination.

c. **Surgical management.** Usually closure of the back lesion is done within 48 h to prevent infection and further loss of function.

d. **Hydrocephalus** is common and often **noncommunicative** secondary to associated **Arnold-Chiari malformation** of the foramen magnum and upper cervical canal (usually type II) with resultant downward displacement of the medulla, pons, and cerebellum and obstruction of cerebrospinal fluid flow.

i. The risk of hydrocephalus is 95% for infants with thoracolumbar, lumbar, and lumbosacral lesions and 63% for those with occipital, cervical, thoracic, or sacral lesions.

ii. In some cases, hydrocephalus may not be evident until after closure of the myelomeningocele, and placement of a **VP shunt** may be required at a later date.

iii. Aggressive treatment with early VP shunt placement may improve cognitive function.

iv. Serial ultrasound scans are necessary to monitor the degree of hydrocephalus because ventricular dilation may occur without rapid head growth or signs of increased intracranial pressure. The hydrocephalus often becomes clinically overt 2–3 weeks after birth.

v. Despite treatment of the myelomeningocele and hydrocephalus, some infants may still succumb to death from complications or associated anomalies.

e. **Urinary tract dysfunction** is one of the major causes of morbidity and mortality after the first year of life.

i. More than 85% of myelomeningoceles located above S2 are associated with neurogenic bladder dysfunction, urinary incontinence, and ureteral reflux. Poor bladder emptying immediately after NTD closure may be temporary ("spinal shock"), and improvement of bladder function may be observed up to 6 weeks after repair.

ii. Without proper management, **hydronephrosis** may develop with progressive scarring and destruction of the kidneys.

iii. Renal ultrasonography and a voiding cystourethrogram may identify patients who may benefit from anticholinergic medication, clean and intermittent catheterization, prophylactic antibiotics, or early surgical intervention.

      iv. Other associated renal anomalies may be present in patients with NTDs including renal agenesis, horseshoe kidneys, and ureteral duplications.

  f. **Orthopedic issues**

      i. With impairment of lower extremity innervation, the risk for atrophy is high.

      ii. Deformities of the foot, knee, hip, and spine are common as a result of muscle imbalance, abnormal in utero positioning, or teratologic factors.

      iii. Hip dislocation or subluxation may occur and is usually evident within the first year of life; common in patients with midlumbar myelomeningocele.

      iv. Treatment of orthopedic abnormalities should be instituted as soon as there is sufficient healing of the back wound.

      v. Physical therapists assist with proper positioning of the extremities to minimize contractures and to maximize function.

  g. **Outcome of aggressive therapy**

      i. The overall **mortality** rate is now <15% by 3–7 years of age. One study revealed a survival rate of infants with spina bifida of 87.2% for the first year. In multivariable analysis, factors associated with increased mortality were low birthweight and high lesions.

      ii. Infants with sacral lesions have essentially no mortality.

      iii. The outcome in regard to the highest potential for ambulation depends largely on the level of the original lesion (see Table 105–1) and is modified by the orthopedic treatment and potential complications (see Section VII, B, 3f).

      iv. A significant percentage of children with lumbar myelomeningocele score within the normal range on **intelligence** and achievement tests. Deficits, possibly progressive, for performance IQ, arithmetic achievement, and visuomotor integration have been reported; reading and spelling may be less affected.

      v. An IQ >80 is found in essentially all patients with lesions below S1.

      vi. Approximately 50% of survivors with thoracolumbar lesions have IQ >80.

      viii. Cognitive function is improved in the presence of favorable socioeconomic and environmental factors.

  h. **Family support groups, educational material and other resources.** Educational material and information regarding existing support groups may be found at the following sites: March of Dimes (www.marchofdimes.com); Spina Bifida Association of America (www.spinabifidaassociation.org); International Federation for Spina Bifida and Hydrocephalus (based in Europe; www.ifglobal.org); National Institute of Neurological Disorders and Stroke (www.ninds.nih.gov). For information about latex allergy and its prevention: American Latex Allergy Association (www.latexallergyresources.org).

4. **Spina bifida occulta**

  a. **Neonatal features.** The presence of spina bifida occulta is suggested by overlying abnormal collections of hair, hemangiomas, pigmented macules, aplasia cutis congenita, skin tags, subcutaneous masses, cutaneous dimples, or tracts.

  b. If undetected in the neonatal period, **clinical presentation later in infancy** may include the following:

      i. Delay in development of sphincter control.

      ii. Delay in walking.

      iii. Development of a foot deformity.

      iv. Recurrent meningitis.

      v. A sudden deterioration may represent vascular insufficiency produced by tension on a tethered cord, angulation of the cord around fibrous or related structures, or cord compression from a tumor or cyst.

  c. **Diagnosis**

      i. **Ultrasonography** is useful for screening. Note that the acoustic window used to diagnose a tethered cord closes at 3–6 months.

    ii. **Magnetic resonance imaging** provides superior anatomic details. An advantage of an MRI is the lack of exposure to radiation; contrast is usually not needed.

  d. Early surgical correction may be necessary to avoid the onset of symptoms. A timely surgical release of a tethered cord or decompression of the spinal cord in patients developing symptoms may completely or partially reverse recently acquired deficits.

VIII. Prognosis. See individual topics in management section.

Selected References

Adzick NS, Walsh DS: Myelomeningocele: prenatal diagnosis, pathophysiology and management. *Semin Pediatr Surg* 2003;12(3):168.

Agarwal SK et al: Outcome analysis of vesicoureteral reflux in children with myelodysplasia. *J Urol* 1997;157:980.

Agarwalla PK et al: Tethered cord syndrome. *Neurosurg Clin N Am* 2007;18(3):531.

American Academy of Pediatrics. Committee on Genetics: Folic acid for the prevention of neural tube defects. *Pediatrics* 1999;104:325.

Bender J: Parental occupation and neural tube defect-affected pregnancies among Mexican Americans. *J Occup Environ Med* 2002;44:650.

Biggio JR Jr et al: Can prenatal ultrasound findings predict the ambulatory status in fetuses with open spina bifida? *Am J Obstet Gynecol* 2001;185:1016.

Birmingham PK et al: Do latex precautions in children with myelodysplasia reduce intraoperative allergic reactions? *J Pediatr Orthop* 1996;16:799.

Bower C et al: Maternal folate status and the risk for neural tube defects. The role of dietary folate. *Ann NY Acad Sci* 1993;678:146.

Brand MC: Examining the newborn with an open spinal dysraphism. *Adv Neonatal Care* 2006;6:181.

Carr MC: Fetal myelomeningocele repair: urologic aspects. *Curr Opin Urol* 2007;17:257.

Centers for Disease Control and Prevention: Knowledge and use of folic acid by women of childbearing age—United States, 1997. *MMWR Morb Mortal Wkly Rep* 1997;46:721.

Dansky LV et al: Mechanisms of teratogenesis: folic acid and antiepileptic therapy. *Neurology* 1992;42(suppl 5):32.

Davis BE et al: Long-term survival of individuals with myelomeningocele. *Pediatr Neurosurg* 2005;41:186.

De Marco P et al: Current perspectives on the genetic causes of neural tube defects. *Neurogenetics* 2006;7(4):201.

Dias MS. Neurosurgical management of myelomeningocele (spina bifida). *Pediatr Rev* 2005;26(2):50.

Doherty D, Shurtleff DB: Pediatric perspective in prenatal counseling for myelomeningocele. *Birth Defects Res A Clin Mol Teratol* 2006;76:645.

Eichholzer M et al: Folic acid: a public-health challenge. *Lancet* 2006;367:1352.

Farmer DL et al: In utero repair of myelomeningocele: experimental pathophysiology, initial clinical experience, and outcomes. *Arch Surg* 2003;138(8):872.

Fraser RK et al: The unstable hip and mid-lumbar myelomeningocele. *J Bone Joint Surg* 1992;74:143.

Honein MA et al: Impact of folic acid fortification of the US food supply on the occurrence of neural tube defects. *JAMA* 2001;285(23):2981.

Kaufmann BA: Neural tube defects. *Pediatr Clin North Am* 2004;51(2):389.

Lew SM, Kothbauer KF: Tethered cord syndrome: an updated review. *Pediatr Neurosurg* 2007;43(2):236.

March of Dimes and the Gallop Organization: *Folic Acid and the Prevention of Birth Defects. A National Survey of Pre-Pregnancy Awareness and Behavior Among Women of Childbearing Age 1995–2001.* White Plains, NY: March of Dimes, 2001.

Medical Research Council Vitamin Study Research Group: Prevention of neural tube defects: results of the Medical Research Council Vitamin Study. *Lancet* 1991;338:131.

Meeropol E et al: Allergic reaction to rubber in patients with myelodysplasia. *N Engl J Med* 1990;323:1072.

Mitchell LE: Epidemiology of neural tube defects. *Am J Med Genet C Semin Med Genet* 2005;135:88.

Mitchell LE et al: Spina bifida. *Lancet* 2004;364:1885.

Morrow JD, Wachs TD: Infants with myelomeningocele: visual recognition memory and sensorimotor abilities. *Dev Med Child Neurol* 1992;34:488.

National Center for Health Statistics: *Trends in Spina Bifida and Anencephalus in the United States, 1991–2005.* Available at: www.cdc.gov/nchs.

Nieto A et al: Efficacy of latex avoidance for primary prevention of latex sensitization in children with spina bifida. *J Pediatr* 2002;140:370.

Norrlin S et al: Factors of significance for mobility in children with meningomyelocele. *Acta Paediatr* 2003;92:204.

Ouyang L et al: Health expenditures of children and adults with spina bifida in a privately insured U.S. population. *Birth Defect Res A Clin Mol Teratol* 2007;79(7):552.

Rasmussen AG et al: A comparison of amniotic fluid alpha-fetoprotein and acetylcholinesterase in the prenatal diagnosis of open neural tube defects and anterior abdominal wall defects. *Prenat Diagn* 1993;13:93.

Recommendations for the use of folic acid to reduce the number of cases of spina bifida and other neural tube defects. *MMWR Morb Mortal Wkly Rep* 1992;41(RR-14):1.

Rodgers WB et al: Surgery of the spine in myelodysplasia. *Clin Orthop Rel Res* 1997;338:1.

Sanders et al: The anocutaneous reflex and urinary continence in children with myelomeningocele. *Br J Urol* 2002;89:720.

Schorah CJ et al: Possible abnormalities of folate and vitamin B_{12} metabolism associated with neural tube defects. *Ann NY Acad Sci* 1993;678: 81.

Shaer CM et al: Myelomeningocele: a review of the epidemiology, genetics, risk factors for conception, prenatal diagnosis, and prognosis for affected individuals. *Obstet Gynecol Surv* 2007; 62(7):471.

Shaw GM et al: Epidemiological characteristics of phenotypically distinct neural tube defects among 0.7 million California births, 1983–1987. *Teratology* 1994;49:143.

Shaw GM et al: Risk of neural tube defect-affected pregnancies among obese women. *JAMA* 1996;275:1093.

Shaw GM et al: Maternal periconceptional vitamin use, genetic variation of infant reduced folate carrier (A80G), and risk of spina bifida. *Am J Med Genet* 2002;108:1.

Shurtleff DB: 44 years experience with management of myelomeningocele: presidential address, Society for Research into Hydrocephalus and Spina Bifida. *Eur J Pediatr Surg* 2000;10(suppl):5.

Stoneking et al: Early evolution of bladder emptying after meningomyelocele closure. *Urology* 2001;58:767.

U.S. Department of Health and Human Services: Recommendations for the use of folic acid to reduce the number of cases of spina bifida and other neural tube defects. *MMWR Morb Mortal Wkly Rep* 1992;41:1.

Wills KE et al: Intelligence and achievement in children with myelomeningocele. *J Pediatr Psychol* 1990;15:161.

Wong LY, Paulozzi LJ: Survival of infants with spina bifida: a population study, 1979–94. *Paediatr Perinat Epidemiol* 2001;15:374.

Wyszynski DF (ed): *Neural Tube Defects: From Origin to Treatment.* New York, NY: Oxford University Press, 2005.

106 Orthopedic and Musculoskeletal Problems

Orthopedic problems are common in neonates. The problems can be isolated deformities or as part of a generalized disorder. Usually these deformities are obvious, but a comprehensive musculoskeletal examination is the key for diagnosis of associated generalized disorders. This chapter provides an overview of the common problems encountered in the neonatal intensive care unit. Many images of these neonatal orthopedic and musculoskeletal conditions, designated by ✿, can be found online by visiting www.neonatologybook.com and clicking on the image tab.

I. **Upper limb and hand anomalies**
   A. **Polydactyly**
      1. **Definition.** Polydactyly is duplication of one or more fingers. It is most common among African Americans. It may be associated with Ellis-van Creveld syndrome or chromosomal anomalies.
         a. **Ulnar polydactyly, postaxial type.** [✿] It may affect the little finger. It has an autosomal dominant inheritance with variable penetration.
         b. **Central polydactyly.** It affects the central three fingers (central polydactyly). It typically has autosomal dominant inheritance.
         c. **Thumb polydactyly, preaxial type.** [✿] It affects the thumb.
      2. **Treatment.** Surgical reconstruction is often indicated.
   B. **Radial club hand**
      1. **Definition.** Radial club hand is a longitudinal partial or complete deficiency of the radius. The typical deformity is radial deviation of the wrist and hand with or without thumb hypoplasia. The ulna is usually short and deformed. It may be associated with thrombocytopenia (TAR [*t*hrombocytopenia with *a*bsent *r*adius] syndrome), Holt-Oram syndrome, Fanconi anemia, Nager syndrome, VACTERAL (*v*ertebral, *a*nal, *c*ardiac, *t*racheal, *e*sophageal, *r*enal dysplasia, *l*imb deformities) syndrome, and other skeletal and cardiac abnormalities.
   C. **Below-elbow amputation (congenital amputation)**
      1. **Definition.** Below-elbow amputation is a transverse deficiency resulting in the complete absence of the forearm just below the elbow. It is the most common form of congenital amputation (1 of 20,000 newborns has a transverse forearm deficiency). The hand or its remnants can be attached to the proximal forearm. Commonly, it is unilateral with no genetic basis or known cause.
      2. **Treatment.** There is no treatment required, although prosthesis fitting may be useful.
   D. **Macrodactyly**
      1. **Definition.** Macrodactyly is an abnormal enlargement of the digits due to an osseous and/or soft tissue enlargement. Generalized enlargement may be due to a complex vascular malformation or neurofibromatosis. Klippel-Trenaunay-Weber syndrome (triad of port-wine stain, varicose veins, and bony and soft tissue hypertrophy involving an extremity) or Proteus syndrome are rare syndromes associated with macrodactyly. There are two varieties of macrodactyly, one presents as a large digit at birth, which grows at a normal growth rate, and in the other, the digit is normal at birth and then grows at a faster rate subsequently.
      2. **Treatment.** Surgical reconstruction is usually indicated.
   E. **Syndactyly**
      1. **Definition.** Syndactyly [✿] is a congenital webbing between the fingers. The fusion may be complete if it extends to the fingertips or complex if it involves

the bony elements of the adjacent digits. It may be an isolated anomaly or associated with chromosomal or genetic disorders (eg, trisomy 21,13,18, Silver syndrome, Prader-Willi syndrome, or focal dermal hypoplasia). It is more common in boys, often with bilateral involvement. Also it is more common in the ring and middle finger than the index and thumb.

  2. **Treatment.** Surgical reconstruction is often indicated in the first year of life to allow for development of hand function.

II. **Spine problems**

  A. **Torticollis**

   1. **Definition.** A lateral tilt of the neck and head typically due to a tight sternocleidomastoid muscle. The head and neck tilt toward the involved side and the chin is turned toward the contralateral side. These are the most common causes:

       a. **Congenital muscular torticollis [✿]** (fibrosis of the sternomastoid muscle, which may be due to a localized compartment syndrome or uterine packing problems).

       b. **Vertebral anomalies.** Klippel-Feil syndrome (congenital anomalies of the cervical spine) or congenital occipitocervical anomalies.

   2. **Diagnosis.** The diagnosis can be made with the observation of the typical deformity as well as palpation of a tight sternocleidomastoid muscle. A palpable mass in the muscle may appear in the postnatal period and resolve later on. Examination of the neonate for other congenital anomalies (developmental dysplasia of hip [DDH], metatarsus adductus) is essential. Radiographs of the cervical spine should be done to rule out any vertebral anomalies when there is no response to stretching exercises of the sternomastoid. Complications include plagiocephaly with facial asymmetry and restriction of neck movement.

   3. **Treatment.** Stretching exercises are successful in 90% of the cases. Surgical correction may be considered in resistant cases after 1 year of age.

  B. **Spina bifida [✿]**

   1. **Definition.** This group of disorders is characterized by congenital malformation of the spinal cord and vertebral column. Whereas the etiology of spina bifida is unknown, inadequate maternal intake of folic acid, gestational diabetes, and history of previously affected siblings with the same partner are contributory factors. There are two types:

       a. **Spina bifida occulta** is a defective formation of the posterior elements with intact skin, normal meninges, and spinal cord.

       b. **Spina bifida cystica** is open skin with abnormal meninges and spinal cord. Spina bifida cystica is further subdivided into three types:

           i. **Meningocele.** The meningeal cyst that herniates through a defect of the posterior elements of the spine but without the spinal cord or roots.

           ii. **Myelocele.** All the neural tissues are exposed without overlying tissues.

           iii. **Myelomeningocele** is the most common type (90%).The spinal cord and the nerve roots protrude outside the spinal canal through a defect in the posterior arch along with the meninges (dura, arachnoid). Other abnormalities of the spinal cord often occur with the myelomeningocele, including duplication of the cord (**diplomyelia**) and vertebral bony anomalies such as defects in segmentation and failure of fusion of vertebral bodies, which cause congenital scoliosis, kyphosis, and kyphoscoliosis.

   2. **Diagnosis.** The diagnosis can be made prenatally by elevated maternal serum α-fetoprotein, by ultrasound, or postnatally by the presence of the lesion in the neonate's back. **A tuft of hair over the neonate's lumbosacral spine or skin dimple may be a sign of underlying anomalies.** Associated conditions are: hydrocephalus, Arnold-Chiari malformation, congenital spinal deformity, and tethered cord syndrome. Ambulation is usually lost in upper thoracic or high lumbar lesions and often preserved in lower lumbar and sacral lesions.

   3. **Treatment.** Surgical repair is usually indicated within 48 h after birth. If hydrocephalus is present, a shunt is required.

III. **Developmental dysplasia of the hip (DDH)** [✿] is a wide spectrum of hip abnormalities ranging from hip instability to frank dislocation. In certain cultures newborn cradling may be an etiologic factor in DDH (eg, using the cradleboard with the hip extended and adducted by American Indians). Hip examinations usually demonstrate hip instability. These tests are used for clinical screening of the neonates:

A. **Ortolani test** (reduction test for the dislocated hip). [✿] The child should be positioned supine with both the knees and hips flexed 90 degrees. The test is then performed with one hand stabilizing the pelvis and the other hand with the thumb over the hip adductors and the index over the greater trochanter. The hip is slowly abducted, so the dislocated femoral head of slips toward the acetabulum creating reduction (audible and palpable). The positive Ortolani test is a sign of dislocated hip.

B. **Barlow test** (provocative test for the dislocatable hip). [✿] The child is positioned as for the **Ortolani test**. The hip is mildly adducted and pressure is applied posteriorly. If the femoral head slips over the posterior rim of the acetabulum and slides back again into the acetabulum when the pressure released, this is considered Barlow positive, which means the hip is dislocatable.

C. **Hip ultrasound** examination is indicated for screening of high-risk neonates (Table 106–1), although some clinical communities do ultrasound screening of all children. **Pavlik harness** is the treatment of choice of neonates with dislocated hips (positive Ortolani test). In the majority of Barlow-positive neonates, the hips stabilize in the postnatal period. Neonates with a positive Barlow test should have a repeat clinical and ultrasound examination after 4 weeks. If the hip is not stable at that time, a Pavlik harness should be used. Surgical treatment is rarely indicated in the postnatal period [✿].

IV. **Neonates with short limbs**

A. **Fibular hemimelia** [✿]

1. **Definition.** This is characterized by congenital complete or partial absence of the fibula. There is no known genetic etiology. The tibia is short with a valgus and procurvatum deformity. There is often a skin dimple at the apex of the deformity. Fibular hemimelia is frequently associated with foot deformities with or without deletion of the lateral foot rays. Equinovalgus foot deformity is the most common associated foot deformity.

2. **Treatment** depends on the foot deformity and degree of limb length discrepancy (LLD). The surgical options are limb reconstruction (lengthening and realignment) or amputation of the deformed foot and fitting of prosthesis.

B. **Proximal focal femoral deficiency (PFFD)** [✿]

1. **Definition.** PFFD is a congenital anomaly of the proximal femur and pelvis resulting in a short femur and hip deformity. There is no known genetic etiology. The femoral segment is short, abducted, flexed, and externally rotated. There may be genu valgum and anterior cruciate ligament deficiency of the knee joint. The deformity is bilateral in 15% of the cases. Fibular hemimelia may be associated with PFFD.

2. **Treatment** is either reconstruction (limb lengthening and realignment) or amputation.

C. **Tibial hemimelia** [✿]

1. **Definition.** This is a congenital partial or complete absence of the tibia. The infant usually presents with a short extremity with a rigid equinovarus, supinated foot deformity. [✿] Preaxial polydactyly is a relatively common associated anomaly.

Table 106–1. RISK FACTORS FOR DEVELOPMENTAL DYSPLASIA OF THE HIP (DDH)

- Breech presentation
- Female gender
- Firstborn infant
- Family history of DDH
- Second infant of identical twin if the other had DDH (34% risk), nonidentical twin (3% risk)

Other congenital anomalies may be associated with tibial hemimelia, such as congenital cardiac anomalies and or spine deformities. It is one of the few congenital limb deformities that have a genetic etiology and is seen with syndromes associated with ectrodactyly (cleft hand and foot deformity).

2. **Treatment.** The surgical options are either reconstruction or knee disarticulation.

D. **Neonate with posteromedial bowing of the tibia**

1. **Definition.** This is a benign condition characterized by a posteromedial bowing of the tibia. It is associated with a calcaneovalgus foot deformity and LLD. The condition should be differentiated from anterolateral bowing of the tibia (associated with congenital pseudarthrosis of the tibia and neurofibromatosis) and from fibular hemimelia.

2. **Treatment.** The natural history is complete resolution of the tibial deformity, although LLD may be significant.

V. **Neonates with hyperextension deformity of the knee (congenital knee dislocation)**

A. **Definition.** It is a rare deformity and varies from a simple hyperextension of the knee to a frank anterior dislocation of the tibia on the femur. It is seen as an isolated deformity and may be associated with other conditions (eg, Larsen syndrome). There is a loss of ability to flex the knee actively or passively. Radiographs are helpful to make the diagnosis and to differentiate simple hyperextension deformities from congenital knee dislocation.

B. **Treatment.** Mild cases respond to serial manipulation and casting. Surgery may be required in severe cases.

VI. **Foot disorders.** Foot disorders are common and require careful assessment for proper diagnosis. Examples of the common foot disorders are noted below and in Table 106–2.

A. **Syndactyly**

1. **Definition.** Syndactyly is a congenital webbing between toes. There are usually no functional problems associated with foot syndactyly. The fusion may be complete if it extends to the toenails or complex if it involves the bony elements of the adjacent digits. It may be associated with polydactyly.

2. **Treatment.** Surgical release is rarely indicated for foot syndactyly.

B. **Cleft foot [✿]**

1. **Definition.** Cleft foot is due to an absence of the central two or three rays of the foot. The cone-shaped cleft of the forefoot tapers proximally. Autosomal inheritance is common in bilateral cases and uncommon in unilateral cases. In bilateral cases, the hand may be affected as well.

2. **Treatment.** Surgery may be indicated to improve shoe fitting.

C. **Macrodactyly [✿]**

1. **Definition.** This is an uncommon deformity due to an enlargement of both soft tissue and osseous elements of the toes; it may affect the great toes or lesser toes. The hand may be affected as well.

2. **Treatment.** Debulking (excision of bone and soft tissues) procedures are usually indicated.

D. **Constriction band syndrome**

1. **Definition.** This syndrome is due to a tight band around the extremity. It can present in different forms: congenital amputations, acrosyndactyly, clubfoot, and craniofacial defects like cleft palate.

2. **Treatment** is a surgical release of the tight band. The band may cause acute vascular compromise, and emergency surgical release of the band may be indicated to preserve the neonate's limb.

E. **Polydactyly [✿]**

1. **Definition.** Polydactyly is characterized by duplication of one or more toes. Preaxial polydactyly refers to a duplication of the great toe; postaxial is a duplication of the fifth toe (the most common type—80%). It is less common in central toes. It is more common in African American children. Fifty percent are bilateral, and

Table 106–2. **DIFFERENTIAL DIAGNOSIS OF COMMON NEONATAL AND NEWBORN FOOT DISORDERS**

Foot Deformity	HF	FF	Missing Rays	Flexibility	Treatment	Comments
FH (Fibular hemimelia) [☼]	Equinovalgus	Normal or abductus	Lateral rays may be missing	Flexible or rigid	Amputation vs reconstruction	Tibia is short and deformed
CF (Clubfoot) [☼]	Equinovarus	1. Adductus, cavus, supination	No			May be associated with DDH or spine anomalies
	Posterior crease	2. Transverse crease of the midfoot crossing longitudinal arch		Rigid	Serial casting	Genetic factors may have role Prenatal diagnosis at 16–20 wk
VT (Vertical talus) [☼]	Equinovalgus	Abductus	No	Very rigid	Serial casting and surgery	Isolated deformity 50% Spine bifida 50% bilateral
MA (Metatarsus adductus) [☼]	Normal	Adductus	No	Flexible	No treatment vs serial casting	Associated with DDH or spine anomalies Related to intrauterine packing
CV (Calcaneovalgus foot) [☼]	Equinovalgus	Normal	No	Flexible	No treatment vs stretching	May be associated with posteromedial bowing tibia

HF, hindfoot; FF, forefoot; equinus, limited ankle dorsiflexion; varus, inversion deformity; valgus, eversion deformity; cavus, increased medial longitudinal arch of the foot; adductus, medial deviation of metatarsus. [☼] **Images can be found at www.neonatologybook.com.**

30% of patients have a positive family history. There is an autosomal dominant inheritance with variable expressivity. Foot polydactyly is commonly an isolated deformity but may be associated with other syndromes like **Ellis-van Creveld** syndrome or trisomy 13. The diagnosis is usually obvious and radiographs are essential to detect the type of polydactyly (which bony structures are duplicated). Preaxial polydactyly may be associated with tibial hemimelia.

   2. **Treatment.** Amputation of the extra digit is the treatment of choice.

V. **Birth trauma. Orthopedic injuries or fractures that occur during birth.** (Table 106–3.)

   A. **Clavicular fractures [✿]**

   1. **Definition.** Clavicular fractures are the most common birth fractures. These typically occur during delivery with shoulder dystocia, complete extension of the arm in breech presentations or with large infants. The neonate may have minimal symptoms and signs, and the diagnosis may be retrospective with palpation of the callus in the second week of life. The neonate may be irritable with tenderness over the clavicle, loss of motion of the affected arm, an asymmetric Moro reflex, and pseudo paralysis. **The radiograph is diagnostic with the fracture at the junction between the middle and outer thirds.** The condition should be differentiated from a humerus fracture or brachial plexus injury. Prognosis is very benign.

   2. **Treatment.** Treatment is immobilization with pinning of the sleeve of the shirt to the chest of the neonate's clothes for 7–10 days.

   B. **Humeral and femoral fractures**

   1. **Definition.** These fractures are less common than the clavicle fracture. **Both are associated with prolonged labor, extension of the injured extremity during breech presentation, with rapid extraction of the infant during fetal distress, and forceps delivery.** The fracture usually occurs through the diaphysis (femur; less commonly the humerus) or through the growth plate (proximal or distal humerus, distal femur). The neonates usually have pain, limitation of movements, pseudo paralysis, tenderness, and crepitus at the fractured ends. Periarticular fractures can be easily overlooked. The diagnosis is made by radiograph.

   2. **Treatment.** Immobilization of the limb with splints for 3 weeks is satisfactory, and the prognosis is excellent. There is a remarkable remodeling potential and rarely residual shortening or angulation.

   C. **Brachial plexus injuries**

   1. **Definition.** Stretching of the cervical nerve roots during delivery results in brachial plexus injuries. **The condition is usually associated with oversized neonates with a vertex presentation and shoulder dystocia, or after a breech presentation.** The fifth and sixth cervical nerve roots are commonly affected and result in an Erb palsy. The arm is adducted and internally rotated with elbow extension and forearm pronation with normal hand function. The extremity sensation is intact, and the Moro reflex and biceps reflex are usually absent in the affected limb. If the lower cervical and first thoracic roots are affected, it is called **Klumpke paralysis.** There is a loss of grasp response of the hand with forearm paralysis, and both are poor prognostic signs. Examination of the other extremities is essential to exclude neonatal quadriplegia. Occasionally it may be bilateral, especially with breech

Table 106–3. **RISK FACTORS FOR ORTHOPEDIC-RELATED BIRTH INJURIES***

- Oversized infants >4 kg
- Premature infants <37 weeks (due to their fragile bones which can be easily fractured)
- Shoulder dystocia with difficult labor
- Cephalopelvic disproportions
- Prolonged labor

*Birth fractures rarely occur below the elbow or below the knee.

deliveries. Full muscle testing is essential 48 h after delivery. **Horner syndrome is usually present on the affected side.** Recovery may occur within 48 h but it may take up to 6 months. Imaging studies includes plain radiograph, computed tomographic myelography and magnetic resonance imaging (MRI). Nerve conduction studies may be helpful to differentiate between root avulsion versus neurapraxia. For upper plexus injuries, the biceps function is a marker of spontaneous recovery. A preserved biceps function has a better prognosis. The prognosis depends on the type of injury to nerve roots (neurapraxia, axonotmesis, or neurotmesis) and the extent of nerve involvement and degree of recovery after initial palsy.

    2. **Treatment.** Surgery is rarely indicated in neonates. Surgical options include a microsurgical repair, tendon transfers to replace the weak muscles, or humeral osteotomy to correct the residual deformities in untreated cases.

VI. **Infection. [✿]** Prematurity, skin infections, and a complicated delivery are known risk factors. Hematogenous spread is the most common route of spread. The organisms may gain access to the circulation through venous or umbilical catheters, intravenous feeding lines, or invasive monitoring. The infection usually starts in the metaphysis of long bones. Because the nutrient vessels cross the growth plate to supply the epiphysis, septic thrombophlebitis of these vessels can lead to a growth plate injury and growth disturbances latter in life. The thin cortex and periosteum of the neonate's bones are poor barriers for infection spread, allowing an infection to be easily spread to the adjacent tissues. When the metaphysis of long tubular bones is intracapsular, these infections usually result in septic arthritis (hip joint, shoulder joints). The osteomyelitis in premature infants or severely ill full-term infants tends to be multifocal with or without septic arthritis (usually two or three sites). **The most common organism is _Staphylococcus aureus_; the least common organism is group B streptococci, although other organisms may be isolated.** Diagnosis may be difficult due to a lack of symptoms and signs especially in mild cases, but limitation of movements or pseudo paralysis and/or local swelling should be taken seriously. Less common presentations are pain on passive motion and abnormal posture of the limb. Once the sepsis is suspected; joint or bone aspiration is indicated to confirm the diagnosis. Laboratory tests include a complete blood count, erythrocyte sedimentation rate, C-reactive protein, and blood culture. Other diagnostic tools include a plain radiograph (usually normal or might only show a soft tissue swelling), ultrasound, bone scan, or MRI. Surgical drainage is indicated when an abscess is formed. The common sites are hip, shoulder, and knee joints. It is considered a surgical emergency to avoid the long-term results of infection.

VII. **Arthrogryposis multiplex congenita [✿]**

    A. **Definition.** It is a syndrome characterized by multiple (at least two or more) joint contractures in multiple body areas (literally the word means "curved joints"). The specific etiology is still unknown. Reduced fetal movement is an etiologic factor. The typical newborn has all the extremities affected. The typical joints contractures are internally rotated shoulders, elbow extension, a pronated forearm, and flexion contractures of the wrist and fingers. Lower extremity contractures include flexion and external contracture of the hip or it may be extended and dislocated. The knee may be extended or flexed, and severe foot deformities are common.

    B. **Treatment.** Stretching and splinting are the treatment of choice in early life to avoid fixed deformities.

Selected References

Bevan WP et al: Arthrogryposis multiplex congenita (amyoplasia): an orthopaedic perspective. _J Pediatr Orthop_ 2007;27(5):594-600.

Bora FW: _The Pediatric Upper Extremity: Diagnosis and Management._ Philadelphia, PA: Saunders, 1986.

Bowen JR, Neto AK: _Developmental Dysplasia of the Hip._ Towson, MD: Data Trace Publishing, 2006.

Fegin RD, Cherry JD: *Textbook of Pediatrics: Infectious Diseases*, 5th ed. Philadelphia, PA: Saunders, 2004.

Herring JA: *Tachdjian's Pediatric Orthopaedics*. Philadelphia, PA: Saunders, 2001.

Knudsen CJ, Hoffman EB: Neonatal osteomyelitis. *J Bone Joint Surg Br* 1990;72(5):846-851.

Mok PM et al: Osteomyelitis in the neonate. Clinical aspects and the role of radiography and scintigraphy in diagnosis and management. *Radiology* 1982;145(3):677-682.

Morrissy RT, Weinstein S: *Lovell and Winter's Pediatric Orthopaedics*, 6th ed. Philadelphia, PA: Lippincott Williams & Wilkins, 2005.

Shenaq SM et al: Management of infant brachial plexus injuries. *Clin Plastic Surg* 2005;32:79-98.

107 Osteopenia of Prematurity

I. **Definition.** Prematurity affects bone mineralization and bone growth. Normal bone is formed by the deposition of minerals, predominantly calcium (Ca^{+2}) and phosphorus (P) onto an organic matrix (osteoid) secreted by the osteoblasts. Osteoclasts play an important role in bone remodelling.

   A. **Osteopenia** refers to a decrease in the amount of organic bone matrix (osteoid) due to a decrease in the thickness or number of trabeculae and/or decreased thickness of the bone cortex. These can be due to either insufficient deposition or increased resorption of the organic bone matrix.

   B. **Osteomalacia** refers to the lack of mineralization of the organic bone matrix resulting in softening of bones. When involving the growth plate, it results in rickets. Bone density and bone mineral content (BMC) are both decreased.

   C. **Osteoporosis** refers to a decrease in bone mineral density <2.5 standard deviations from the norm (adults). There is no accepted definition of osteoporosis in infants.

II. **Incidence.** Due to improvements in nutritional management such as initiation of early feedings, changes in nutritional formulas, and other clinical practices, the current incidence of osteopenia is difficult to estimate. It is now more commonly seen in extreme prematurity and preterm infants with chronic illnesses like bronchopulmonary dysplasia and necrotizing enterocolitis.

   Previously, osteopenia has been reported in 23% of very low birthweight infants (VLBW) and in 55–60% in extremely low birthweight infants <1000 g. It was more commonly reported in breast-fed (40%) compared to formula-fed (16%) infants. Fractures have been reported in up to 10% of VLBW infants but are likely to be less common now.

III. **Pathophysiology**

   A. **An increase in trabecular thickness and bone volume occurs faster in utero compared to ex utero.** After birth, bone growth is due to cyclical bone formation and resorption. In the first year, bone growth occurs by increases in length and diameter but with a decrease in cortical thickness; however, there is an overall threefold increase in bone strength. This adaptation occurs earlier in preterm infants than in term infants. Mineral retention is affected more than linear growth, contributing to a reduction in bone density following preterm birth. In preterm infants, the bone mineral content remains lower at term-equivalent than for full-term infants.

   B. **Approximately 99% of body Ca^{+2} and 80% of P is in the skeleton at term birth,** and nearly 80% of this transfer occurs between 25 weeks' gestation and term. Fetal accretion rate for Ca^{+2} and P cannot be met ex utero. Further, inadequate intake (Ca^{+2} and P) in the face of increased growth demands result in nutrient deficiency.

C. **Vitamin D hydroxylation** is fully functional at 24 weeks' gestation, and preterm infants can form 1,25 dihydroxy vitamin D.

D. **Genetics and bone disease.** In adults and in VLBW infants, osteoporosis is associated with polymorphisms involving VDR, ER, and COLIA1 genes. In VLBW infants, homozygous allelic variants of ERα genotype with low number of thymidine-adenine repeat [(TA)n] were correlated with high urinary pyridinoline crosslink levels (indicating increased bone resorption) and with the development of metabolic bone disease. The locus interaction between VDR and COLIA1 was found to be protective in the development of bone disease.

IV. **Risk factors**

A. **Fetal and neonatal causes**

1. **Prematurity and birthweight.** Preterm birth results in Ca^{+2} and P deficiency. The frequency of osteopenia is inversely related to gestational age and birthweight. Both conditions predispose these infants to mineral deficiencies in face of increased nutritional and growth requirements.

2. **Feeding practices.** Delayed enteral feeding, prolonged use of parenteral nutrition, use of unfortified human milk, enteral feeding restrictions, and malabsorption states can result in mineral deficiencies.

3. **Human milk is low in P,** and donor milk content is even lower compared with preterm maternal milk. Prolonged use can result in low serum phosphate levels and decreased incorporation into the organic bone matrix. Unfortified human milk cannot match the mineral accretion that can be achieved across the placenta.

4. **Drugs.** Corticosteroids, furosemide, and methylxanthines commonly used in preterm infants cause mobilization of Ca^{+2} from the bone, resulting in decreased bone mineral content.

5. **Lack of mechanical stimulation.** Bone growth requires mechanical stimulation that is interrupted by preterm birth, illness, sedation, and paralysis. Neurologically impaired infants with spina bifida or arthrogryposis have limited mobility and poor bone growth.

6. **Vitamin D.** Preterm infants can absorb vitamin D and convert 25-OH to 1, 25 dihydroxy vitamin D. Vitamin D is also converted to 1, 25-dihydrocholecalciferol in the *placenta,* which is important in the transfer of phosphate to the fetus. Postnatal Vitamin D deficiency may occur in breast-fed infants without fortification due to low levels (25–50 IU/L) in breast milk. Other causes of vitamin D deficiency in preterm infants include the following:

   a. Renal (osteodystrophy) disorders.

   b. Drugs like phenytoin and phenobarbital increase vitamin D metabolism.

   c. Pseudo-vitamin D deficiency (absence of 1-α hydroxylase enzyme that converts 25 (OH) to 1,25 dihydroxy vitamin D or type I, or tissue resistance to 1,25 dihydroxy vitamin D or type II).

7. **Aluminum contamination of parenteral nutrition.**

8. **Malabsorption of vitamin D and Ca^{+2}** can occur in infants with prolonged cholestasis and short gut syndrome.

B. **Maternal factors**

1. **Maternal deficiency of vitamin D** results in low fetal levels.

2. **Maternal vitamin D deficiency** in Europe, particularly in the winter, is associated with a low total BMC and a decreased intrauterine long bone growth.

3. **Maternal smoking, thin body habitus,** low Ca^{+2} intake, and increased physical activity in the third trimester result in a decreased BMC in the fetus.

4. **Exposure to high doses of magnesium** in utero, preeclampsia, chorioamnionitis, and placental infections are associated with osteopenia.

5. **Higher incidence of postnatal rickets** is seen in infants with intrauterine growth restriction (chronic damage to the placenta may alter phosphate transport).

6. **Increased maternal parity and boys** have higher incidence.

7. **Placental hormones** including estrogen and parathyroid hormone (PTH) and parathyroid hormone-related protein also play a role.

V. **Clinical presentation.** Clinically, osteopenia manifests between 6 and 12 weeks of age and is usually asymptomatic; however, severe manifestations may include the following:
  A. **Severe manifestations**
    1. Poor weight gain and growth failure.
    2. Rickets (growth retardation, frontal bossing, craniotabes, prominence of the costochondral junction (rachitic rosary), and epiphyseal widening.
    3. Fractures may manifest as pain on handling.
    4. Respiratory difficulties or failure to wean off ventilatory support due to poor chest wall compliance.
  B. **Consequences of osteopenia.** Osteopenia can result in myopia of prematurity due to alterations in the shape of the skull. In childhood, infants remain thinner and shorter with a decreased total BMC and density. Increased urinary calcium excretion has also been reported.
VI. **Diagnosis**
  A. **Radiographs** are subjective. Most commonly, osteopenia is recognized on radiographs. Objective changes are not seen until a 20–40% decrease in bone mineralization occurs. Thin "washed-out" bones, cupping, fraying, and rarefaction of the end of long bones may occur. Subperiosteal new bone formation and fractures may also be visible. Serial radiographs in 3–4 weeks may be useful for follow-up.
  B. **Biochemical markers of bone turnover**
    1. **Markers of bone activity**
      a. **Calcium.** Calcium levels may remain normal until late in the course.
      b. **Phosphorous.** Serum phosphate levels are low (< 3 mg/dL). Low phosphate levels have low sensitivity but high specificity. Low levels of inorganic phosphate (P_i) <1.8 mmol/L with elevated alkaline phosphatase may be more specific for diagnosing inadequate intake.
      c. **Alkaline phosphatase (ALP).** Serum ALP is the sum of three isoforms (liver, intestine, and bone). The bone isoform contributes to the largest proportion (90%). ALP in infants can be up to five times the normal adult values. Elevated levels can be due to both osteoblastic and osteoclastic activity. The use of bone-specific isoform has not been found to improve sensitivity for predicting the development of osteopenia.
        i. **Elevated levels of ALP** can be seen with normal growth, healing rickets, fractures, or with Copper deficiency.
        ii. **Low levels** are seen with zinc deficiency, severe malnutrition, and congenital hypophosphatasia.
        iii. **ALP is also negatively correlated with phosphate levels;** high levels (>1200 units/L) have been associated with short stature in childhood.
        iv. **Isolated elevation in ALP** without Ca^{+2} and P may occur with transient hyperphosphatasemia of infancy.
      d. **C-terminal procollagen peptide** or propeptide of type I collagen correlates with collagen turnover and bone formation in premature infants.
      e. **1, 25 dihydroxy vitamin D levels** are elevated with osteopenia.
      f. **Routine serum vitamin D and PTH levels** are not needed.
      g. **Osteocalcin** may be elevated.
    2. **Markers of bone resorption**
      a. **Urinary calcium and phosphorous.** Extreme prematurity is associated with a low phosphate threshold and an increased excretion even with low serum phosphate levels. High tubular resorption of phosphate suggests inadequate intake. Urinary calcium excretion >1.2 mmol/L and an inorganic phosphorus at >0.4 mmol/L suggest a high bone mineral accretion.
      b. **Cross-linked carboxy-terminal telopeptide of type I collagen (ICTP),** urinary pyridinium crosslink products, cross linked N-telopeptides of type I collagen, and pyridinoline crosslinks of collagen are markers for bone resorption but are in limited clinical use.

C. **Dual energy X-ray absorptiometry** (DXA) is well validated and the gold standard used to assess bone mineral status and can also predict a risk of fractures in newborn infants. However, limitations in its use and interpretation of data preclude wide clinical application.

D. **Quantitative computed tomography** measures true volumetric bone density. Limitations are similar to DXA.

E. **Ultrasound.** Quantitative ultrasound, using broadband ultrasound measurement, speed of sound (SOS), or bone transmission time, has been used.

1. **Ultrasound** offers several advantages including easy accessibility and lack of exposure to ionizing radiation. It uses peripheral sites such as the calcaneus and tibia. It measures both qualitative and quantitative bone properties, such as bone mineralization and cortical thickness, respectively.

2. **Most commonly, SOS is used.** The SOS decreases in preterm infants from birth to term (corrected age) and is suggestive of decreased BMC. Inverse correlation between tibial SOS at birth and serum ALP has also been noted.

F. **Single and dual photon absorptiometry** are used to assess bone mineral content but are of limited clinical use.

VII. **Management**

A. **Feeding and nutritional practices.** Establishment of early enteral feeding, decreasing length of parenteral nutrition, fortification of human milk, and using specialized preterm formula can limit osteopenia. Postdischarge use of specially designed preterm or transitional formulas (see also Chapter 9 on nutrition) and human milk fortification promotes mineralization. Ca^{+2} and P supplementation to achieve adequate *retention* levels range from 60–90 mg/kg/day (provide 100–160 mg/kg/day to ensure adequate bioavailability) to 60–90 mg/kg/day of phosphate. Care should be taken to avoid adding them directly to milk to prevent precipitation. Adequate vitamin D intake is also essential.

B. **Vitamin D** sufficiency in mothers is important to prevent deficiency in the fetus. Requirements have been reported to vary between 150 and 1000 IU per day of vitamin D.

C. **Stimulation.** Mechanical stimulation by passive exercises to improve bone mineralization has yielded conflicting outcomes. Improved BMC, bone length, and bone area have been reported in individual studies. Current evidence does not justify the standard use of physical activity programs in preterm infants.

D. **Minimize use of furosemide and corticosteroids.** The use of thiazide diuretics, although of theoretical advantage, has not been shown to prevent osteopenia.

E. **Malabsorption.** Infants at risk of cholestasis and malabsorption may benefit from additional supplementation with fat-soluble vitamins and use of a specialized formula to facilitate fat absorption.

VIII. **Prognosis.** Osteopenia of prematurity appears to be decreasing with improved prevention and treatment practices. Bone mineral content remains 25–70% lower at term in the extremely premature infants. Catchup mineralization occurs by 6 months of age. Long-term follow-up suggests that bone growth and adult height may also be impacted in these infants.

Selected References

Atkinson SA, Tsang RC: Calcium, magnesium, phosphorous, and vitamin D. In Tsang RC et al (eds): *Nutrition of the Preterm Infant: Scientific Basis and Practical Guidelines,* 2nd ed. Cincinnati, OH: Digital Education Publishing, 2005:245-275.

Avila-Díaz M et al: Increments in whole body bone mineral content associated with weight and length in pre-term and full-term infants during the first 6 months of life. *Arch Med Res* 2001;32:288-292.

Backstrom MC et al: Bone isoenzyme of serum alkaline phosphatase and serum inorganic phosphate in metabolic bone disease of prematurity. *Acta Pediatr* 2000;89: 867-873.

Crofton PM et al: Bone and collagen markers in preterm infants: relationship with growth and bone mineral content over the first 10 weeks of life. *Pediatr Res* 1999;46:581-587.

Faerk J et al: Bone mineralization in premature infants cannot be predicted from serum alkaline phosphatase or serum phosphate. *Arch Dis Child Fetal Neo Ed* 2002;87:133-136.

Fewtrell MS et al: Neonatal factors predicting childhood height in preterm infants: evidence for a persisting effect of early metabolic bone disease? *J Pediatr* 2000;137:668-673.

Funke S et al: Influence of genetic polymorphisms on bone disease of preterm infants. *Pediatr Res* 2006;60:607-612.

Harrison CM et al: Osteopenia of prematurity: a national survey and review of practice. *Acta Pediatr* 2008;97:407-413.

Lapillone A et al: Bone turnover assessments in infants. *Acta Pediatr* 2000;89:772-774.

Lapillone A et al: Bone mineralization and growth are enhanced in preterm infants fed isocaloric, nutrient enriched preterm formula through term. *Am J Clin Nutr* 2004;80:1595-1603.

McDevitt H, Ahmed SF: Quantitative ultrasound assessment of bone health in the neonate. *Neonatology* 2007;91:2-11.

Rauch F, Schoenau E: Skeletal development in premature infants: a review of bone physiology beyond nutritional aspects. *Arch Dis Child Fetal Neo Ed* 2002;86:F82-F5.

Rigo J et al: Bone mineral metabolism in the micropremie. *Clin Perinatol* 2000;27:147-170.

Rigo J et al: Enteral calcium, phosphate and vitamin D requirements and mineralization in preterm infants. *Acta Pediatr* 2007;96:969-974.

Schulzke SM et al: Physical activity programs for promoting bone mineralization and growth in preterm infants. *Cochrane Database Syst Rev* 2007;2:CD005387.

Seibold-Weiger K et al: Plasma concentrations of the carboxyterminal propeptide of Type I procollagen in preterm neonates from birth to term. *Pediatr Res* 2000;48:104-108.

Tomlison C et al: Longitudinal changes in bone health as assessed by the speed of sound in very low birth weight preterm infants. *J Pediatr* 2006;148:450-455.

Wedig KE et al: Skeletal demineralization and fractures caused by fetal magnesium toxicity. *J Perinatol* 2006;26:371-374.

108 Parvovirus B19 Infection

I. **Definition.** Human parvovirus B19 (PB19) is a small single-stranded, nonenveloped DNA virus.

II. **Incidence.** An infection with PB19 is common worldwide. Infection occurs mostly among school-aged children where the major manifestation is erythema infectiosum (fifth disease). The prevalence of immunoglobulin G (IgG) antibodies directed against PB19 ranges from 15–60% in children 6–19 years old. About 35–45% of women of child-bearing age do not possess protective IgG antibodies against PB19 and therefore are susceptible to primary infection. Annual seroconversion rates in pregnant women in the United States range from 1–1.5%.

III. **Pathophysiology.** The only known natural host cell of PB19 is the human erythroid progenitor cells. PB19 is a potent inhibitor of hematopoiesis. The cellular receptor for PB19 is globoside or P-antigen, which is found on erythrocyte progenitor cells, synovium, placental tissue, fetal myocardium, and endothelial cells. Infection with PB19 is usually acquired through respiratory droplets, but the virus can also be transmitted by blood or blood products and vertically from mother to fetus. In children and adults, viremia develops 2 days after exposure and reaches its peak at ~1 week. During the phase of viral replication and shedding, the patient is generally asymptomatic. When the characteristic rash (also known as **erythema infectiosum**) or arthralgias develop, the patient is no longer infectious to others. Symptoms during pregnancy are nonspecific and include a flulike syndrome with a low-grade fever, sore throat, generalized malaise, and headache. The fetus may become infected during the maternal viremic stage. Because of active erythropoiesis in the fetus with a shortened red cell life span, marked fetal anemia, high-output cardiac failure, and fetal hydrops may develop. Myocarditis may be a contributing factor to fetal cardiac failure. PB19 is nonteratogenic with no congenital malformations syndromes attributed to this infection.

IV. **Risk factors.** For the pregnant woman, the risk of acquiring PB19 infection is highest in those who have school-aged children at home.

V. **Clinical presentation**

    A. **During pregnancy** the mother may report a history of exposure to a child with erythema infectiosum. More commonly, the mother does not recall such exposure and the diagnosis is made based on ultrasound findings. Fortunately, most maternal infections are associated with normal pregnancy outcomes. The risk of adverse outcomes after primary infection is probably <5% despite transplacental transmission rate of 33–50%. Adverse outcomes include the following:

        1. **Fetal death.** Infection in the first trimester may result in fetal loss or miscarriage. Cases of fetal death due to PB19 infection have been described mostly between 20 and 24 weeks' gestation. Fetuses that die in the third trimester (stillborn) are usually nonhydropic.

        2. **Nonimmune hydrops fetalis.** The observed risk of PB19-induced hydrops fetalis is 3.9% after maternal infection throughout pregnancy, with a maximum of 7.1% when infection occurred between 13 and 20 weeks' gestation.

    B. **Neonatal period.** The newborn infant may present with anemia, especially if maternal infection occurred in the third trimester. Few cases of encephalopathy, meningitis, and severe central nervous system abnormalities following intrauterine PB19 infection have been reported.

VI. **Diagnosis**

    A. **Laboratory studies**

        1. **Serologic tests.** PB19 **IgG** and **IgM** antibodies are first ordered when PB19 infection is suspected. PB19-specific IgM antibodies become detectable in maternal serum within 7–10 days after infection, sharply peak at 10–14 days, and then rapidly decrease within 2 or 3 months. IgG antibodies rise considerably more slowly and reach a plateau at 4 weeks after infection. Measurement of maternal IgM is highly sensitive and specific. However, at the time of clinically overt hydrops fetalis, IgM levels may already have become low or (rarely) even undetectable. In contrast to maternal testing, serologic examination of fetal and neonatal blood samples is highly unreliable.

        2. **Polymerase chain reaction (PCR)** to detect PB19 DNA is extremely sensitive. This method is especially useful in patients lacking an adequate antibody-mediated immune response, immunocompromised or immunosuppressed individuals, and fetuses. Using standard procedures, detection of PB19-specific IgM in fetal blood has a sensitivity of 29% compared with almost 100% for PCR. However, low viral DNA levels may persist for years after acute infection, and therefore low-positive PCR results do not prove recent infection.

    B. **Ultrasound and Doppler velocimetry** are very useful noninvasive measures to monitor the pregnant woman who is exposed to PB19. Ultrasound is used to monitor for hydrops and fluid accumulation in fetal body cavities. Doppler velocimetry is used to detect blood flow pattern in the fetal middle cerebral artery (MCA). An increase in the MCA peak systolic velocity (MCA-PSV) is a very sensitive measure to identify fetal anemia.

VII. **Management.** Isolation precautions for all infectious diseases, including maternal and neonatal precautions, breast-feeding, and visiting issues, can be found in Appendix F.

A. **Monitoring of the exposed pregnant woman.** Women who have been exposed or symptomatic should be assessed by determining their PB19 IgG and IgM status. If the woman is immune to PB19 (IgG positive, IgM negative), she can be reassured that recent exposure will not result in adverse consequences in her pregnancy. If there is no immunity to the virus and seroconversion has not taken place after 1–2 weeks, the woman is not infected but remains at risk. If the woman has been infected with PB19 (IgM positive), the fetus should be monitored for the development of hydrops fetalis by ultrasound examination and Doppler assessment of MCA-PSV, preferably weekly until 10–12 weeks postexposure.

B. **Intrauterine blood transfusion (IUT).** If the fetus subsequently develops hydrops and/or anemia (increase in MCA-PSV), periumbilical blood sampling and IUT (PUBS-IUT) should be considered. PUBS-IUT is an invasive procedure and carries a complication rate of 2–5% but can be lifesaving. It should be considered only for fetuses that are symptomatic. In most cases, one transfusion is sufficient for fetal recovery. When preparing for fetal transfusion, both packed red blood cells (PRBC) and platelets must be available because some fetuses have thrombocytopenia in addition to anemia. Platelet transfusion may help if the fetus develops a hemorrhagic complication secondary to the procedure.

C. **Packed red blood cell (PRBC) transfusion** may be indicated for the symptomatic anemic newborn patient.

D. **Antiviral agents.** No antiviral agents are effective against PB19.

VI. **Prognosis.** Mortality with parvovirus-related fetal hydrops is better than the generally reported mortality for nonimmune fetal hydrops (50–98%).With treatment, the long-term prognosis is good.

Selected References

de Jong EP et al: Parvovirus PB19 infection in pregnancy. *J Clin Virol* 2006;36:1-7.

Koch WC: Fifth (human parvovirus) and sixth (herpesvirus 6) diseases. *Curr Opin Infect Dis* 2001;14:343-356.

Malm G, Engman ML: Congenital cytomegalovirus infections. *Semin Fetal Neonatal Med* 2007;12:154-159.

Ramirez MM, Mastrobattista JM: Diagnosis and management of human parvovirus PB19 infection. *Clin Perinatol* 2005;32:697-704.

Skjoldebrand-Sparre L et al: Parvovirus PB19 infection: association with third-trimester intrauterine fetal death. *Br J Obstet Gynaecol* 2000;107:476-480.

von Kaisenberg CS, Jonat W: Fetal parvovirus PB19 infection. *Ultrasound Obstet Gynecol* 2001;18:280-288.

Young NS, Brown KE: Parvovirus PB19. *N Engl J Med* 2004;350:586-597.

109 Patent Ductus Arteriosus

I. **Definition.** The ductus arteriosus is a large vessel that connects the main pulmonary trunk (or proximal left pulmonary artery) with the descending aorta, some 5–10 mm distal to the origin of the left subclavian artery. In the fetus, it serves to shunt blood away from the lungs and is essential (closure in utero may lead to fetal demise or pulmonary hypertension). In full-term healthy newborns, functional closure of the ductus occurs rapidly after birth. Final functional closure occurs in almost half of full-term infants by 24 h of age, in 90% by 48 h, and in all by 96 h after birth. Patent ductus arteriosus (PDA) refers to the failure of the closure process and continued patency of this fetal channel.

II. **Incidence.** The incidence varies according to means of diagnosis (eg, clinical signs vs echocardiography).

    A. **Factors associated with increased incidence of PDA:**

        1. **Prematurity.** The incidence is inversely related to gestational age. PDA is found in ~45% of infants <1750 g; in infants weighing <1000 g, the incidence is closer to 80%.

        2. **Respiratory distress syndrome (RDS) and surfactant treatment.** The presence of RDS is associated with an increased incidence of a PDA, and this is correlated with the severity of RDS. After surfactant treatment, there is an increased risk of a clinically symptomatic PDA; moreover, surfactant may lead to an earlier clinical presentation of a PDA.

        3. **Fluid administration.** An increased intravenous fluid load in the first few days of life is associated with an increased incidence of PDA.

        4. **Asphyxia.**

        5. **Congenital syndromes.** PDA is present in 60–70% of infants with congenital rubella syndrome. Trisomy 13, trisomy 18, Rubinstein-Taybi syndrome, and XXXXX (Penta X) syndrome are associated with an increased incidence of PDA.

        6. **High altitude.** Infants born at a high altitude have an increased incidence of PDA.

        7. **Congenital heart disease.** A PDA may occur as part of a congenital heart disease (eg, coarctation, pulmonary atresia with intact septum, transposition of the great vessels, or total anomalous pulmonary venous return).

    B. **Factors associated with a decreased incidence of PDA:**

        1. Antenatal steroid administration.

        2. Intrauterine growth restriction (IUGR).

        3. Prolonged rupture of membranes.

III. **Pathophysiology.** In the fetus, the ductus is essential to divert blood flow from the high-resistance pulmonary circulation to the descending aorta. After birth, functional closure of the ductus occurs within hours (but up to 3–4 days). Complete anatomic closure with fibrosis and permanent sealing of the lumen takes up to 2–3 weeks. An increase in PaO_2, as occurs with ventilation after birth, constricts the ductus in mature animals. Other factors, such as the release of vasoactive substances (eg, acetylcholine), may contribute to the postnatal closure of the ductus under physiologic conditions. Of paramount importance, however, is the dilatory effects of prostaglandins (E_1 and E_2) and prostacyclin on the ductus. Inhibitors of prostaglandin synthesis produce constriction of the ductus. Thus the patency or closure of the ductus depends on the balance between the various constricting effects (eg, of oxygen) and the relaxing effects of various prostaglandins. The effects of oxygen and prostaglandins vary at different gestational ages. Oxygen has less of a constricting effect with decreasing gestational age.

However, the sensitivity of the ductus to the relaxing effects of prostaglandin E_2 is greatest in immature animals (and decreases with advancing gestational age). In term infants, responsiveness is lost shortly after birth, but this does not occur in the immature ductus. Indomethacin constricts the immature ductus more than it does in the close-to-term ductus. The magnitude and direction of the ductus shunt are related to the vessel size (diameter and length), the pressure difference between the aorta and the pulmonary artery, and the ratio between the systemic and pulmonary vascular resistances. The clinical features associated with a left-to-right ductal shunt depend on the magnitude of the shunt and the ability of the infant to handle the extra volume load. Left ventricular output is increased by the extra volume return. The increase in pulmonary venous return causes an increase in ventricular diastolic volume (preload). Left ventricular dilation will result, with an increase in left ventricular end-diastolic pressure and a secondary increase in left atrial pressure. This may eventually result in left heart failure with pulmonary edema. Eventually, these changes may lead to right ventricular failure. With a PDA, there is also a redistribution of systemic blood flow secondary to retrograde aortic flow (ductal steal, or "runoff"). Renal and mesenteric blood flows are thus reduced, as is cerebral blood flow.

IV. **Risk factors.** See Section II.

V. **Clinical presentation.** The initial presentation may be at birth but is usually on days 1–4 of life. The cardiopulmonary signs and symptoms are as follows:

A. **Heart murmur.** The murmur is usually systolic and heard best in the second or third intercostal space at the left sternal border. The murmur may also be continuous and sometimes heard only intermittently. Frequently, it may be necessary to disconnect the infant from mechanical ventilation to appreciate the murmur.

B. **Hyperactive precordium.** The increased left ventricular stroke volume may result in a hyperactive precordium.

C. **Bounding peripheral pulses and increased pulse pressure.** The increased stroke volume with diastolic runoff through the PDA may lead to these signs.

D. **Hypotension.** A PDA is associated with a decreased mean arterial blood pressure. In some infants (particularly those of extremely low birthweight), hypotension may be the earliest clinical manifestation of a PDA, sometimes without a murmur (ie, the "silent" PDA).

E. **Respiratory deterioration.** Respiratory deterioration after an initial improvement in a small premature infant with RDS should arouse suspicion of a PDA. The deterioration may be gradual (days) or brisk (hours) but is usually not sudden (as in pneumothorax). PDA may similarly complicate the respiratory course of chronic lung disease.

F. **Other signs.** These may include tachypnea, crackles, or apneic spells. If the PDA is untreated, the left-to-right shunt may lead to heart failure with frank pulmonary edema and hepatomegaly.

VI. **Diagnosis**

A. **Echocardiography.** Two-dimensional echocardiography combined with Doppler ultrasonography is by far the most sensitive means of diagnosing a PDA. The ductus can be directly visualized, and the direction of flow may be demonstrated. In addition, echocardiography can assess the secondary effects of the PDA (eg, left atrial and ventricular size) and contractility. The echocardiogram will also rule out alternative or additional cardiac diagnoses.

B. **Radiologic studies.** On initial presentation, the chest film may be unremarkable, especially if the PDA has occurred against a background of preexisting RDS. Later, pulmonary plethora and increased interstitial fluid may be noted with subsequent florid pulmonary edema. True cardiomegaly is usually a later sign, but a gradual increase in heart size may often be appreciated if serial films are available. An increase in pulmonary fluid in an infant with a previously improving or stable respiratory status should raise the possibility of a PDA.

VII. **Management**

A. **Ventilatory support.** Respiratory distress secondary to a PDA may require intubation and mechanical ventilation. If the infant is already ventilated, the PDA may lead to increased ventilatory requirements. These should be determined by blood gases. Increasing positive end-expiratory pressure is helpful in controlling pulmonary edema.

B. **Fluid restriction.** Decreasing fluid intake as far as possible decreases the PDA shunt as well as the accumulation of fluid in the lungs. Increased fluid intake in the first few weeks of life is associated with an increased risk of patency of the ductus in premature infants with RDS.

C. **Increasing hematocrit (Hct).** Increasing the Hct above 40–45% will decrease the left-to-right shunt. Frequently, an increase in Hct abates some of the signs of the PDA (eg, the murmur may disappear).

D. **Indomethacin** is a prostaglandin synthetase inhibitor that has proved to be effective in promoting ductal closure. Its effectiveness is limited to premature infants and also decreases with increasing postnatal age; thus it has limited efficacy beyond 3–4 weeks of age, even in premature infants. There are essentially three approaches to administering indomethacin for ductal closure in premature infants: prophylactic, early symptomatic, and late symptomatic. (*Note:* There are minor variations in dosage regimens, and what follows are guidelines.)

1. **Prophylactic indomethacin.** Indomethacin, 0.1 mg/kg/dose, is given intravenously (infused over 20 min) every 24 h from the first day of life for 6 days. In this regimen, indomethacin is given prophylactically to all infants <1250 g birthweight who have received surfactant for RDS (before any clinical signs suggestive of PDA). It would also be appropriate to limit this regimen to infants with RDS who are <1000 g birthweight. Clinical trials have shown that this treatment is safe and effective in reducing the incidence of symptomatic PDA in these infants. The major drawback is that up to 40% of these infants probably would never have had a symptomatic PDA and hence did not require treatment. A study in 2000 by Narayanan et al found that indomethacin given prophylactically for the first 3 days of life had a greater rate of permanent ductus closure.

2. **Early symptomatic indomethacin.** Infants are given indomethacin, 0.2 mg/kg intravenously (infused over 20 min). Second and third doses are given 12 and 36 h after the first dose. The second and third doses are 0.1 mg/kg/dose if the infant is <1250 g birthweight and <7 days old. If the infant is either >7 days old or >1250 g, the second and third doses are also 0.2 mg/kg/dose. Indomethacin is given if there is any clinical sign of a PDA (eg, a murmur) and before there are signs of overt failure. This is usually on days 2–4 of life.

3. **Late symptomatic indomethacin.** Infants are given indomethacin when signs of congestive failure appear (usually at 7–10 days). Dosage is as described in Section VII, D, 2. The problem with this approach is that if indomethacin fails to constrict the ductus significantly, there is less opportunity for a second trial of indomethacin, and the infant is likely to require surgery.

4. **Ductus reopening and indomethacin failure.** In 20–30% of infants, the ductus reopens after the first course of indomethacin. In such cases, a second course of indomethacin may be worthwhile because a significant proportion of these infants have their PDA closed with this course. The ductus is more likely to reopen in infants of very low gestational age and in those who had received a greater amount of fluids previously. Infection and necrotizing enterocolitis (NEC) are also risk factors for ductus reopening (and may be contraindications for indomethacin).

5. **Complications of indomethacin**
   a. **Renal effects.** Indomethacin causes a transient decrease in the glomerular filtration rate and urine output. In such cases, fluid intake should be reduced to correct for the decreased urine output, which should improve with time (usually within 24 h).
   b. **Gastrointestinal bleeding.** Stools may be heme-positive after indomethacin. This is transient and usually of no clinical significance. Indomethacin is a mesenteric vasoconstrictor, but the PDA itself also decreases mesenteric blood flow. In the trials of indomethacin, there is no increased incidence of NEC in the infants treated with this drug.
   c. **Platelet function.** Indomethacin impairs platelet function for 7–9 days regardless of platelet number. In the various trials of indomethacin, there is no increased incidence of intraventricular hemorrhage (IVH) associated with the drug, and there is no evidence that it extends the degree of preexisting IVH. Nevertheless, it may be unwise to impose additional platelet dysfunction in infants who are also significantly thrombocytopenic.

6. **Contraindications for indomethacin**
   a. Serum creatinine >1.7 mg/dL.
   b. Frank renal or gastrointestinal bleeding or generalized coagulopathy.
   c. Necrotizing enterocolitis (NEC).

   d. **Sepsis.** All anti-inflammatory drugs should be withheld if there is sepsis. Indomethacin may be given once this is under control.

E. **Ibuprofen** is another nonselective cyclo-oxygenase inhibitor that closes the ductus in animals. Clinical studies have shown that ibuprofen is as effective as indomethacin for the treatment of PDA in preterm infants. It has an advantage in that it does not reduce mesenteric and renal blood flow as much as indomethacin, and is associated with fewer renal side effects. Urine output is higher and serum creatinine is lower in infants treated with ibuprofen compared with those treated with indomethacin. However, in trials comparing indomethacin with ibuprofen, no differences were found in incidence of significant clinical side effects (eg, NEC, renal failure, IVH, etc.). Choice of one drug over the other is largely a matter of institutional preference and may be often based on physiologic rather than clinical considerations. The dose used is an initial dose of 10 mg/kg followed by two doses of 5 mg/kg each after 24 and 48 h.

F. **Surgery.** Surgery should be performed in patients with a hemodynamically significant PDA in whom medical treatment has failed or in whom there is a contraindication to the use of indomethacin. Surgical mortality is low (<1%). However, recent observational studies have suggested that surgical ligation is associated with an increased risk of chronic lung disease and neurosensory impairment in extremely premature infants. It is not clear whether this association is causal or whether the need for ligation served as a marker for a higher-risk subgroup of patients.

G. **PDA in the full-term infant.** PDA accounts for ~10% of all congenital heart disease in full-term infants. The PDA in a full-term infant is structurally different, which may explain why it does not respond appropriately to the various stimuli for closure. Indomethacin is usually ineffective. The infant should be monitored carefully, and surgical ligation should be considered at the earliest signs of significant congestion. Even without signs of failure, the PDA should be ligated before 1 year of age to prevent endocarditis and pulmonary hypertension.

H. **Should the ductus be treated?** *Controversial.* The issues of when and, in fact, whether at all, to treat the PDA in the preterm infant is a matter of ongoing controversy. There is no doubt that there is an association between the PDA and various morbidities of the premature infant. However, there is a debate whether this relation is a causal one, and, hence, whether treatment is likely to be of benefit. Numerous controlled trials have failed to show clinical benefit to the pharmacologic closure of the symptomatic PDA in terms of duration of mechanical ventilation, incidence of chronic lung disease, NEC, retinopathy of prematurity, or length of hospitalization. Early pharmacologic closure is, unsurprisingly, associated with a decreased need for later surgical ligation (and, hence, surgical morbidities). Meta-analyses have confirmed these findings. The only beneficial effect of very early prophylactic treatment with indomethacin appears to be a reduction in the incidence of severe pulmonary hemorrhage and of severe IVH; and even this does not necessarily translate into improved long-term neurodevelopmental outcome. Moreover, indomethacin's ability to reduce the incidence of severe IVH is independent of its effect on the PDA, and this effect has not been observed with ibuprofen. A differing overview and analysis of the clinical trials carried out to date has suggested, however, that exposure to a symptomatic PDA for ≥6 days is associated with a prolonged need for supplemental oxygen or mechanical ventilation. Studies in premature baboons have shown diminished alveolar development and impaired pulmonary mechanics in animals exposed to a moderate PDA for 14 days. The impaired alveolarization and pulmonary mechanics were attenuated by pharmacologic closure of the PDA (but not by surgical ligation). It is thus possible that the adverse effects of the ductus would be primarily seen in those infants destined to have either a PDA with a sizable shunt and/or prolonged exposure to significant ductal patency. Thus only a subgroup of neonates may require treatment. However, it is difficult to assess quantitatively the degree of shunt through the PDA, and it is unknown which measures or risk factors might selectively identify those infants with a PDA who would benefit from PDA closure in terms of improved clinical outcomes. No outcome-based controlled trials have been done in which treatment was based on quantitative measures of ductal shunt size or established markers of patient-specific risk.

VIII. **Prognosis** is excellent in those infants who only have a PDA. Studies show that premature infants <30 weeks have a spontaneous closure of the PDA 72% of the time. Conservative treatment (with medication) has a closure rate of ~94%.

Selected References

Aranda JV, Thomas R: Systematic review: intravenous ibuprofen in preterm newborns. *Semin Perinatol* 2006;30:114-120.

Bose CL, Laughon MM: Patent ductus arteriosus: lack of evidence for common treatments. *Arch Dis Child Fetal Neonatal Ed* 2007;92:F498-F502.

Chorn N et al: Patent ductus arteriosus and its treatment as risk factors for neonatal and neurodevelopmental morbidity. *Pediatrics* 2007;119:1165-1174.

Corff KE, Sekar KC: Clinical considerations for the pharmacologic management of patent ductus arteriosus with cyclooxygenase inhibitors in premature infants. *J Pediatr Pharmacol Ther* 2007;12:147-157.

Clyman RI: Mechanisms regulating the ductus arteriosus. *Biol Neonate* 2006;89:330-335.

Clyman RI, Chorne N: Patent ductus arteriosus: evidence for and against treatment. *J Pediatr* 2007;150:216-219.

Evans N: Diagnosis of patent ductus arteriosus in the preterm newborn. *Arch Dis Child* 1993;68:58–61.

Hermes-DeSantis ER, Aranda JV: Clinical experience with intravenous ibuprofen lysine in the pharmacologic closure of patent ductus arteriosus. *J Pediatr Pharmacol Ther* 2007;12:171-182.

Kabra NS et al: Neurosensory impairment after surgical closure of patent ductus arteriosus in extremely low birth weight infants: results from the trial of indomethacin prophylaxis in preterms. *J Pediatr* 2007;150:229-234.

Knight DB: The treatment of patent ductus arteriosus in preterm infants: a review and overview of randomized trials. *Semin Neonatol* 2001;6:63-73.

McNamara PJ, Sehgal A: Towards rational management of the patent ductus arteriosus: the need for disease staging. *Arch Dis Child Fetal Neonatal Ed* 2007;92:424-427.

Van Overmeire B: Common clinical and practical questions on the use of intravenous ibuprofen lysine for the treatment of patent ductus arteriosus. *J Pediatr Pharmacol Ther* 2007;12: 194-206.

110 Perinatal Asphyxia

I. Definition
   A. **Perinatal asphyxia or hypoxic ischemic encephalopathy (HIE)** is a condition of impaired blood gas exchange during the intrapartum period that, if it persists, leads to progressive hypoxemia and hypercapnia with a metabolic acidosis. **HIE is a subset of neonatal encephalopathy (NE).**
   B. **Neonatal encephalopathy (NE)** is clinically defined as a disturbance in neurologic function demonstrated by difficulty in maintaining respirations, hypotonia, altered level

of consciousness, reflexes, seizures, and poor feeding. NE does not imply HIE. **NE may represent a metabolic disorder, infection, drug exposure, or neonatal stroke and is the preferred terminology to describe a depressed newborn at the time of birth.**

C. **Definition of perinatal asphyxia**
  1. **The definition of perinatal asphyxia** is imprecise. Essential criteria required to define an acute intrapartum event include:
     a. Evidence of a metabolic acidosis in fetal umbilical cord arterial blood obtained at delivery (pH <7.00 and base deficit ≥12 mmol/L).
     b. Early onset of severe or moderate neonatal encephalopathy in infants born at ≥34 weeks' gestation.
     c. Exclusion of other identifiable etiologies such as trauma, coagulation disorders, infections, or genetic disorders.
  2. **Criteria that collectively suggest an intrapartum event,** but individually do not, include:
     a. A sentinel hypoxic event occurring immediately before or during labor.
     b. A sudden and sustained fetal bradycardia or the absence of fetal heart rate variability in the presence of persistent, late, or variable decelerations.
     c. Apgar scores of 0–3 >5 min of life.
     d. Onset of multiorgan involvement within the first 3 days of life.
     e. Early imaging study showing evidence of acute nonfocal cerebral abnormality.
D. **Biochemical indices.** There is no specific blood test to diagnose perinatal asphyxia.
  1. **Fetal acidemia.** Neonatal morbidity increases as umbilical arterial pH falls below 7.0. The metabolic component (base deficit and bicarbonate) is more important than the respiratory component (PCO_2). Isolated respiratory acidosis is not typically associated with neonatal complications. The precise value that is required to define damaging acidemia is not known. A pH <7.0 realistically represents clinically significant acidosis. Acidemia alone does not establish that hypoxic injury has occurred.
  2. **Umbilical artery PO_2 levels** are not predictive of adverse neonatal outcome.
E. **Apgar score**
  1. It is a poor tool for assessing asphyxia. Low Apgar scores are unlikely to be the cause of morbidity but rather the results of prior causes.
  2. An infant with an Apgar score of 0–3 at 5 min, improving to ≥4 by 10 min, has >99% chance of not having cerebral palsy (CP) at 7 years of age; 75% of children who develop CP have normal Apgar scores at birth.
  3. A 1996 revised American Academy of Pediatrics/American College of Gynecologists and Obstetricians statement emphasized that the Apgar score *alone* should not be used as evidence that neurologic damage was caused by hypoxia resulting in neurologic injury or by inappropriate intrapartum management.
II. **Incidence.** The incidence of HIE is 2–9 in 1000 live term births. The incidence of CP has not fallen despite improved obstetric and neonatal interventions and remains at 1–2 in 1000 live term births. Only 8–17% of CP in term infants is associated with adverse perinatal events suggestive of asphyxia; the cause of ≥90% of cases remains unknown. **One cannot state with a reasonable degree of medical certainty that CP in a given child was due to intrapartum asphyxia merely because the physician can find no other explanation.** The death rate in term infants with HIE is ~11%, and ~0.3 in 1000 live term births are severely affected. The incidence of HIE, deaths, and disability rates are all significantly higher for premature infants.
III. **Pathophysiology**
  A. **Mechanisms of neonatal encephalopathy during antepartum period**
     1. **Maternal thyroid disease has been associated with NE.** The effect may be mediated by a hormonal, drug, or autoimmune mechanism.
     2. **Intrauterine growth restriction may lead to NE independent of HIE.** Prolonged placental insufficiency in the third trimester can result in severe gliosis in the cerebral cortex and reduced myelination in the subcortical white matter.

Impairment in fetal growth can have a causative effect on neonatal brain injury apart from predisposing toward an intrapartum event.

B. **Mechanisms of neonatal encephalopathy during intrapartum period (labor and delivery), and the immediate postpartum period**
   1. **Interruption of the umbilical circulation** (tight nuchal cord, cord prolapse).
   2. **Inadequate perfusion of the maternal side of the placenta** (maternal hypotension, hypertension, preeclampsia, abruptio placenta, abnormal uterine contractions).
   3. **Impaired maternal oxygenation** (cardiopulmonary disease, anemia).
   4. **Impaired fetal oxygenation or perfusion** (fetomaternal hemorrhage, fetal thrombosis).
   5. **Maternal fever.** Clinical chorioamnionitis associated with elevated cytokines (IL-6, IL-8) play an important role in NE. Infants who subsequently developed CP have elevated cytokines in umbilical cord blood. Chorioamnionitis could predispose to HIE or could potentiate the brain injury of HIE. Infants with an intrapartum fever >100.4°F are more likely to develop newborn hypotonia, newborn seizures, and need for resuscitation.
   6. **Failure of the neonate to accomplish lung inflation** and successful transition from fetal to neonatal cardiopulmonary circulation.

C. **Adaptive responses of the fetus or newborn to asphyxia.** The fetus and neonate are much more resistant to asphyxia than adults. In response to asphyxia, the mature fetus redistributes blood flow to the heart, brain, and adrenals to ensure adequate oxygen and substrate delivery to these vital organs.
   1. **Impairment of cerebrovascular autoregulation** results from direct cellular injury and cellular necrosis from prolonged acidosis and hypercarbia.
   2. **The majority of neuronal disintegration occurs** *after* **termination of the asphyxial insult** because of persistence of abnormal energy metabolism and low adenosine triphosphate (ATP) levels **(primary energy failure).** A cascade of deleterious events is triggered, resulting in formation of free radicals, increased extracellular glutamate, increased cytosolic Ca^{2+}, and delayed cell death.
   3. **Major circulatory changes** *during* **asphyxia (reperfusion phase)**
      a. **Loss of cerebrovascular autoregulation** under conditions of hypercapnia, hypoxemia, or acidosis cerebral blood flow (CBF) becomes "pressure passive," leaving the infant at risk for cerebral ischemia with systemic hypotension and cerebral hemorrhage with systemic hypertension.
      b. **Increase in cerebral blood flow (occurs in phase of secondary energy failure)** secondary to redistribution of cardiac output, initial systemic hypertension, loss of cerebrovascular autoregulation, and local accumulation of vasodilator factors (H^+, K^+, adenosine, and prostaglandins).
      c. **In prolonged asphyxia,** there is a decrease in cardiac output, hypotension, and a corresponding fall in CBF. In general, brain injury occurs only when the asphyxia is severe enough to impair CBF.
      d. **The postasphyxial human newborn is in a persistent state of vasoparalysis and cerebral hyperemia,** whose severity is correlated with the severity of the asphyxial insult. Cerebrovascular hemorrhage may occur on reperfusion of the ischemic areas of the brain. However, when there has been prolonged and severe asphyxia, local tissue recirculation may not be restored because of collapsed capillaries in the presence of severe cytotoxic edema.
   4. **Neurophysiology**
      a. **Cerebral edema** is a *consequence* of extensive cerebral necrosis rather than a cause of ischemic cerebral injury.
      b. **Regional central nervous system (CNS) vulnerability** changes with postconceptional age (PCA) and as the infant matures.
         i. Periventricular white matter is most severely affected in infants <34 weeks' PCA. The "watershed" areas between the anterior and middle cerebral

arteries and between the middle and posterior cerebral arteries are predominantly involved in term infants.

    ii. Areas of brain injury in profound asphyxia correlate temporally and topographically with the progression of myelinization and of metabolic activity within the brain at the time of the injury. White matter, therefore, is more susceptible to hypoxic injury.

    iii. The topography of brain injury observed in vivo corresponds closely to the topography of glutamate receptors.

    iv. When cerebral blood flow is increased in response to asphyxia, regional differences exist such that there is relatively more blood flow to the brainstem than to higher cerebral structures.

  5. **Neuropathology.** Experimental models in animal studies have been used extensively in the study of human asphyxia to establish the basic physiology of the CNS injury. Findings in humans include the following:

    a. **Cortical changes.** Cortical edema, with flattening of cerebral convolutions, is followed by cortical necrosis until finally a healing phase results in gradual cortical atrophy. Cortical atrophy, if severe, may result in **microcephaly.**

    b. **Selective neuronal necrosis** is the most common type of injury observed in neonatal HIE. The pathogenesis most likely involves hypoperfusion and reperfusion with injury promulgated by glutamate.

    c. **Other findings seen in term infants** include status marmoratus of the basal ganglia and thalamus (the marbled appearance is a result of the characteristic feature of hypermyelinization) and parasagittal cerebral injury (bilateral and usually symmetric, with the parieto-occipital regions affected more often than those regions anteriorly).

    d. **Periventricular leukomalacia (PVL)** is hypoxic-ischemic necrosis of periventricular white matter resulting from cerebral hypoperfusion and the vulnerability of the oligodendrocyte within the white matter to free radicals, excitotoxin neurotransmitters, and cytokines. Injury to the periventricular white matter is the most significant problem contributing to long-term neurologic deficit in the premature infant, although it does occur in sick full-term infants as well. The incidence of PVL increases with the length of survival and the severity of postnatal cardiorespiratory disturbances. PVL involving the pyramidal tracts usually results in spastic diplegic or quadriplegic CP. Visuoperception deficits may result from involvement of the optic radiation.

    e. **Porencephaly, hydrocephalus, hydranencephaly, and multicystic encephalomalacia** may follow focal and multifocal ischemic cortical necrosis, PVL, or intraparenchymal hemorrhage.

    f. **Brainstem damage** is seen in the most severe cases of hypoxic-ischemic brain injury and results in permanent respiratory impairment.

IV. **Risk factors.** Previous stillbirth or neonatal death, membranes ruptured for >12 h prior to delivery, meconium staining, maternal fever, antepartum hemorrhage, fetal heart rate abnormalities, prolonged first and second stages of labor, cesarean delivery, preterm delivery, and postterm delivery. (See also pathophysiology.)

V. **Clinical presentation**

  A. The *majority* of infants who experience intrauterine hypoxic-ischemic insults do *not* exhibit overt neonatal neurologic features or subsequent neurologic evidence of brain injury. It is generally accepted that after acute perinatal asphyxia there should be an acute encephalopathy, often accompanied by multiorgan malfunction.

  B. **Occurrence of neonatal encephalopathy** shortly after birth is a sine qua non for recent (ie, intrapartum) insult. Prenatal insult *may* also have occurred. The primary signs of CNS injury in the term infant include seizures, abnormal respiratory patterns (apnea), posturing and movement disorders, impaired suck, and jitteriness. The absence of this neonatal neurologic syndrome rules out intrapartum insult as the cause of major brain injury.

C. **The severity of hypoxic ischemic encephalopathy** correlates with the duration and severity of the asphyxial insult. A constellation of neurologic signs evolves over the first 72 h of life best characterized by Sarnat and Sarnat in 1976.

   1. Stage I NE is characterized by hyperalertness and uninhibited Moro and stretch reflexes lasting <24 h.
   2. In stage II, the NE progresses to obtundation, hypotonia, decreased spontaneous movements with or without seizures.
   3. Newborns reaching stage III become stuporous and flaccid with depressed brainstem responses and have seizures. Depressed reflexes and cranial nerve palsies are common findings. Presentation of hypertonicity and irritability generally are not noted until the second week of life.

D. **Occurrence of seizures within the first 12–24 h after birth** is not unusual and may be indicative of intrapartum insult. Seizures may also be secondary to hypoglycemia, inborn error of metabolism, or perinatal stroke.

E. **Hypoxic-ischemic spinal cord injury.** Ischemic injury to anterior horn cells within the spinal cord gray matter is relatively common among hypotonic and hyporeflexic neonates after severe perinatal hypoxia-ischemia. Electromyographic examinations show injury to the lower motor neuron above the level of the dorsal root ganglion.

F. **Clinical presentation** may be further obscured by the coexistence of skull fracture, subdural hematoma, or subarachnoid hemorrhage resulting from traumatic delivery.

G. **Multiple organ involvement.** Involvement of one or more organs occurs in 82% of infants with perinatal asphyxia. The CNS was the organ most frequently involved (72%). Severe CNS injury always occurred with involvement of other organs, although moderate CNS involvement was isolated in 20% of the infants. Other organ system involvement includes renal in 42%, pulmonary in 26%, cardiac in 29%, and gastrointestinal involvement in 29%. Fifteen percent of neonates experienced renal failure, and 19% had respiratory failure. All of the infants in this study with an Apgar score <5 at 5 min had severe involvement of at least one organ, whereas 90% of the infants with an Apgar score ≥5 at 5 min did not have severe involvement of any organ. Acute intrapartum asphyxia (uterine rupture or maternal arrest) in contrast to evolving intrapartum asphyxia may not demonstrate multiple organ injury apart from a brain injury alone.

   1. **Cardiovascular system.** Shock, hypotension, tricuspid insufficiency, myocardial necrosis, congestive heart failure, and ventricular dysfunction.
   2. **Renal function.** Oliguria or anuria, acute tubular or cortical necrosis (hematuria, proteinuria), and renal failure.
   3. **Hepatic function.** Elevated serum g-glutamyl transpeptidase activity, ammonia and indirect bilirubin, and decreased clotting factors at 3–4 days of age in moderate to severe asphyxia.
   4. **Gastrointestinal tract.** Paralytic ileus or delayed (5–7 days); necrotizing enterocolitis.
   5. **Lungs.** Respiratory distress syndrome (see Chapter 89) of surfactant deficiency or dysfunction, pulmonary hemorrhage, shock lung, and persistent pulmonary hypertension (see Chapter 111).
   6. **Hematologic system.** Thrombocytopenia can result from shortened platelet survival or disseminated intravascular coagulopathy. Increased numbers of nucleated red blood cells have been reported (see later discussion).
   7. **Metabolic.** Acidosis (elevated lactate), hypoglycemia (hyperinsulinism), hypocalcemia (increased phosphate load, correction of metabolic acidosis), and hyponatremia/syndrome of inappropriate antidiuretic hormone secretion (SIADH).
   8. **Acute Perinatal Asphyxia Scoring System.** A simple scoring system can be used to identify those newborns depressed at birth that are at greatest risk for multiple organ system sequelae. The scoring system is composed of the 5-min Apgar, umbilical artery base deficit, and fetal heart rate (FHR) monitor tracing. Multiple organ system morbidity was more likely to occur when the score >6.

VI. **Diagnosis.** Recognition of NE depends principally on information gained from a careful maternal (prior pregnancy loss, thyroid disease, fever, drug use, infection) and family history (thromboembolic disorders, seizure disorder), examination of the placenta, and a thorough physical examination. Cord arterial blood should be obtained for pH and blood gas analysis. Neurodiagnostic and neuroimaging studies can help determine the extent of the injury and may also be of value prognostically.

A. **Intrapartum indicators of uteroplacental insufficiency or fetal compromise** (see also Chapter 1) may include the following:

1. **Reactive FHR and subsequent prolonged FHR deceleration** suggestive of a sudden catastrophic event (pattern of acute asphyxia).

2. **Reactive FHR, which, during labor, becomes nonreactive, associated with rising FHR baseline and repetitive late decelerations** (pattern of intrapartum asphyxia).

3. **A persistent nonreactive FHR tracing with a fixed baseline rate, from admission until delivery,** is suggestive of prior neurologic injury. This FHR pattern is often associated with reduced fetal movement, old passage of meconium, oligohydramnios, and abnormal fetal pulmonary vasculature (persistent pulmonary hypertension).

4. **FHR patterns are not always specific,** with a substantial false-positive rate. Improving the predictive value of FHR pattern in detecting intrapartum asphyxia may require supplementary tests:

   a. **Fetal vibroacoustic stimulation.**

   b. **Fetal pulse oximetry** is not helpful in timing delivery of a suspected fetus in distress or improving the condition of the newborn at the time of birth.

   c. **Abnormal biophysical profile score** demonstrated by nonreactive nonstress test and decreased fetal heart rate variability or a nonreactive nonstress test associated with absent fetal tone or absent fetal breathing or absent fetal breathing associated with decreased amniotic fluid volume.

   d. **Umbilical artery end-diastolic blood flow velocity.** Evidence indicates that decreased umbilical artery end-diastolic blood flow velocity reflects increasing placental vascular resistance in the fetal circulation due to placental pathology. However, the absence of end-diastolic blood flow velocity does not correlate with hypoxemia and acidosis at delivery.

5. **ACOG cautions against using terms such as *asphyxia, hypoxia,* and *fetal distress* when applied to continuous electronic fetal monitoring or auscultation.**

B. **Electroencephalogram (EEG)** consisting of low voltage, electocerebral inactivity or burst-suppression pattern suggests moderate to severe NE. Evolution of EEG changes may provide information on the severity of the asphyxial injury, and the type of EEG abnormality may be indicative of a specific pathologic variety. EEG background abnormalities correlate with magnetic resonance imaging (MRI) abnormalities.

C. **Amplitude-integrated electroencephalography (aEEG).** Standard EEG background findings correlate with aEEG. The advantage of aEEG is that it can be readily applied at the bedside and involves a single-channel EEG signal obtained from biparietal electrodes. Identification of abnormal aEEG patterns within the first hours after delivery may be helpful in selecting infants for treatment with neuroprotective agents. In contrast, Sarkar et al demonstrated a poor sensitivity and a low negative predictive value between a normal aEEG and an abnormal MRI at 1 week of age. Worrisome voltage patterns include:

1. Discontinuous background with minimum amplitude variable but <5 μV and maximum amplitude >10 μV.

2. Burst suppression discontinuous with minimum amplitude without variability at 0–1 μV with bursts with amplitude >25 μV.

3. Continuous background with very low voltage ≤ 5 μV.

4. Inactive, flat trace with background <5 μV.

D. **Computed tomography scan** in the assessment of diffuse cortical neuronal injury is of most value *several weeks* after severe asphyxial insults. It is of particular value in the identification of brain calcifications suggestive of an antepartum insult or hemorrhagic lesions associated with birth trauma or perinatal stroke.

E. **Magnetic resonance imaging (MRI)** is the technique of choice for evaluation of NE in term newborns. MRI can differentiate periventricular white matter injury, arterial infarction, brain malformations, and HIE. Diffusion-weighted MRI images can detect brain lesions within hours after a hypoxic-ischemic insult. Poor prognosis is seen with abnormal apparent diffusion coefficient at the level of the posterior limb of the internal capsule. MRI demonstrates the structural sequelae of asphyxial injury on follow-up and has prognostic value. Repeat MRI at 3 months of age usually shows the full extent of brain injury. MRI can help differentiate between partial asphyxia and anoxia.

1. **Partial asphyxia.** Injury is caused primarily by mild or moderate hypoxia or hypotension. Regions of the brain with the most tenuous perfusion are affected, and susceptibility varies as the infant matures (ie, periventricular white matter in premature infants and "watershed" areas in term infants). Deep gray matter structures of the cerebrum are typically spared.

2. **Anoxia.** Injury is the result of a cardiorespiratory arrest or profound hypotension. The volume of damaged brain varies with the duration of the injury. An arrest of long duration (≥25 min) damages nearly the entire brain. Arrests of shorter duration show specific patterns that vary with PCA: at 26–32 weeks, the lateral thalami are primarily affected; at 34–36 weeks, the lentiform nucleus and hippocampus and the perirolandic cortex are affected; and by 40 weeks, the corticospinal tracts from the internal capsule to the perirolandic cortex are affected. More severe or prolonged events result in injury to the optic radiation.

F. **Evoked electrical potentials** (auditory, visual, and somatosensory) have prognostic value in defining areas of CNS damage. Persistence of deficits beyond the neonatal period correlates with persistence of other signs of brain injury.

G. **Potentially useful techniques** that may be clinically useful in the future include **magnetic resonance spectroscopy (MRS), proton MRS, and near infrared spectroscopy.**

VII. **Management**

A. **Optimal management is prevention.** The first goal is to identify the fetus being subjected to or likely to experience hypoxic-ischemic insults with labor and delivery. Interruption of an unfavorable intrauterine environment is the most effective way to reduce or prevent HIE. **Despite meticulous obstetrical care, many cases of perinatal asphyxia are unanticipated and unpreventable.**

B. **Immediate resuscitation.** Any newborn that is apneic at birth must be promptly resuscitated because it cannot be determined whether the infant is in primary or secondary apnea. Drying and warming the infant per standard neonatal Advanced Neonatal Life Support guidelines may change in light of potential neuroprotective effects of cerebral hypothermia (see later discussion). In addition to assigning Apgar scores, document when heart rate >100 beats/min, the time spontaneous respirations begin, and when tone returns. Ensure that cord gases are collected and that the placenta is sent for pathologic examination.

C. **Maintenance of adequate ventilation.** Use an assisted ventilatory rate to maintain physiologic levels of Pco_2. Hypercarbia can further increase cerebral intracellular acidosis and impair cerebrovascular autoregulation, whereas hypocarbia ($Paco_2$ <20–25 mm Hg) is associated with PVL in preterm infants and late-onset sensorineural hearing loss in full-term infants.

D. **Maintenance of adequate oxygenation** (Pao_2 >40 in premature infants and Pao_2 >50 in term infants). Avoid hyperoxia (see later discussion), which may lead to additional brain injury from possible reduction in CBF and vaso-obliterative changes. Any infant requiring high levels of inspired oxygen should be evaluated for pulmonary hypertension and cardiac function with an echocardiogram.

E. **Maintenance of adequate perfusion.** Maintain arterial blood pressure in the "normal" range for gestational age and weight. Volume expanders and inotropic support to maintain blood pressure should be used cautiously. With the loss of cerebrovascular autoregulation, it is important to avoid systemic hypotension and hypertension.

F. **Correct metabolic acidosis** with cautious use of volume expanders. The primary objective is to sustain tissue perfusion. With effective cardiopulmonary resuscitation (CPR), metabolic acidosis typically resolves within 30–60 min despite an initial washout effect secondary to improved perfusion and transient increase in lactic acid levels. Bicarbonate administration may lead to hypercarbia and intracellular acidosis and increase lactate. Use bicarbonate only when CPR is prolonged and the infant remains unresponsive. Consider an inborn error of metabolism if the degree of acidosis seems out of proportion to history and presentation and if the metabolic acidosis persists despite vigorous therapy.

G. **Maintain a normal serum glucose level** (~75–100 mg/dL). Hypoglycemia is not unusual in a depressed, severely acidotic full-term infant who requires resuscitation. Avoid hyperglycemia to prevent hyperosmolality and a possible increase in brain lactate levels.

H. **Control of seizures.** May exacerbate secondary neuronal injury.

1. **Phenobarbital is the drug of choice.** It is usually continued until the EEG is normal and there are no clinical seizures for ≥2 months. Prophylactic therapy prior to the onset of seizures is not a benefit.

2. If seizures persist despite therapeutic phenobarbital levels, diazepam, lorazepam, and phenytoin may be used (for dosages and other pharmacologic information, see Chapter 132).

I. **Prevention of cerebral edema. The cornerstone of prevention of serious brain swelling is avoidance of fluid overload.** The main contribution of cerebral edema results from cytotoxic injury rather than vasogenic edema. Maintain slight to moderate fluid restriction (eg, 60 mL/kg) and reduce fluids further in the presence of renal dysfunction. Monitor urine output and observe the infant for SIADH. A single dose of theophylline within the first hour of life in term HIE patients may improve renal function. Glucocorticoids and osmotic agents are not recommended.

J. **Potential new therapies should aim at preventing delayed neuronal death once an asphyxial insult has occurred.** There is a 6- to 12-h window of opportunity after acute asphyxia whereby administration of a neuroprotective agent or a combination of neuroprotective strategies could reduce or prevent brain damage. Protecting the brain from injury would depend on the baseline fetal brain status.

1. **Resuscitation with room air.** Using 100% oxygen when resuscitating a depressed newborn with an acute intrapartum sentinel event (25% of HIE; ie, cord prolapse, uterine rupture, or complete abruption) activates reactive oxygen species known to contribute to brain injury. **Newborns recover more quickly when resuscitated with room air.** Keep in mind that oxygen saturations normally increase slowly in healthy newborns. Although it is *controversial*, avoid oxygen initially with acute intrapartum HIE and adjust inspired oxygen only if the infant remains bradycardic.

2. **Resuscitation without supplemental heat (strive to prevent hyperthermia in that excessive warming after HIE may be deleterious). Is there a potential role for hypothermia?** Neuroprotective effects of cerebral hypothermia may keep **secondary energy failure** at bay, by maintaining cerebral energy state, diminishing excitatory neurotransmitter release, inhibiting apoptosis, reducing free oxygen radicals, and modulating microglial activation.

Two large multicenter trials of cerebral hypothermia for NE, begun within 6 h of birth and continued for 72 h, have been completed using selective head cooling (Cool cap) with mild systemic hypothermia (34–35°F) and whole body cooling with moderate systemic hypothermia (33.5°F). The Cool cap study showed improvement in neurodevelopmental outcome (<50% reduction) in a subgroup of NE patients without an aEEG marked by severe abnormality. The whole body cooling study, which did not use aEEG, demonstrated significant reduction in death or disability in the hypothermic group (44% vs 62%).

Other large clinical trials in progress include the Total Body Cooling Trial (TOBY) using aEEG, and a feasibility study; Infant Cooling Evaluation (ICE), using "hot-cold" gel packs at 10°C around the infant's head and over the chest.

The optimal mode of cooling is unknown and long-term outcome needs to be continued. If therapeutic hypothermia is to be implemented, the study center should adhere to strict published protocol to ensure developmental outcome.

3. **N-methyl-D-aspartate receptor antagonist: Use of magnesium.** Magnesium can block the glutamate-controlled NMDA receptor and competitively blocks Ca^{2+} entry through voltage-dependent Ca^{2+} channels during hypoxia. Magnesium has anticonvulsive properties and prevents membrane depolarization resulting from injury to the Na-K-ATP-dependent pump. Multicenter randomized, controlled trials are needed to determine dose, timing, and control of side effects (hemodynamic instability and need for mechanical ventilation) along with long-term follow-up.

4. **Other pharmacologic agents to prevent free oxygen radical formation** (allopurinol, inhibitors of nitric oxide production), neuroprotection directed toward Ca^{2+} intraneuronal entry (calcium channel blockers), neurotropins, and apoptosis inhibition remain investigational.

K. **Ethics.** Decision making is often difficult, but it is easier if the medical team and families communicate openly and clearly. (See Chapters 20 and 44.) Shared decision making creates a partnership between parents and the physician and potentially reduces conflicts. Discussing best and worst case outcomes may help define the range of potential outcome.

L. **Medicolegal issues**

1. **Fetal monitoring.** In the presence of a reactive FHR pattern and normal fetal movement, the key is to monitor the baseline rate. A rise or fall in FHR baseline should alert the labor and delivery team to impending fetal asphyxia.

2. **Timing of asphyxia to the intrapartum period** may be the cause of CP if there is no evidence of antenatal injury (clinically or by neuroimaging studies), classic criteria for severe asphyxia are present, and all other causes of neonatal encephalopathy have been excluded. Acute intrapartum asphyxia typically leads to CP of the spastic quadriplegic type.

3. **Persistent nonreactive FHR pattern** from admission to delivery is suggestive of brain injury remote to the intrapartum period. This FHR pattern is associated with high numbers of nucleated red blood cells and lower platelet counts in brain-damaged newborns.

4. **When asked whether an identified event led to a subsequent adverse outcome,** it is important to realize that the baseline fetal brain status is unknown.

VIII. **Prognosis.** Most survivors of perinatal asphyxia do not have major sequelae.

A. **Predicting probable death or neurologic disability in the first 6 h of life to identify eligible encephalopathic newborns for neuroprotective therapies.**

1. Shah et al used three variables, which consisted of cardiac compressions >1 min, onset of breathing >30 min, and base deficit >16. Forty-six percent of encephalopathic newborns had adverse outcomes with none of the three variables present, increasing to 64% with one variable, 76% with two variables, and 93% with all three of the variables present.

2. Ambalavanan et al analyzed HIE infants who participated in their National Institute of Child Health and Human Development whole body hypothermia trial. They used a classification and regression tree model to predict death or disability. Positive predictive value increases if the umbilical artery cord pH <6.7, if associated with no spontaneous activity, and if the base deficit in the first postnatal blood gas was ≥16. The neurologic findings of abnormal posture, absent spontaneous activity, and absent suck were the most useful components of the neurologic examination. In their model, infants with a cord pH >6.7, base deficit ≤18.5 mmol/L, and normal to decreased spontaneous activity had better outcomes if the cord P_{CO_2} was >87 mm Hg compared to a cord P_{CO_2} <87 mm Hg. This underscores the importance of obtaining all the components of the cord blood gas.

B. **Predicting long-term neurologic sequelae**
1. **Severity of the neonatal encephalopathy.** Severe HIE (Sarnat stage III) carries a mortality rate of ~80%, and survivors often have multiple disabilities, including spastic CP, severe or profound mental retardation, cortical blindness, or seizure disorder. Moderately affected (Sarnat stage II) patients have outcomes that vary with their overall clinical course and duration of their neurologic condition. Sarnat stage II continuing >5 days is a poorer prognostic sign.
2. **Presence of neonatal seizures,** especially if they occur within the first 12 h after birth and are difficult to control.
3. **An abnormal MRI** obtained in the first 24–72 h (alterations in the basal ganglia and thalami, absence of a normal signal at the level of the posterior limb of the internal capsule, or injury to the hippocampus) is associated with a poor outcome, irrespective of birth variables. An abnormal signal in the posterior limb of the internal capsule predicted an unfavorable outcome in 33 of 36 infants with Sarnat stage II HIE.
4. **Severity and duration of EEG abnormalities.** Normal EEG background within the first days after delivery is significantly correlated with normal outcomes, and moderately to severely abnormal EEG patterns are significantly related to abnormal outcomes. A burst-suppression or isoelectric pattern on any day and prolonged EEG depression after day 12 are associated with a poor outcome. Recovery of normal EEG background by day 7 is associated with a normal outcome. The early presence (within the first days after birth) of a normal or near-normal EEG, even in a "comatose" child, is a strong predictor of a good neurologic outcome.
5. **Abnormal visual evoked potentials (VEPs).** Abnormal VEP throughout the first week of life or an absent VEP at any time guaranteed an abnormal outcome in asphyxiated full-term infants.
6. **Subsequent hearing is normal in most children who have suffered perinatal or postnatal asphyxia.** Children with residual neurodevelopmental deficits have more frequent peripheral hearing loss and more abnormalities of the central components of auditory evoked potentials than those who do not have neurodevelopmental deficits, suggestive of residual dysfunction in the rostral brainstem.
7. **Microcephaly** at 3 months of age or an abnormal neurologic exam at 12 months of age predict poor neurodevelopmental outcome at 5 years of age. A decrease in head circumference (HC) ratios (actual HC/mean HC for age × 100%) of >3.1% between birth and 4 months of age is highly predictive of the eventual development of microcephaly before 18 months of age. Suboptimal rate of head growth associated with moderate cerebral white matter changes on MRI may be a better predictor of poor neurodevelopmental outcome.
8. **The presence of optic atrophy** is an indicator of poor visual outcome. Many children with postasphyxial CNS abnormalities have lower visual acuity scores and smaller visual fields.
C. **Nondisabled survivors of moderate HIE** have delayed skills in reading, spelling, or arithmetic and have more difficulties with attention and short-term recall than survivors of mild HIE and normal individuals.

Selected References

Ambalavanan N et al: Predicting outcomes of neonates diagnosed with hypoxemic-ischemic encephalopathy. *Pediatrics* 2006;118:2084-2093.

Andres RL et al: Association between umbilical blood gas parameters and neonatal morbidity and death in neonates with pathologic fetal acidemia. *Am J Obstet Gynecol* 1999;18:867-871.

Ankarcrona M et al: Glutamate-induced neuronal death: a succession of necrosis or apoptosis depending on mitochondrial function. *Neuron* 1995;15:961-973.

Badawi N et al: Antepartum risk factors for newborn encephalopathy: the Western Australian case-control study. *Brit Med J* 1998;317:1549-1553.

Behrman RE et al: Distribution of circulation in the normal and asphyxiated fetal primate. *Am J Obstet Gynecol* 1970;108:956-969.

Berger R, Garnier Y: Pathophysiology of perinatal brain damage. *Brain Res Brain Res Rev* 1999;30:107-134.

Bhat MA et al: Theophylline for renal function in term neonates with perinatal asphyxia: a randomized, placebo-controlled trial. *J Pediatr* 2006;149:180-184.

Blackmon LR, Stark AR; The Committee on Fetus and Newborn, AAP: Hypothermia: a neuroprotective therapy for neonatal hypoxic-ischemic encephalopathy. *Pediatrics* 2006;117:942-948.

Bloom SL et al: Fetal pulse oximetry and cesarean delivery. *N Engl J Med* 2006;355:2195-2202.

Boichot C et al: Term neonate prognoses after perinatal asphyxia: contributions of MR imaging, MR spectroscopy, relaxation times, and apparent diffusion coefficients. *Radiology* 2006;239:839-848.

Bukowski R et al: Impairment of fetal growth potential and neonatal encephalopathy. *Am J Obstet Gynecol* 2003;188:1011-1015.

Carter BS et al: Prospective validation of a scoring system for predicting neonatal morbidity after perinatal asphyxia. *J Pediatr* 1998;132:619-632.

Cheong JLY et al: Proton MR spectroscopy in neonates with perinatal cerebral hypoxic-ischemic injury: metabolite peak-area ratios, relaxation times, and absolute concentrations. *Am J Neuroradiol* 2006;27:1546-1554.

Clancy RR et al: Hypoxic-ischemic spinal cord injury following perinatal asphyxia. *Ann Neurol* 1989;25:185-189.

Cordes I et al: Early prediction of the development of microcephaly after hypoxic-ischemic encephalopathy in the full-term newborn. *Pediatrics* 1994;93:703-707.

De Hann HH et al: Brief repeated umbilical cord occlusions cause sustained cytotoxic cerebral edema and focal infarcts in near-term fetal lambs. *Pediatr Res* 1997;41:96-104.

de Vries LS, Toet MC: Amplitude integrated electroencephalography in the full-term newborn. *Clin Perinatol* 2006;33:619-623.

Edwards AD, Nelson KB: Neonatal encephalopathies: time to reconsider the cause of encephalopathies. *Brit Med J* 1998;317:1537–1538.

El-Ayouty M et al: Relationship between electroencephalography and magnetic resonance imaging findings after hypoxic-ischemic encephalopathy. *Am J Perinatol* 2007;8: 467-473.

Evans DJ et al: Anticonvulsants for preventing mortality and morbidity in full term newborns with perinatal asphyxia. *Cochrane Database Syst Rev* 2007;3:CD001240.

Ferriero DM: Neonatal brain injury. *N Engl J Med* 2004;351:1985-1995.

Gluckman PD et al: Selective head cooling with mild systemic hypothermia after neonatal encephalopathy: multicentre randomized trial. *Lancet* 2005;365:663-670.

Goldaber KG et al: Pathologic fetal acidemia. *Obstet Gynecol* 1991;78:1103-1107.

Greene CL, Goodman SI: Catastrophic metabolic encephalopathies in the newborn period. Evaluation and management. *Clin Perinatol* 1997;24:773-786.

Gunn AJ, Gunn TR: The 'pharmacology' of neuronal rescue with cerebral hypothermia. *Early Hum Dev* 1998;53:19-35.

Jacobs MM, Phibbs RH: Prevention, recognition, and treatment of perinatal asphyxia. *Clin Perinatol* 1989;16:785-807.

Jiang ZD, Tierney TS: Long term effect of perinatal and postnatal asphyxia on developing human auditory brainstem responses: brainstem impairment. *Int J Pediatr Otorhinolaryngol* 1996;34:111-127.

Kamlin CO et al: Oxygen saturation in healthy infants immediately after birth. *J Pediatr* 2006;148:569-570.

Korst LM et al: Acute fetal asphyxia and permanent brain injury: a retrospective analysis of current indicators. *J Matern Fetal Med* 1999;8:101-106.

Lieberman E et al: Intrapartum fever and neonatal outcome. *Pediatrics* 2000;105:8-13.

Lorek A et al: Delayed ("secondary") cerebral energy failure after acute hypoxic-ischemia in the newborn piglet: continuous 48-hour studies by phosphorus magnetic resonance spectroscopy. *Pediatr Res* 1994;36:699-706.

Luna B et al: Grating acuity and visual field development in infants following perinatal asphyxia. *Dev Med Child Neurol* 1995;37:330-344.

Mallard EC et al: Effects of chronic placental insufficiency on brain development in fetal sheep. *Pediatr Res* 1998;43:262-270.

Manning FA et al: The abnormal fetal biophysical profile score. V. Predictive accuracy according to score composition. *Am J Obstet Gynecol* 1990;162:918-924.

Martín-Ancel A et al: Multiple organ involvement in perinatal asphyxia. *J Pediatr* 1995;127:786-793.

Martin E et al: Diagnostic and prognostic value of cerebral ^{31}P magnetic resonance spectroscopy in neonates with perinatal asphyxia. *Pediatr Res* 1996;40:749-758.

Ment LR et al: Practice parameter: neuroimaging of the neonate. Report of the Quality Standards Subcommittee of the American Academy of Neurology and the Practice Committee of the Child Neurology Society. *Neurology* 2002;58:1726-1738.

Mercuri E et al: Head growth in infants with hypoxic-ischemic encephalopathy: correlation with neonatal magnetic resonance imaging. *Pediatrics* 2000;106(2 Pt 1):235-243.

Miller SP et al: Patterns of brain injury in term neonatal encephalopathy. *J Pediatr* 2005;146:453-460.

Muttit SC et al: Serial visual evoked potentials and outcome in term birth asphyxia. *Pediatr Neurol* 1991;7:86-90.

Myers RE: Experimental models of perinatal brain damage; relevance to human pathology. In Gluck L (ed): *Intrauterine Asphyxia in the Developing Fetal Brain*. Chicago, IL: Yearbook Medical Publishers, 1977:37-97.

Myers RE et al: Brain swelling in the newborn rhesus monkey following severe in utero partial asphyxia. *Neurology* 1975;25:516-521.

Nelson KB: Perinatal ischemic stroke. *Stroke* 2007;38:742-745.

Nelson KB, Ellenberg JH: Apgar scores as predictors of chronic neurologic disability. *Pediatrics* 1981;68:36-44.

Nicklin SE: Perinatal ischemic stroke. *Stroke* 2007;38:742-745.

Nicklin SE et al: The light still shines, but not that brightly? The current status of perinatal near infrared spectroscopy. *Arch Dis Child Fetal Neonatal Ed* 2003;88:F263-F268.

Papadopoulos VG et al: Vibroacoustic stimulation in abnormal biophysical profile: verification of facilitation of fetal well-being. *Early Hum Dev* 2007;83:191-197.

Pattinson RC et al: Obstetric and neonatal outcome in fetuses with absent end-diastolic velocities of the umbilical artery: a case-controlled study. *Am J Perinatol* 1993;10:135-138.

Phelan JP, Kim JO: Fetal heart rate observations in the brain damaged infant. *Semin Perinatol* 2000;24:221-229.

Phelan JP et al: Neonatal nucleated red blood cell and platelet counts in asphyxiated neonates sufficient to result in permanent neurologic impairment. *J Matern Fetal Neonatal Med* 2007;20:377-380.

Ranck JB, Windle WF: Brain damage in the monkey, Macaca mulatta by asphyxia neonatorum. *Exp Neurol* 1959;1:130-154.

Robertson CM, Finer NN: Long-term follow-up of term neonates with perinatal asphyxia. *Clin Perinatol* 1993;20:483-500.

Rutherford MA et al: Abnormal magnetic resonance signal in the internal capsule predicts poor neurodevelopmental outcome in infants with hypoxic-ischemic encephalopathy. *Pediatrics* 1998;102(2 Pt 1):323-328.

Salhab WA et al: Initial hypoglycemia and neonatal brain injury in term infants with severe fetal acidemia. *Pediatrics* 2004;114:361-366.

Sarkar S et al: Should amplitude-integrated electroencephalography be used to identify infants suitable for hypothermic neuroprotection? *J Perinatol* 2008;28:117-122.

Sarnat HB, Sarnat MS: Neonatal encephalopathy following fetal distress. A clinical and electroencephalographic study. *Arch Neurol* 1976;33:696-705.

Saugstad OD: Oxygen for newborns: How much is too much? *J Perinatol* 2005;25(suppl 2):S45-S49.

Scalais E et al: Multimodality evoked potentials as a prognostic tool in term asphyxiated newborns. *Electroencephalogr Clin Neurophysiol* 1998;108:199-207.

Schifrin BS et al: Fetal heart rate patterns and the timing of fetal injury. *J Perinatol* 1194;14:174-181.

Shah PS et al: Postasphyxial hypoxic-ischemic encephalopathy in neonates: outcome prediction rule within 4 hours of birth. *Arch Pediatr Adolesc Med* 2006;160:729-736.

Shakaran S, Laptook AR: Hypothermia as a treatment of birth asphyxia. *Clin Obstet Gynecol* 2007;50:624-635.

Shakaran S et al: Acute neonatal morbidity and long-term central nervous system sequelae of perinatal asphyxia in term infants. *Early Hum Dev* 1991;25:135-148.

Shalak LF et al: Clinical chorioamnionitis, elevated cytokines, and brain injury in term infants. *Pediatrics* 2002;110:673-680.

Shankaran S et al: Whole body-hypothermia for neonates with hypoxic-ischemic encephalopathy. *N Engl J Med* 2005;353:1574-1584.

Van Lieshout HB et al: The prognostic value of the EEG in asphyxiated newborns. *Acta Neurol Scand* 1995;91:203-207.

Volpe JJ: *Neurology of the Newborn,* 4th ed. Philadelphia, PA: Saunders, 2001.

Williams CE et al: Outcome after ischemia in the developing sheep brain: an electroencephalogram and histological study. *Ann Neurol* 1992;31:14-21.

Wolf RL et al: Quantitative apparent diffusion coefficient measurements in term neonates for early detection of hypoxic-ischemic brain injury initial experience. *Radiology* 2001;218:825-833.

Zimmerman RA, Bilaniuk T: Neuroimaging evaluation of cerebral palsy. *Clin Perinatol* 2006;33:517-544.

111 Persistent Pulmonary Hypertension of the Newborn

I. **Definition.** Persistent pulmonary hypertension of the newborn (PPHN) is a condition characterized by marked pulmonary hypertension resulting from elevated pulmonary vascular resistance (PVR) and altered pulmonary vasoreactivity, leading to right-to-left extrapulmonary shunting of blood across the foramen ovale and the ductus arteriosus, if it is patent. It is associated with a wide array of cardiopulmonary disorders that may also cause intrapulmonary shunting. When this disorder is of unknown cause and is the primary cause of cardiopulmonary distress, it is often called "idiopathic PPHN" or persistent fetal circulation.

II. **Incidence** is 2-6 per 1000 live births.

III. **Pathophysiology.** PPHN may be the result of underdevelopment of the lung together with its vascular bed (eg, congenital diaphragmatic hernia and hypoplastic lungs), maladaptation of the pulmonary vascular bed to the transition occurring around the time of birth (eg, various conditions of perinatal stress, hemorrhage, aspiration, hypoxia, and hypoglycemia); and maldevelopment of the pulmonary vascular bed in utero from a known or unknown cause. It is convenient to think in terms of this basic pathologic classification. However, the clinical manifestations of PPHN are often not attributable to a single physiologic or structural entity, and many disorders exhibit more than one underlying pathology. Often, even when there is evidence of perinatal or postnatal stress (eg, meconium aspiration), the underlying cause of PPHN had been secondary to an in utero process of some duration.

Preacinar arteries are already present in the lungs by 16 weeks' gestation; thereafter, respiratory units are added with further growth of the appropriate arteries. Muscularization of the peripheral pulmonary arteries is related to differentiation of pericytes and to recruitment of fibroblasts and is influenced by numerous trophic factors (eg, neuropeptides, fibroblast growth factors, and insulin-like growth factors). In addition, the growth, differentiation, and adaptation of the pulmonary vascular bed are also influenced by changes that occur in the connective tissue matrix (eg, elastin and collagen). The lungs of infants with PPHN contain many undilated precapillary arteries, and pulmonary arterial medial thickness is increased. There may be extension of muscle in small and peripheral arteries that are normally nonmuscular. After a few days, there is already evidence of structural remodeling with connective tissue deposition.

In the fetus, PVR is high, and only 5–10% of the combined cardiac output flows into the lungs, with most of the right ventricular output crossing the ductus arteriosus to the aorta. After birth, with expansion of the lungs, there is a sharp drop in PVR and pulmonary blood flow increases about 10-fold. The factors responsible for maintaining high PVR in the fetus and for effecting the acute reduction in PVR that occurs after birth are incompletely understood. Fetal and neonatal pulmonary vascular tone is modulated through a balance between vasoconstrictive and vasodilatory stimuli. Vasoconstrictive stimuli possibly include various products of arachidonic acid metabolism (eg, thromboxane, leukotrienes, and isoprostanes), Rho/Rho kinase, and the endothelins (ETs). The hemodynamic effect of the ETs are mediated by at least two receptors; ET-A and ET-B. There are at least three isoforms of endothelin. ET-1, the most studied of these, constricts pulmonary arteries from various animals, but the intrapulmonary infusion of ET-1 has a biphasic response: initially dilating the vascular bed of the intact fetal lamb. This vasodilatory effect is transient and followed by a return to baseline tone when the infusion is continued. The biphasic response to ET-1 is likely due to initial activation of ET-B receptors (which stimulate release of nitric oxide), followed by activation of the ET-A receptors, which mediate vasoconstriction. Selective ET-A blockade causes fetal pulmonary vasodilatation, and upregulation of ET-1 contributes to pulmonary hypertension. RhoA is a GTPase, and rho-kinase is its effector protein. These have been identified as key regulators of vascular tone and structure. Rho-kinase phosphorylates and inactivates myosin light chain phosphatase, increasing calcium sensitivity of vascular smooth muscle, and thus promotes vasoconstriction. Prolonged treatment with rho-kinase inhibitors prevents the development of pulmonary hypertension in some animal models. There is an interaction between the rho-kinase and the nitric oxide signaling pathway, and inhibition of rho-kinase also prevents vasoconstriction caused by inhibition of nitric oxide production. Strong experimental data support the potential role for ET antagonists and rho-kinase inhibitors in future therapy for PPHN. The fetal lung also produces a number of cyclo-oxygenase (COX)-dependent metabolites that function as pulmonary vasodilators (eg, PGI-2, PGE-1, and PGE-2). It has also become clear that the endothelium (and its interaction with vascular smooth muscle cells) plays a crucial role in regulating pulmonary vascular tone. Nitric oxide (NO), a potent vasodilator, is synthesized from L-arginine by endothelial nitric oxide synthase (eNOS). NO stimulates soluble guanylate cyclase (sGC), which produces cGMP and causes vasodilation. cGMP, in turn, is hydrolyzed by cyclic nucleotide phosphodiesterases (PDEs), and manipulation of these control the intensity and duration of cGMP action. Various isoenzymes of PDE have been identified and inhibition of PDE-5 (by, eg, sildenafil) causes pulmonary vasodilation.

In summary, for successful pulmonary circulatory transition to occur, various mechanical, physiologic, and biochemical factors, which maintain high fetal PVR, must be eliminated or reversed. Major events are the replacement of the fluid-filled lung of the fetus with the air-filled postnatal lung, the increase in oxygen tension, and the increase in pulmonary blood flow (which increases shear stress and thereby increases NO). At the same time, changes occur in the synthesis and release of various biochemical modulators of vascular tone and there are interactions between the mechanical and biochemical events surrounding birth. Disturbances in this cascade of events may lead to PPHN. At the same time, manipulation of these pathways enables us to treat it.

IV. **Risk factors.** The following factors or conditions may be associated with PPHN:

A. **Lung disease.** Meconium aspiration, respiratory distress syndrome (RDS), pneumonia, pulmonary hypoplasia, cystic lung disease, including congenital cystic adenomatoid malformation and congenital lobar emphysema, diaphragmatic hernia, and congenital alveolar capillary dysplasia.

B. **Systemic disorders.** Polycythemia, hypoglycemia, hypoxia, acidosis, hypocalcemia, hypothermia, and sepsis.

C. **Congenital heart disease.** Particularly, total anomalous venous return, hypoplastic left heart syndrome, transient tricuspid insufficiency (transient myocardial ischemia), coarctation of the aorta, critical aortic stenosis, endocardial cushion defects, Ebstein anomaly, transposition of the great arteries, endocardial fibroelastosis, and cerebral venous malformations.

D. **Perinatal factors.** Asphyxia, perinatal hypoxia, and maternal ingestion of aspirin or indomethacin.

E. **Miscellaneous.** Central nervous system disorders, neuromuscular disease, and upper airway obstruction. An observational case control study has suggested that the use of selective serotonin reuptake inhibitors during the last half of pregnancy may be associated with PPHN in the newborn.

V. **Clinical presentation.** The primary finding is respiratory distress with cyanosis (confirmed by demonstrating hypoxemia). This may occur despite adequate ventilation. Other clinical findings are highly variable and depend on the severity, stage, and other associated disorders (particularly pulmonary and cardiac diseases).

A. **Respiratory.** Initial respiratory symptoms may be limited to tachypnea, and onset may be at birth or within 4–8 h of age. In addition, in an infant with pulmonary disease, PPHN should be suspected as a complicating factor when there is marked lability in oxygenation. These infants may have significant decreases in pulse oximetry readings with routine nursing care or minor stress (eg, movement or noise). Furthermore, a minor decrease in inspired oxygen concentration may lead to a surprisingly large decrease in arterial oxygenation (eg, the $AaDo_2$ gradient changes more rapidly and is more labile than that seen in the normal course of progression of uncomplicated RDS or other pulmonary disease).

B. **Cardiac signs.** Physical findings may include a prominent right ventricular impulse, a single second heart sound, and a murmur of tricuspid insufficiency. In extreme cases, there may be hepatomegaly and signs of heart failure.

C. **Radiography.** The chest film may show either cardiomegaly or a normal-sized heart. If there is no associated pulmonary disease, the film may show normal or diminished pulmonary vascularity. If there is also a parenchymal lung disorder, the degree of hypoxemia may be out of proportion to the radiographic measure of severity of the pulmonary disease.

D. **Other.** Thrombocytopenia has been reported to be present in as many as 60% of infants with PPHN. The specificity of this finding is unknown. Once the diagnosis is suspected, certain tests are either strongly suggestive or supportive of PPHN.

VI. **Diagnosis.** PPHN is essentially a diagnosis of exclusion.

A. **Differential oximeter readings.** In the presence of right-to-left shunting of blood via the PDA, the Pao_2 in preductal blood (eg, from the right radial artery) is higher than that in the postductal blood (obtained from left radial, umbilical, or tibial arteries).

Hence simultaneous preductal and postductal monitoring of oxygen saturation is a useful indicator of right-to-left shunting at the ductal level. However, it is important to note that PPHN cannot be excluded if no difference is found because the right-to-left shunting may be predominantly at the atrial level (or the ductus may not be patent at all). A difference >5% between preductal and postductal oxygen saturations is considered indicative of a right-to-left ductal shunt. A difference >10–15 mm Hg between preductal and postductal Pao_2 is also considered suggestive of a right-to-left ductal shunt. Preductal and postductal oxygenation should be assessed simultaneously.

B. **Hyperventilation test.** PPHN should be considered if marked improvement in oxygenation (>30 mm Hg increase in Pao_2) is noted on hyperventilating the infant (lowering $Paco_2$ and increasing pH). When a "critical" pH value is reached (often ~7.55 or greater), PVR decreases, there is less right-to-left shunting, and Pao_2 increases. This test may differentiate PPHN from cyanotic congenital heart disease. Little or no response is expected in infants with the latter diagnoses. It has been suggested that infants subjected to this test should be hyperventilated for 10 min. Prolonged hyperventilation is not recommended, however, particularly in premature infants (see later discussion).

C. **Radiography.** Clear lung fields or only minor disease in the face of severe hypoxemia is strongly suggestive of PPHN, if cyanotic congenital heart disease has been ruled out. In an infant with significant pulmonary parenchymal disease, a chest film is of little help in diagnosing PPHN (although it is indicated for other reasons). In an infant with rapidly worsening oxygenation, the major value of a chest film is in the exclusion of alternative diagnosis (eg, pneumothorax or pneumopericardium).

D. **Echocardiography** is often essential in distinguishing cyanotic congenital heart disease from PPHN because the latter is frequently a diagnosis of exclusion. Furthermore, whereas all the other previously mentioned signs and tests are suggestive, echocardiography (together with Doppler studies) can provide confirmatory evidence that is often diagnostic. The first question that needs to be answered is whether the heart is structurally normal. Then the pulmonary artery pressure can be assessed indirectly by measuring the acceleration time of the systolic flow in the main pulmonary artery, by measuring the velocity of the tricuspid regurgitant jet, and by measuring ductal shunt velocities. A flattened interventricular septum, or one that is bowing into the left ventricle, also support the diagnosis of PPHN. Echocardiography (with Doppler) also provides information about shunting at the atrial and ductal levels. Echocardiography can also be used to assess ventricular output and contractility (both of which may be depressed in infants with PPHN).

VII. **Management**

A. **Prevention.** Adequate resuscitation and support from birth may presumably prevent or ameliorate, to some degree, PPHN when it may occur superimposed on a preexisting condition. An example is adequate and timely ventilation of an asphyxiated infant with appropriate attention to temperature control.

B. **General management.** Infants with PPHN clearly require careful and intensive monitoring. Fluid management is important because hypovolemia aggravates the right-to-left shunt. However, once normovolemia can be assumed, there is no known benefit to be gained from repeated administration of either colloids or crystalloids. Normal serum glucose and calcium should be maintained because hypoglycemia and hypocalcemia aggravate PPHN. Temperature control is also crucial. Significant acidosis should be avoided. It is useful to use two pulse oximeters: one preductal and one postductal.

C. **Minimal handling.** Because infants with PPHN are extremely labile with significant deterioration after seemingly "minor" stimuli, this aspect of care deserves special mention. Endotracheal tube suctioning, in particular, should be performed only if indicated and not as a matter of routine. Noise level and physical manipulation should be kept to a minimum.

D. **Mechanical ventilation** is often needed to ensure adequate oxygenation and should first be attempted using "conventional" ventilation. The goal is to maintain adequate and stable oxygenation using the lowest possible mean airway pressures. The lowest possible positive end-expiratory pressure should also be sought. However, atelectasis should be avoided because it may aggravate pulmonary hypertension and also impair effective delivery of inhaled nitric oxide (iNO) to the lungs. Hyperventilation should, if possible, be avoided and, as a guide, arterial P_{CO_2} values should be kept >30 mm Hg if possible; and levels of 40–50 mm Hg, or even higher, are also acceptable if there is no associated compromise in oxygenation. Initially, it would be wise to ventilate with 100% inspired oxygen concentration. Weaning should be gradual and in small steps. In those infants who cannot be adequately oxygenated with conventional ventilation, high-frequency oscillatory ventilation (HFOV) should be considered early. In the presence of parenchymal lung disease, infants treated with HFOV combined with iNO were less likely to be referred for ECMO than those treated with either therapy alone.

E. **Surfactant.** In infants with RDS, administration of surfactant is associated with a fall in PVR. Surfactant may also be of benefit in various other pulmonary disorders (eg, meconium aspiration), although it is unknown whether its actions in these is related to a reduction in PVR. There is evidence for surfactant deficiency in some patients with PPHN.

F. **Pressor agents.** Some infants with PPHN have reduced cardiac output. In addition, increasing systemic blood pressure reduces the right-to-left shunt. Hence at least normal blood pressure should be maintained, and some recommend maintaining blood pressure of ≥40 mm Hg. Dopamine is the most commonly used drug for this purpose. Dobutamine has the disadvantage, in this context, that, although it may improve cardiac output, it has less of a pressor effect than dopamine. Milrinone, a type 3 phosphodiesterase inhibitor, is also sometimes employed to treat hypotension and improve cardiac output. A simple nonpharmacologic measure to increase systemic vascular resistance is to inflate blood pressure cuffs on all four extremities. In a small study using this technique, inflating the blood pressure cuffs was associated with a 10–25 mm Hg increase in arterial oxygen tension.

G. **Sedation.** The lability of these infants has been mentioned previously, and hence sedation is commonly used. Nembutal (1–5 mg/kg) or Versed (0.1 mg/kg) is frequently used, and analgesia with morphine (0.05–0.2 mg/kg) is also used.

H. **Inhalational nitric oxide (iNO).** See also Chapter 132.

1. **Background.** Controlled clinical trails have shown that NO, when given by inhalation, reduces PVR and improves oxygenation and outcomes in a significant proportion of term and near-term neonates with PPHN. The drug is currently approved by the U.S. Food and Drug Administration for this indication in newborns ≥35 weeks' gestation. The administration of iNO to infants with PPHN reduces the number requiring extracorporeal membrane oxygenation (ECMO) without increasing morbidity at 2 years of age. In another large multicenter trial, iNO was demonstrated to reduce both the need for ECMO and the incidence of chronic lung disease. Oxygenation can also improve during iNO therapy via mechanisms additional to its effect of reducing extrapulmonary right-to-left shunting. Inhaled NO can also improve oxygenation by redirecting blood from poorly aerated or diseased lung regions to better aerated distal air spaces (which are better exposed to the inhaled drug), thereby improving ventilation-perfusion mismatching. Although the benefits of iNO have been demonstrated in full- and near-term neonates with pulmonary hypertension, iNO treatment of preterm infants is more *controversial*. In preterm neonates, the hope was that iNO would decrease the incidence of chronic lung disease and, possibly, mitigate other morbidities. However, results of clinical trials have been conflicted, and respiratory distress in premature infants is regarded as a *controversial* indication for which further studies are necessary.

2. **Physiology.** NO is a colorless gas with a half-life of seconds. Exogenous inhaled NO diffuses from alveoli to pulmonary vascular smooth muscle and produces

vasodilation. Excess NO diffuses into the bloodstream, where it is rapidly inactivated by binding to hemoglobin and subsequent metabolism to nitrates and nitrites. This rapid inactivation thereby limits its action to the pulmonary vasculature. Dosage of inhaled NO (iNO) is measured as ppm (parts per million) of gas.

3. **Toxicity.** NO reacts with oxygen to form other oxides of nitrogen and, in particular, NO_2 (nitrogen dioxide). The latter may produce toxic effects and hence must be removed from the respiratory circuit (which can be done by using an adsorbent). When NO combines with hemoglobin, it forms methemoglobin, and this is also of potential concern. In the several large trials that have been completed, methemoglobinemia has not been a significant complication at NO doses <20 ppm. The rate of accumulation of methemoglobin depends on both the dose and duration of NO administration. Even when using doses >20 ppm, clinically significant methemoglobinemia does not appear to be a frequent complication. NO inhibits platelet adhesion to endothelium. Hence another potential complication is the prolongation of bleeding time described at NO doses of 30–300 ppm. NO may also have an adverse effect on surfactant function, but this appears to require much higher doses than those relevant in clinical applications. On the contrary, low-dose NO also has antioxidant effects, and these may be potentially beneficial. Because of these potential complications, when administering NO, NO_2 levels should be monitored. Also, blood methemoglobin concentration should be measured. Follow-up studies in infants receiving iNO have not shown any adverse effects.

4. **Dosage and administration.** Available evidence supports the use of doses of iNO beginning at 20 ppm. Among infants with a positive response to iNO, the response time is rapid. There is no agreement, however, about the duration of treatment and criteria for discontinuation; these vary and often reflect institutional preferences. Thus some recommend weaning once arterial Po_2 is >50 mmHg; others suggest an oxygenation index <10 as an indications for weaning. Moreover, no evidence suggests the superiority of one weaning regimen over another. However, some observations are available to assist in weaning considerations. One point is, however, beyond contention: weaning should be done under careful and intensive monitoring of each step. Particular note should be made of the observation that sudden discontinuation of iNO can be associated with "rebound" pulmonary hypertension (see 4b).

   a. **Initial dose.** Start treatment with iNO at 20 ppm. Little is to be gained by administering higher doses because, at most, only a few patients will respond to these higher doses after not having responded to a dose of 20 ppm. Higher doses may significantly increase the rate of methemoglobinemia. Also, initial treatment with subtherapeutic low-dose iNO may diminish the subsequent response to iNO at 20 ppm. Among infants with a positive response to iNO, the response time is rapid.

   b. **Weaning.** Wean inspired oxygen concentration until FIO_2 <0.6. Then start weaning iNO concentrations in steps of 5 ppm until iNO is 5 ppm. Weaning may be initiated as early as 4–6 h after starting treatment, or later, and should be attempted at least once per day, but may be done as frequently as every 30 min. Hemodynamic stability and adequate oxygenation should be monitored closely 30–60 min after each weaning step. Significant deterioration should be an indication of reversing the previous weaning step. Once iNO is at 5 ppm, weaning should be continued at a slower pace, in steps of 1 ppm, until iNO is 1 ppm. Once the patient has demonstrated stability at iNO of 1 ppm for a few hours, iNO may be discontinued. Some decline in oxygen saturation should be anticipated, and an increase of 10–20% in required inspired oxygen concentration may be considered reasonable when discontinuing iNO and need not be an indication for reinstating therapy. However, if an FIO_2 >0.75 is required to maintain adequate oxygenation, the patient may benefit from being placed back on iNO. *Caution:* Although there are various weaning regimens of iNO, evidence suggests that iNO should be discontinued from a dose of 1 ppm and not from a higher one. The rate of success is higher when discontinuation is done from a dose of 1 ppm than from 5 ppm or higher. Moreover, the phenomenon of rebound pulmonary hypertension should be kept in mind after discontinuation of iNO. Sudden discontinuation of iNO can be associated with "rebound" pulmonary hypertension and this rebound can be severe and may occur even in infants who had initially failed to respond to iNO treatment when it was initiated. We should emphasize that this protocol is merely a suggestion and is compatible with data derived from trials and experience with the use of iNO. Many other regimens would be just as reasonable.

5. **Failure to respond to iNO or the need for prolonged administration.** Patients not responding to iNO or those in whom iNO cannot be weaned after 5 days of treatment, merit a re-evaluation. Effective therapy requires adequate lung inflation, and an infant who fails to respond should be evaluated by chest radiograph for airway obstruction and atelectasis. Lung volume recruitment strategies may be required as may surfactant treatment in appropriate circumstances. Pressor support or volume administration may be required because impaired cardiac output may render iNO treatment ineffective. An echocardiogram is warranted to rule out cardiac anomalies that may have been missed and to assess cardiac function. Consideration should be directed toward lung diseases that respond poorly to iNO, such as alveolar-capillary dysplasia or those associated with pulmonary hypoplasia. Less than 35% of infants with congenital diaphragmatic hernia respond to iNO or survive without ECMO.

I. **Sildenafil.** The phosphodiesterase PDE5 is abundantly expressed in lung tissue and degrades cGMP. Sildenafil, a PDE5 inhibitor, prolongs the half-life of cGMP and would be expected to enhance the actions of both endogenous and exogenous nitric oxide. Uncontrolled studies of this drug indicated that it reduces pulmonary artery pressure in patients with pulmonary hypertension and is synergistic with iNO. In case reports, sildenafil was noted to attenuate rebound pulmonary hypertension following withdrawal of iNO therapy in patients with congenital heart disease, and there were various anecdotal reports of its successful use in neonates with PPHN. A small randomized controlled study was done using oral sildenafil, 1 mg/kg every 6 h, in infants with PPHN. In the treatment group, oxygenation index improved within 6–30 h without affecting systemic blood pressure. Survival was significantly greater in the sildenafil group. Concern has been raised about possible adverse effects of this drug in those infants at risk for retinopathy of prematurity, although the putative association has been questioned. Larger trials will be required to address issues of risk and benefits. Sildenafil is sometimes used as an adjunct to iNO in infants with insufficient response to iNO and as a treatment to facilitate weaning from iNO. Trials of safety and efficacy in these contexts are lacking.

J. **Prostacyclin.** Prostacyclin (PGI_2) is a short-acting, potent vasodilator of both the pulmonary and systemic circulations. It also has antithrombotic and antiproliferative effects. The greatest experience of its use is as a continuous intravenous (IV) infusion of epoprostenol. Trials in adults and older children with pulmonary hypertension have shown an improvement in symptoms and mortality. However, epoprostenol treatment is associated with various limitations. The drug has a very short half-life and requires continuous infusion. There are special storage requirements, and side effects include systemic hypotension. Aerosolized PGI_2, in contrast, results in selective pulmonary vasodilation and can also improve ventilation-perfusion matching, much like iNO. The use of inhaled prostacyclin was reported in four neonates with PPHN refractory to iNO. All four infants showed a rapid improvement. One neonate subsequently deteriorated and was found to have alveolar-capillary dysplasia. No systemic vascular effects were noted.

K. **Bosentan.** ET-1 is a potent vasoconstrictor and is increased in newborns with PPHN. Bosentan is an endothelin receptor antagonist that improves hemodynamics and quality of life in adults with pulmonary hypertension. Up to 10% of patients are affected by liver toxicity. Bosentan improved hemodynamics in a study of its use in pediatric patients with pulmonary hypertension. Its use also enabled a reduction of the epoprostenol dose. There is, however, little information on the use of bosentan in neonates with PPHN. A case report describes its use, together with epoprostenol, in an infant with severe chronic lung disease and pulmonary hypertension. The combined treatment decreased RV systolic pressure. Bosentan is sometime used anecdotally for refractory pulmonary hypertension in infants with congenital diaphragmatic hernia, severe chronic lung disease, and congenital heart diseases. There are no systematic data on its use and safety in neonates, either as a single therapy or as an adjunct in combination therapy. Bosentan is a nonselective inhibitor of both ET-A and ET-B receptors. This is a potential drawback because ET-B releases NO and mediates vasodilation. Sitaxsentan, a selective ET-A antagonist, has been used successfully in adults with pulmonary hypertension; the patients exhibited functional improvement with no evidence of hepatic toxicity.

L. **Paralyzing agents.** The use of these agents is **controversial.** Their use has been advocated in infants who have not responded to sedation and are still labile or who appear to "fight" the ventilator. In a retrospective survey, the use of paralysis was associated with increased mortality, although a causal relation cannot be inferred. Pancuronium is the drug most commonly used, although it may increase PVR to some extent and worsen ventilation-perfusion mismatch. Vecuronium (0.1 mg/kg) has also been used.

M. **Alkalinization.** In the past, it had been noted that hyperventilation, with the resulting hypocapnia, improved oxygenation secondary to pulmonary vasodilation. Subsequently, it was shown, in animal studies, that the beneficial effect of hypocapnia was actually a result of the increased pH rather than of the low $Paco_2$ values achieved. Furthermore, follow-up of infants with PPHN had suggested that hypocapnia was related to poor neurodevelopmental outcome (especially sensorineural hearing loss). Hypocapnia is known to reduce cerebral blood flow. There are no adequately controlled trials on the use of alkali infusion to alleviate PPHN. A retrospective survey of treatment of PPHN, prior to approval of iNO as treatment, showed no association between alkali administration and improved outcome. If alkalinization is employed, it may be advisable to increase pH using an infusion of sodium bicarbonate (0.5–1 mEq/kg/h) if possible. Serum sodium should be monitored to avoid hypernatremia. Improvement in oxygenation has been anecdotally reported with arterial pH 7.50–7.55 (sometimes levels as high as 7.65 are required).

N. **Intravenous pulmonary vasodilators.** Various IV pulmonary vasodilators have been tried in the past (tolazoline, prostaglandin E_1, prostacyclin, nitroglycerin, nitroprusside, and others). All of these are also systemic vasodilators and often cause systemic hypotension with little, if any, net benefit.

1. **Tolazoline** is an α-adrenergic antagonist with histaminergic action. It is given as a loading dose of 1–2 mg/kg followed by continuous infusion of 1–2 mg/kg/h. It should be given with both volume support and pressor drugs close at hand in case systemic hypotension occurs. Some advocate its use only in conjunction with simultaneous infusion of pressors as a prophylactic measure. Side effects of tolazoline are hypotension, oliguria, seizures, thrombocytopenia, and gastrointestinal hemorrhage, but some of these effects may have resulted from the severity of the infant's underlying condition. It is possible that a lower dosage of tolazoline may be effective as a pulmonary vasodilator while reducing the incidence of dose-related side effects. A loading dose of 0.5 mg/kg has been recommended, followed by infusion of 0.5 mg/kg/h. Tolazoline is effective in 10–50% of newborns with PPHN, but the rate of complications is close to 70% and treatment response is not correlated with ultimate survival. Endotracheal tolazoline may produce more selective pulmonary vasodilation. **The drug, however, is now off the market and thus trials are unlikely.**

2. **Two IV drugs that have been reported** as successful pulmonary vasodilators are **magnesium sulfate** and **adenosine.** The experience with **magnesium sulfate** has

been uncontrolled, and some animal studies have shown other findings. Nevertheless, magnesium appears to be worthy of further study. Adenosine has been tried in full-term infants with PPHN in a controlled randomized study. It was found to improve oxygenation in some of the infants in whom it was tried and was without detrimental systemic hemodynamic effects. It thus appears promising.

    O. **Extracorporeal membrane oxygenation (ECMO)** (see Chapter 13). ECMO may be indicated for term or near-term infants with PPHN who fail to respond to conventional therapy and who meet ECMO entry criteria. The survival rate with ECMO is reportedly >80%, although only the most severely afflicted infants are referred for this treatment.

VIII. **Prognosis.** The overall survival rate is >70–75%. There is, however, a marked difference in survival and long-term outcome according to the cause of the PPHN. More than 80% of term or near-term neonates with PPHN are expected to have an essentially normal neurodevelopmental outcome. Abnormal long-term outcome in PPHN survivors (and a high incidence of sensorineural hearing loss) has been reported to correlate with duration of hyperventilation. However, the relationship may not be causal because prolonged hyperventilation may simply be a marker for the severity of PPHN and hypoxic insult. Survivors of idiopathic PPHN usually have no residual lung or heart disease. Very low birthweight infants with PPHN accompanying severe RDS have a much higher rate of mortality, and there are few data on the long-term outcome of the survivors.

Selected References

Abman SH: Recent advances in the pathogenesis and treatment of persistent pulmonary hypertension of the newborn. *Neonatology* 2007;91:283-290.

American Academy of Pediatrics, Committee on Fetus and Newborn: Use of inhaled nitric oxide. *Pediatrics* 2000;106:344-345.

Baquero H et al: Oral sildenafil in infants with persistent pulmonary hypertension of the newborn: a pilot randomized blinded study. *Pediatrics* 2006;117:1077-1083.

Davidson D et al: Safety of withdrawing inhaled nitric oxide therapy in persistent pulmonary hypertension of the newborn. *Pediatrics* 1999;104:231-236.

Kelly LK et al: Inhaled prostacyclin for term infants with persistent pulmonary hypertension refractory to inhaled nitric oxide. *J Pediatr* 2002;141:830-832.

Kinsella JP, Abman SH: Inhaled nitric oxide and high frequency oscillatory ventilation in persistent pulmonary hypertension of the newborn. *Eur J Pediatr* 1997;157(suppl 1):S28-S30.

Leibovitch L et al: Therapeutic applications of sildenafil citrate in the management of paediatric pulmonary hypertension. *Drugs* 2007;67:57-73.

Ostrea EM Jr et al: Persistent pulmonary hypertension of the newborn. *Pediatr Drugs* 2006;8:179-188.

Rhodes J et al: Effect of blood pressure cuffs on neonatal circulation: their potential application to newborns with persistent pulmonary hypertension. *Pediatr Cardiol* 1995;16:20-23.

Rugolotto S et al: Weaning of epoprostenol in a small infant receiving concomitant bosentan for severe pulmonary arterial hypertension secondary to BPD. *Minerva Pediatr* 2006;58:491-494.

Sokol GM et al: Changes in arterial oxygen tension when weaning neonates from inhaled nitric oxide. *Pediatr Pulmonol* 2001;32:14-19.

Steinhorn RH, Porta NFM: Use of inhaled nitric oxide in the preterm infant. *Curr Opin Pediatr* 2007;19:137-141.

The Neonatal Inhaled Nitric Oxide Study Group: Inhaled nitric oxide in term and near-term infants: neurodevelopmental follow-up of the neonatal inhaled nitric oxide study group (NINOS). *J Pediatr* 2000;136:611-617.

Walsh-Sukys MC et al: Persistent pulmonary hypertension of the newborn in the era before nitric oxide: practice variation and outcomes. *Pediatrics* 2000;105:14-20.

112 Polycythemia and Hyperviscosity

I. **Definitions.** Polycythemia is an increased total red blood cell (RBC) mass. Polycythemic hyperviscosity is an increased viscosity of the blood resulting from, or associated with, increased numbers of RBCs.

   A. **Polycythemia** of the newborn is defined as a central venous hematocrit >65%. The clinical significance of this value results from the curvilinear relationship between the circulating RBC volume (hematocrit) and whole blood viscosity. Above a hematocrit of 65%, blood viscosity, as measured in vitro, rises exponentially.

   B. **Hyperviscosity** is defined as a viscosity >14 cP at a shear rate of 11.5/s measured by a viscometer. (*Note:* Normal serum viscosity units are reported as centipoises [cP]). Hyperviscosity is the cause of clinical symptoms in infants presumed to be symptomatic from polycythemia. Many polycythemic infants are also hyperviscous, but this is not invariably the case. The terms **polycythemia** and **hyperviscosity** are not interchangeable.

II. **Incidence**

   A. **Polycythemia.** Polycythemia occurs in 2–4% of the general newborn population. Half of these patients are symptomatic, although it is not at all certain whether their symptoms are caused by polycythemia.

   B. **Hyerviscosity.** Hyperviscosity without polycythemia occurs in 1% of normal (nonpolycythemic) newborns. In infants with a hematocrit of 60–64%, a fourth have hyperviscosity.

III. **Pathophysiology.** Clinical signs attributed to hyperviscosity may result from the regional effects of hyperviscosity, including tissue hypoxia, acidosis, and hypoglycemia, and from the formation of microthrombi within the microcirculation. An important caveat, however, is that the same clinical signs may result from coexisting perinatal circumstances in the presence or absence of hyperviscosity. Potentially affected organs include the central nervous system, the kidneys and adrenal glands, the cardiopulmonary system, and the gastrointestinal tract. Blood viscosity depends on the interaction of frictional forces in whole blood. These forces are defined as **shear stress** (refers to frictional forces within a fluid) and **shear rate** (a measure of blood flow velocity). The shear rate in the aorta is 230/s and only 11.5/s in the small arterioles and venules. As the viscosity increases, such as in the microcirculation, blood with a high hematocrit may virtually cease flowing. The frictional forces identified within whole blood and their relative contributions to hyperviscosity in the newborn include the following:

   A. **Hematocrit.** An increase in the hematocrit is the most important single factor contributing to hyperviscosity in the neonate. An increased hematocrit results from either an absolute increase in circulating RBC volume or a decrease in plasma volume.

   B. **Plasma viscosity.** A direct linear relationship exists between plasma viscosity and the concentration of plasma proteins, particularly those of high molecular weight, such as fibrinogen. Term infants and, to a greater degree, preterm infants have low plasma fibrinogen levels compared with adults. Consequently, except for the rare case of primary hyperfibrinogenemia, plasma viscosity does not contribute to an increased whole blood viscosity in the neonate. Under normal conditions, low plasma fibrinogen levels and, correspondingly, low plasma viscosity actually may protect the microcirculation of the neonate by facilitating perfusion and contributing to low whole blood viscosity.

   C. **RBC aggregation.** Aggregation of erythrocytes occurs only in areas of low blood flow and is usually limited to the venous microcirculation. Because fibrinogen levels are typically low in term and preterm infants, RBC aggregation does not contribute significantly to whole blood viscosity in newborn infants. There is some concern that the use of adult fresh-frozen plasma for partial exchange transfusion in neonates might critically alter the concentration of fibrinogen and paradoxically raise whole blood viscosity within the microcirculation.

D. **Deformability of RBC membrane.** There are apparently no differences among term infants, preterm infants, and adults in terms of the membrane deformability of erythrocytes.

IV. **Risk factors**
A. **Conditions that alter incidence**
   1. **Altitude.** There is an absolute increase in RBC mass as part of physiologic adaptation to high altitude.
   2. **Neonatal age.** The normal pattern of fluid shifts during the first 6 h of life is away from the intravascular compartment. The period of maximum physiologic increase in the hematocrit occurs at 2–4 h of age.
   3. **Obstetric factors.** A delay in cord clamping beyond 30 s or stripping of the umbilical cord, if that is the prevailing practice, results in a higher incidence of polycythemia.
   4. **High-risk delivery.** A high-risk delivery is associated with an increased incidence of polycythemia, particularly if precipitous or uncontrolled.
B. **Perinatal processes**
   1. **Enhanced fetal erythropoiesis.** Elevated erythropoietin levels result from a direct stimulus, usually related to fetal hypoxia, or from an altered regulation of erythropoietin production.
      a. **Placental insufficiency**
         i. Maternal hypertensive disease (preeclampsia/eclampsia) or primary renovascular disease.
         ii. Abruptio placentae (chronic recurrent).
         iii. Postmaturity.
         iv. Cyanotic congenital heart disease.
         v. Intrauterine growth restriction (IUGR).
         vi. Maternal cigarette smoking.
      b. **Endocrine disorders.** Increased oxygen consumption is the suggested mechanism by which hyperinsulinism or hyperthyroxinemia creates fetal hypoxemia and stimulates erythropoietin production.
         i. Infant of a diabetic mother (>40% incidence of polycythemia).
         ii. Infant of a mother with gestational diabetes (>30% incidence of polycythemia).
         iii. Congenital thyrotoxicosis.
         iv. Congenital adrenal hyperplasia.
         v. Beckwith-Wiedemann syndrome (secondary hyperinsulinism).
      c. **Genetic trisomies** (trisomies 13, 18, and 21).
   2. **Hypertransfusion.** Conditions that enhance placental transfusion at birth may create hypervolemic normocythemia, which evolves into hypervolemic polycythemia as the normal pattern of fluid shift occurs. A larger transfusion may create hypervolemic polycythemia at birth, with signs present in the infant. Conditions associated with hypertransfusion include the following:
      a. **Delay in cord clamping.** Placental vessels contain up to a third of the fetal blood volume, half of which is returned to the infant within 1 min after birth. Representative blood volumes for term infants with a variable delay in cord clamping are as follows:
         • **15-s delay,** 75–78 mL/kg.
         • **60-s delay,** 80–87 mL/kg.
         • **120-s delay,** 83–93 mL/kg.
         The risks associated with delayed cord clamping are probably negligible compared with the benefits that are in the term infant: reduction in the rate of iron deficiency in the first 2 years of life and in the sick preterm, decreased need for blood transfusions, inotrope support, and intraventricular hemorrhage.

b. **Gravity.** Positioning the infant below the placental bed (>10 cm below the placenta) enhances placental transfusion via the umbilical vein. Elevation of the infant >50 cm above the placenta prevents placental transfusion.

c. **Maternal use of medications.** Drugs that enhance uterine contractility—specifically oxytocin—do not significantly alter the gravitational effects on placental transfusion during the first 15 s after birth. With further delay in clamping of the cord, however, blood flow toward the infant accelerates to a maximum at 1 min of age.

d. **Cesarean delivery.** In cesarean delivery, there is usually a lower degree of placental transfusion if the cord is clamped early because of the absence of active uterine contractions in most cases and because of gravitational effects.

e. **Twin-twin transfusion.** Interfetal transfusion (**parabiosis syndrome**) is observed in monochorionic twin pregnancy with an incidence of 15%. The recipient twin, on the venous side of the anastomosis, becomes polycythemic, and the donor, on the arterial side, becomes anemic. Simultaneous venous hematocrits obtained after delivery differ by >12–15%, and both twins have a high risk of intrauterine or neonatal death and increased neurologic morbidity.

f. **Maternal-fetal transfusion.** Approximately 10–80% of normal newborn infants receive a small volume of maternal blood at the time of delivery. The "reverse" Kleihauer-Betke acid elution technique documents maternal RBC "ghosts" on a neonatal blood smear. With large transfusions, the test is positive for several days. Because various conditions may lead to a false-negative test result, new and more accurate flow cytometry techniques can be used when the index of suspicion for fetomaternal transfusions is elevated.

g. **Intrapartum asphyxia.** Prolonged fetal distress enhances the net umbilical blood flow toward the infant until cord clamping occurs, and acidosis may encourage capillary leak and reduced plasma volume.

V. **Clinical presentation.** Clinical signs observed in polycythemia are nonspecific and reflect the regional effects of hyperviscosity within a given microcirculation. The conditions listed next may occur independently of polycythemia or hyperviscosity and must be considered in the differential diagnosis.

A. **Central nervous system.** There may be an altered state of consciousness, including lethargy and decreased activity, hyperirritability, proximal muscle hypotonia, vasomotor instability, and vomiting. Seizures, thromboses, and cerebral infarction are extraordinarily rare.

B. **Cardiopulmonary system.** Respiratory distress and tachycardia may be present. Congestive heart failure with cardiomegaly may be seen but is rarely clinically prominent. Pulmonary hypertension may occur but is not usually severe unless other predisposing factors are present.

C. **Gastrointestinal tract.** Feeding intolerance occurs occasionally. Necrotizing enterocolitis has been reported but rarely without other factors (eg, IUGR), which casts doubt on the primary cause.

D. **Genitourinary tract.** Oliguria, acute renal failure, renal vein thrombosis, or priapism may occur.

E. **Metabolic disorders.** Hypoglycemia, hypocalcemia, or hypomagnesemia may be seen.

F. **Hematologic disorders.** There may be hyperbilirubinemia, thrombocytopenia, or reticulocytosis (with enhanced erythropoiesis only).

VI. **Diagnosis**

A. **Venous (not capillary) hematocrit.** Polycythemia is present when the central venous hematocrit is ≥65%.

B. **The following screening studies may be used:**

1. A cord blood hematocrit >56% suggests polycythemia.

2. A warmed capillary hematocrit ≥65% suggests polycythemia.

VII. **Management.** Clinical management of the polycythemic infant is more expectant now than a decade ago. Studies and reviews have created much doubt about any long-term benefits of partial exchange transfusion (PET). Consequently, PET should probably be performed only on infants in whom significant morbidity is in question.

A. **Asymptomatic infants.** Only expectant observation is required for virtually all asymptomatic infants. The possible exception is an infant with a central venous hematocrit of >75%, but even in this group the risks of central catheter insertion probably outweigh the benefits of PET.

B. **Symptomatic infants.** When the central venous hematocrit is ≥65%, PET with normal saline may ameliorate acute signs of polycythemia or hyperviscosity. Whether treatment of a self-limited problem justifies the risks of central catheter insertion and an exchange procedure is debatable, however. For the procedure for partial exchange transfusion, see Chapter 29.

VIII. **Prognosis.** The long-term outcome of infants with polycythemia or hyperviscosity and response to PET is as follows:

A. A causal relationship exists between PET and an increase in gastrointestinal tract disorders and necrotizing enterocolitis.

B. Older randomized controlled prospective studies of polycythemic and hyperviscous infants indicate that PET may reduce but not eliminate the risk of neurologic sequelae. More recent data suggest that no benefits accrue from PET.

C. Infants with "asymptomatic" polycythemia have an increased risk for neurologic sequelae, but normocythemic controls with the same perinatal histories have a similarly increased risk.

Selected References

Dempsey EM, Barrington K: Crystalloid or colloid for partial exchange transfusion in neonatal polycythemia: a systematic review and meta-analysis. *Acta Paediatr* 2005;94:1650.

Dempsey EM et al: Short and long term outcomes following partial exchange transfusion in the polycythaemic newborn: a systematic review *Arch Dis Child Fetal Neonatal* 2006;91:F2.

Mercer JS et al. Delayed cord clamping in very preterm infants reduces the incidence of intraventricular hemorrhage and late-onset sepsis: a randomized, controlled trial. *Pediatrics* 2006;117:1235.

Oh W: Timing of umbilical cord clamping at birth in full-term infants. *JAMA* 2007;11:1257.

Rosenkrantz TS: Polycythemia and hyperviscosity in the newborn. *Sem Thromb Hemost* 2003;29:515.

Seng YC et al: Twin-twin transfusion syndrome: a five year review. *Arch Dis Child Fetal Neonatal Ed* 2000;83:168.

113 Renal Failure (Acute)

I. **Definition.** In neonates, acute renal failure is defined as the absence of urinary output (anuria) or as urine output of <0.5 mL/kg/24 h (oliguria) with an associated increase in serum creatinine. One hundred percent of infants void by 24 h (for average times from birth to first voiding, see Table 61–1).

II. **Incidence.** In some studies, as many as 23% of neonates have some form of renal failure; prenatal factors are identified as the cause in 73%. In a recent study causes included cardiac (27%), prematurity (27%), septic (10%), hepatic (9%), renal (9%), and other (18%) causes. Twelve infants needed transient dialysis treatment.

III. **Pathophysiology.** Normal urine output is ~1–3 mL/kg/h in newborns. The normal newborn kidney has poor concentrating ability. Renal failure leads to problems with volume overload, hyperkalemia, acidosis, hyperphosphatemia, and hypocalcemia. Acute renal failure is traditionally divided into three categories:

A. **Prerenal failure.** Prerenal failure is due to decreased renal perfusion. Causes include dehydration (poor feeding or increased insensible losses referable to radiant warmers), perinatal asphyxia, and hypotension (septic shock, hemorrhagic shock, or cardiogenic shock resulting from congestive heart failure).

B. **Intrinsic renal failure.** If poor renal perfusion persists, acute tubular necrosis with intrinsic renal failure may result. Other causes are nephrotoxins such as aminoglycosides, nonsteroidal anti-inflammatory medications and methoxyflurane anesthesia, congenital anomalies (eg, renal agenesis or polycystic kidney disease), disseminated intravascular coagulation (DIC), renal vein or renal artery thrombosis, and isolated cortical necrosis.

C. **Postrenal failure.** All of the causes involve obstruction of urinary outflow. These include bilateral ureteropelvic obstruction, bilateral ureterovesical obstruction, posterior urethral valves, urethral diverticulum or stenosis, large ureterocele, neurogenic bladder, blocked urinary drainage tubes, and extrinsic tumor compression.

IV. **Risk factors.** Dehydration, sepsis, asphyxia, and administration of nephrotoxic drugs to the neonate are risk factors for acute renal failure. Maternal diabetes may increase the risk for renal vein thrombosis and subsequent renal insufficiency.

V. **Clinical presentation**

A. **Decreased or absent urine output.** Low or absent urine output is usually the presenting problem. Virtually all infants void by 24 h (see Table 61–1).

B. **Family history.** A history of urinary tract disease in other family members should be sought as well as a history of oligohydramnios, which frequently accompanies urinary outflow obstruction or severe renal dysplasia or agenesis.

C. **Physical examination.** The following abnormalities on physical examination are significant:

1. **Abdominal mass,** suggesting a distended bladder, polycystic kidneys, or hydronephrosis.

2. **Potter facies,** associated with renal agenesis.

3. **Meningomyelocele,** associated with neurogenic bladder.

4. **Pulmonary hypoplasia,** resulting from severe oligohydramnios in utero secondary to inadequate urinary output.

5. **Urinary ascites,** which may be seen with posterior urethral valves.

6. **Prune belly** (hypoplasia of the abdominal wall musculature and cryptorchidism), associated with urinary abnormalities.

VI. **Diagnosis**

A. **Bladder catheterization.** Perform bladder catheterization, using a 5F or 8F feeding tube to confirm inadequate urine output (see Chapter 25). Immediate passage of large volumes of urine suggests obstruction (eg, posterior urethral valves) or a hypotonic (neurogenic) bladder.

B. **Laboratory studies**

1. **Blood urea nitrogen and creatinine levels**

a. A **blood urea nitrogen level** 15–20 mg/dL suggests dehydration or renal insufficiency.

b. **Creatinine level.** Normal serum creatinine values are 0.8–1.0 mg/dL at 1 day, 0.7–0.8 mg/dL at 3 days, and <0.6 mg/dL by 7 days of life. Higher values suggest renal disease except in low birthweight infants, in whom a creatinine level of <1.6 mg/dL is considered normal. (Rule of thumb: If the creatinine doubles, then 50% of the renal function has been lost.)

2. **Urinary indices** of acute renal failure are listed in Table 113–1. Order a spot urine osmolality, a serum and spot urine sodium, and serum and urine creatinine, and calculate the fractional excretion of sodium (FENa) and the renal failure index (RFI).

Table 113–1. **RENAL FAILURE INDICES IN THE NEONATE**

	Prerenal	Renal
Urine osmolality (mOsm)	>400	<400
Urine sodium (mEq/L)	31 ± 19	63 ± 35
Urine/plasma creatinine	29 ± 16	10 ± 4
Fractional excretion of sodium	<2.5	>2.5
Renal failure index	<3.0	>3.0

These indices are of limited value if measured while the effects of diuretics such as furosemide are present.

$$FENa = \frac{Urine\ Na \times Plasma\ Cr}{Urine\ Cr \times Plasma\ Na} \times 100$$

$$RFI = \frac{Urine\ Na \times Serum\ Cr}{Urine\ Cr}$$

3. **Complete blood cell count and platelet count** may reveal thrombocytopenia, seen with sepsis or renal vein thrombosis.
4. **Serum potassium levels** should be monitored to rule out hyperkalemia.
5. **Urinalysis** may reveal hematuria (associated with renal vein thrombosis, tumors, or DIC; see the discussion of hematuria) or pyuria, suggesting urinary tract infection as either the cause of renal insufficiency (sepsis) or the result of mechanical obstruction.
C. **Diagnostic fluid challenge.** If the patient does not have clinical volume overload or congestive failure, give a fluid challenge. Administer normal saline or colloid solution, 5–10 mL/kg as an intravenous bolus, and repeat once as needed. If there is no response, give furosemide, 1 mg/kg. If there is still no increase in urine output, obstruction above the level of the bladder must be ruled out by ultrasound examination. If there is no evidence of obstruction and the patient does not respond to these maneuvers, the most likely cause of anuria or oliguria is intrinsic renal failure.
D. **Radiologic studies**
   1. **Abdominal ultrasonography** can delineate hydronephrosis, dilated ureters, abdominal masses, a distended bladder, or renal vein thrombosis.
   2. **Intravenous urography** has limited usefulness in the neonatal period because of the poor concentrating ability of the kidney. It is of limited value in the setting of renal failure.
   3. **Abdominal radiograph studies** may show spina bifida or an absent sacrum, which can cause neurogenic bladder. Displaced bowel loops suggest the presence of a space-occupying mass.
   4. **Radionuclide scanning** can delineate functioning renal parenchyma (using dimercaptosuccinic acid [DMSA]) and give some indication of renal flow and function (using diethyltriamine penta-acetic acid [DTPA]). MAG-3 scanning has largely replaced these two scans, however, because it can image the parenchyma and determine function.
VII. **Management**
   A. **General management**
      1. **Replace insensible fluid losses** (preterm, 50–70 mL/kg/day; term, 30 mL/kg/day) plus fluid output (urine and gastrointestinal tract).
      2. **Keep strict intake and output and frequent weight records.**
      3. **Monitor serum sodium and potassium levels** frequently, and replace losses cautiously as needed. Infants with renal failure should never be given intravenous

fluids containing potassium because hyperkalemia, if it occurs, may be lethal. If hyperkalemia does occur, treat as outlined in Chapter 53.

4. **Restrict protein** to <2 g/kg/day, and ensure adequate nonprotein caloric intake. Breast milk or formulas such as Similac PM 60/40 are frequently used for infants with renal failure.

5. **Hyperphosphatemia and hypocalcemia frequently coexist, and phosphate binders such as aluminum hydroxide**, 50–150 mg/kg/day orally, should be used to normalize the phosphate. Once the phosphate is normal, calcium with or without vitamin D supplements is usually needed.

6. **For tetany or convulsions,** acute intravenous calcium replacement with 10% calcium gluconate, 40 mg/kg, or 10% calcium chloride will increase the serum calcium 1 mg/dL. Monitor ionized calcium, if available in your laboratory.

7. **Metabolic acidosis may require chronic oral bicarbonate supplementation.** Blood pressures should be monitored serially because these infants are always at risk for chronic hypertension. Intravenous bicarbonate therapy should be given if the pH is <7.25 or the serum bicarbonate (HCO_3) is <12 mEq.

$$HCO_3 \text{ deficit} = (24 - \text{observed}) \ 0.5 \times \text{body weight (kg)}$$

B. **Definitive management**
1. **Prerenal failure** is treated by correcting the specific cause (see Section III, A).
2. **Postrenal failure.** Acute management involves bypassing the obstruction with a bladder catheter or by percutaneous nephrostomy drainage, depending on the level of the obstruction. Surgical correction is usually indicated at some point.
3. **Intrinsic renal disease.** If renal disease is caused by toxins or acute tubular necrosis, renal function may recover to some extent with time.
4. **Dialysis.** If recovery of renal function is expected or if renal transplantation is considered an option when the child is older, peritoneal dialysis is the treatment most commonly used in the neonate. On occasion, hemodialysis, ultrafiltration, and continuous venovenous hyperfiltration may be required.

VIII. **Prognosis.** The prognosis from acute renal failure depends on the underlying cause. The main concern is the development of renal failure later on. Mortality and morbidity are increased in newborns with multiorgan failure. Factors that increase mortality are hypotension, need for mechanical ventilation, dialysis, use of pressors, hemodynamic instability, and multiorgan failure. Follow-up is especially important in this group of newborns to monitor their renal function, blood pressure, and urine studies.

Selected References

Andreoli SP: Acute renal failure in the newborn. *Semin Perinatol* 2004;28:112-123.

Farhat W et al: The natural history of neonatal vesicoureteral reflux associated with antenatal hydronephrosis. *J Urol* 2000;164:1057.

Herndon CDA et al: Consensus on the prenatal management of antenatally detected urological abnormalities. *J Urol* 2000;164:1052.

Matthew OP et al: Neonatal renal failure: usefulness of diagnostic indices. *Pediatrics* 1980;65:57.

Moghal NE, Embleton ND: Management of acute renal failure in the newborn. *Semin Fetal Neonatal Med* 2006;11:207-213.

Norman ME, Asadi FK: A prospective study of acute renal failure in the newborn infant. *Pediatrics* 1979;63:475.

Stapleton FB et al: Acute renal failure in neonates: incidence, etiology and outcome. *Pediatr Nephrol* 1987;1:314.

Wedekin M et al: Aetiology and outcome of acute and chronic renal failure in infants. *Nephrol Dial Transplant* 2008;23(5):1575-1580.

114 Respiratory Syncytial Virus (RSV)

I. **Definition.** Respiratory syncytial virus (RSV) is a large, enveloped RNA paramyxovirus. Two major strains (groups A and B) have been identified and often circulate concurrently .

II. **Incidence.** Almost all children are infected at least once by 2 years of age. Humans are the only source of infection. Initial infection occurs most commonly during the child's first year. Reinfection throughout life is common. In the United States, RSV usually occurs in annual epidemics during winter and early spring (predominantly November through March). It is a common cause of nosocomial infection. It can survive up to 6 h on nonporous surfaces. Most cases of bronchiolitis in infants are caused by RSV.

III. **Pathophysiology.** The disease is limited to the respiratory tract. The inoculation of the virus occurs in the upper respiratory tract where it spreads to the lower tract by cell-to-cell transfer. In infants the disease usually involves the lower respiratory tract and manifests itself as bronchiolitis or pneumonia.

IV. **Risk factors.** Risk factors include premature infants, infants born with lung disease, infants <2 years of age with heart disease, infants with a birthweight <2500 g, infants with school-age siblings, infants who attend daycare, family history of asthma, regular exposure to secondhand smoke or air pollution, multiple birth babies, peak RSV season (fall to end of spring), being male, <1 month or no breast-feeding and others sharing the bedroom with the infant. High altitude increases the risk of RSV hospitalization. **Risk factors for more severe or fatal RSV disease** include a premature infant, an infant with cyanotic or complicated congenital heart disease (CHD) especially those that cause pulmonary hypertension, an infant with pulmonary disease, especially bronchopulmonary dysplasia (chronic lung disease [CLD]), those infants with immunodeficiency with lymphopenia, or therapy causing immunosuppression. Asthma is associated with an increased susceptibility to severe RSV disease.

V. **Clinical presentation.** RSV usually begins in the nasopharynx with coryza and congestion. During the first 2–5 days, it may progress to the lower respiratory tract with development of cough, dyspnea, and wheezing. RSV is the most important cause of bronchiolitis and pneumonia. Lethargy, irritability, and poor feeding often accompanied by apneic episodes may be the presenting manifestations in young infants. Most previously healthy infants infected with RSV do not require hospitalization. Characteristics that increase the risk of severe or fatal RSV infection are preterm birth without or especially with CLD of prematurity; hemodynamically significant CHD especially if associated with cyanosis or pulmonary hypertension; and T-cell immunodeficiency disease or therapy causing immunosuppression. RSV infection predisposes to reactive airway disease and recurrent wheezing during the first decade of life.

VI. **Diagnosis**

A. **Enzyme-linked immunoabsorbent assay (ELISA) and direct fluorescent antibody tests (DFA)** have sensitivity (in comparison with culture) in the range of 80–90%. These rapid tests detect RSV antigen in epithelial cells obtained by nasopharyngeal washings.

B. **Chest radiograph** usually reveals infiltrates or hyperinflation.

C. **Blood gas analysis** may show hypoxemia and occasionally hypercarbia. Development of hypercarbia is an ominous sign of impending respiratory failure.

VII. **Management.** Isolation precautions for all infectious diseases, including maternal and neonatal precautions, breast-feeding, and visiting issues, can be found in Appendix F.

A. **Immunization**

1. **Passive. Palivizumab (Synagis)** provides passive immunity. It is a humanized RSV monoclonal antibody and administered intramuscularly (15 mg/kg) monthly during RSV season. It is well tolerated with infrequent or minimal side effects.

According to the American Academy of Pediatrics guidelines, palivizumab should be considered for:

   a. **Infants and children <2 years with CLD** who have required medical therapy (supplemental oxygen, bronchodilator, diuretic, or corticosteroid therapy) for CLD within 6 months before the anticipated start of the RSV season.

   b. **Infants born at 28 weeks' gestation or earlier during their first RSV season** whenever that occurs during the first 12 months of life. Infants born at 29–32 weeks' gestation may benefit most from prophylaxis up to 6 months of age. For infants between 32 and 35 weeks' gestation, palivizumab should be considered only if two or more risk factors are present. Risk factors include child care attendance, school-aged siblings, exposure to environmental air pollutants, congenital abnormalities of the airways, or severe neuromuscular disease.

   c. **Children who are ≤24 months of age with hemodynamically significant cyanotic and acyanotic CHD.** Infants and children with hemodynamically insignificant heart disease (eg, secundum atrial septal defect, small ventricular septal defect, pulmonic stenosis, uncomplicated aortic stenosis, mild coarctation of the aorta, and patent ductus arteriosus) are not at increased risk from RSV and generally should not receive immunoprophylaxis.

2. **Active.** Two novel recombinant RSV vaccines with multiple mutations are being studied. A preliminary trial showed both vaccines to be well tolerated and likely to be protective in young infants.

B. **Ribavirin** has in vitro antiviral activity against RSV, but ribavirin aerosol treatment for RSV is not recommended routinely.

C. **Surfactant.** A recent small randomized study shows that surfactant therapy improves gas exchange and respiratory mechanics and shortens mechanical ventilation days and intensive care unit stay in infants with severe RSV-induced respiratory failure.

D. β-**Adrenergic agents** are not recommended for routine care of first-time wheezing associated with RSV bronchiolitis. If an inhaled bronchodilator is tried, repeated doses should be tried only in the small number of infants with well-documented improvement in respiratory function soon after the first dose.

E. **Antibiotics, theophylline, and corticosteroids** have not been shown to be helpful in the treatments of RSV.

F. **Isolation.** Contact precautions are recommended for the duration of the illness. Infected secretions remain viable for up to six hours on countertops. Gowns, gloves, and scrupulous handwashing practices are required. Patients with RSV infection should be cared for in a single room or placed in a cohort.

VIII. **Prognosis.** The prognosis is generally excellent; however, infants with underlying cardiac or pulmonary conditions can have an increased risk of complications. In premature born infants with CLD and hospitalization in the first two years of life, there is a reduced airway calibre at school age. There is a bidirectional association between severe RSV and asthma. Asthma is associated with an increased susceptibility for RSV, and RSV infection is associated with a short term increase in asthma. It is not yet determined if these infants infected with RSV are at an increased risk for asthma later in life.

Selected References

American Academy of Pediatrics: Respiratory syncytial virus. In Pickering LK et al (eds): *Red Book: 2006 Report of the Committee on Infectious Diseases,* 27th ed. Elk Grove Village, IL: American Academy of Pediatrics, 2006:560-566.

Greenough A et al: School age outcome of respiratory syncytial virus hospitalization of prematurely born infants. *Thorax* 2009. [Epub ahead of print]

Greenough A, Broughton S: Chronic manifestations of respiratory syncytial virus infection in premature infants. *Pediatr Infect Dis J* 2005;24:S184-S187.

Karron RA et al: Identification of a recombinant live attenuated respiratory syncytial virus vaccine candidate that is highly attenuated in infants. *J Infect Dis* 2005;191:1093-1104.

Luchetti M et al: Multicenter, randomized, controlled study of porcine surfactant in severe respiratory syncytial virus-induced respiratory failure. *Pediatr Crit Care Med* 2002;3:261-268.

Stensballe LG et al: The causal direction in the association between respiratory syncytial virus hospitalization and asthma. *J Allergy Clin Immunol* 2009;123(1):131-137.

Simões EA: RSV disease in the pediatric population: epidemiology, seasonal variability, and long-term outcomes. *Manag Care* 2008;17(11 Suppl 12):3-6, discussion 18-9. Review.

Welliver RC: Review of epidemiology and clinical risk factors for severe respiratory syncytial virus (RSV) infection. *J Pediatr* 2003;143:S112-S117.

115 Rh Incompatibility

I. **Definition.** Isoimmune hemolytic anemia of variable severity may result when Rh incompatibility develops between an Rh-negative mother previously sensitized to the Rh (D) antigen and her Rh-positive fetus. The onset of clinical disease begins in utero as the result of active placental transfer of maternal IgG-Rh antibody. It is manifested as a partially compensated, moderate to severe hemolytic anemia at birth, with unconjugated hyperbilirubinemia developing in the early neonatal period.

II. **Incidence.** Historically, Rh hemolytic disease of the newborn accounted for up to a third of symptomatic cases seen and was associated with detectable antibody in ~15% of Rh-incompatible mothers. The use of Rh immunoglobulin (RhoGAM) prophylaxis has reduced the incidence of Rh sensitization to <1% of Rh-incompatible pregnancies. Other alloimmune antibodies have become relatively more important as a cause of hemolysis. Anti-c, Kell (K and k), Duffy (Fya), Kidd (Jka and Jkb), MNS (M,N,S and s) and less commonly anti-C and anti-E may cause severe hemolytic disease of the newborn. This cannot be prevented by the use of D antigen–specific Rh immunoglobulin.

III. **Pathophysiology.** Initial exposure of the mother to the Rh antigen occurs most often during parturition, miscarriage, abortion, and ectopic pregnancy. Invasive investigative procedures such as amniocentesis, chorionic villus sampling, and fetal blood sampling also increase the risk of fetal transplacental hemorrhage and alloimmunization. Recognition of the antigen by the immune system ensues after initial exposure, and reexposure to the Rh antigen induces a maternal anamnestic response and elevation of specific IgG-Rh antibody. Active placental transport of this antibody and immune attachment to the Rh antigenic sites on the fetal erythrocyte are followed by extravascular hemolysis of erythrocytes within the fetal liver and spleen. The rate of the hemolytic process is proportionate in part to the levels of the maternal antibody titer but is more accurately reflected in the antepartum period by elevation of the amniotic fluid bilirubin concentration and in the postpartum period by the rate of rise of unconjugated bilirubin. In contrast to ABO incompatibility, the greater antigenicity and density of the Rh antigen loci on the fetal erythrocyte facilitates progressive, rapid clearance of fetal erythrocytes from the circulation. A demonstrable phase of spherocytosis will be absent. Compensatory reticulocytosis and shortening of the erythrocyte generation time, if unable to match the often high rate of hemolysis in utero, results in anemia in the newborn infant and a risk of multiple systemic complications.

IV. **Risk factors**

A. **Birth order.** The firstborn infant is at minimum risk (<1%) unless sensitization has occurred previously. Once sensitization has occurred, subsequent pregnancies are at a progressive risk for fetal disease.

B. **Fetomaternal hemorrhage.** The volume of fetal erythrocytes entering the maternal circulation correlates with the risk of sensitization. The risk is ~8% with each pregnancy but ranges from 3–65%, depending on the volume of fetal blood (3% with 0.1 mL compared with 22% with >0.1 mL) that passes into the maternal circulation.

C. **ABO incompatibility.** Coexistent incompatibility for either the A or B blood group antigen reduces the risk of maternal Rh sensitization to 1.5–3.0%. Rapid immune clearance of these fetal erythrocytes after their entry into the maternal circulation exerts a partial protective effect. It confers no protection once sensitization has occurred.

D. **Obstetric factors.** Cesarean delivery or trauma to the placental bed during the third stage of labor increases the risk of significant fetomaternal transfusion and subsequent maternal sensitization.

E. **Gender.** Male infants are reported to have an increased risk of more severe disease than females, although the basis for this observation is unclear.

F. **Ethnicity.** Approximately 15% of whites are Rh negative compared with 7% of blacks and almost 0% in Asiatic Chinese and Japanese. The risk to the fetus varies accordingly.

G. **Maternal immune response.** A significant proportion of Rh-negative mothers (10–50%) fail to develop specific IgG-Rh antibody despite repeated exposure to Rh antigen.

V. **Clinical presentation**

A. **Symptoms and signs**

1. **Jaundice.** Unconjugated hyperbilirubinemia is the most common presenting neonatal sign of Rh disease, usually appearing within the first 24 h of life.

2. **Anemia.** A low cord blood hemoglobin at birth reflects the relative severity of the hemolytic process in utero and is present in ~50% of cases.

3. **Hepatosplenomegaly.** Enlargement of the liver and spleen is seen in severe hemolysis, sometimes occurring in association with ascites, with an increased risk for splenic rupture.

4. **Hydrops fetalis.** Severe Rh disease has a historical association with hydrops fetalis and at one time was its most common cause. Clinical features in the fetus include progressive hypoalbuminemia with ascites, pleural effusion, or both; severe chronic anemia with secondary hypoxemia; and cardiac failure. There is an increased risk of late fetal death, stillbirth, and intolerance of active labor. The neonate frequently has generalized edema, notably of the scalp, which can be detected by antepartum ultrasonography, cardiopulmonary distress often involving pulmonary edema and severe surfactant deficiency, congestive heart failure, hypotension and peripheral perfusion defects, cardiac rhythm disturbances, and severe anemia with secondary hypoxemia and metabolic acidosis. Currently, nonimmune conditions are more commonly associated with hydrops fetalis. Secondary involvement of other organ systems may result in hypoglycemia or thrombocytopenic purpura.

VI. **Diagnosis.** Obligatory screening in an infant with unconjugated hyperbilirubinemia includes the following studies:

A. **Blood type and Rh type (mother and infant).** These studies establish the likelihood of Rh incompatibility and exclude the diagnosis if the infant is Rh negative, with one exception (see Section VI, C, on the direct Coombs test).

B. **Reticulocyte count.** Elevated reticulocyte levels, adjusted for the degree of anemia and gestational age in preterm infants, reflect the degree of compensation and support a diagnosis of an ongoing hemolytic process. Normal values are 4–5% for term infants and 6–10% for preterm infants (30–36 weeks' gestational age). In symptomatic Rh disease, expected values are 10–40%.

C. **Direct antiglobulin (Coombs) test.** A strongly positive direct Coombs test indicates that fetal red blood cells (RBCs) are coated with antibodies and is diagnostic of Rh incompatibility in the presence of the appropriate setup and an elevated reticulocyte count. If Rh immunoglobulin was given at 28 weeks' gestation, subsequent passive transfer of antibody will result in a false-positive direct Coombs test without associated reticulocytosis. Very rarely, a strongly positive direct Coombs test is associated with a falsely Rh-negative infant when all fetal RBC Rh antigenic sites are covered by a high titer of maternal antibodies.

D. **Blood smear.** Polychromasia and normoblastosis proportionate to the reticulocyte count are typically present. Spherocytes are not usually present. The nucleated RBC count is often >10 per 100 white blood cells.

E. **Bilirubin levels.** Progressive elevation of unconjugated bilirubin on serial testing provides an index of the severity of the hemolytic process. An elevated direct fraction is most likely to be secondary to a laboratory artifact in the first 3 days of life and should not be subtracted from the total bilirubin when making management decisions. In the most severely affected infant, particularly those who are hydropic, the intense extramedullary erythropoiesis may cause hepatocellular dysfunction and biliary canalicular obstruction with significant elevated direct bilirubin by 5–6 days of age.

F. **Bilirubin-binding capacity tests.** Correlation between measurements of serum albumin, free bilirubin, bilirubin saturation index, and reserve binding capacity and outcome has been variable. The role of these values in directing the management of patients remains unclear.

G. **Glucose and blood gas levels** should be monitored closely.

H. **Supplementary laboratory studies.** Supportive diagnostic studies may be required when the basis of the hemolytic process remains unclear.

1. **Direct Coombs test in the mother.** This study should be negative in Rh disease. This test can be positive in the presence of maternal autoimmune hemolytic disease, particularly collagen vascular disease.

2. **Indirect antiglobulin titer (indirect Coombs test).** This test detects the presence of antibodies in the maternal serum. Rh-positive RBCs are incubated with the serum being tested for the presence of anti-D. If present, the RBCs now coated with anti-D are agglutinated by an antihuman globulin serum reflecting a positive indirect antiglobulin (Coombs) test result. The reciprocal of the highest dilution of maternal serum that produces agglutination is the indirect antiglobulin titer.

3. **Carbon monoxide (CO).** The severity of Rh disease may be determined by measurement of endogenous CO production. When heme is catabolized to bilirubin, CO is produced in equimolar amounts. Hemoglobin binds the CO to form carboxyhemoglobin (CO Hb) and then is finally excreted in the breath. CO Hb levels are increased in neonates with hemolysis. CO Hb levels >1.4% have correlated with an increased need for exchange transfusion.

VII. **Management**

A. **Antepartum treatment.** Verification of the Rh-negative status at the first prenatal visit may be obtained by the following measures:

1. **Maternal antibody titer.** Once an IgG-Rh antibody has been identified, it is important to determine the titer. Serial antibody titer determinations are required every 1–4 weeks (depending on the gestational age) during pregnancy. Invasive fetal testing becomes indicated when the titer is above a critical level, usually between 1:8 and 1:16. A negative antibody screen (indirect Coombs test) signifies absence of sensitization. This test should be repeated at 28–34 weeks' gestation.

2. **RhoGAM.** Current obstetric guidelines suggest giving immunoprophylaxis at 28 weeks' gestation in the absence of sensitization.

3. **Amniocentesis.** If maternal antibody titers indicate a risk of fetal death (usual range, 1:16–1:32), amniocentesis should be performed to assess fetal Rh genotype and assess severity. Fetal Rh-genotype determination can also be made from fetal cell free DNA found in maternal plasma. To reasonably predict the risk of moderate to severe fetal disease, serial determinations of amniotic fluid bilirubin levels present photometrically at 450 nm are plotted on standard graphs according to gestational age (known as the **Liley curve**). Readings falling into very high zone II or zone III indicate that hydrops will develop within 7–10 days. Zone I indicates no fetal hemolytic disease or no anemia.

4. **Ultrasonography.** As a screening study in pregnancies at risk, serial fetal ultrasound examinations allow detection of scalp edema, ascites, or other signs of developing hydrops fetalis. Peak systolic middle cerebral artery velocity can reliably

detect moderate and predict severe fetal anemia and thus reduce the need for more invasive diagnostic procedure such as amniocentesis and cordocentesis.

5. **Intrauterine transfusion.** Based on the studies just mentioned, intrauterine transfusion may be indicated because of possible fetal demise or the presence of fetal hydrops. This procedure must be performed by an experienced team. The goal is maintenance of effective erythrocyte mass within the fetal circulation and maintenance of the pregnancy until there is a reasonable chance for successful extrauterine survival of the infant.

6. **Glucocorticoids.** If premature delivery is anticipated, glucocorticoids should be given to accelerate fetal lung maturation.

7. **Reduction of maternal antibody level.** Intensive maternal plasma exchange and high-dose intravenous immunoglobulins (IVIGs) have been reported of value in the severely alloimmunized pregnant woman to reduce circulating maternal antibodies levels by >50%.

B. **Postpartum treatment**

1. **Resuscitation.** Moderately to severely anemic infants with or without hydropic features are at risk for high-output cardiac failure, hypoxemia secondary to decreased oxygen-carrying capacity or surfactant deficiency, and hypoglycemia. These infants may require immediate single-volume exchange blood transfusion at delivery to improve oxygen-carrying capacity, mechanical support of ventilation, and an extended period of monitoring for hypoglycemia.

2. **Cord blood studies.** A cord blood bilirubin level >4 mg/dL, a cord hemoglobin <12 g/dL, or both usually suggests moderate to severe disease. The cord blood is used for these and initial screening studies, including blood typing, Rh typing, and Coombs test.

3. **Serial unconjugated bilirubin studies.** Determination of the rate of increase in unconjugated bilirubin levels provides an index of the severity of the hemolytic process and the need for exchange transfusion. Commonly used guidelines include a rise of >0.5 mg/dL/h or >5 mg/dL over 24 h within the first 2 days of life or projection of a serum level that will exceed a predetermined "exchange level" for a given infant (usually 20 mg/dL in term infants).

4. **Phototherapy.** In severe Rh hemolytic disease, phototherapy is used only as an adjunct to exchange transfusion. Phototherapy decreases bilirubin levels and reduces the number of total exchange transfusions required. Phototherapy should be started if bilirubin rises 0.5 mg/dL/h or if total bilirubin exceeds 10, 12, or 14 mg/dL at 12, 18, or 24 h of life, respectively.

5. **Exchange transfusion.** (For the procedure, see Chapter 29.) Exchange transfusion is indicated if the unconjugated bilirubin level is likely to reach a predetermined "exchange level" for that patient. Optimally, exchange transfusion is done well before this exchange level is reached to minimize the risk of entry of unconjugated bilirubin into the central nervous system. Consideration should be given to irradiation of blood before the transfusion is given, particularly in preterm infants or infants expected to require multiple transfusions, to reduce the risk of graft-versus-host disease. The process removes 70–90% of the fetal red cells but only 25% of the total bilirubin because most of the bilirubin is in the extravascular space. A rapid rebound of serum bilirubin is common after re-equilibration, and thus additional exchange transfusions may be required.

6. **Heme oxygenase inhibitors (Stannsoporfin).** These metalloporphyrins are currently investigational. The enzyme heme oxygenase catalyzes the rate-limiting step in bilirubin production, the conversion of heme to biliverdin.

7. **IVIG.** Postnatal treatment may be effective by blocking neonatal reticuloendothelial Fc receptors and thus decrease hemolysis of the antibody-coated Rh-positive RBCs.

C. **RhoGAM prophylaxis.** Most cases of incompatibility involve the D antigen. RhoGAM given at 28 weeks' gestation, within 72 h of suspected Rh antigen exposure, or both reduces the risk of sensitization to <1%; the recommended dosage (300 mcg) should be well in excess of the amount of Rh antigen transfused (300 mcg for every 25 mL of fetal blood in maternal circulation. The amount of fetal blood entering the maternal circulation may be estimated using the Kleihauer-Betke acid elution technique (page 407) during the immediate postpartum period.

No treatment equivalent to RhoGAM is available for maternal Rh sensitization to non-D antigens, notably C and E antigens. These antigens, however, are significantly less antigenic than the D antigen, clinical manifestations of incompatibility are frequently milder, and the risk of severe disease is considerably less.

D. **Hydrops fetalis.** Skilled resuscitation and anticipation of selective systemic complications may prevent early neonatal death.

1. **Isovolumetric partial exchange transfusion** with type O Rh-negative packed erythrocytes raises the hematocrit and improves the oxygen-carrying capacity (see Chapter 29).

2. **Central arterial and venous catheterization** may be performed to provide the following measures:

   a. **Isovolumetric exchange transfusion.**

   b. **Monitoring of arterial blood gas levels and central venous and systemic blood pressures.**

   c. **Monitoring of fluid and electrolyte balance,** particularly renal and hepatic function, calcium-to-phosphorus ratio, and serum albumin levels as well as appropriate hematologic studies and serum bilirubin levels.

3. **Positive-pressure mechanical ventilation.** This measure may include increased levels of positive end-expiratory pressure, if pulmonary edema is present, as a means of stabilizing alveolar ventilation. Treatment with exogenous surfactant may be considered in particular when the infant is judged to be not fully mature.

4. **Therapeutic paracentesis or thoracentesis** may be performed to remove fluid that may further compromise respiratory effort. Excessive removal of ascitic fluid may lead to systemic hypotension.

5. **Volume expanders** may be necessary, in addition to erythrocytes, to improve peripheral perfusion defects. This should be done with caution because most hydropic infants are hypotensive or poorly perfused because of hypoxic heart failure rather than hypovolemia, or both.

6. **Drug treatment** may include diuretics such as furosemide for pulmonary edema and pressor agents such as dopamine (for dosages, see Chapter 132). In the case of cardiac rhythm disturbances, appropriate drugs may be used if indicated.

7. **Electrocardiography or echocardiography** may be needed to determine whether cardiac abnormalities are present.

VIII. **Prognosis.** Prenatal mortality for infants at risk of anti-D Rh isoimmunization is currently ~1.5% and has decreased significantly over the past two decades. Antenatal immune prophylaxis and improved management techniques, including amniotic fluid spectrophotometry, intrauterine transfusion, and advances in neonatal intensive care, have been largely responsible for this reduction. Isolated cases of severe isoimmunization still occur because of isoimmunization by other than anti-D antibody or failure to receive immune prophylaxis and may exhibit the full spectrum of disease, including an increased risk of stillbirths and early neonatal morbidity and mortality.

Selected References

Abrams ME et al: Hydrops fetalis: a retrospective review of cases reported to a large national database and identification of risk factors associated with death. *Pediatrics* 2007;120(1):84-89.

Moise KJ Jr: Management of rhesus alloimmunization in pregnancy. *Obstet Gynecol* 2008;112(1):164-176.

Wagle S et al: Hemolytic disease of the newborn. Available at: http://emedicine.medscape.com/article/ 974349-overview. Accessed February 22, 2009.

116 Seizures in the Neonate

I. **Definition.** A seizure is defined clinically as a paroxysmal alteration in neurologic function (ie, behavioral, motor, or autonomic function).

II. **Incidence.** Neonatal seizures are relatively common and affect ~1% of all neonates.

III. **Pathophysiology.** The neurons within the CNS undergo depolarization as a result of inward migration of sodium. Repolarization occurs via efflux of potassium. A seizure occurs when there is excessive depolarization, resulting in excessive synchronous electrical discharge. Volpe (2001) proposed the following four possible reasons for excessive depolarization: failure of the sodium-potassium pump because of a disturbance in energy production, a relative excess of excitatory versus inhibitory neurotransmitter, a relative deficiency of inhibitory versus excitatory neurotransmitter, and alteration in the neuronal membrane, causing inhibition of sodium movement. The basic mechanisms of neonatal seizures, however, are unknown. There are numerous causes of neonatal seizures, but relatively few account for most cases (Table 116–1). Therefore, only common causes of seizures are discussed here.

A. **Perinatal asphyxia** is the most common cause of neonatal seizures. These occur within the first 24 h of life in most cases and may progress to overt status epilepticus. In premature infants, seizures are of the generalized tonic type, whereas in full-term infants they are of the multifocal clonic type. Accompanying subtle seizures are usually present in both types.

B. **Intracranial hemorrhage,** whether subarachnoid, periventricular, or intraventricular, may occur as a result of hypoxic insults that can lead to neonatal seizures. Subdural hemorrhage, usually a result of trauma, can cause seizures.

1. **Subarachnoid hemorrhage.** In primary subarachnoid hemorrhage, convulsions often occur on the second postnatal day, and the infant appears quite well during the interictal period.

2. **Periventricular or intraventricular hemorrhage** arising from the subependymal germinal matrix is accompanied by subtle seizures, decerebrate posturing, or generalized tonic seizures, depending on the severity of the hemorrhage.

3. **Subdural hemorrhage** over the cerebral convexities leads to focal seizures and focal cerebral signs.

C. **Metabolic disturbances**

1. **Hypoglycemia** is frequently seen in infants with intrauterine growth retardation and in infants of diabetic mothers (IDMs). The duration of hypoglycemia and the time lapse before initiation of treatment determine the occurrence of seizures. Seizures are less frequent in IDMs, perhaps because of the short duration of hypoglycemia.

2. **Hypocalcemia** has been noted in low birthweight infants, IDMs, asphyxiated infants, infants with DiGeorge syndrome, and infants born to mothers with hyperparathyroidism. Hypomagnesemia is a frequent accompanying problem.

3. **Hyponatremia** occurs because of improper fluid management or as a result of the syndrome of inappropriate antidiuretic hormone (SIADH).

4. **Hypernatremia** is seen with dehydration as a result of inadequate intake in breast-fed infants, excessive use of sodium bicarbonate, or incorrect dilution of concentrated formula.

5. **Other metabolic disorders**

a. **Pyridoxine dependency** leads to seizures resistant to anticonvulsants. Infants with this disorder experience intrauterine convulsions and are born with meconium staining. They resemble asphyxiated infants.

b. **Amino acid disorders.** Seizures in infants with amino acid disturbances are invariably accompanied by other neurologic manifestations. Hyperammonemia and acidosis are commonly present in amino acid disorders.

Table 116–1. CAUSES OF NEONATAL SEIZURES

Perinatal asphyxia
Intracranial hemorrhage
   Subarachnoid hemorrhage
   Periventricular or intraventricular hemorrhage
   Subdural hemorrhage
Metabolic abnormalities
   Hypoglycemia
   Hypocalcemia
   Electrolyte disturbances: hyponatremia and hypernatremia
Amino acid disorders
Congenital malformations
Infections
   Meningitis
   Encephalitis
   Syphilis, cytomegalovirus infections, toxoplasmosis
   Cerebral abscess
Drug withdrawal
Toxin exposure (particularly local anesthetics)
Inherited seizure disorders
   Benign familial epilepsy
   Tuberous sclerosis
   Zellweger syndrome
Pyridoxine dependency

D. **Infections.** Intracranial infection secondary to bacterial or nonbacterial agents may be acquired by the neonate in utero, during delivery, or in the immediate perinatal period.

  1. **Bacterial infection.** Meningitis resulting from **group B streptococcus, _Escherichia coli,_ or _Listeria monocytogenes_** infection is accompanied by seizures during the first week of life.

  2. **Nonbacterial infection.** Nonbacterial causes such as toxoplasmosis and infection with herpes simplex, cytomegalovirus, rubella, and coxsackie B viruses lead to intracranial infection and seizures.

E. **Drug withdrawal.** Three categories of drugs used by the mother lead to passive addiction and drug withdrawal (sometimes accompanied by seizures) in the infant. These are **analgesics** such as heroin, methadone, and propoxyphene (Darvon); **sedative-hypnotics** such as secobarbital; and **alcohol.** Current studies revealed that antidepressant exposure was associated with an increased risk for infant seizures, especially selective serotonin reuptake inhibitor (SSRI) exposure.

F. **Toxins.** Inadvertent injection of local anesthetics into the fetus at the time of delivery (paracervical, pudendal, or saddle block anesthesia) may cause generalized tonic-clonic seizures. Mothers often notice the absence of pain relief during delivery.

IV. **Risk factors.** See pathophysiology.

V. **Clinical presentation.** It is important to understand that **seizures in the neonate are different from those seen in older children.** The differences are perhaps due to the neuroanatomic and neurophysiologic developmental status of the newborn infant. In the neonatal brain, glial proliferation, neuronal migration, establishment of axonal and dendritic contacts, and myelin deposition are incomplete. **Four types of seizures,** based on clinical presentation, are recognized: **subtle, clonic, tonic, and myoclonic.**

A. **Subtle seizures.** These seizures are not clearly clonic, tonic, or myoclonic and are more common in premature than in full-term infants. Subtle seizures are more commonly associated with an electroencephalographic seizure in premature infants than in full-term infants. They consist of tonic horizontal deviation of the eyes with or without jerking; eyelid blinking or fluttering; sucking, smacking, or drooling; "swimming," "rowing," or "pedaling" movements; and apneic spells. Apnea accompanied by electroencephalographic abnormalities has been called **convulsive apnea.** It is differentiated from nonconvulsive apnea (which is due to sepsis, lung disease, or metabolic abnormalities) by the absence of electroencephalographic abnormalities. Apnea as a manifestation of seizures is usually accompanied or preceded by other subtle manifestations. In premature infants, apnea is less likely to be a manifestation of seizures.

B. **Clonic seizures** are more common in full-term infants than in premature infants and commonly associated with an electroencephalographic seizure. There are two types of clonic seizures:

1. **Focal seizures.** Well-localized, rhythmic, slow, jerking movements involving the face and upper or lower extremities on one side of the body or the neck or trunk on one side of the body. Infants are usually not unconscious during or after the seizures.

2. **Multifocal seizures.** Several body parts seize in a sequential, nonjacksonian fashion (eg, left arm jerking followed by right leg jerking).

C. **Tonic seizures** occur primarily in premature infants. Two types of tonic seizures are seen.

1. **Focal seizures.** Sustained posturing of a limb, asymmetric posturing of the trunk or neck, or both. These are commonly associated with an electroencephalographic seizure.

2. **Generalized seizures.** Most commonly, these occur with a tonic extension of both upper and lower extremities (as in decerebrate posturing) but may also present with tonic flexion of the upper extremities with extension of the lower extremities (as in decorticate posturing). It is uncommon to see electroencephalographic seizure disorders.

D. **Myoclonic seizures** are seen in both full-term and premature infants and are characterized by single or multiple synchronous jerks. Three types of myoclonic seizures are seen.

1. **Focal seizures** typically involve the flexor muscles of an upper extremity and are not commonly associated with electroencephalographic seizure activity.

2. **Multifocal seizures** exhibit asynchronous twitching of several parts of the body and are not commonly associated with electroencephalographic seizure activity.

3. **Generalized seizures** present with bilateral jerks of flexion of the upper and sometimes the lower extremities. They are more commonly associated with electroencephalographic seizure activity.

Note: It is important to distinguish jitteriness from seizures. Jitteriness is not accompanied by abnormal eye movements, and movements cease on application of passive flexion. In jitteriness, movements are stimulus sensitive and are not jerky.

VI. **Diagnosis**

A. **History.** Although it is often difficult to obtain a thorough history in infants transported to tertiary-care facilities from other hospitals, the physician must make a concerted effort to elicit pertinent historical data.

1. **Family history.** A positive family history of neonatal seizures is usually obtained in cases of metabolic errors and benign familial neonatal convulsions.

2. **Maternal drug history** is critical in cases of narcotic withdrawal syndrome.

3. **Delivery.** Details of the delivery provide information regarding maternal analgesia, the mode and nature of delivery, the fetal intrapartum status, and the resuscitative measures used. Information regarding maternal infections during pregnancy points toward an infectious basis for seizures in an infant.

B. **Physical examination**

1. A thorough **general physical examination** should precede a well-planned neurologic examination. Determine the following:

a. **Gestational age.**

b. **Blood pressure.**

c. **Presence of skin lesions.**

d. **Presence of hepatosplenomegaly.**

2. **Neurologic evaluation** should include assessment of the level of alertness, cranial nerves, motor function, primary neonatal reflexes, and sensory function. Some of the specific features to look for are the size and "feel" of the fontanelle, retinal hemorrhages, chorioretinitis, pupillary size and reaction to light, extraocular movements, changes in muscle tone, and status of primary reflexes.
3. **Notation of the seizure pattern.** When seizures are noted, they should be described in detail, including the site of onset, spread, nature, duration, and level of consciousness. Recognition of subtle seizures requires special attention.
C. **Laboratory studies.** In selecting and prioritizing laboratory tests, use the information obtained by history taking and physical examination and look for common and treatable causes.
   1. **CBC and differential.** To rule out infection and polycythemia.
   2. **Serum chemistries.** Estimations of serum glucose, calcium, sodium, blood urea nitrogen, and magnesium and blood gas levels must be performed. They may reveal the abnormality causing the seizures.
   3. **Spinal fluid examination.** Evaluation of the cerebrospinal fluid (CSF) is essential because the consequences of delayed treatment or nontreatment of bacterial meningitis are grave. CSF PCR for herpes simplex virus if suspected.
   4. **Metabolic disorders.** (See also Chapter 93.) With a family history of neonatal convulsions, a peculiar odor about the infant, milk intolerance, acidosis, alkalosis, or seizures not responsive to anticonvulsants, other metabolic causes should be investigated.
      a. **Blood ammonia levels** should be checked.
      b. **Amino acids** should be measured in urine and plasma. The urine should be tested for reducing substances.
         i. **Urea cycle disorders.** Respiratory alkalosis is seen as a result of direct stimulation of the respiratory center by ammonia.
         ii. **Maple syrup urine disease.** With 2,4-dinitrophenylhydrazine (2,4-DNPH) testing of urine, a fluffy yellow precipitate is seen in cases of maple syrup urine disease.
D. **Radiologic studies**
   1. **Ultrasonography of the head** is performed to rule out intraventricular hemorrhage (IVH) or periventricular hemorrhage.
   2. **Computed tomography (CT) scanning of the head** provides detailed information regarding intracranial disease. CT scanning is helpful in looking for evidence of infarction, hemorrhage, calcification, and cerebral malformations. Experience with this technique suggests that valuable information is obtained in term infants with seizures, especially when seizures are asymmetric.
   3. **Magnetic resonance imaging (MRI).** A cranial MRI is the most sensitive test to determine the etiology of seizures in the neonate. It is difficult to do in an unstable infant and is a test that requires a lot of time.
E. **Other studies**
   1. **Electroencephalography.** Electroencephalograms (EEGs) obtained during a seizure are abnormal. Interictal EEGs may be normal. However, an order to obtain an ictal EEG should not delay other diagnostic and therapeutic steps. The diagnostic value of an EEG is greater when it is obtained in the first few days because diagnostic patterns indicative of unfavorable prognosis disappear thereafter. Electroencephalography is valuable in confirming the presence of seizures when manifestations are subtle or when neuromuscular paralyzing agents have been given. EEGs are of prognostic significance in full-term infants with recognized seizures. For proper interpretation of EEGs, it is important to know the clinical status of the infant (including the sleep state) and any medications given. Video EEG monitoring can be done when infrequent seizures occur. Continuous EEG monitoring with amplitude integrated electroencephalography (aEEG) has improved seizure detection and is useful in full term infants with hypoxia-ischemia.

VII. **Management.** Because repeated seizures may lead to brain injury, **urgent treatment is indicated. The method of treatment depends on the cause.** Neurologic consultation is recommended. Optimal treatment for neonatal seizures is *controversial* and highly variable between centers especially concerning the use of anticonvulsants.

A. **Hypoglycemia.** Hypoglycemic infants with seizures should receive 10% dextrose in water, 2–4 mL/kg intravenously (IV), followed by 6–8 mg/kg/min by continuous infusion. (See Chapter 55.)

B. **Hypocalcemia** is treated with slow IV infusion of calcium gluconate (for dosage and other information, see Chapters 78 and 132). If serum magnesium levels are low (<1.52 mEq/L), magnesium should be given. (See Chapter 99.)

C. **Anticonvulsant therapy.** Conventional anticonvulsant treatment is used when no underlying metabolic cause is found. Loading doses of phenobarbital and phenytoin control 85% of neonatal seizures.

1. **Phenobarbital** is usually given first (for dosage and other pharmacologic information, see Chapter 132). A recent review of treatment in 31 United States pediatric hospitals verified that most treated infants received phenobarbital. Neither gestational age nor birthweight seems to influence the loading or maintenance dose of phenobarbital. When phenobarbital alone fails to control seizures, another agent is used. Gilman et al (1989) found that sequentially administered phenobarbital controlled seizures in term and preterm newborns in 77% of cases. If seizures are not controlled at a serum phenobarbital level of 40 mcg/mL, Gilman et al recommend administering a second agent (eg, phenytoin [Dilantin]).

2. **Phenytoin (Dilantin)** is usually used next by many practitioners. Fosphenytoin may be a preferred form. (For dosage and other pharmacologic information, see Chapter 132.)

3. **If seizures still persist, then the third medication usually given is a benzodiazepine.**
   a. **Diazepam** has been used as single or repeated doses. Because of its very rapid brain clearance, it is more effective if given by continuous infusion of 0.3 mg/kg/h.
   b. **Lorazepam**, given IV, can be repeated four to six times in a 24-h period. It is advantageous to use over diazepam because it causes less sedation and respiratory depression and has a less rapid brain clearance. It has been quite effective and safe. (For dosage and other pharmacologic information, see Chapter 132.)

4. **If seizures are still present, then three disorders need to be ruled out before more medications are given:**
   a. **Pyridoxine-dependent seizures.** A trial of pyridoxine (vitamin B_6), 50–100 mg, given IV with EEG monitoring is now recommended. With pyridoxine dependency, the seizures stop quickly after the medication is given. Some institutions wait to give this after three medications have been given; some try this after two medications have been given.
   b. **Folinic acid responsive seizures (rare).** Obtain CSF neurotransmitter studies. Then folinic acid is given at 2.5 mg twice daily (up to 4 mg/kg/day initially) in two doses. After 24 h of treatment, seizures may stop. Folinic acid can be given for 48 h as a trial.
   c. **De Vivo syndrome (glucose transporter deficiency).** Treatment is a ketogenic diet.

5. **If seizures still persist, the following drugs may be used depending on institutional preference:**
   a. **High-dose phenobarbital** (>30 mg/kg to achieve serum level >60 mcg/mL) was effective in one review.
   b. **Midazolam**, IV, and is also given intranasally. The IV dose is 0.2 mg/kg, then 0.1–0.4 mg/kg/h.
   c. **Pentobarbital**, 10 mg/kg IV, then 1 mg/kg/h.
   d. **Thiopental**, 10 mg/kg IV, then 2–4 mg/kg/h.
   e. **Clonazepam**, 0.1 mg/kg orally.
   f. **Valproic acid**, 10–25 mg/kg, then 20 mg/kg per day in three doses.

    g. Chlormethiazole (not available in United States). Initial infusion rate of 0.08 mg/kg/min.

    h. Paraldehyde, given rectally, (IV preparation no longer available in United States), used as a last effort.

    i. Lidocaine. Dose, 2 mg/kg IV, then 6 mg/kg/h with cardiac monitoring. New infusion doses are used to decrease cardiac arrhythmias. Not recommended in infants who have been treated with phenytoin or who have congenital heart disease.

    6. Newer medications under study: lamotrigine, vigabatrin, zonisamide, topiramate, and levetiracetam.

  D. Duration of anticonvulsant therapy. The optimal duration of anticonvulsant therapy has not been established. Although some clinicians recommend continuation of phenobarbital for a prolonged period, others recommend stopping it after seizures have been absent for 2 weeks.

VIII. Prognosis. The etiology of the seizure is critical in deciding the outcome and prognosis. Recent evidence suggests that neonatal seizures impair normal brain development. In infants with transient or metabolic disorders that can be corrected, the outcome is usually favorable. In infants with CNS infections, hypoxic-ischemic encephalopathy, or brain malformations, the outcome is not as favorable. The type of seizure can also dictate outcome. In one study, pure clonic seizures without facial involvement in term infants suggested favorable outcome, whereas generalized myoclonic seizures in preterm infants were associated with mortality. Prognosis is usually better for term infants than preterm infants. In one study of 34,615 infants, 90 were noted to have seizures by strict clinical classification. Of the 90 children, 27% of survivors had epilepsy, 25% had cerebral palsy, 20% had mental retardation, and 27% had a learning disorder. Poor prognosis was associated with severe encephalopathy, complicated IVH, infections in preterm neonates, abnormal interictal EEG, cerebral dysgenesis, and the use of multiple drugs to treat the seizures.

Selected References

Blume HK et al: Neonatal seizures: treatment and treatment variability in 31 United States pediatric hospitals. *J Child Neurol* 2009;24(2):148-154.

Dimmick JE, Kalousek DK: *Developmental Pathology of the Embryo & Fetus.* Philadelphia, PA: Lippincott, 1992.

Dlugos D, Sirven JI: Prognosis of neonatal seizures: "It's the etiology, stupid"—or is it? *Neurology* 2007;6;69(19):1812-1813.

Donn SM et al: Prevention of intraventricular hemorrhage with phenobarbital therapy: now what? *Pediatrics* 1986;77:779.

Gilman JT et al: Rapid sequential phenobarbital treatment of neonatal seizures. *Pediatrics* 1989;83:674.

Kaempf JW et al: Antenatal phenobarbital for the prevention of periventricular and intraventricular hemorrhage: a double-blind, randomized, placebo-controlled, multihospital trial. *J Pediatr* 1990;117:933.

Riviello J Jr: Pharmacology review: Drug therapy for neonatal seizures: Part 1. *NeoReviews* 2004;5:e215-e220.

Riviello J Jr: Pharmacology review: drug therapy for neonatal seizures: Part 2. *NeoReviews* 2004;5:e262-e268.

Ronen GM et al: Long-term prognosis in children with neonatal seizures: a population-based study. *Neurology* 2007;69(19):1812-1813.

Rooij L et al: Cardiac arrhythmias in neonates receiving lidocaine as anticonvulsive treatment. *Eur J Pediatr* 2004;163(11):637-641.

Shankaran S et al: Antenatal phenobarbital therapy and neonatal outcome: I. Effect on intracranial hemorrhage. *Pediatrics* 1996a;97:644.

Shankaran S et al: Antenatal phenobarbital therapy and neonatal outcome: II. Neurodevelopmental outcome at 36 months. *Pediatrics* 1996b;97:649.

Shankaran S et al: The effect of antenatal phenobarbital therapy on neonatal intracranial hemorrhage in preterm infants. *N Engl J Med* 1997;337:466.

Shany E: Comparison of continuous drip of midazolam or lidocaine in the treatment of intractable neonatal seizures. *J Child Neurol* 2007;22(3):255-259.

Silverstein FS, Ferriero DM: Off-label use of antiepileptic drugs for the treatment of neonatal seizures. *Pediatr Neurol* 2008;39(2):77-79.

Silverstein FS et al: Improving the treatment of neonatal seizures: National Institute of Neurological Disorders and Stroke workshop report. *J Pediatr* 2008;153(1):12-15.

Stafstrom CE: Neonatal seizures. *Pediatr Rev* 1995;16:248.

Thibeault-Eybalin MP et al: Neonatal seizures: do they damage the brain? *Pediatr Neurol* 2009;40(3):175-180.

Toet MC, Lemmers PM: Brain monitoring in neonates. *Early Hum Dev* 2009;85(2):77-84.

Volpe JJ: Neonatal seizures: current concepts and revised classification. *Pediatrics* 1989b;84:422.

Volpe JJ: *Neurology of the Newborn,* 4th ed. Philadelphia, PA: Saunders, 2001.

117 Sepsis

I. **Definition.** Neonatal sepsis is a clinical syndrome of systemic illness accompanied by bacteremia occurring in the first month of life.

II. **Incidence.** The incidence of primary sepsis is 1–5 per 1000 live births. The incidence is much higher for very low birthweight (VLBW) infants (BW <1500 g) with early-onset sepsis of 15–19 per 1000 and late-onset nosocomial sepsis at 21% according to data from the National Institute of Child Health and Human Development Neonatal Research Network. The mortality rate is high (13–25%); higher rates are seen in premature infants and in those with early fulminant disease.

III. **Pathophysiology.** Neonatal sepsis can be classified into two relatively distinct syndromes based on the age of presentation: early-onset and late-onset sepsis.

    A. **Early-onset sepsis (EOS)** presents in the first 5–7 days of life and is usually a multi-system fulminant illness with prominent respiratory symptoms. Typically, the infant has acquired the organism during the intrapartum period from the maternal genital tract. In this situation, the infant is colonized with the pathogen in the perinatal period. Several infectious agents, notably treponemes, viruses, *Listeria,* and probably *Candida,* can be acquired transplacentally via hematogenous routes. Acquisition of other organisms is associated with the birth process. With rupture of membranes, vaginal flora or various bacterial pathogens may ascend to reach the amniotic fluid and the fetus. Chorioamnionitis develops, leading to fetal colonization and infection. Aspiration of infected amniotic fluid by the fetus or neonate may play a role in the resultant respiratory symptoms. Finally, the infant may be exposed to vaginal flora as it passes through the birth canal. The primary sites of colonization tend to be the skin, nasopharynx, oropharynx, conjunctiva, and umbilical cord. Trauma to these mucosal surfaces may lead to infection. Early-onset disease is characterized by a sudden onset and fulminant course that can progress rapidly to septic shock and death.

    B. **Late-onset sepsis (LOS)** may occur as early as 5 days of age. LOS is usually more insidious but it can be fulminant at times. It is usually not associated with early obstetric complications. In addition to bacteremia, these infants may have an identifiable focus, most often meningitis in addition to sepsis. Bacteria responsible for LOS and meningitis include those acquired after birth from the maternal genital tract as well as organisms acquired after birth from human contact or from contaminated equipment (nosocomial). Therefore, horizontal transmission appears to play a significant role in late-onset disease. The reasons for delay in development of clinical illness, the predilection for central nervous system (CNS) disease, and the less severe systemic and cardiorespiratory symptoms are unclear. Transplacental transfer of maternal antibodies to the mother's own vaginal flora may play a role in determining which exposed infants become infected, especially in the case of group B streptococcal infections. In case of nosocomial spread, the pathogenesis is related to the underlying illness and debilitation of the infant, the flora in the neonatal intensive care (NICU) environment, and invasive monitoring and other techniques used in the NICU. Breaks in the natural barrier function of the skin and intestine allow opportunistic organisms to invade and overwhelm the neonate. Infants, especially the premature ones, have an increased susceptibility to infection because of underlying illnesses and immature immune defenses that are less efficient at localizing and clearing bacterial invasion.

C. **Microbiology.** The principal pathogens involved in EOS have tended to change with time. Before 1965, *Staphylococcus aureus* and *Escherichia coli* used to be the most commonly isolated organisms. In the late 1960s, group B streptococcus (GBS) emerged as the most common microorganism. Currently, most centers continue to report GBS as the most common microorganism even though the incidence has decreased considerably after the widespread adoption of universal antenatal screening for GBS colonization at 35 to 37 weeks' gestation and intrapartum prophylaxis with penicillin or ampicillin for colonized women. The incidence of EOS secondary to GBS decreased from 1.7 per 1000 live births in 1993 to 0.34 per 1000 in 2004. The second most common bacteria are Gram-negative enteric organisms, especially *E. coli*. An increase in the incidence of *E. coli* has been recently noted in EOS in VLBW infants to the extent that *E. coli* is currently the predominant microorganism in this group of patients. Whether this increase is linked to the widespread use of intrapartum antibiotics is not clear. Other pathogens causing EOS include *Listeria monocytogenes, Staphylococcus, Enterococci,* anaerobes, *Haemophilus influenzae,* and *Streptococcus pneumoniae.* The pathogens that cause LOS or nosocomial sepsis tend to vary in each nursery; however, coagulase-negative *Staphylococci* (CoNS), especially *Staphylococcus epidermidis,* are the most predominant. Other microorganisms causing LOS include Gram-negative rods (including *Pseudomonas, Klebsiella, Serratia,* and *Proteus*), *S. aureus,* GBS, and fungal organisms.

IV. **Risk factors**
   A. **Prematurity and low birthweight.** Prematurity is the single most significant factor correlated with sepsis. The risk increases in proportion to the decrease in birthweight.
   B. **Rupture of membranes.** Premature or prolonged (>18 h) rupture of membranes.
   C. **Maternal peripartum fever (≥38°C/100.4°F) or infection.** Chorioamnionitis (foul-smelling or cloudy amniotic fluid), urinary tract infection (UTI), vaginal colonization with GBS, previous delivery of a neonate with GBS disease, perineal colonization with *E. coli,* and other obstetric complications.
   D. **Resuscitation at birth.** Infants who had fetal distress, were born by traumatic delivery, or were severely depressed at birth and required intubation and resuscitation.
   E. **Multiple gestation.**
   F. **Invasive procedures.** Invasive monitoring (fetal scalp electrodes), intravascular catheterization (percutaneous inserted central catheters [PICC] and umbilical catheters) and respiratory (endotracheal intubation) or metabolic support (total parenteral nutrition).
   G. **Infants with galactosemia** (predisposition to *E. coli* sepsis), immune defects, or asplenia.
   H. **Other factors.** Males are four times more affected than females, and the possibility of a sex-linked genetic basis for host susceptibility is postulated. Variations in immune function may play a role. Bottle-feeding (as opposed to breast-feeding) may

predispose to infection. Low socioeconomic status is often reported as an additional risk factor, but this may be explained by low birthweight. NICU staff and family members are often vectors for the spread of microorganisms, primarily as a result of improper handwashing.

V. **Clinical presentation.** The initial diagnosis of sepsis is, by necessity, a clinical one because it is imperative to begin treatment before the results of culture are available. Clinical signs and symptoms of sepsis are nonspecific, and the differential diagnosis is broad. Some signs are subtle or insidious, and therefore a high index of suspicion is required to identify and evaluate infected neonates. Clinical signs and symptoms most often mentioned include the following:

A. **Temperature irregularity.** Hypothermia is more common than fever as a presenting sign for bacterial sepsis. Hyperthermia is more common if viral agents (eg, herpes) are involved.

B. **Change in behavior.** Lethargy, irritability, or change in tone.

C. **Skin.** Poor peripheral perfusion, cyanosis, mottling, pallor, petechiae, rashes, sclerema, or jaundice.

D. **Feeding problems.** Feeding intolerance, vomiting, diarrhea, or abdominal distention with or without visible bowel loops.

E. **Cardiopulmonary.** Tachypnea, respiratory distress (grunting, flaring, and retractions), apnea within the first 24 h of birth or of new onset (especially after 1 week of age), tachycardia, or hypotension, which tends to be a late sign.

F. **Metabolic.** Hypoglycemia, hyperglycemia, or metabolic acidosis.

G. **Focal infections** may precede or accompany LOS. Look for cellulitis, impetigo, soft tissue abscesses, omphalitis, conjunctivitis, otitis media, meningitis, or osteomyelitis.

VI. **Diagnosis**

A. **Differential diagnosis.** Because signs and symptoms of neonatal sepsis are nonspecific, noninfectious etiologies need to be considered. If the infant is presenting with respiratory symptoms, respiratory distress syndrome, transient tachypnea of the newborn, meconium aspiration, and aspiration pneumonia are considered. If the infant is showing CNS symptoms, then intracranial hemorrhage, drug withdrawal, and inborn errors of metabolism are considered. Patients with feeding intolerance and bloody stool may have necrotizing enterocolitis, gastrointestinal perforation, or obstruction. Some nonbacterial infections like disseminated herpes simplex virus can be indistinguishable from bacterial sepsis and should be considered in the differential diagnosis especially if the infant has fever.

B. **Laboratory studies**

1. **Cultures.** Blood and other normally sterile body fluids (urine, spinal fluid, and tracheal aspirate) should be obtained for culture. (In neonates <24 h of age, a sterile urine specimen is not necessary, given that the occurrence of UTIs is exceedingly rare in this age group.) Positive bacterial cultures confirm the diagnosis of sepsis. Computer-assisted automated blood culture systems identify up to 94–96% of all microorganisms by 48 h of incubation. Results may vary because of a number of factors, including maternal antibiotics administered before birth, organisms that are difficult to grow and isolate (ie, anaerobes), and sampling error with small sample volumes (the optimal amount is 1–2 mL/sample). One blood culture is typically obtained in cases of EOS and two blood cultures (one from PICC and one peripheral) in cases of LOS. In many clinical situations, infants are treated for "presumed" sepsis despite negative cultures, with apparent clinical benefit. Some **controversy** currently exists as to whether a lumbar puncture (LP) is needed in asymptomatic newborns being worked up for early-onset presumptive sepsis. Many institutions perform LPs only on infants who are clinically ill, infants who have CNS symptoms like apnea or seizures, or in cases of documented positive blood cultures. LP should be part of the routine evaluation for LOS. Meningitis is likely to happen without sepsis in VLBW infants, and therefore LP should be considered strongly in this group.

Tracheal aspirate cultures should be obtained in intubated neonates with a clinical picture suggestive of pneumonia; if the mother developed chorioamnionitis with overwhelming EOS of the newborn; or when the quality and volume of tracheal secretions change substantially.

2. **Gram stain of various fluids.** Gram staining is especially helpful for the study of CSF. Gram-stained smears and cultures of amniotic fluid are helpful in diagnosing chorioamnionitis.

3. **Adjunctive laboratory tests**

   a. **White blood cell count with differential.** These values alone are very nonspecific. There are reference values for total white blood cell count and absolute neutrophil count as a function of postnatal age in hours (see Chapter 66, particularly Tables 66–1 and 66–2). Neutropenia may be a significant finding with an ominous prognosis when associated with sepsis. However, neutropenia has been described commonly as an incidental finding in otherwise healthy growing VLBW infants. The presence of immature forms is more specific but still rather insensitive. Ratios of bands to segmented forms >0.3 and of bands to total polymorphonuclear cells >0.1 have good predictive value, if present. A variety of conditions other than sepsis can alter neutrophil counts and ratios, including maternal hypertension and fever, neonatal asphyxia, maternal intrapartum oxytocin, hypoglycemia, stressful labor, meconium aspiration syndrome, pneumothorax, and even prolonged crying. Serial white blood cell counts several hours apart may be helpful in establishing a trend.

   b. **Platelet count.** A decreased platelet count is usually a late sign and very nonspecific.

   c. **Acute-phase reactants (APRs)** are a complex multifunctional group comprising complement components, coagulation proteins, protease inhibitors, C-reactive protein (CRP), and others that rise in concentration in the serum in response to inflammation. The inflammation may be secondary to infection, trauma, or other processes of cellular destruction. An elevated APR does not distinguish between infectious and noninfectious causes of inflammation. Except for CRP, most of APRs are not commercially available for routine testing.

      i. **CRP** is an acute phase reactant that increases the most in the presence of inflammation caused by infection or tissue injury. The highest concentrations of CRP are reported in patients with bacterial infections, whereas moderate elevations typify chronic inflammatory conditions. Synthesis of acute phase proteins by hepatocytes is modulated by cytokines. Interleukin-1b (IL-1b), IL-6, IL-8, and tumor necrosis factor (TNF) are the most important regulators of CRP synthesis. CRP secretion starts within 4–6 h after the inflammatory stimulus and peaks at ~36–48 h. The biologic half-life of CRP is 19 h, with a 50% reduction daily after the acute-phase stimulus resolves. CRP demonstrates high sensitivity and negative predictive value. A single normal value cannot rule out infection because the sampling may have preceded the rise in CRP. Serial determinations, therefore, are indicated. CRP elevations in noninfected neonates have been seen with fetal hypoxia, respiratory distress syndrome (RDS), meconium aspiration, after trauma/surgery, and postimmunizations. A false-positive rate of 8% has been found in healthy neonates. Nonetheless, CRP is a valuable adjunct in the diagnosis of sepsis, monitoring the response to treatment as well as guiding duration of treatment.

      ii. **Cytokines IL-6, IL-8, and TNF** are produced primarily by activated monocytes and macrophages and are major mediators of the systemic response to infection. Studies have shown that combining cytokines with CRP may be better than using CRP alone. IL-6, IL-8, and procalcitonin may be better than CRP in the diagnosis and follow-up of neonatal sepsis secondary to CoNS.

      iii. **Procalcitonin (PCT)** is a propeptide of calcitonin that increases markedly with sepsis. It may not be useful to screen for early sepsis because it normally rises in the first 48 h of life. However, PCT is a sensitive marker for LOS and may be superior to CRP.

      iv. **Neutrophil surface antigen CD11 and CD64** are promising markers of early infection that correlate well with CRP but peak earlier.

       d. Serum apolipoprotein–A (Apo-A). Recent studies state that Apo-A may be a useful marker for detection of neonatal LOS.

       e. Miscellaneous tests. Abnormal values for bilirubin, glucose, and sodium may, in the proper clinical situation, provide supportive evidence for sepsis.

   C. Radiologic studies

      1. A chest radiograph should be obtained in cases with respiratory symptoms, although it is often impossible to distinguish GBS or *Listeria* pneumonia from uncomplicated RDS. One distinguishing feature is the presence of pleural effusion, which occurs in 67% of cases of pneumonia.

      2. Urinary tract imaging. Imaging with renal ultrasound examination, renal scan, or voiding cystourethrography should be part of the evaluation when UTI accompanies sepsis. Sterile urine for culture must be obtained by either a suprapubic tap (Chapter 24) or catheterized specimen (Chapter 25). Bag urine samples should not be used to diagnose UTI.

   D. Other studies. Examination of the placenta and fetal membranes may disclose evidence of chorioamnionitis and thus an increased potential for neonatal infection.

VII. Management. Isolation precautions for all infectious diseases, including maternal and neonatal precautions, breast-feeding, and visiting issues, can be found in Appendix F.

   A. GBS prophylaxis. Because of the widespread use of intrapartum antibiotic prophylaxis, EOS secondary to GBS has been reduced by 80%. Approximately 10–30% of pregnant women are colonized with GBS in the vaginal or rectal area. Consensus guidelines regarding management of GBS were published by the Centers for Disease Control and Prevention (CDC) initially in 1996 and were later revised in 2002. These guidelines are supported by the American Academy of Pediatrics (AAP) and the American College of Obstetricians and Gynecologists (ACOG). The guidelines recommended that all pregnant women should be screened at 35–37 weeks' gestation for vaginal and rectal GBS colonization. At the time of labor or rupture of membranes, intrapartum chemoprophylaxis should be given to all pregnant women identified as GBS carriers. Women with GBS isolated from the urine in any concentration during their current pregnancy should receive intrapartum chemoprophylaxis because such women usually are heavily colonized with GBS and are at increased risk of delivering an infant with early-onset GBS disease. Women who have previously given birth to an infant with invasive GBS disease should receive intrapartum chemoprophylaxis as well. Penicillin is the drug of choice, but ampicillin is an acceptable alternative. Cefazolin or vancomycin may be used for penicillin-allergic women. The risk-based approach is no longer acceptable except for circumstances in which screening results are not available before delivery. Culture techniques that maximize the likelihood of GBS recovery are required for prenatal screening. To ensure appropriate treatment for neonates born to mothers who receive antibiotics for fever and presumed chorioamnionitis, as well as for those born to mothers who receive intrapartum antibiotic prophylaxis because of GBS colonization, we are clinically using an algorithm in our hospital based on the CDC guidelines (Figure 117–1).

   B. Initial therapy. Treatment is most often begun before a definite causative agent is identified. It consists of a **penicillin,** usually **ampicillin,** plus an **aminoglycoside** such as gentamicin. In nosocomial sepsis, the flora of the NICU must be considered; however, generally, staphylococcal coverage with **vancomycin plus an aminoglycoside** such as gentamicin or amikacin is usually begun. Third-generation cephalosporins should be avoided as an empirical therapy because they are associated with increased risk for antibiotic resistance and invasive fungal infections. Dosages are presented in Chapter 132.

   C. Continuing therapy is based on culture and sensitivity results, clinical course, and other serial laboratory studies (eg, CRP). Monitoring for antibiotic toxicity is important as well as monitoring levels of aminoglycosides and vancomycin. When GBS is documented as the causative agent, a penicillin is the drug of choice; however, an aminoglycoside is often given as well because of documented synergism in vitro.

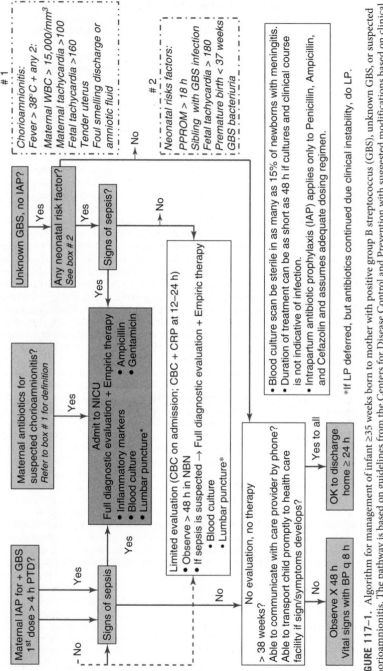

FIGURE 117–1. Algorithm for management of infant ≥35 weeks born to mother with positive group B streptococcus (GBS), unknown GBS, or suspected chorioamnionitis. The pathway is based on guidelines from the Centers for Disease Control and Prevention with suggested modifications based on clinical experience. IAP, intrapartum antibiotic prophylaxis.

D. **Complications and supportive therapy**
1. **Respiratory.** Ensure adequate oxygenation with blood gas monitoring, and initiate oxygen therapy or ventilator support if needed.
2. **Cardiovascular.** Support blood pressure and perfusion to prevent shock. Use volume expanders like normal saline, and monitor the intake and output of fluids. Inotropes such as dopamine or dobutamine may be needed (see Chapter 132).
3. **Hematologic**
   a. **Disseminated intravascular coagulation (DIC).** With DIC, one may observe generalized bleeding at puncture sites, the gastrointestinal tract, or CNS sites. In the skin, large-vessel thrombosis may cause gangrene. Laboratory parameters consistent with DIC include thrombocytopenia, increased prothrombin time, and increased partial thromboplastin time. There is an increase in fibrin split products or d-dimers. Treatment options include fresh-frozen plasma, 10 mL/kg; vitamin K (Chapter 132); platelet infusion; and possible exchange transfusion (Chapter 29).
   b. **Neutropenia.** Multiple factors contribute to the increased susceptibility of neonates to infection, including developmental quantitative and qualitative neutrophil defects. Colony-stimulating factors (CSFs) comprise a group of cytokines that are central to the hematopoiesis of blood cells, as well as to the maintenance of homeostasis and overall immune competence. Granulocyte-CSF (G-CSF) and granulocyte-macrophage-CSF (GM-CSF) have been used in neonates with established sepsis associated with neutropenia, in neutropenic infants without sepsis, and prophylactically in neonates at risk for sepsis. Limited data suggest that CSF treatment may reduce mortality when systemic infection is accompanied by severe neutropenia. However, a recent review suggested there is insufficient evidence to support the widespread introduction of either G-CSF or GM-CSF into neonatal practice. Intravenous immunoglobulin (IVIG) does not appear useful either as a prophylactic or as an adjunct to antibiotic therapy in serious neonatal infection.
4. **Central nervous system (CNS).** Implement seizure control measures (use phenobarbital, 20 mg/kg loading dose for established seizures), and monitor for the syndrome of inappropriate antidiuretic hormone (decreased urine output, hyponatremia, decreased serum osmolarity, and increased urine specific gravity and osmolarity).
5. **Metabolic.** Monitor for and treat hypoglycemia or hyperglycemia. Metabolic acidosis may accompany sepsis and is treated with bicarbonate and fluid replacement.

E. **Future developments.** Immunotherapy progress continues in the development of vaccines as well as various hyperimmune globulins and synthetic monoclonal antibodies to the specific pathogens causing neonatal sepsis (ie, antistaphylococcal antibodies). They may prove to be significant adjuvants to the routine use of antibiotics for the treatment of sepsis. Research is also ongoing into blocking some of the body's own inflammatory mediators that result in significant tissue injury, including endotoxin inhibitors, cytokine inhibitors, nitric oxide synthetase inhibitors, and neutrophil adhesion inhibitors. Finally, studies are ongoing to test if probiotics with or without lactoferrin will be helpful in the prevention or modulation of neonatal sepsis.

VIII. **Prognosis.** With early diagnosis and treatment, most infants will recover and not have any long-term problems. However, the mortality rate is still significant. For early-onset disease, the mortality rate is 5–10%, for late-onset disease, the rate is 2–6%. For premature and low birthweight infants with early-onset disease, the fatality rate is higher.

Selected References

Bernstein HM et al: Administration of recombinant granulocyte colony-stimulating factor to neonates with septicemia: a meta-analysis. *J Pediatr* 2001;138:917-920.

Carr R et al: G-CSF and GM-CSF for treating or preventing neonatal infections. *Cochrane Database Syst Rev* 2003;3:CD003066.

Cotten CM et al: The association of third-generation cephalosporin use and invasive candidiasis in extremely low birth-weight infants. *Pediatrics* 2006;118:717-722.

Edwards MS: Postnatal bacterial infections. In Martin RJ et al (eds): *Fanaroff and Martin's Neonatal-Perinatal Medicine*, 8th ed. Philadelphia, PA: Mosby Elsevier, 2006:791-829.

Franz AR et al: Measurement of interleukin 8 in combination with C-reactive protein reduced unnecessary antibiotic therapy in newborn infants: a multicenter, randomized, controlled trial. *Pediatrics* 2004;114:1-8.

Gordon A, Isaacs D: Late-onset infection and the role of antibiotic prescribing policies. *Curr Opin Infect Dis* 2004;17:231-236.

Kumar Y et al: Time to positivity of neonatal blood cultures. *Arch Dis Child Fetal Neonatal Ed* 2001;85:F182-186.

Mohan P, Abrams SA. Oral lactoferrin for the treatment of sepsis and necrotizing enterocolitis in neonates. Cochrane Database Syst Rev. 2009 Jan 21;(1):CD007138.

Ng PC et al: Neutrophil CD64 is a sensitive diagnostic marker for early-onset neonatal infection. *Pediatr Res* 2004;56:796-803.

Nupponen I et al: Neutrophil CD11b expression and circulating interleukin-8 as diagnostic markers for early-onset neonatal sepsis. *Pediatrics* 2001;108:E12.

Omar SA et al: Late-onset neutropenia in very low birth weight infants. *Pediatrics* 2000;106:E55.

Pourcyrous M et al: Primary immunization of premature infants with gestational age <35 weeks: cardiorespiratory complications and C-reactive protein responses associated with administration of single and multiple separate vaccines simultaneously. *J Pediatr* 2007;151:167-172.

Ray B et al: Is lumbar puncture necessary for evaluation of early neonatal sepsis? *Arch Dis Child* 2006;91:1033-1035.

Schrag S et al: Prevention of perinatal group B streptococcal disease. Revised guidelines from CDC. *MMWR Recomm Rep* 2002 16;51(RR-11):1-22.

Schrag SJ, Stoll BJ: Early-onset neonatal sepsis in the era of widespread intrapartum chemoprophylaxis. *Pediatr Infect Dis J* 2006;25:939-940.

Stoll BJ et al: Late-onset sepsis in very low birth weight neonates: the experience of the NICHD Neonatal Research Network. *Pediatrics* 2002;110:285-291.

Stoll BJ et al: To tap or not to tap: high likelihood of meningitis without sepsis among very low birth weight infants. *Pediatrics* 2004;113:1181-1186.

Stoll BJ et al: Very low birth weight preterm infants with early onset neonatal sepsis: the predominance of Gram-negative infections continues in the National Institute of Child Health and Human Development Neonatal Research Network, 2002–2003. *Pediatr Infect Dis J* 2005;24:635-639.

Suri M et al: Immunotherapy in the prophylaxis and treatment of neonatal sepsis. *Curr Opin Pediatr* 2003;15:155-160.

Tettelin H et al: Towards a universal group B Streptococcus vaccine using multistrain genome analysis. *Expert Rev Vaccines* 2006;5:687-694.

Vazzalwar R et al: Procalcitonin as a screening test for late-onset sepsis in preterm very low birth weight infants. *J Perinatol* 2005;25:397-402.

Verboon-Maciolek MA et al: Inflammatory mediators for the diagnosis and treatment of sepsis in early infancy. *Pediatr Res* 2006;59:457-461.

Weinberg GA, D'Angio CT: Laboratory aids for diagnosis of neonatal sepsis. In Remington JS et al (eds): *Infectious Diseases of the Fetus and Newborn Infant*. Philadelphia, PA: Elsevier Saunders, 2006:1207.

Weitkamp JH, Aschner JL: Diagnostic use of C-reactive protein (CRP) in assessment of neonatal sepsis. *NeoReviews* 2005:e508-e515. Available at: http://neoreviews.aappublications.org/. Accessed February 23, 2009.

Yildiz B et al. Diagnostic values of lipid and lipoprotein levels in late onset neonatal sepsis. *Scand J Infect Dis* 2009:1-6.

118 Surgical Diseases of the Newborn: Abdominal Masses

RENAL MASSES

In most clinical series, the majority of abdominal masses in neonates are renal in origin. They may be unilateral or bilateral, solid or cystic. After physical examination, evaluation begins with ultrasonography, which is simple and safe to perform. Ultrasonography should define the solid or cystic nature of the mass, determine the presence or absence of normal kidneys, and yield information on other intra-abdominal abnormalities. In selected instances, more involved procedures such as renal scan, computed tomography (CT) scan, retrograde pyelography, venography, and arteriography may be needed to define the problem and plan appropriate therapy.

I. **Multicystic kidney** is a form of renal dysplasia and the most common renal cystic disease of the newborn. Fortunately, it is usually unilateral. Ultrasonography can define the nature of the disorder, and CT/nuclear renal scans are useful in assessing the remainder of the urinary system. Nephrectomy is appropriate treatment.

II. **Hydronephrosis.** Urinary obstruction, depending on its location, can cause unilateral or bilateral flank and abdominal masses. Treatment is by correction of the obstructing lesion or decompression proximal to it. A kidney rendered nonfunctional by back pressure is usually best removed. Obstructive uropathy may be one category of lesion suitable for in utero intervention. Surgery on the developing fetus to decompress the obstructed urinary system may improve the postnatal status and increase survival. (See Chapter 123.)

III. **Infantile polycystic kidney disease.** Inherited in an autosomal recessive fashion, this entity involves both kidneys and carries a grim prognosis.

IV. **Renal vein thrombosis.** The typical presentation is one or more flank masses and hematuria, usually within the first 3 days of life. Risk factors are maternal diabetes and dehydration. In general, conservative nonoperative management is recommended.

V. **Wilms tumor.** See Chapter 122.

OVARIAN MASSES

Simple ovarian cyst is a frequent cause of a palpable abdominal mass in the female neonate. It presents as a relatively mobile, smooth-walled abdominal mass. It is not associated with cancer, and excision with preservation of any ovarian tissue is curative. Smaller lesions ($\leq$5 cm) may be followed with serial ultrasound until gone over the first year of life as long as they continue to get smaller.

HEPATIC MASSES

The liver can be enlarged, often to grotesque proportions, by a variety of problems. When physical examination, ultrasonography, and other radiographic studies suggest hepatic origin, magnetic resonance imaging (MRI) or CT should be performed. These studies may be diagnostic and will aid in surgical planning. Lesions include the following:

I. **Hepatic cysts.** Congenital solitary non-parasitic cysts of the liver are extremely rare in newborns.

II. **Solid, benign tumors**

A. **Hamartomas** commonly have a cystic component. They are characterized by fine internal septations without calcifications. Surgical removal or marsupialization of the cysts are options.

III. **Vascular tumors**
   A. **Hemangiomas** of the liver may cause heart failure, thrombocytopenia, and anemia. Therapeutic options include digitalis, corticosteroid administration, embolization, hepatic artery ligation, and liver resection.
   B. **Hemangioendothelioma.** Now reliably diagnosed with MRI or contrast CT. The infant has normal α-fetoprotein levels. Treatment is reserved only for symptomatic lesions (eg, Kasabach-Merritt syndrome) and includes interferon, systemic corticosteroids, vincristine, or cyclophosphamide. Hepatic resection and even liver transplantation has been described for select lesions.
IV. **Malignant tumors.** Hepatoblastoma is by far the most common liver cancer in the neonate. The serum α-fetoprotein is usually elevated. Although surgical resection remains the key to achieving a cure, new chemotherapeutic protocols (cisplatin and doxorubicin) have improved the formerly dismal prognosis for infants with this tumor. Hepatic transplantation for unresectable lesions is associated with improved cure rates.

GASTROINTESTINAL MASSES

Palpable abdominal masses that arise from the gastrointestinal tract are very unusual and tend to be cystic, smooth walled, and mobile (depending on the size). Causes include intestinal duplication and mesenteric cyst.

Selected References

Albanese CT (ed): Abdominal masses in the newborn. *Semin Pediatr Surg* 2000;9:107.

Grosfeld JL et al (eds): *Pediatric Surgery,* 6th ed. St. Louis, MO: Mosby-Year Book, 2006.

Hayes-Jordan A: Surgical management of the incidentally identified ovarian mass. *Semin Pediatr Surg* 2005;14(2):106-110.

Leclair MD et al; French Pediatric Urology Study Group: The outcome of prenatally diagnosed renal tumors. *J Urol* 2005;173(1):186-189.

O'Neill, JA et al: *Principles of Pediatric Surgery,* 2nd ed. St. Louis, MO: Mosby, 2004.

119 Surgical Diseases of the Newborn: Abdominal Wall Defects

GASTROSCHISIS

I. **Definition.** Gastroschisis is a centrally located, full-thickness abdominal wall defect with two distinctive anatomic features.
   A. **The extruded intestine never has a protective sac covering it.**
   B. **The umbilical cord is an intact structure** at the level of the abdominal skin, just to the left of the defect. Typically, the opening in the abdominal wall is 2–4 cm in diameter, and the solid organs (the liver and spleen) reside in the peritoneal cavity.
II. **Pathophysiology.** Exposure of unprotected intestine to irritating amniotic fluid in utero results in its edematous, indurated, foreshortened appearance. Because of these intestinal abnormalities, development of appropriate peristalsis and effective absorption is

significantly delayed, usually by several weeks. Fortunately, associated congenital anomalies are rare in patients with gastroschisis.

III. **Clinical presentation.** The infant is born with varying amounts of extruded intestine via the defect. The intestine is swollen and friable. There is an association with atresias from blood supply disruption in utero.

IV. **Diagnosis.** The key differential diagnosis is ruptured omphalocele, although the diagnosis is readily apparent in most cases. Increasingly, prenatal ultrasonography identifies gastroschisis.

V. **Management**
   A. **General considerations.** All agree that infants with gastroschisis should be delivered at a neonatal center equipped and staffed to provide definitive care. Less certain is the recommended mode of delivery. Some experts argue that an abdominal wall defect is an indication for cesarean delivery. However, other investigators note that, in the absence of other factors, vaginal delivery does not increase the mortality, morbidity, or length of hospital stay for newborns with gastroschisis.
   B. **Specific measures**
      1. **Temperature regulation.** Immediate attention should be directed toward maintenance of normal body temperature. The tremendous intestinal surface area exposed to the environment puts these infants at great risk for hypothermia.
      2. **Protective covering/position.** It is best not to keep replacing moist, saline-soaked gauze over the exposed intestine because doing so promotes evaporative heat loss. It is better to apply a dry (or moist) protective dressing and then wrap the abdomen in layers of cellophane. A warm, controlled environment should be provided. The infant should be laid on its side so the vascular pedicle of the intestine is not "kinked" while awaiting surgical intervention.
      3. **Nasogastric decompression** is helpful.
      4. **Broad-spectrum antibiotic coverage** is appropriate, given the unavoidable contamination.
      5. **Total parenteral nutrition.** A protracted ileus is to be expected, and appropriate intravenous nutritional support must be provided.
      6. **Surgical correction.** As soon as the infant's condition permits, operative correction should be undertaken. Complete reduction of herniated intestine, with primary closure of the abdominal wall, or placement of unreduced intestine in a protective prosthetic silo, with subsequent staged reduction over 7–14 days, is usually performed. Gastroschisis is associated with long (weeks) periods of ileus so central venous access is also usually part of the surgical intervention.

OMPHALOCELE

I. **Definition.** An omphalocele is a herniation of abdominal contents into the base of the umbilical cord. The gross appearance of omphalocele differs from that of gastroschisis in two important respects:
   A. **A protective membrane encloses the malpositioned abdominal contents** (unless rupture has occurred, eg, during the birth process).
   B. **Elements of the umbilical cord course individually over the sac and come together at its apex to form a normal-appearing umbilical cord.**

II. **Associated anomalies.** Significant associated congenital anomalies occur in ~25–40% of infants with omphalocele. Problems include chromosomal abnormalities, congenital diaphragmatic hernia, and a variety of cardiac defects.

III. **Clinical presentation.** There are different sizes of omphaloceles. The smaller ones typically contain only intestine; large or giant omphaloceles contain liver and spleen as well as the gastrointestinal tract. The peritoneal cavity in infants with large or giant omphaloceles is very small because growth has proceeded without the solid organs in proper position.

IV. **Diagnosis.** The anomaly is usually apparent. A ruptured omphalocele may be confused with a gastroschisis; both defects are characterized by exposed intestine, but infants with omphalocele do not possess an intact umbilical cord at the level of the abdominal wall to the left of the defect. Careful studies to identify associated congenital anomalies should be performed.

V. **Management.** Reduction, even in stages over a lengthy period, may be very difficult to achieve. Therapeutically, infants with omphalocele fall into two main groups:

A. **Ruptured sac.** Infants with ruptured sacs resemble those with gastroschisis. The unprotected intestine should be cared for as described for gastroschisis (see Gastroschisis, Section V, B, 2), and the problem should be corrected surgically on an emergent basis.

B. **Intact sac.** Intact omphalocele is a less urgent surgical problem. The protective membrane conserves heat and in most cases allows effective peristalsis. This sac should be carefully protected. Some surgeons favor daily dressing changes with gauze pads impregnated with povidone-iodine until the sac toughens and desiccates. The timing of surgery is influenced by a number of factors, including the dimensions of the defect, size of the infant, and presence of other anomalies. Nonoperative staged reduction using compressive dressings has been described. Skin coverage as a temporary measure to allow growth of the abdominal cavity and repair of the midline hernia defect later is also acceptable.

INGUINAL HERNIA AND HYDROCELE

I. **Definition.** Persistence of a patent processus vaginalis (related to testicular descent) is responsible for an inguinal hernia and hydrocele in the neonate.

A. **Inguinal hernia.** The opening of the patent processus at the internal ring is large enough to allow a loop of intestine to extrude from the abdominal cavity with an increase in intra-abdominal pressure.

B. **Hydrocele.** The patent processus is too narrow to permit egress of intestine; peritoneal fluid drips down along the course of the narrow patent processus and accumulates in the scrotum. Hydroceles may be communicating (processus stays open) or noncommunicating (closes spontaneously) without need for operative correction.

II. **Diagnosis**

A. **Inguinal hernias** tend to present as lumps or bulges that come and go at the pubic tubercle. Less commonly, they descend into the scrotum.

B. **Hydroceles** typically are scrotal in location, transilluminate, and not reducible.

III. **Management**

A. **Inguinal hernia** carries a 5–15% risk of incarceration during the first year of life. Accordingly, they are usually surgically repaired when the infant's general medical condition permits.

B. **Hydrocele** frequently resolves without specific treatment because the obliteration of the narrow patent processus continues after birth. Persistence of hydrocele beyond 6–12 months is an indication for surgical repair.

UMBILICAL HERNIA

I. **Definition.** This hernia is a skin-covered fascial defect at the umbilicus that allows protrusion of intra-abdominal content.

II. **Diagnosis.** Transmission of intra-abdominal pressure via fascial defect at the umbilicus establishes the diagnosis.

III. **Management.** In infancy, surgical intervention for an umbilical hernia is seldom warranted. Complications such as incarceration and skin breakdown are exceedingly rare. The natural history is one of gradual closure of the umbilical fascial defect, often leading to complete resolution of the problem. Surgical correction should be considered if defect persists after the second birthday.

Selected References

Langer JC: Gastroschisis and omphalocele. *Semin Pediatr Surg* 1996;5:124.

Ledbetter DJ: Gastroschisis and omphalocele. *Surg Clin North Am.* 2006;86(2):249-260.

O'Neill, JA et al: *Principles of Pediatric Surgery,* 2nd ed. St. Louis, MO: Mosby, 2004.

Snyder CL: Current management of umbilical abnormalities and related anomalies. *Semin Pediatr Surg* 2007;16(1):41-49.

120 Surgical Diseases of the Newborn: Alimentary Tract Obstruction

ESOPHAGEAL ATRESIA WITH TRACHEOESOPHAGEAL FISTULA

I. **Definition.** **Type C tracheoesophageal (TE) fistula** is the most common type of esophageal atresia (85%). The esophagus ends blindly ~10–12 cm from the nares and the distal esophagus communicates with the posterior trachea (distal tracheoesophageal fistula [TEF]). **Type A "pure" esophageal atresia** has a similar presentation without the distal gastrointestinal air. This implies esophageal atresia without TEF (10% of cases).

II. **Pathophysiology.** Prime morbidity is pulmonary. Complete esophageal obstruction results in inability of the infant to handle his or her own secretions, producing "excess salivation" and aspiration of pharyngeal contents. More important, the direct communication between the stomach and the tracheobronchial tree via the distal TEF allows the crying newborn to greatly distend the stomach with air; impairment of diaphragmatic excursion promotes basilar atelectasis and subsequent pneumonia. Additionally, the distal TEF permits reflux of gastric secretions directly into the tracheobronchial tree, causing chemical pneumonitis, which may be complicated by bacterial pneumonia.

III. **Clinical presentation.** The pregnancy may have been complicated by polyhydramnios. After delivery, the infant typically is unable to swallow saliva, which drains from the corners of the mouth and requires frequent suctioning. Attempts at feeding result in prompt regurgitation, coughing, choking, and cyanosis.

IV. **Diagnosis.** It is established by attempting to pass a nasogastric tube and meeting resistance at 10–12 cm from the nares followed by chest radiograph for confirmation. Chest radiograph will show the tube to end or coil in the region of the thoracic inlet. You can improve the sensitivity of the test by insufflating 20–30 mL of air into the tube as the radiograph is being taken. The radiograph should also be examined for possible skeletal anomalies, pulmonary infiltrates, cardiac size and shape, and abdominal bowel gas patterns. The tube in the proximal pouch with the presence of air in the gastrointestinal (GI) tract confirms diagnosis. Careful contrast radiograph of the proximal esophageal pouch can also be performed to delineate the precise length of the proximal pouch and to rule out the rare proximal TEF.

V. **Management**

    A. **Preoperative treatment** should focus on protecting the lungs by evacuating the proximal esophageal pouch with an indwelling Repogle tube or frequent suctioning and by placing the infant in a relatively upright (45-degree) position to lessen the likelihood of reflux of gastric contents up the distal esophagus into the trachea. **Broad-spectrum antibiotics** should be administered.

    B. **Surgical therapy.** The steps and timing of surgical therapy must be individualized. Some surgeons perform preliminary gastrostomy to decompress the stomach and provide additional protection against reflux. Single-step ligation of the TEF and esophageal anastomosis via a thoracotomy or thoracoscopy is the preferred intervention if the clinical status of the neonate allows single-stage closure.

C. **Type A "pure" esophageal atresia.** Surgical management differs somewhat because pure esophageal atresia is associated with a higher incidence of long gaps between the proximal and distal esophageal segments. Delayed surgical correction may be an option to allow growth of the segments and thus permit easier approximation.

DUODENAL OBSTRUCTION

I. **Definition.** Obstruction of the lumen of the duodenum may be complete or partial, preor postampullary, and caused by either intrinsic or extrinsic problems.

II. **Pathophysiology**

A. **Duodenal atresia** results in complete obstruction of the lumen of the duodenum, whereas symptoms of partial obstruction result from a stenotic lesion. Duodenal atresia is associated with trisomy 21.

B. **Annular pancreas** is a congenital anomaly of pancreatic development, which results in an encircling "napkin ring" of pancreatic tissue about the descending duodenum. It can result in either complete or, more commonly, partial duodenal obstruction.

C. **Malrotation** may cause complete or partial duodenal obstruction in one of two ways. In uncomplicated malrotation, peritoneal attachments (Ladd bands) may compress the duodenum, resulting in total or, more commonly, partial obstruction. Midgut volvulus may complicate nonrotation and nonfixation of the intestine. The entire midgut may twist on the pedicle of its blood supply, the superior mesenteric artery, resulting in duodenal obstruction and eventual nonviability of the midgut.

III. **Clinical presentation**

A. **General.** Infants with duodenal obstruction typically experience vomiting (often bilious). Abdominal distention is not usually a prominent feature. Polyhydramnios may be evident.

B. **Duodenal atresia.** The presence of Down syndrome, esophageal atresia, or imperforate anus should make one worry about the presence of duodenal atresia.

C. **Midgut volvulus** typically presents with symptoms of duodenal obstruction (bilious vomiting) and evidence of intestinal ischemia (mucoid bloody stools), usually in an infant who for days or weeks has eaten and stooled normally.

IV. **Differential diagnosis** includes duodenal atresia (stenosis), annular pancreas, and malrotation with or without the complication of midgut volvulus.

V. **Diagnosis.** The exact cause of the obstruction may not be known until a laparotomy is performed.

A. **Abdominal radiographic study.** In complete duodenal obstruction, the pathognomonic radiographic finding is a **"double bubble."** Two large gas collections, one in the stomach and the other in the first portion of duodenum, are the only lucencies in the GI tract.

B. **Radiologic contrast studies**

1. **Partial obstructions** probably require an upper GI series to identify the site of difficulty.

2. **Malrotation.** It is important to eliminate malrotation as a possibility because its complication, midgut volvulus, is a true surgical emergency. This is best done by an upper GI (UGI) series, identifying a transverse portion of the duodenum leading to a fixed ligament of Treitz, or by barium enema, localizing the cecum to its normal right lower quadrant position. The gold standard is the UGI.

VI. **Management**

A. **Duodenal atresia or annular pancreas.** In cases of atresia or annular pancreas, gastric suction controls vomiting and allows "elective" surgical correction.

B. **Malrotation mandates immediate surgical intervention** because the viability of the intestine from the duodenum to the transverse colon may be at risk from midgut volvulus.

C. **Unknown proximal obstruction.** In cases where the source of the obstruction is unsure, early surgical exploration is warranted after resuscitation to prove that the obstruction is not being caused by a lesion causing ischemia to the entire bowel.

PROXIMAL INTESTINAL OBSTRUCTION

I. **Definition.** Proximal intestinal obstruction is obstruction of the jejunum.
II. **Pathophysiology.** Jejunal obstruction typically results from atresia of that segment of the bowel, usually caused by a vascular accident in utero.
III. **Clinical presentation.** Infants with jejunal obstruction usually have bilious vomiting associated with minimal abdominal distention because only a few loops of intestine are involved in the obstructive process.
IV. **Diagnosis.** A plain **abdominal radiograph** reveals only a few dilated small bowel loops with no gas distally. It may be hard to distinguish between jejunal atresia and midgut volvulus by plain films alone.
V. **Management.** Surgical correction is required.

DISTAL INTESTINAL OBSTRUCTION

I. **Definition.** The term **distal intestinal obstruction** denotes partial or complete obstruction of the distal portion of the GI tract. It may be either small bowel (ileum) or large bowel obstruction. It may be a physical obstruction (meconium disease, atresia) or a functional obstruction (small left colon syndrome, Hirschsprung disease). The list of causes includes the following:
   A. **Jejunal/Ileal atresia.** May be single or multiple. Usually complete obstruction.
   B. **Meconium ileus**
      1. **Uncomplicated (simple) obstruction of the terminal ileum** by pellets of inspissated meconium.
      2. **Complicated meconium ileus,** implying compromise of bowel viability either prenatally or postnatally.
   C. **Colonic atresia.**
   D. **Meconium plug–hypoplastic left colon syndrome.**
   E. **Hirschsprung disease** (congenital aganglionic megacolon).
II. **Clinical presentation.** Infants with obstructing lesions in the distal intestine have similar signs and symptoms. They typically have distended abdomens, fail to pass meconium, and vomit bilious material.
III. **Diagnosis**
   A. **Abdominal radiographic studies** show multiple dilated loops of intestine; the site of obstruction (distal small bowel vs colon) cannot be determined on plain films.
   B. **Contrast radiologic studies.** The preferred diagnostic test is contrast enema. It may identify colonic atresia, outline microcolon (which may signify complete distal small bowel obstruction), or suggest a transition zone (which may signify Hirschsprung disease). The procedure can identify and treat meconium plug–hypoplastic left colon syndrome. If the test is normal, ileal atresia, meconium ileus, and Hirschsprung disease are possibilities.
   C. **Cystic fibrosis (CF) evaluation.** A sweat test may be needed to document cystic fibrosis in cases of meconium ileus (unlikely to be helpful in the first few weeks of life). A CF gene screen may identify CF before a sweat test is practical.
   D. **Mucosal rectal biopsy** for histologic detection of ganglion cells is the safest and most widely available screening test for Hirschsprung disease. However, laparotomy is often necessary to determine the exact nature of the problem in infants with normal results of barium enema.
IV. **Management**
   A. **Nonoperative management** in cases of meconium plug and hypoplastic left colon is accomplished with stimulation and is "curative" by either water contrast enema(s) or digital stimulation.

1. **Passage of time and colonic stimulation by digital examination and rectal enemas** promote return of effective peristalsis.
2. **In infants who achieve apparently normal bowel function**, rule out Hirschsprung disease by mucosal rectal biopsy; a small percentage of patients with meconium plug prove to have aganglionosis.
3. **Interestingly, uncomplicated meconium ileus, if identified, can often be treated by nonoperative means.** Repeated enemas with Hypaque or acetylcysteine (Mucomyst) may disimpact the inspissated meconium in the terminal ileum and relieve the obstruction.

B. **Surgical therapy.** Urgent surgical intervention is required for atresia of the ileum or colon, for complicated meconium ileus, and when the diagnosis is in doubt. Hirschsprung disease (HD) is always treated surgically. There are three accepted times for surgical intervention for HD. Laparoscopic, open, and transanal procedures are described for each of these timed procedures:

1. Delayed repair with colostomy through ganglionic bowel in the neonatal period.
2. One-stage pull-through procedure while the infant is in the neonatal intensive care unit.
3. Delay one-stage repair until the infant has doubled its birthweight. Therapeutic irrigations/enemas are used to keep the distal colon decompressed.

IMPERFORATE ANUS

I. **Definition.** Imperforate anus is the lack of an anal opening of proper location or size. There are two types: high and low.

A. **High imperforate anus.** The rectum ends above the puborectalis sling, the main muscle responsible for maintaining fecal continence. There is never an associated fistula to the perineum. In males, there may be a rectourinary fistula, and in females, a rectovaginal fistula. High imperforate anus is much more common in males.

B. **Low imperforate anus.** The rectum has traversed the puborectalis sling in the correct position. Variants include anal stenosis, imperforate anus with perineal fistula, and imperforate anus without fistula.

II. **Diagnosis** is by inspection and calibration of any perineal opening that emits meconium. All patients with imperforate anus should have radiographic studies of the lumbosacral spine and urinary tract because there is a high incidence of dysmorphism in these areas.

III. **Management.** Surgical therapy in the neonate consists of colostomy for high anomalies and perineal anoplasty or dilation of fistula for low lesions. If the level is not known, colostomy is preferable to blind exploration of the perineum. If colostomy is done, a contrast radiographic study of the distal limb should be performed to ascertain the level at which the rectum ends and to determine the presence or absence of an associated fistula.

NECROTIZING ENTEROCOLITIS

I. **Definition.** In most centers, necrotizing enterocolitis (NEC) is the most common indication for operation in neonates. It is caused by a combination of mucosal injury, relative hypoxia, and infection of the intestinal wall. It is presented in detail in Chapter 104.

II. **Diagnosis.** Clinical diagnosis of "true" NEC is made in the presence of pneumatosis of the intestinal wall and/or the presence of portal venous air only. Abdominal distention, bloody bowel movements, and intolerance of feeds in an infant who previously tolerated feeds are all signs of NEC. However, the diagnosis can only be confirmed with these radiographic findings or a pathology specimen from the affected intestine.

III. **Management**

A. **Nonoperative management.** Intestinal decompression with a Replogle-style nasogastric or orogastric tube, aggressive resuscitation, broad-spectrum antibiotics to include anaerobic coverage, and inotropic support as necessary.

B. **Surgical therapy.** Abdominal exploration is usually reserved for infants with full-thickness necrosis of the intestine, usually manifested by pneumoperitoneum (best identified by serial left lateral decubitus radiographs). Other, less common indications for surgery include cellulitis and erythema of the abdominal wall and an unchanging abdominal mass. Delayed stricture formation, which is most common on the left side of the colon, complicates NEC in 15–25% of cases.

Selected References

Bianchi A: One stage neonatal reconstruction without stoma for Hirschsprung's disease. *Semin Pediatr Surg* 1998;7:170.

Chwals WJ et al: Surgery-associated complications in necrotizing enterocolitis: a multi-institutional study. *J Pediatr Surg* 2001;36:1722.

Grosfeld et al (eds): *Pediatric Surgery,* 6th ed. St. Louis, MO: Mosby-Year Book, 2006.

Levitt MA, Peña A: Outcomes from the correction of anorectal malformations. *Curr Opin Pediatr* 2005;17(3):394-401.

Moss RL et al: A meta-analysis of peritoneal drainage versus laparotomy for perforated necrotizing enterocolitis. *J Pediatr Surg* 2001;36:1210.

O'Neill, JA et al: *Principles of Pediatric Surgery,* 2nd ed. St. Louis, MO: Mosby, 2004.

121 Surgical Diseases of the Newborn: Diseases of the Airway, Tracheobronchial Tree, and Lungs

INTRINSIC ABNORMALITIES OF THE AIRWAY

I. **Definition.** Abnormalities of, or within, the airway that cause partial obstruction fall into this category. Examples include laryngomalacia, paralyzed vocal cord, subglottic web, and hemangioma.

II. **Pathophysiology.** These lesions result in partial obstruction of the airway and cause stridor and respiratory distress of varying severity.
   A. **Laryngomalacia.** Delayed development of the supraglottic pharynx.
   B. **Congenital paralyzed vocal cords.** Can be congenital or acquired (birth trauma, patent ductus arteriosus [PDA] ligation), rarely bilateral.
   C. **Subglottic web.** Congenital web that may be partial or complete.
   D. **Hemangioma.** Can occur below glottis, engorge, and obstruct with agitation.

III. **Clinical presentation.** Can vary from mild respiratory stridor to complete airway obstruction depending on the exact variant.

IV. **Diagnosis.** The diagnosis is established by endoscopy of the airway with careful visualization of the entire airway to establish diagnosis.

V. **Management** is individualized. Some problems, such as laryngomalacia, will be outgrown if the child can be supported through the period of acute symptoms. Other lesions, such as subglottic webs and hemangiomas, may be amenable to endoscopic resection or laser therapy.

CHOANAL ATRESIA

I. **Definition.** Choanal atresia is a congenital blockage of the posterior nares caused by a persistence of a bony septum (90%) or a soft tissue membrane (10%).

II. **Pathophysiology.** Unilateral or bilateral obstruction at the posterior nares may be secondary to soft tissue or bone. True choanal atresia is complete and bilateral, and it is one cause of respiratory distress immediately after delivery. The effects of upper airway obstruction are compounded because neonates are obligate nose breathers and do not "think" to breathe through the mouth. Unilateral defects may be well tolerated and go unnoticed.

III. **Clinical presentation.** Respiratory distress resulting from partial or total upper airway obstruction is the mode of presentation.

IV. **Diagnosis** is based on an **inability to pass a catheter into the nasopharynx via either side of the nose.**

V. **Management.** Simply making the infant cry and thereby breathe through the mouth temporarily improves breathing. Insertion of an oral airway maintains the ability to breathe until the atresia is surgically corrected. Definitive management requires resection of the soft tissue or bony septum in the nasopharynx.

PIERRE ROBIN SYNDROME

I. **Definition.** This anomaly consists of mandibular hypoplasia (micrognathia) in association with cleft palate.

II. **Pathophysiology.** Airway obstruction is produced by posterior displacement of the tongue associated with the small size of the mandible.

III. **Clinical presentation.** Severity of symptoms varies, but most infants manifest a high degree of partial upper airway obstruction.

IV. **Management**
   A. **Infants with mild involvement** can be cared for in the prone position and fed through a special Breck nipple. Adjustment to the airway compromise occurs over weeks to months as the mandible grows relatively faster and the degree of obstruction lessens with growth.
   B. **More severe cases** require nasopharyngeal tubes or surgical procedures to hold the tongue in an anterior position. Tracheostomy is generally a last resort.

LARYNGOTRACHEAL ESOPHAGEAL CLEFT

I. **Definition.** Laryngotracheal esophageal cleft is a rare congenital anomaly in which there is an incomplete separation of the larynx (and sometimes the trachea) from the esophagus, resulting in a common channel of esophagus and airway. This communication may be short or may extend almost the entire length of the trachea.

II. **Pathophysiology.** The persistent communication between the larynx (and occasionally a significant portion of the trachea) and the esophagus results in recurring symptoms of aspiration and respiratory distress with feeding.

III. **Clinical presentation.** Respiratory distress during feeding is the presenting symptom.

IV. **Diagnosis.** Contrast swallow may suggest the anomaly, but endoscopy is essential in firmly establishing the diagnosis and delineating the extent of the defect.

V. **Management.** Laryngotracheal esophageal cleft is treated by surgical correction, which is difficult and often unsuccessful.

VASCULAR RING

I. **Definition.** **Vascular ring** denotes a variety of anomalies of the aortic arch and its branches that create a "ring" of vessels around the trachea and esophagus.

II. **Pathophysiology.** Partial obstruction of the trachea or the esophagus, or both, may result from extrinsic compression by the encircling ring of vessels.

III. **Clinical presentation.** Dysphagia or stridor (respiratory insufficiency), or both, are the modes of presentation. Airway compromise is rarely severe and usually presents as stridor.

IV. **Diagnosis** is by barium swallow, which identifies extrinsic compression of the esophagus in the region of the aortic arch.

V. **Management** consists of surgical division of a portion of the constricting ring of vessels. The specific surgical plan must be tailored to the particular type of aortic arch anomaly present.

H-TYPE TRACHEOESOPHAGEAL FISTULA (TYPE-E TEF)

I. **Definition.** This anomaly is the third most common type of tracheoesophageal fistula (TEF), making up 5% of cases. Esophageal continuity is intact, but there is a fistulous communication between the posterior trachea and the anterior esophagus.

II. **Pathophysiology.** If the fistula is small, as is usually the case, "silent" aspiration occurs during feedings with resulting pneumonitis. If the fistula is unusually large, coughing and choking may accompany each feeding.

III. **Clinical presentation.** Symptoms, as noted previously, depend on the size of the fistula. This is the subtype of tracheoesophageal (TE) fistula that may escape diagnosis in the newborn period.

IV. **Diagnosis.** Barium swallow is the initial diagnostic study and may identify the fistula but also may miss it. The sensitivity of the test can be increased with a "pull back" upper gastrointestinal (UGI) series. Here, a nasogastric tube placed in the distal esophagus is pulled out slowly while instilling water-soluble contrast. The most accurate procedure, however, is bronchoscopy (perhaps combined with esophagoscopy); this should allow discovery and perhaps cannulation of the fistula.

V. **Management.** Surgical correction is required. The approach (via the neck or chest) is determined by location of the fistula.

CONGENITAL LOBAR EMPHYSEMA

I. **Definition. Lobar emphysema** is a term used to denote hyperexpansion of the air spaces of a segment or lobe of the lung.

II. **Pathophysiology.** Inspired air is trapped in an enclosed space. As the cyst of entrapped air enlarges, the normal lung is increasingly compressed. Cystic problems are more common in the upper lobes.

III. **Clinical presentation.** Small cysts may cause few or no symptoms and are readily seen on radiograph. Giant cysts may cause significant respiratory distress, with mediastinal shift and compromise of the contralateral lung.

IV. **Diagnosis.** Usually, the cysts are easily seen on plain chest radiographs. However, the radiologic findings may be confused with those of tension pneumothorax.

V. **Management.** Therapeutic options include observation for small asymptomatic cysts, repositioning of the endotracheal tube to ventilate the uninvolved lung selectively for 6–12 h, bronchoscopy for endobronchial lavage, and operative resection of the cyst with or without the segment or lobe from which it arises.

CYSTIC ADENOMATOID MALFORMATION

I. **Definition.** The term **cystic adenomatoid malformation** encompasses a spectrum of congenital pulmonary malformations involving varying degrees of cyst formation. They communicate with the normal tracheobronchial tree. There are three types depending on the size of the cysts within the malformation.

II. **Pathophysiology.** Severity of symptoms is related to the amount of lung involved and particularly to the degree to which the normal ipsilateral and contralateral lung is compressed.

III. **Clinical presentation.** Signs of respiratory insufficiency such as tachypnea and cyanosis are modes of presentation.

IV. **Diagnosis.** The characteristic pattern on chest radiograph is multiple discrete air bubbles, occasionally with air-fluid levels, involving a region of the lung. The radiographic appearance can mimic that of congenital diaphragmatic hernia (CDH).

V. **Management.** Treatment is surgical resection of the involved lobe of lung, allowing reexpansion of compressed normal pulmonary tissue. If small and without symptoms, the surgical management can wait until the infant is several months of age.

PULMONARY SEQUESTRATION

I. **Definition.** Masses of abnormal tissue with aberrant blood supply arising from systemic and not pulmonary source. May be intralobar or extralobar. Intralobar sequestrations have abnormal connections to the tracheobronchial tree. Extralobar sequestrations have separate pleura and no connections to the tracheobronchial tree.

II. **Pathophysiology.** Sequestrations are usually not recognized in the neonate. Intralobar sequestrations are found after frequent recurrent infections. Extralobar are masses that are usually not associated with infections.

III. **Clinical presentation.** Lung mass found with or without frequent recurrent infections.

IV. **Diagnosis.** Chest radiograph and computed tomography scan.

V. **Management.** Surgical resection. Aberrant blood supply may originate from below the diaphragm.

CONGENITAL DIAPHRAGMATIC HERNIA (CDH)

I. **Definition.** A patent pleuroperitoneal canal through the foramen of Bochdalek is the most common defect in CDH. A central anterior defect of the diaphragm (Morgagni hernia) is less common and usually not associated with lung hypoplasia.

II. **Pathophysiology**

A. **Prenatal.** The abnormal communication between the peritoneal and pleural cavities allows herniation of intestine into the pleural space as the developing GI tract returns from its extracoelomic phase at 10–12 weeks' gestation. Depending on the degree of pulmonary compression by herniated intestine, there may be marked diminution of bronchial branching, limited multiplication of alveoli, and persistence of muscular hypertrophy in pulmonary arterioles. These anatomic abnormalities are most notable on the side of the CDH (usually the left); they are also present to some degree in the contralateral lung.

B. **Postnatal.** After delivery, the anatomic anomaly may contribute to the development of either or both of the following pathologic conditions:

1. **Pulmonary parenchymal insufficiency.** Infants with CDH have an abnormally small functional lung mass. Some have so few conducting air passages and developed alveoli—a condition known as **pulmonary parenchymal insufficiency**—that survival is unlikely.

2. **Pulmonary hypertension.** Infants with CDH are predisposed anatomically to pulmonary hypertension of the newborn (PHN), also known as persistent fetal circulation. In this condition, blood is shunted around the lungs through the foramen ovale and PDA. Shunting promotes acidosis and hypoxia, both of which are potent stimuli to additional pulmonary vasoconstriction. Thus a vicious cycle of clinical deterioration is established.

III. **Clinical presentation.** Most infants with CDH exhibit significant respiratory distress within the first few hours of life.

IV. **Diagnosis.** Prenatal diagnosis can reliably be made by ultrasonography. Delivery should occur in a neonatal center with full resuscitation capability including extracorporeal membrane oxygenation (ECMO). Afflicted infants tend to have scaphoid abdomens because there is a paucity of the GI tract located in the abdomen. Auscultation reveals diminished breath sounds on the affected side. Diagnosis is established by a chest radiograph that reveals a bowel gas pattern in one hemithorax, with shift of mediastinal structures to the other side and compromise of the contralateral lung.

V. **Management**

A. **Indwelling arterial catheter.** Blood gas levels should be monitored by an arterial catheter.

B. **Supportive care.** Intubation with positive-pressure ventilation should be initiated immediately. CDH lungs are surfactant deficient, and replacement therapy appears to be helpful. Several different strategies for appropriate respiratory and metabolic support have been described. These include permissive hypercapnia with conventional ventilation, oscillator ventilation, and/or the addition of inhaled nitric oxide. All these therapies are aimed at providing maximal pulmonary vasodilatation with minimal secondary lung injury due to barotrauma.

C. **Nasogastric intubation** should be performed to lessen gaseous distention of the stomach and intestine. Care must be taken to make sure the tube remains functional and does not clog.

D. **Surgical correction** is by reduction of intrathoracic intestine and closure of the diaphragmatic defect. Surgical intervention is obviously an essential element of treatment, but it is not the key to survival. Most authorities favor a delayed approach, allowing the newborn to stabilize a hyperreactive pulmonary vascular bed and to improve pulmonary compliance. If indicated, ECMO can be instituted, and repair of the hernia defect performed immediately after stabilization on ECMO, when the infant is ready to wean from ECMO, or after successful decannulation from ECMO.

E. **Extracorporeal membrane oxygenation (ECMO)** is used in the treatment of neonates with severe respiratory failure. Exposure of venous blood to the extracorporeal circuit allows correction of PO_2 and PCO_2 abnormalities as the lungs recover from the trauma associated with positive-pressure ventilation (see Chapter 13).

VI. **Prognosis.** Mortality rates for infants with CDH are still in the range of 50%. This high rate has prompted a search for other modes of treatment in addition to the expensive, labor-intensive modality ECMO.

A. **Fetal surgery** has been performed successfully on a case study basis, with the idea that in utero intervention will lessen the risk for development of pulmonary hypoplasia, which may be incompatible with life after delivery. However, trials of fetal tracheal occlusion and complete fetal correction have been abandoned due to high mortality.

B. **Medications.** Another major area of research is the attempt to develop a pharmacologic agent to decrease pulmonary vascular resistance selectively. To date, early promising data on inhaled nitric oxide have been tempered with realization that it does not reverse PHN. Now, sildenafil (0.5–1mg/kg every 6 h) is reported to lower pulmonary hypertension in neonates with PHN.

Selected References

Dimmitt RA et al: Venoarterial versus venovenous extracorporeal membrane oxygenation in congenital diaphragmatic hernia: the extracorporeal life support organization registry, 1990–1999. *J Pediatr Surg* 2001;36:1199.

Greenholz SK: Congenital diaphragmatic hernia: an overview. *Semin Pediatr Surg* 1996;5:216.

Grosfeld JL et al (eds): *Pediatric Surgery,* 6th ed. St. Louis, MO: Mosby-Year Book, 2006.

Harting MT, Lally KP: Surgical management of neonates with congenital diaphragmatic hernia. *Semin Pediatr Surg* 2007;16(2):109-114.

Logan JW et al: Congenital diaphragmatic hernia: a systematic review and summary of best-evidence practice strategies. *J Perinatol* 2007;27(9):535-549.

Nuchtern JG, Harberg FJ: Congenital lung cysts. *Semin Pediatr Surg* 1994;3:233.

O'Neill JA et al: *Principles of Pediatric Surgery*, 2nd ed. St. Louis, MO: Mosby, 2004.

Skinner SC et al: Extracorporeal life support. *Semin Pediatr Surg* 2006;15(4):242-250.

Wong JT et al: Congenital diaphragmatic hernia: survival treated with very delayed surgery, spontaneous respiration and no chest tube. *J Pediatr Surg* 1995;30:406.

122 Surgical Diseases of the Newborn: Retroperitoneal Tumors

NEUROBLASTOMA

I. **Definition.** Neuroblastoma is a primitive malignant neoplasm that arises from neural crest tissue. It is the most common congenital tumor and is usually located in the adrenal gland but can occur anywhere where there are neural crest cells. Estimates are about 1 per 8000–10,000 children in the United States.

II. **Clinical presentation.** This tumor typically presents as a firm, fixed, irregular mass extending obliquely from the costal margin, occasionally across the midline and into the lower abdomen.

III. **Diagnosis**

A. **Laboratory studies.** A 24-h urine collection should be analyzed for vanillylmandelic acid and other metabolites.

B. **Radiologic studies.** A plain abdominal radiograph may reveal calcification within the tumor. A computed tomography (CT) scan typically shows extrinsic compression and inferolateral displacement of the kidney. Search for possible metastatic deposits involves bone marrow aspiration and biopsy, bone scan, chest radiograph, and chest CT scan.

IV. **Management.** Treatment is based on stage. Complete surgical resection is still the best hope for cure unless the infant has type 4S disease, which is associated with spontaneous regression without resection. Planned therapy should take into account this well-recognized but poorly understood fact. Advanced tumors require multimodality therapy with surgery, radiation, and chemotherapy, but this is uncommon in neonates.

MESOBLASTIC NEPHROMA

I. **Definition.** Embryonic solid renal tissue that is not usually malignant.

II. **Clinical presentation.** Palpable mass or solid kidney mass seen on prenatal ultrasound.

III. **Diagnosis**

A. **Physical examination.** Mass present on examination in the newborn period, usually apparent in first few months of life if not felt in the nursery.

B. **Radiologic studies.** Ultrasonography if there is a solid mass in the neonate.

IV. **Management**

A. **Surgery.** Nephrectomy is the first step in treatment and includes lymph node sampling in the event of rare malignant degeneration of the mass.

WILMS TUMOR (NEPHROBLASTOMA)

I. **Definition.** Wilms tumor is an embryonal renal neoplasm in which blastemic, stromal, and epithelial cell types are present. Renal involvement is usually unilateral but may be bilateral (5% of cases).

II. **Clinical presentation.** A palpable abdominal mass extending from beneath the costal margin is the usual mode of presentation.

III. **Risk factors.** Aniridia, hemihypertrophy, certain genitourinary anomalies, and a family history of nephroblastoma.

IV. **Diagnosis**
   A. **Laboratory studies.** There is no tumor marker for Wilms tumor.
   B. **Radiologic studies.** Ultrasonography is generally followed by CT scan, which reveals intrinsic distortion of the caliceal system of the involved kidney. The possibility of tumor thrombus in the renal vein and inferior vena cava should be evaluated by ultrasonography and venography, if necessary.

V. **Management**
   A. **Unilateral renal involvement.** Nephrectomy is the first step in treatment. Surgical staging determines the administration of radiotherapy and chemotherapy; both are very effective.
   B. **Bilateral renal involvement.** Treatment of bilateral Wilms tumor is highly individualized.

TERATOMA

I. **Definition.** Teratoma is a neoplasm containing elements derived from all three germ cell layers: endoderm, mesoderm, and ectoderm. Teratomas in the neonate are primarily sacrococcygeal in location and believed to represent a type of abortive caudal twinning.

II. **Clinical presentation.** This tumor is usually grossly evident as a large external mass in the sacrococcygeal area. Occasionally, however, it may be presacral and retroperitoneal in location and may present as an abdominal mass.

III. **Diagnosis.** See Section II. Digital rectal examination of the presacral space is important.

IV. **Management.** Because the incidence of malignancy in these tumors increases with age, prompt surgical excision is required.

Selected References

DeMarco RT et al: Congenital neuroblastoma: a cystic retroperitoneal mass in a 34-week fetus. *J Urol* 2001;166(6):2375.

Grosfeld JL et al (eds): *Pediatric Surgery,* 6th ed. St. Louis, MO: Mosby-Year Book, 2006.

Maris JM et al: Neuroblastoma. *Lancet* 2007;369(9579):2106-2120.

O'Neill JA et al: *Principles of Pediatric Surgery,* 2nd ed. St. Louis, MO: Mosby, 2004.

123 Surgical Diseases of the Newborn: Urologic Disorders

UNDESCENDED TESTIS (CRYPTORCHIDISM)

I. **Definition.** Cryptorchidism, or undescended testis, is the positioning of one or both testes outside the scrotum.

II. **Clinical presentation.** Boys present with an empty scrotum, and testes may be nonpalpable or palpable in the prescrotal region, perineum (considered ectopic), or the inguinal region (near the external ring, in the superficial inguinal pouch or within the inguinal

canal). The ipsilateral scrotum may be hypoplastic, and a hernia or hydrocele may also
be present. Cryptorchidism may be associated with other anomalies such as disorders of
sexual development (DSD), especially in presence of hypospadias, Prune-belly syndrome,
bladder exstrophy, pituitary disorders, and multiple other syndromes.

III. **Diagnosis.** Careful examination in a warm room is required, although testes are rarely
retractile in the neonatal period. Note should be made of a palpable hernia.

    A. **Palpable testes.** Extrascrotal testes must be distinguished from other inguinal
swellings such as a hernia, hydrocele, or portion of epididymis.

    B. **Nonpalpable testes.** If a testis is nonpalpable, imaging studies are rarely indicated
initially, although ultrasound (US) may identify a small inguinal testis or a clinical
hernia. If both testes are nonpalpable, a karyotype should be performed to rule out
congenital adrenal hyperplasia, even if penile development is normal.

IV. **Management.** Observation is indicated until 6 months of age or later to assess for spontaneous descent. Surgery is indicated if a clinical hernia is present or a testis fails to descend.
For nonpalpable testes, laparoscopy is indicated to localize the testis or identify the characteristic blind-ending spermatic artery associated with an absent or "vanished" testis. If
both testes remain nonpalpable at 2–3 months of age, serum gonadotropins, testosterone,
and anti-Müllerian hormone should be obtained to confirm presence of testicular tissue
during the spontaneous hormonal surge of infancy.

SCROTAL AND TESTICULAR MASSES

I. **Definition.** Causes of an abnormal testicular examination or scrotal swelling in the newborn period include the following:

    A. **Hydrocele.** Fluid within the tunica vaginalis and/or along the spermatic cord.

    B. **Hernia (inguinal).** Protrusion of intra-abdominal content through a patent proces-
sus vaginalis along the spermatic cord.

    C. **Testicular torsion.** Twisting of the spermatic cord with reduction or cessation of tes-
ticular blood flow.

    D. **Testicular tumor (rare).**

II. **Clinical presentation.** Scrotal hydroceles are often noncommunicating. Both scrotal and
inguinal swelling may indicate a hernia or abdominoscrotal hydrocele. Scrotal discoloration and testicular induration without significant swelling is typical of perinatal testicular torsion. Boys are usually asymptomatic unless an incarcerated hernia is present,
which is associated with crankiness and vomiting.

III. **Diagnosis** is based on physical examination and scrotal transillumination. Ultrasound
can identify patency of the processus vaginalis, identify tumors, and assess for testicular
blood flow and calcification in cases of torsion. Yolk sac tumors may occur in infancy;
α-fetoprotein (AFP) is normally high until several months after birth and cannot be used
as a tumor marker in the newborn period.

IV. **Management.** Hernias and persistently communicating hydroceles should be repaired
when diagnosed and when nonfluctuating hydroceles are observed. Inguinal orchiec-
tomy is indicated for tumors. Perinatal torsion should be explored urgently and contralateral testicular fixation performed (***controversial***).

HYPOSPADIAS

I. **Definition.** Hypospadias is a failure of complete development of the anterior urethra.

II. **Clinical presentation.** The defect is usually identified at the time of neonatal examinations due to frequent presence of a dorsal hooded foreskin, ventral chordee, and/or penile
torsion. Milder forms may be discovered after a dorsal slit is performed for circumcision. Occasional patients present later in life with a urinary tract infection (UTI) or voiding difficulty.

III. **Diagnosis.** Severity is typically defined as glanular, coronal, subcoronal, distal shaft,
penile, penoscrotal, or perineal. About 10% of patients also have cryptorchidism, and up

to half of these may have disorders of sexual development. Karyotyping should be performed with proximal hypospadias and cryptorchidism, and additional endocrine testing and imaging (pelvic US, genitogram/voiding cystourethrogram) performed in selected cases. The risk of an enlarged utricle, which may complicate catheterization or present a source for UTI, is positively correlated with the severity of hypospadias.

IV. **Management.** Newborn circumcision should be avoided in any infant with abnormal penile development. Repair is not urgent because medical complications are rare. The defect is typically repaired in one stage at 6 months of age; more severe forms are likely to require more than one surgery due to the significantly higher risk of complications. Milder forms of distal glanular hypospadias not associated with significant chordee or meatal stenosis do not require repair.

EPISPADIAS

I. **Definition.** Epispadias is incomplete development of the dorsal urethra.

II. **Clinical presentation.** Epispadias presents at birth, usually in association with classical bladder exstrophy but also as an isolated anomaly. All but mild cases are typically associated with a partial ventral foreskin and dorsal chordee in males and bifid clitoris in females.

III. **Diagnosis.** Associated widening of the pubic symphysis on plain abdominal films (>1 cm) and a widened bladder neck are often present and associated with dribbling incontinence. Voiding cystourethrography is indicated to assess vesicourethral anatomy.

IV. **Management.** Surgical repair is performed in the first year of life and includes urethroplasty and correction of chordee. Anti-incontinence surgery is performed at or after the expected time of toilet training, but multiple procedures and persistent incontinence are not uncommon.

CLASSICAL BLADDER EXSTROPHY

I. **Definition.** Exstrophy of the bladder represents failure of closure of the bladder plate, dorsal urethra, and overlying structures.

II. **Clinical presentation.** The anomaly may be identified prenatally or at birth, and it occurs more commonly in males (3–6:1). The abdominal wall below the umbilical cord is open, and the bladder plate and urethra are visualized.

III. **Diagnosis.** Associated anomalies are rare but may occasionally include renal anomalies or obstruction. Vesicoureteral reflux is almost always present. Epispadias is present, the penis is broad and short, and there is dorsal chordee. In females, the clitoris is bifid and the mons is absent. The anus may be anteriorly placed, and inguinal hernias are frequently present.

IV. **Management.** A renal US is obtained after birth, and the bladder plate is protected with a thin plastic covering. Bladder closure is best performed in the first few days of life with or without pelvic osteotomies to facilitate ventral closure. Staged repair was used exclusively for many years, with epispadias repair and bladder neck reconstruction following months or years after initial bladder closure. More recently, single staged closure of the bladder and urethra has been recommended. Sequelae of initial closure that may require additional surgery include urinary incontinence, persistent vesicoureteral reflux, and urethral abnormalities (hypospadias, fistula, and chordee) related to the anomaly itself or to complications of closure.

CLOACAL EXSTROPHY

I. **Definition.** Failure of closure of the bladder plate, urethral plate, and ileocecal junction in combination with omphalocele and separation of the penis.

II. **Clinical presentation** is at birth or via prenatal US showing the abdominal wall defect, absent bladder filling and/or abnormal umbilical cord. At birth, the open bladder plate is noted inferiorly, the elongated terminal ileum on the left side and open cecum on the right, and the omphalocele superiorly.

III. **Diagnosis.** Associated anomalies are common and include renal anomalies of position or fusion, obstructive uropathy, Müllerian fusion anomalies, intestinal anomalies, hip or limb defects, and myelodysplasia. The genitalia are splayed and may appear ambiguous.

IV. **Management.** The open plate should be covered with light plastic wrap soon after birth for protection. Imaging should include renal and spinal US and skeletal imaging. Karyotyping should be performed if the sex of the infant is not clear. Reconstructive surgery is usually performed soon after birth, but the timing depends on the severity of gastrointestinal and neural anomalies. Osteotomies are often used to facilitate bladder closure. Genital reconstruction is performed as possible; gender reassignment, performed in the past, carries the risk of future discordant gender identity. Long-term issues are significant and common, and they include short gut syndrome, psychosocial issues, incontinence, neurologic issues related to myelodysplasia, and abnormal sexual function.

PRUNE BELLY (EAGLE-BARRETT OR TRIAD) SYNDROME

I. **Definition.** The triad consists of deficient abdominal musculature, bilateral cryptorchidism, and urinary tract anomalies (eg, dilated prostatic urethra, renal dysplasia, hydroureteronephrosis).

II. **Clinical presentation.** "Prune belly" refers to the classic appearance of abdominal wall wrinkling and budging flanks caused by varying degrees of abdominal wall deficiency. Ninety five percent of patients are male. Bilateral cryptorchidism is the rule and talipes equinovarus and hip dislocation are found. Marked oligohydramnios due to severe renal dysplasia or bladder outlet obstruction with pulmonary hypoplasia and skeletal anomalies (Potter sequence) may be present and may be incompatible with life in the most extreme forms.

III. **Diagnosis.** Clinical diagnosis is based on the classic triad.

IV. **Management.** Early UTI prophylaxis (amoxicillin or trimethoprim) and early circumcision to reduce the incidence of UTI should be considered. Urinary tract reconstruction (eg, ureteral reimplantation) is *controversial* due to the potential for improvement or resolution, stabilization of function, or need for eventual renal transplantation. Early intervention may be warranted with progressive/ severe hydronephrosis, progressive renal failure, or recurrent UTIs and may include temporary cutaneous vesicostomy or bilateral cutaneous pyelostomies. Abdominal wall reconstruction for cosmesis may help pulmonary and bladder function.

POSTERIOR URETHRAL VALVES

I. **Definition.** A posterior urethral valve (PUV) is a partial obstruction of the urethra by folds extending distal to the verumontanum of the prostate.

II. **Clinical presentation.** The presentation of PUV encompasses a wide spectrum, from bladder outlet obstruction without upper tract changes to severe obstructive uropathy with renal failure and pulmonary hypoplasia. The majority of cases of PUV present prenatally with bilateral hydroureteronephrosis, retention of bladder urine, and a vesicourethral keyhole sign and/or oligohydramnios. Cases diagnosed in the neonatal period may be associated with bladder distension, weak urinary stream, and UTI with possible sepsis.

III. **Diagnosis.** Voiding cystourethrogram (VCUG) is critical for diagnosis and classically shows bladder trabeculation with or without vesicoureteral reflux (VUR), bladder neck hypertrophy, a dilated posterior urethra, a typical valvular defect distal to the verumontanum, and distal urethral narrowing. Renal US and renogram are indicated to assess the status of the renal parenchyma, degree of hydronephrosis, and differential renal function.

IV. **Management.** Initial treatment consists of indwelling catheterization and serial chemistries to assess renal function. Nadir serum creatinine in the newborn period or first year of life of ≤0.8 suggests a better long-term prognosis. Primary valve ablation is the treatment of choice; in rare cases, upper tract diversion is performed but may not improve ultimate outcome. Antimicrobial prophylaxis is indicated initially and is continued in patients with VUR. Risk of renal failure is increased with complicating factors such as VUR and UTI.

HYDRONEPHROSIS (PRENATAL AND POSTNATAL)

I. **Definition.** Dilation of the fetal renal collecting system seen on maternal ultrasonography and confirmed on postnatal imaging is antenatal hydronephrosis. When limited to the renal pelvis alone, the more appropriate term is *pyelectasis* or *pelviectasis.*

II. **Clinical presentation** is at any stage of gestation, unilateral or bilateral, with or without bladder distension, oligohydramnios and/or renal duplication. The anterior-posterior renal pelvic diameter is the basic unit of measurement; a repeat US is typically performed if ≥5–7 mm.

III. **Diagnosis.** Persistent dilation is evaluated postnatally as indicated:
   A. **Renal/bladder US** is usually performed after the first few days of age to avoid false negatives unless bladder outlet obstruction is suspected. Significant caliceal dilation may indicate obstruction at the ureteropelvic junction (UPJ), ureterovesical junction (UVJ), or urethra (eg, posterior urethral valves). Severe ureterectasis may indicate ectopic ureter or ureterocele.
   B. **Voiding cystourethrography (VCUG)** is indicated in cases of significant or bilateral hydronephrosis, or ureterectasis. VUR is associated with 10–15% of mild to moderate pyelectasis cases; the need for screening remains **controversial**.
   C. **Radionuclide renal scans** are used selectively to assess function; cortical scans are used to assess primary nephropathy in cases of VUR, and diuretic renography can assess upper tract drainage with suspected obstructive uropathy.

IV. **Management.** The risk of postnatal complications is correlated to the severity of prenatal dilation.
   A. **Prophylactic antibiotics** are given prior to VCUG and are continued if VUR is present. The overall risk of VUR is 10–15%.
   B. **Serial US imaging** is used to document stabilization/improvement of mild-to-moderate dilation. Normal postnatal US precludes the need for additional studies.
   C. **Surgery** is indicated for PUV; UPJO with reduced renal function, abdominal mass, and/or UTI; and duplication anomalies with severe dilation.

Selected References

Baskin LS, Ebbers MB: Hypospadias: anatomy, etiology, and technique. *J Pediatr Surg* 2006;41:463-472.

Braga LH et al: Outcome analysis of isolated male epispadias: single center experience with 33 cases. *J Urol* 2008;179(3):1107-1112.

Cuervo JL et al: Perinatal testicular torsion: a unique strategy. *J Pediatr Surg* 2007;42:699-703.

Gearhart JP et al: Results of bladder neck reconstruction after newborn complete primary repair of exstrophy. *J Urol* 2007;178:1619-1622; discussion 1622.

Ghanem MA, Nijman RJ: Long-term followup of bilateral high (sober) urinary diversion in patients with posterior urethral valves and its effect on bladder function. *J Urol* 2005;173:1721-1724.

Ismaili K et al: Primary vesicoureteral reflux detected in neonates with a history of fetal renal pelvis dilatation: a prospective clinical and imaging study. *J Pediatr* 2006;148:222-227.

Lau ST et al: Current management of hernias and hydroceles. *Semin Pediatr Surg* 2007;16:50-57.

Lee RS et al: Antenatal hydronephrosis as a predictor of postnatal outcome: a meta-analysis. *Pediatrics* 2006;118:586-593.

Levy DA et al: Neonatal testis tumors: a review of the Prepubertal Testis Tumor Registry. *J Urol* 1994;151:715-717.

MacLellan DL, Diamond DA: Recent advances in external genitalia. *Pediatr Clin North Am* 2006;53:449-464, vii.

Mathews R, Gearhart JP: Modern staged reconstruction of bladder exstrophy—still the gold standard. *Urology* 2005;65:2-4.

McHoney M et al: Cloacal exstrophy: morbidity associated with abnormalities of the gastrointestinal tract and spine. *J Pediatr Surg* 2004;39:1209-1213.

Merlini L et al: Postnatal management of isolated mild pelvic dilatation detected in antenatal period. *Acta Paediatr* 2007;96:1131-1134.

Mieusset R, Soulie M: Hypospadias: psychosocial, sexual, and reproductive consequences in adult life. *J Androl* 2005;26:163-168.

Mitchell ME: Bladder exstrophy repair: complete primary repair of exstrophy. *Urology* 2005;65:5-8.

Natale R, Erhard M: *Prune Belly (Eagle-Barrett or Triad) Syndrome in 5 Minute Urology Consult.* In Gomella LG (ed). 2nd ed. Philadelphia, PA: Lippincott Williams & Wilkins, 2009 (in press)

Nijs SM et al: Nonpalpable testes: is there a relationship between ultrasonographic and operative findings? *Pediatr Radiol* 2007;37:374-379.

Perovic SV, Djinovic RP: New insight into surgical anatomy of epispadiac penis and its impact on repair. *J Urol* 2008;179:689-695; discussion 695-696.

Reiner WG, Gearhart JP: Discordant sexual identity in some genetic males with cloacal exstrophy assigned to female sex at birth. *N Engl J Med* 2004;350:333-341.

Ritzen EM et al: Nordic consensus on treatment of undescended testes. *Acta Paediatr* 2007;96:638-643.

Sarhan O et al: Long-term outcome of prenatally detected posterior urethral valves: single center study of 65 cases managed by primary valve ablation. *J Urol* 2008;179:307-312; discussion 312-313.

Schober JM et al: The ultimate challenge of cloacal exstrophy. *J Urol* 2002;167:300-304.

van Eerde AM et al: Vesico-ureteral reflux in children with prenatally detected hydronephrosis: a systematic review. *Ultrasound Obstet Gynecol* 2007;29:463-469.

Virtanen HE et al: Cryptorchidism: classification, prevalence and long-term consequences. *Acta Paediatr* 2007;96:611-616.

Wilcox D, Snodgrass W: Long-term outcome following hypospadias repair. *World J Urol* 2006;24:240-243.

Yerkes EB et al: Management of perinatal torsion: today, tomorrow or never? *J Urol* 2005;174:1579-1582; discussion 1582-1583.

Ylinen E et al: Prognostic factors of posterior urethral valves and the role of antenatal detection. *Pediatr Nephrol* 2004;19:874-879.

124 Syphilis

I. **Definition.** Syphilis is a sexually transmitted disease caused by *Treponema pallidum.* **Early congenital syphilis** (CS) is when clinical manifestations occur at <2 years of age; **late congenital syphilis** is when manifestations occur at >2 years of age. In 1990, a new surveillance case definition for congenital syphilis was adopted by the Centers for Disease Control and Prevention (CDC) to improve reporting of congenital syphilis by public health agencies. It calls for reporting all infants (and stillbirths) born to women with untreated or inadequately treated syphilis at delivery, regardless of neonatal symptoms or findings.

II. **Incidence.** The incidence of CS parallels that of primary and secondary syphilis in the general population. The most recent incidence in the United States is 8.8 cases per 100,000 live births. Worldwide, syphilis continues to represent a serious public health problem especially in developing countries. The World Health Organization estimates that a million pregnancies a year are adversely affected by maternal syphilis with 460,000 such pregnancies resulting in abortion or perinatal death and 270,000 infants born with CS.

III. **Pathophysiology.** Treponemes appear able to cross the placenta at any time during pregnancy, thereby infecting the fetus. Syphilis can cause preterm delivery, stillbirth (30–40% of fetuses with CS are stillborn), congenital infection, or neonatal death, depending on the stage of maternal infection and duration of fetal infection before delivery. Untreated infection in the first and second trimesters often leads to significant fetal morbidity, whereas with third-trimester infection many infants are asymptomatic. The most common cause of fetal death is placental infection associated with decreasing blood flow to the fetus, although direct fetal infection also plays a role. Infection can also be acquired by the neonate via contact with infectious lesions during passage through the birth canal. Kassowitz law states that the risk of vertical transmission of syphilis from an infected, untreated mother decreases as maternal disease progresses. Thus transmission ranges from 70–100% in primary syphilis, 40% for early latent syphilis to 10% for late latent disease. CS can cause placentomegaly and congenital hydrops.

IV. **Risk factors.** Infants whose mothers received no or inadequate treatment (dose was unknown, inadequate, or undocumented), the mother received a nonpenicillin treatment during pregnancy for syphilis, or the mother was treated within 28 days of the infant's birth. Infants of high-risk mothers (drug use, especially cocaine use, low socioeconomic levels, HIV infection, teen pregnancy, lack of prenatal care) are at increased risk for syphilis. Lack of prenatal care is the strongest predictor of CS.

V. **Clinical presentation.** CS is a multiorgan infection that may cause neurologic or skeletal disabilities or death in the fetus or newborn. However, when mothers with syphilis are treated early in pregnancy, the disease is almost entirely preventable. Spirochetes can cross the placenta and infect the fetus from ~14 weeks' gestation, with the risk of fetal infection increasing with advancing gestation. About two thirds of liveborn neonates with CS are asymptomatic at birth but have low birthweight. Clinical manifestations after birth are arbitrarily divided into early CS (<2 years of age) and late CS (>2 years old).

A. **Early manifestations** include nasal discharge (snuffles) and maculopapular or vesiculobullous rash that appears on the palms and soles. The rash may be associated with desquamation. Other early stigmata include abnormal bone radiographs, hepatosplenomegaly, petechiae, lymphadenopathy, jaundice, osteochondritis, pseudoparalysis, and central nervous system (CNS) abnormalities.

B. **Late manifestations** are characterized by chronic granulomatous inflammation. The sites most often involved include bones, teeth, and the nervous system. Hutchinson triad (blunted upper incisors, interstitial keratitis, and eighth nerve deafness) and saddle nose are distinct complications. A poor response to antibiotic treatment is often noted.

VI. **Diagnosis**

A. **Laboratory studies.** Patients with congenital or acquired syphilis produce several different antibodies, which are grouped as **nonspecific, nontreponemal antibody (NTA) tests,** and **specific antitreponemal antibody (STA) tests.** NTA tests (including Venereal Disease Research Laboratory [VDRL], rapid plasma reagin [RPR], and automated reagin test) are inexpensive, rapid, and convenient screening tests that may indicate disease activity. They test a patient's serum or cerebrospinal fluid (CSF) for its ability to flocculate a suspension of a cardiolipin-cholesterol lecithin antigen. They are used as initial screening tests and quantitatively to monitor a patient's response to treatment and to detect reinfection and relapse. False-positive reactions can be secondary to autoimmune disease, intravenous (IV) drug addiction, aging, pregnancy, and many infections, such as hepatitis, mononucleosis, measles, and endocarditis. The interpretation of NTA and STA tests can be confounded by maternal immunoglobulin G antibodies that are passed transplacentally to the fetus.

1. **Nonspecific reagin antibody tests.** The two most often used of these nonspecific screening tests are **VDRL** and **RPR.** A titer of at least two dilutions (fourfold) higher in the infant than in the mother signifies probable active infection. Titers should be monitored and repeated. If titers decrease in the first 8 months of life, the infant is probably not infected. VDRL (not RPR) should be used on CSF. A normal test result is negative, and any positive test should be followed up with a specific treponemal test. When NTA tests are used to monitor treatment response, the same specific test (eg, VDRL or RPR) must be used throughout the follow-up period, preferably by the same laboratory, to ensure comparability of results.

2. **Specific treponemal tests (STA)** verify a diagnosis of current or past infection. These tests should be performed if NTA test results are positive. These antibody tests do not correlate with disease activity and are not quantified. They are useful for diagnosing a first episode of syphilis and for distinguishing a false-positive result of NTA tests. However, they have limited use for evaluating response to therapy and possible reinfections. Once the STA test is positive, it will stay positive for life.

   a. **FTA-ABS (fluorescence treponemal antibody absorption) test.** This test may be positive in the infant secondary to maternal transfer of IgG, but if results remain positive after 6–12 months, the infant is most likely infected.

   b. **Microhemagglutination test for *T. pallidum*** uses less serum and is easier than FTA to perform.

   c. **IgM FTA-ABS.** This test measures antibody to the treponeme developed by the infant. It is not as specific as initially thought because false-positive results may occur. The test is not commercially available.

   d. **Newer diagnostic tests.** Direct antigen tests for *T. pallidum,* include enzyme-linked immunosorbent assay, which uses monoclonal antibody to the organism's surface proteins, and polymerase chain reaction (PCR), which detects the organism in CSF, amniotic fluid, and other specimens. These tests are being evaluated and could become commercially available.

3. **Microscopic dark-field examination** can be performed on appropriate lesions for spirochetes.

4. **Lumbar puncture.** CNS disease may be detected by positive serologic tests (VDRL or FTA-ABS), dark-field examination positive for spirochetes, elevated monocyte count, or elevated spinal fluid protein levels. VDRL is most commonly used, but some experts recommend the FTA-ABS test as well. FTA-ABS may be more sensitive but less specific than VDRL. PCRs on CSF may prove useful.

B. **Radiologic studies.** Radiographic abnormalities may be noted in 65% of the cases. These manifestations include periostitis, osteitis, and sclerotic metaphyseal changes. Infants may also present with pseudoparalysis or pathologic fractures.

VII. **Management.** Isolation precautions for all infectious diseases, including maternal and neonatal precautions, breast-feeding, and visiting issues, can be found in Appendix F.

A. **Infants with proven or highly probable disease** (abnormal physical examination consistent with congenital syphilis, a serum quantitative NTA titer that is fourfold higher than the mother's titer, or a positive dark-field or fluorescent antibody test of a body fluid). The recommended treatment according to the recent CDC guidelines is **Aqueous crystalline penicillin G** 100,000–150,000 units/kg/day, administered as 50,000 units/kg/dose IV every 12 h during the first 7 days of life and every 8 h thereafter for a total of 10 days *or* **procaine penicillin G,** 50,000 units/kg/dose intramuscularly (IM) in a single daily dose for 10 days. If >1 day of therapy is missed, the entire course should be restarted. Data are insufficient regarding the use of other antimicrobial agents (eg, ampicillin). When possible, a full 10-day course of penicillin is preferred, even if ampicillin was initially provided for possible sepsis. The use of agents other than penicillin requires close serologic follow-up to assess adequacy of therapy.

B. **Asymptomatic infants** who have normal physical examination and a serum quantitative NTA titer the same or less than fourfold the maternal titer should be managed according to the status of maternal treatment:

1. **Maternal treatment uncertain.** The mother was not treated, inadequately treated, or has no documentation of having received treatment; the mother was treated with erythromycin or other nonpenicillin regimen; or the mother received treatment <4 weeks before delivery. These infants should be fully evaluated and treated as described in Section VII, A. Alternatively, **benzathine penicillin G,** 50,000 units/kg as a single **IM** dose, is acceptable provided adequate follow up is ensured.

2. **Maternal treatment in pregnancy is adequate** (given >4 weeks before delivery and the mother has no evidence of infection or relapse). No evaluation is needed; however, a single **IM** dose of **benzathine penicillin G,** 50,000 units/kg, is recommended.

3. **Maternal treatment before pregnancy is adequate and mother's NTA titer remained low and stable during delivery and at delivery.** No evaluation or therapy is needed for the infant.

C. **Isolation procedures.** Precautions regarding drainage, secretions, and blood and body fluids are indicated for all infants with suspected or proven CS until therapy has been given for 24 h.

D. **Follow-up care.** The infant should have repeated quantitative NTA tests at 3, 6, and 12 months. Most infants have a negative titer with adequate treatment. A rising titer requires further investigation and retreatment.

VIII. **Prognosis.** Infants infected early in the pregnancy are usually stillborn. Infants infected through the birth canal have a better prognosis. Prognosis is excellent in early treated CS.

Selected References

American Academy of Pediatrics: Syphilis. In Pickering LK et al (eds): *Red Book: 2006 Report of the Committee on Infectious Diseases,* 27th ed. Elk Grove Village, IL: American Academy of Pediatrics, 2006:631-644.

Centers for Disease Control and Prevention; Workowski KA, Berman SM: Sexually transmitted diseases treatment guidelines, 2006. *MMWR Recomm Rep* 2006;4;55(RR-11):1-94.

Chakraborty R, Luck S: Managing congenital syphilis again? The more things change . . . *Curr Opin Infect Dis* 2007;20:247-252.

Doroshenko A et al: Syphilis in pregnancy and the neonatal period. *Int J STD AIDS* 2006;17:221-227.

Rasool MN, Govender S: The skeletal manifestations of congenital syphilis. A review of 197 cases. *J Bone Joint Surg Br* 1989;71:752-755.

Walker GJ, Walker DG: Congenital syphilis: a continuing but neglected problem. *Semin Fetal Neonatal Med* 2007;12:198-206.

Wicher V, Wicher K: Pathogenesis of maternal–fetal syphilis revisited. *Clin Infect Dis* 2001;33:354-363.

125 Thrombocytopenia and Platelet Dysfunction

I. **Definition.** Thrombocytopenia is defined as a platelet count <150,000/μL, although a few normal neonates may have counts as low as 100,000/μL in the absence of clinical disease. The best measure of platelet function is the standardized (Ivy) bleeding time (1.5–5.5 min). During the first week of life, bleeding times are shorter than those in adults (<3.5 min).

II. **Incidence. Thrombocytopenia is the most common hematologic abnormality among preterm infants.** In healthy term infants the incidence is ~1%. In neonatal intensive care unit (NICU) patients, the incidence is as high as 35%; in low birthweight preterm infants, it is 15–20%; and in extremely low birthweight infants, it is 73%. Approximately 25% of the cases are severe (<50,000/µL); 75% are considered mild to severe.

III. **Pathophysiology**

   A. **Normal platelets.** The rate of platelet production and turnover in neonates is similar to that of older children and adults. The platelet life span is 7–10 days, and the mean platelet count is >200,000/µL. Platelet counts are slightly lower in low birthweight infants, in whom platelet counts <100,000/µL have occasionally been observed in the absence of a clinical disorder. Low platelet counts should nonetheless be investigated in low birthweight infants. Platelet counts vary according to the method of determination. Phase microscopy determinations are generally 25,000–50,000/µL lower than those obtained by direct microscopy.

   B. **Etiology of thrombocytopenia**

   1. **Maternal disorders causing thrombocytopenia in infant:**

      a. Chronic intrauterine hypoxia. This is the most frequent cause of thrombocytopenia in preterm neonates in the first 72 h of life. This is seen in cases of placenta insufficiency such as diabetes and pregnancy induced hypertension.

      b. Drug use (eg, heparin, quinine, hydralazine, tolbutamide, and thiazide diuretics).

      c. Infections (eg, TORCH [*t*oxoplasmosis, *o*ther infections, *r*ubella, *c*ytomegalovirus, and *h*erpes simplex] infections, bacterial or viral infections).

      d. Disseminated intravascular coagulation (DIC).

      e. Pregnancy-induced hypertension (in particular with HELLP syndrome (*h*emolysis, *e*levated *l*iver enzymes, *l*ow *p*latelet count).

      f. Antiplatelet antibodies

         i. Antibodies against maternal and fetal platelets (autoimmune thrombocytopenia):

            (a) Idiopathic thrombocytopenic purpura (ITP).

            (b) Drug-induced thrombocytopenia.

            (c) Systemic lupus erythematosus.

            (d) Gestational or *incidental* thrombocytopenia.

         ii. Antibodies against fetal platelets (isoimmune thrombocytopenia):

            (a) Neonatal alloimmune thrombocytopenia (mostly anti-HPA-1a alloantibodies).

            (b) Isoimmune thrombocytopenia associated with erythroblastosis fetalis.

   2. **Placental disorders causing thrombocytopenia in infant (rare):**

      a. Chorioangioma.

      b. Vascular thrombi.

      c. Placental abruption.

   3. **Neonatal disorders causing thrombocytopenia:**

      a. Decreased platelet production or congenital absence of megakaryocytes.

         i. Isolated.

         ii. Thrombocytopenia and absent radius (TAR) syndrome.

         iii. Fanconi anemia.

         iv. Rubella syndrome.

         v. Congenital leukemia.

         vi. Trisomies 13, 18, 21 or Turner syndrome.

         vii. Inherited metabolic disorders (methylmalonic, propionic, and isovaleric acidemia, ketotic glycinemia).

         viii. Congenital amegakaryocytic thrombocytopenia.

      b. Increased platelet destruction

         i. Increased platelet consumption occurs in many sick infants not associated with any specific pathologic state. This form of thrombocytopenia is the most common hemostatic abnormality in the newborn admitted to the NICU. About 20% of newborns admitted to the NICU experience thrombocytopenia; for 20% of those, counts are <50,000/μL. This form of thrombocytopenia, generally present by 2 days of life, reaches a nadir by 4 days and usually recovers to normal by 10 days of life.

    ii. Pathologic states associated with increased platelet destruction.

      (a) Bacterial and *Candida* sepsis.

      (b) Congenital infections. TORCH infections especially CMV. Neonates with HIV and Enterovirus frequently have thrombocytopenia.

      (c) Thrombosis (renal vein, intracardiac, vascular).

      (d) DIC.

      (e) Intrauterine growth retardation.

      (f) Birth asphyxia.

      (g) Necrotizing enterocolitis (NEC).

      (h) Platelet destruction associated with giant hemangioma (Kasabach-Merritt syndrome).

C. Platelet dysfunction

  1. Drug-induced platelet dysfunction:

    a. Maternal use of aspirin.

    b. Indomethacin.

  2. Metabolic disorders:

    a. Phototherapy-induced metabolic abnormalities.

    b. Acidosis.

    c. Fatty acid deficiency.

    d. Maternal diabetes.

  3. Inherited thrombasthenia (Glanzmann disease).

IV. Risk factors. Low birthweight, lower gestational age, small for gestational age, growth restriction, hypoxia at birth, umbilical line placement, respiratory assistance, hyperbilirubinemia, phototherapy, prematurity, respiratory distress syndrome, low 5-min Apgar score (<7), sepsis especially by *Candida* infection, meconium aspiration, NEC, mother with ITP, preterm infants of hypertensive mothers. **Risk factors for preterm infants** includes growth restriction, lower gestational age at delivery, and low 5-min Apgar score(<7).

V. Clinical presentation

  A. Symptoms and signs. It is important to assess the general condition of the infant carefully. A "sick"-appearing newborn implies a very different approach for the investigation and treatment of thrombocytopenia (such as sepsis) than the infant who otherwise appears healthy (such as with most cases of alloimmune thrombocytopenia).

    1. Generalized superficial petechiae are often present, particularly in response to minor trauma or pressure or increased venous pressure. Platelet counts are usually <60,000/μL.

    2. Gastrointestinal bleeding, mucosal bleeding, or spontaneous hemorrhage in other sites may be occurring with platelet counts <20,000/μL.

    3. Intracranial hemorrhage may occur with severe thrombocytopenia.

    4. Large ecchymoses and muscle hemorrhages are more likely to be due to coagulation disturbances than to platelet disturbances.

    5. Petechiae in normal infants tend to be clustered on the head and upper chest, do not recur, and are associated with normal platelet counts. They are a result of a transient increase in venous pressure during birth.

  B. History

    1. There may be a family history of thrombocytopenia or history of intracranial hemorrhage in a sibling.

    2. Maternal drug ingestion may be a factor.

    3. A history of infection should be noted.

    4. Previous episodes of bleeding may have occurred.

  C. Placental examination. The placenta should be carefully examined for evidence of chorioangioma, thrombi, or abruptio placentae.

  D. Physical examination

    1. Petechiae and bleeding should be noted.

2. Physical malformations may be present in TAR syndrome, rubella syndrome, giant hemangioma, or trisomy syndromes.
3. Hepatosplenomegaly may be caused by viral or bacterial infection or congenital leukemia.

VI. **Diagnosis**
  A. **Laboratory studies**
    1. **Newborn studies**
      a. Neonatal platelet count: Thrombocytopenia diagnosed from a capillary sample should be confirmed by a repeated count from a sample obtained from a peripheral vein and by careful examination of a peripheral blood smear.
      b. Complete blood count.
      c. Blood typing.
      d. Coombs test.
      e. Coagulation studies: prothrombin time, activated partial thromboplastin time, fibrinogen, and d-dimer level.
      f. Other studies (if indicated).
        i. TORCH titers.
        ii. Bacterial cultures.
        iii. Bone marrow studies if decreased platelet production is present.
      g. **New studies.** Because of the difficulty of bone marrow studies in neonates, new blood tests are being developed to evaluate platelet production. Many have shown promising results (serum or plasma thrombopoietin (THPO, TPO) concentrations, megakaryocyte progenitors, reticulated platelet percentages (RP%) and glycocalicin concentrations). The immature platelet fraction (IPF) is already available and being used in some institutions. IPF values are increased in conditions associated with increased platelet destruction and decreased in conditions due to decreased platelet production.
    2. **Maternal studies**
      a. Test for maternal thrombocytopenia. A low maternal count suggests autoimmune thrombocytopenia or inherited thrombocytopenia (X-linked recessive thrombocytopenia or autosomal dominant thrombocytopenia).
      b. Maternal serum and whole blood sample for rapid HPA-1a (Pl^{A1}) phenotyping plus screen for anti-HPA-1a (Pl^{A1}) alloantibodies.
  B. **Decreased platelet production versus increased platelet destruction**
    1. **Decreased platelet production:**
      a. Platelet size is normal.
      b. Platelet survival time is normal.
      c. Megakaryocytes are decreased in a bone marrow sample.
      d. A sustained increase in the platelet count over a period of 4–7 days is seen after platelet transfusion.
    2. **Increased platelet destruction:**
      a. Platelet size is increased (>10.8 fL)
      b. Platelet survival time is decreased.
      c. Megakaryocytes in the bone marrow are normal or increased.
      d. There is little or no sustained increase in platelet count after platelet transfusion.

VII. **Management**
  A. **Obstetric management of maternal autoimmune thrombocytopenia**
    1. The occurrence of fetal hemorrhage (in utero) is very rare compared with the risk of such hemorrhage in alloimmune thrombocytopenia (10%).
    2. Treatment is aimed at prevention of an intracranial hemorrhage during vaginal delivery.
    3. There is an increased risk of severe neonatal thrombocytopenia and intracranial hemorrhage if antibody is present in the maternal plasma, if fetal scalp platelet counts are <50,000/μL.
    4. Cesarean delivery may be indicated.

B. **Management of maternal alloimmune thrombocytopenia**
   1. After a pregnancy has been affected by alloimmune thrombocytopenia, the proportion of subsequent pregnancies affected mostly depends on the father's genotype. If the father is heterozygous (HPA-1a/HPA-1b), the risk is 50% and close to 100% if homozygous (HPA-1a/HPA-1a). The history of intracranial hemorrhage in a previous sibling is predictive of the presence severe thrombocytopenia for the next fetus. In subsequent pregnancies, administering corticosteroids and intravenous immune globulin (IVIG) during the third trimester coupled with transfusions of platelets to the fetus using ultrasound-guided intraumbilical cord infusion has been described.
   2. Vaginal delivery is allowed when fetal platelet count is known to be >50,000/µL and presentation and labor is normal. Otherwise cesarean delivery is indicated.
C. **Treatment of infants with thrombocytopenia**
   1. Treat the underlying cause (eg, sepsis). If drugs are the cause, stop administration.
   2. Platelet transfusions are indicated if active bleeding is occurring with any degree of thrombocytopenia or if there is no active bleeding but platelet counts are <20,000/µL. It may be desirable to transfuse "sick" premature infants if the platelet count is <50,000/µL. Random donor platelets are given in a dosage of 10–20 mL/kg of standard platelet concentrates. The plasma in platelets should be ABO and Rh compatible with the infant's red blood cells. The platelet count should increase to >100,000/µL. Platelet count should be repeated 1 h posttransfusion. Failure to achieve or sustain a rise in platelet count suggests a destructive process. Washed maternal platelets or platelets from a HPA-compatible donor (in general HPA-1a negative platelets) may need to be used for infants with alloimmune thrombocytopenia. When not available a random donor platelet transfusion combined with IVIG may achieve a transient rise.
   3. IVIG, 400 mg/kg/day for 3–5 consecutive days, or a single dose of 1000 mg/kg on 2 consecutive days is given for immune thrombocytopenia.
   4. Prednisone, 2 mg/kg/day, may also be beneficial in immune thrombocytopenia.
VIII. **Prognosis.** Etiology of the thrombocytopenia dictates the outcome and prognosis.

Selected References

Chakravorthy S et al: Neonatal thrombocytopenia. *Early Hum Dev* 2005;81:35.

Murray NA: Evaluation and treatment of thrombocytopenia in the neonatal intensive care. *Acta Paediatr Suppl* 2002;438:74.

Sola M et al: Developmental aspects of platelets and disorders of platelets in the neonatal period. In Christensen RD (ed): *Hematologic Problems of the Neonate*. Philadelphia, PA: Saunders, 2000:273.

Sola-Visner M et al: New insights into the mechanisms of nonimmune thrombocytopenia in neonates. *Semin Perinatol* 2009;33(1):43-51.

126 Thyroid Disorders

Disorders of thyroid function in neonates often present a diagnostic dilemma. The initial signs and symptoms are often subtle or misleading. A good understanding of the unique thyroid physiology and the assessment of thyroid function is necessary to recognize, diagnose, and treat thyroid disorders.

GENERAL CONSIDERATIONS

I. **Fetal and neonatal thyroid function**

    A. **Embryogenesis** begins in the third week of gestation with thyroglobulin synthesis and continues through 10–12 weeks' gestation. At that time, thyroid-stimulating hormone (TSH) can be detected. Thyroid activity remains low until midgestation and then increases slowly until term.

    B. **Thyroid hormones** undergo rapid and dramatic changes in the immediate postnatal period.

        1. **An acute release of TSH occurs within minutes after birth.** Peak values of 80 mU/L are seen at 30–90 min. Levels decrease to <10 mU/L by the end of the first postnatal week.

        2. **Stimulated by the TSH surge,** thyroxine (T_4), free T_4 (FT_4), and triiodothyronine (T_3) rapidly increase, reaching peak levels by 24 h. Levels decrease slowly over the first few weeks of life.

    C. **Thyroid function in the premature infant.** Identical changes in TSH, T_4, and T_3 are seen in premature infants; however, absolute values are lower. TSH levels return to normal by 3–5 days of life regardless of gestational age.

II. **Physiologic action of thyroid hormones.** Thyroid hormones have profound effects on growth and neurologic development. They also influence oxygen consumption, thermogenesis, and the metabolic rate of many processes. Maternal T_4 is critical for normal central nervous system maturation in the fetus.

III. **Biochemical steps to thyroid hormone synthesis.** Thyroid hormone production includes the stages of iodide transport, thyroglobulin synthesis, organization of iodide, monoiodotyrosine and diiodotyrosine coupling, thyroglobulin endocytosis, proteolysis, and deiodination.

IV. **Assessment of thyroid function.** Thyroid tests are intended to measure the level of thyroid activity and to identify the cause of thyroid dysfunction.

    A. **T_4 concentration** is an important parameter in the evaluation of thyroid function. More than 99% of T_4 is bound to thyroid hormone–binding proteins. Therefore, changes in these proteins may affect T_4 levels. Serum levels for term newborn infants range between 6.4 and 23.2 mcg/dL.

    B. **Free T_4** reflects the availability of thyroid hormone to the tissues. Serum levels vary widely by gestational age: newborn term infants (2.0–5.3 ng/dL) and infants of 25–30 weeks' gestation (0.6–3.3 ng/dL).

    C. **TSH measurement** is a valuable test in evaluating thyroid disorders, particularly for primary hyperthyroidism. Serum levels over all gestational ages of 25–42 weeks range from 2.5–18.0 mU/L.

    D. **T_3 concentration** is useful in the diagnosis and treatment of hyperthyroidism. Serum levels of T_3 are very low in the fetus and cord blood samples (20–75 ng/dL). Shortly after birth, levels exceed 100 ng/dL to ~400 ng/dL. In hyperthyroid states, levels may exceed 400 ng/dL. In sick preterm infants, a very low T_3 (hypothyroid range) may signal the euthyroid sick syndrome, also known as the nonthyroidal illness syndrome.

    E. **Thyroid-binding globulin (TBG)** can be measured directly by radioimmunoassay. T_3 resin uptake provides an indirect measurement of TBG and is now considered an outdated test, unless it is factored with the T_4 level to give an FT_4 index, using the infant's T_4 level and T_3 uptake against a normal control T_3 uptake.

    F. **The thyrotropin-releasing hormone (TRH) stimulation test** can assess pituitary and thyroid responsiveness. It is used to differentiate between secondary and tertiary hypothyroidism.

    G. **Thyroid imaging**

        1. **Thyroid scanning** with ^{123}I (preferred isotope) is performed to identify functional thyroid tissue.

        2. **Color doppler ultrasonography** has shown improved sensitivity in detecting ectopic thyroid tissue in recent studies.

CONGENITAL HYPOTHYROIDISM

   I. **Definition.** Congenital hypothyroidism is defined as a significant decrease in, or the absence of, thyroid function present at birth.

  II. **Incidence.** The overall incidence is 1 in 3500 to 1 in 4500 births. Sporadic cases account for 85% of patients diagnosed; 15% are hereditary. It is more prevalent among females than males by a ratio of 2:1. It is more common in Hispanic and Asian infants (1 in 3000 births) and less common in blacks (1 in 32,000 births). The incidence is significantly increased in Down syndrome (1 in 140).

 III. **Pathophysiology**

    A. **Primary hypothyroidism**

      1. Developmental defects such as ectopic thyroid (most common), thyroid hypoplasia, or agenesis.

      2. Inborn errors of thyroid hormone synthesis.

      3. Maternal exposure to radioiodine, propylthiouracil, or methimazole during pregnancy.

      4. Iodine deficiency (endemic cretinism).

    B. **Secondary hypothyroidism:** TSH deficiency.

    C. **Tertiary hypothyroidism:** TRH deficiency.

    D. **Hypopituitary hypothyroidism:** associated with other hormonal deficiencies.

 IV. **Risk factors.** Genetic/family history, birth defects, female gender, and gestational age >40 weeks.

  V. **Clinical presentation.** Symptoms are usually absent at birth; however, subtle signs may be detected during the first few weeks of life.

    A. **Early manifestations.** Signs at birth include prolonged gestation, large size for gestational age, large fontanelles, and respiratory distress syndrome. Manifestations that may be seen by 2 weeks include hypotonia, lethargy, hypothermia, prolonged jaundice, and feeding difficulty.

    B. **Late manifestation.** Classic features usually appear after 6 weeks and include puffy eyelids, coarse hair, large tongue, myxedema, and hoarse cry. Late manifestations in borderline hypothyroidism detected in screening programs can present as significant hearing impairment with speech delays.

 VI. **Diagnosis**

    A. **Screening.** Newborn screening for congenital hypothyroidism in addition to the profound clinical benefit is cost effective.

      1. **Method.** The screening strategies include primary TSH, backup T_4 (may miss TBG deficiency, hypothalamic-pituitary hypothyroidism, and hypothyroxinemia with delayed TSH elevation), primary T_4, backup TSH (will miss delayed TSH elevation with initial normal T_4), and primary T_4 and TSH (ideal screening approach).

      2. **Timing.** The ideal time for screening is by 48 h to 4 days of age. Infants discharged before 48 h should be screened before discharge; however, this increases the number of false-positive TSH elevations. A repeat test at 2 to 6 weeks identifies ~10% of cases.

      3 **Results.** Accurate screening results depend on good quality of blood spots. A low T_4 level and TSH concentrations >40 mU/L are indicative of congenital hypothyroidism. **The update of newborn screening and therapy for congenital hypothyroidism (June 2006) by the American Academy of Pediatrics, American Thyroid Association, and Lawson Wilkins Pediatric Endocrine society provides a useful algorithm and is recommended reading.**

    B. **Diagnostic studies**

      1. **Serum** for confirmatory measurements of T_4 and TSH concentrations should be tested. If an abnormality of TBG is suspected, FT_4 and TBG concentrations should also be evaluated.

      2. **Thyroid scan** remains the most accurate diagnostic modality to determine the cause of congenital hypothyroidism.

VII. **Management**
   A. **Consultation** with a pediatric endocrinologist is recommended.
   B. **Treatment.** Levothyroxine (LT_4) is the treatment of choice. The average starting dose is 10–15 mcg/kg/day. The pill should be crushed and suspended in breast-milk, formula, or water. Care should be taken to avoid concomitant administration of soy, fiber, or iron. The goal of therapy is to maintain T_4 concentration in the upper normal range (10–16 mcg/dL), FT_4 (1.4–2.3 ng/dL), and low-normal serum TSH (0.5–2 mU/L) during the first 3 years of life.
   C. **Follow-up.** Frequent clinical evaluations of thyroid function, growth, and development and laboratory measurements of T_4 and TSH are required to ensure optimal treatment. Recommended follow-up is as follows:
      1. **2 and 4 weeks** after initiation of therapy.
      2. **Every 1–2 months** during the 6 months.
      3. **Every 3–4 months** between 6 months and 3 years.
      4. **Follow-up at more frequent intervals is recommended** with dose change, abnormal values, and with compliance concerns.
VIII. **Prognosis.** Prognosis depends on prudent initiation of therapy and subsequent management in an effort to mitigate the deficits in neurocognitive areas. Best outcome is for treatment started by 2 weeks at a dose of 9.5 mcg/kg of LT_4, or more, per day.

NEONATAL THYROTOXICOSIS

I. **Definition.** Neonatal thyrotoxicosis is defined as a hypermetabolic state resulting from excessive thyroid hormone activity in the newborn.
II. **Incidence.** This is a rare disorder occurring in only ~1 of 70 thyrotoxic pregnancies (autoimmune disease). The incidence of maternal thyrotoxicosis in pregnancy is 1–2 per 1000 pregnancies.
III. **Pathophysiology**
   A. This disorder usually results from transplacental passage of thyroid-stimulating immunoglobulin from a mother with Graves disease or Hashimoto thyroiditis.
   B. Congenital nonautoimmune hyperthyroidism has been identified as a result of activating mutations in the TSH receptor, stimulatory G protein, and the McCune-Albright syndrome.
IV. **Risk factors.** Mother with active or inactive Graves disease or Hashimoto thyroiditis.
V. **Clinical presentation.** Fetal tachycardia in the third trimester may be the first manifestation. Signs are usually apparent within hours after birth through the first 10 days of life. Delayed presentation up to 45 days may occur if there are coexisting maternal blocking and stimulating antibodies. Thyrotoxic signs include irritability, tachycardia, hypertension, flushing, tremor, poor weight gain, thrombocytopenia, hepatomegaly, and arrhythmias. A goiter is usually present and may be large enough to cause tracheal compression. Eye signs such as lid retraction and exophthalmos, as well as craniosynostosis, may also be present.
VI. **Diagnosis**
   A. **History and physical examination.** A maternal past history of thyrotoxicosis and the presence of maternal thyroid-stimulating antibodies in the last trimester correlate well with the development of neonatal thyrotoxicosis. The features on physical examination are discussed in Section V.
   B. **Laboratory studies.** Diagnosis is confirmed by demonstrating increased levels of T_4, FT_4, and T_3 with suppressed levels of TSH.
VII. **Management.** Although the disorder is usually self-limited, therapy depends on the severity of the symptoms and is a life threatening emergency in its most severe form.
   A. **Mild.** Close observation is required. Therapy is not necessary.
   B. **Moderate.** Administer one of the following antithyroid medications:
      1. **Lugol solution (8.3 mg iodide/drop),** 1 drop every 8 h.
      2. **Propylthiouracil,** 5–10 mg/kg/day in three divided doses.
      3. **Methimazole,** 0.5–1 mg/kg/day in three divided doses.

C. **Severe.** In addition to the medications just listed, during extreme conditions, prednisone, 2 mg/kg/day; propranolol, 1–2 mg/kg/day in two to four divided doses; and digitalis (in preventing cardiovascular collapse) may be used.

D. **Nonautoimmune hyperthyroidism** requires thyroid gland ablation or near-total thyroidectomy.

VIII. **Prognosis.** The disorder is usually self-limited and disappears spontaneously within 2–4 months. Mortality in affected infants is ~15% if the disorder is not recognized and treated properly.

EUTHYROID SICK SYNDROME

I. **Definition.** Transient alteration in thyroid function associated with a severe nonthyroidal illness.

II. **Incidence.** The syndrome is frequently seen in premature infants because of their increased susceptibility to neonatal morbidity. Preterm infants with respiratory distress syndrome have been the most frequently reported patients with this disorder.

III. **Diagnosis.** A low T_3 level is usually present, associated with low or normal T_4 and normal TSH. Infants are euthyroid (normal TSH).

IV. **Treatment.** Treatment has not been shown to be beneficial. Abnormal thyroid functions return to normal as the sick infant improves.

TRANSIENT HYPOTHYROXINEMIA OF PREMATURITY

I. **Definition.** Decreased thyroid levels without elevated TSH, but not as low as congenital hypothyroidism.

II. **Incidence.** All preterm infants have some degree of hypothyroxinemia (>50% have T_4 levels <6.5 mcg/dL).

III. **Pathophysiology.** The condition is presumed to be related to immaturity of the hypothalamic-pituitary axis that cannot compensate for the loss of maternal thyroid hormone.

IV. **Diagnosis** is low T_4 and FT_4 with normal TSH and normal response to the TRH stimulation test.

V. **Treatment.** Attempts to supplement preterm infants born before 30 weeks' gestation with thyroxine to improve neurologic outcome have been unsuccessful. There is some suggestion that treatment effect is variable at different gestational ages.

Selected References

Adams LM et al: Reference ranges for newer thyroid function tests in premature infants. *J Pediatr* 1995;126:122-127.

American Academy of Pediatrics; Rose SR; Section on Endocrinology and Committee on Genetics, American Thyroid Association, et al: Update of newborn screening and therapy for congenital hypothyroidism. *Pediatrics* 2006;117:2290-2303.

Biswas S et al: A longitudinal assessment of thyroid hormone concentrations in preterm infants younger than 30 weeks' gestation during the first 2 weeks of life and their relationship to outcome. *Pediatrics* 2002;109:222-227.

Djemli A et al: Congenital hypothyroidism: from Paracelsus to molecular diagnosis. *Clin Biochem* 2006;39:511-518.

Fisher DA: Thyroid function and dysfunction in premature infants. *Pediatr Endocrinol Rev* 2007;4:317-328.

Forghani N, Aye T: Hypothyroxinemia and prematurity. *NeoReviews* 2008;9:e66-e71.

Hunter MK et al: Follow-up of newborns with low thyroxine and non-elevated thyroid-stimulating hormone-screening concentrations: results of the 20-year experience in the Northwest Regional Newborn Screening Program. *J Pediatr* 1998;132:70-74.

Knobel RB: Thyroid hormone levels in term and preterm neonates. *Neonatal Netw* 2007;26:253-259.

LaFranchi S: Congenital hypothyroidism: etiologies, diagnosis, and management. *Thyroid* 1999;9:735-740.

Osborn DA, Hunt RW: Postnatal thyroid hormones for preterm infants with transient hypothyroxinemia. *Cochrane Database Syst Rev* 2007;1:CD005945.

Peters CJ, Hindmarsh PC: Management of neonatal endocrinopathies—best practice guidelines. *Early Hum Dev* 2007;83:553-561.

Polk DH, Fisher DA: Fetal and neonatal thyroid physiology. In Polin RA et al (eds): *Fetal and Neonatal Physiology*, 3rd ed. Philadelphia, PA: Saunders, 2004:1926-1933.

Skuza KA et al: Prediction of neonatal hyperthyroidism in infants born to mothers with Graves disease. *J Pediatr* 1996;128:264-268.

Van Wassenaer AG et al: Thyroid function in very preterm newborns: possible implications. *Thyroid* 1999;9:85-91.

Williams FL et al: Developmental trends in cord and postpartum serum thyroid hormones in preterm infants. *J Clin Endocrinol Metab* 2004;89:5314-5320.

Zimmerman D: Fetal and neonatal hyperthyroidism. *Thyroid* 1999;9:727-733.

127 TORCH Infections (Toxoplasmosis, Rubella, Cytomegalovirus, and Herpes Simplex Virus)

TORCH is an acronym that denotes a chronic nonbacterial perinatal infection. It stands for *t*oxoplasmosis; *o*ther infections; *r*ubella virus; *c*ytomegalovirus (CMV); and *h*erpes simplex virus (HSV). "Other" infections include syphilis, hepatitis B, coxsackievirus, Epstein-Barr, varicella-zoster virus (VZV), and human parvovirus B-19. Herpetic disease in the neonate does not fit the pattern of chronic intrauterine infection but is traditionally grouped with the others. This group of infections may present in the neonate with similar clinical and laboratory findings (ie, small for gestational age, hepatosplenomegaly, rash, central nervous system [CNS] manifestations, early jaundice, and low platelets), hence the usefulness of the TORCH concept. Isolation precautions for all infectious diseases, including maternal and neonatal precautions, breast-feeding, and visiting issues, can be found in Appendix F.

TOXOPLASMOSIS

I. **Definition.** Toxoplasmosis is caused by *Toxoplasma gondii,* an intracellular parasitic protozoan capable of causing intrauterine infection.

II. **Incidence.** The incidence of congenital infection is 1–10 per 10,000 live births. An estimated number of 400–4000 cases of congenital toxoplasmosis occur each year in the United States. Serologic surveys demonstrate that worldwide exposure to *T. gondii* is high (30% in the United States and 50–80% in Europe).

III. **Pathophysiology.** *T. gondii* is a coccidian parasite ubiquitous in nature. The primary natural host is the cat family. The organism exists in three forms: **oocyst, tachyzoite,** and **tissue cyst** (bradyzoites). Cats generally acquire the infection by feeding on infected animals such as mice or uncooked household meats. The parasite replicates sexually in the feline intestine. Cats may begin to excrete **oocysts** in their stool for 7–14 days after infection. After excretion, oocysts require a maturation phase (sporulation) of 24–48 h before they become infective by oral route. Intermediate hosts (sheep, cattle, and pigs) can have tissue cysts within organs and skeletal muscle. These cysts can remain viable for the lifetime of the host. The pregnant woman usually becomes infected by consumption of raw or undercooked meat that contains cysts or by the accidental ingestion of sporulated oocysts from soil or contaminated food. Ingestion of oocysts and cysts is followed by penetration of gastrointestinal mucosa by sporozoites and circulation of **tachyzoites**, the ovoid unicellular organism characteristic of acute infections. There are reports of transmission of toxoplasmosis through contaminated municipal water, blood transfusion, organ donation, and occasionally as a result of a laboratory accident. Actual transmission to the fetus is by the transplacental-fetal hematogenous route. In the chronic form of the disease, organisms invade certain body tissues, especially those of the brain, eye, and striated muscle, forming bradyzoites.

Acute infection in the adult is often subclinical (90% of the cases). If symptoms are present, they are generally nonspecific: mononucleosis-like illness with fever, painless lymphadenopathy, fatigue, malaise, myalgia, fever, skin rash, and splenomegaly. The vast majority of congenital toxoplasmosis cases are a result of acquired maternal primary infection during pregnancy; however, toxoplasmic reactivations can occur in immunosuppressed pregnant women and result in fetal infection. About 84% of women of childbearing age in the United States are seronegative and thereby are at risk to acquire *T. gondii* infection during gestation. Placental infection occurs and persists throughout pregnancy. The infection may or may not be transmitted to the fetus. The later in pregnancy that infection is acquired, the more likely is transmission to the fetus (first trimester, 17%; second trimester, 25%; and third trimester, 65% transmission). Infections transmitted earlier in gestation are likely to cause more severe fetal effects (abortion, stillbirth, or severe disease with teratogenesis). Those transmitted later are more likely to be subclinical. Rarely, the parasite may be transmitted via an infected placenta during parturition. Infection in the fetus or neonate usually involves the CNS or the eyes with or without disseminated systemic infection. Approximately 70–90% of infants with congenital infection are asymptomatic at birth; however, visual impairment, learning disabilities, or mental impairment becomes apparent in a large percentage of children months to several years later.

IV. **Risk factors.** Several epidemiologic studies have identified some risk factors for acquiring toxoplasmosis during pregnancy. These risk factors include eating or contact with raw or undercooked meat, cleaning the cat litter box, eating unwashed raw vegetables or fruits, exposure to soil, and travel outside the United States, Europe, or Canada. Interestingly, cat ownership by itself is not linked to toxoplasmosis. Premature infants have a higher incidence of congenital toxoplasmosis than term infants (25–50% of cases in most series).

V. **Clinical presentation.** Congenital toxoplasmosis may be manifested as clinical neonatal disease, disease in the first few months of life, late sequelae or relapsed infection, or subclinical disease. Subclinical disease occurs in the majority of cases.

A. **Clinical disease.** Those with evident clinical disease may have disseminated illness or isolated CNS or ocular disease. Late sequelae are primarily related to ocular or CNS disease. **Obstructive hydrocephalus, chorioretinitis, and diffuse intracranial calcifications** form the **classic triad** of toxoplasmosis. New eye lesions can develop many years after birth.

B. **Prominent signs and symptoms** in infants with congenital toxoplasmosis include chorioretinitis, abnormalities of CSF (high protein content), anemia, seizures, intracranial calcifications, direct hyperbilirubinemia, fever, hepatosplenomegaly, lymphadenopathy, vomiting, microcephaly or hydrocephalus, diarrhea, cataracts, eosinophilia, bleeding diathesis, hypothermia, glaucoma, optic atrophy, microphthalmos, rash, and pneumonitis.

C. **Associated findings.** Toxoplasmosis is associated with congenital nephrosis, various endocrinopathies (secondary to hypothalamic or pituitary effects), myocarditis, erythroblastosis with hydrops fetalis, and isolated mental retardation.

VI. **Diagnosis**

A. **Laboratory studies.** The maternal diagnosis of toxoplasmosis during pregnancy is primarily made by the use of serologic tests. Presence or absence of symptoms or a detailed epidemiologic history suggesting exposures to *T. gondii* are not useful tools to decide whether laboratory testing should be performed. The diagnosis of congenital toxoplasmosis in the newborn is most often based on clinical suspicion plus serologic tests; however, most cases of neonatal disease are asymptomatic and, therefore, without a screening test, will be missed. Many hospital-based and commercial laboratories' serologic tests are inaccurate and frequently misinterpreted. Therefore, establishing the diagnosis of congenital toxoplasmosis can be challenging. This is particularly true of the indirect fluorescence test for immunoglobulin IgG and IgM antibodies and of enzyme-linked immunosorbent assay (ELISA) systems for quantitation of IgM specific antibodies. In 1997, a Food and Drug Administration warning was issued about the misinterpretation of IgM serologies. The recommendation is that all IgM-positive results be confirmed by a toxoplasma reference laboratory like the one present at the Palo Alto Medical Foundation (PAMF-TSL; http://www.pamf.org/serology).

1. **Direct isolation of the organism from body fluids or tissues** requires inoculating blood, body fluids, or placental tissue into mice or tissue culture and is not readily available. Isolation of the organism from placental tissue correlates strongly with fetal infection.

2. **Serologic tests** with toxoplasma-specific IgG and IgM are usually done through commercial laboratories. IgG achieves a peak concentration 1–2 months after infection and remains positive indefinitely. IgM usually becomes positive within 1–2 weeks of infection and persists for months or years, especially when very sensitive assays are used. Negative results in IgG and IgM tests essentially indicate that the patient has not been exposed. If IgG is positive and IgM is negative, it usually indicates past exposure without current active infection. Rarely, IgM titers can normalize if the infection happened early in the first trimester and the test was not done until late in the third trimester of pregnancy. If IgM is positive, it may indicate acute infection, especially if titers are high. However, positive IgM results need confirmation with multiple markers (IgM, IgA, and IgE) through a reference laboratory. A toxoplasma serologic profile (TSP), which consists of the dye test, IgM ELISA, IgA ELISA, IgE ELISA, and AC/HS (differential agglutination) test is commonly used. The TSP has been successfully used at the PAMF-TSL to establish whether a pregnant woman has been infected with the parasite. Researchers at PAMF-TSL have shown the ability to decrease the rate of unnecessary abortions by approximately 50% among women with initial positive IgM done by outside laboratories. Sometimes, when IgM results are equivocal, more specialized testing like the IgG avidity test are used to help discriminate between past and recently acquired infection.

3. **Perinatal diagnosis** can be made by using polymerase chain reaction (PCR) amplification of *T. gondii* DNA in a sample of amniotic fluid. Cordocentesis has been largely abandoned because of its inherently higher risk for fetal injury and lower yield for the diagnosis of congenital infection when compared with amniocentesis for PCR examination. Because IgM and IgA antibodies do not cross the placenta, they form the basis of serodiagnosis of congenital infection in the live newborn. Toxoplasma-specific IgM and IgA should be done in a reference laboratory as discussed earlier. Toxoplasma DNA PCR can be done on body fluids (peripheral blood, urine, and CSF) obtained from suspected infants.

4. **CSF examination** should be performed in suspected cases. The most characteristic abnormalities are xanthochromia, mononuclear pleocytosis, and a very high protein level. Tests for PCR and CSF IgM to toxoplasmosis may also be performed.

B. **Radiologic studies**

1. **A cranial ultrasonogram or computed tomography (CT) scan of the head** may demonstrate characteristic diffuse intracranial calcifications (speckled throughout the CNS, including the meninges).

2. **Long-bone films** may show abnormalities, specifically metaphyseal lucency and irregularity of the line of calcification at the epiphyseal plates without periosteal reaction.

C. **Other studies. Ophthalmologic examination** characteristically shows chorioretinitis.
VII. **Management. Congenital toxoplasmosis** is a treatable infection, although at present it is not curable. Therapeutic agents are effective in killing the tachyzoite phase of the parasite but are not capable of eradicating encysted bradyzoites. Treatment of acute maternal toxoplasmosis appears to reduce the risk of fetal wastage and decreases the likelihood of congenital infection. However, the efficacy of maternal treatment to prevent congenital toxoplasmosis has been questioned. A recent meta-analysis found weak evidence for an association between early treatment and reduced risk of congenital toxoplasmosis.
   A. **Treatment** of symptomatic infants is indicated and consists of **sulfadiazine** (50 mg/kg, twice daily), **pyrimethamine** (2 mg/kg/day for 2 days, then 1 mg/kg/day for 2–6 months, then 1 mg/kg/day three times a week), and **folinic acid** (10 mg, three times weekly) for a minimum of 12 months. Serial follow-up to gauge the response of the infant to therapy should include neuroradiology, ophthalmologic examinations, and CSF analysis if indicated. A follow-up study of a cohort of 120 children with severe congenital *T. gondii* infection found an improved outcome in children receiving 1 year of treatment with sulfadiazine and pyrimethamine compared with historical controls. Corticosteroids are somewhat *controversial;* prednisone (1 mg/kg/day, in two divided doses) has been used when CSF protein is >1g/dL and when active chorioretinitis threatens vision. Prednisone is continued until resolution of CSF protein elevation and active chorioretinitis. Infants treated with pyrimethamine and sulfadiazine require weekly blood counts (including platelets), and urine microscopy to detect any adverse drug effects. The treatment of asymptomatic infants identified through newborn screening is controversial because proper randomized, controlled trials are lacking.
   B. **Prevention.** Primary prevention should be done through education. Pregnant women should be counseled that toxoplasma infection can be prevented in large part by cooking meat to a safe temperature (ie, one sufficient to kill toxoplasma); peeling or thoroughly washing fruits and vegetables before eating; cleaning cooking surfaces and utensils after they have contacted raw meat, poultry, seafood, or unwashed fruits or vegetables; avoiding changing cat litter or, if necessary, using gloves, then washing hands thoroughly; not feeding raw or undercooked meat to cats; and keeping cats inside to prevent acquisition of toxoplasma by eating infected prey. Secondary prevention by serologic screening of the pregnant woman and the newborn infant is done in some countries but is not widely used in the United States.
VIII. **Prognosis.** Maternal toxoplasmosis acquired during the first and second trimesters is associated with stillbirth (35%) and perinatal death (7%). Infants with congenital toxoplasmosis have a mortality rate as high as 12% and are at risk for many other problems later in life (seizures, visual impairment, learning disabilities, deafness, mental retardation and spasticity).

RUBELLA

I. **Definition.** Rubella is a viral infection capable of causing chronic intrauterine infection and damage to the developing fetus. Rubella is classified as a member of the togavirus family.
II. **Incidence.** Rubella vaccination has virtually eliminated the majority of cases of congenital rubella syndrome (CRS) in the developed world. In the United States, only two cases of CRS were reported in 2003 and 2004. Rubella remains prevalent in developing countries and in nonvaccinated immigrant populations.
III. **Pathophysiology.** Rubella virus is an RNA virus that typically has an epidemic seasonal pattern of increased frequency in the spring. In developing countries with no vaccination programs, epidemics have occurred at 4- to 7-year intervals, and major pandemics, every 10–30 years. Humans are the only known hosts, with an incubation period of ~18 days after contact. Virus is spread by respiratory secretions and also from stool, urine, and cervical secretions. A live virus vaccine has been available since 1969. In places with no

vaccination, 15–20% of women of childbearing age are susceptible to rubella. There is a high incidence of subclinical infections. Maternal viremia is a prerequisite for placental infection, which may or may not spread to the fetus. Most cases occur after primary disease, although a few cases have been described after reinfection.

The fetal infection rate varies according to the timing of maternal infection during pregnancy. If infection occurs at 1–12 weeks and is associated with maternal rash, there is an 81% risk of fetal infection; at 13–16 weeks, 54%; at 17–22 weeks, 36%; at 23–30 weeks, 30%; there is a rise to 60% at 31–36 weeks; and 100% in the last month of pregnancy. No correlation exists between the severity of maternal rubella and teratogenicity. However, the incidence of fetal effects is greater the earlier in gestation that infection occurs, especially at 1–12 weeks when 85% of infected fetuses will have congenital defects. Infection during weeks 13–16 results in 35% of fetuses having congenital defects; infection at later gestational ages rarely causes deafness or congenital malformations. The virus sets up chronic infection in the placenta and fetus. Placental or fetal infection may lead to resorption of the fetus, spontaneous abortion, stillbirth, fetal infection with multisystem disease, congenital anomalies, or unapparent infection. Spontaneous abortion may occur in up to 20% of cases when rubella occurs in the first 8 weeks of pregnancy.

The disease involves angiopathy as well as cytolytic changes. Other viral effects include chromosome breakage, decreased cell multiplication time, and mitotic arrest in certain cell types. There is little inflammatory reaction.

IV. **Risk factors.** Women of childbearing age who are rubella nonimmune are at risk. Laboratory confirmation of rubella infection is required because a clinical diagnosis is unreliable. Rubella is indistinguishable clinically from other infections that present with a rash, such as parvovirus B19, measles, human herpesvirus (HHV)-6, HHV-7, enterovirus, and group A streptococcus infections.

V. **Clinical presentation.** Congenital rubella has a wide spectrum of presentations, ranging from acute disseminated infection to deficits not evident at birth.

A. **Systemic transient manifestations** include low birthweight, hepatosplenomegaly, meningoencephalitis, thrombocytopenia, with or without purpura, and bony radiolucencies. These are probably a consequence of extensive virus infection and usually resolve spontaneously within days or weeks. Infants with these abnormalities usually fail to thrive during infancy.

B. **Systemic permanent manifestations** include heart defects (eg, patent ductus arteriosus, pulmonary artery stenosis, pulmonary arterial hypoplasia), eye defects (eg, cataracts, iris hypoplasia, microphthalmos, retinopathy), CNS problems (eg, mental retardation, psychomotor retardation, speech defects/language delay), microcephaly, and sensorineural or central auditory deafness (unilateral or bilateral). More than half of those children infected during the first 8 weeks of gestation have heart defects. PDA is the most common of heart lesions and occurs alone in ~30% of cases. Of the eye defects, a "salt and pepper" retinopathy is the most common. A cataract occurs in about a third of all cases of CRS and in about half of these they are bilateral. Deafness is a major disabling abnormality and may occur alone.

C. **Developmental and late-onset abnormalities.** Rubella is a progressive disease due to the persistence of the viral infection and the defective immune response to the virus. Existing manifestations, such as deafness and CNS disease, may progress, and some abnormalities may not be detected until the second year of life or later. These include hearing, developmental and eye defects, diabetes mellitus (DM), thyroid disorders, behavioral and educational difficulties, and progressive panencephalitis. Insulin-dependent DM is the most frequent endocrine abnormality, occurring in ~20% of the cases.

VI. **Diagnosis**

A. **Laboratory studies**

1. **Open cultures.** The virus can be cultured for up to 1 year despite measurable antibody titer. The best specimens for viral recovery are from nasal pharyngeal swabs, conjunctival scrapings, urine, and CSF (in decreasing order of usefulness).

2. **CSF examination** may reveal encephalitis with an increased protein and cell count.

3. **Serologic studies** are the mainstay of rubella diagnosis. CRS is diagnosed by the detection of rubella-specific IgM in a serum or oral fluid taken before 3 months of age. IgM testing is less reliable after 3 months of age as levels of specific IgM decline. However, if sensitive assays are used, specific IgM may be detected in 85% of symptomatic infants at 3–6 months and >30% at 6–12 months of age. A negative result by IgM-capture enzyme immunosorbent assay in the first 3 months of age virtually excludes congenital infection. It is also possible to make a diagnosis by demonstrating persistence of rubella IgG in sera taken between 6 and 12 months of age. It is no longer possible to make a serologic diagnosis of congenital rubella after rubella vaccination. Testing of oral-fluid samples as an alternative to serum has been used and standardized. It offers many advantages for surveillance of CRS in developing countries. Serologic tests for detection of rubella-specific IgM in oral-fluid samples are accurate. CRS may also be diagnosed by detection of viral RNA by nested reverse transcriptase polymerase chain reaction (RT-PCR) in nasopharyngeal swabs, urine, oral fluid, CSF, lens aspirate, and EDTA-blood.

B. **Radiologic studies.** Long-bone films may show metaphyseal radiolucencies that correlate with metaphyseal osteoporosis.

VII. **Management.** There is no specific treatment for rubella. Long-term follow-up is needed secondary to late-onset symptoms. Prevention consists of vaccination of the susceptible population (especially young children). Vaccine should not be given to pregnant women. Pregnancy should be avoided for 28 days after vaccination. Inadvertent vaccination of pregnant women does not cause CRS, although there is a 3% chance of congenital infection. Passive immunization does not prevent fetal infection when maternal infection occurs. Children with congenital rubella should be considered contagious until they are at least 1 year of age, unless nasopharyngeal and urine cultures are repeatedly negative for the virus. Rubella vaccine virus can be isolated from breast milk in lactating women who have received the vaccine. However, breast-feeding is not a contraindication to vaccination because no evidence indicates that the vaccine virus is in any way harmful to the infant.

VIII. **Prognosis.** Infection in the first or second trimester can cause growth restriction and deafness. Consequences of congenital rubella may present later (inguinal hernia, motor and mental retardation, hearing and communication disorders, and microcephaly).

CYTOMEGALOVIRUS

I. **Definition.** CMV is a DNA virus and a member of the herpesvirus group.

II. **Incidence.** CMV is the most common cause of congenital infection in the United States and occurs in ~0.2–2.2% of all live births. This results in ~40,000 new cases in the United States per year.

III. **Pathophysiology.** CMV is a ubiquitous virus that may be transmitted in secretions, including saliva, tears, semen, urine, cervical secretions, blood (white blood cells), and breast milk. The seroprevalence increases with age and is influenced by many factors such as hygienic circumstances, socioeconomic factors, breast-feeding, and sexual contacts. In developed countries, CMV seroprevalence varies inversely with socioeconomic status, with 40–80% of women of childbearing age in the United States having serologic evidence of past CMV infection. Seroconversion and initial infection can occur around the time of puberty, and shedding of the virus may continue for a long time. CMV can also become latent and reactivate periodically. CMV is capable of penetrating the placental barrier as well as the blood-brain barrier. During early pregnancy, CMV has a teratogenic potential in the fetus. CMV infections may result in neuronal migration disturbances in the brain. Both primary and recurrent maternal CMV can lead to transmission of the virus to the fetus. When primary maternal infection occurs during pregnancy, the virus is transmitted to the fetus in ~35% of cases. Infection in early pregnancy causes more severe fetal infection with significant CNS sequelae. During recurrent infection, transmission rate is only 0.2–1.8%. More than 90% of infants born with CMV have a subclinical infection. Symptomatic infants are usually born to women with a primary infection. **Symptomatic infants have a mortality rate of 20–30%.** Maternal virus-infected leukocytes are the proposed vehicle of transplacental transmission to the fetus. Fetal viremia is spread by the hematogenous route. The primary target organs are the CNS, eyes, liver, lungs, and kidneys. Characteristic histopathologic features of CMV include focal necrosis, inflammatory response, formation of enlarged cells with intranuclear inclusions (cytomegalic cells), and the production of multinucleated giant cells. CMV may also be transmitted to the infant at delivery (with cervical colonization), via breast milk, and via transfusion of seropositive blood to an infant whose mother is seronegative. CMV infection acquired during delivery or via breast milk has no effect on future neurodevelopmental outcome in full-term infants. A sepsis-like illness has been described in premature infants. There is no definite evidence of CMV transmission among hospital personnel.

IV. **Risk factors.** CMV infection in neonates is associated with nonwhite race, lower socioeconomic status, drug abuse, and neonatal intensive care unit admittance. Premature infants are more often affected than full-term infants. Transfusion with unscreened blood is an additional risk factor for neonatal disease.

V. **Clinical presentation**

   A. **Subclinical infection** occurs in 85–90% of the cases. Despite being asymptomatic at birth, these infants are at risk for sensorineural hearing loss (SNHL) during the first 5 years of life.

   B. **Low birthweight.** Maternal CMV infection is associated with low birthweight and small for gestational age infants even when the infant is not infected.

   C. **Classic CMV inclusion disease** occurs in 10–15% of the cases and consists of intrauterine growth retardation, hepatosplenomegaly with jaundice, abnormal liver function tests (LFTs), thrombocytopenia with or without purpura, and severe CNS disease (CNS and sensory impairments are seen in 50–90% of symptomatic newborns). Neurologic complications include microcephaly, intracerebral calcifications (most characteristically in the subependymal periventricular area), chorioretinitis, and progressive SNHL (10–20% of cases). Other symptoms include hemolytic anemia and pneumonitis. The most severely affected infants have a mortality rate of ~30%. Deaths are usually due to hepatic dysfunction, bleeding, disseminated intravascular coagulation, or secondary bacterial infection. Factors associated with poor outcome in symptomatic infants include microcephaly, abnormal findings on head CT scan, and increased viral load.

   D. **Late sequelae.** About 10–20% of children with congenital CMV infections, regardless of symptoms, exhibit neurologic damage when followed up. SNHL occurs in 22–65% of symptomatic and 6–23% of asymptomatic infants. CMV-related SNHL may be present at birth or occur later in childhood. Repeated auditory evaluation during the first 5 years of life is strongly recommended. Visual impairment and strabismus are common in children with clinically symptomatic CMV infection. Visual complications may occur secondary to chorioretinitis, pigmentary retinitis, macular scarring, optic atrophy, and central cortical defects.

VI. **Diagnosis**

   A. **Laboratory studies**

      1. **Culture for demonstration of the virus.** The **gold standard** for the diagnosis of congenital CMV is urine or saliva culture obtained before 3 weeks of age. Most urine specimens from infants with congenital CMV are positive within 48–72 h, especially if shell vial tissue culture techniques are used. Shell vial assay detects CMV-induced antigens by monoclonal antibodies, allowing for identification of the virus within 48 h compared with the standard tissue culture, which takes 2–4 weeks. Studies evaluating a rapid assay for detection of CMV in saliva as a screening method for congenital infection have shown it to be at least as sensitive a method

for detecting congenital infection as for detection of viruria. Given that saliva can be collected with less difficulty and expense, it may eventually replace the current use of urine screening.

2. **Polymerase chain reaction (PCR)** for CMV DNA is as sensitive as a urine culture for the detection of CMV infection. PCR has been used successfully in retrospective diagnosis of congenital CMV beyond 3 weeks of age through CMV DNA analysis of dried blood spots (Guthrie cards).

3. **Serologic tests** based on the detection of IgM should not be used to diagnose congenital CMV because they are less sensitive and more subject to false-positive results than culture or PCR. Only 70% of neonates infected with congenital CMV have IgM antibodies at birth.

4. **Other** laboratory tests that are indicated in the workup include complete blood count, LFT, disseminated intravascular coagulation (DIC) panel, and CSF analysis, culture, and PCR.

B. **Radiologic studies.** Skull films, ultrasound, or CT scans of the head may demonstrate characteristic periventricular calcifications.

VII. **Management**

A. **Prevention and treatment of maternal infection during pregnancy.** Possible approaches to preventing and treating congenital CMV infections during pregnancy include changes in hygienic behavior for seronegative pregnant women, administration of CMV hyperimmune globulin (HIG) to pregnant women with a primary infection, administering antiviral therapy to women with primary infection, and vaccines administered to girls or women well before pregnancy. Hygienic studies have shown that instructing mothers who are pregnant on frequent handwashing, wearing gloves for specific child-care tasks, and avoiding various types of intimate contact with their children in day-care setting reduces their chances of acquiring congenital CMV infection. To test the efficacy of HIG, a multicenter nonrandomized study in Italy enrolled pregnant women with primary congenital CMV infection diagnosed before 21 weeks' gestation. The study demonstrated that HIG (100 units/kg) given monthly until delivery reduces congenital infection in the newborn infants (16% vs 40%) compared with mothers who refused therapy. HIG was safe, and therefore this therapy should be strongly considered for mothers diagnosed with primary CMV during the first half of gestation. Use of antiviral therapy for the infected pregnant woman has not been studied in controlled trials. The most effective preventive strategy is developing a vaccine against CMV. Work is in progress to develop such vaccines, and phase II clinical trials are underway.

B. **Antiviral agents.** No antiviral agent is yet approved for treatment of congenital CMV infection. Ganciclovir has been used to treat infants who have symptomatic disease. In a randomized, placebo-controlled phase III clinical trial in infants with congenital CMV and CNS involvement, treatment with intravenous ganciclovir for 6 weeks at a dose of 6 mg/kg/day resulted in improved hearing compared with controls after 6 months follow-up. In addition, 68% of controls had deterioration of hearing at 1-year follow-up compared with 21% of treated children. During therapy the viral excretion in urine decreases but returns to near pretreatment levels after cessation of therapy. The antiviral therapy may suppress virus replication temporarily but may not prevent long-term sequelae. No effect on long-term neurodevelopmental outcome has been reported yet. Ganciclovir was associated with significant side effects, especially neutropenia, which occurred in 60% of the recipients. Based on the results of this study, some experts suggest that ganciclovir therapy may be offered to CMV-infected neonates who manifest CNS disease for prevention of hearing impairment. Another possible indication is chorioretinitis, which involves the macula and may result in blindness. A third possible indication is the critically ill preterm infant who acquires the infection natally or postnatally. Such infants have life-threatening CMV infection manifested by pneumonitis, hepatitis, or encephalitis, and ganciclovir may modify the course of the disease. Other agents under investigation are valganciclovir and foscarnet.

VIII. **Prognosis.** Congenital CMV is the leading cause of SNHL. For symptomatic infants at birth, mortality is up to 30%, and 90% will have late complications (intellectual or developmental impairment, hearing loss, spasticity). With asymptomatic, congenitally infected infants, the prognosis is uncertain but they are at a risk for SNHL.

HERPES SIMPLEX VIRUSES

I. **Definition.** HSV-1 and HSV-2 are enveloped, double-stranded DNA viruses. They are part of the herpes group, which also includes CMV, Epstein-Barr virus, VZV, and HHV-6 and HHV-7). HSV infection is among the most prevalent of all viral infections encountered by humans.

II. **Incidence.** The incidence of neonatal HSV is estimated to range from 1 in 3000 to 1 in 20,000 live births. Seroprevalence of HSV-1 and HSV-2 in pregnant women in the United States is ~63% and 22%, respectively.

III. **Pathophysiology.** Two serologic subtypes can be distinguished by antigenic and serologic tests: HSV-1 (usually affects face and skin above the waist) and HSV-2 (genitalia and skin below the waist). Three quarters of neonatal herpes infections are secondary to HSV-2. HSV-1, however, can be the cause of maternal genital herpes infections in 9% of the cases and its rate appears to be increasing. HSV infection of the neonate can be acquired at one of three times: intrauterine, intrapartum, or postnatal. Most infections (85%) are acquired in the intrapartum period as ascending infections with ruptured membranes (4–6 h is considered a critical period for this to occur) or by delivery through an infected cervix or vagina. An additional 10% of infected neonates acquire the virus postnatally (eg, from someone shedding HSV from the mouth who then kisses the infant). The final 5% of neonatal HSV infections occur in utero. The usual portals of entry for the virus are the skin, eyes, mouth, and respiratory tract. Once colonization occurs, the virus may spread by contiguity or via a hematogenous route. The incubation period is from 2–20 days. Three general patterns of neonatal HSV infection are recognized: disease localized to the skin, eyes, and mouth (SEM); CNS involvement (with or without SEM involvement); and disseminated disease (which also may include signs of the first two groups). Maternal infection can be classified as either *first-episode* or *recurrent* infections. First-episode infections are further classified as either *primary* or *first-episode nonprimary* based on type-specific serologic testing. *Primary infections* are those in which the mother is experiencing a new infection with either HSV-1 or HSV-2 and has not already been infected with the other virus type. *First-episode nonprimary* infections are those in which the mother has a new infection with one virus type, usually HSV-2, but has antibodies to the other virus type, usually HSV-1. Infants born vaginally to mothers with a true primary infection are at highest risk, with transmission rates of 50%. Those born to a mother with a first-episode nonprimary infection are at a somewhat lower risk of 30%. The lowest risk (<2%) infants are those who are born to a mother with recurrent infections. Maternal antibody is not always protective in the fetus.

IV. **Risk factors.** The risk of genital herpes infection may vary with maternal age, socioeconomic status, and number of sexual partners. Only ~12% of pregnant women who test seropositive for HSV-2 give a clinical history suggestive of the disease. The first-episode infection may stay "active" with asymptomatic cervical shedding for as long as 2 months. Besides a first-episode infection (primary or nonprimary), additional risk factors for neonatal HSV infection include the use of a fetal-scalp electrode and maternal age <21 years.

V. **Clinical presentation.** The disease may be localized or disseminated. Humoral and cellular immune mechanisms appear important in preventing initial HSV infections or limiting their spread. Infants with disseminated and SEM disease generally present at 10–12 days of life, whereas patients with CNS disease usually presents at 16–19 days of life. More than 20% of infants with disseminated disease and 30–40% of infants with encephalitis never have skin vesicles.

A. **Localized infections.** In the era of acyclovir therapy, HSV disease localized to the skin, eyes, or oral cavity accounts for ~45% of the cases. **Skin lesions** vary from discrete vesicles to large bullous lesions and denuded the skin. There is skin involvement in 80–85% of SEM cases. Assertive **mouth lesions** (~10% of SEM cases) with or without cutaneous involvement can be seen. **Ocular findings** include keratoconjunctivitis and chorioretinitis.

B. **Disseminated disease** carries the worst prognosis with respect to mortality and long-term sequelae. Patients commonly present with fever, lethargy, apnea, and a septic shock-like picture, including respiratory collapse, liver failure, and DIC. Approximately half of these cases also have localized disease as described previously, and 60–75% have CNS involvement. More than 20% of infants with disseminated disease will not develop cutaneous vesicles during the course of their illness. Infants with disseminated HSV infection account for 25% of all cases of neonatal herpes infection.

C. **Encephalitis.** CNS involvement can present with or without SEM lesions. Clinical manifestations of encephalitis include seizures (focal and generalized), lethargy, irritability, tremors, poor feeding, temperature instability, a bulging fontanelle, and pyramidal tract signs. These infants usually present at 16–19 days of age, and 30–40% have no herpetic skin lesions. CSF findings are variable and typically show a mild pleocytosis, increased protein, and a slightly low glucose.

VI. **Diagnosis**

A. **Laboratory studies**

1. **Viral cultures.** Isolation of HSV by culture remains the definitive diagnostic method of documenting HSV infection. Skin or mucous membrane lesions or surfaces are scraped and transferred in appropriate viral transport media on ice. Specimens for viral culture from multiple body sites (with the exception of CSF) may be combined before plating in cell culture to decrease costs. With the exception of CNS involvement, the important information gathered from such cultures is the presence or absence of the replicating virus, rather than its precise location. Preliminary results may become available in 24–72 h. Cultures are usually obtained from conjunctiva, throat, feces, urine, and nasopharynx. Surface cultures obtained before 24–48 h of life may indicate exposure (contamination from maternal secretion) without infection.

2. **Immunologic assays** to detect HSV antigen in lesion scrapings, usually using monoclonal anti-HSV antibodies in either an ELISA or fluorescent microscopy assay, are very specific and 80–90% sensitive.

3. **Polymerase chain reaction (PCR)** is an important tool in the diagnosis of HSV infection. PCR has been used to detect HSV DNA in CSF and blood specimen. PCR is especially useful for the diagnosis of HSV encephalitis. Overall sensitivities of CSF PCR in neonatal HSV disease have ranged from 75–100% with overall specificities ranging from 71–100%. PCR is especially important in monitoring therapy of CNS disease with discontinuation of therapy only when PCR is negative.

4. **Serologic tests** are not helpful in the diagnosis of neonatal infection but are helpful in diagnosing and classifying maternal disease (primary versus secondary).

5. **Lumbar puncture** should be performed in all suspected cases. Evidence of hemorrhagic CNS infection with increased white and red blood cells and protein is found. PCR should always be performed on CSF.

B. **Radiologic studies.** **CT scan of the head** may be useful in the diagnosis of CNS disease, but **magnetic resonance imaging** and an electroencephalogram (multiple independent foci of periodic slow and sharp wave discharge) are probably better for detecting earlier disease.

VII. **Management**

A. **Antepartum.** The history of genital herpes in a pregnant woman or in her partner(s) should be solicited and recorded in the prenatal record. If a positive history is obtained, the following steps may be taken:

1. **Antiviral therapy.** **Acyclovir** or **valacyclovir** may be given to pregnant women who have a primary episode of genital HSV as well as to women with an active

infection (primary or secondary) near or at the time of delivery. A recent meta-analysis of published trials indicates that prophylactic **acyclovir** beginning at 36 weeks' gestation reduces the risk of clinical HSV recurrence at delivery, cesarean delivery, and the risk of HSV viral shedding at delivery. **Valacyclovir** in randomized studies also demonstrated similar results. These studies did not identify any neonatal side effects from maternal suppressive therapy. These infants will need to be monitored closely because the risk of neonatal HSV infection is not totally eliminated.

2. **If there are no visible lesions** at the onset of labor or prodromal symptoms, vaginal delivery is acceptable.

3. **Delivery by cesarean is recommended** in women who have clinically apparent HSV infection. Debate exists if membranes have already been ruptured for >6 h. Most experts still recommend cesarean delivery. All neonates delivered by cesarean should be monitored closely because neonatal HSV infections have occasionally occurred despite delivery before the membranes rupture.

4. **The ultimate preventive strategy** might be the development of a **vaccine** to prevent HSV infection in the pregnant woman and her newborn infant. An inactivated glycoprotein-D-adjuvant vaccine has been evaluated and shown to be 70% effective in seronegative women (for both HSV-1 and HSV-2), but it is not effective in men or seropositive women.

B. **Neonatal treatment**

1. **Infants born to mothers with a genital lesion.** If it is a known recurrent lesion and the infant is asymptomatic, the infection rate is 1–3%. Educate the parents regarding the signs and symptoms of early herpes infection. Consider surface screen cultures of the infant at 24–48 h of age. Treat if symptoms develop or if the culture is positive. If the maternal infection is primary, or the first episode nonprimary, the risk to the infant is high (57% for primary and 25% for the first-episode nonprimary), and most clinicians recommend empirical acyclovir therapy at birth after cultures have been obtained.

2. **Pharmacologic therapy.** Neonates with HSV disease should be treated with intravenous acyclovir at 60 mg/kg/day, divided, every 8 h (20 mg/kg/dose). The dosing interval of intravenous acyclovir may need to be increased in premature infants, based on their creatinine clearance. Duration of therapy is 21 days for patients with disseminated or CNS disease and 14 days for SEM disease. All patients with CNS involvement should have a repeat lumbar puncture at the end of intravenous acyclovir therapy to determine if CSF is PCR-negative. Those infants who remain PCR-positive should receive intravenous acyclovir therapy until PCR-negativity is achieved. Absolute neutrophil counts should be followed twice weekly during the course of therapy. Lower dose acyclovir is associated with a higher morbidity and mortality and should be avoided. Trifluridine is the treatment of choice for ocular HSV infection in the neonate.

3. **Breast-feeding.** The infant may breast-feed as long as no breast lesions are present on the mother, and the mother should be instructed in good handwashing technique.

4. **Parents with orolabial herpes** should wear a mask when handling the newborn and should not kiss or nuzzle the infant.

VIII. **Prognosis.** Antiviral therapy, especially high-dose acyclovir (60 mg/kg/day) has greatly reduced **mortality** for neonatal HSV infection. In the pre-antiviral era, 85% of patients with disseminated neonatal HSV disease died by 1 year of age, as did 50% of patients with CNS disease. With current antiviral therapy, 12-month mortality has been reduced to 29% for disseminated disease and to 4% for CNS disease. Predictors of mortality include disease severity (pneumonia, DIC, seizures, and hepatitis), virus type (HSV-1 in systemic disease, HSV-2 in CNS disease), and prematurity. Systemic infection in premature infants is associated with near 100% mortality. Improvements in **morbidity** rates have not been as dramatic as with mortality. The proportion of survivors of disseminated neonatal HSV disease who have normal neurologic development has increased from 50% in the pre-antiviral era to 83% today. In the case of CNS disease, morbidity in survivors has not changed, with only ~30% of them developing normally by 12 months of age. In contrast to the disseminated or CNS disease, morbidity following SEM disease has dramatically improved during the antiviral era with <2% of acyclovir recipients having developmental delays. Survivors of neonatal HSV infections should undergo **developmental assessments** regularly. Cutaneous recurrences are relatively common, especially for SEM disease. Suppressive oral acyclovir therapy may have a role in decreasing those recurrences.

Selected References

TOXOPLASMOSIS

American Academy of Pediatrics: *Toxoplasma gondii* infections. In Pickering LK et al (eds): *Red Book: 2006 Report of the Committee on Infectious Diseases,* 27th ed. Elk Grove Village, IL: American Academy of Pediatrics, 2006:666-671.

Guerina NG et al: Neonatal serologic screening and early treatment for congenital *Toxoplasma gondii* infection. *N Engl J Med* 1994;330:1858-1863.

Liesenfeld O et al: Confirmatory serologic testing for acute toxoplasmosis and rate of induced abortions among women reported to have positive Toxoplasma immunoglobulin M antibody titers. *Am J Obstet Gynecol* 2001;184:140-145.

Lopez A et al: Preventing congenital toxoplasmosis. *MMWR Recomm Rep* 2000;49(RR-2):59-68.

McLeod R et al: Outcome of treatment for congenital toxoplasmosis, 1981–2004: The National Collaborative Chicago-Based, Congenital Toxoplasmosis Study. *Clin Infect Dis* 2006;15(42):1383-1394.

Montoya JG, Rosso F: Diagnosis and management of toxoplasmosis. *Clin Perinatol* 2005;32:705-726.

Remington J et al: Toxoplasmosis. In Remington JS et al (eds): *Infectious Diseases of the Fetus and Newborn Infant.* Philadelphia, PA: Elsevier Saunders, 2006:947-1091.

Sensini A: *Toxoplasma gondii* infection in pregnancy: opportunities and pitfalls of serological diagnosis. *Clin Microbiol Infect* 2006;12:504-512.

SYROCOT (Systematic Review on Congenital Toxoplasmosis) study group; Thiebaut R et al: Effectiveness of prenatal treatment for congenital toxoplasmosis: a meta-analysis of individual patients' data. *Lancet* 2007;13(369):115-122.

Wallon M et al: Long-term ocular prognosis in 327 children with congenital toxoplasmosis. *Pediatrics* 2004;113:1567-1572.

RUBELLA

American Academy of Pediatrics: Rubella. In Pickering LK et al (eds): *Red Book: 2006 Report of the Committee on Infectious Diseases,* 27th ed. Elk Grove Village, IL: American Academy of Pediatrics, 2006:574-579.

Banatvala JE, Brown DW: Rubella. *Lancet* 2004;363:1127-1137.

Best JM: Rubella. *Semin Fetal Neonatal Med* 2007;12:182-192.

Cooper L, Alford C: Rubella. In Remington JS et al (eds): *Infectious Diseases of the Fetus and Newborn Infant.* Philadelphia, PA: Elsevier Saunders, 2006:893-926.

Cooray S et al: Improved RT-PCR for diagnosis and epidemiological surveillance of rubella. *J Clin Virol* 2006;35:73-80.

da Silva e Sá G et al: Seroepidemiological profile of pregnant women after inadvertent rubella vaccination in the state of Rio de Janeiro, Brazil, 2001–2002. *Rev Panam Salud Publica* 2006;19:371-378.

Reef SE et al: The epidemiological profile of rubella and congenital rubella syndrome in the United States, 1998–2004: the evidence for absence of endemic transmission. *Clin Infect Dis* 2006;1(43):S126-S132.

Vijaylakshmi P et al: Evaluation of a commercial rubella IgM assay for use on oral fluid samples for diagnosis and surveillance of congenital rubella syndrome and postnatal rubella. *J Clin Virol* 2006;37:265-268.

CYTOMEGALOVIRUS

Adler SP et al: Recent advances in the prevention and treatment of congenital cytomegalovirus infections. *Semin Perinatol* 2007;31:10-18.

Fowler KB, Boppana SB: Congenital cytomegalovirus (CMV) infection and hearing deficit. *J Clin Virol* 2006;35:226-231.

Kenneson A, Cannon MJ: Review and meta-analysis of the epidemiology of congenital cytomegalovirus (CMV) infection. *Rev Med Virol* 2007;17:253-276.

Kimberlin DW et al: Effect of ganciclovir therapy on hearing in symptomatic congenital cytomegalovirus disease involving the central nervous system: a randomized, controlled trial. *J Pediatr* 2003;143:16-25.

Lazzarotto T et al: New advances in the diagnosis of congenital cytomegalovirus infection. *J Clin Virol* 2008;41(3):192-197.

Malm G, Engman ML: Congenital cytomegalovirus infections. *Semin Fetal Neonatal Med* 2007;12:154-159.

Nigro G et al: Passive immunization during pregnancy for congenital cytomegalovirus infection. *N Engl J Med* 2005;353:1350-1362.

Noyola DE et al: Early predictors of neurodevelopmental outcome in symptomatic congenital cytomegalovirus infection. *J Pediatr* 2001;138:325-331.

Pass RF et al: Congenital cytomegalovirus infection following first trimester maternal infection: symptoms at birth and outcome. *J Clin Virol* 2006;35:216-220.

Schleiss MR, Heineman TC: Progress toward an elusive goal: current status of cytomegalovirus vaccines. *Expert Rev Vaccines* 2005;4:381-406.

Stagno S, Britt B: Cytomegalovirus. In Remington JS et al (eds): *Infectious Diseases of the Fetus and Newborn Infant.* Philadelphia, PA: Elsevier Saunders, 2006:739-781.

Stehel EK, Sánchez PJ: Cytomegalovirus infection in the fetus and neonate. *NeoReviews* 2005;6:e38-e45.

van der Knaap MS et al: Pattern of white matter abnormalities at MR imaging: use of polymerase chain reaction testing of Guthrie cards to link pattern with congenital cytomegalovirus infection. *Radiology* 2004;230:529-536.

Walter S et al: Congenital cytomegalovirus: association between dried blood spot viral load and hearing loss. *Arch Dis Child Fetal Neonatal Ed* 2008;93(4):F280-F285.

HERPES SIMPLEX VIRUSES

American Academy of Pediatrics: Herpes simplex. In Pickering LK et al (eds): *Red Book: 2006 Report of the Committee on Infectious Diseases,* 27th ed. Elk Grove Village, IL: American Academy of Pediatrics, 2006:361-371.

American College of Obstetricians and Gynecologists; ACOG practice bulletin: Management of herpes in pregnancy. *Int J Gynecol Obstet* 2000;68:165-174.

Arvin AM et al: Herpes simplex virus infections. In Remington JS et al (eds): *Infectious Diseases of the Fetus and Newborn Infant.* Philadelphia, PA: Elsevier Saunders, 2006:845-865.

Baker DA: Consequences of herpes simplex virus in pregnancy and their prevention. *Curr Opin Infect Dis* 2007;20:73-76.

Brown ZA et al: Effect of serologic status and cesarean delivery on transmission rates of herpes simplex virus from mother to infant. *JAMA* 2003;289:203-209.

Kimberlin DW: Herpes simplex virus infections of the newborn. *Semin Perinatol* 2007;31:19-25.

Kimberlin DW et al: Natural history of neonatal herpes simplex virus infections in the acyclovir era. *Pediatrics* 2001;108:223-229.

Kimberlin DW et al: The safety and efficacy of high-dose intravenous acyclovir in the management of neonatal herpes simplex virus infections. *Pediatrics* 2001;108:230-238.

Leone P et al: Seroprevalence of herpes simplex virus-2 in suburban primary care offices in the United States. *Sex Transm Dis* 2004;31:311-316.

O'Riordan DP et al: Herpes simplex virus infections in preterm infants. *Pediatrics* 2006;118(6):e1612-e1620.

Sheffield JS et al: Acyclovir prophylaxis to prevent herpes simplex virus recurrence at delivery: a systematic review. *Obstet Gynecol* 2003;102:396-403.

Sheffield JS et al: Valacyclovir prophylaxis to prevent recurrent herpes at delivery: a randomized clinical trial. *Obstet Gynecol* 2006;108:141-147.

Stanberry LR et al: Glycoprotein-D-adjuvant vaccine to prevent genital herpes. *N Engl J Med* 2002;347:1652-1661.

Xu F et al: Seroprevalence of herpes simplex virus types 1 and 2 in pregnant women in the United States. *Am J Obstet Gynecol* 2007;196:43.e1-e6.

128 Transient Tachypnea of the Newborn

I. **Definition.** Transient tachypnea of the newborn (TTN) is also known as wet lung or type II respiratory distress syndrome (RDS). It is a benign disease of near-term, term, or large premature infants who have respiratory distress shortly after delivery that usually resolves within 3–5 days.

II. **Incidence.** The incidence of TTN is ~1–2% of all newborns.

III. **Pathophysiology.** Its true cause is unknown, but three factors are involved.

   A. **Delayed resorption of fetal lung fluid.** TTN is thought to occur because of delayed resorption of fetal lung fluid from the pulmonary lymphatic system. The increased fluid volume causes a reduction in lung compliance and increased airway resistance. This results in tachypnea and retractions. Infants delivered by elective cesarean delivery are at risk because of lack of the normal vaginal thoracic squeeze, which forces lung fluid out.

   B. **Pulmonary immaturity.** One study noted that a mild degree of pulmonary immaturity is a central factor in the cause of TTN. The authors found a mature L-S ratio but negative phosphatidylglycerol (the presence of phosphatidylglycerol indicates completed lung maturation) in infants with TTN. Infants who were closer to 36 weeks' gestation than to 38 weeks had an increased risk of TTN.

   C. **Mild surfactant deficiency.** One hypothesis is that TTN may represent a mild surfactant deficiency in these infants.

IV. **Risk factors**

   A. **Elective cesarean delivery without preceding labor (especially with gestational age <38 weeks).**

   B. **Male sex.**

   C. **Macrosomia.**

   D. **Excessive maternal sedation.**

   E. **Prolonged labor.**

   F. **Negative amniotic fluid phosphatidylglycerol.**

   G. **Birth asphyxia.**

   H. **Fluid overload to the mother, especially with oxytocin infusion.**

   I. **Maternal asthma.**

    J. Delayed clamping of the umbilical cord. Optimal time is 45 s.

    K. Breech delivery.

    L. Fetal polycythemia.

    M. Infant of a diabetic mother.

    N. Prematurity (can occur but is less frequent).

    O. Infant of drug-dependent mother (narcotics).

    P. Very low birthweight neonates.

    Q. Exposure to B-mimetic agents.

    R. Precipitous delivery.

    S. Multiple gestations.

V. Clinical presentation. The infant is usually near term, term, or large and premature and shortly after delivery has tachypnea (>60 breaths/min and can be up to 100–120 breaths/min). The infant may also have grunting, nasal flaring, rib retraction, and varying degrees of cyanosis. The infant often appears to have the classic "barrel chest" secondary to the increased anteroposterior diameter. There are usually no signs of sepsis. Some infants may have edema and a mild ileus on physical examination. One can also see tachycardia with usually a normal blood pressure.

VI. Diagnosis

    A. Laboratory studies

        1. Prenatal testing. A mature L-S ratio with the presence of phosphatidylglycerol in the amniotic fluid may help rule out HMD.

        2. Postnatal testing

            a. Arterial blood gas on room air shows some degree of mild hypoxia. Hypocarbia is usually present. Hypercarbia, if it exists, is usually mild (PCO_2 >55 mm Hg). Extreme hypercarbia is rare and, if present, another diagnosis should be considered.

            b. Complete blood cell count with differential is normal in TTN but should be obtained if one is considering an infectious process. The hematocrit will also rule out polycythemia.

            c. Urine and serum antigen test may help rule out certain bacterial infections.

            d. Plasma endothelin-1 levels (ET-1). One study revealed that plasma ET-1 levels were higher in patients with RDS compared with those with TTN. This test may prove useful in differentiating RDS from TTN.

            e. Interleukin-6 (IL-6). Studies have shown that an initial IL-6 can distinguish proven and clinical sepsis from TTN. This may make it possible to avoid antibiotics in this group of infants.

    B. Radiologic studies

        1. Chest radiograph. (See example in Figure 10–15A and B.) The typical findings in TTN are as follows:

            a. Hyperexpansion of the lungs, a hallmark of TTN.

            b. Prominent perihilar streaking (secondary to engorgement of periarterial lymphatics).

            c. Mild to moderately enlarged heart.

            d. Depression (flattening) of the diaphragm, best seen on a lateral view of the chest.

            e. Fluid in the minor fissure and perhaps fluid in the pleural space.

            f. Prominent pulmonary vascular markings.

        2. Lung sonography. Recently an ultrasound sign (**double lung point**) was found to be diagnostic of TTN. Lung ultrasound shows a difference in lung echogenicity between the upper and lower lung areas. It was also noted that very compact comet-tail artifacts were in the inferior fields and not in the superior fields. This finding is the "**double lung point**" and was seen in infants **with TTN** and not seen in RDS, atelectasis, pneumothorax, pneumonia, pulmonary hemorrhage, or in healthy infants.

    C. Other tests. Any infant who is hypoxic on room air must have a **100% oxygen test** to rule out heart disease. (This test is described on page 436)

VII. **Management**
  A. **General**
    1. **Oxygenation.** Initial management consists of providing adequate oxygenation. Start with hood oxygen and deliver enough to maintain normal arterial saturation. These infants typically require only hood oxygen, usually <60%. If the oxygen needs to be increased and 100% hood oxygenation does not work, change to nasal continuous positive airway pressure. If these maneuvers are not effective, intubate the infant and proceed with mechanical ventilation. If the infant requires 100% oxygen or endotracheal intubation with ventilator support, another disease process should be suspected.
    2. **Antibiotics.** Most infants are initially treated with broad-spectrum antibiotics until the diagnosis of sepsis or pneumonia is excluded.
    3. **Feeding.** Because of the risk of aspiration, an infant should not be fed by mouth if the respiratory rate is >60 breaths/min. If the respiratory rate is <60 breaths/min, oral feeding is permissible. If the rate is 60–80 breaths/min, feeding should be by nasogastric tube. If the rate is >80 breaths/ min, intravenous nutrition is indicated.
    4. **Fluid and electrolytes.** Fluid status should be monitored and hydration maintained.
    5. **Diuretics.** Two randomized trials using furosemide showed an increase in weight loss in the treated group but no difference in decrease or duration of respiratory symptoms or length of hospital stay.
  B. **Confirm the diagnosis.** TTN is often a diagnosis of exclusion, and other causes of tachypnea should be excluded first. The usual causes of tachypnea include the following:
    1. **Pneumonia/sepsis.** If the infant has pneumonia/sepsis, the prenatal history usually suggests infection. There may be maternal chorioamnionitis, premature rupture of membranes, and fever. The blood cell count may show evidence of infection (neutropenia or leukocytosis with abnormal numbers of immature cells). The urine antigen test may be positive if the infant has group B streptococcal infection. Remember that it is best to give broad-spectrum antibiotics if there is any suspicion or evidence of infection. The antibiotics can always be discontinued if the cultures are negative in 3 days.
    2. **Heart disease.** The 100% oxygen test should be done to rule out heart disease (see page 436). Cardiomegaly may be seen.
    3. **Hyaline membrane disease (HMD).** The infant is normally premature or has some reason for delayed lung maturation, such as maternal diabetes. The chest radiograph is helpful because it shows the typical HMD reticulogranular pattern with air bronchograms and underexpansion (atelectasis) of the lungs.
    4. **Cerebral hyperventilation.** This disorder is seen when CNS lesions cause overstimulation of the respiratory center, resulting in tachypnea. The CNS lesions can include meningitis or hypoxic-ischemic insult. Arterial blood gas measurements show respiratory alkalosis.
    5. **Metabolic disorders.** Infants with hypothermia, hyperthermia, or hypoglycemia may have tachypnea.
    6. **Polycythemia and hyperviscosity.** This syndrome may present with tachypnea with or without cyanosis.
VIII. **Prognosis.** TTN is self-limited and usually lasts only 2–5 days. Recent studies have revealed that TTN is associated with the development of wheezing syndromes in early childhood and subsequent diagnosis of childhood asthma, especially in males of nonwhite race, whose mothers lived at an urban address and did not have asthma.

Selected References

Behrman RE et al: *Nelson Textbook of Pediatrics,* 16th ed. Philadelphia, PA: Saunders, 2002.

Birnkrant DJ et al: Association of transient tachypnea of the newborn and childhood asthma. *Pediatr Pulmonol* 2006;41(10):978-984.

Copetti R, Cattarossi L: The 'double lung point': an ultrasound sign diagnostic of transient tachypnea of the newborn. *Neonatology* 2007;91(3):203-209.

Fanaroff AA, Martin RJ (eds): *Neonatal-Perinatal Medicine—Diseases of the Fetus and Infant,* 6th ed. St. Louis, MO: Mosby, 2002.

Källman J: Contribution of interleukin-6 in distinguishing between mild respiratory disease and neonatal sepsis in the newborn infant. *Acta Paediatr* 1999;88(8):880-884.

Kao B et al: Inhaled epinephrine for the treatment of transient tachypnea of the newborn. *J Perinatol* 2008;28(3):205-210.

Karabayir, Nalan: Kavuncuoglu, Sultan, Intravenous frusemide for transient tachypnoea of the newborn: A randomised controlled trial. *Journal of Paediatrics and Child Health* 2006;42(10):640-2.

Kuo CY et al: Study of plasma endothelin-1 concentrations in Taiwanese neonates with respiratory distress. *Chang Gung Med J* 2001;24:239.

Levine EM et al: Mode of delivery and risk of respiratory diseases in newborns. *Obstet Gynecol* 2001;97:439.

Malloy MH, Freeman DH: Respiratory distress syndrome mortality in the United States, 1987 to 1995. *J Perinatol* 2000;20:414.

Miller MJ et al: Respiratory disorders in preterm and term infants. In Fanaroff AA, Martin RJ (eds): *Neonatal-Perinatal Medicine: Diseases of the Fetus and Infant,* 7th ed. St. Louis, MO: Mosby, 2002.

Newman B: Neonatal imaging. *Radiol Clin North Am* 1999;37:1049.

Schatz M et al: Increased transient tachypnea of the newborn in infants of asthmatic mothers. *Am J Dis Child* 1991;145:156.

129 *Ureaplasma Urealyticum* Infection

I. **Definition.** *Ureaplasma* belongs to the Mycoplasmataceae family. These are small pleomorphic bacteria that characteristically lack a cell wall.

II. **Incidence.** *Ureaplasma urealyticum* is frequently present in the lower genital tract of sexually active women with a colonization rate ranging between 40% and 80%. Vertical transmission to the newborn is high, especially in premature infants <1000 g birthweight where transmission rate approaches 90%.

III. **Pathophysiology.** *U. urealyticum* has been implicated in a variety of obstetric and neonatal diseases including preterm labor, preterm premature rupture of membranes (PPROM), chorioamnionitis, congenital pneumonia, and bronchopulmonary dysplasia (BPD). The presumed mechanisms of infection include fetal exposure to ascending intrauterine infection, passage through an infected birth canal, and hematogenous dissemination through the placenta into umbilical vessels. This exposure leads to colonization of the skin, mucosal membranes, and respiratory tract, and sometimes leads to dissemination into the bloodstream and CNS. Phospholipases and cytokines produced through the inflammatory response can trigger uterine contractions and premature birth. Ureaplasmal infection of the respiratory tract in the newborn promotes a proinflammatory cytokine cascade with increase in tumor necrosis factor alpha, interleukin (IL)-1β, and IL-8. These cytokines recruit neutrophils to the lungs and intensify the inflammatory cascade, which damages the premature lung and impairs future alveolar development .

IV. **Risk factors.** *Ureaplasma* colonization is associated with preterm labor, chorioamnionitis, birthweight <1000 g, and gestational age <30 weeks.

V. **Clinical presentation**
    A. **Preterm labor, PPROM, and chorioamnionitis.** *Ureaplasmas* can invade the amniotic fluid early in pregnancy and are the single most common organisms that can be

isolated from inflamed placentas. *Ureaplasmas* can persist in the amniotic fluid subclinically for several weeks. A recent study showed preterm labor to occur in 58.6% of women with a positive polymerase chain reaction (PCR) assay for *Ureaplasmas* at 15–17 weeks of gestation as compared with only 4.4% of women with negative results.

B. **Congenital pneumonia.** Evidence that suggests *Ureaplasma* as a cause of congenital pneumonia includes isolation of the organism in pure culture from amniotic fluid and tracheal aspirate of neonates <24 h after birth in the midst of an acute inflammatory response with radiographic changes. These infants develop early interstitial pulmonary infiltrates with cystic/dysplastic changes as early as 10–14 days of age.

C. **Predisposition to chronic lung disease.** Multiple cohort studies have linked the development of BPD with colonization of the airways with *Ureaplasma*.

VI. **Diagnosis**
   A. **Laboratory studies**
      1. **Culture.** Specimens for culture require specific transport media with refrigeration at 4°C. Dacron or calcium alginate swabs should be used instead of cotton swabs.
      2. **Other tests.** Several sensitive PCR assays have been developed, but they are not available routinely. Serologic assays are of limited value.

VII. **Management.** Isolation precautions for all infectious diseases, including maternal and neonatal precautions, breast-feeding, and visiting issues, can be found in Appendix F.

   A. **Treatment of the colonized pregnant mother.** Treatment of pregnant women who present with PPROM with a 10-day course of **erythromycin** has been shown in a large randomized study to prolong pregnancy, reduce neonatal treatment with surfactant, decrease infant oxygen dependency at ≥28 days of age, and result in fewer major cerebral abnormalities on ultrasonography before discharge. Those same benefits were not accrued if the mother presented with preterm labor but with intact membranes.

   B. **Treatment of the colonized newborn infant** is controversial. Limited current evidence does not demonstrate a reduction in BPD or other long-term neonatal morbidities when *Ureaplasma* colonized and intubated preterm infants are treated with erythromycin. For infants with congenital pneumonia, some experts recommend treatment with erythromycin if there is a radiographic evidence of early interstitial pneumonitis and when *Ureaplasma* is the only microorganism isolated from the respiratory tract.

VIII. **Prognosis.** *Ureaplasma* infection or colonization may be a risk factor for development of BPD (see Chapter 77).

Selected References

American Academy of Pediatrics: Ureaplasma urealyticum infections. In: Pickering LK et al (eds): *Red Book: 2006 Report of the Committee on Infectious Diseases,* 27th ed. Elk Grove Village, IL: American Academy of Pediatrics, 2006:709-710.

Gerber S et al: Detection of *Ureaplasma urealyticum* in second-trimester amniotic fluid by polymerase chain reaction correlates with subsequent preterm labor and delivery. *J Infect Dis* 2003;187:518-521.

Kenyon SL et al: ORACLE Collaborative Group. Broad spectrum antibiotics for preterm, prelabour rupture of fetal membranes: The ORACLE I randomized trial. ORACLE Collaborative Group. *Lancet* 2001;357:979-988.

Mabanta CG et al: Erythromycin for the prevention of chronic lung disease in intubated preterm infants at risk for, or colonized or infected with *Ureaplasma urealyticum*. *Cochrane Database Syst Rev* 2003;4:CD003744.

Schelonka RL, Waites KB: Ureaplasma infection and neonatal lung disease. *Semin Perinatol* 2007;31:2-9.

Waites KB et al: Mycoplasmas and ureaplasmas as neonatal pathogens. *Clin Microbiol Rev* 2005;18:757-789.

130 Urinary Tract Infection

I. **Definition.** Urinary tract infection (UTI) is the presence of pathogenic bacteria or fungus in the urinary tract with or without symptoms of infection. A definitive diagnosis is made by culture of any organism in a urine specimen that has been properly collected by suprapubic bladder aspiration (>10,000 col), ideally, or by gentle catheterization (>100,000 col).

II. **Incidence.** Various series report an incidence of 0.5–1.0% in term infants weighing >2500 g and higher rates (3–5%) in premature infants or infants weighing <2500 g. (*Note*: In the neonatal period, there is a greater incidence among males than females.) The predominant organisms are Gram-negative rods; *Escherichia coli* is the most common. In neonates, UTIs are most frequently acquired by hematogenous spread.

III. **Pathophysiology.** The three routes with which the urinary tract can become infected are retrograde ascent of fecal-perineal bacteria, introduction of bacteria into urinary system by instrumentation (eg, catheter insertion), or urinary tract involvement as part of a systemic infection (may see Gram-positive species). When a UTI is present in an infant <1 year of age, an associated urinary tract abnormality is found in ~50% of neonates. Associated anomalies that may give rise to a UTI include neurogenic bladder, posterior urethral valves, vesicoureteral reflux, and ureteropelvic junction obstruction.

IV. **Risk factors** include indwelling urinary catheters, systemic sepsis with hematogenous seeding of the urinary tract, urinary tract obstruction, neurogenic bladder (myelodysplasia), and male newborns. Evidence suggests that uncircumcised males may be at higher risk for UTIs. Ritual (religious) circumcision performed by nonphysicians may be a risk factor for male UTI.

V. **Clinical presentation**
   A. **Signs of sepsis.** The infant may have frank signs of sepsis (respiratory distress, apnea, bradycardia, hypoglycemia, or poor perfusion) or abdominal distention.
   B. **Nonspecific findings.** The signs are often subtle and may include lethargy, irritability, poor feeding, vomiting, jaundice, or failure to thrive.

VI. **Diagnosis**
   A. **Laboratory studies**
      1. **Urine culture.** Suprapubic aspiration or bladder catheterization is mandatory for a dependable urine culture in a neonate. Some clinicians consider "bag" urine inadequate to achieve reliable culture results.
      2. **Blood cultures** should be obtained before starting antibiotic therapy.
      3. **Urinalysis.** Microscopic examination may show white blood cells, but the presence of bacteria is a more reliable sign of UTI in the neonate, especially when urine is collected by suprapubic aspiration.
      4. **The complete blood cell count** may show leukocytosis.
      5. **Serum bilirubin** may be elevated and increased bilirubin levels in neonates with an UTI are related to pathological findings (renal cortex changes) when technetium-99m DMSA renal scintigraphy is performed.
   B. **No other studies are indicated.**

VII. **Management**
   A. **Initial antibiotic treatment.** Initial antibiotic therapy usually consists of broad-spectrum intravenous antibiotics, usually ampicillin and gentamicin, or third-generation cephalosporins, until definitive urine and blood culture results are reported. (For dosages and other pharmacologic information, see Chapter 132.)
   B. **Further investigations.** Further tests are necessary to rule out anatomic abnormalities in the neonate. Tests such as renal/bladder ultrasonography, contrast voiding cystourethrogram, and renal scan are indicated; at times, an intravenous pyelogram is required for complex problems. Urologic consultation is usually recommended.

VIII. **Prognosis.** Up to a one-fourth of infants can have a recurrent UTI within the first year of life. Effective use of long-term suppressive antibiotics (in the presence of vesicoureteral reflux) along with any indicated corrective surgery has dramatically reduced the long-term incidence of renal scarring and renal insufficiency.

Selected References

Ginsburg CM, McCracken GH: Urinary tract infections in young infants. *Pediatrics* 1982;69:409.

Holliday MA, Bennett TM (eds): *Pediatric Nephrology,* 3rd ed. Philadelphia, PA: Williams & Wilkins, 1994.

Lee JH et al: Nonrefluxing neonatal hydronephrosis and the risk of urinary tract infection. *J Urol* 2008;179(4):1524-1528.

Ma JF, Shortliffe LM: Urinary tract infection in children: etiology and epidemiology. *Urol Clin N Am* 2004; 31:517-526.

Prais D et al: Is ritual circumcision a risk factor for neonatal urinary tract infections? *Arch Dis Child* 2008. [Epub ahead of print]

Sweeney B et al: Reflux nephropathy in infancy: a comparison of infants presenting with and without urinary tract infection. *J Urol* 2001;166:648.

Xinias I et al: Bilirubin levels predict renal cortical changes in jaundiced neonates with urinary tract infection. *World J Pediatr* 2009;5(1):42-45.

131 Varicella-Zoster Infections

Varicella-zoster virus (VZV) is a member of the herpesvirus family. Primary maternal VZV infection (chickenpox) can result in fetal or neonatal infection; however, reactivation infection (zoster) does not result in fetal infection. Primary maternal VZV infection during the last trimester can cause pneumonia with significant morbidity and mortality. Three forms of varicella-zoster infections involve the neonate: fetal, congenital, and postnatal.

FETAL VARICELLA-ZOSTER SYNDROME (FVZS)

I. **Definition.** This form occurs when the mother has her first exposure to VZV during the first half of pregnancy.
II. **Incidence.** This form is fortunately rare; the incidence of varicella during pregnancy is estimated at 1.6–4.6 per 1000. The incidence of embryopathy and fetopathy after maternal varicella infection in the first 20 weeks is ~1% . Recent evidence suggests that the incidence is much lower than previously estimated.
III. **Pathophysiology.** Maternal transmission of the virus probably occurs via respiratory droplets or direct contact with chickenpox or zoster lesions. The virus replicates in the oropharynx, and viremia results, before the onset of rash, with transplacental passage to the fetus. Almost all cases reported have involved exposure between the 8th and 20th weeks of pregnancy. From the pattern of defects seen in the fetal varicella syndrome, particularly the scarring and limb hypoplasia, it has been suggested that fetal varicella syndrome is the result of intrauterine herpes zoster. The extremely short latent period between fetal infection and reactivation is the consequence of the lack of cell-mediated immunity in the fetus before 20 weeks' gestation. The defects probably result from viral replication and destruction of developing fetal ectodermal tissue.

IV. **Risk factors.** A mother with her first exposure to VZV during the first half of pregnancy (usually exposure between the 8th and 20th week). One study found the risk was higher if the maternal rash onset was between 13 and 20 weeks of pregnancy.

V. **Clinical presentation.** Sauerbrei and Wutzler summarized the main symptoms of FVZS after studying 124 cases reported in the literature as the following:

A. **Skin lesions (72%)** involve cicatricial scars and skin loss.

B. **Central nervous system defects or disease (62%):** microcephaly, seizures, encephalitis, cortical atrophy and spinal cord atrophy, mental retardation, and cerebral calcifications.

C. **Eye diseases (52%):** microphthalmia, endo-ophthalmia, chorioretinitis, cataracts, optic atrophy, and Horner syndrome (ptosis, miosis, and enophthalmos).

D. **Limb hypoplasia and other skeletal defects (44%).**

E. **Intrauterine growth restriction (35%).**

VI. **Diagnosis.** Alkalay et al proposed the following criteria for the diagnosis of FVZS in the newborn:

A. **Appearance of maternal varicella** during pregnancy.

B. **Presence of congenital skin lesions** in dermatomal distribution and/or neurologic defects, eye disease, or limb hypoplasia.

C. **Proof of intrauterine VZV infection** by detection of viral DNA in the infant by polymerase chain reaction (PCR); presence of VZV-specific immunoglobulin (Ig)M; persistence of VZV IgG beyond 7 months of age, or appearance of zoster during early infancy.

VZV DNA PCR (both from fetal blood or amniotic fluid) appears to be sensitive and accurate in detecting fetal infection; however, most of the "infected" fetuses are morphologically normal (ie, not affected by FVZS). Prenatal diagnosis is most often done by detailed ultrasound searching for typical anomalies and VZV-specific PCR in amniotic fluid. At least a 5-week interval is advised between onset of maternal rash and obtaining the ultrasound. An initial ultrasound is recommended at 17–21 weeks' gestation with a follow-up study done 4–6 weeks later.

VII. **Management.** Isolation precautions for all infectious diseases, including maternal and neonatal precautions, breast-feeding, and visiting issues, can be found in Appendix F.

A. **Mother.** If the mother is exposed to VZV infection in the first or second trimester, treat the mother with **varicella-zoster immune globulin (VZIG)** if her past history of varicella is negative or uncertain. (For dosage, see Chapter 132.) VZIG should be given within 72–96 h and appears to protect both mother and fetus. The only U.S.-licensed VZIG was discontinued by the manufacturer in 2004. Since February 2006, an investigational (not licensed) VZIG called VariZIG became available under an investigational new drug (IND) protocol and can be requested by calling the 24-hour toll-free number at FFF Enterprises (800-843-7477). If VariZIG is not available, then intravenous immunoglobulin (IVIG) can be considered; however, there are no data demonstrating its effectiveness in postexposure prophylaxis. If chickenpox is diagnosed during pregnancy, antiviral therapy with acyclovir should be strongly considered. This therapy has not been associated with increased congenital abnormalities compared with the general population.

B. **Infant.** Supportive care of the infant is required because there is usually profound neurologic impairment. Acyclovir therapy may be helpful to stop the progression of eye disease.

C. **Isolation.** Isolation is not necessary.

VIII. **Prognosis.** Approximately 30% of these infants die in the first months of life, often because of secondary infections. Survivors usually suffer profound mental retardation and major neurologic disabilities. These infants are also at risk for developing zoster (shingles) in the first year of life.

CONGENITAL VARICELLA INFECTION

I. **Definition.** This is the form of the disease that occurs when a pregnant woman suffers chickenpox during the last 3 weeks of pregnancy or within the first few days postpartum. Disease begins in the neonate just before delivery or within the first 10–12 days of life.

II. **Incidence.** Although the congenital form is more common than the teratogenic form, it is still rare. Only about 1 per 1000 pregnant women develop chickenpox in the third trimester.

III. **Pathophysiology.** Maternal chickenpox near term or soon after delivery may cause severe or fatal illness in the newborn. Maternal varicella can infect the baby by transplacental viremia, ascending infection during birth, or respiratory droplet/direct contact with infectious lesions after birth. Neonatal chickenpox occurring in the first 10–12 days of life has to be caused by intrauterine transmission of VZV because of the incubation period of varicella. Chickenpox after the 10th to 12th day of the neonatal period is most likely acquired by postnatal VZV infection. If the onset of maternal disease is between 5 days before delivery or 2 days postpartum, there is a high attack rate (up to 50%) with significant associated mortality (up to 30%). If the maternal rash happens >5 days before delivery, there is enough maternal anti-VZV IgG production with subsequent transplacental transfer that protects the newborn and results in a milder case of chickenpox.

IV. **Risk factors.** A mother with chickenpox during the last 3 weeks of pregnancy or within the first few days postpartum. (There is a higher risk of mortality if the onset of maternal disease is 5 days before delivery or 2 days postpartum.)

V. **Clinical presentation** is variable. There may be only mild involvement of the infant, with vesicles on the skin, or the following may be seen:
   A. **Skin.** A centripetal rash (beginning on the trunk and spreading to the face and scalp, sparing the extremities) begins as red macules and progresses to vesicles and encrustation. Lesions are more common in the diaper area and skin folds. There may be two or three lesions or thousands of them. The differential diagnosis includes herpes simplex virus and enterovirus. The main complication is staphylococcal and streptococcal secondary skin infections.
   B. **Lungs.** Lung involvement is seen in all fatal cases. It usually appears 2–4 days after the onset of the rash but may be seen up to 10 days after. Signs include fever, cyanosis, rales, and hemoptysis. Chest radiograph shows a diffuse nodular-miliary pattern, especially in the perihilar region.
   C. **Other organs.** Focal necrosis may be seen in the liver, adrenals, intestines, kidneys, and thymus. Glomerulonephritis, myocarditis, encephalitis, and cerebellar ataxia are sometimes seen.

VI. **Diagnosis**
   A. **Polymerase chain reaction (PCR)** is the most sensitive and specific method for detection of VZV DNA in clinical specimens. This is the method of choice for investigation of skin swabs, biopsies, and amniotic fluid for diagnosis of infections. Culture is not usually recommended.
   B. **Serum testing of VZV antibody.** Detection of IgM/IgA class antibodies is the most convincing for active infection.

VII. **Management**
   A. **VariZIG**
      1. **Perinatal infection.** Infants of mothers who develop VZV infection within 5 days before or 2 days after delivery should receive 125 units of VariZIG as soon as possible and not later than 96 h (see Chapter 132). IVIG should be use if VariZIG is not available. Infants treated with immunoglobulins should be placed in strict respiratory isolation for 28 days because immunoglobulin treatment may prolong the incubation period. VariZIG is not expected to reduce the clinical attack rate in treated newborns; however, they tend to develop milder infections than the untreated neonates.
      2. **Maternal rash occurring >7 days before delivery.** These infants do not need VZIG. It is believed that infants will have received antibodies via the placenta.
   B. **Acyclovir** therapy, 10–15 mg/kg every 8 h for 5–7 days, should be considered in symptomatic neonates.
   C. **Use antibiotics** if secondary bacterial skin infections occur.

VIII. **Prognosis.** Prognosis is good if the onset of maternal varicella occurs >5 days before delivery because the mother has enough time to develop antibodies and pass these to the infant. In these cases, the infant has a mild case of varicella with excellent prognosis. If the mother has onset of disease within 5 days before delivery or 2 days after, the infant is exposed with no antibodies. In these cases the disease is usually severe with dissemination. Overwhelming sepsis and multiple organ failure can lead to a mortality rate as high as 30%. The usual cause of death is pneumonia and fulminant hepatitis.

POSTNATAL CHICKENPOX

I.   **Definition.** This form of the disease presents on days 12–28 of life. It does not represent transplacental infection from the mother.

II. **Incidence.** There has been a significant decline in the incidence since the introduction of the vaccine in 1995 (by 85-90%).

III. **Pathophysiology.** Postnatal VZV infection occurs by droplet transmission. It is more common than congenital chickenpox. This disease is usually mild because of passive protection from maternal antibodies. Placental antibody transfer is lower in preterm infants, which makes them more susceptible compared with term infants.

IV. **Risk factors.** Seronegative mother, delivery before 28 weeks, birthweight <1.5 kg, immunocompromised neonates (sepsis, steroids, etc.).

V.   **Clinical presentation.** The typical chickenpox rash is seen with centripetal spread, beginning on the trunk and spreading to the face and scalp and sparing the extremities. All stages of the rash may appear at the same time, from red macules to clear vesicles to crusting lesions. Complications of this form of the disease are rare but may include secondary infections and varicella pneumonia. In older children, necrotizing fasciitis secondary to group A streptococcal infections is particularly worrisome and may be associated with ibuprofen use.

VI. **Diagnosis.** Same as for congenital varicella (see the previous section). Diagnosis is usually made based on clinical grounds.

VII. **Management.** For the full-term infant in community setting, the disease is usually mild. Therefore, acyclovir therapy is ***controversial***. For nosocomial chickenpox in the intensive care nursery:

   A. **VariZIG** is recommended for infants of <28 weeks' gestational age or weighing ≤1000 g regardless of the maternal history. It is also recommended in premature infants whose mothers do not have a history of chickenpox.

   B. **Infants of >28 weeks' gestation** should have sufficient transplacental antibodies, if the mother is immune, to protect them from the risk of complications.

   C. **Isolation.** Exposed infants should be placed in strict isolation for 10–21 days after the onset of the rash in the index case. Exposed infants who receive VariZIG should be in strict respiratory isolation for 28 days.

   D. **Acyclovir** is recommended for infants who develop breakthrough lesions. Therapy should be continued for 48 h after the last new lesions have appeared. Duration of 7 days is usually sufficient.

VIII. **Prognosis.** This form of the disease is mild, and death is extremely rare. Normal term infants who develop postnatal chickenpox have the same risk of complications of chickenpox as older children. The risk of complications for infants <28 weeks who develop postnatal chickenpox is unknown.

Selected References

Alkalay AL et al: Fetal varicella syndrome. *J Pediatr* 1987;111:320-323.

American Academy of Pediatrics: Varicella-zoster infections. In Pickering LK et al (eds): *Red Book: 2006 Report of the Committee on Infectious Diseases*, 27th ed. Elk Grove Village, IL: American Academy of Pediatrics, 2006:711-725.

Birthistle K, Carrington D: Fetal varicella syndrome—a reappraisal of the literature. *J Infect* 1998;36:25-29.

Centers for Disease Control and Prevention: Prevention of varicella. Recommendations of the Advisory Committee on Immunization Practices (ACIP). *MMWR Recomm Rep* 2007;56(RR-4):1-40.

Enders G et al: Consequences of varicella and herpes zoster in pregnancy: prospective study of 1739 cases. *Lancet* 1994 18;343:1548-1551.

Frangides CY, Pneumatikos I: Varicella-zoster virus pneumonia in adults: Report of 14 cases and review of the literature. *Eur J Intern Med* 2004;15:364-370.

Harger JH et al: Frequency of congenital varicella syndrome in a prospective cohort of 347 pregnant women. *Obstet Gynecol* 2002;100:260-265.

Lesko SM et al: Invasive group A streptococcal infection and nonsteroidal antiinflammatory drug use among children with primary varicella. *Pediatrics* 2001;107:1108-1115.

Linder N et al: Placental transfer and decay of varicella-zoster virus antibodies in preterm infants. *J Pediatr* 2000;137:85-89.

Miller E et al: Outcome in newborn babies given anti-varicella-zoster immunoglobin after perinatal maternal infection with varicella-zoster virus. *Lancet* 1989;2:371-373.

Mouly F et al: Prenatal diagnosis of fetal varicella-zoster virus infection with polymerase chain reaction of amniotic fluid in 107 cases. *Am J Obstet Gynecol* 1997;177:894-898.

Sauerbrei A, Wutzler P: Neonatal varicella. *J Perinatol* 2001;21:545-549.

Sauerbrei A, Wutzler P: Herpes simplex and varicella-zoster virus infections during pregnancy: current concepts of prevention, diagnosis and therapy. Part 2: Varicella-zoster virus infections. *Med Microbiol Immunol* 2007;196:95-102.

Stone KM et al: Pregnancy outcomes following systemic prenatal acyclovir exposure: conclusions from the International Acyclovir Pregnancy Registry, 1984–1999. *Birth Defects Res A Clin Mol Teratol* 2004;70:201-207.

Tan MP, Koren G: Chickenpox in pregnancy: revisited. *Reprod Toxicol* 2006;21:410-420.

132 Commonly Used Medications

This section provides a description of commonly used drugs used in the contemporary care of sick newborn infants. It is not intended to be an exhaustive list of all drugs available for infants, nor is it intended to be an in-depth source of information about neonatal pharmacology. Readers are encouraged to consult with their institutional pharmacists regarding issues of pharmacokinetics, drug interactions, drug elimination and metabolism, and monitoring drug serum levels. Information on medications and breast-feeding and pregnancy can be found in Chapter 133.

ACETAMINOPHEN (APAP) (LIQUIPRIN, TEMPRA, TYLENOL)

INDICATIONS AND USE: Analgesic, antipyretic.

ACTIONS: Analgesic effect is caused by inhibition of prostaglandin synthesis in the CNS and peripherally, which blocks pain impulse generation. Reduction of fever is produced by direct action on the hypothalamic heat-regulating center.

SUPPLIED: Suppositories, elixir, liquid, drops (preferred).

ROUTE: PO, PR.

DOSAGE:

- **Neonates:** 10–15 mg/kg/dose PO/PR every 6–8 hours as needed.
- **Preterm infants 28–32 weeks:** 10–12 mg/kg/dose PO every 6–8 hours or 20 mg/kg/dose PR every 12 hours. **Maximum daily dose:** 40 mg/kg/day.
- **Preterm infants 32–36 weeks < 10 days:** 10–15 mg/kg/dose PO every 6 hours or 30 mg/kg PR loading dose; then 15 mg/kg/dose every 8 hours. **Maximum daily dose:** 60 mg/kg.
- **Term infants ≥10 days:** 10–15 mg/kg/dose PO every 4–6 hours or 30 mg/kg PR loading dose; then 20 mg/kg/dose every 6–8 hours. **Maximum daily dose:** 90 mg/kg.

ADVERSE EFFECTS: Hepatic necrosis with overdosage, rash, and blood dyscrasias (neutropenia, pancytopenia, leukopenia, and thrombocytopenia). Renal injury may occur with chronic use.

ACETAZOLAMIDE (DIAMOX)

INDICATIONS AND USE: Mild diuretic or an anticonvulsant in refractory neonatal seizures. To decrease cerebrospinal fluid (CSF) production in posthemorrhagic hydrocephalus; also used in the treatment of renal tubular acidosis.

ACTIONS: Competitive, reversible, carbonic anhydrase inhibitor. Retards abnormal discharge from CNS neurons. Beneficial effects may be related to direct inhibition of carbonic anhydrase or may be due to the acidosis produced. Produces urinary alkalosis, useful in the treatment of renal tubular acidosis.

SUPPLIED: Injection, tablets (suspension can be compounded by the pharmacist).

ROUTE: IV, PO.

DOSAGE:

- **Diuretic:** 5 mg/kg/dose IV/PO daily.
- **Anticonvulsant:** 4–16 mg/kg/day PO divided every 6–8 hours not to exceed 30 mg/kg/day or 1 g/day.
- **Alkalinize urine:** 5 mg/kg/dose PO 2–3 times over 24 hours.
- **Decrease CSF production:** 5 mg/kg/dose IV/PO every 6 hours; increased by 25 mg/kg/day to a maximum of 100 mg/kg/day. Furosemide has been used in combination.

PHARMOCOKINETICS: Unchanged in urine. Half-life is 4–10 hours.

ADVERSE EFFECTS: Gastrointestinal (GI) irritation, anorexia, transient hypokalemia, hyperchloremic metabolic acidosis, growth retardation, bone marrow suppression, thrombocytopenias, hemolytic anemia, pancytopenia, agranulocytosis, leucopenia, drowsiness, and paresthesias.

COMMENTS: Limited clinical experience in neonates. Questionable efficacy to slow progression of hydrocephalus in neonates and infants. Used as an adjunct to other medications in refractory seizures. Tolerance to diuretic effect may occur with long-term use.

ACYCLOVIR (ZOVIRAX)

INDICATIONS AND USE: Treatment and prophylaxis of herpes simplex virus (HSV-1 and HSV-2) infections, herpes simplex encephalitis, herpes zoster infections, and varicella zoster infections.

ACTION: Antiviral agent that inhibits viral DNA synthesis and viral replication. It is preferentially taken up by infected cells. Generally demonstrates poor activity against Epstein-Barr virus and cytomegalovirus. Cerebrospinal fluid (CSF) concentrations are 50% of those of plasma.

SUPPLIED: Injection, suspension.

ROUTE: IV, PO.

DOSAGE:
- **Congenital herpes simplex:** Birth to 3 months of age: 20 mg/kg/dose IV every 8 hours for 21 days for disseminated infection or 14 days for mucous membrane or skin disease (Centers for Disease Control and Prevention [CDC] recommendations). Prolong dosing interval to every 12 hours for premature infants <34 weeks and in patients with significant renal impairment or hepatic failure.
- **Herpes simplex encephalitis:** 3 months to 12 years of age: 20 mg/kg/dose IV every 8 hours for 14 to 21 days.
- **Varicella zoster infection:**
  - **Immunocompromised children <12 years of age:** 20 mg/kg/dose IV every 8 hours for 7 days.
  - **Immunocompetent children:** 20 mg/kg/dose PO every 6 hours for 5 days.

ADVERSE EFFECTS: Generally well tolerated. Thrombophlebitis and inflammation of injection site. Neutropenia, thrombocytopenia, anemia, thrombocytosis, leukocytosis, and neutrophilia. Neutropenia may necessitate reduction in dose or treatment with granulocyte colony-stimulating factor (G-CSF) if absolute neutrophil count (ANC) remains <500/mm^3.

COMMENTS: Maintain adequate hydration to prevent renal tubular crystallization. It is important to infuse dose over 1 hour using a concentration <7 mg/mL to avoid vein irritation.

ADENOSINE (ADENOCARD)

INDICATIONS AND USE: Acute treatment of sustained paroxysmal supraventricular tachycardia for conversion to normal sinus rhythm. Repeat doses may be used without risk of accumulation.

ACTIONS: A purine nucleoside naturally occurring in all human cells. Slows conduction time through the atrioventricular (AV) node and interrupts reentry pathways through the AV node to restore normal sinus rhythm. Effects are mediated by depression of calcium slow-channel conduction, an increase in potassium conductance, and possibly indirect antiadrenergic effects.

SUPPLIED: Injection.

ROUTE: IV.

DOSAGE: 0.05–0.2 mg/kg by rapid IV push over 1–2 seconds. Repeat bolus doses at 2 minutes intervals by increasing increments of 0.05 mg/kg until sinus rhythm is achieved or until a maximum dose of 0.3 mg/kg is reached. Infuse as close as possible to IV site and immediately flush IV with saline to ensure dose enters circulation. For doses <0.2 mL, prepare dilution using normal saline (NS) to final concentration of 300 mcg/mL.

ADVERSE EFFECTS: Do not use in second- or third-degree AV block. May produce a short-duration first-, second-, or third-degree heart block; hypotension; brief dyspnea; and facial flushing. Half-life is <10 seconds; duration is 20–30 seconds. Methylxanthines (eg, caffeine and theophylline) are competitive antagonists; larger adenosine doses may be required.

ALBUMIN, HUMAN

INDICATIONS AND USE: Plasma volume expander, treatment of hypovolemia and maintenance of cardiac output in cases of shock, and hypoproteinemia associated with acute nephritic syndrome or in premature infants. Not recommended for initial volume expansion; use isotonic crystalloid solutions (Pediatric Advanced Life Support [PALS] and Neonatal Resuscitation Program [NRP] guidelines).

ACTIONS: Increases intravascular oncotic pressure, which causes a mobilization of fluid from the interstitial spaces into the intravascular space. Serves as a carrier for many substances, such as bilirubin.

SUPPLIED: Injection, 50 mg/mL (5%), 250 mg/mL (25%) (contains 130–160 mEq of sodium/liter).

ROUTE: IV.

DOSAGE: 0.5–1 g/kg IV (or 10–20 mL/kg of 5% IV bolus) repeated as necessary. **Maximum:** 6 g/kg/day. 5% solutions should be used in hypovolemic or intravascularly depleted patients; 25% solutions should be used in cases of fluid or sodium restriction. Up to 1.5 g/kg/day has been added to hyperalimentation solutions.

ADVERSE EFFECTS: Infrequent. Rapid infusion may cause vascular overload and precipitation of congestive heart failure. Hypersensitivity reactions may include chills, fever, nausea, and urticaria. A blood product derivative increases risk of infection. Use 25% concentration with extreme caution and infuse slowly in premature neonates due to increased risk of intraventricular hemorrhage. A 5% concentration is osmotically equivalent to equal volume of plasma, and 25% concentration is osmotically equivalent to 5 times its volume of plasma.

COMMENTS: If unavailable, 5% solutions can be prepared by diluting the 25% solution with NS or 5% dextrose in water (D$_5$W). *Do not use sterile water* to prepare dilution; this may cause hypotonic-associated hemolysis, which can be fatal.

ALBUTEROL (PROVENTIL, VENTOLIN)

INDICATIONS AND USE: Manage bronchospasm in reversible airway obstruction, increase maximal expiratory flow in infants with respiratory distress syndrome (RDS), and improve lung mechanics in ventilator-dependent infants and those with bronchopulmonary dysplasia (BPD). Also may be used for treatment of hyperkalemia.

ACTIONS: Primarily β_2-adrenergic stimulation (bronchodilation and vasodilation) with minor β_1 stimulation (increased myocardial contractility and conduction). Duration of action is ~3–8 hours.

SUPPLIED: Solution for nebulization, aerosol for oral inhalation.

ROUTE: Nebulization, inhalation.

DOSAGE:
- **Nebulization:** 0.1 to 0.5 mg/kg/dose (minimum of 2.5 mg) every 2 to 6 hours as needed.
- **Inhalation:** Metered dose inhaler (MDI) 90 mcg/spray: 1 to 2 puffs every 2 to 6 hours as needed.

ADVERSE EFFECTS: Tachycardia, tremors, CNS stimulation, hypokalemia, hyperglycemia, and hypertension.
COMMENTS: Titrate the dose according to the effect on heart rate and improvement in respiratory symptoms.

ALPROSTADIL (PROSTAGLANDIN E₁) (PROSTIN VR)

INDICATIONS AND USE: Any state in which blood flow must be maintained through the ductus arteriosus to sustain either pulmonary or systemic circulation until corrective or palliative surgery can be performed. Examples are pulmonary atresia, pulmonary stenosis, tricuspid atresia, transposition of the great arteries, aortic arch interruption, coarctation of the aorta, and severe tetralogy of Fallot (TOF).
ACTIONS: Vasodilator and platelet aggregation inhibitor. Smooth muscle of the ductus arteriosus is especially sensitive to its effects, responding to the drug with marked dilatation. Decreased response after 96 hours of infusion. Maximal improvement in PaO_2, usually within 30 minutes in cyanotic infants, 1.5–3 hours in acyanotic infants.
SUPPLIED: Injection.
ROUTE: IV.
DOSAGE:
- **Initial:** 0.05 to 0.1 mcg/kg/minute by continuous infusion. Gradually titrate to maintain acceptable oxygen levels without adverse effects. Use the lowest rate to maintain improved oxygenation response.
- **Maintenance:** 0.01 to 0.4 mcg/kg/minute.

ADVERSE EFFECTS: Cutaneous vasodilation, seizure-like activity, jitteriness, temperature elevation, hypocalcemia, hypoglycemia, thrombocytopenia, bradycardia, and hypotension. May cause apnea. Have an intubation kit at the bedside if the patient is not already intubated.
COMMENTS: Use cautiously in infants with bleeding tendencies.

ALTEPLASE, RECOMBINANT (ACTIVASE, CATHFLO ACTIVASE, TISSUE PLASMINOGEN ACTIVATOR [t-PA])

INDICATIONS AND USE: Used to restore patency of occluded central venous catheters and for the lysis of large-vessel thrombus (systemic use).
ACTIONS: Alteplase is a thrombolytic. It enhances conversion of plasminogen to plasmin, which then cleaves fibrin, fibrinogen, factor V, and factor VIII, resulting in clot dissolution.
SUPPLIED: Injection.
ROUTE: Intracatheter, IV.
DOSAGE:
- **Occluded central venous catheter:**
  - ≤2.5 kg: 0.25 mg diluted in normal saline (NS) to volume required to fill line.
  - 2.5–10 kg: 0.5 mg diluted in NS to volume required to fill line.
  - **Note:** Check catheter product literature or manufacturer for catheter volume.

  Instill into lumen of catheter slowly and carefully so as not to inject the drug into the systemic circulation. Dwell time is 2–4 hours. Concentration: 0.5–1 mg/mL in dextrose or saline. Check for catheter malposition with radiograph before alteplase administration. (See Choi et al: The use of alteplase to restore patency of central venous lines in pediatric patients: a cohort study. *J Pediatr* 2001;139:152.)
- **Lysis of large vessel thrombus (systemic use):** Dose is *controversial,* ranging from 0.1 to 0.6 mg/kg/hour for hours to days. Dose must be titrated to effect.

ADVERSE EFFECTS:
- **Large-vessel thrombus (systemic use):** Not recommended with preexisting intraventricular hemorrhage or cerebral ischemic changes. Correct hypertension before use. May cause puncture site or internal bleeding. Severe bleeding complications may occur. Monitoring methods are *controversial;* the following have been used by various investigators: frequent reassessment of thromboses usually by ultrasonography; daily cranial sonography; after fibrin/fibrinogen degradation products and/or d-dimers; and after fibrinogen with a lower limit of usually 100 mg/dL, but >150 mg/dL in one study (*J Pediatr* 1998;133:133).
- **Occluded central venous catheter:** Bleeding may occur if excessive tissue plasminogen activator (t-PA) is inadvertently injected into the systemic circulation. Excessive pressure on instillation may force the clot into the systemic circulation.

COMMENTS: Increases risk of bleeding in infants concurrently on heparin, warfarin (Coumadin), or indomethacin. Failure of thrombolytic agents in newborns/neonates may occur due to the low plasminogen concentrations (~50 to 70% of adult levels); administration of fresh-frozen plasma may possibly help.

AMIKACIN SULFATE (AMIKIN)

ACTION AND SPECTRUM: Primarily bactericidal against Gram-negative organisms by inhibiting protein synthesis. Active against Gram-negative bacteria, including most *Pseudomonas* and *Serratia* spp. No activity against anaerobic organisms.
SUPPLIED: Injection.

ROUTE: IM, IV (infuse over 30 minutes).
DOSAGE: Dosage should be monitored and adjusted by use of pharmacokinetics.
Initial empirical dosing based on body weight:
- **Neonates: 0–4 weeks, < 1.2 kg:** 7.5 mg/kg/dose every 18–24 hours.
- **Postnatal age ≤7 days:**
  - 1.2 kg–2 kg: 7.5 mg/kg/dose every 12 hours.
  - >2 kg: 7.5–10 mg/kg/dose every 12 hours.
- **Postnatal age >7 days:**
  - 1.2 kg–2 kg: 7.5–10 mg/kg/dose every 8–12 hours.
  - >2 kg: 10 mg/kg/dose every 8 hours.

PHARMACOKINETICS: Renal elimination (glomerular filtration); half-life is 4–8 hours; volume of distribution is 0.6 L/kg.
ADVERSE EFFECTS: Possible nephrotoxicity and ototoxicity. Toxicities may be potentiated when used with furosemide, vancomycin, and neuromuscular blockade increased if used with pancuronium or with coexisting hypermagnesemia.
COMMENTS: Lowest overall resistance of all the aminoglycosides and thus should be reserved for infections with organisms resistant to other aminoglycosides. Adjust the dosage according to serum peak and trough levels. Draw serum levels at about the fourth maintenance dose (draw a serum trough sample 30 minutes to just before the dose and a serum peak sample 30 minutes after infusion is complete). Therapeutic peak level is 25–35 mcg/mL, and trough level is ≤10 mcg/mL. Nephrotoxicity is associated with serum trough concentrations >10 mcg/mL; ototoxicity, with serum peak concentrations >35–40 mg/mL (more cochlear damage than vestibular).

AMINOPHYLLINE-THEOPHYLLINE

INDICATIONS AND USE: To reduce the frequency and severity of apnea of prematurity. May be used to help wean from mechanical ventilation or as a bronchodilator in the treatment of bronchopulmonary dysplasia. Caffeine is more effective and safer for the treatment of apnea of prematurity. Caffeine also has the advantage of once-a-day dosing. Aminophylline/theophylline has greater bronchodilator effects.
ACTIONS: Theophylline, the active component of aminophylline causes relaxation of bronchial smooth muscle; increases the force of contraction of the diaphragmatic muscles; dilates the pulmonary, coronary, and renal arteries; causes mild diuretic action; causes increased sensitivity of the CNS medullary respiratory centers to CO_2; stimulates central respiratory drive and peripheral chemoreceptors; and increases sensitivity to catecholamines resulting in increased cardiac output and improved oxygenation.
SUPPLIED: Injection, elixir.
ROUTE: IV (Aminophylline), PO (Aminophylline and Theophylline).
DOSAGE:
- **IV loading dose:** 5–8 mg/kg, infused slowly over 30 minutes. IV maintenance dosage follows as 1.5–3.0 mg/kg/dose every 8 to 12 hours starting 8 to 12 hours after loading dose.
- **PO loading doses:** Same as IV. PO maintenance dose as theophylline is 4 to 22 mg/kg/day divided every 6 to 8 hours. Older infants may need higher doses as clearance rate increases with increased postnatal age possibly up to 25 to 30 mg/kg/day. Aminophylline is ~80% theophylline. Neonates have a unique ability to convert theophylline to caffeine in a ratio of 1:0.3. Caffeine may account for as much as 50% of the theophylline level.

ADVERSE EFFECTS: Hyperglycemia, dehydration, diuresis, and feeding intolerance. CNS effects include jitteriness, hyperreflexia, and seizures. Most common side effects are cardiovascular with tachycardia (heart rate ≥180 beats/min) and other tachyarrhythmias.
COMMENTS: Therapeutic levels for apnea are 7–12 mcg/mL, and for bronchospasm 10–20 mcg/mL. Toxicity is usually attributed to levels of ≥20 mcg/mL. Monitor serum levels as a peak 1 hour after IV dosing or 2 hours after PO dosing. Ideally trough levels would be taken 30 minutes before next dose. Serum levels of caffeine and theophylline should be monitored anytime toxicity is suspected or when apnea spells are increasing in number.

AMIODARONE (CORDARONE)

INDICATIONS AND USE: Treatment of resistant life-threatening ventricular arrhythmias unresponsive to other agents; prevention and suppression of supraventricular arrhythmias (especially those associated with Wolff-Parkinson-White [WPW] syndrome) and postoperative junctional ectopic tachycardia (JET).
ACTIONS: An iodinated benzofuran that prolongs the action potential and increases the effective refractory period. It decreases afterload (causes peripheral and coronary vasodilation), demonstrates α- and β-blocking properties and calcium channel inhibition. It slows the heart rate (decreases atrioventricular [A-V] node and sinus node conduction-negative inotropic effects).
SUPPLIED: Injection [contains benzyl alcohol and polysorbate 80], tablets.
DOSAGE: Limited data is available. Generally not used as first-line agent due to high incidence of adverse effects. Recommend consultation with pediatric cardiologist prior to use.
- **IV loading dose:** 5 mg/kg over 30 to 60 minutes, central venous access is recommended. May repeat dose up to 15 mg/kg.
- **Maintenance:** May give a single daily dose of 5 mg/kg or a continuous infusion of 5 mcg/kg/minute gradually increasing as needed to 15 mcg/kg/minute.

- **PO loading dose:** 10 to 15 mg/kg/day divided in 1–2 doses per day for 4–14 days or until adequate control of arrhythmia is achieved or significant adverse effects occur. Reduce dose to 5 mg/kg/day given once daily for several weeks. Attempt to reduce dose to lowest possible without the recurrence of arrhythmia: 2.5 mg/kg/day.

PHARMACOKINETICS: Onset of oral antiarrhythmic effects may take up to 3 to 6 weeks. Duration of antiarrhythmic effects may persist for 30 to 90 days or longer following discontinuation of therapy. Protein binding: 96%. Metabolized in liver.

ADVERSE EFFECTS: Bradycardia and hypotension (may be related to rate of infusion), proarrhythmias (including torsade de pointes), heart block, congestive heart failure (CHF), and paroxysmal ventricular tachycardia. Hyperthyroidism or hypothyroidism partially inhibits the peripheral conversion of T_4 to T_3; serum T_4 and RT_3 concentrations may be increased, and serum T_3 may be decreased. Amiodarone HCl contains 37% iodine by weight and is a potential source of iodine ~3 mg of inorganic iodine per 100 mg of amiodarone is released into the circulation. Elevated liver enzymes, elevated bilirubin. Phlebitis and local injection site irritation: Avoid concentrations >2 mg/mL, administer through central vein.

COMMENTS: Potential drug–drug interactions may occur. Amiodarone inhibits certain cytochrome P450 enzymes and may increase serum levels of digoxin, flecainide, lidocaine, theophylline, procainamide, quinidine, warfarin, and phenytoin. To avoid toxicities with these agents, dosage reduction and serum concentration monitoring is recommended. Dosage reductions of 30 to 50% have been recommended. Concurrent administration of amiodarone with β-blockers, digoxin or calcium channel blockers may result in bradycardia, sinus arrest, and heart block.

AMPHOTERICIN B (AMPHOCIN), AMPHOTERICIN B, LIPOSOMAL (AMBISOME), AMPHOTERICIN B LIPID COMPLEX (ABELCET)

ACTION AND SPECTRUM: Antifungal agent that acts by binding to sterols and disrupting the fungal cell membranes. Broad spectrum of activity against *Candida* spp. and other fungi.

SUPPLIED: Injection.

ROUTE: IV.

DOSAGE:

- **Conventional Amphotericin B:**
  - **Initial dose:** 0.25–0.5 mg/kg IV over 4–6 hours. Use a 0.1 mg/mL concentration in 5% dextrose in water (D_5W). Incompatible with NaCl.
  - **Maintenance:** 0.5–1mg/kg IV every 24 to 48 hours for 2 to 6 weeks or longer, but a lower dose may suffice. In general, infusions should be given over 2–6 hours, but infusion over 1–2 hours may be used if tolerated.
  - **Intrathecal or intraventricular:** Reconstitute with sterile water at 0.25 mg/mL; dilute with CSF and reinfuse. **Usual dose:** 25 to 100 mcg every 48 to 72 hours increase as tolerated to 500 mcg.
- **Liposomal amphotericin B:** 5 to 7 mg/kg/dose IV infused over 2 hours. Concentrates in liver and spleen, but penetrates the CNS less than conventional amphotericin B. Used when refractory to or intolerant of conventional amphotericin B.
- **Amphotericin B lipid complex:** 5 mg/kg/dose IV every 24 hours infused over 2 hours. Used when refractory to or intolerant of conventional amphotericin B. Less nephrotoxic than conventional amphotericin B.

PHARMACOKINETICS: Slow renal excretion.

ADVERSE EFFECTS: Fewer adverse effects in neonates as compared to adults. May cause fever, chills, vomiting, thrombophlebitis at injection sites, renal tubular acidosis, renal failure, hypomagnesemia, hypokalemia, bone marrow suppression with reversible decline in hematocrit, hypotension, hypertension, wheezing, and hypoxemia.

COMMENTS: Protect the solution from light. Monitor serum potassium, magnesium, blood urea nitrogen (BUN), creatinine, and urine output at least every other day until the dosage is stabilized, then every week. Monitor complete blood cell count (CBC) and liver function every week. Discontinue if BUN is >40 mg/dL, serum creatinine is >3 mg/dL, or liver function tests are abnormal.

AMPICILLIN (POLYCILLIN, OTHERS)

ACTION AND SPECTRUM: Semisynthetic penicillinase-sensitive penicillin that is bactericidal and acts by inhibiting the late stages of cell wall synthesis. As effective as penicillin G in pneumococcal, streptococcal, and meningococcal infections; and also active against many strains of *Salmonella* spp., *Shigella* spp., *Proteus mirabilis*, *Escherichia coli*, and *Listeria* spp. as well as most strains of *Haemophilus influenzae*. Inactivated by staphylococcal and *H. influenzae* β-lactamases.

SUPPLIED: Injection, powder for oral suspension.

ROUTE: PO, IM, IV.

DOSAGE:

- **Postnatal age ≤7 days:**
  - ≤2000 g: 50 mg/kg/day IM, IV divided every 12 hours. **Meningitis:** 100 mg/kg/day divided every 12 hours.
  - >2000 g: 75 mg/kg/day IM, IV divided every 8 hours. **Meningitis:** 150 mg/kg/day divided every 8 hours.
  - **Group B streptococcal meningitis:** 200 mg/kg/day IM, IV divided every 8 hours.

- **Postnatal age >7 days:**
  - **<1200 g:** 50 mg/kg/day divided every 12 hours. **Meningitis:** 100 mg/kg/day divided every 12 hours.
  - **1200–2000 g:** 75 mg/kg/day divided every 8 hours. **Meningitis:** 150 mg/kg/day divided every 8 hours.
  - **>2000 g:** 100 mg/kg/day divided every 6 hours. **Meningitis:** 200 mg/kg/day divided every 6 hours.
  - **Group B streptococcal meningitis:** 300 mg/kg/day divided every 6 hours.
- **Infants and children:** 100–200 mg/kg/day IM, IV divided every 6 hours.
  - **Meningitis:** 200–400 mg/kg/day IM, IV divided every 6 hours. **Maximum dose:** 12 g/day.
  - **Oral dosing:** 50–100 mg/kg/day PO divided every 6 hours. **Maximum dose:** 2–3 g/day.

ADVERSE EFFECTS: Hypersensitivity, rash, abdominal discomfort, nausea, vomiting, diarrhea, interstitial nephritis and eosinophilia. Large doses may cause CNS excitation or convulsions.

COMMENTS: The penicillin of choice in combination with an aminoglycoside in the prophylaxis and treatment of infections with group B streptococci, group D streptococci (enterococci), and *Listeria monocytogenes*. Contains 3 mEq of sodium per gram.

AMPICILLIN SODIUM/SULBACTAM SODIUM (UNASYN)

ACTION AND SPECTRUM: Combination β-lactamase inhibitor and β-lactam agent with the bactericidal spectrum of ampicillin that is extended by the addition of sulbactam, a β-lactamase inhibitor, to include β-lactamase-producing strains of *Staphylococcus aureus*, *Staphylococcus epidermidis*, enterococci, *Haemophilus influenzae*, *Branhamella catarrhalis*, and *Klebsiella* spp., including *K. pneumoniae*. Also has good activity against *Bacteroides fragilis*, making it a suitable choice for single-drug treatment of intra-abdominal and pelvic infections caused by susceptible organisms.
SUPPLIED: Injection.
ROUTE: IV, IM.
DOSAGE: (based on ampicillin component)
- **Preterm infants and neonates during the first week of life 0–7 days:** 100 mg ampicillin/kg/day IM/IV divided every 12 hours.
- **Neonates >7 days:** 100 mg ampicillin/kg/day IM/IV divided every 6–8 hours.
  - **Infants ≥ 1 month:** 100–150 mcg ampicillin/kg/day divided every 6 hours.
    - **Meningitis:** 200–300 mg ampicillin/kg/day divided every 6 hours.

ADVERSE EFFECTS: elevated BUN and serum creatinine. See Ampicillin.
COMMENTS: Modify dosage in patients with renal impairment.

ARGININE HCL (R-GENE)

INDICATIONS AND USE: Treatment of severe metabolic alkalosis after other treatment has failed, pituitary function test (stimulant for the release of growth hormone), and treatment of certain neonatal-onset urea cycle disorders.
ACTIONS: Corrects severe hypochloremic metabolic alkalosis resulting from the chloride content of arginine. Arginine stimulates pituitary release of growth hormone and prolactin and the pancreatic release of glucagon and insulin.
SUPPLIED: Injection: 10% = 100 mg/mL (contains 0.475 mEq chloride)
ROUTE: IV, PO.
DOSAGE: IV, PO
- **Metabolic alkalosis: infants, children:**
  - Arginine hydrochloride dose (g) = weight (kg) × 0.1 × [HCO_3^- − 24] where HCO_3^- = the patient's serum bicarbonate concentration in mEq/L. Give 1/2 to 2/3 of calculated dose and re-evaluate.
- **To correct hypochloremia: infants and children:**
  - **Arginine hydrochloride dose** (mEq) = 0.2 × weight (kg) × [103 − Cl⁻] where Cl⁻ = the patient's serum chloride concentration in mEq/L; give 1/2 to 2/3 of the calculated dose, then reevaluate. IV: May use undiluted (irritating to tissues) or dilute with saline or dextrose administration through a central line is recommended. Infuse over at least 30 minutes or over 24 hours in maintenance IV. **Maximum:** 1 g/kg/hour (= 10 mL/kg/hour of 10% solution). PO: May use the injectable form, diluted.
- **Growth hormone reserve test:** IV 500 mg/kg (= 5 mL/kg of the 10% solution) infused IV over 30 minutes. (Use only IV, not PO administration for this test.)
- **Urea cycle disorders:** Consult specialists in metabolic disorders and specialized references if a urea cycle disorder is suspected (see Urea Cycle Disorders Conference Group: Consensus statement from a conference for the management of patients with urea cycle disorders. *J Pediatr* 2001;138:S1).

ADVERSE EFFECTS: Not a first-line treatment for metabolic alkalosis and should never be used as initial therapy; try sodium, potassium, or ammonium chlorides first. May be toxic in infants with arginase deficiency. Do not use in patients sensitive to arginine HCl or in those with hepatic or renal failure. May cause hyperchloremic metabolic acidosis, elevated gastrin, glucagon, and growth hormone; flushing and GI upset with rapid IV administration; hyperglycemia, hypoglycemia, hyperkalemia; tissue necrosis on extravasation, vein irritation; allergic reactions; elevated BUN and creatinine.
COMMENTS: Monitor IV site, blood glucose, chloride, and blood pressure.

ATROPINE SULFATE

INDICATIONS AND USE: Sinus bradycardia, cardiopulmonary resuscitation (CPR) unresponsive to epinephrine, and in conjunction with neostigmine for the reversal of nondepolarizing neuromuscular blockade. Used preoperatively to inhibit salivation and reduce excessive secretions of the respiratory tract.

ACTIONS: A competitive antagonist of acetylcholine at parasympathetic sites in smooth muscle, cardiac muscle, and various glandular cells, leading to increased heart rate, increased cardiac output, reduced GI motility and tone, urinary retention, cycloplegia, and decreased salivation and sweating.

SUPPLIED: Injection, ophthalmic ointment, ophthalmic solution.

ROUTE: IV, IM, subcutaneous, PO, intratracheal.

DOSAGE:

- **Bradycardia in infants and children:** 0.02–0.03 mg/kg/dose every 5 minutes as needed. **Minimum dose:** 0.1 mg. **Maximum dose:** 1 mg.
- **Preanesthetic:** 0.02 mg/kg/dose 30–60 minutes pre-op, then every 4–6 hours as needed; use a minimum dosage of 0.1 mg.
- **With neostigmine for reversal of neuromuscular blockade:** Neostigmine 0.06 mg/kg/dose with atropine 0.02 mg/kg/dose.
- **Endotracheal:** 0.01 mg–0.03 mg/kg/dose immediately followed by 1 mL of normal saline.
- **PO:** Initial dose: 0.02 mg/kg/dose given every 4 to 6 hours. May increase gradually to 0.09 mg/kg/dose

ADVERSE EFFECTS: Xerostomia, blurred vision, mydriasis, tachycardia, palpitations, constipation, urinary retention, ataxia, tremor, and hyperthermia. Toxic effects are especially likely in children receiving low doses.

COMMENTS: Contraindicated in thyrotoxicosis, tachycardia secondary to cardiac insufficiency, and obstructive GI disease. In low doses, it may cause paradoxic bradycardia secondary to its central actions.

AZT (See Zidovudine)

Aztreonam (Azactam)

ACTION AND SPECTRUM: Monobactam antibiotic with antibacterial activity resulting from inhibition of mucopeptide synthesis in the cell wall. Bactericidal against most Enterobacteriaceae, *Pseudomonas aeruginosa*, *Escherichia coli, Klebsiella pneumoniae, Proteus mirabilis, Serratia, Haemophilus influenzae, and Citrobacter species;* but little or no activity against Gram-positive aerobic or anaerobic bacteria.

SUPPLIED: Injection.

ROUTE: IV or IM.

DOSAGE:

- **Neonates postnatal age ≤7 days:**
  - **≤2 kg:** 30 mg/kg/dose every 12 hours.
  - **>2 kg:** 30 mg/kg/dose every 8 hours.
- **Neonates postnatal age > 7 days:**
  - **<1.2 kg:** 30 mg/kg/dose every 12 hours.
  - **1.2–2 kg:** 30 mg/kg/dose every 8 hours.
  - **>2 kg:** 30 mg/kg/dose every 6 hours.
- **Children >1 month:** 90 to 120 mg/kg/day divided every 6 to 8 hours.

PHARMACOKINETICS: Eliminated renally as unchanged drug. Half-life is 3 to 9 hours in neonates.

ADVERSE EFFECTS: Diarrhea, nausea, vomiting, rash, hypoglycemia, irritation at the infusion site. May cause transient eosinophilia, leukopenia, thrombocytopenia, hypoglycemia, and elevated liver enzymes.

COMMENTS: Demonstrates synergistic activity with aminoglycosides against most strains of *P. aeruginosa,* many strains of Enterobacteriaceae and other Gram-negative aerobic bacilli.

BERACTANT (SURVANTA)

INDICATIONS AND USE: Prevention and treatment of respiratory distress syndrome in preterm infants.

ACTIONS: A natural bovine lung extract containing phospholipids, neutral lipids, fatty acids, and surfactant-associated proteins to which dipalmitoylphosphatidylcholine (DPPC), palmitic acid, and tripalmitin are added to mimic the surface tension–lowering properties of natural lung surfactant. Surfactant lowers surface tension on alveolar surfaces during respiration and stabilizes the alveoli against collapse.

SUPPLIED: Suspension in single-use vials containing 25 mg of phospholipids per mL. Refrigerate.

ROUTE: Intratracheal using a no. 5F end-hole catheter.

DOSAGE: 4 mL/kg (100 mg of phospholipids/kg) birthweight. Divide dose into 4 aliquots, repositioning the infant with each dose. Inject each aliquot gently into the catheter over 2–3 seconds. Ventilate the infant after each 1/4 dose for at least 30 seconds or until stable. Four doses of 4 mL/kg can be given in the first 48 hours of life, no more frequently than every 6 hours. Wean ventilator settings rapidly after administration.

ADVERSE EFFECTS: Most adverse effects are associated while administering the beractant to the infant: transient bradycardia, oxygen desaturation, endotracheal tube (ET) reflux, pallor, vasoconstriction, hypotension, endotracheal blockage, hypertension, hypocarbia, hypercarbia, and apnea. Pulmonary hemorrhage has been reported, especially in very low birthweight infants.

BUMETANIDE (BUMEX)

INDICATIONS AND USE: Bumetanide is a potent loop diuretic used for the management of edema associated with congenital heart disease, congestive heart failure, and hepatic or renal disease.

ACTIONS: Inhibition of sodium and chloride in the ascending loop of Henle and proximal renal tubule. Urinary excretion of sodium, chloride, potassium, hydrogen, calcium, magnesium, ammonium, phosphate, and bicarbonate increases with bumetanide-induced diuresis. Renal blood flow increases substantially as a result of renovascular dilation and increases prostaglandin secretion.

SUPPLIED: Injection, 0.25 mg/mL(caution contains 10 mg/mL benzyl alcohol); tablets.

ROUTE: PO, IV, IM.

DOSAGE:

- **Neonates:** 0.005 to 0.05 mg/kg/dose every 6 to 24 hours.
- **Infants and children:** 0.015 mg/kg/dose up to 0.1 mg/kg/dose every 6 to 24 hours (maximum dose is 10 mg/kg/day).

ADVERSE EFFECTS: Hypokalemia, hypochloremia, hyponatremia, metabolic alkalosis, and hypotension. Potentially ototoxic but less than furosemide.

COMMENTS: Patients refractory to furosemide may respond to bumetanide for diuretic therapy. Although patients may respond differently, bumetanide is ~40 times more potent on a mg/mg basis than furosemide.

CAFFEINE CITRATE

INDICATIONS AND USE: Treatment of apnea of prematurity; postextubation and postanesthesia apnea.

ACTIONS: Similar to those of other methylxanthine drugs (eg, aminophylline and theophylline). Caffeine appears to be more active on and less toxic to the CNS and the respiratory system. Proposed mechanisms of action include increased production of adenosine 3'5' cyclic monophosphate (cAMP) alterations of intracellular calcium concentrations. Stimulates the CNS, which increases the medullary respiratory center sensitivity to carbon dioxide, stimulates central inspiratory drive, and improves diaphragmatic contractility. Caffeine exerts a positive inotropic effect on the myocardium, increases renal blood flow and glomerular filtration rate, and stimulates glycogenolysis and lipolysis.

SUPPLIED: Injection, oral solution: 20 mg/mL as caffeine citrate (10 mg/mL as caffeine base).

ROUTE: IV (not IM), PO.

DOSAGE:

- **Loading dose:** 20 mg of caffeine citrate (10 mg caffeine base) IV or PO.
- **Maintenance:** 5–8 mg/kg/day caffeine citrate (2.5–4 mg/kg/day caffeine base) as a single daily dose.

ADVERSE EFFECTS: Nausea, vomiting, gastric irritation, agitation, tachycardia (if heart rate >180 beats/minute may consider holding dose), and diuresis. Symptoms of overdosage include arrhythmias and tonic-clonic seizures.

COMMENTS: Therapeutic serum trough levels are 5–25 mcg/mL; severe toxicity is associated with levels >50 mcg/mL. Trough level should be drawn on day 5 of treatment. The serum half-life in neonates range from 40 to 230 hours and decreases with increased postnatal age; infants >9 months ~5 hours.

CALCIUM CHLORIDE (VARIOUS)

INDICATIONS AND USE: The acute treatment of symptomatic hypocalcemia; prevention of hypocalcemia; treatment of hypermagnesemia, cardiac disturbances of hyperkalemia, hypocalcemia, or calcium channel blocker toxicity.

ACTIONS: Calcium is essential for the functional integrity of the nervous, muscular, skeletal, and cardiac systems and for clotting function.

SUPPLIED: Injection, 100 mg/mL (10%, 10 mL), contains 27.2 mg (1.36 mEq) of elemental calcium and 1.35 mEq of chloride per mL.

ROUTE: IV, PO.

DOSAGE:

- **Cardiac arrest (last resort):** 20–30 mg/kg/dose (10% solution) IV every 10 minutes as needed.
- **Maintenance in infants:** 75–300 mg/kg/day IV as a continuous infusion.

ADVERSE EFFECTS: Arrhythmias (in particular, bradycardia) and deterioration of cardiovascular function. Extravasation may cause severe tissue damage (sloughing and necrosis). May potentiate digoxin-related arrhythmias. The administration of calcium chloride increases the amount of chloride intake and may increase risk of acidosis.

COMMENTS: Contraindicated in ventricular fibrillation or hypercalcemia. Use with caution in digitalized patients. Chloride salt is preferred to the gluconate form (see Calcium Gluconate) during cardiac arrest because the calcium in the chloride is already ionized, and the gluconate requires metabolism to release the calcium ion. Precipitates when mixed with sodium bicarbonate.

CALCIUM GLUCONATE

INDICATIONS AND USE: Treatment and prevention of hypocalcemia and prevention of hypocalcemia during exchange transfusion.

ACTIONS: See Calcium Chloride. Calcium gluconate must be metabolized to release calcium ion.
SUPPLIED: Injection 10% = 100 mg/mL (9.3 mg [0.46 mEq] of elemental calcium per mL).
ROUTE: IV, PO.
DOSAGE:

- **Acute treatment of symptomatic hypocalcemia:** 100 to 200 mg/kg/dose IV diluted in appropriate fluid and administered over 10 to 30 minutes.
- **Maintenance IV:** 200–800 mg/kg/day divided every 6 hours or as infusion; **maximum rate:** 50–100 mg/minute of calcium salt (gluconate). Continuous infusion is more efficacious then intermittent infusion due to less renal calcium loss.
- **Maintenance PO:** 200–800 mg/kg/day divided every 6 hours mixed in feedings.
- **Exchange transfusion:** 100 mg (1 mL of 10% solution) per 100 mL of citrated blood exchanged infused over 10 minutes.

ADVERSE EFFECTS: See Calcium Chloride. Oral administration may cause GI irritation. Dilute and use with caution in infants at risk for necrotizing enterocolitis.

CALFACTANT (INFASURF)

INDICATIONS AND USE: Prevention and treatment of neonatal respiratory distress syndrome (RDS).
ACTIONS: Natural, preservative-free calf lung extract that contains phospholipids, neutral lipids, fatty acids and surfactant-associated proteins B and C. Each milliliter of Infasurf contains 35 mg of total phospholipids and 0.65 mg of proteins (0.26 mg of protein B). Calfactant decreases the surface tension on alveolar surfaces, stabilizing the alveoli, preventing collapse. This results in improved ventilation, lung compliance, and gas exchange.
SUPPLIED: Preservative free suspension in 3 mL and 6 mL single-use vials. Store under refrigeration (2° to 8°C or 36° to 46°F).
ROUTE: Intratracheal administration through a side port adapter or through a 5F feeding catheter inserted into the endotracheal tube. Allow to warm to room temperature prior to administration. Do not shake; swirl vial to resuspend particles.
DOSAGE: **Prophylactic initial dose for respiratory distress syndrome (RDS):** As soon as possible after birth, give 3 mL/kg/dose, divided into two 1.5–mL/kg aliquots. After the instillation of each aliquot, the infant should be positioned either on the right or left side. Ventilation is continued during administration over 20 to 30 seconds. The two aliquots should be separated by a pause to evaluate respiratory status and reposition the patient. The initial dose may be followed by three subsequent doses of 3 mL/kg/dose at 12 hour intervals, if necessary.
ADVERSE EFFECTS: Bradycardia, cyanosis, airway obstruction, pneumothorax, pulmonary hemorrhage and apnea. Most adverse effects occur during administration of dose.
COMMENTS: Following administration, lung compliance and oxygenation often rapidly improve. Patients should be closely monitored and appropriate changes in ventilatory support should be made as clinically indicated.

CAPTOPRIL (CAPOTEN)

INDICATIONS AND USE: Congestive heart failure (reduction of afterload) and hypertension.
ACTIONS: Competitive inhibitor of angiotensin-converting enzyme. Causes a decrease in angiotensin II and aldosterone levels; increases plasma and tissue renin activity; decreases systemic vascular resistance without reflex tachycardia and augmentation of cardiac output.
SUPPLIED: Tablets. (Tablets can be dissolved in water and administered PO within 30 minutes, or an oral suspension can be compounded by the pharmacist.)
ROUTE: PO.
DOSAGE:

- **Newborns and premature neonates: Initial dose:** 0.01 to 0.05 mg/kg/dose every 8–12 hours; titrate dose and interval based on response.
- **Neonates: Initial dose:** 0.05–0.1 mg/kg/dose every 8 to 24 hours; titrate dose up to 0.5 mg/kg/dose every 6 to 24 hours.
- **Infants: Initial dose:** 0.15–0.3 mg/kg/dose; titrate dose up to 6 mg/kg/day divided in 1–4 doses.

ADVERSE EFFECTS: Hypotension, rash, fever, eosinophilia, neutropenia, gastrointestinal (GI) disturbances, and hyperkalemia. A low initial dose is used because some neonates experience a dramatic drop in blood pressure. Significant decreases in cerebral and renal blood flow have occurred in premature infants who have chronic hypertension and received higher doses (0.15 to 0.3 mg/kg/dose). These adverse effects have resulted in neurologic complications including seizures, apnea and lethargy, and oliguria.
COMMENTS: Administer 1 hour before or 2 hours after feedings if possible, food decreases absorption. Captopril is contraindicated in patients with bilateral renovascular disease. Use with caution in patients with low renal perfusion pressure. Reduce the dose with renal impairment and in sodium- and water-depleted patients (use with caution if on concurrent diuretic therapy).

CARBAMAZEPINE (TEGRETOL)

INDICATIONS AND USE: Anticonvulsant. Treatment of partial (especially complex partial), primary generalized tonic-clonic seizures and mixed partial or generalized seizures.
ACTIONS: Reduces polysynaptic responses and blocks the post-tetanic potentiation.

SUPPLIED: Suspension, 20 mg/mL.
ROUTE: PO. No parenteral form available.
DOSAGE: 10–20 mg/kg/day PO, initially divided four times a day. May increase weekly to optimal response, then to a maximum of 35 mg/kg/day if needed. Administer the daily dose in 3–4 divided doses. Administer with feedings.
PHARMACOKINETICS: Absorbed slowly from the gastrointestinal (GI) tract. Protein binding is 76%. Metabolized in the liver to active epoxide by cytochrome P450 3A4. Induces liver enzymes and increases its own metabolism. Eliminated 72% in urine and 28% in feces. Half-life in neonates is 8–28 hours. Therapeutic range is 4–12 mcg/mL.
ADVERSE EFFECTS:
• **Gastrointestinal:** Nausea and vomiting.
• **Hematologic:** Leukopenia, thrombocytopenia, aplastic anemia, and agranulocytosis.
• **Cardiovascular:** Congestive heart failure, heart block, and cardiovascular collapse.
• **CNS:** Dystonia, drowsiness, and behavioral changes.
• **Ophthalmic:** Eyes—scattered punctate cortical lens opacities.
• **Endocrine/metabolic:** Syndrome of inappropriate antidiuretic hormone (SIADH) and hyponatremia.
• **Hepatic:** Hepatitis and cholestasis.
• **Dermatologic:** Rash and Stevens-Johnson syndrome.
• **Genitourinary:** Urine retention, azotemia, oliguria, and anuria.
Monitor complete blood cell count (CBC), liver function, and urinalysis; perform periodic eye exam. Do not discontinue abruptly because seizures may result in epileptic patients.
COMMENTS: Avoid switching between Tegretol and generic carbamazepine if possible, because changes in carbamazepine serum concentration and seizure activity may result; monitor serum concentrations. Interactions are numerous. Erythromycin, isoniazid, and cimetidine may inhibit hepatic metabolism of carbamazepine, resulting in increased carbamazepine serum concentrations. Concurrent phenobarbital may lower carbamazepine serum levels. Carbamazepine may induce metabolism of warfarin, phenytoin, theophylline, benzodiazepines, and corticosteroids. Thyroid function tests may show decreased values with carbamazepine.

CEFAZOLIN SODIUM (ANCEF, KEFZOL)

ACTION AND SPECTRUM: Cefazolin is a first-generation cephalosporin. It is a broad-spectrum semisynthetic β-lactam antibiotic that exerts its bactericidal activity by virtue of its inhibition of cell wall synthesis. It demonstrates good activity against Gram-positive cocci (except enterococci), including penicillinase-producing staphylococci; Gram-negative coverage includes *Escherichia coli*, most *Klebsiella* spp., many strains of *Haemophilus influenzae*, and indole-positive *Proteus* spp. Organism resistance is primarily due to elaboration of β-lactamases, which inactivate the antibiotic through hydrolysis.
SUPPLIED: Injection.
ROUTE: IM, IV (infuse over 20–30 minutes).
DOSAGE:
• **Neonates:**
  • **Postnatal age ≤7 days:** 40 mg/kg/day divided every 12 hours.
  • **Postnatal age >7 days:**
    • **≤2000 g:** 40 mg/kg/day divided every 12 hours.
    • **>2000 g:** 60 mg/kg/day divided every 8 hours.
• **Infants and children:** 50–100 mg/kg/day divided every 8 hours; **maximum dose:** 6 g/day.
PHARMOCOKINETICS: 80 to 100% excreted unchanged in urine. Half-life is 3 to 5 hours in neonates.
ADVERSE EFFECTS: Infrequent except for allergic reactions, including fever, rash, and urticaria. May cause leukopenia, thrombocytopenia, and a positive Coombs test reaction. Excessive dosage (especially in renal impairment) may result in CNS irritation with seizure activity.
COMMENTS: Use with caution in patients with a history of severe allergic reactions to penicillins. Dosage reduction is required in moderate to severe renal failure. Contains 2 mEq of sodium/g.

CEFOTAXIME SODIUM (CLAFORAN)

ACTION AND SPECTRUM: Cefotaxime is a third-generation cephalosporin with a mechanism of action identical to that of other β-lactam antibiotics, and it is bactericidal. Chiefly active against Gram-negative organisms (except *Pseudomonas* spp.), including *Escherichia coli*, *Enterobacter* spp., *Klebsiella* spp., *Haemophilus influenzae* (including ampicillin-resistant strains), *Proteus mirabilis*, and indole-positive *Proteus* spp., *Serratia marcescens*, *Neisseria gonorrhoeae*, and *Neisseria meningitidis*. Generally poor activity against Gram-positive aerobic organisms.
SUPPLIED: Injection.
ROUTE: IM, IV (infuse over 30 minutes).
DOSAGE:
• **Neonates: 0–4 weeks: <1200 g:** 100 mg/kg/day divided every 12 hours.
• **Postnatal age ≤7 days:**
  • **1200–2000 g:** 100 mg/kg/day divided every 12 hours.
  • **>2000 g:** 100–150 mg/kg/day divided every 8–12 hours.

- **Postnatal age >7 days:**
  - **1200–2000 g:** 150 mg/kg/day divided every 8 hours.
  - **>2000 g:** 150–200 mg/kg/day divided every 6–8 hours.
- **Infants and children 1 month to 12 years:**
  - **<50 kg:** 100–200 mg/kg/day divided every 6–8 hours.
  - **Meningitis:** 200 mg/kg/day divided every 6 hours; 225–300 mg/kg/day divided every 6–8 hours has been used to treat invasive pneumococcal meningitis.
  - **≥50 kg:**
    - **Moderate to severe infection:** 1–2 g every 6–8 hours.
    - **Life-threatening infection:** 2 g/dose every 4 hours.
    - **Maximum dose:** 12 g/day.
- **Disseminated gonococcal infection and scalp abscesses:** The Centers for Disease Control and Prevention recommends cefotaxime as an alternative to ceftriaxone in the treatment of disseminated gonococcal infection and gonococcal scalp abscesses in newborns. The dose of cefotaxime is 25 mg/kg in a single daily dose IM or IV for 7 days; duration is 10 to 14 days for meningitis.
- **Gonococcal ophthalmia prophylaxis in newborns of mothers with gonorrhea at delivery:** 100 mg/kg IV or IM as a single dose (topical antibiotic therapy alone is inadequate).

PHARMACOKINETICS: Excreted principally unchanged in the urine. Half-life in neonates is 1 to 4 hours.

ADVERSE EFFECTS: Hypersensitivity reactions, serum sickness–like reaction with prolonged administration, and positive Coombs test. Leukopenia, eosinophilia, granulocytopenia. Hepatic and renal dysfunction have been reported.

COMMENTS: Should be reserved for suspected or documented Gram-negative meningitis or sepsis. When used as empiric therapy, combine with ampicillin or aqueous penicillin G to provide Gram-positive coverage (ie, group B streptococci, pneumococci, and *Listeria monocytogenes*). High degree of stability to β-lactamases. Third-generation cephalosporins have been proven to induce the emergence of multidrug-resistant bacteria when used excessively and without proper clinical indications. Contains 2.2 mEq of sodium/g.

CEFOXITIN (MEFOXIN)

INDICATIONS AND USE: Treatment of infections from Gram-negative enteric organisms, ampicillin-resistant *Haemophilus influenzae*, and anaerobic bacteria, including *Bacteroides fragilis* spp.

ACTIONS: A second-generation cephalosporin with bactericidal activity that inhibits bacterial cell wall synthesis by binding to one or more of the penicillin-binding proteins. Cefoxitin exhibits enhanced activity against anaerobic bacteria.

SUPPLIED: Vials, powder for injection.

ROUTE: IV, IM.

DOSAGE:
- **Neonates:** 90–100 mg/kg/day divided every 8 hours.
- **Infants ≥3 months and children:**
  - **Mild-moderate infection:** 80–100 mg/kg/day divided every 6–8 hours.
  - **Severe infection:** 100–160 mg/kg/day divided every 4–6 hours; **maximum dose:** 12 g/day.

PHARMACOKINETICS: Highly protein bound and renally excreted essentially unchanged.

ADVERSE EFFECTS: Usually well tolerated. May cause rash, thrombophlebitis, a positive direct Coombs test, eosinophilia, and increase in liver enzymes.

COMMENTS: Not inactivated by β-lactamase. Has poor CNS penetration.

CEFTAZIDIME (FORTAZ, TAZIDIME)

ACTION AND SPECTRUM: A broad-spectrum third-generation cephalosporin with bactericidal activity due to its inhibition of bacterial cell wall synthesis. It possesses good activity against Gram-negative aerobic bacteria, including *Neisseria meningitidis*, *Haemophilus influenzae*, and most of the Enterobacteriaceae. It exhibits excellent activity against *Pseudomonas aeruginosa*, which is superior to other third-generation cephalosporins. Aminoglycosides act synergistically with ceftazidime against *Pseudomonas*. It exhibits poor Gram-positive activity compared with first-generation cephalosporins and little activity against *Listeria monocytogenes* and enterococci.

SUPPLIED: Injection.

ROUTE: IM, IV (infuse over 20–30 minutes).

DOSAGE:
- **Neonates:**
  - **0–4 weeks:** <1200 g: 100 mg/kg/day divided every 12 hours.
  - **Postnatal age ≤7 days:**
    - **1200–2000 g:** 100 mg/kg/day divided every 12 hours.
    - **>2000 g:** 100–150 mg/kg/day divided every 8–12 hours.
  - **Postnatal age >7 days:** ≥1200 g: 150 mg/kg/day divided every 8 hours.
- **Infants and children 1 month to 12 years:** 100–150 mg/kg/day divided every 8 hours; **maximum dose:** 6 g/day.
  - **Meningitis:** 150 mg/kg/day divided every 8 hours; maximum dose, 6 g/day.

PHARMACOKINETICS: Renal (glomerular filtration), 80–90% excreted unchanged. Half-life is 2.2–4.7 hours.
ADVERSE EFFECTS: Infrequent except for allergic reactions, including fever, rash, and urticaria. May cause transient leukopenia, neutropenia, and thrombocytopenia; a direct positive Coombs test; and transient elevation in the liver function test.
COMMENTS: Penetrates well into cerebral spinal fluid (CSF); concentrations ~25–50% of serum concentrations. Also may be used as an alternative to aminoglycosides for *P. aeruginosa* therapy, particularly in patients with renal failure.

CEFTRIAXONE SODIUM (ROCEPHIN)
ACTION AND SPECTRUM: Third-generation cephalosporin, with a mechanism of action is identical to that of other β-lactam antibiotics. High degree of stability to β-lactamases and good activity against both Gram-negative and Gram-positive organisms except *Pseudomonas* spp., enterococci, methicillin-resistant staphylococci, and *Listeria monocytogenes*. Has longest serum half-life of all currently available cephalosporins.
SUPPLIED: Injection.
ROUTE: IM, IV (infuse over 30 minutes).
DOSAGE:

- **Neonates:**
  - **Postnatal age ≤7 days:** 50 mg/kg/day given every 24 hours.
  - **Postnatal age >7 days:**
    - **≤2000 g:** 50 mg/kg/day given every 24 hours.
    - **>2000 g:** 50–75 mg/kg/day given every 24 hours.
  - **Gonococcal prophylaxis:** 25–50 mg/kg as a single dose (dose not to exceed 125 mg).
  - **Gonococcal infection:** 25–50 mg/kg/day (maximum dose: 125 mg) given every 24 hours for 7 days, up to 10–14 days if meningitis is documented. (*Note:* Use cefotaxime in place of ceftriaxone in hyperbilirubinemic neonates.)
- **Infants and children:** 50–75 mg/kg/day divided every 12–24 hours.
  - **Meningitis:** 80–100 mg/kg/day divided every 12–24 hours; loading dose of 75 mg/kg may be administered at the start of therapy; **maximum dose:** 4 g/day.

PHARMACOKINETICS: Both biliary and renal excretion. Half-life is 5–19 hours.
ADVERSE EFFECTS: Mild diarrhea and eosinophilia are most common. May also cause neutropenia, rash, thrombophlebitis, and bacterial (gastrointestinal) or fungal overgrowth. Rare reports of increased prothrombin times. Increases free and erythrocyte-bound bilirubin in premature infants with hyperbilirubinemia; use with caution in infants with hyperbilirubinemia.
COMMENTS: *Warning:* Ceftriaxone is incompatible with calcium-containing solutions. Calcium-containing solutions or products must not be administered within 48 hours of the ceftriaxone dose due to the fatal reaction involving calcium-ceftriaxone precipitates in the lungs and kidneys of neonates. Many clinical studies support once-daily dosing. Do not use as the sole drug in infections caused by staphylococci or pseudomonas. Combine with ampicillin for initial empiric therapy of meningitis (ceftriaxone has poor activity against *Listeria* spp.). Generally, no dosage reduction is required in renal or hepatic dysfunction. Contains 3.6 mEq of sodium/g.

CEFUROXIME SODIUM (KEFUROX, ZINACEF)
ACTION AND SPECTRUM: Second-generation cephalosporin with a mechanism of action identical to that of other β-lactam antibiotics. Active against both Gram-positive and Gram-negative organisms, including streptococci (except enterococci), both penicillinase-producing and nonpenicillinase-producing staphylococci (not including methicillin-resistant staphylococci), *Escherichia coli*, *Haemophilus influenzae* (including ampicillin-resistant strains), *Klebsiella* spp., *Neisseria gonorrhoeae*, *Neisseria meningitidis*, *Proteus mirabilis*, *Salmonella* spp., *Shigella* spp., and *Enterobacter* spp.
SUPPLIED: Injection.
ROUTE: IM, IV (IV preferred; infuse over 30 minutes).
DOSAGE: IM, IV:

- **Neonates:** 50–100 mg/kg/day divided every 12 hours.
- **Children:** 75–150 mg/kg/day divided every 8 hours; maximum dose: 6 g/day.
- **Meningitis:** Not recommended due to reports of treatment failures and slower bacteriologic response time.

PHARMACOKINETICS: Primarily excreted unchanged in the urine. Half-life is 5.1–5.8 hours in infants <3 days old and 1–4.2 hours in infants >8 days of age.
ADVERSE EFFECTS: Generally free of adverse effects; but may cause hypersensitivity reactions, thrombophlebitis, elevated serum transaminases, mildly elevated blood urea nitrogen (BUN), diarrhea, and, rarely, blood dyscrasias (transient neutropenia, leukopenia, and thrombocytopenia).
COMMENTS: Provides no activity against *Listeria* spp., so ampicillin should be added in initial empiric therapy. Has added Gram-negative coverage over first-generation cephalosporins while retaining very good Gram-positive coverage. Decrease the dosage in renal failure. Contains 2.4 mEq of sodium/g. Limited experience in neonates.

CHLORAL HYDRATE (AQUACHLORAL SUPPRETTES, NOCTEC)

ACTIONS: CNS depressant. Mechanism of action not completely understood. Usual doses produce mild CNS depression and quiet, deep sleep; higher doses can result in general anesthesia with concurrent respiratory depression.

SUPPLIED: Syrup (contains sodium benzoate; benzoic acid [benzoate] is a metabolite of benzyl alcohol), suppositories.

ROUTE: PO, PR.

DOSAGE: Use the lowest effective dose.

• Usual dose: 25–50 mg/kg/dose PO or PR every 6–8 hours as needed.

• Sedation prior to electroencephalography and other procedures: 25–75 mg/kg/dose once PO or PR. Usually, 50 mg/kg/dose once, with orders to repeat with 25 mg/kg/dose once if needed.

ADVERSE EFFECTS: Gastrointestinal irritation resulting in nausea, vomiting, and diarrhea; paradoxic excitation; and respiratory depression, particularly if administered with opiates and barbiturates. May cause direct hyperbilirubinemia with chronic use (active metabolite 2,2,2 Trichloroethanol [TCE]); competes with bilirubin for glucuronide conjugation in the liver); overdose can be lethal.

COMMENTS: Contraindicated with marked renal or hepatic impairment.

CHLORAMPHENICOL (CHLOROMYCETIN)

ACTION AND SPECTRUM: A broad-spectrum antimicrobial bacteriostatic agent. Interferes with or inhibits protein synthesis. May be bactericidal for *Haemophilus influenzae* and *Neisseria meningitidis*. Bacteriostatic for *Escherichia coli; Klebsiella* spp.; *Serratia* spp.; *Enterobacter* spp.; *Salmonella* spp.; *Shigella* spp.; *Neisseria gonorrhoeae;* staphylococci; *Streptococcus pneumoniae;* and groups A, B, C, nonenterococcal D, and G streptococci.

SUPPLIED: Injection.

ROUTE: IV push over 5 minutes at a maximum concentration of 100 mg/mL; IV intermittent infusion over 15–30 minutes at a final concentration of < 20 mg/mL. IM not recommended.

DOSAGE:

• Neonates:

• Loading dose: 20 mg/kg IV.

• Maintenance dose: 12 hours after the loading dose.

• ≤7 days: 25 mg/kg/day once every 24 hours.

• >7 days, ≤2000 g: 25 mg/kg/day once every 24 hours.

• >7 days, >2000 g: 50 mg/kg/day divided every 12 hours.

• Infants and children:

• Meningitis: 75–100 mg/kg/day IV divided every 6 hours.

• Other infections: Usual dose: 50–75 mg/kg/day IV divided every 6 hours. Maximum daily dose: 4 g/day.

PHARMACOKINETICS: Metabolized by the liver. Half-life is 10–24 hours.

ADVERSE EFFECTS: Idiosyncratic reactions result in aplastic anemia (irreversible and rare), reversible bone marrow suppression (dose-related), allergy (rash and fever), diarrhea, vomiting, stomatitis, glossitis, *Candida* superinfection, and "gray baby" syndrome (early signs are hyperammonemia and unexplained metabolic acidosis; other signs are abdominal distention, hypotonia, gray skin color, and cardiorespiratory collapse). Use with extreme caution in neonates.

COMMENTS: Avoid use where possible. Must monitor serum levels. Desired peak is 10–25 mcg/mL; levels >50 mcg/mL are strongly associated with "gray baby" syndrome. Monitor complete blood count (CBC) with differential, platelet count, and reticulocyte count every 3 days.

CHLOROTHIAZIDE (DIURIL)

INDICATIONS AND USE: Fluid overload, pulmonary edema, and hypertension.

ACTIONS: The thiazide diuretics inhibit sodium reabsorption in the distal renal tubules. Sodium, potassium, bicarbonate, magnesium, phosphate, and chloride excretion are increased, whereas calcium excretion is decreased. Duration of action of chlorothiazide and hydrochlorothiazide is 6–12 hours; onset of action is within 2 hours and peak action is at 3–6 hours.

SUPPLIED: Suspension, injection.

ROUTE: PO, IV.

DOSAGE: *Note:* IV dosage in infants and children has not been established. These IV doses in infants and children are based on anecdotal reports. The lower IV dosing regimens have been extrapolated from the oral dosing regimens and the fact that only 10% to 20% of an oral dose is absorbed.

• Neonates and infants <6 months: Oral: 20 to 40 mg/kg/day PO divided every 12 hours; maximum: 375 mg/day. IV: 2 to 8 mg/kg/day IV divided every 12 hours; doses up to 20 mg/kg/day have been used.

• Infants >6 months and children: Oral: 20 mg/kg/day PO divided every 12 hours; maximum: 1 g/day. IV: 4 mg/kg/day IV divided in 1–2 doses; doses up to 20 mg/kg/day have been used.

ADVERSE EFFECTS: Hypokalemia, hypochloremic alkalosis, dehydration and prerenal azotemia, hyperuricemia, hyperglycemia, hypermagnesemia, hyperlipidemia.

COMMENTS: Do not use in patients with anuria or hepatic dysfunction.

CHOLESTYRAMINE RESIN (QUESTRAN)

INDICATIONS AND USE: A resin-binding agent in patients with chronic diarrhea and short-gut syndrome to decrease fecal output.

ACTION: Cholestyramine resin binds to bile acids in the intestine, forms a nonabsorbable complex preventing the reabsorption and enterohepatic recirculation of bile salts, and releases chloride ions in the process.

SUPPLIED: Powder.

ROUTE: PO.

DOSAGE: Children: 240 mg/kg/day in 3 divided doses. Titrate dose depending on the indication.

PHARMACOKINETICS: Not absorbed; excreted in the feces.

ADVERSE EFFECTS: Constipation. High doses can cause hyperchloremic acidosis and increase urinary calcium excretion.

COMMENTS: May bind concurrent oral medications, in particular levothyroxine.

CIMETIDINE (TAGAMET)

INDICATIONS AND USE: Prevention and treatment of duodenal and gastric ulcers, gastroesophageal reflux, esophagitis and hypersecretory conditions.

ACTIONS: A histamine (H_2) receptor antagonist; competitively inhibits the action of histamine on the gastric parietal cells, decreasing gastric acid secretion.

SUPPLIED: Oral liquid, injection.

ROUTE: IV, PO.

DOSAGE:

- **Neonates:** 5–10 mg/kg/day IV/PO divided every 8–12 hours.
- **Infants:** 10–20 mg/kg/day IV/PO divided every 6–12 hours.
- **Children:** 20–40 mg/kg/day IV/PO divided every 6 hours.

ADVERSE EFFECTS: CNS toxicity such as agitation and alterations in consciousness, antiandrogenic effects; elevated AST, ALT and creatinine levels.

Cimetidine reduces the hepatic metabolism of drugs metabolized by the cytochrome P450 pathway, which may result in decreased elimination of diazepam, theophylline, phenytoin, metronidazole, propranolol, carbamazepine, and metoclopramide. Doses of these drugs may need to be decreased.

COMMENTS: Limited use in neonates. May add daily IV dose to the parenteral nutrition solution and infuse over 24 hours to avoid the need intermittent administration.

CITRATE AND CITRIC ACIDS SOLUTIONS (SHOHL'S SOLUTION, MODIFIED)

INDICATIONS AND USE: Treatment of metabolic acidosis or as a urinary alkalinizing agent for conditions that require the maintenance of alkaline urine.

ACTIONS: Sodium and potassium citrate salts have the capability to buffer gastric acidity (pH >2.5) and are metabolized to bicarbonate and act as systemic alkalinizers.

SUPPLIED:

- Oral solutions:
  - **Bicitra and Oracit:** 1 mEq of sodium and 1 mEq of bicarbonate equivalent per mL.
  - **Polycitra:** 1 mEq of sodium and 1 mEq of potassium and 2 mEq of bicarbonate equivalents per mL.
  - **Polycitra-K:** 2 mEq of potassium and 2 mEq of bicarbonate equivalents per mL.

ROUTE: Oral.

DOSAGE: 2–3 mEq/kg/day in divided doses 3–4 times per day with water.

ADVERSE EFFECTS: Tetany, metabolic alkalosis, hypernatremia (if sodium salt used), hypocalcemia, hyperkalemia (if potassium salt used), diarrhea, nausea, vomiting.

COMMENTS: Conversion to bicarbonate may be impaired in patients with hepatic failure.

CLINDAMYCIN (CLEOCIN)

ACTION AND SPECTRUM: Inhibits protein synthesis; bacteriostatic (primarily) or bactericidal activity depending on drug concentration, infection site, and organism. Active against both aerobic and anaerobic streptococci (except enterococci), most staphylococci (except methicillin-resistant strains), *Bacteroides* spp. (except *Bacteroides melaninogenicus*), *Fusobacterium* spp., *Actinomyces israelii, Clostridium perfringens,* and *Clostridium tetani.* Chiefly used against the above anaerobes. Ineffective against Gram-negative organisms or many clostridial species.

SUPPLIED: Injection, oral solution.

ROUTE: PO, IM, IV (infuse over 10–20 minutes).

DOSAGE:

- **Neonates:**
  - **Postnatal age ≤7 days:**
    - **≤2000 g:** 10 mg/kg/day IM/IV divided every 12 hours.
    - **>2000 g:** 15 mg/kg/day IM/IV divided every 8 hours.
  - **Postnatal age >7 days:**
    - **<1200 g:** 10 mg/kg/day IM/IV divided every 12 hours.

- **1200–2000 g:** 15 mg/kg/day IM/IV divided every 8 hours.
- **>2000 g:** 20–30 mg/kg/day IM/IV divided every 6–8 hours.
- **Infants and children:** 10–30 mg/kg/day PO divided every 6–8 hours; maximum dose: 1.8 g/day or 25–40 mg/kg/day IM/IV divided every 6–8 hours; doses as high as 4.8 g/day have been given IV in life-threatening situations.

PHARMACOKINETICS: Primarily hepatic metabolism.

ADVERSE EFFECTS: Sterile abscess formation at the IM injection site. Vomiting and diarrhea frequently occur. Pseudomembranous colitis resulting from suppression of normal flora and overgrowth of *Clostridium difficile* is uncommon but potentially fatal (treated with oral vancomycin or metronidazole). Rash, glossitis, and pruritus occur occasionally. Serum sickness, anaphylaxis, hematologic (granulocytopenia and thrombocytopenia), and hepatic abnormalities rarely occur.

COMMENTS: Does not cross the blood-brain barrier; therefore, do not use to treat meningitis.

CLONAZEPAM (KLONOPIN)

INDICATIONS AND USE: For the treatment of petit mal, Lennox-Gastaut, infantile spasms, and akinetic and myoclonic seizures, either as a single agent or as adjunctive therapy.

ACTIONS: Depresses all levels of the CNS including the limbic and reticular formation by binding to the benzodiazepine site on the gamma-aminobutyric acid (GABA) receptor complex; suppresses the spike-and-wave discharge in absence seizures by depressing nerve transmission in the motor cortex.

SUPPLIED: Tablets, orally disintegrating wafer. (An oral suspension may be prepared by pharmacist.)

ROUTE: Oral.

DOSAGE: Seizure disorders:

- **Infants and children <10 years or 30 kg:**
  - **Initial daily dose:** 0.01–0.03 mg/kg/day PO (maximum 0.05 mg/kg/day) given in 2–3 divided doses; increase by no more than 0.5 mg every third day until seizures are controlled or adverse effects occur.
  - **Maintenance:** 0.1–0.2 mg/kg/day PO divided into three doses; do not exceed 0.2 mg/kg/day.

PHARMACOKINETICS: Cytochrome P450 isoenzyme CYP3A3/4 substrate CNS depressants increase sedation; phenytoin, carbamazepine, rifampin, or barbiturates increase clonazepam clearance; drugs that inhibit cytochrome P450 isoenzyme CYP3A3/4 may increase levels and effects of clonazepam (monitor for altered benzodiazepine response); concurrent use with valproic acid may result in absence status.

ADVERSE EFFECTS: Hypotension, drowsiness, hypotonia, thrombocytopenia, anemia, leukopenia, eosinophilia, tremor, choreiform movements, bronchial hypersecretion, respiratory depression.

COMMENTS: Use with caution in patients with chronic respiratory disease, hepatic disease, or impaired renal function. Abrupt discontinuation of clonazepam may precipitate withdrawal symptoms, status epilepticus, or seizures. (Withdraw gradually when discontinuing therapy in children, the clonazepam dose may be safely reduced by ≤0.04 mg/kg/week and discontinued when the daily dose is ≤0.04 mg/kg/day.) Worsening of seizures may occur when clonazepam is added to patients with multiple seizure types.

CLONIDINE (CATAPRES; CATAPRES-TTS)

INDICATIONS AND USE: Management of hypertension (not commonly used in infants), neonatal abstinence syndrome, and iatrogenic narcotic dependency and an aid in the diagnosis of pheochromocytoma and growth hormone deficiency. Although preliminary data show that clonidine produces a dramatic reduction in the severity of neonatal withdrawal symptoms, more experience is needed before clonidine is routinely used to treat opioid withdrawal in infants. Use with caution and monitor infant for hypotension.

ACTIONS: Stimulates CNS α_2-adrenergic receptors. Results in decreased sympathetic outflow, peripheral vascular resistance, systolic and diastolic blood pressure, and heart rate. Clonidine reduces circulating plasma renin levels. Single doses of the drug produce pronounced increase in growth hormone concentration in normal children, but not in growth hormone–deficient children.

SUPPLIED: Tablet; an oral suspension can be prepared by the pharmacist.

ROUTE: PO, transdermal.

DOSAGE: Use the lowest effective dose. Reduce dose in renal dysfunction.

- **Hypertension:** 5–10 mcg/kg/day PO divided every 8–12 hours. May increase dose gradually if needed, allowing 5–7 days between dose adjustments, to 5–25 mcg/kg/day in divided doses every 6 hours; **maximum dose:** 0.9 mg/day.

- **Opioid withdrawal:** 3 to 5 mcg/kg/day divided every 4 to 6 hours. **Maximum dose:** 5 mcg/kg/day PO divided every 6 hours. **Weaning:** wean gradually over 1–2 weeks. Adjust the dose to avoid hypotension and oversedation; individualize dose per patient tolerance.

- **Growth hormone provocation test:** 0.1–0.15 mg/m^2 PO as a single dose. Levels for growth hormone are usually drawn in blood samples 30, 60, and 90 minutes after PO clonidine. Monitor for drowsiness, pallor, and hypotension.

- **Transdermal:** Children may be switched to the transdermal delivery system after oral therapy is titrated to an optimal and stable dose; a transdermal dose equal to the total oral daily dose may be used. Patches are applied at bedtime to a clean, hairless area of the upper arm or chest; rotate sites weekly; children may need the patch changed more frequently (eg, every 3–5 days). *Note:* Transdermal patch is a membrane-controlled system; do not cut the patch to deliver partial doses; rate of drug delivery, reservoir contents, and adhesion may be affected if cut; if partial dose is needed, surface area of patch can be blocked proportionally using adhesive bandage.

ADVERSE EFFECTS: Hypotension, bradycardia; severe rebound hypertension with abrupt discontinuation (or missing several consecutive doses) discontinue gradually over more than a week; drowsiness, weakness, anxiety, hypothermia; dry mouth, gastrointestinal upset; urine retention; decrease in plasma renin activity in hyperreninemic patients; rash; thrombocytopenia (rare); transient weight gain resulting from sodium and water retention. Infants and children may be especially sensitive to the effects of clonidine; use with caution.

COMMENTS: Overdose can cause CNS depression, apnea, bradycardia, arrhythmia, profound hypotension, transient hypertension, hyporeflexia, hypothermia, miosis, irritability, and dry mouth. Observe for excessive CNS and/or respiratory depression. Monitor blood pressure, heart rate, and rhythm. Ensure that the drug is not abruptly discontinued.

COSYNTROPIN (CORTROSYN)

INDICATIONS AND USE: Aid in the diagnosis of adrenocortical insufficiency; used in the diagnosis of congenital adrenal hyperplasia.

ACTIONS: Stimulates the adrenal cortex to secrete cortisol (hydrocortisone and cortisone), androgenic substances, and a small amount of aldosterone.

SUPPLIED: Injection, 0.25 mg/vial; dilution: 0.25 mg/mL.

ROUTE: IM, IV (infuse initial dilution over 2 minutes).

DOSAGE:

- **Adrenocortical insufficiency:**
  - **Preterm neonates:** Not well defined; 0.1 mcg/kg, 0.2 mcg/kg and 3.5 mcg/kg used.
  - **Neonates:** 0.015 mg/kg (1 dose only).
  - **Children ≤2 years:** 0.125 mg.
- **Congenital adrenal hyperplasia evaluation:** 1 mg/m^2/dose up to a maximum of 1 mg.

COMMENTS: For rapid diagnostic screening of adrenocortical insufficiency, plasma cortisol concentrations should be measured immediately before and exactly 30 minutes after administration of cosyntropin; 0.25 mg of cosyntropin = 25 USP units of corticotropin.

DEXAMETHASONE (DECADRON)

INDICATIONS: Treatment of airway edema prior to extubation. Used in infants with bronchopulmonary dysplasia to facilitate weaning from the ventilator.

ACTIONS: Long-acting, potent glucocorticoid without mineralocorticoid properties that prevents or suppresses inflammation and immune responses when administered at pharmacological doses. Actions include inhibition of leukocyte infiltration at the site of inflammation, interference in the function of mediators of inflammatory response, and suppression of humoral immune responses. Some of the net effects include reduction in edema, scar tissue, reversal of increased capillary permeability, and a general suppression in immune response. The degree of clinical effect is normally related to the dose administered.

SUPPLIED: Injection; oral solution.

ROUTE: IV, IM, PO.

DOSAGE:

- **Neonates:**
  - **Airway edema or extubation:**
    - **Usual dose:** 0.25 mg/kg/dose IV given ~4 hours prior to scheduled extubation and then every 8 hours for 3 doses total.
    - **Range:** 0.25–1 mg/kg/dose for 1–3 doses.
    - **Maximum dose:** 1 mg/kg/day.
    - *Note:* A longer duration of therapy may be needed with more severe cases.
  - **Bronchopulmonary dysplasia (to facilitate ventilator weaning):**
    - **Numerous dosing schedules** have been proposed.
    - **Range:** 0.5–0.6 mg/kg/day given in divided doses PO or IV every 12 hours for 3–7 days, then taper over 1–6 weeks.

ADVERSE EFFECTS: With long-term use, increased susceptibility to infection, osteoporosis, growth retardation, hyperglycemia, fluid and electrolyte disturbances, cataracts, myopathy, gastrointestinal perforation and hemorrhage, hypertension, and acute adrenal insufficiency. Dexamethasone use for low birthweight infants has come under close scrutiny because of increasing numbers of reports indicating neurodevelopmental compromise (see Comments).

COMMENTS: Please review the important statement from the American Academy of Pediatrics, Committee on Fetus and Newborn, and Canadian Pediatric Society, Fetus and Newborn Committee: Postnatal corticosteroids to treat or prevent chronic lung disease in preterm infants. *Pediatrics* 2002;109:330-338.

DIAZEPAM (VALIUM)

INDICATIONS: Alternative choice to lorazepam for the treatment of status epilepticus. Treatment of seizures refractory to other combined anticonvulsant agents. Reduces anxiety, and can use as a preoperative sedation.

ACTIONS: Exact action is unknown; appears to act as a CNS depressant producing sedation, hypnotic, skeletal muscle relaxant, and anticonvulsant effects. Like other benzodiazepines, diazepam increases the activity of the inhibitory neurotransmitter gamma-aminobutyric acid (GABA) by binding the benzodiazepine receptor sites in the CNS.

SUPPLIED: Injection, oral solution.

ROUTE: IV, PO.

DOSAGE:
- **Status epilepticus:**
  - **Neonates:** (Not recommended as first line; injection contains benzoic acid, benzyl alcohol, and sodium benzoate) 0.1–0.3 mg/kg/dose IV given over 3–5 minutes, every 15–30 minutes to a maximum total dose of 2 mg.
  - **Infants >30 days and children <5 years:** 0.05–0.3 mg/kg/dose given over 3–5 minutes, every 15–30 minutes to a maximum total dose of 5 mg or 0.2–0.5 mg/dose every 2–5 minutes to a maximum total dose of 5 mg; repeat in 2–4 hours as needed.
- **Conscious sedation for procedures:** 0.1–0.3 mg/kg IV or PO (maximum dose: 10 mg) 45–60 minutes prior to procedure.
- **Sedation or muscle relaxation or anxiety:**
  - **Oral:** 0.12–0.8 mg/kg/day in divided doses every 6–8 hours
  - **IV:** 0.04–0.3 mg/kg/dose every 2–4 hours to a maximum of 0.6 mg/kg within an 8-hour period if needed.

ADVERSE EFFECTS: May cause rash, vasodilation, bradycardia, respiratory arrest, and hypotension. Use with caution in patients receiving other CNS depressants, may have additive CNS and respiratory depressant effects.

COMMENTS: Observe for and be prepared to manage respiratory arrest. Rapid IV push may cause sudden respiratory depression, apnea, or hypotension. Use of the rectal gel formulation in infants <6 months is not recommended; use in children <2 years, the safety and efficacy have not been studied.

DIAZOXIDE (HYPERSTAT IV, PROGLYCEM)

INDICATIONS AND USE: Persistent hyperinsulinemic neonatal hypoglycemia (oral) and hypertensive crisis (IV).

ACTIONS: Nondiuretic thiazide with antihypertensive and hyperglycemic effects. Inhibits the release of insulin from the pancreas and reduces total peripheral vascular resistance by direct relaxation of arteriolar smooth muscle which results in a decrease in blood pressure and reflex increase in heart rate and cardiac output.

SUPPLIED: Oral suspension, injection.

ROUTE: IV, PO.

DOSAGE:
- **Hyperinsulinemic hypoglycemia:** 8–15 mg/kg/day PO in 2–3 divided doses every 8–12 hours.
- **Hypertensive crisis:** 1–3 mg/kg/dose IV may repeat every 5–15 minutes until blood pressure adequately reduced. (Maximum 5 mg/kg/dose.) Repeat every 4–24 hours; monitor blood pressure closely. Maximum total 150 mg/dose.

ADVERSE EFFECTS: When given for short periods, adverse effects are rare. Tachycardia; sodium and fluid retention is common. May cause bilirubin displacement from albumin, hypotension, hyperglycemia, hyperuricemia, rash, fever, leukopenia, thrombocytopenia, and ketosis. May cause pain, burning, cellulitis/phlebitis upon extravasation. (The pH of parenteral solution is 11.6.)

DIGIBIND (DIGOXIN IMMUNE FAB)

INDICATIONS AND USE: Treatment of potentially life-threatening digoxin or digitoxin toxicity in carefully selected patients; use in life-threatening ventricular arrhythmias secondary to digoxin, acute digoxin ingestion (ie, >4 mg in children), and hyperkalemia (serum potassium >5 mEq/L) in the setting of digoxin toxicity.

ACTIONS: Binds with molecules of free (unbound) digoxin or digitoxin and then is removed from the body by renal excretion.

SUPPLIED: Injection, powder for reconstitution—Digibind, 38 mg.

ROUTE: IV.

DOSAGE:
- **Determine the dose by determining the total body load of digoxin (TBL) using either method 1 or method 2.**
  - **Method 1:** An approximation of the amount ingested:
    - TBL of digoxin (in mg) = C (in ng/mL) × 5.6 × body weight (in kg)/1000 or TBL = mg of digoxin ingested (as tablets or elixir) × 0.8.
    - Dose of Digibind (in mg) IV = TBL × 76.
    - Dose of digoxin immune Fab (Digibind) (number of vials) IV = TBL/0.5.
  - **Method 2:** A postdistribution serum digoxin concentration C determination.
    - Dose estimates of digoxin immune Fab based on serum digoxin concentration infants and children:

Patient weight 1 kg and serum digoxin concentration:	Patient weight 3 kg and serum digoxin concentration:	Patient weight 5 kg and serum digoxin concentration:
1 ng/mL: 0.4 mg^2	1 ng/mL: 1 mg^2	1 ng/mL: 2 mg^2
2 ng/mL: 1 mg^2	2 ng/mL: 2–2.5 mg^2	2 ng/mL: 4 mg
4 ng/mL: 1.5 mg^2	4 ng/mL: 5 mg	4 ng/mL: 8 mg
8 ng/mL: 3 mg	8 ng/mL: 9–10 mg	8 ng/mL: 15–16 mg
12 ng/mL: 5 mg	12 ng/mL: 14 mg	12 ng/mL: 23–24 mg
16 ng/mL: 6–6.5 mg	16 ng/mL: 18–19 mg	16 ng/mL: 30–32 mg
20 ng/mL: 8 mg	20 ng/mL: 23–24 mg	20 ng/mL: 38–40 mg

- **Acute digoxin toxicity:**
  - Ingestion of known amount of digoxin, each vial (38 mg) IV binds ~0.5 mg digoxin.
  - Bioavailability of digoxin is 0.8 for 0.25 mg tablets OR 1 for 0.2 Lanoxicaps.
  - Use the following formula:
    Dose (in vials) = digoxin ingested (mg) × bioavailability/0.5 mg of digoxin bound per vial.
- **Chronic digoxin toxicity:**
  - Infants and small children: single vial (38 mg) IV initially.
  - *Or* use the following formula:
    Number of vials needed = (serum digoxin concentration in ng/mL) × (wt in kg)/100, then dose (in mg) = number of vials × 38 mg per vial.

PHARMACOKINETICS:
- Distribution:
  - V$_d$: Digibind®: 0.3 L/kg.
- Half-life:
  - Renal impairment prolongs the half-life of both agents.
  - Digibind: 15–20 hours.
- Onset of action:
  - Improvement in signs and symptoms occurs within 2–30 minutes following IV infusion.

ADVERSE EFFECTS: Use with caution in renal or cardiac failure; allergic reactions possible; epinephrine should be immediately available; patients may deteriorate due to withdrawal of digoxin and may require IV inotropic support (eg, dobutamine) or vasodilators. Hypokalemia has been reported to occur following reversal of digitalis intoxication; monitor serum potassium levels closely.

DIGOXIN (LANOXIN)

INDICATIONS AND USE: Treatment of congestive heart failure, atrial fibrillation or flutter, and supraventricular tachycardia.

ACTIONS: Exerts a positive inotropic effect (increased myocardial contractility). Its negative chronotropic effects (antiarrhythmic actions/decrease in heart rate) are due to the slowing of conduction through the sinoatrial (SA) and atrioventricular (AV) nodes caused by vagal stimulation.

SUPPLIED: Pediatric injection, 100 mcg/mL; elixir, 50 mcg/mL.

ROUTE: IV, PO, IM.

DOSAGE:
- **Total digitalizing dose (TDD)** to be divided 1/2, 1/4, and 1/4 every 8 hours. *Note:* Oral doses (elixir) are ~25% higher than IV doses listed below.
- **Preterm neonates:**
  - **TDD:** 15–25 mcg/kg IV or 20–30 mcg/kg PO.
  - **Daily maintenance dose:** 4–6 mcg/kg/dose IV every 24 hours or 5–7.5 mcg/kg/dose PO every 24 hours
- **Full-term neonates:**
  - **Total digitalizing dose:** 20–30 mcg/kg IV, 25–35 mcg/kg PO.
  - **Daily maintenance dose:** 5–8 mcg/kg/day IV divided every 12 hours or 6–10 mcg/kg/day PO divided every 12 hours.
- **1 month to 2 years:**
  - **Total digitalizing dose:** 30–50 mcg/kg IV or 35–60 PO mcg/kg.
  - **Daily maintenance dose:** 7.5–12 mcg/kg/day IV or 10–15 mcg/kg/day PO divided every 12 hours.
- **Therapeutic levels:** 0.5–2.0 ng/mL. Considerable overlap exists between toxic and therapeutic serum levels. Digoxin-like immunoreactive substance (DLIS) may cross-react with digoxin immunoassay and falsely increase serum concentrations; DLIS has been found in neonates.

ADVERSE EFFECTS: Persistent vomiting is usually the most common sign of digoxin toxicity in infants. Other adverse effects are anorexia, feeding intolerance, nausea, and dysrhythmias (paroxysmal ventricular contractions, bradycardia, tachycardia). Toxicity is markedly enhanced by hypokalemia. To manage toxicity, see Digibind. Give potassium chloride (KCl) if hypokalemic.

COMMENTS: Contraindicated in second- and third-degree block, idiopathic hypertrophic subaortic stenosis, and atrial flutter or fibrillation with slow ventricular rates.

DOBUTAMINE HYDROCHLORIDE (DOBUTREX)

INDICATIONS AND USE: To increase cardiac output during states of depressed contractility, such as septic shock, organic heart disease, or cardiac surgical procedures. To treat hypotension and hypoperfusion related to myocardial dysfunction.

ACTIONS: A direct β_1-agonist that increases myocardial contractility, oxygen delivery, and oxygen consumption; actions on β_2- and α-adrenergic receptors are much less marked than those of dopamine. Unlike dopamine, dobutamine does not cause release of endogenous norepinephrine, nor does it have any effect on dopaminergic receptors.

SUPPLIED: Injection, 250 mg/20 mL.

ROUTE: IV.

DOSAGE: 2–15 mcg/kg/minute by continuous infusion and titrate to desired response. **Maximum:** 40 mcg/kg/minute.

ADVERSE EFFECTS: Tachycardia and arrhythmias at higher doses, hypotension if patient is hypovolemic, ectopic heart beats, and elevated blood pressure.

COMMENTS: Correct hypovolemia prior to initiation of therapy; contraindicated in idiopathic subaortic stenosis and atrial fibrillation.

DOPAMINE HYDROCHLORIDE (DOPASTAT, INTROPIN)

INDICATIONS AND USE: To increase cardiac output, blood pressure, renal perfusion and glomerular filtration rate (GFR) (low dosages), which persists despite volume resuscitation.

ACTIONS: Actions are dose dependent. Low doses act directly on dopaminergic receptors to produce renal and mesenteric vasodilation. In moderate doses, β_1-adrenergic effects become prominent, resulting in a positive inotropic effect on the myocardium. High doses stimulate α-adrenergic receptors, producing increased peripheral resistance and renal vasoconstriction.

SUPPLIED: Injection.

ROUTE: IV by continuous infusion.

DOSAGE: *Note:* Dose–effect relationship is speculative in neonates.

• **Low:** 1–5 mcg/kg/minute may increase renal perfusion.
• **Moderate:** 5–15 mcg/kg/minute facilitates increased cardiac output.
• **High:** >15 mcg/kg/minute causes systemic vasoconstriction.

ADVERSE EFFECTS: Dopamine may cause ectopic heartbeats, tachycardia, hypertension, and azotemia. Gangrene of the extremities has occurred with high doses over prolonged periods. Extravasation may cause tissue necrosis and sloughing of surrounding tissues; if this occurs, infiltrate area with a small amount (1 mL) of phentolamine, made by diluting 2.5–5 mg in 10 mL preservative free NS; do not exceed 0.1 mg/kg or 2.5 mg total for neonates and 0.1 to 0.2 mg/kg or 5 mg total for infants.

COMMENTS: Administration of phenytoin IV to patients receiving dopamine may result in severe hypotension and bradycardia; therefore, use with extreme caution. Do not infuse through umbilical arterial catheter or other arterial catheter.

DOXAPRAM HYDROCHLORIDE (DOPRAM)

INDICATIONS AND USE: Apnea of prematurity unresponsive to methylxanthine therapy.

ACTIONS: Stimulates respiration through action on central respiratory centers and reflex stimulation of carotid, aortic or other peripheral chemoreceptors; decreases P_{CO_2} and increases minute ventilation and tidal volume without changing respiratory rate or inspiratory and expiratory times.

SUPPLIED: Injection, 20 mg/mL (contains 0.9% benzyl alcohol).

ROUTE: IV.

DOSAGE:

• **Loading dose:** 2.5–3 mg/kg IV over 30 minutes (follow by maintenance dose).
• **Maintenance:** IV infusion of 0.5–1.5 mg/kg/hour (maximum: 2.5 mg/kg/hour); decrease the infusion rate when control of apnea is achieved.
• **Therapeutic range:** 1.5–3 mcg/mL (<5 mcg/mL). Assay unavailable in most centers.

ADVERSE EFFECTS: Increases in blood pressure, heart rate, cardiac output, and skeletal muscle hyperactivity may occur. Abdominal distention, increased gastric residuals, vomiting, jitteriness, hyperglycemia, glycosuria, and seizures have been reported in neonates.

COMMENTS: Efficacy of doxapram in premature neonates with severe idiopathic apnea resistant to theophylline has been documented. Use cautiously because of its side effects. Should not be given during the first few days of life, when hypertensive episodes may be associated with an increased risk of intraventricular hemorrhage. Has a narrow therapeutic range, and its use warrants serum drug level monitoring. Contraindicated in cardiovascular and seizure disorders. Benzyl alcohol is contained in the formulation, which may accumulate to toxic levels after prolonged use.

ENALAPRIL (PO)/ENALAPRILAT (IV) (VASOTEC)

INDICATIONS AND USE: Manage hypertension and heart failure by reducing left ventricular preload and afterload.

ACTIONS: An angiotensin-converting enzyme (ACE) inhibitor that acts by inhibiting the conversion of angiotensin I to angiotensin II and the breakdown of bradykinin, causing vasodilation. Enalapril decreases aldosterone, increases sodium and fluid loss, and increases serum potassium.

SUPPLIED: Injection: 1.25 mg/mL, tablet: an oral suspension can be compounded by the pharmacist.

ROUTE: IV, PO.

DOSAGE:

- **IV:** 5–10 mcg/kg/dose every 8–24 hours. The frequency depends on blood pressure response. Monitor patient closely.
- **PO:** 100 mcg/kg/dose as a single daily dose. Increase gradually every few days as needed to a maximum of 500 mcg/kg/day PO. Titrate dose and interval based on amount and duration of response. May need to dose as frequently as every 6 hours.

ADVERSE EFFECTS: Hypotension, hyperkalemia, decreased renal function, oliguria, cough, decreased hemoglobin and hematocrit, and (rarely) bone marrow depression, neutropenia, and thrombocytopenia.

COMMENTS: Reduce the dose in renal dysfunction. Use a low initial dose to avoid a profound drop in blood pressure, especially in patients on diuretics who are hyponatremic or hypovolemic. Monitor blood pressure hourly for the first 12 hours.

Note that the IV dose is much smaller than the PO dose. Use caution to adjust the dose when changing route of administration. Use with caution and reduce dosage in patients with renal impairment. A profound decrease in blood pressure may occur with initial dose, especially with patients on diuretics, with hyponatremia and/or hypovolemia. Use lowest initial dose.

ENOXAPARIN (LOVENOX)

INDICATIONS AND USE:

Prophylaxis and treatment of thromboembolic disorders.

ACTIONS: Low molecular weight heparin that potentiates the action of antithrombin III and inactivates coagulation factor Xa and factor IIa (thrombin). Compared with standard heparin, enoxaparin has much less activity against thrombin. Low antithrombin plasma concentration reduces the efficacy in neonates. Enoxaparin is less likely to cause thrombocytopenia and osteoporosis.

SUPPLIED: Injection.

ROUTE: For subcutaneous use only; do not administer IM or IV; administer by deep SQ injection; do not rub injection site after subcutaneous administration, because bruising may occur.

DOSAGE:

- **Initial treatment:**
  - **Infants <2 months:** 1.5 mg/kg subcutaneous every 12 hours.
  - **Infants >2 months and children ≤18 years:** 1 mg/kg subcutaneous every 12 hours.
  - **Maintenance:** Adjust dose to maintain antifactor Xa level between 0.5 and 1.0 units/mL. It may take several days to reach target range. Preterm infants may require higher doses to maintain antifactor Xa levels in target range: **mean dose** of 2 mg/kg every 12 hours, **range** of 0.8 to 3 mg/kg every 12 hours.
- **Initial prophylaxis:**
  - **Infants <2 months:** 0.75 mg/kg subcutaneous every 12 hours.
  - **Infants >2 months and children ≤18 years:** 0.5 mg/kg subcutaneous every 12 hours.
  - **Maintenance:** Adjust to maintain antifactor Xa level between 0.1 and 0.4 units/mL.

PHARMACOKINETICS: Measure antifactor Xa levels 4 hours after a dose. After target level is reached, dosage adjustments may be required once or twice a month. Preterm infants and infants with hepatic or renal dysfunction may require more frequent adjustments.

ADVERSE EFFECTS: Bleeding, hemorrhage, thrombocytopenia (incidence of heparin-induced thrombocytopenia is less than with heparin therapy).

Hematoma, irritation, ecchymosis, and erythema can occur at the injection site.

EPINEPHRINE

INDICATIONS AND USE: Bradycardia, cardiac arrest, cardiogenic shock, anaphylactic reactions, and bronchospasm.

ACTIONS: Acts directly on both α- and β-adrenergic receptors; β_2 effects predominate at lower doses. Exerts both positive chronotropic and inotropic effects on the heart and relaxes bronchial smooth muscle. The α-adrenergic stimulation increases systolic blood pressure and constricts renal blood vessels.

SUPPLIED: Injection, solution for oral inhalation.

ROUTE: IV, endotracheal, nebulization.

DOSAGE:

- **IV bolus:** (Use 1:10,000) 0.1–0.3 mL/kg/dose every 3–5 minutes PRN.
- **IV infusion:** Use 1:1000 for preparation of infusion. Start with 0.1 mcg/kg/minute and titrate to desired response to a maximum of 1 mcg/kg/minute.

- **Intratracheal:** 0.3–1 mL/kg/dose immediately followed by 1 mL NS.
- **Nebulization:** 0.25–0.5 mL of 2.25% racemic epinephrine diluted in 3 mL of NS.

ADVERSE EFFECTS: Hypertension, tachycardia, nausea, pallor, tremor, cardiac arrhythmias, increased myocardial oxygen consumption, and decreased renal and splanchnic blood flow.

ERYTHROMYCIN (ILOSONE, OTHERS)

INDICATION AND USE: Treatment of mild to moderately severe infections due to susceptible bacteria as listed below; routine eye prophylaxis for gonococcal ophthalmia in all infants at birth; prokinetic agent for GI motility disorders.

ACTION AND SPECTRUM: Macrolide antibiotic that acts by suppression of protein synthesis. Action may be bactericidal or bacteriostatic depending on the tissue concentration of drug and the microorganism. Spectrum of activity is broad and includes the streptococci (except enterococci), *Staphylococcus aureus, Clostridium* spp., *Corynebacterium diphtheriae, Listeria monocytogenes, Haemophilus influenzae, Bordetella pertussis, Brucella* spp., *Campylobacter fetus, Branhamella catarrhalis, Neisseria gonorrhoeae, Legionella micdadei, Legionella pneumophila, Rickettsia* spp., *Mycoplasma pneumoniae, Chlamydia trachomatis, Treponema pallidum,* and some *Bacteroides* spp.

SUPPLIED: Oral suspension, injection, ophthalmic ointment.

ROUTE: PO, IV >60 minutes, ophthalmic.

DOSAGE:

- **Neonates: oral ethylsuccinate form.**
  - **Postnatal age:**
    - **≤7 days:** 20 mg/kg/day in divided doses every 12 hours.
    - **>7 days, <1200 g:** 20 mg/kg/day in divided doses every 12 hours.
    - **>7 days, 1200–2000 g:** 30 mg/kg/day in divided doses every 8 hours.
    - **>7 days, >2000 g:** 30–40 mg/kg/day in divided doses every 6–8 hours.
  - **IV lactobionate** 5–10 mg/kg every 6 hours for severe infections or when PO route is unavailable.
  - **Chlamydial conjunctivitis and pneumonia: Oral: Ethylsuccinate:** 50 mg/kg/day divided every 6 hours for 14 days.
- **Infants and children: Oral:**
  - **Base and ethylsuccinate:** 30–50 mg/kg/day PO divided every 6–8 hours; do not exceed 2 g/day (as base) or 3.2 g/day (as ethylsuccinate). *Note:* Due to differences in absorption, 200 mg erythromycin ethylsuccinate produces the same serum levels as 125 mg erythromycin base.
  - **Stearate:** 30–50 mg/kg/day PO divided every 6 hours; do not exceed 2 g/day.
  - *Chlamydia trachomatis:* **Child <45 kg:** 50 mg/kg/day PO divided every 6 hours for 14 days; maximum dose: 2 g/day.
  - **Pertussis:** 40–50 mg/kg/day divided every 6 hours for 14 days. Maximum dose: 2 g/day (not preferred agent for infants <1 month).
  - **IV lactobionate:** 15–50 mg/kg/day IV divided every 6 hours, not to exceed 4 g/day.
- **Ophthalmic prophylaxis:** 0.5–1 cm ribbon in each eye once.
- **Ophthalmic for acute infection:** 0.5–1 cm ribbon in each eye every 6 hours.
- **Gastrointestinal motility disorders:** 10 mg/kg/dose PO every 8 hours, 30 minutes before feedings; may be given IV but PO is preferred route.

PHARMACOKINETICS: Hepatic metabolism, excreted via the bile and kidneys. Half-life is 1.5–3 hours (prolonged in renal failure).

ADVERSE EFFECTS: Stomatitis, epigastric distress, and oral or perianal candidiasis. Transient cholestatic hepatitis and allergic reactions occur rarely. May cause increased serum levels of theophylline, digoxin, and carbamazepine. Infantile hypertrophic pyloric stenosis (IHPS) with symptoms of nonbilious vomiting or irritability with feeding has been reported in 5% of infants who received erythromycin for pertussis prophylaxis. Also exposure to high antimicrobial doses (30–50 mg/kg/day) for ≥14 days in neonates up to 2 weeks old has been associated with a 10-fold increase in the risk of hypertrophic pyloric stenosis. Cardiac toxicity requiring CPR may occur with IV erythromycin; reduce risk of arrhythmias by slowly infusing over 1 hour.

COMMENTS: Parenteral forms are painful and irritative; dilute to 5 mg/mL and infuse >60 minutes. Do not use IM.

ERYTHROPOIETIN/EPOETIN ALFA (EPOGEN, PROCRIT) [EPO, rEpo]

INDICATIONS AND USE: To stimulate erythropoiesis and decrease the need for erythrocyte transfusions rhEpo in preterm infants; treatment of anemia of prematurity.

ACTIONS: Epoetin alfa (EPO) induces erythropoiesis by stimulating the division and differentiation of committed erythroid progenitor cells. It induces the release of reticulocytes from the bone marrow into the bloodstream where they mature to erythrocytes (dose–response relationship), resulting in an increase in reticulocyte counts followed by a rise in hematocrit and hemoglobin levels. Noticeable effects on hematocrit and reticulocyte counts occur within 2 weeks.

SUPPLIED: Injection.

ROUTE: Subcutaneous, IV.

DOSAGE: 200 to 400 units/kg/dose, 3 to 5 times per week, for 2 to 6 weeks. **Total dose per week:** 600 to 1400 units/kg/week. **Short course:** 300 units/kg/dose daily × 10 days.

ADVERSE EFFECTS: May cause hypertension, edema, fever, rash, possible seizures, transient early thrombocytosis and late neutropenia, polycythemia, and local skin reaction at injection site.
COMMENTS: EPO is usually administered with iron; optimal response is achieved when iron stores are adequate. Iron supplementation is given orally as ferrous sulfate drops if tolerated or IV as iron dextran. EPO should be used in conjunction with restrictive transfusion guidelines and minimizing of phlebotomy losses. EPO is not a substitute for emergency blood transfusion. Do not use in patients with uncontrolled hypertension.

ETHACRYNIC ACID (EDECRIN)

INDICATIONS AND USE: Use when prompt diuresis is needed in patients refractory to other diuretics. Use other diuretics first because ethacrynic acid is more toxic.
ACTIONS: Loop diuretic. Inhibits reabsorption of sodium and chloride in the ascending loop of Henle and distal tubules causing increased excretion of water, sodium, chloride, magnesium, and calcium. Inhibits sodium reabsorption to a greater degree than other diuretics. Does not appear to have a direct effect on the pulmonary vasculature, as furosemide does.
SUPPLIED: Injection, 50 mg in 50-mL vials for reconstitution; tablet, 25 mg (scored). Oral suspension can be compounded by pharmacist.
ROUTE: PO, IV.
DOSAGE:

- **IV:** 0.5–1 mg/kg/dose repeat doses are not routinely recommended; however, if indicated, repeat doses every 8–12 hours.
- **PO:** 1 mg/kg/dose once daily; increase at intervals of 2–3 days to a maximum of 3 mg/kg/day.

ADVERSE EFFECTS: Inject the IV dose slowly over several minutes. May cause hypotension, dehydration, electrolyte depletion, diarrhea, GI bleeding, hearing loss, rash, local irritation and pain, hematuria, and, rarely, hypoglycemia and neutropenia.

FAMOTIDINE (PEPCID)

INDICATIONS AND USE: Prevention and short-term treatment of gastroesophageal reflux disease, stress, gastric and duodenal ulcers, and gastrointestinal hemorrhage.
ACTIONS: Inhibits gastric acid secretion by reversible, competitive antagonism of histamine on the H_2 receptor of the gastric parietal cells.
SUPPLIED: Tablet, powder for oral suspension, injection (contains benzyl alcohol).
ROUTE: IV, PO.
DOSAGE:

- **Neonates and infants < 3 months:** 0.25 to 0.5 mg/kg/dose every 24 hours slow IV push.
- **GERD:**
  - **<3 months:** 0.5 mg/kg PO once daily.
  - **3–12 months:** 0.5 mg/kg PO twice daily.

PHARMACOKINETICS: Onset of GI effect is within 1 hour. Duration is 10–12 hours. Elimination of 65% to 70% is unchanged in urine.
ADVERSE EFFECTS: Hypotension and cardiac arrhythmias with rapid IV administration; bradycardia, tachycardia, hypertension, thrombocytopenia, elevated liver enzymes, cholestatic jaundice, elevated blood urea nitrogen (BUN) and creatinine, and proteinuria.
COMMENTS: Limited experience in infants and children. Famotidine does not inhibit cytochrome P450.

FENTANYL (SUBLIMAZE)

INDICATIONS AND USE: Analgesia, anesthesia, and sedation.
ACTIONS: A synthetic opiate agonist that binds to the opioid mu-receptors within the CNS, increases the pain threshold, alters pain reception, and inhibits ascending pain pathway. Acts similarly to morphine and meperidine but without the cardiovascular effects of those drugs and with shorter respiratory depressant effects.
SUPPLIED: Injection, 50 mcg/mL.
ROUTE: IV.
DOSAGE:

- **Neonates:**
  - **Analgesia:** International Evidence-Based Group for Neonatal Pain recommendations (Anand KJS: Consensus statement for the prevention and management of pain in the newborn. *Arch Pediatr Adolesc Med* 2001;155(2): 173-180.)
    - **Intermittent doses:** Slow IV push: 0.5–3 mcg/kg/dose.
    - **Continuous infusion:** 0.5–2 mcg/kg/hour.
- **Neonates and younger infants:**
  - **Analgesia/sedation:** 1–4 mcg/kg/dose slow IV push every 2–4 hours as needed.
  - **Continuous analgesia/sedation:** Initial 1–2 mcg/kg IV bolus then 0.5–1mcg/kg/hour; titrate upward.
  - **Continuous sedation/analgesia during extracorporeal membrane oxygenation (ECMO):** Initial IV bolus: 5–10 mcg/kg slow IV push over 10 minutes, then 1–5 mcg/kg/hour; titrate upward; tolerance may develop; higher doses (up to 20 mcg/kg/hour) may be needed by day 6 of ECMO.
  - **Anesthesia:** 5–50 mcg/kg/dose.

ADVERSE EFFECTS: CNS and respiratory depression; bradycardia; Skeletal muscle and chest wall rigidity with reduced pulmonary compliance, apnea, and laryngospasm. Reversible with naloxone. Tolerance and withdrawal symptoms reported with continuous use. Urinary retention, gastrointestinal symptoms, and biliary spasms may occur.

COMMENTS: Potency is 0.1 mg of fentanyl IM = 10 mg of morphine IM. Concurrent ventilatory assistance is suggested with its use. Tachyphylaxis occurs after several days of therapy. Adheres to ECMO filter membranes; may have to adjust the dose.

FERROUS SULFATE (20% ELEMENTAL IRON)

INDICATIONS AND USE: Treatment and prevention of iron deficiency anemia; supplemental therapy for patients receiving epoetin alfa.

ACTIONS: Iron is needed for the production of heme proteins. Iron is released from the plasma and replenishes the depleted stores in the bone marrow where it is incorporated into hemoglobin.

SUPPLIED: Drops (preferred), 75 mg/0.6 mL (15 mg of elemental iron); elixir, 220 mg/5 mL (44 mg of elemental iron). *Note:* The product Fer-in-sol changed its concentration to 15 mg of elemental iron per mL.

ROUTE: PO.

DOSAGE: Recommendations of the American Academy of Pediatrics (AAP) for treatment and prevention of iron deficiency; dosages are for elemental iron.

* **Term infants:** 1–2 mg elemental iron/kg/day divided every 12–24 hours.
* **Preterm infants:** 2–4 mg elemental iron/kg/day divided every 12–24 hours. Begin therapy after 2 weeks of age.
* **Iron deficiency anemia:** 6 mg/kg/day in 3 divided doses.
* **Iron supplementation with erythropoietin:** 6 mg/kg/day in 1 or 2 divided doses.

ADVERSE EFFECTS: Gastrointestinal irritation (vomiting, diarrhea, constipation, and darkened stool color).

COMMENTS: The use of iron-fortified formulas during the first year of life usually prevents iron deficiency anemia in both the preterm and term infants. Iron-fortified formulas can be fed safely to preterm infants. Of the ferrous salts available (sulfate, fumarate, and gluconate), sulfate is preferred. Caution parents to guard against iron poisoning from accidental ingestion. Antidote is chelation with deferoxamine; consult specialized references and regional Poison Control Center for further information.

FILGRASTIM (GRANULOCYTE COLONY-STIMULATING FACTOR [G-CSF])

INDICATIONS AND USE: For the reduction of neutropenia in neonates with sepsis.

ACTIONS: Stimulates the production, maturation, and activation of neutrophil granulocytes and activates neutrophils to enhance both their migration and cytotoxicity.

SUPPLIED: Neupogen: 300 mcg/mL (1 mL, 1.6 mL vial).

ROUTE: Subcutaneous: Administer undiluted solution. **Continuous infusion:** Dilute dose in 10 mL D_5W and infuse at a rate of 10 mL/24 hours. Administer IV over 15–60 minutes or as a continuous IV infusion at a final concentration of at least 15 mcg/mL in D_5W. If the final concentration of granulocyte colony-stimulating factor (G-CSF) in D_5W is <15 mcg/mL, add 2 mg albumin/mL to IV fluid; the solution is stable for 24 hours; albumin acts as a carrier molecule to prevent drug adsorption to the IV tubing. Albumin should be added to the D_5W prior to addition of G-CSF; final concentration of G-CSF for administration <5 mcg/mL is not recommended; to avoid foaming, do not shake solution.

DOSAGE: Neonates: 5–10 mcg/kg/day once daily for 3–5 days has been administered to neutropenic neonates with sepsis. Refer to individual protocols.

PHARMACOKINETICS: Onset of action: Immediate transient leukopenia with the nadir occurring 5–15 minutes after an IV dose or 30–60 minutes after a subcutaneous dose followed by a sustained elevation in neutrophil levels within the first 24 hours reaching a plateau in 3–5 days. **Duration:** Upon discontinuation of G-CSF, absolute neutrophil count (ANC) decreases by 50% within 2 days and returns to pretreatment levels within 1 week; white blood cell (WBC) counts return to normal range in 4–7 days.

ADVERSE EFFECTS: Thrombocytopenia, leukocytosis, transient decrease in blood pressure.

FLUCONAZOLE (DIFLUCAN)

INDICATIONS AND USE: Antifungal agent for treatment of susceptible fungal infections including oropharyngeal and esophageal candidiasis; treatment of systemic candidal infections including urinary tract infection, peritonitis, cystitis, and pneumonia. Strains of *Candida* with decreased in vitro susceptibility to fluconazole are being isolated with increasing frequency. Fluconazole is more active against *Candida albicans* than other candidal strains like *Candida parapsilosis, Candida glabrata,* and *Candida tropicalis;* alternative to amphotericin B in patients with preexisting renal impairment or when requiring concomitant therapy with other potentially nephrotoxic drugs. Advantages over amphotericin B are once-a-day dosing, good absorption after oral administration; good cerebral spinal fluid (CSF) penetration after both oral and IV administration, and fewer adverse effects. Check the sensitivity of the organism.

ACTIONS: Interferes with fungal cytochrome P450 and sterol C-14 α-demethylation, resulting in a fungistatic effect.

SUPPLIED: PO; injection.

ROUTE: PO, IV.

DOSAGE:
- **Systemic infections, including meningitis:**
  - **<29 weeks' gestation:**
    - **Postnatal age 0–14 days:** 12 mg/kg loading dose, then 6 mg/kg IV/PO every 72 hours.
    - **Postnatal age >14 days:** 12 mg/kg loading dose, then 6 mg/kg IV/PO every 48 hours.
  - **30–36 weeks' gestation:**
    - **Postnatal age 0–14 days:** 12 mg/kg loading dose, then 6 mg/kg IV/PO every 48 hours.
    - **Postnatal age >14 days:** 12 mg/kg loading dose, then 6 mg/kg IV/PO every 24 hours.
  - **37–44 weeks' gestation:**
    - **Postnatal age 0–7 days:** 12 mg/kg loading dose, then 6 mg/kg IV/PO every 48 hours.
    - **Postnatal age >7 days:** 12 mg/kg loading dose, then 6 mg/kg IV/PO every 24 hours.
  - **≥45 weeks' gestation:** 12 mg/kg loading dose, then 6mg/kg IV/PO every 24 hours.
- **Neonates >14 days, infants, and children:**
  - **Oropharyngeal candidiasis IV or PO:** day 1: 6 mg/kg IV/PO, then 3 mg/kg IV/PO minimum 14 days.
  - **Esophageal candidiasis IV or PO:** as above but 21-day minimum.
  - **Prophylaxis:** 3 mg/kg/dose IV infusion twice weekly has been used in extremely low birthweight (ELBW) infants at increased risk of invasive fungal infection.

ADVERSE EFFECTS: Usually well tolerated. Vomiting, diarrhea, rash, and elevations in liver transaminases.

COMMENTS: Reduce the dose in renal dysfunction. Use caution in preexisting renal dysfunction. Monitor liver function tests. Cimetidine and rifampin decrease fluconazole levels. Hydrochlorothiazide increases fluconazole area under the curve (AUC). Fluconazole interferes with the metabolism of barbiturates, theophylline, midazolam, phenytoin, and zidovudine.

FLUCYTOSINE (ANCOBON)

ACTION AND SPECTRUM: Antifungal agent that penetrates fungal cells and is converted to fluorouracil, which competes with uracil interfering with fungal RNA and protein synthesis. In combination with amphotericin B in the treatment of serious candidal or cryptococcal pulmonary or urinary tract infections, sepsis, meningitis, or endocarditis (resistance emerges if flucytosine is used as a single agent); used in combination with another antifungal agent for treatment of chromomycosis and aspergillosis.

SUPPLIED: Capsules (pharmacist can compound an oral liquid: 10 mg/mL).

ROUTE: PO.

DOSAGE:
- **Neonates:** Initial: 50–100 mg/kg/day in divided doses every 12–24 hours.
- **Infants and children:** 50–150 mg/kg/day PO divided every 6 hours.
- **Renal impairment:** 12.5–25 mg/kg/day divided as follows:
  - **Creatinine clearance of 20–40 mL/minute:** every 12 hours.
  - **Creatinine clearance of 10–20 mL/minute:** every 24 hours.
  - **Creatinine clearance of <10 mL/minute:** every 24–48 hours.

PHARMACOKINETICS: Desired peak serum concentrations: 25–100 mcg/mL. Half-life, neonates: 4–34 hours. Renal elimination.

ADVERSE EFFECTS: Vomiting, diarrhea, rash, anemia, leukopenia, thrombocytopenia, elevated liver enzymes and bilirubin, increased blood urea nitrogen (BUN) and creatinine, and CNS disturbances.

COMMENTS: Toxicities related to serum concentration above 100 mcg/mL and usually reversible when drug is discontinued or dose is reduced. Amphotericin B may increase toxicity by decreasing renal excretion.

FLUDROCORTISONE (FLORINEF)

INDICATIONS AND USE: Used for partial replacement therapy for adrenocortical insufficiency and treatment of salt-losing forms of congenital adrenogenital syndrome, usually used with concurrent hydrocortisone.

ACTIONS: Fludrocortisone is a potent mineralocorticoid with glucocorticoid activity that acts on the distal tubule to increase loss of potassium and hydrogen ion and increases reabsorption of sodium with subsequent water retention.

SUPPLIED: Scored tablet: 0.1 mg/tablet (100 mcg/tablet).

ROUTE: PO.

DOSAGE:
- **Usual:** 0.05–0.1 mg/day (50–100 mcg/day) as a single daily dose. (**Note:** Doses are the same regardless of patient weight or age. Newborns are insensitive to the drug and may require larger doses than adults). May administer with feedings.
- **Congenital adrenal hyperplasia (salt losers): Maintenance:** range of 0.05–0.3 mg/day (American Academy of Pediatrics Section on Endocrinology and Committee on Genetics Technical Report: Congenital Adrenal Hyperplasia. *Pediatrics* 2000; 106(6):1511-1518. Reaffirmed May 1 2005.)

ADVERSE EFFECTS: Hypertension, congestive heart failure, gastrointestinal upset, hypokalemia, growth suppression, hyperglycemia, salt and water retention, edema, hypothalamic-pituitary-adrenal suppression, osteoporosis, and muscle weakness resulting from excessive potassium loss. Rarely causes anaphylaxis and rash. Monitor serum electrolytes (particularly sodium and potassium).

COMMENTS: Fludrocortisone 0.1 mg has a sodium retention activity equal to deoxycorticosterone acetate (DOCA) 1 mg.

FOLIC ACID (FOLATE, FOLVITE)

INDICATIONS AND USE: Treatment of anemia due to nutritional deficit, prematurity, megaloblastic anemia, or macrocytic anemia.

ACTIONS: Required for formation of a number of coenzymes in many metabolic systems, specifically for purine and pyrimidine synthesis, nucleoprotein synthesis and maintenance of erythropoiesis. Also stimulates white blood cell (WBC) and platelet production in folate deficiency anemia.

SUPPLIED: Injection (contains benzyl alcohol), tablets. Pharmacist may compound an oral solution using the injection. Not contained in oral multivitamin drops due to instability.

ROUTE: Oral, IM, IV, subcutaneous.

DOSAGE:

- **Recommended daily allowance:**
  - **Premature neonates:** 50 mcg PO/day (~15 mcg/kg/day).
  - **Neonates to 6 months:** 25–35 mcg PO/day.
  - **Children, 6 months–3 years:** 50 mcg PO/day.
- **Folic acid deficiency** PO, IM, IV, subcutaneous.
  - **Infants:** 15 mcg/kg/dose daily or 50 mcg/day.
  - **Children:** 1 mg/day initial dose, maintenance 0.1–0.4 mg/day.

PHARMACOKINETICS: Absorbed in the proximal portion of small intestine. Metabolized in the liver.

ADVERSE EFFECTS: Generally well tolerated. High doses of folic acid are considered nontoxic.

FOLINIC ACID (LEUCOVORIN, LEUCOVORIN CALCIUM)

CAUTION: May be confused with folic acid.

INDICATION: Adjunctive treatment with sulfadiazine and pyrimethamine to prevent hematologic toxicity, antidote for folic acid antagonist overdosage, reduces toxic effects of methotrexate.

ACTIONS: Folinic acid is a derivative of tetrahydrofolic acid, a reduced form of folic acid; enables purine and thymidine synthesis, required for normal erythropoiesis.

SUPPLIED: Injection, tablet.

ROUTE: IV or PO.

DOSAGE:

- **Folic acid antagonist overdosage** (eg, pyrimethamine, trimethoprim): 5–15 mg/day PO for 3 days or until blood counts are normal or 5 mg every 3 days; doses of 6 mg/day are needed for patients with platelet counts <100,000/mm³.
- **Adjunctive treatment with sulfadiazine** to prevent hematologic toxicity (for toxoplasmosis): **Infants children:** 5–10 mg PO/IV once daily; repeat every 3 days.

PHARMACOKINETICS:

- Onset of action:
  - Oral: Within 30 minutes.
  - IV: Within 5 minutes.
- Absorption:
  - Oral, IM: rapid.
- Metabolism: Rapidly converted to (5MTHF) 5-methyl-tetrahydrofolate (active) in the intestinal mucosa and by the liver.

ADVERSE EFFECTS: Thrombocytosis.

FOSPHENYTOIN (CEREBYX)

INDICATIONS AND USE: Management of generalized convulsive status epilepticus; used for short-term parenteral administration of phenytoin, prevention and management of seizures.

ACTIONS AND SPECTRUM: Fosphenytoin is a water-soluble prodrug of phenytoin that is rapidly converted by phosphatases in blood and tissues.

SUPPLIED: Injection, solution: 75 mg/mL (2 mL, 10 mL vials), equivalent to phenytoin sodium 50 mg/mL.

ROUTE: IV or IM.

DOSAGE: Phenytoin equivalent (PE).

- **Loading dose:** 15 to 20 mg PE/kg IM or IV infusion over at least 10 minutes
- **Maintenance dose:** 4 to 8 mg PE/kg every 24 hours IM or IV slow push. Start maintenance dose 24 hours after loading dose.
- **Term infants > 1 week of age:** may require doses up to 8 mg PE/kg/dose every 8 to 12 hours.

PHARMACOKINETICS: Conversion to phenytoin half-life is ~7 minutes. Fosphenytoin is highly protein bound. (Caution in neonates with hyperbilirubinemia: Both fosphenytoin and bilirubin displace phenytoin from protein-binding sites, which result in increased serum free phenytoin concentrations.)

ADVERSE EFFECTS: Hypotension (with rapid IV administration), vasodilation, tachycardia, bradycardia, drowsiness.

COMMENTS: Dilute with D_5W or NS to 1.5–25 mg PE/mL. Maximum rate of infusion is 1.5 mg PE/kg/minute. Flush IV with saline pre- and postadministration. Monitor blood pressure during infusion.

FUROSEMIDE (LASIX)

INDICATIONS AND USE: Fluid overload, pulmonary edema, congestive heart failure, and hypertension.
ACTIONS: Inhibits reabsorption of sodium and chloride in the ascending limb of the loop of Henle and distal rental tubule. Furosemide-induced diuresis results in enhanced excretion of sodium, chloride, potassium, calcium, magnesium, bicarbonate, ammonium, hydrogen, and possibly phosphate. Nondiuretic effects include decreased pulmonary transvascular fluid filtration and improved pulmonary function.
SUPPLIED: Oral solution, 10 mg/mL; injection, 10 mg/mL.
ROUTE: PO, IV, IM.
DOSAGE:

- **Neonates, premature:**
  - **PO:** 1–4 mg/kg/dose 1–2 times a day as initial dose has been used, and increase slowly if needed; highly variable oral bioavailability.
  - **IV or IM:** 1 mg/kg/dose every 12–24 hours.
- **Infants and children:**
  - **Oral:** 2 mg/kg PO once daily; if effective, may increase in increments of 1–2 mg/kg/dose every 6–8 hours; not to exceed 6 mg/kg/dose. In most cases, it is unnecessary to exceed individual doses of 4 mg/kg or a dosing frequency of once or twice daily.
  - **IM, IV:** 1–2 mg/kg/dose every 6–12 hours
  - **Continuous infusion:** 0.05 mg/kg/hour; titrate dosage to clinical effect.

ADVERSE EFFECTS: Hypokalemia, hypocalcemia, and hyponatremia; hypercalciuria, with prolonged use, nephrocalcinosis and hypochloremic metabolic alkalosis. Ototoxicity is possible especially in association with concurrent use of aminoglycosides.

GANCICLOVIR

INDICATIONS AND USE: Symptomatic congenital cytomegalovirus infection (CMV) for the prevention of progressive hearing loss.
ACTIONS AND SPECTRUM: An acyclic nucleoside structurally related to acyclovir, possesses antiviral activity against herpes viruses. Ganciclovir is a prodrug that is phosphorylated to a substrate which inhibits viral DNA synthesis by competitive inhibition of viral DNA polymerases and incorporation into viral DNA resulting in eventual termination of viral DNA elongation. Ganciclovir is preferentially metabolized in virus-infected cells.
SUPPLIED: Injection, powder for reconstitution, 500 mg vial. Capsule: 250 mg, 500 mg (an oral suspension may be compounded by pharmacist).
ROUTE: IV.
DOSAGE: Neonates: 6 mg/kg/dose every 12 hours IV, infused over 1 hour. Treat for a minimum of 6 weeks. Reduce dose by half for significant neutropenia (< 500 cells/mm^3).
ADVERSE EFFECTS:

- **Cardiovascular:** Edema, arrhythmias, hypertension.
- **Central nervous system:** Seizures, sedation.
- **Gastrointestinal:** Loss of appetite, vomiting, diarrhea.
- **Hematologic:** Neutropenia (oral ganciclovir is associated with less neutropenia and fewer bacterial infections than IV ganciclovir); thrombocytopenia, leukopenia, anemia, eosinophilia.
- **Hepatic:** Elevated liver enzymes.
- **Local:** Phlebitis.
- **Ocular:** Retinal detachment in patients with CMV retinitis.
- **Renal:** Hematuria, elevated blood urea nitrogen (BUN), and serum creatinine.
- **Respiratory:** Dyspnea.

PHARMACOKINETICS:

- **Absorption:** Oral is poor, bioavailability of oral ganciclovir is lower in children than adults.
- **Elimination:** Renal excretion is the major route of elimination. Most of drug is excreted unchanged in the urine via glomerular filtration and active tubular secretion.

COMMENTS: Handle and dispose according to guidelines issued for cytotoxic drugs; avoid direct contact of skin or mucous membranes with the powder contained in capsules or the IV solution. Dosage adjustment or interruption of ganciclovir therapy may be necessary in patients with neutropenia and/or thrombocytopenia and patients with impaired renal function.

GENTAMICIN SULFATE (GARAMYCIN)

ACTION AND SPECTRUM: Aminoglycoside exerts its bactericidal activity by the inhibition of bacterial protein synthesis. Active chiefly against Gram-negative aerobic bacteria, including most *Pseudomonas, Proteus,* and *Serratia* spp. Some activity against coagulase-positive staphylococci but ineffective against anaerobes and streptococci. Provides some synergistic effect against group D streptococci (enterococci) when used in combination with a penicillin.

SUPPLIED: Injection, intrathecal injection, ophthalmic solution, ointment.
ROUTE: IM, IV (preferred, infuse over 30 minutes), ophthalmic.
DOSAGE: Base the initial dose on body weight, then monitor levels and adjust using pharmacokinetics.

- **<29 weeks postmenstrual age (PMA):**
  - **0 to 7 days:** 5 mg/kg/dose every 48 hours.
  - **8 to 28 days:** 4 mg/kg/dose every 36 hours.
  - **≥29 days:** 4 mg/kg/dose every 24 hours.
- **30 to 34 weeks PMA:**
  - **0 to 7 days:** 4.5 mg/kg/dose every 36 hours.
  - **>7 days:** 4 mg/kg/dose every 24 hours.
- **≥35 weeks PMA:** 4 mg/kg/dose every 24 hours.
- **Intrathecal or intraventricular** (use preservative free):
  - **Newborns:** 1 mg/day.
  - **Infants >3 months and children:** 1–2 mg/day.
- **Ophthalmic solution:** 1 drop into each eye every 4 hours.
- **Ophthalmic ointment:** apply 2–3 times a day.

PHARMACOKINETICS: Renal excretion by glomerular filtration. Half-life is 3–11.5 hours initially.
ADVERSE EFFECTS: Ototoxicity (may be associated with high serum aminoglycoside concentrations persisting for prolonged periods) with tinnitus, hearing loss; early toxicity usually affects high-pitched sound, Nephrotoxicity (high trough levels) with proteinuria, elevated serum creatinine, oliguria, and macular rash.
COMMENTS: Desired serum peak is 4–12 mcg/mL (sample obtained 30 minutes after infusion has been completed), and desired serum trough is 0.5–2 mcg/mL (sample obtained 30 minutes to just before next dose). Obtain serum levels if treating for >48 hours. Monitor serum creatinine. Aminoglycosides should not be used alone against Gram-positive pathogens.

GLUCAGON

INDICATIONS AND USE: Management of hypoglycemia unresponsive to routine treatment.
ACTIONS: Glucagon, a hormone produced by the α cells of the pancreas, stimulates synthesis of cAMP, hepatic glycogenolysis, and gluconeogenesis, causing an increase in blood glucose levels; it inhibits small bowel motility and gastric acid secretion.
SUPPLIED: Injection, 1-mg (1-unit) vials.
ROUTE: Subcutaneous, IM, IV.
DOSAGE: 0.02–0.30 mg/kg/dose; may repeat in 20 minutes as needed. **Maximum single dose:** 1 mg.
ADVERSE EFFECTS: Hypersensitivity, nausea, and vomiting.
COMMENTS: Incompatible with electrolyte-containing solutions, precipitates with chloride solutions; compatible with dextrose solutions. *Caution:* Do not delay initiation of glucose infusion while observing for glucagon effect.

HEPARIN SODIUM

INDICATIONS AND USE: Prophylaxis and treatment of thromboembolic disorders and maintain patency of arterial or venous catheters.
ACTIONS: Activates antithrombin III (heparin cofactor) and inactivates coagulation factors IX, X, XI, and XII and thrombin, inhibiting the conversion of fibrinogen to fibrin. Heparin also stimulates release of lipoprotein lipase (lipoprotein lipase hydrolyzes triglycerides to glycerol and free fatty acids).
SUPPLIED: Injection.
ROUTE: Subcutaneous, IV.
DOSAGE:

- **Treatment of thrombosis: Loading dose:** 75 units/kg as IV bolus given over 10 minutes, followed by 28 units/kg/hour as continuous infusion; adjust dose to maintain activated partial thromboplastin time (APTT) of 60–85 seconds (assuming this reflects an antifactor Xa level of 0.3–0.7).
- **Maintain catheter patency:** Heparinize fluid with a usual final concentration of 0.5–1 unit/mL.
- **Line flushing:** When using daily flushes of heparin to maintain patency of single- and double-lumen central catheters, 10 units/mL is commonly used for younger infants (eg, <10 kg); 100 units/mL is used for older infants and children.

ADVERSE REACTIONS: Thrombocytopenia, bleeding tendency, hemorrhage, fever, rash, and abnormal liver function tests (LFT's).
COMMENTS: Clearance in neonates is more rapid than in children or adults; half-life is dose-dependent, but the average is 1 to 3 hours. Antidote: protamine sulfate, refer to monograph for dosing.

HEPATITIS B IMMUNE GLOBULIN (HBIG)

INDICATIONS AND USE: Provide prophylactic passive immunity to hepatitis B infection.
ACTIONS: Passive immunization agent. Immune serum provides protection against the hepatitis B virus by directly providing specific antibody to hepatitis B surface antigen (HBsAg). The duration of immunity is short (1–3 months).

SUPPLIED: Injection.

ROUTE: IM only into anterolateral thigh.

DOSAGE: Administer 0.5 mL as soon after birth as possible (within 12 hours; efficacy decreases significantly if treatment is delayed >48 hours); hepatitis B vaccine series to begin at the same time; if this series is delayed for as long as 3 months, the HBIG dose may be repeated.

ADVERSE EFFECTS: Swelling, warmth, erythema, and soreness at the injection site. Rarely, rash, fever, and urticaria.

COMMENTS: Administer with caution in patients with immunoglobulin (Ig) A deficiency, thrombocytopenia, or coagulopathy. Do not administer IV.

HEPATITIS B VACCINE (HEPTAVAX-B, RECOMBIVAX HB, ENGERIX-B)

INDICATIONS AND USE: Immunization against infection caused by all known subtypes of hepatitis B virus, in individuals considered at high risk of potential exposure to hepatitis B virus.

ACTIONS: Promotes immunity to hepatitis B virus by inducing the production of specific antibodies to the virus.

SUPPLIED: Injection 0.5 mL IM (Recombivax HB, 5 mcg; Engerix-B, 10 mcg).

ROUTE: IM only; administer in the anterolateral thigh.

DOSAGE: Recommended schedule: 0.5 mL/dose in 3 total doses.

- **Infants born of hepatitis B surface antigen (HB_sAg) positive mothers:** First dose within the first 12 hours of life, even if premature and regardless of birthweight (hepatitis immune globulin should also be administered at the same time/different site); second dose at 1–2 months of age; and third dose at 6 months of age. Check anti-hepatitis B surface antigen (anti-HB_s) and HB_sAg at 9–15 months of age. If anti-HB_s and HB_sAg are negative, reimmunize with 3 doses 2 months apart and reassess. *Note:* Premature infants <2000 g should receive 4 total doses at 0, 1, 2–3, and 6–7 months of chronological age.

- **Infants born of HB_sAg negative mothers:** First dose prior to discharge; however, the first dose may be given at 1–2 months of age. Another dose is given 1–2 months later, and a final dose at 6 months of age. A total of 4 doses of vaccine may be given if a "birth dose" is administered and a combination vaccine is used to complete the series. *Note:* Premature infants <2000 g may have the initial dose deferred up to 30 days of chronological age.

- **Infants born of mothers whose HB_sAg status is unknown at birth:** First dose within 12 hours of birth even if premature regardless of birthweight, second dose following 1–2 months later; the third dose at 6 months of age; if the mother's blood HB_sAg test is positive, the infant should receive hepatitis immune globulin as soon as possible (no later than age 1 week).

ADVERSE EFFECTS: Swelling, warmth, erythema, soreness at the injection site, and, rarely, vomiting, rash, and low-grade fever.

COMMENTS: Do not give IV or intradermally.

HYALURONIDASE

INDICATIONS AND USE: Treatment of extravasation injuries.

ACTIONS: An enzyme that temporarily hydrolyses hyaluronic acid (one of the chief components of tissue cement) and thereby allows the infiltrated drug or solution to be absorbed over a larger surface area. This speeds absorption and reduces tissue contact time with the irritant substance.

SUPPLIED: Injection, 150 units/mL solution, refrigerate.

ROUTE: Subcutaneous.

DOSAGE: Using a 25- or 26-gauge needle, inject 5 separate 0.2 mL subcutaneous injections around the periphery of the extravasation site. Change the needle after each injection, Elevate the extremity. Do not apply heat. Repeat as needed. Some use 5 separate 0.2 mL subcutaneous injections of a dilution, 15 units/mL.

ADVERSE EFFECTS: Usually well tolerated. Urticaria (rare). Administer hyaluronidase within 1 hour of the extravasation, if possible.

HYDRALAZINE HYDROCHLORIDE (APRESOLINE HYDROCHLORIDE)

INDICATIONS AND USE: For the management of moderate to severe hypertension and as an afterload reducing agent to treat congestive heart failure.

ACTIONS: Causes direct relaxation of smooth muscle in the arteriolar resistance vessels; decreases systemic vascular resistance and increases cardiac output; increases renal, coronary, cerebral and splanchnic blood flow.

SUPPLIED: Injection; tablets (oral liquid can be compounded by the pharmacist).

ROUTE: IM, IV, PO.

DOSAGE:

- **IM or IV:** 0.1–0.5 mg/kg/dose every 6–8 hours (maximum: 2 mg/kg/dose).
- **PO:** 0.25–1 mg/kg/dose every 6–8 hours.

ADVERSE EFFECTS: Most frequent are tachycardia and hypotension; most serious is a reversible lupus-like syndrome. Tachyphylaxis often occurs on chronic therapy. Occasionally, gastrintestinal bleeding, or diarrhea.

COMMENTS: Contraindicated in mitral valve rheumatic heart disease.

HYDROCHLOROTHIAZIDE (VARIOUS)

INDICATIONS AND USE: Mild to moderate edema and hypertension.

ACTIONS: Inhibits sodium reabsorption in the distal tubules causing increased excretion of sodium and water as well as potassium, hydrogen, magnesium, phosphate, calcium, and bicarbonate ions.

SUPPLIED: Solution, 50 mg/5 mL; oral solution contains sodium benzoate; benzoic acid (benzoate) is a metabolite of benzyl alcohol.

ROUTE: PO.

DOSAGE:

- **Edema:**
  - **Neonates and infants <6 months:** 2–3.3 mg/kg/day in 2 divided doses; **maximum dose:** 37.5 mg/day.
  - **Infants >6 months and children:** 2 mg/kg/day in 2 divided doses; **maximum dose:** 200 mg/day.
- **Hypertension:**
  - **Infants and children:** Initially, administer 1 mg/kg/day once daily; increase to maximum 3 mg/kg/day if needed; not to exceed 50 mg/day.

ADVERSE EFFECTS: Hypokalemia, hyperglycemia, hyperuricemia, hypochloremic metabolic alkalosis.

HYDROCORTISONE

INDICATIONS AND USE: Management of acute adrenal insufficiency, congenital adrenal hyperplasia, and vasopressor-resistant hypotension. Adjunctive treatment for persistent hypoglycemia.

ACTIONS: The short-acting adrenal corticosteroid that possesses glucocorticoid activity, anti-inflammatory activity, and some mineralocorticoid effects; most effects probably result from modification of enzyme activity, thus affecting almost all body systems. Promotes protein catabolism, gluconeogenesis, renal excretion of calcium, capillary wall permeability and stability, and red blood cell production; suppresses immune and inflammatory responses.

SUPPLIED: Injection, tablet (pharmacist can compound an oral suspension).

ROUTE: PO, IV, IM.

DOSAGE:

- **Acute adrenal insufficiency:** 1–2 mg/kg/dose IV bolus; then 25–150 mg/day divided every 6–8 hours.
- **Congenital adrenal hyperplasia (American Academy of Pediatrics Recommendations):**
  - **Initial:** 10–20 mg/m^2/day PO in 3 divided doses.
  - **Usual requirement:**
    - **Infants:** 2.5–5 mg 3 times/day.
    - **Children:** 5–10 mg 3 times/day.
  - **Physiologic replacement:** 7 to 9 mg/m^2/day IV or PO divided into 2 or 3 doses.
  - **Stress doses (treatment-resistant hypotension):** 20 to 30 mg/m^2 IV divided into 2 or 3 doses; alternatively 1 mg/kg/dose every 8 hours.

ADVERSE EFFECTS AND COMMENTS: Hypertension, hypothalamo-pituitary-axis (HPA) suppression, hypokalemia, hyperglycemia, growth suppression, sodium and water retention, decreased bone mineral density, and immunosuppression.

Note: Morning dose should be administered as early as possible; tablets may result in more reliable serum concentrations than oral liquid formulation; individualize dose by monitoring growth, hormone levels, and bone age; mineralocorticoid (eg, fludrocortisone) and sodium supplement may be required in salt losers.

IBUPROFEN (MOTRIN, OTHERS)

INDICATIONS AND USE: Treatment of mild to moderate pain, fever, and inflammatory diseases. Oral Ibuprofen may be a safe alternative for patent ductus arteriosus (PDA) closure; recent studies have shown this, but larger studies are needed.

ACTIONS: Inhibits prostaglandin synthesis by decreasing the activity of the enzyme, cyclooxygenase.

SUPPLIED: Oral suspension, 100 mg/5mL; infant drops, 40 mg/mL.

ROUTE: PO.

DOSAGE: To reduce the risk of adverse cardiovascular and gastrointestinal (GI) effects, use the lowest effective dose for the shortest period of time.

- **Infants and children:**
  - **Analgesic:** 4–10 mg/kg/dose PO every 6 to 8 hours; maximum daily dose is 40 mg/kg/day.
  - **Antipyretic:** 6 months to 12 years, maximum daily dose is 40 mg/kg/day.
    - **Temperature <102.5°F (39°C):** 5 mg/kg/dose; every 6 to 8 hours.
    - **Temperature ≥102.5°F (39°C):** 10 mg/kg/dose; every 6 to 8 hours.
  - **PDA closure:** 10 mg/kg/body weight for the first dose, followed at 24 hours intervals by 2 doses of 5 mg/kg each on the second and third day of life.

PHARMACOKINETICS: Hepatic metabolism. Primarily renally excreted.

ADVERSE EFFECTS: Edema, hypertension, fluid retention, GI bleed, GI perforation, neutropenia, anemia, inhibition of platelet aggregation, elevated liver enzymes, acute renal failure.

COMMENTS: May increase risk of GI irritation, ulceration, bleeding, and perforation; may compromise existing renal function; use with caution in patients with decreased liver function.

IBUPROFEN LYSINE (NEOPROFEN)

INDICATIONS AND USE: Pharmacologic closure of patent ductus arteriosus. Not indicated for intraventricular hemorrhage prophylaxis.

ACTIONS: Nonsteroidal anti-inflammatory drug (NSAID) with analgesic and antipyretic properties. Action is principally by inhibition of prostaglandin synthesis, thus inhibiting cyclooxygenase, an enzyme that catalyzes the formation of prostaglandin precursors (endoperoxides) from arachidonic acid.

SUPPLIED: Injection.

ROUTE: IV only.

DOSAGE: 10 mg/kg, initially followed by two doses of 5 mg/kg at 24 and 48 hours intervals after the initial dose.

ADVERSE EFFECTS: Anemia, fluid retention, edema, tachycardia, hepatic dysfunction, decreased urine output, elevated blood urea nitrogen (BUN) and serum creatinine (renal effects are less severe and less frequent than with indomethacin); may inhibit platelet aggregation; monitor for signs of bleeding. Use with caution in infants when total bilirubin is elevated (ibuprofen may displace bilirubin from albumin-binding sites). Feeding intolerance, gastrointestinal irritation, ileus.

COMMENTS: NeoProfen is contraindicated in preterm neonates with infection, active bleeding, thrombocytopenia or coagulation defects, necrotizing enterocolitis (NEC), significant renal dysfunction, and congenital heart disease with ductal-dependent systemic blood flow.

IMMUNE GLOBULIN, INTRAVENOUS (IVIG)

INDICATIONS AND USE: Neonatal alloimmune thrombocytopenia, hemolytic jaundice, adjuvant treatment of fulminant neonatal sepsis (*controversial*) and immunodeficiency syndromes.

ACTIONS: The pooled, heterogenous immunoglobulin G (IgG) present in IVIG provides a plethora of antibodies capable of opsonization and neutralization of many toxins and microbes as well as complement activation. Although the amount of each IgG subclass in the parenteral products is similar to that of human plasma, the titers against specific antigens vary from manufacturer to manufacturer. The passive immunity imparted by IVIG is capable of attenuating or preventing infectious diseases or deleterious reactions from toxins, *Mycoplasma,* parasites, bacteria, and viruses. IVIG is thought to promote blockade of Fc receptors in macrophages (preventing phagocytosis of circulating opsonized platelets or cells tagged with autoantibodies).

SUPPLIED: Injection.

ROUTE: IV only.

DOSAGE: Usual dosage ranges from 400 mg/kg/dose to 1 g/kg/dose infused over 2 to 6 hours. Many different products available; consult specific product insert for information regarding dosing, preparation, administration, storage, and so forth.

ADVERSE EFFECTS: Hypotension, transient tachycardia and anaphylaxis. If either occurs, the rate of infusion should be decreased or stopped until resolved, then resumed at a slower rate as tolerated. Contraindicated in IgA deficiency (except with the use of Gammagard S/D or Polygam S/D).

INDOMETHACIN (INDOCIN IV)

INDICATIONS AND USE: Pharmacologic closure of patent ductus arteriosus (PDA). May provide prophylaxis for intraventricular hemorrhage (IVH) in low birthweight infants.

ACTIONS: Nonsteroidal anti-inflammatory drug (NSAID) with analgesic and antipyretic properties. Inhibits of prostaglandin synthesis by decreasing cyclooxygenase activity, an enzyme that catalyzes the formation of prostaglandin precursors (endoperoxides) from arachidonic acid. Decreases cerebral blood flow.

SUPPLIED: Powder for injection.

ROUTE: IV.

DOSAGE:

- **Patent ductus arteriosus:**
  - **Neonates:** Initially, 0.2 mg/kg IV, followed by 2 doses depending on postnatal age (PNA):
    - **PNA at first dose <48 hours:** 0.1 mg/kg at 12- to 24-hour intervals.
    - **PNA at first dose 2–7 days:** 0.2 mg/kg at 12- to 24-hour intervals.
    - **PNA at first dose >7 days:** 0.25 mg/kg at 12- to 24-hour intervals.
    - **Dosing interval:**
      - **12-hour dosing** interval if urine output >1 mL/kg/hour after prior dose.
      - **24-hour dosing** interval if urine output is <1 mL/kg/hour but >0.6 mL/kg/hour.
      - **Hold dose** if patient has oliguria (urine output <0.6 mL/kg/hour) or anuria.
- **Prophylaxis for IVH:** 0.1 mg/kg IV/dose every 24 hours for 3 doses; give first dose at 6 to 12 hours of age.

ADVERSE EFFECTS: May cause decreased platelet aggregation, transient oliguria (decreased glomerular filtration rate), increased serum creatinine, and increased serum concentration of renally excreted drugs such as gentamicin. May also cause hyponatremia, hyperkalemia, and hypoglycemia. Gastrointestinal perforations are known to occur if used concurrently with corticosteroids.

COMMENTS: Contraindicated in premature neonates with necrotizing enterocolitis (NEC), severe renal impairment (urine output <0.6 mL/kg/hour or serum creatinine ≥1.8 mg/dL), thrombocytopenia, active bleeding; or if there has been intraventricular bleeding within the preceding 7 days (*controversial*).

INSULIN, REGULAR

INDICATIONS AND USE: Hyperglycemia, hyperkalemia, and increasing caloric intake in infants with glucose intolerance on parenteral nutrition (PN).

ACTIONS: Hormone derived from the β cells of the pancreas and the principal hormone required for glucose utilization. In skeletal and cardiac muscle and adipose tissue, insulin facilitates transport of glucose into these cells. Stimulates lipogenesis and protein synthesis and inhibits lipolysis and release of free fatty acids from adipose cells. Promotes intracellular shift of potassium and magnesium.

SUPPLIED: Injection, 100 units/mL; Humulin R (human insulin prepared using recombinant DNA technology). *Note:* Should be diluted with sterile water or NS by the pharmacy to 1 unit/mL or 10 unit/mL to improve accuracy in measurement and avoid overdose.

ROUTE: IV, subcutaneous.

DOSAGE:

- **Continuous IV infusion** 0.01–0.1 unit/kg/hour (titrate with hourly determinations of blood glucose until stable, then every 4 hours).
- **Intermittent:** 0.1 to 0.2 unit/kg/dose subcutaneous every 6 to 12 hours.

ADVERSE EFFECTS: Hypoglycemia (may cause coma and severe CNS injury), hyperglycemic rebound (Somogyi effect), urticaria, and anaphylaxis.

COMMENTS: To minimize absorption of insulin to IV solution bag or tubing: If new tubing is not needed, wait a minimum of 30 minutes between the preparation of the solution and the initiation of the infusion. If new tubing is needed, after receiving the insulin continuous infusion solution, the administration set should be attached to the IV container and the line should be flushed with the insulin solution; wait 30 minutes, then flush the line again with the insulin solution prior to initiating the infusion. Because of adsorption, the actual amount of insulin being administered could be substantially less than the apparent amount. Therefore, adjustment of the insulin drip rate should be based on the effect and not solely on the apparent insulin dose.

IPRATROPIUM BROMIDE (ATROVENT)

INDICATIONS AND USE: Bronchodilator for adjunctive treatment of acute bronchospasm.

ACTIONS: Anticholinergic drug that acts by antagonizing the action of acetylcholine at the parasympathetic receptor sites, thereby producing bronchodilation.

SUPPLIED: Solution for nebulization, 500 mcg/2.5 mL.

ROUTE: Nebulization. Metered dose inhaler (MDI) use not recommended for neonates.

DOSAGE:

- **Neonates:** 25mcg/kg/dose nebulized every 8 hours.
- **Infants:** 125–250 mcg/dose nebulized every 8 hours. Dilute to 3 mL with normal serum or concurrent albuterol.

ADVERSE EFFECTS: Rebound airway hyperresponsiveness after discontinuation. Nervousness, dizziness, nausea, blurred vision, dry mouth, exacerbation of symptoms, airway irritation, cough, palpitations, rash, and urinary retention. Use with caution in narrow-angle glaucoma or bladder neck obstruction.

COMMENTS: Compatible when admixed with albuterol if given within 1 hour. Bronchodilator effect may be potentiated when given with β-2 agonist (ie, albuterol).

IRON DEXTRAN (INFED, DEXFERRUM)

INDICATIONS AND USE: Used to treat iron deficiency anemia, as an iron supplement for infants on epoetin, and for infants on long-term parenteral nutrition (PN). Oral iron is much safer than the parenteral form; the parenteral form is usually reserved for patients who cannot take oral iron.

ACTIONS: Iron is a component in the formation of hemoglobin, and adequate amounts are necessary for erythropoiesis and oxygen transport capacity of blood.

SUPPLIED: Injection: 50 mg Fe/mL.

ROUTE: IV.

DOSAGE:

- **Iron deficiency anemia:** Calculate total deficit or required dose in mg of iron:
  - Dose Fe (mg/kg) = (12 g/dL—Hgb [g/dL]) × 4.5.
  - Divide this total dose into daily increments (or less frequently), usually not >25 mg Fe/day for infants weighing <5 kg and 50 mg Fe/day for infants 5–10 kg.
- **Anemia of prematurity:** IV: 0.2–1 mg/kg/day or 20 mg/kg/week with epoetin alfa therapy.
- **Parenteral nutritional addition:** Admixed in the PN solution (solution must contain at least 2% amino acids): 0.4–1 mg/kg/day (or 3–5 mg/kg as a single weekly dose).

ADVERSE EFFECTS: Iron accumulation in patients with serious liver dysfunction; anaphylaxis, fever, and arthralgia. IV use: Pain and redness at IV site, rash, shivering; hypotension and flushing with rapid infusion.

ISONIAZID (INH)

INDICATIONS AND USE: Treatment of susceptible *Mycobacterium* spp. (eg, *M. tuberculosis, M. kansasii,* and *M. avium*) and for prophylaxis for individuals exposed to tuberculosis.

ACTION AND SPECTRUM: Antimycobacterial agent which is bactericidal for both extracellular and intracellular organisms. Inhibits mycolic acid synthesis resulting in disruption of the bacterial cell wall.

SUPPLIED: Injection, oral solution.

ROUTE: PO, IM.

DOSAGE: Perinatal tuberculosis—10–15 mg/kg/day divided every 12 hours with rifampin (see rifampin for dosage) for 3–12 months. If skin test conversion is positive, treat with 10–15 mg/kg/day PO every 24 hours for 9–12 months.

ADVERSE EFFECTS: Peripheral neuropathy, seizures, encephalopathy, blood dyscrasias, nausea, vomiting, and diarrhea (associated with administration of syrup formulation) and hypersensitivity reactions. May be hepatotoxic, follow liver function tests at regular intervals during treatment.

ISOPROTERENOL (ISUPREL, OTHERS)

INDICATIONS AND USE: Low cardiac output or vasoconstrictive shock states, cardiac arrest, ventricular arrhythmias resulting from AV block, and bronchospasm.

ACTIONS: Stimulates both β_1- and β_2-adrenergic receptors with minimal or no effect on α receptors in therapeutic doses. Relaxes bronchial smooth muscle, cardiac stimulation (inotropic and chronotropic), and peripheral vasodilation (reduces cardiac afterload).

SUPPLIED: Injection 0.2 mg/mL(1:5000) solution in 1- and 5-mL ampules.

ROUTE: IV, inhalation.

DOSAGE:

• **IV:** 0.05–0.5 mcg/kg/minute IV continuous infusion; maximum dose is 2 mcg/kg/minute. Correct acidosis before initiating therapy.

• **Nebulized:** 0.1–0.25 mL (0.5–1.25 mg) of 0.5% solution. Dilute with NS to 3 mL. Dose: every 3–4 hours.

ADVERSE EFFECTS: Tremor, vomiting, hypertension, tachycardia, cardiac arrhythmias, hypotension, and hypoglycemia.

COMMENTS: Contraindicated in hypertension, hyperthyroidism, tachycardia caused by digoxin toxicity, and preexisting cardiac arrhythmias. Increases cardiac oxygen consumption disproportional to the increase in cardiac oxygen output. Not considered an inotropic agent of choice.

KANAMYCIN SULFATE (KANTREX)

ACTION AND SPECTRUM: Aminoglycoside with a mechanism of action that is similar to that of gentamicin sulfate. Active primarily against Gram-negative aerobic bacteria, including *Escherichia coli; Klebsiella, Enterobacter, Serratia,* and *Proteus* spp.; and some *Pseudomonas* spp. Some activity against staphylococci and mycobacteria. Not active against other Gram-positive organisms or anaerobes.

SUPPLIED: Injection.

ROUTE: IV (infuse over 30 minutes), IM.

DOSAGE: Base the initial dose on body weight, then monitor levels and adjust using pharmacokinetics.

• **0 to 4 weeks of age and <1.2 kg:** 7.5 mg/kg/dose every 18–24 hours.

• **1.2–2 kg:**
  • **0–7 days old:** 7.5 mg/kg/dose every 12–18 hours.
  • **>7 days old:** 7.5 mg/kg/dose every 8–12 hours.

• **>2 kg:**
  • **0–7 days old:** 10 mg/kg/dose every 12 hours.
  • **>7 days old:** 10 mg/kg/dose every 8 hours.

PHARMACOKINETICS: Primarily renally excreted by glomerular filtration. Half-life is 4–8 hours.

ADVERSE EFFECTS:

• **Nephrotoxicity:** (U.S. boxed warning): May cause nephrotoxicity; usual risk factors include preexisting renal impairment, concomitant nephrotoxic medications, and dehydration. Discontinue treatment if signs of nephrotoxicity occur; renal damage is usually reversible.

• **Neurotoxicity:** (U.S. boxed warning): May cause neurotoxicity; usual risk factors include preexisting renal impairment, concomitant neuro-/nephrotoxic medications, and dehydration.

• **Ototoxicity** (auditory and vestibular) is proportional to the amount of drug given and the duration of treatment. Tinnitus or vertigo may be indications of vestibular injury and impending bilateral irreversible damage. Discontinue treatment if signs of ototoxicity occur.

COMMENTS: Desired serum peak is 15–35 mcg/mL (sample obtained 30 minutes after infusion is complete), and serum trough is <10 mcg/mL (sample obtained 30 minutes to just before next dose). In general, a set of serum peak and trough levels should be obtained at about the fourth maintenance dose. Monitor serum creatinine every 3–4 days. Excessive serum peak levels are associated with ototoxicity; excessive trough levels, with nephrotoxicity.

KETOCONAZOLE (NIZORAL)

ACTION AND SPECTRUM: A broad-spectrum antifungal agent that acts by disrupting cell membranes. Fungicidal against *Blastomyces dermatitidis, Candida* spp., *Coccidioides immitis, Histoplasma capsulatum, Paracoccidioides brasiliensis,* and *Phialophora* spp.

SUPPLIED: Tablet, oral suspension may be prepared by the pharmacist.

ROUTE: PO.

DOSAGE: 3.3–6.6 mg/kg/day once daily; administer with food to decrease nausea and vomiting; administer 2 hours prior to antacids, proton pump inhibitors, or H_2-receptor antagonists to prevent decreased ketoconazole absorption; shake suspension well before use.

PHARMACOKINETICS: Hepatic metabolism.

ADVERSE EFFECTS: Gastric distress is the most common side effect. Has been associated with hepatotoxicity, including some fatalities (U.S. boxed warning); perform periodic liver function tests, use with caution in patients with impaired hepatic function; high doses of ketoconazole may depress adrenocortical function and decrease serum testosterone concentrations.

COMMENTS: Penetration into cerebrospinal fluid (CSF) is poor, so do not use in the treatment of fungal meningitis. Minimum period of treatment for candidiasis is 1–2 weeks, but duration should be based on clinical response. Monitor liver function tests. Limited experience in neonates.

KETAMINE HYDROCHLORIDE (KETALAR)

INDICATIONS AND USE: Ketamine is a rapid-acting general anesthetic agent for short diagnostic and minor surgical procedures that do not require skeletal muscle relaxation.

ACTIONS: Produces dissociative anesthesia by direct action on the cortex and limbic system; does not usually impair pharyngeal or laryngeal reflexes Induces coma, analgesia, and amnesia. The patient appears to be awake but is immobile and unresponsive to pain. Increases cerebral blood flow and cerebral oxygen consumption; improves pulmonary compliance and relieves bronchospasm.

SUPPLIED: Injection.

ROUTE: IV, IM, PO.

DOSAGE:

- IV: 0.5–2 mg/kg/dose; use smaller doses (0.5–1 mg/kg) for sedation for minor procedures.
- **Usual induction dose:** 1–2 mg/kg IV. IM: 3–7 mg/kg/dose. PO: 6–10 mg/kg/dose 30 minutes prior to procedure. Dilute before administration. Repeat doses are 1/2 of the initial dose. Reduce dose in hepatic dysfunction.
- **Continuous IV infusion: Sedation:** 5–20 mcg/kg/minute; start at lower dosage listed and titrate to effect.

PHARMACOKINETICS: IV acts in 30 seconds and lasts 5–10 minutes. IM acts 3–4 minutes and lasts 12–25 minutes. Amnesia lasts for 1–2 hours. Concurrent narcotics or barbiturates prolong recovery time.

ADVERSE EFFECTS: Avoid use of ketamine in patients with increased intracranial pressure, cerebral blood flow, cerebrospinal fluid (CSF) pressure, cerebral metabolism, or if significant elevation in blood pressure may present a risk.

- **Cardiovascular:** Elevated blood pressure (frequent), tachycardia, arrhythmia, hypotension, bradycardia, increased cerebral blood flow, and decreased cardiac output may occur.
- **Respiratory:** Respiratory depression, and apnea after rapid IV administration of high doses; laryngospasm; and hypersalivation. Increased airway resistance, cough reflex may be depressed, decreased bronchospasm.
- **Ophthalmic:** Nystagmus, increased intraocular pressure.
- **CNS:** Emergence reactions (psychic disturbances such as hallucinations and delirium lasting up to 24 hours). Minimize by reducing verbal, tactile, and visual simulation in the recovery period. These occur less commonly in pediatric patients than in adults. Severe reactions can be treated with a benzodiazepine. Increased muscle tone that may resemble seizures and extensor spasm with opisthotonos may occur in infants receiving high, repeated doses.
- **Dermatologic:** Rash as well as pain and redness at the IM injection site.

COMMENTS: Pretreatment with a benzodiazepine 15 minutes before ketamine may reduce side effects such as psychic, increased intracranial pressure and cerebral blood flow, tachycardia, and jerking movements. Monitor heart rate, respiratory rate, blood pressure, and pulse oximetry. Observe for CNS side effects during the recovery period. Have equipment for resuscitation available.

LABETALOL HYDROCHLORIDE (NORMODYNE)

INDICATIONS AND USE: Treatment of mild to severe hypertension. IV form is used in case of hypertension emergencies.

ACTIONS: Causes a dose-related decrease in blood pressure through α-, β_1- and β_2-adrenergic receptor blockade without causing significant reflex tachycardia or a decrease in heart rate. Reduces elevated renin levels.

SUPPLIED: Injection, tablet.

ROUTE: IV, PO.

DOSAGE: Limited experience in neonates; labetalol should be initiated cautiously, carefully monitor blood pressure, heart rate, and electrocardiogram, and adjust the dose accordingly. Use the lowest effective dose. IV intermittent bolus doses: 0.2–0.5 mg/kg/dose over 2–3 minutes every 4–6 hours; with a range of 0.2–1 mg/kg/dose have been suggested; maximum dose: 20 mg/dose.

- **Treatment of pediatric hypertensive emergencies:** Continuous IV infusion: 0.4–1 mg/kg/hour with a maximum of 3 mg/kg/hour have been used; one study used initial bolus dose of 0.2–1 mg/kg (maximum dose: 20 mg, mean: 0.5 mg/kg) followed by a continuous infusion of 0.25–1.5 mg/kg/hour (mean: 0.78 mg/kg/hour).
- **Oral:** Some centers use initial PO doses of 4 mg/kg/day in 2 divided doses. Reported oral doses have started at 3 mg/kg/day and 20 mg/kg/day and have increased up to 40 mg/kg/day.

PHARMACOKINETICS: Peak effect with PO is 1–4 hours after the dose while peak effect with IV is 5–15 minutes. Metabolized in the liver by glucuronidation. Oral labetalol has a bioavailability of only 25% because of extensive first-pass effect. Oral absorption is improved by taking with food. Concomitant oral cimetidine may increase the bioavailability of oral labetalol.

ADVERSE EFFECTS: Orthostatic hypotension, bronchospasm, nasal congestion, edema, congestive heart failure, bradycardia, myopathy, and rash. Intensifies atrioventricular (AV) block. Reversible hepatic dysfunction (rare).

COMMENTS: Do not discontinue chronic labetalol abruptly; rather, discontinue gradually over 1–2 weeks. Contraindicated in patients with asthma, overt cardiac failure, heart block, cardiogenic shock, or severe bradycardia. May cause a paradoxic increase in blood pressure in patients with pheochromocytoma. Use with caution in hepatic dysfunction. Incompatible with sodium bicarbonate.

LEVETIRACETAM (KEPPRA)

INDICATIONS AND USE: Adjunctive therapy in the treatment of partial onset seizures in children ≥4 years of age.

ACTIONS AND SPECTRUM: The exact antiepileptic effects are unknown. The results of several studies suggest that one or more of the following central pharmacologic effects may be involved: inhibition of voltage-dependent N-type calcium channels; blockade of gabanergic inhibitory transmission through displacement of negative modulators; reversal of the inhibition of glycine currents; reduction of delayed rectifier potassium current; and/or binding to synaptic proteins which modulate neurotransmitter release.

SUPPLIED: Injection, oral solution, tablet.

ROUTE: IV, PO.

DOSAGE: Not approved for use in infants 6 months of age to children 4 years; limited information available. Initial dose: 5 to 10 mg/kg/day PO/IV given in 2 or 3 divided doses; may increase every week by 10 mg/kg/day, if tolerated, to maximum of 60 mg/kg/day. *Note:* When switching from oral to IV formulation, the total daily dose should be the same.

PHARMACOKINETICS: Oral absorption is rapid and complete, oral bioavailability 100%.

ADVERSE EFFECTS: Somnolence, nervousness.

COMMENTS: Limited information from small clinical trials, there are neonatal pharmacokinetic studies and pilot trials in progress at this time.

LEVOTHYROXINE SODIUM (T₄) (SYNTHROID, LEVOXYL, OTHERS)

INDICATIONS AND USE: Replacement or supplemental therapy in congenital or acquired hypothyroidism.

ACTIONS: The exact mechanism of action is unknown; however, it is believed the thyroid hormone exerts its many metabolic effects through control of DNA transcription and protein synthesis. Thyroid hormones increase the metabolic rate of body tissues, noted by increases in oxygen consumption; respiratory rate; body temperature; cardiac output; heart rate; blood volume; rates of fat, protein, and carbohydrate metabolism; and enzyme system activity, growth, and maturation. Thyroid hormones are very important in CNS development. Deficiency in infants results in growth retardation and failure of brain growth and development.

SUPPLIED: Injection; tablets may be crushed and mixed with water or a small amount of infant formula and administered immediately after mixing. Discard the unused portion.

ROUTE: IV, IM, PO.

DOSAGE: *Note:* IV, IM use 50% to 75% of the oral dose.

• **Neonates, infants, and children:**
  • **0–3 months:** 10–15 mcg/kg PO; if the infant is at risk for development of cardiac failure, use a lower starting dose ~25 mcg/day; if the initial serum T_4 is very low (<5 mcg/dL), begin treatment at a higher dosage, ~50 mcg/day.
  • **>3–6 months:** 8–10 mcg/kg or 25–50 mcg.
  • **>6–12 months:** 6–8 mcg/kg or 50–75 mcg.
• **Alternate dosing:** 8–10 mcg/kg/day PO has been recommended for infants from birth to 1 year.

ADVERSE EFFECTS: Adverse effects are usually due to excessive dose. If the following occur, discontinue and reinstitute at a lower dose: tachycardia, cardiac arrhythmias, tremors, diarrhea, weight loss, and fever.

LIDOCAINE (XYLOCAINE, OTHERS)

INDICATIONS AND USE: IV lidocaine is used almost exclusively for the short-term control of ventricular arrhythmias (premature beats, tachycardia, and fibrillation) or for prophylactic treatment of such arrhythmias. Also used as a local anesthetic.

ACTIONS: Class IB antiarrhythmic agent, suppresses spontaneous depolarization of the ventricles during diastole by a direct action on the tissues; blocks both the initiation and conduction of nerve impulses by decreasing the neuronal membrane's permeability to sodium ions; inhibits of depolarization and results in blockade of conduction.

SUPPLIED: IV forms: injection; solution for local anesthesia.

ROUTE: IV, subcutaneous, intratracheal and topical.

DOSAGE:

- **Initial:** 0.5–1 mg/kg/dose as IV bolus over 5 minutes. May repeat dose every 10 minutes as necessary to control arrhythmia to a maximum total bolus dose of 5 mg/kg.
- **Maintenance IV infusion:** 10–50 mcg/kg/minute Use lowest possible dose for preterm infants.
- **Endotracheal:** 2–3 mg/kg; flush with 5 mL of normal saline and follow with 5 assisted manual ventilations.

PHARMACOKINETICS: Primarily metabolized by the liver.

ADVERSE EFFECTS: Drowsiness, dizziness, tremulousness, paresthesias, muscle twitching, seizures, and coma; respiratory depression and or arrest. Hypotension and heart block can occur.

COMMENTS: Therapeutic levels: 1–5 mcg/mL with toxic levels >6 mcg/mL. Adjust dosage in liver failure. Contraindicated in sinoatrial or atrioventricular (AV) nodal block and Wolff-Parkinson-White syndrome. Avoid using with epinephrine.

LIDOCAINE/PRILOCAINE CREAM (EMLA)

INDICATIONS AND USE: Topical anesthetic for use on intact skin for minor procedures such as insertion of intravenous catheters, venipuncture, and lumbar puncture in infants ≥37 weeks' gestational age.

ACTIONS: EMLA (eutectic mixture of local anesthetics) contains two local anesthetics: lidocaine and prilocaine. Local anesthetics inhibit conduction of nerve impulses from sensory nerves by changing the cell membrane's permeability to ions.

SUPPLIED: Cream: Lidocaine 2.5% with prilocaine 2.5% and Tegaderm™ dressings; disc and gel.

ROUTE: Topical.

DOSAGE: Maximum EMLA dose, application area and application time:

- **0–3 months or <5 kg:** Maximum 1 g over 10 cm² for 1 hour.
- **3–12 months and >5 kg:** Maximum 2 g over 20 cm² for 4 hours.
- **1–6 years and >10 kg:** Maximum 10 g over 100 cm² for 4 hours.

ADVERSE EFFECTS: Not for use on mucous membranes or ophthalmic use. May cause methemoglobinemia. Not for use in infants <37 weeks' gestational age or infants <12 months old receiving concurrent methemoglobin-inducing agents (sulfonamides, acetaminophen, nitroprusside, nitric oxide, phenobarbital, phenytoin). Reduce amounts if infant has hepatic and/or renal dysfunction.

COMMENT: Do not rub into skin; cover with occlusive dressing.

LINEZOLID (ZYVOX)

INDICATIONS AND USE: Treatment of community- and hospital-acquired pneumonia; complicated and uncomplicated skin and soft tissue infections; bacteremia caused by susceptible vancomycin-resistant *Enterococcus faecium* (VREF), *Enterococcus faecalis, Streptococcus pneumoniae* including multidrug resistant strains, *Staphylococcus aureus* including methicillin-resistant *Staphylococcus aureus* (MRSA), *Streptococcus pyogenes*, or *Streptococcus agalactiae. Note:* There have been reports of vancomycin-resistant *E. faecium* and MRSA developing resistance to linezolid during its clinical use.

ACTIONS AND SPECTRUM: Linezolid inhibits initiation of protein synthesis by binding to a site on the bacterial 23S ribosomal RNA of the 50S subunit preventing the formation of a functional 70S initiation complex, which is an essential component of the bacterial translation process.

SUPPLIED: Injection, oral suspension and tablet.

ROUTE: IV, PO.

DOSAGE: *Note:* No dosage adjustment needed when switching from IV to oral.

- **Neonates 0–4 weeks and birthweight <1200 g:**
  - Oral, IV: 10 mg/kg/dose every 8–12 hours.
  - *Note:* Use 12 hours in patients <34 weeks' gestation and <1 week of age.
- **Neonates <7 days and birthweight ≥1200 g:**
  - Oral, IV: 10 mg/kg/dose every 8–12 hours.
  - *Note:* Use every 12 hours in patients <34 weeks' gestation and <1 week of age.
- **Neonates ≥7 days and birthweight ≥1200 g (infants and children):**
  - **Complicated skin and skin structure infections, nosocomial or community-acquired pneumonia including concurrent bacteremia:** 10 mg/kg/dose PO/IV every 8 hours for 10–14 days.
  - **VREF:** Oral, IV—10 mg/kg/dose every 8 hours for 14–28 days.
  - **Uncomplicated skin and skin structure infections:** Children <5 years: 10 mg/kg/dose PO every 8 hours for 10–14 days.

PHARMACOKINETICS: Orally well absorbed, and distributed to well perfused tissues.

ADVERSE EFFECTS: Thrombocytopenia, anemia, leukopenia, and pancytopenia have been reported in patients receiving linezolid and may be dependent on duration of therapy (generally >2 weeks of treatment); monitor patients' complete blood cell count (CBC) weekly during linezolid therapy; discontinuation of therapy may be required in patients who develop or have worsening myelosuppression. *C. difficile*–associated colitis has been reported; fluid and electrolyte management, protein supplementation, antibiotic treatment, and surgical evaluation may be indicated. Peripheral and optic neuropathy with vision loss have been reported primarily in patients treated for longer then 28 days with linezolid. Cases of lactic acidosis in which patients experienced repeated episodes of nausea and vomiting, acidosis, and low bicarbonate levels have been reported. Elevated transaminases, rash, and diarrhea.

COMMENTS: Therapeutic linezolid concentrations were inconsistently achieved or maintained in the CSF of pediatric patients with ventriculoperitoneal shunts, use of linezolid for the empiric treatment of pediatric CNS infections is not recommended. Linezolid is not approved for the treatment of catheter-related bloodstream, catheter-site, or Gram-negative infections. Linezolid is a reversible, nonselective inhibitor of monoamine oxidase: Enhanced vasopressor effects if used with sympathomimetic agents such as dopamine, epinephrine; myelosuppressive drugs (may increase risk of myelosuppression with linezolid).

LORAZEPAM (ATIVAN)

INDICATIONS AND USE: Treatment of status epilepticus resistant to conventional anticonvulsant therapy (ie, phenobarbital or phenytoin); sedation.

ACTIONS: A benzodiazepine that binds to the gamma-aminobutyric acid (GABA) receptor complex and facilitates the inhibitory effect of GABA on the CNS.

SUPPLIED: Oral solution; injection.

ROUTE: PO, IM, IV.

DOSAGE:

- Status epilepticus:
  - Neonates: 0.05 mg/kg/dose IV over 2–5 minutes. If no response after 10–15 minutes, may repeat the dose; dilute with an equal volume of sterile water, normal saline, or D$_5$W.
  - Infants and children: 0.1 mg/kg slow IV over 2–5 minutes, do not exceed 4 mg/single dose; may repeat second dose of 0.05 mg/kg slow IV in 10–15 minutes if needed; dilute with an equal volume of sterile water, NS, or D$_5$W.
  - Sedation, anxiety: 0.02–0.1 mg/kg/dose IV or PO every 4–8 hours as needed; not to exceed 2 mg/dose.

ADVERSE EFFECTS: May cause respiratory depression, apnea, hypotension, bradycardia, cardiac arrest, and seizure-like activity. Paradoxic CNS stimulation may occur, usually early in therapy. Some preterm infants may exhibit myoclonic activity. The drug should be discontinued if any CNS effect occurs. Overdose may be reversed using flumazenil (Romazicon), 5–10 mcg/kg/dose IV. Reversal agent may trigger seizures.

COMMENTS: Note: IV preparations contain benzyl alcohol, propylene glycol, and polyethylene glycol. Contraindicated for infants with pre-existing CNS, hepatic or renal disease.

MAGNESIUM SULFATE

INDICATIONS AND USE: Treatment and prevention of hypomagnesemia and refractory hypocalcemia.

ACTIONS: Magnesium is important as a cofactor in many enzymatic reactions in the body. In the CNS, magnesium prevents or controls seizures by blocking neuromuscular transmission and decreasing the amount of acetylcholine liberated. It also has a depressant effect on the CNS. In the heart, magnesium acts as a calcium channel blocker and acts on cardiac muscle to slow sinoatrial nodal impulse formation and prolong conduction time. Magnesium is necessary for the maintaining of serum potassium and calcium levels due to its effect on the renal tubule.

SUPPLIED: Injection.

ROUTE: IM and IV.

DOSAGE:

- Hypomagnesemia:
  - Neonates: 25–50 mg/kg/dose (0.2–0.4 mEq/kg/dose) IV every 8–12 hours for 2–3 doses until magnesium level is normal or symptoms resolve.
    - Maintenance: 0.25–0.5 mEq/kg/24 hours IV (add to infusion or give IV).
  - Children: 25–50 mg/kg/dose (0.2–0.4 mEq/kg/dose) IM/IV every 4–6 hours for 3–4 doses; maximum single dose: 2000 mg (16 mEq).

ADVERSE EFFECTS: Adverse effects with magnesium therapy are primarily related to the magnesium serum level; hypotension, flushing, depression of reflexes, depressed cardiac function, and CNS and respiratory depression.

COMMENTS: Contraindicated in renal failure. Monitor serum magnesium, calcium, and phosphate levels. For intermittent infusion: Dilute to a concentration of 0.5 mEq/mL (60 mg/mL) of magnesium sulfate; maximum concentration: 1.6 mEq/mL, 200 mg/mL of magnesium sulfate); infuse magnesium sulfate over 2–4 hours and do not exceed 1 mEq/kg/hour.

MEROPENEM (MERREM)

INDICATIONS AND USE: Specifically active against pneumococcal and pseudomonas meningitis, extended-spectrum beta-lactamase producing Klebsiella pneumoniae. Treatment of serious infections caused by multidrug-resistant Gram-negative organisms and Gram-positive aerobic and anaerobic pathogens susceptible to meropenem.

ACTIONS: A broad spectrum antibiotic of the carbapenem family that penetrates well into cerebrospinal fluid (CSF) and most body tissues. Inhibits bacterial cell wall synthesis.

SUPPLIED: Injection.

ROUTE: IV. Infuse drug over 15–30 minutes.
DOSAGE:
- **Neonates:**
  - **Postnatal age 0–7 days:** 20 mg/kg/dose IV every 12 hours.
  - **Postnatal age >7 days:**
    - **Weight 1200–2000 g:** 20 mg/kg/dose IV every 12 hours.
    - **Weight >2000 g:** 20 mg/kg/dose IV every 8 hours.
  - **Meningitis and infection caused by *Pseudomonas* species:** 40 mg/kg/dose IV every 8 hours.
- **Children ≥3 months:**
  - **Complicated skin and skin structure infection:** 10 mg/kg/dose every 8 hours; maximum dose 500 mg.
  - **Intra-abdominal infection:** 20 mg/kg/dose every 8 hours; maximum dose: 1 g.
  - **Meningitis:** 40 mg/kg/dose every 8 hours; maximum dose: 2 g.

ADVERSE EFFECTS: Gastrointestinal effects such as diarrhea, vomiting, and rarely pseudomembranous colitis. *Note:* compatible with amphotericin: fungal overgrowth a risk. Thrombocytosis and eosinophilia have been noted. Monitoring liver enzymes is recommended. Some cautionary reports have noted seizure like episodes in a few preterm infants.

COMMENT: Serum half-life of meropenem is relatively short in infants (3 hours or less).

METHADONE HYDROCHLORIDE (DOLOPHINE)

INDICATIONS AND USE: Long-acting narcotic analgesic used for the treatment of neonatal abstinence syndrome.
ACTIONS: CNS opiate receptor agonist resulting in analgesia and sedation; produces generalized CNS depression.
SUPPLIED: Injection; oral solution.
ROUTE: IV, PO.
DOSAGE: **Neonatal abstinence syndrome:** 0.05–0.2 mg/kg/dose PO/IV given every 12–24 hours or 0.5mg/kg/day divided every 8 hours. Individualize dose and tapering schedule to control symptoms of withdrawal; usually taper dose by 10% to 20% per week over 1 to 1 1/2 months. *Note:* Due to long elimination half-life, tapering is difficult; consider alternate agent like morphine.
ADVERSE EFFECTS: Respiratory depression, bronchospasm, gastric residuals, abdominal distension, constipation, hypotension, bradycardia, CNS depression, sedation, increased intracranial pressure, urinary tract spasm, urine retention, biliary tract spasm, and dependence with prolonged use.
COMMENTS: *Caution:* Methadone may accumulate; reassess for the need to adjust the dose downward after 3–5 days to avoid overdose. Smaller doses or less frequent administration may be required in renal and hepatic dysfunction. Rifampin and phenytoin increase metabolism of methadone and may precipitate withdrawal symptoms. Methadone 10 mg IM = morphine 10 mg IM.

METHICILLIN SODIUM (STAPHCILLIN)

ACTION AND SPECTRUM: Mechanism of action identical to that of other β-lactam antibiotics, active primarily against penicillinase-positive and penicillinase-negative staphylococci and less effective than penicillin G against other Gram-positive cocci. Does not demonstrate any activity against enterococci. Other anti-staphylococcal penicillins such as nafcillin and oxacillin are used more commonly in the United States.
SUPPLIED: Injection.
ROUTE: IM, IV (infuse over 20 minutes).
DOSAGE:
- **Meningitis:**
  - **<2000 g and 0–7 days old:** 100 mg/kg/day divided every 12 hours.
  - **<2000 g and >7 days old:** 150 mg/kg/day divided every 8 hours.
  - **>2000 g and 0–7 days old:** 150 mg/kg/day divided every 8 hours.
  - **>2000 g and >7 days old:** 200 mg/kg/day divided every 6 hours.
- **Other indications:**
  - **<2000 g and 0–7 days old:** 50 mg/kg/day divided every 12 hours.
  - **<2000 g and >7 days old:** 75 mg/kg/day divided every 8 hours.
  - **>2000 g and 0–7 days old:** 75 mg/kg/day divided every 8 hours.
  - **>2000 g and >7 days old:** 100 mg/kg/day divided every 6 hours.

PHARMACOKINETICS: Renal excretion. Half-life is variable (60–120 minutes or longer).
ADVERSE EFFECTS: Nephrotoxicity (interstitial nephritis) occurs more often with methicillin than with other penicillins. May cause hypersensitivity reactions, anemia, leukopenia, thrombocytopenia, phlebitis at the infusion site, and hemorrhagic cystitis (in poorly hydrated patients).
COMMENTS: In cases of methicillin resistance, vancomycin becomes the antistaphylococcal drug of choice. Dosage adjustment is necessary in renal impairment. Monitor serum urea nitrogen and creatinine. Contains 2.9 mEq of sodium/g.

METOCLOPRAMIDE HYDROCHLORIDE (REGLAN)

INDICATIONS AND USE: In neonates and infants, the drug is used to facilitate gastric emptying and gastrointestinal (GI) motility. May improve feeding intolerance and gastroesophageal reflux.

ACTIONS: Dopamine receptor antagonist acting on the CNS. Metoclopramide improves GI motility by releasing acetylcholine from the myenteric plexus resulting in contraction of the smooth muscle. Metoclopramide's effects on the GI tract include the following:

• Increased resting esophageal sphincter tone.
• Improved gastric tone and peristalsis.
• Relaxes pyloric sphincter
• Augmented duodenal peristalsis.

The combined effect of metoclopramide on the GI tract leads to increased gastric emptying and a decrease in the transit time through the duodenum, jejunum, and ileum.

SUPPLIED: Injection, syrup.

ROUTE: IM, IV, PO.

DOSAGE: Gastroesophageal reflux in neonates, infants, and children—0.1–0.2 mg/kg/dose PO/IM/IV given every 6 hours 30 minutes before feedings.

ADVERSE EFFECTS: CNS effects include restlessness, drowsiness, and fatigue. Extrapyramidal reactions may occur but usually subside 24 hours after discontinuation of the drug. These reactions occur most frequently in children following IV administration of high doses.

COMMENTS: Contraindicated with bowel obstruction and seizure disorders.

METRONIDAZOLE (FLAGYL)

ACTION AND SPECTRUM: Bactericidal antibiotic that causes loss of helical DNA structure and strand breakage, which halt protein synthesis resulting in cell death. Good activity against anaerobic protozoa, including *Trichomonas vaginalis, Entamoeba histolytica, Giardia lamblia,* and *Balantidium coli.* Good activity also against Gram-positive bacteria (*Clostridium, Peptococcus, Peptostreptococcus,* and *Veillonella* spp.) and anaerobic Gram-negative bacteria (*Bacteroides* and *Fusobacterium* spp.). Nonsporulating Gram-positive bacilli are often resistant (eg, *Propionibacterium* and *Actinomyces* spp.), and the drug has minimal activity against aerobic and facultative anaerobic bacteria.

SUPPLIED: Injection.

ROUTE: IV (infuse over 30–60 minutes).

DOSAGE:

• **Neonates, anaerobic infections:**
  • **0–4 weeks, <1200 g:** 7.5 mg/kg PO/IV every 48 hours.
  • **Postnatal age ≤7 days:**
    • **1200–2000 g:** 7.5 mg/kg/day PO/IV given every 24 hours.
    • **>2000 g:** 15 mg/kg/day in PO/IV divided doses every 12 hours.
  • **Postnatal age >7 days:**
    • **1200–2000 g:** 15 mg/kg/day PO/IV in divided doses every 12 hours.
    • **>2000 g:** 30 mg/kg/day PO/IV in divided doses every 12 hours.
• **Infants and children:**
  • **Anaerobic infections:** 30 mg/kg/day PO/IV in divided doses every 6 hours; maximum dose: 4 g/day.
• **Antibiotic-associated pseudomembranous colitis:** 30 mg/kg/day PO divided every 6 hours for 7–10 days.

PHARMACOKINETICS: Hepatic metabolism with final excretion via the urine and feces. Large volume of distribution (penetrates into all body tissues and fluids).

ADVERSE EFFECTS: Occasional vomiting, diarrhea, insomnia, weakness, rash, discoloration of urine (dark or reddish brown), phlebitis at the injection site, and (rarely) leukopenia.

COMMENTS: Use of metronidazole is contraindicated during the first trimester of pregnancy. Some texts recommend an initial loading dose of 15 mg/kg, with the first maintenance dose either 48 hours later (for premature infants <2000 g) or 24 hours later (for the infant >2000 g at birth). Effectively penetrates into the CSF and, therefore, is indicated for meningitis resulting from susceptible anaerobic pathogens. *Note:* Some centers use for empiric coverage with ampicillin and gentamicin for NEC. Use of metronidazole in NEC remains *controversial.*

MIDAZOLAM HYDROCHLORIDE (VERSED)

INDICATIONS AND USE: Anxiolytic and antiepileptic agent. Can be used as a sedative before procedures and given IV continuously to sedate intubated or mechanically ventilated patients.

ACTIONS: Short-acting benzodiazepine; depresses CNS by binding to the benzodiazepine site on the gamma-aminobutyric acid (GABA) receptor complex and increasing GABA, which is a major inhibitory neurotransmitter in the brain.

SUPPLIED: Injection, oral syrup (contains sodium benzoate).

ROUTE: PO, IV, IM, intranasal, sublingual.

DOSAGE:

• **Intermittent:** 0.05–0.15 mg/kg/dose IV/IM every 2–4 hours as needed.
• **Continuous infusion:**
  • **<32 weeks:** Initial 0.03 mg/kg/hour (0.5 mcg/kg/minute).
  • **>32 weeks:** Initial 0.06 mg/kg/hour (1 mcg/kg/minute).

- **Dosage ranges from 0.01 to 0.06 mg/kg/hour.** May need to increase dose after several days of therapy due to tolerance or increased clearance. *Note:* Do not use IV loading doses in neonates; for faster achievement of sedation, infuse the continuous infusion at a faster rate for the first several hours; use the smallest dose possible.
- **Oral:** 0.25 mg/kg/dose using oral syrup.
- **Intranasal:** 0.2 to 0.3 mg/kg/dose using 5 mg/mL injectable form; may repeat in 5–15 minutes.
- **Sublingual:** 0.2 mg/kg/dose using 5 mg/mL injectable form mixed with small amount of flavored syrup.

ADVERSE EFFECTS: Respiratory depression and cardiac arrest with excessive doses or rapid IV infusions. May cause hypotension and bradycardia. Myoclonic activity has been reported in preterm infants as well as other seizure-like activity.

COMMENT: Infuse IV slowly. Benzodiazepine withdrawal may occur if abruptly discontinued in patients receiving prolonged IV continuous infusions; doses should be tapered slowly with prolonged use. Contraindicated if pre-existing CNS depression.

MILRINONE (PRIMACOR)

INDICATIONS AND USE: Short-term (<72 hours) treatment of acute low cardiac output due to septic shock or following cardiac surgery.

ACTIONS AND SPECTRUM: Inhibits phosphodiesterase III (PDE III), the major PDE in cardiac and vascular tissues. Inhibition of PDE III increases cyclic adenosine monophosphate (cAMP), which potentiates the delivery of calcium to myocardial contractile systems and results in a positive inotropic effect. Inhibition of PDE III in vascular tissue results in relaxation of vascular muscle and vasodilatation. Unlike catecholamines, milrinone does not increase myocardial oxygen consumption.

SUPPLIED: Injection.

ROUTE: IV.

DOSAGE:

- **Neonates, infants, and children:** A limited number of studies have used different dosing schemes. Two studies propose per kg doses for pediatric patients with septic shock that are greater than those recommended for adults and in infants and children after cardiac surgery Further pharmacodynamic studies are needed to define pediatric milrinone guidelines. Several centers use the following guidelines:
  - **Loading dose:** 50 mcg/kg administered over 15 minutes followed by a continuous infusion of 0.5 mcg/kg/minute; range: 0.25–0.75 mcg/kg/minute; titrate to effect.
  - **Pediatric Advanced Life Support (PALS) Guidelines 2005:** Loading dose: 50–75 mcg/kg IV or IO (or intraosseous) administered over 15 minutes followed by a continuous infusion of 0.5–0.75 mcg/kg/minute.

PHARMACOKINETICS: With renal impairment, half-life is prolonged and clearance is decreased. Excreted in urine as unchanged drug (83%) and glucuronide metabolite (12%).

ADVERSE EFFECTS: Hypokalemia, thrombocytopenia, abnormal liver function tests, ventricular arrhythmias, and hypotension.

COMMENTS: Use with caution and modify dosage in patients with impaired renal function; adequate intravascular volume is necessary prior to initiating therapy.

MORPHINE SULFATE (VARIOUS)

INDICATIONS AND USE: Analgesia, preoperative sedation, supplement to anesthesia, treatment of opioid withdrawal and relief of dyspnea associated with pulmonary edema.

ACTIONS: Morphine sulfate is a pure opioid agonist, selective to the mu receptor in the CNS. The interaction with these opioid receptors results in effects that mimic the actions of enkephalins, β-endorphin and other exogenous ligands.

SUPPLIED: Injection, oral solution.

ROUTE: IM, IV, subcutaneous, PO.

DOSAGE:

- **Neonates** (use preservative free form):
  - **Initial:** 0.05 mg/kg IM, IV, subcutaneous every 4–8 hours; titrate carefully to effect; maximum dose: 0.1 mg/kg/dose.
  - **Continuous infusion:** Initial: 0.01 mg/kg/hour (10 mcg/kg/hour); do not exceed infusion rates of 0.015–0.02 mg/kg/hour due to decreased elimination, increased CNS sensitivity, and adverse effects; may need to use slightly higher doses, especially in neonates who develop tolerance.
  - **International evidence-based group for neonatal pain recommendations** (Anand: *Arch Pediatr Adolesc Med* 2001; 155(2):173-180):
    - **Intermittent dose:** 0.05–0.1 mg/kg/dose.
    - **Continuous infusion:** Range: 0.01–0.03 mg/kg/hour
  - **Neonatal narcotic abstinence:** 0.03–0.1 mg/kg/dose PO every 3–4 hours. Taper dose by 10–20% every 2–3 days based on abstinence scoring.
  - **Infants and children:** Oral: 0.2–0.5 mg/kg/dose every 4 to 6 hours as needed.

ADVERSE EFFECTS: Dose-dependent side effects include miosis, respiratory depression, drowsiness, bradycardia, and hypotension. Constipation, sedation, gastrointestinal upset, urinary retention, histamine release, and sweating may occur. Causes physiologic dependence; taper the dose gradually after long-term use to avoid withdrawal.

Mupirocin (Bactroban)

INDICATIONS AND USE: Topical treatment of impetigo resulting from *Staphylococcus aureus* (including methicillin-resistant strains), β-hemolytic *Streptococcus* spp., and *Streptococcus pyogenes*. Used for minor bacterial skin infections resulting from susceptible organisms and eradication of *S. aureus* from nasal and perineal carriage sites.
ACTIONS: Inhibits protein and RNA synthesis by binding to bacterial isoleucyl-tRNA synthetase.
SUPPLIED: 2% Topical ointment and cream.
ROUTE: Topical.
DOSAGE:

- **Intranasal:**
  - **Children:** Apply sparingly 2–4 times a day for 5–14 days. Reevaluate in 5 days if no response.
- **Topical:**
  - **Cream, infants ≥3 months:** Apply small amount 3 times/day for 10 days.
  - **Ointment, infants ≥2 months:** Apply a small amount 3–5 times/day for 5–14 days.

ADVERSE EFFECTS: Burning, rash, erythema, and pruritus.
COMMENTS: Use with caution in burn patients and patients with impaired renal function. Avoid contact with eyes; not for ophthalmic use. When applied to extensive open wounds or burns, the possibility of absorption of the polyethylene glycol vehicle, resulting in serious renal toxicity, should be considered.

NAFCILLIN SODIUM (UNIPEN)

ACTION AND SPECTRUM: Semisynthetic penicillinase-resistant penicillin with bactericidal activity against susceptible bacteria due the interference with bacterial cell wall synthesis. Treatment of bacterial infections such as osteomyelitis, septicemia, endocarditis, and CNS infections due to susceptible penicillinase-producing strains of *Staphylococcus*.
SUPPLIED: Injection.
ROUTE: IV (infuse over 15–60 minutes), IM.
DOSAGE:

- **Neonates:**
  - **0–4 weeks, <1200 g:** 50 mg/kg/day IM/IV in divided doses every 12 hours.
  - **≤7 days:**
    - **1200–2000 g:** 50 mg/kg/day IM/IV in divided doses every 12 hours.
    - **>2000 g:** 75 mg/kg/day IM/IV in divided doses every 8 hour.
  - **>7 days:**
    - **1200–2000 g:** 75 mg/kg/day IM/IV in divided doses every 8 hours.
    - **>2000 g:** 100–140 mg/kg/day IM/IV in divided doses every 6 hours.
- **Children:**
  - **Mild to moderate infections:** 50–100 mg/kg/day IM/IV in divided doses every 6 hours.
  - **Severe infections:** 100–200 mg/kg/day IM/IV in divided doses every 4–6 hours; maximum dose, 12 g/day.
  - **Staphylococcal endocarditis native valve:** 200 mg/kg/day IM/IV in divided doses every 4–6 hours for 6 weeks.

PHARMACOKINETICS: Hepatic metabolism; concentrated in bile.
ADVERSE EFFECTS: Thrombophlebitis, hypersensitivity, granulocytopenia, and agranulocytosis. Severe tissue injury after IV extravasation.
COMMENTS: Avoid IM use if possible. Contains 3.33 mEq of sodium/g.

NALOXONE HYDROCHLORIDE (NARCAN)

INDICATIONS AND USE: Reverses CNS and respiratory depression in suspected narcotic overdose; neonatal opiate depression; adjunct in the treatment of septic shock.
ACTIONS: An opiate antagonist that competes and displaces narcotics at narcotic receptor sites. It has little to no agonistic activity. Onset of action is within 1–2 minutes after IV injection and 2–5 minutes after IM injection. Duration of action is generally 20–60 minutes.
SUPPLIED: Injection.
ROUTE: IV, IM.
DOSAGE:

- **Usual dose:** 0.1 mg/kg and may repeat in 3–5 minutes, or
- **Alternative dosing to avoid sudden hemodynamic effects from opioid reversal:** 0.01–0.03 mg/kg and repeat every 2–3 minutes as needed.

ADVERSE EFFECTS: Hypertension, hypotension, tachycardia, and ventricular arrhythmias.
COMMENTS: Avoid in infants of narcotic-addicted mothers because naloxone may precipitate acute withdrawal syndrome. Infants must be monitored for reappearance of respiratory depression and the need for repeated doses.

NEOMYCIN SULFATE

ACTION AND SPECTRUM: Aminoglycoside that acts by interfering with bacterial protein synthesis. Inactive against anaerobic organisms. Indicated in the treatment of diarrhea resulting from enteropathogenic *Escherichia coli* and as preoperative prophylaxis before intestinal surgery. As an adjunct therapy in hepatic encephalopathy.
SUPPLIED: Oral solution (contains benzoic acid), powder, tablet.
ROUTE: PO.
DOSAGE: 50–100 mg/kg/day PO divided every 6–8 hours.
PHARMACOKINETICS: Renal excretion if systemic absorption occurs; otherwise, fecally excreted.
ADVERSE EFFECTS: Sensitization with allergic reaction. May cause renal toxicity or ototoxicity.
COMMENTS: Poorly absorbed from the gastrointestinal tract.

NEOSTIGMINE METHYLSULFATE (PROSTIGMIN)

INDICATIONS AND USE: Improvement of muscle strength in the treatment of myasthenia gravis. May be used to reverse nondepolarizing neuromuscular blockers (eg, tubocurarine and pancuronium).
ACTIONS: Neostigmine competitively inhibits hydrolysis of acetylcholine by acetylcholinesterase facilitating transmission of impulses across the myoneural junction and producing cholinergic activity.
SUPPLIED: Injection.
ROUTE: IM, IV, subcutaneous, PO.
DOSAGE:

- **Myasthenia gravis:**
  - **Diagnosis:** 0.025–0.04 mg/kg/dose IM once. (Discontinue all cholinesterase medications at least 8 hours before; atropine should be administered IV immediately prior to or IM 30 minutes before neostigmine.)
  - **Treatment:** 0.01–0.04 mg/kg/dose IM, IV, or subcutaneous every 2–4 hours as needed or 1 mg PO given 2 hours prior to feeding.
- **Reversal of nondepolarizing neuromuscular blockade:** 0.025–0.1 mg/kg/dose. (Use with atropine: 0.01–0.04 mg/kg or 0.4 mg of atropine for each 1 mg of neostigmine.)

ADVERSE EFFECTS: Cholinergic crisis, which may include bronchospasm, increased bronchial secretions, vomiting, diarrhea, bradycardia, respiratory depression and seizures.
COMMENTS: Antidote is atropine, 0.01–0.04 mg/kg/dose. Reversal of the blocking agent should not be attempted for at least 30 minutes after a dose of pancuronium or tubocurarine.

NETILMICIN SULFATE (NETROMYCIN)

ACTION AND SPECTRUM: Aminoglycoside used for the treatment of infections caused by aerobic Gram-negative bacilli such as *Pseudomonas, Klebsiella,* and *Escherichia coli.* Usually used in combination with a β-lactam antibiotic.
SUPPLIED: Injection.
ROUTE: IM, IV (infuse over 30 minutes).
DOSAGE: Monitor and adjust by pharmacokinetics. Initial empiric dosing is based on body weight.

- **Neonates, premature, and normal gestational age (0 to 1 week of age):** 3 mg/kg IV or IM every 12 hours.
- **Neonates and infants over 1 week of age:** 2.5 to 3 mg/kg IV or IM every 8 hours.
- **Children:** 2 to 2.5 mg/kg IV or IM every 8 hours.

PHARMACOKINETICS: Renal excretion. Half-life is 4–8 hours.
ADVERSE EFFECTS: Vestibular and auditory ototoxicity is associated with serum peak concentrations >12 mcg/mL; nephrotoxicity is associated with serum trough concentrations >4 mcg/mL. **The addition of other nephrotoxic and/or ototoxic medications may increase these adverse effects.**
COMMENTS: Therapeutic range is 5 to 12 mcg/mL (sample obtained 30 minutes after the infusion is completed); serum trough concentrations are <3 mcg/mL (sample obtained 30 minutes to just before the next dose). Obtain an initial set of serum peak and trough levels at about the fourth maintenance dose. Monitor serum creatinine every 3–4 days. Limited experience in neonates.

NITRIC OXIDE (INOMAX FOR INHALATION; NO, INHALED NITRIC OXIDE [iNO])

INDICATIONS AND USE: iNO is indicated for the treatment of term and near-term (≥34 weeks) neonates with hypoxic respiratory failure associated with clinical or echocardiographic evidence of persistent pulmonary hypertension of the newborn (PPHN).
ACTIONS: iNO is a selective pulmonary vasodilator without significant effects on the systemic circulation that decreases extrapulmonary right-to-left shunting. Nitric oxide relaxes vascular smooth muscle by binding to the heme moiety of cytosolic guanylate cyclase, activating guanylate cyclase and increasing intracellular levels of cyclic guanosine 3,' 5'-monophosphate, which leads to vasodilation and an increase in the partial pressure of arterial oxygen.
SUPPLIED: Medical-grade gas cylinders.
ROUTE: Given as a gas by inhalation.
DOSAGE:

- **Term infants or >34 weeks' gestation:** Begin at 20 ppm. Reduce dose to lowest possible level. **Maximum:** Per manufacturer, doses >20 ppm are usually not used because of the increased risk of methemoglobinemia and elevated NO_2. Maintain treatment up to 14 days or until the underlying oxygen desaturation has resolved and the infant is ready to be weaned from iNO. Abrupt discontinuation may lead to worsening hypotension, oxygenation, and increasing pulmonary artery pressure (PAP). Further diagnostic testing should be sought for infants who are unable to be weaned off iNO after 4-day of therapy.

ADVERSE EFFECTS: Do not use in neonates dependent on right-to-left shunting of blood. Direct pulmonary injury from excess levels of NO_2 and ambient air contamination may occur. May cause methemoglobinemia and elevated NO_2. Risk of adverse effects increases when iNO is given at doses >20 ppm. Conflicting data have been published on whether or not iNO inhibits platelet aggregation and prolongs bleeding time. Monitor methemoglobin levels, iNO, NO_2, and O_2 levels. iNO therapy should be directed by physicians qualified by education and experience in its use and offered only at centers that are qualified to provide multisystem support, generally including on-site ECMO capability or with a collaborating ECMO center. Consult the manufacturer's product literature and specialized references for complete information on the use of iNO.

NITROPRUSSIDE SODIUM (NIPRIDE, NITROPRESS)

INDICATIONS AND USE: Severe hypertension and hypertension crisis, congestive heart failure, and congenital heart lesions that have resulted in pulmonary hypertension with increased pulmonary vascular resistance.

ACTIONS: Direct-acting vasodilator (arterial and venous) that reduces peripheral vascular resistance (afterload). Venous return is reduced (preload), increases cardiac output by decreasing afterload. Acts within seconds to lower blood pressure; when discontinued, the effect dissipates within minutes. Rapidly metabolized to thiocyanate, which is eliminated by the kidneys.

SUPPLIED: Injection.

ROUTE: Continuous IV infusion.

DOSAGE:

• **Initial:** 0.25–0.5 mcg/kg/minute; titrate dose every 20 minutes to the desired response.
• **Usual dose:** 3 mcg/kg/minute; rarely need >4 mcg/kg/minute; maximum dose: 8–10 mcg/kg/ minute.

ADVERSE EFFECTS: Generally related to a very rapid reduction in blood pressure. Thiocyanate may accumulate, especially in patients receiving high doses or those who have impaired renal function. Cyanide toxicity can develop abruptly if large doses are administered rapidly. Cyanide causes early persistent acidosis. Thiocyanate toxicity appears at plasma levels of ~35–100 mcg/ mL; levels >200 mcg/mL have been associated with death. Thiocyanate levels should be monitored in any patient receiving 3 mcg/kg/minute or more of nitroprusside, especially those with renal impairment. Toxicity is treated with IV sodium thiosulfate.

COMMENTS: Contraindicated with decreased cerebral perfusion, hypertension secondary to arteriovenous shunts, or coarctation of the aorta. May add sodium thiosulfate to infusion solution at a 10:1 ratio to minimize thiocyanate toxicity. Protect from light.

NOREPINEPHRINE BITARTRATE (LEVARTERENOL BITARTRATE) (LEVOPHED)

INDICATIONS AND USE: Treatment of shock, which persists after adequate fluid volume replacement; severe hypotension; cardiogenic shock.

ACTIONS: Stimulates β_1-adrenergic receptors and α-adrenergic receptors causing increased contractility and heart rate as well as vasoconstriction, thereby increasing systemic blood pressure and coronary blood flow; clinically, α effects (vasoconstriction) are greater than β effects (inotropic and chronotropic effects).

SUPPLIED: Injection.

ROUTE: Continuous IV infusion.

DOSAGE: 0.02–0.1 mcg/kg/minute initially, titrated to attain desired perfusion. Not to exceed 2 mcg/kg/minute.

ADVERSE EFFECTS: Respiratory distress, arrhythmias, bradycardia or tachycardia, hypertension, chest pain, headache and vomiting. Organ ischemia (due to vasoconstriction of renal and mesenteric arteries).

COMMENTS: Ischemic necrosis may occur after extravasation. Administer phentolamine, 0.1–0.2 mg/kg subcutaneous, infiltrated into the area of extravasation within 12 hours to minimize damage.

NYSTATIN (MYCOSTATIN, NILSTAT)

ACTION AND SPECTRUM: Fungistatic and fungicidal in vitro against a wide variety of yeasts and yeast-like fungi. Acts by disrupting fungal cell membranes. Neonatal indications include oral candidiasis (thrush), *Candida* diaper rash, and benign mucocutaneous candidiasis.

SUPPLIED: Oral suspension, 100,000 units/mL; topical cream; powder; ointment.

ROUTE: PO, topical.

DOSAGE:

• **Oral thrush:**
  • **Neonates:** 0.5–1 mL to each side of the mouth four times a day after feedings for 7–10 days.
  • **Infants:** 1–2 mL to each side of mouth four times a day after feedings for 7–10 days.
• **Diaper rash:** Topical cream/ointment/powder applied 3–4 times a day for 7–10 days.

PHARMACOKINETICS: Poorly absorbed. Most is passed unchanged in the stool.

ADVERSE EFFECTS: Side effects are uncommon but may cause diarrhea, local irritation, contact dermatitis, rash, pruritus and Stevens-Johnson syndrome.

OCTREOTIDE (SANDOSTATIN)

INDICATIONS AND USE: Short-term management of persistent hyperinsulinemic hypoglycemia of the newborn. Useful in the management of chylothorax. Chyle accumulation usually decreases after 24 hours of continuous infusion. Has also been used to treat hypersecretory diarrhea and fistulas in infants. Significant reductions in stool or ileal output were achieved with this drug.

ACTIONS: A synthetic polypeptide that mimics natural somatostatin by inhibiting serotonin release, and the secretion of gastrin, vasoactive intestinal peptide (VIP), insulin, glucagon, secretin, motilin, thyrotropin, cholecystokinin; reduces splanchnic blood flow, decreases gastrointestinal motility and inhibits intestinal secretion of water and electrolytes Duration of action (subcutaneous) is 6–12 hours with immediate release formulation.

SUPPLIED: Injection, refrigerate.

ROUTE: IV, IM and subcutaneous.

DOSAGE:

- **Persistent hyperinsulinemic hypoglycemia of infancy:** Initial dose is 2–10 mcg/kg/day divided every 6–12 hours; up to 40 mcg/kg/day divided every 6–8 hours. Adjust the dose to maintain symptomatic control.
- **Diarrhea:** 1–10 mcg/kg/dose IV/subcutaneous given every 12 hours. Adjust the dose to maintain symptomatic control.
- **Chylothorax:** IV continuous infusion: 0.5–4 mcg/kg/hour titrate dose to response; case reports of effective dosage ranging between 0.3–40 mcg/kg/hour; treatment duration is usually 1–2 weeks but may vary with clinical response.

ADVERSE EFFECTS: Possible growth retardation during long-term treatment, flushing, hypertension, insomnia, fever, chills, seizures, Bell's palsy, hair loss, bruising, rash, hypoglycemia, hyperglycemia, galactorrhea, hypothyroidism, diarrhea, abdominal distention, constipation, hepatitis, jaundice, local injection site pain, thrombophlebitis, muscle weakness, increased creatine kinase, muscle spasm, tremor, oliguria, shortness of breath, and rhinorrhea.

COMMENTS: Tachyphylaxis may occur.

OMEPRAZOLE (PRILOSEC)

INDICATIONS AND USE: Short-term (less than 8 weeks) treatment of reflux esophagitis, duodenal ulcer refractory to conventional therapy.

ACTIONS: Inhibits gastric acid secretion by inactivating the parietal cell membrane enzyme (H^+/K^+)-ATPase or proton pump; demonstrates antimicrobial activity against *Helicobacter pylori*.

SUPPLIED: Tablet and capsule (delayed release). Pharmacist may compound a 2 mg/mL suspension.

ROUTE: PO.

DOSAGE:

- **Neonates:** 0.7 mg/kg once daily in the morning as the initial dose increasing to 1.4 mg/kg once daily after 7 to 14 days. Some neonates may require 2.8 mg/kg once daily.
- **1 month to 2 years:** 0.7 mg/kg once daily increase to 3mg/kg once daily if necessary (maximum dose 20 mg).
- **10 to 20 kg body weight:** 10 mg once daily as initial dose; increase to 20 mg if necessary.

PHARMACOKINETICS: Cytochrome P450 isoenzyme CYP1A2 inducer; isoenzyme CYP2C8, CYP2C18, CYP2C19, and CYP3A3/4 substrate; isoenzyme CYP2C9, CYP3A3/4, CYP2C8, and CYP2C19 inhibitor. **Maximum secretory inhibition:** 4 days. Extensive first-pass metabolism in the liver. **Bioavailability:** 30% to 40%; improves slightly with repeated administration.

ADVERSE EFFECTS: Mild elevation of liver enzymes, diarrhea.

COMMENTS: Lack of data regarding the safety of long-term use in children.

OPIUM TINCTURE

HIGH ALERT MEDICATION: May also be confused with camphorated tincture of opium (Paregoric). Opium tincture is 25 times as potent as paregoric. Avoid the use of the abbreviation DTO.

INDICATIONS AND USE: A **25-fold dilution with water (final concentration 0.4 mg/mL)** can be used to treat neonatal abstinence syndrome (opiate withdrawal).

ACTIONS: Contains many narcotic alkaloids including morphine; inhibition of GI motility due to morphine content; decreases digestive secretions increases GI muscle tone.

SUPPLIED: Liquid: 10% (0.6 mL equivalent to morphine 6 mg; contains alcohol 19%).

ROUTE: PO.

DOSAGE: Neonates (full-term): Neonatal abstinence syndrome (opiate withdrawal): **Use a 25-fold dilution with water of opium tincture (final concentration: 0.4 mg/mL morphine). Initial dose:** Give 0.1 mL/kg of the 25-fold dilution per dose with feedings every 3–4 hours; increase as needed by 0.1 mL/kg of the 25-fold dilution every 3–4 hours until withdrawal symptoms are controlled. **Usual dose:** 0.2–0.5 mL of the 25-fold dilution per dose given every 3–4 hours; it is rare to exceed 0.7 mL of the 25-fold dilution per dose; stabilize withdrawal symptoms for 3–5 days, then gradually decrease the dosage (keeping the same dosage interval) over a 2- to 4-week period.

PHARMACOKINETICS: Metabolized in liver and eliminated in urine and bile.

ADVERSE EFFECTS: Hypotension, bradycardia, peripheral vasodilation, CNS depression, drowsiness, sedation, urinary retention, constipation, respiratory depression, and histamine release.

COMMENTS: Observe for excessive sedation and respiratory depression. Do not abruptly discontinue. Monitor for the resolution of withdrawal symptoms (such as irritability, high-pitched cry, stuffy nose, rhinorrhea, vomiting, poor feeding, diarrhea, sneezing, yawning etc), and signs of overtreatment (such as bradycardia, lethargy, hypotonia, irregular respirations, respiratory depression etc). An abstinence scoring system (eg, Finnegan abstinence scoring system) should be used to more objectively assess neonatal opiate withdrawal symptoms and the need for dosage adjustment. Use 25-fold dilution with water for the treatment of neonatal abstinence syndrome.

OXACILLIN SODIUM (BACTOCILL, PROSTAPHLIN)

ACTION AND SPECTRUM: Semisynthetic penicillinase-resistant penicillin that has bactericidal activity against susceptible bacteria as a result of interfering with bacterial cell wall synthesis. Treatment of bacterial infections such as osteomyelitis, septicemia, endocarditis, and CNS infections due to susceptible penicillinase-producing strains of *Staphylococcus*.
SUPPLIED: Injection.
ROUTE: IM, IV (infuse over 10–30 minutes).
DOSAGE:

- **Neonates:**
  - **<1200 g and ≤4 weeks old:** 50 mg/kg/day IM/IV divided every 12 hours.
  - **1200–2000 g and ≤7 days old:** 50–100 mg/kg/day IM/IV divided every 12 hours.
  - **1200–2000 g and >7 days old:** 75–150 mg/kg/day IM/IV divided every 8 hours.
  - **>2000 g and ≤7 days old:** 75–150 mg/kg/day divided IM/IV every 8 hours.
  - **>2000 g and >7 days old:** 100–200 mg/kg/day divided IM/IV every 6 hours.
- **Infants and children:**
  - **Mild to moderate infections:** 100–150 mg/kg/day IM/IV in divided doses every 6 hours; maximum 4 g/day.
  - **Severe infections:** 150–200 mg/kg/day IM/IV in divided doses every 4–6 hours; maximum 12 g/day.

PHARMACOKINETICS: Metabolized chiefly in the liver and excreted in bile; dosage modification required in patients with renal impairment.
ADVERSE EFFECTS: Hypersensitivity reactions (rash), thrombophlebitis, mild leukopenia, acute interstitial nephritis, hematuria, azotemia, and elevation in AST. *Clostridium difficile* colitis has been reported.
COMMENTS: Avoid IM injection.

PALIVIZUMAB (SYNAGIS)

INDICATIONS AND USE: Immunoprophylaxis against severe respiratory syncytial virus (RSV) lower respiratory tract infections in high risk infants and children:

- <2 years of age with chronic lung disease who have required medical therapy for their chronic lung disease within 6 months before the anticipated RSV season.
- Prevention of serious RSV disease in patients with a history of prematurity (≤28 weeks' gestation) up to 12 months of age or infants born at 29–32 weeks' gestation up to 6 months of age.
- Prophylaxis may be considered in infants (<6 months of age) born between 32 and 35 weeks of gestation who are at greatest risk of severe infection (risk factors include childcare attendance, school-age siblings, exposure to environmental air pollutants, congenital abnormalities of the airways, or severe neuromuscular disease; see American Academy of Pediatrics Red Book, 2006).
- Prevention of serious RSV disease in children with hemodynamically significant congenital heart disease; prophylaxis of infants with severe immune deficiency exposed to RSV.

ACTIONS AND SPECTRUM: Humanized monoclonal antibody directed to an epitope in the A antigenic site of the respiratory syncytial virus F protein resulting in neutralizing and fusion-inhibitory activity against RSV.
SUPPLIED: Injection.
ROUTE: IM (anterolateral aspect of the thigh is preferred).
DOSAGE: 15 mg/kg/dose IM once a month during the RSV season. The first dose should be administered before the start of the RSV season.
PHARMACOKINETICS: The mean half-life of Palivizumab is ~20 days and adequate antibody titers are maintained for 30 days. Time to achieve adequate serum antibody titers: 48 hours.
ADVERSE EFFECTS: Upper respiratory tract infection, otitis media, fever and rhinitis. Rash, injection site reaction, erythema, induration. Rare cases of anaphylaxis (<1 case/100,000 patients) and severe hypersensitivity reactions(<1 case/1000 patients) have been reported.
COMMENTS: A complete course of prophylaxis should continue through the entire RSV season. Palivizumab is not indicated for the treatment of RSV infections.
Palivizumab does not interfere with the response to routine childhood vaccines and therefore may be administered concurrently.

PANCURONIUM BROMIDE (PAVULON)

INDICATIONS AND USE: Produces skeletal muscle relaxation during surgery, increases pulmonary compliance during assisted mechanical respiration, and facilitates endotracheal intubation.
ACTIONS: Nondepolarizing neuromuscular blocking agent that produces skeletal muscle paralysis mainly by causing a decreased response to acetylcholine at the myoneural junction. Pancuronium may cause an increase

in heart rate and changes in blood pressure. The onset of action is generally 30–60 seconds, with duration of action of ~40–60 minutes, but it may be much longer in neonates.
SUPPLIED: Injection.
ROUTE: IV.
DOSAGE: Neonates and infants: 0.1 mg/kg IV every 30–60 minutes as needed; **maintenance dose:** 0.04–0.15 mg/kg IV every 1–4 hours as needed to maintain paralysis or as **continuous IV infusion:** 0.02–0.04 mg/kg/hour or 0.4–0.6 mcg/kg/minute.
ADVERSE EFFECTS: Tachycardia, hypertension, hypotension, excessive salivation and bronchospasm may occur.
COMMENTS: Neonates are particularly sensitive to its actions; prolonged paralysis may be noted. Potentiation by aminoglycosides, electrolyte abnormalities, severe hyponatremia, severe hypocalcemia, severe hypokalemia, hypermagnesemia, neuromuscular diseases, acidosis, renal failure, hepatic failure Antagonism by alkalosis, hypercalcemia, hyperkalemia, and epinephrine. Ventilation must be supported during neuromuscular blockade. Many centers place a sign over the patient's bedside to alert all medical personnel that the infant is paralyzed. Neostigmine methylsulfate and atropine sulfate are used for reversal. Sensation remains intact; analgesia should be used with painful procedures.

PAPAVERINE HYDROCHLORIDE (VARIOUS)
INDICATIONS AND USE: Peripheral arterial spasms.
ACTIONS: Directly relaxes vascular smooth muscle and results in vasodilation.
SUPPLIED: Injection.
ROUTE: IM, IV (infuse over 1–2 minutes).
DOSAGE: 6 mg/kg/24 hours in 4 divided doses.
COMMENTS: IV infusion should be performed under a physician's supervision because arrhythmias and fatal apnea may result from rapid injection. *Note:* Not FDA approved for use in children. Limited experience in neonates.

PENICILLIN G (AQUEOUS), PARENTERAL
ACTION AND SPECTRUM: Inhibits bacterial wall synthesis. Effective mainly against streptococci, some community-acquired staphylococci (except methicillin-resistant and penicillinase-producing strains), *Neisseria gonorrhoeae*, *Neisseria meningitidis*, *Bacillus anthracis*, *Clostridium tetani*, *Clostridium perfringens*, *Bacteroides* (oropharyngeal strains), *Leptospira* spp., and *Treponema pallidum*.
SUPPLIED: Injection, as the potassium or sodium salt.
ROUTE: IM, IV (infuse over 15–30 minutes).
DOSAGE:
- **Neonates postnatal age ≤7 days:**
  - **≤2000 g:** 50,000 units/kg/day IM/IV in divided doses every 12 hours.
    - **Meningitis:** 100,000 units/kg/day IM/IV in divided doses every 12 hours.
  - **>2000 g:** 75,000 units/kg/day IM/IV in divided doses every 8 hours.
    - **Meningitis:** 150,000 units/kg/day IM/IV in divided doses every 8 hours.
  - **Congenital syphilis:** 100,000 units/kg/day IM/IV in divided doses every 12 hours.
  - **Group B streptococcal meningitis:** 250,000–450,000 units/kg/day IM/IV in divided doses every 8 hours.
- **Neonates postnatal age >7 days:**
  - **<1200 g:** 50,000 units/kg/day IM/IV in divided doses every 12 hours.
    - **Meningitis:** 100,000 units/kg/day IM/IV in divided doses every 12 hours.
  - **1200–2000 g:** 75,000 units/kg/day IM/IV in divided doses every 8 hours.
    - **Meningitis:** 150,000 units/kg/day IM/IV in divided doses every 8 hours.
  - **>2000 g:** 100,000 units/kg/day IM/IV in divided doses every 6 hours.
    - **Meningitis:** 200,000 units/kg/day IM/IV in divided doses every 6 hours.
  - **Congenital syphilis:** 150,000 units/kg/day IM/IV in divided doses every 8 hours.
  - **Group B streptococcal meningitis:** IV: 450,000 units/kg/day IV in divided doses every 6 hours.
- **Infants and children:**
  - **Usual dose:** 100,000 to 250,000 units/kg/day IM/IV in divided doses every 4–6 hours.
  - **Severe infections:** 250,000–400,000 units/kg/day IM/IV in divided doses every 4–6 hours; maximum dose: 24 million units/day.

PHARMACOKINETICS: Penetration across the blood-brain barrier is poor with uninflamed meninges, excreted in urine mainly by tubular secretion.
ADVERSE EFFECTS: Allergic reactions, rash, fever, change in bowel flora, *Candida* superinfection, diarrhea, and hemolytic anemia. Acute interstitial nephritis. Bone marrow suppression with granulocytopenia. Very large doses may cause seizures. Rapid IV push of potassium penicillin G may cause cardiac arrhythmias and arrest because of the potassium component. Infuse slowly over 30 minutes.
COMMENTS: 1600 units = 1 mg. Some strains of group B streptococci are penicillinase producers, thus requiring the addition of an aminoglycoside antibiotic for synergistic bactericidal effect. Good activity against anaerobes. Drug of choice for tetanus neonatorum. Penicillin G potassium contains 1.7 mEq potassium per million units and Penicillin G sodium contains 2 mEq sodium per million units.

PENICILLIN G BENZATHINE (BICILLIN L-A)

ACTION AND SPECTRUM: See Penicillin G (Aqueous), Parenteral. A drug of choice in the treatment of asymptomatic congenital syphilis.
SUPPLIED: Injection.
ROUTE: IM only. (Viscosity requires ≥23-gauge needle.)
DOSAGE:

• **Asymptomatic congenital syphilis:** A single dose of 50,000 units/kg IM.
• **Congenital syphilis:** 50,000 units/kg IM every week for 3 weeks; **maximum dose:** 2.4 million units/dose.

PHRMACOKINETICS: Renally excreted over a prolonged interval owing to slow absorption from the injection site.
ADVERSE EFFECTS AND COMMENTS: See Penicillin G (Aqueous), Parenteral. 1211 units = 1 mg. Not often used.

PENICILLIN G PROCAINE (WYCILLIN)

ACTION AND SPECTRUM: See Penicillin G (Aqueous), Parenteral. A drug of choice in the treatment of symptomatic or asymptomatic congenital syphilis.
SUPPLIED: Injection.
ROUTE: IM only. (Viscosity requires ≥23-gauge needle.)
DOSAGE: 50,000 units/kg/dose IM every 24 hours.
PHRMACOKINETICS: See Penicillin. (Aqueous, Parenteral.)
ADVERSE EFFECTS: See Penicillin G (Aqueous), Parenteral. May also cause sterile abscess formation at the injection site. Contains 120 mg of procaine per 300,000 units, which may cause allergic reactions, myocardial depression, or systemic vasodilation. There is cause for much greater concern about these effects in the neonate than in older patients and therefore not recommended for use in neonates.
COMMENTS: 1000 units = 1 mg. Not often used.

PENTOBARBITAL SODIUM (NEMBUTAL)

INDICATIONS AND USE: Sedative/hypnotic. Used for agitation, for pre-procedure sedation, or as an anticonvulsant.
ACTIONS: Short-acting barbiturate.
SUPPLIED: Injection, 50 mg/mL, solution contains propylene glycol 40% and alcohol 10%, irritating to veins, pH is 9.5; suppositories. (Suppositories should be used for the older, larger infant only because 30 mg is the smallest size available, and it is recommended that they not be divided.)
ROUTE: IV, IM, PR.
DOSAGE:

• **Sedative:** 2–6 mg/kg/day divided every 8 hours. Maximum: 100 mg/day.
• **Hypnotic and anticonvulsant:** 3–5 mg/kg/dose. Maximum: 100 mg/dose.

ADVERSE EFFECTS: Inject the IV dose slowly in fractional doses. Observe the IV site closely during administration because this drug may cause extravasation injury. Tolerance and physical dependence may occur with continued use. May cause somnolence, apnea, bradycardia, rash, pain on IM injection, thrombophlebitis, osteomalacia from prolonged use (rare), and excitability. May increase reaction to painful stimuli. Rapid IV administration may cause hypotension and apnea.

PHENOBARBITAL

INDICATIONS AND USE: Treatment of neonatal seizures; used to treat neonatal abstinence symptoms; may also be used for prevention and treatment of neonatal hyperbilirubinemia and lowering of bilirubin in chronic cholestasis.
ACTIONS: Anticonvulsant that limits the spread of seizure activity, increases the threshold for electrical stimulation of the motor cortex and depresses CNS activity by binding to barbiturate site at gamma-aminobutyric acid (GABA)–receptor complex enhancing GABA activity; In neonates, the initial half-life is 100–120 hours or longer, gradually declining to 60–70 hours at 3–4 weeks of age. Reduction in serum bilirubin levels is attributed to increased levels of glucuronyl transferase, stimulates bile flow and increases the concentration of the Y-binding protein involved in the uptake of bilirubin by hepatocytes. Observed reductions usually require 2–3 days of treatment.
SUPPLIED: Injection, elixir.
ROUTE: IV, IM, PO.
DOSAGE:

• **Anticonvulsant, status epilepticus:**
  • **Neonates: Loading dose:** 15–20 mg/kg IV in a single or divided dose. *Note:* In select patients, may give additional 5 mg/kg/dose every 15–30 minutes until seizure is controlled or a total dose of 30 mg/kg is reached; be prepared to support respirations.
• **Anticonvulsant maintenance.** *Note:* Maintenance dose usually starts 12 hours after loading dose:
  • **Neonates:** 3–4 mg/kg/day PO/IV given once daily; assess serum concentrations; increase to 5 mg/kg/day if needed (usually by second week of therapy).
  • **Infants:** 5–6 mg/kg/day in 1–2 divided doses.

- **Hyperbilirubinemia:** 3–8 mg/kg/day PO in 2–3 divided doses up to 12mg/kg/day have been used; but dose not clearly established.
- **Neonatal abstinence syndrome:** 5–10 mg/kg/day in 1 to 4 divided doses. Monitor serum concentrations coincident to abstinence scores.

ADVERSE EFFECTS: Sedation, lethargy, paradoxic excitement, hypotension, gastrointestinal distress, ataxia, rash, and phlebitis. Drug accumulation may occur if treating concurrently with phenytoin. Monitor drug levels. Respiratory depression can occur at levels exceeding 40 mcg/mL.
COMMENT: Contraindicated if porphyria suspected. Maintenance serum levels usually fall between 15–40 mcg/mL. Abrupt withdrawal may precipitate status epilepticus.

PHENTOLAMINE (REGITINE)

INDICATIONS AND USE: Treatment of extravasation from IV α-adrenergic drugs (dobutamine, dopamine, epinephrine, norepinephrine or phenylephrine). Helps prevent dermal necrosis and sloughing.
ACTIONS: Phentolamine blocks α-adrenergic receptors and reverses the severe vasoconstriction from the extravasation of α-adrenergic drugs.
SUPPLIED: Injection.
ROUTE: Subcutaneous.
DOSAGE:

- **Neonate:** Infiltrate area with small amount of solution (~1 mL) made by diluting 2.5–5 mg in 10 mL of preservative free normal saline within 12 hours of extravasation- do not exceed 0.1 mg/kg or 2.5 mg total.
- **Infants and children:** Infiltrate area with small amount of solution (~1 mL) made by diluting 5–10 mg in 10 mL of preservative free normal saline within 12 hours of extravasation; do not exceed 0.1–0.2 mg/kg or 5 mg maximum.

ADVERSE EFFECTS: Hypotension, tachycardia, cardiac arrhythmias, flushing, and gastrointestinal upset.

PHENYTOIN (DILANTIN)

INDICATIONS AND USE: Seizures unresponsive to phenobarbital.
ACTIONS: Stabilizes neuronal membranes and decreases seizure activity by increasing efflux or decreasing influx of sodium ions across cell membranes in the motor cortex during generation of nerve impulses.
SUPPLIED: Injection and oral suspension.
ROUTE: IV, PO.
DOSAGE:

- **Loading dose:** 15–20 mg/kg IV at a rate not to exceed 0.5 mg/kg/minute.
- **Maintenance:** 12 hours after loading, 5–8 mg/kg/day PO/IV divided every 12 hours; some patients may require dosing every 8 hours.

PHARMACOKINETICS: Bilirubin displaces phenytoin from albumin binding sites thereby increasing unbound drug levels and complicating dosage to serum level interpretations. Neonates absorb phenytoin poorly from gastrointestinal tract.
ADVERSE EFFECTS: Local tissue damage if extravasation occurs. High serum levels can precipitate seizures. Other CNS complications included drowsiness, lethargy, ataxia, and nystagmus. Cardiovascular affects can be arrhythmias, hypotension, or cardiovascular collapse with too rapid an infusion. Reactions also include hypersensitivity rash or Stevens-Johnson syndrome. Other complications include hepatic dysfunction, pancreatic dysfunction with hyperglycemia and hypoinsulinemia, and blood dyscrasias.
COMMENTS: Therapeutic levels are 10 to 20 mcg/mL; lower levels preferred for preterm infants. Multiple drug interactions include corticosteroids, carbamazepine, cimetidine, digoxin, furosemide, phenobarbital, and heparin (especially in central lines causing precipitation).

PHOSPHORUS (VARIOUS)

INDICATIONS AND USE: Treatment of hypophosphatemia, provision of maintenance phosphorus in parenteral nutrition (PN) solutions, and treatment of nutritional rickets of prematurity.
ACTIONS: Phosphorus is an intracellular ion required for formation of energy-transfer enzymes such as adenosine diphosphate (ADP) and adenosine triphosphate (ATP). Phosphorus is also needed for bone metabolism and mineralization.
SUPPLIED: Injection, sodium phosphates: 3 mmol of elemental phosphorus/mL and 4 mEq of sodium/mL; potassium phosphates: 3 mmol of elemental phosphorus/mL and 4.4 mEq of potassium/mL.
ROUTE: IV, PO.
DOSAGE:

- **Severe hypophosphatemia:** 0.15–0.3 mmol/kg/dose (= 5–9 mg of elemental phosphorus/kg/dose). Infuse slowly over several hours or dilute in daily 24 hour maintenance IV solution (preferred).
- **Maintenance:** 0.5–2 mmol/kg/day (= 16–63 mg of elemental phosphorus/kg/day). For oral use, may use parenteral form and give PO in divided doses, diluted in infant's feedings.

ADVERSE EFFECTS: Hyperphosphatemia, hypocalcemia, and hypotension. Gastrointestinal discomfort may occur with oral administration. Rapid IV bolus of potassium phosphates can cause cardiac arrhythmias.

PIPERACILLIN SODIUM (PIPRACIL)

ACTION AND SPECTRUM: Semisynthetic extended-spectrum penicillin with increased activity against *Pseudomonas aeruginosa* and many strains of *Klebsiella, Serratia, Escherichia coli, Enterobacter, Citrobacter, and Proteus.* Also demonstrates activity against Group B *Streptococcus.*
SUPPLIED: Injection.
ROUTE: IM, IV (infuse over 30 minutes).
DOSAGE:

• **Neonates:**
  • **≤ 7 days:** 150 mg/kg/day divided every 8 hours.
  • **>7 days:** 200 mg/kg/day divided every 6 hours.
• **Intants and children:** 200–300 mg/kg/day in divided doses every 4–6 hours; **maximum dose:** 24 g/day.
PHARMACOKINETICS: Excreted unchanged in the urine.
ADVERSE EFFECTS: Hemolytic anemia, eosinophilia, neutropenia, prolonged bleeding time, thrombocytopenia; elevated liver enzymes, cholestatic hepatitis; acute interstitial nephritis, thrombophlebitis, and hypokalemia.
COMMENTS: Avoid IM use where possible. Contains 1.85 mEq (42.5 mg) of sodium/g.

PNEUMOCOCCAL 7-VALENT CONJUGATE VACCINE (PREVNAR)

INDICATIONS AND USE: For active immunization of infants and toddlers against *Streptococcus pneumoniae* invasive disease caused by the 7 capsular serotypes in the vaccine for all children 2–23 months of age. It is also recommended for certain children 24–59 months of age. *S. pneumoniae* causes invasive infections such as bacteremia and meningitis, pneumonia, otitis media, and sinusitis (see Advisory Committee on Immunization Practices [ACIP]) guidelines for the most current recommendations).
ACTIONS: The vaccine is a sterile solution of saccharides of the capsular antigens of *S. pneumoniae* serotypes 4, 6B, 9V, 14, 18C, 19F, and 23F conjugated to diphtheria CRM_{197} protein. CRM_{197} protein is a nontoxic variant of diphtheria toxin. These 7 serotypes cause about 80% of invasive pneumococcal disease in children <6 years of age in the United States.
SUPPLIED: Injection.
ROUTE: IM.
DOSAGE: 0.5 mL/dose as a single dose IM at 2, 4, 6, and 12–15 months of age. Shake well before administration. Refer to the current AAP/ACIP immunization recommendations. The schedule usually begins at 2 months of age, but as young as 6 weeks of age is acceptable. Three doses of 0.5 mL each are ideally given at ~2-month intervals, but a dosing interval of 4 to 8 weeks is acceptable. These doses are followed by a fourth dose of 0.5 mL at 12 months to 15 months of age. Give the fourth dose at least 2 or more months after the third dose.
ADVERSE EFFECTS: May cause decreased appetite, drowsiness, irritability, fever, and injection site local tenderness, redness, and edema. This vaccine is not a treatment of active infection. Do not give if patient is hypersensitive to any component of the vaccine. Immune response in preterm infants has not been studied. Use of this vaccine does not replace the use of the 23-valent pneumococcal polysaccharide vaccine in children ≥24 months old with sickle cell disease, chronic illness, asplenia, HIV, or immunocompromise. May be administered simultaneously vaccines as part of the routine immunization schedule.

PORACTANT ALFA (CUROSURF)

INDICATIONS AND USE: Treatment of neonatal respiratory distress syndrome (RDS).
ACTIONS: An extract of natural porcine lung surfactant, that contains phospholipids, neutral lipids, fatty acids, and surfactant-associated proteins B and C. It replaces deficient or ineffective endogenous lung surfactant in neonates with RDS; surfactant prevents the alveoli from collapsing during expiration by lowering surface tension between air and alveolar surfaces.
SUPPLIED: Preservative free intratracheal suspension. Each mL contains 80 mg of total phospholipids, 1 mg of protein including 0.3 mg of surfactant protein-B (SP-B).
ROUTE: Intratracheal administration through a side port adapter or through a 5F feeding catheter inserted into the endotracheal tube. Allow to warm to room temperature prior to administration. Do not shake, swirl vial to resuspend particles. Inspect for discoloration, normal color is creamy white. Discard unused drug.
DOSE: **Initial dose** is 2.5 mL/kg intratracheally, divided into 2 aliquots, followed by up to 2 doses of 1.25 mL/kg administered at 12 hours intervals as needed to infants that continue to require mechanical ventilation and oxygen supplementation.
ADVERSE EFFECTS: Transient bradycardia, hypotension, endotracheal tube blockage, and oxygen desaturation.

COMMENTS: Following administration, lung compliance and oxygenation often improve rapidly. Patients should be closely monitored and appropriate changes in ventilatory support should be made as clinically indicated.

POTASSIUM CHLORIDE (KCL)

INDICATIONS AND USE: Treatment of hypokalemia and as a supplement to maintain adequate serum potassium levels. Also corrects hypochloremia.

ACTIONS: Potassium is the major intracellular cation. Potassium is essential for maintaining intracellular tonicity; transmission of nerve impulses; contraction of cardiac, skeletal, and smooth muscle; and maintenance of normal renal function.

SUPPLIED: Injection, oral liquid.

ROUTE: IV, PO.

DOSAGE:

- **Acute treatment of hypokalemia:** 0.5 to 1 mEq/kg/dose IV over 1 hour. **Maximum dose/rate:** 1 mEq/kg/hour; continuous electrocardiograph monitoring should be used for intermittent doses >0.5 mEq/kg/hour.

- **Maintenance:** 2–6 mEq/kg/day (usually 2–3 mEq/kg/day) diluted in 24 hour maintenance IV solution. Higher doses are often required in infants receiving diuretics. Monitor serum potassium levels and adjust dose as needed.

- **Oral supplementation:** 2–6 mEq/kg/day (usually 2–3 mEq/kg/day) in divided doses and diluted with feedings. The injectable form of the drug may be given in divided doses PO and diluted in the infant's formula.

ADVERSE EFFECTS: Avoid rapid IV injection. Excessive dose or rate of infusion may cause cardiac arrhythmias (peaked T waves, widened QRS, flattened P waves, bradycardia, and heart block), respiratory paralysis, and hypotension. Monitor renal function, urine output, and serum potassium levels; hyperkalemia may result with renal dysfunction.

COMMENTS: Causes severe vein irritation; do not give undiluted in a peripheral vein. Dilute to 0.04 mEq/mL for a peripheral line, maximum of 0.08 mEq/mL for a central line with maximum of 0.15 mEq/mL.

PREDNISONE (LIQUID PRED, PREDNISONE INTENSOL CONCENTRATE)

INDICATIONS AND USE: Used chiefly as an anti-inflammatory or immunosuppressive agent. Prednisone is an intermediate-acting glucocorticoid that has four times the antiinflammatory potency of hydrocortisone, and half the mineralocorticoid potency.

SUPPLIED: Tablets, oral solution, 5 mg/5 mL (5% alcohol) and 5 mg/mL (30% alcohol).

ROUTE: PO.

DOSAGE: 0.5–2 mg/kg/day given as a single daily dose or divided every 6 to 12 hours.

ADVERSE EFFECTS: Cataracts, leukocytosis, peptic ulcer, nephrocalcinosis, myopathy, osteoporosis, diabetes, growth failure, hyperlipidemia, hypocalcemia, hypokalemic alkalosis, sodium retention and hypertension, and increased susceptibility to infection. Withdraw the dose gradually after prolonged therapy to prevent acute adrenal insufficiency.

PROCAINAMIDE HYDROCHLORIDE (VARIOUS)

INDICATIONS AND USE: Used for the treatment of ventricular tachycardia, premature ventricular contractions, paroxysmal atrial tachycardia, and atrial fibrillation; to prevent recurrence of ventricular tachycardia, paroxysmal supraventricular tachycardia, atrial fibrillation or flutter. **Note:** Due to proarrhythmic effects, use should be reserved for life-threatening arrhythmias.

ACTIONS: Class I antiarrhythmic agent that increases the effective refractory period of the atria and ventricles of the heart. Partially metabolized by the liver to the active metabolite N-acetylprocainamide (NAPA).

SUPPLIED: Capsules, tablets, injection.

ROUTE: PO, IV.

DOSAGE: Consider consult with pediatric cardiologist prior to use.

- **Initial bolus dose:** (monitor electrocardiogram, heart rate and blood pressure): 3 to 10 mg/kg (dilute to 20 mg/mL) IV over 10–30 minutes, then continuous infusion of 20–80 mcg/kg/minutes, maximum dose is 2 g/day. Use lowest dose in preterm neonates.

- **PO:** 15 to 50 mg/kg divided every 3 to 6 hours, maximum 4 g/day.

ADVERSE EFFECTS: Serious toxic effects if given rapidly IV, including asystole, myocardial depression, ventricular fibrillation, hypotension, and reversible lupus-like syndrome. May cause nausea, vomiting, diarrhea, anorexia, skin rash, tachycardia, agranulocytosis, and hepatic toxicity.

COMMENTS:

- **Therapeutic levels:**
  - Procainamide, 4–10 mcg/mL: Toxicity associated with levels >12 mcg/mL.
  - NAPA, 6–20 mcg/mL: Toxicity associated with levels >30 mcg/mL.

Contraindicated in second- or third-degree heart block, bundle-branch block, digitalis intoxication, and allergy to procaine. Do not use in atrial fibrillation or flutter until the ventricular rate is adequately controlled to avoid a possible paradoxic increase in ventricular rate. Phenylephrine should be available to treat severe hypotension caused by IV procainamide. QRS or QT prolongation >35% of baseline is an indication to withhold further doses of procainamide. **Do not administer with amiodarone, may cause severe hypotension and prolongation of QT interval.**

PROPRANOLOL (INDERAL)

INDICATIONS AND USE: Hypertension, supraventricular tachycardia, especially if associated with Wolff-Parkinson-White syndrome, tachyarrhythmias, and tetralogy of Fallot spells. Adjunctive therapy for neonatal thyrotoxicosis.

ACTIONS: Nonselective β-adrenergic blocking agent that inhibits adrenergic stimuli by competitively blocking β-adrenergic receptors within the myocardium and bronchial and vascular smooth muscle. Propranolol decreases heart rate, myocardial contractility, blood pressure and myocardial oxygen demand.

SUPPLIED: Oral liquid, injection.

ROUTE: PO, IV.

DOSAGE:

- **Arrhythmias:**
  - **IV:** 0.01–0.15 mg/kg/dose IV to a maximum of 1 mg/dose as slow push over 10 minutes; may repeat every 6 to 8 hours as needed; increase slowly to maximum (neonates) of 0.15 mg/kg/dose every 6 to 8 hours; maximum dose 1 mg (infants) and 3 mg (children).
  - **PO:** Neonates: 0.25 mg/kg/dose PO every 6 to 8 hours. Increase slowly as needed to 5 mg/kg/day. Children: Initially 0.5 to 1 mg/kg/day in divided doses every 6 to 8 hours titrate dosage upward every 3–5 days. Usual dose: 2–4 mg/kg/day; higher doses may be needed; do not exceed 16 mg/kg/day or 60 mg/day.
- **Hypertension:** 0.5–1 mg/kg/day PO in divided doses every 6–12 hours. May increase gradually every 5–7 days; usual dose is 1 to 5 mg/kg/day PO; maximum dose is 8 mg/kg/day PO.
- **Tetralogy spells:**
  - **IV:** 0.01–0.02 mg/kg/dose IV over 10 minutes; maximum initial dose: 1 mg. Some centers use 0.15–0.25 mg/kg/dose slow IV; may repeat in 15 minutes
  - **Oral palliation:** Initial—0.25 mg/kg/dose every 6 hours; if ineffective within first week, may increase by 1 mg/kg/day every 24 hours to maximum of 5 mg/kg/day; if patient refractory may increase slowly to a maximum of 10–15 mg/kg/day but must carefully monitor heart rate, heart size, and cardiac contractility. Some centers use an initial: 0.5–1 mg/kg/dose every 6 hours.
- **Thyrotoxicosis, neonates:** 2 mg/kg/day PO in divided doses every 6–12 hours; occasionally higher doses may be required.

ADVERSE EFFECTS: Generally dose-related hypotension and related to ß-adrenergic blockage; nausea, vomiting, bronchospasm, increased airway resistance, heart block, depressed myocardial contractility, hypoglycemia and inhibition of warning signs of hypoglycemia.

COMMENTS: Contraindicated in obstructive pulmonary disease, asthma, heart failure, shock, second- or third-degree heart block, and hypoglycemia. Use with caution in renal or hepatic failure.

PROTAMINE SULFATE

INDICATIONS AND USE: Treatment of heparin overdose, neutralize heparin during surgery.

ACTIONS: Combines with heparin, forming a stable salt complex, neutralizing the anticoagulation activity of both drugs. Effect on heparin is rapid (~5 minutes) and persists for ~2 hours.

SUPPLIED: Injection.

ROUTE: IV.

DOSAGE:

- **Heparin overdosage:** Blood heparin concentrations decrease rapidly after heparin administration, adjust the protamine dosage depending upon the duration of time since heparin administration as follows:
  - **Time since last heparin <30 minutes:** 1 mg protamine needed to neutralize 100 units of heparin.
  - **Time since last heparin 30–60 minutes:** 0.5–0.75 mg protamine needed to neutralize 100 units of heparin.
  - **Time since last heparin >60–120 minutes:** 0.375–0.5 mg protamine needed to neutralize 100 units of heparin.
  - **Time since last heparin: >120 minutes:** 0.25–0.375 mg protamine needed to neutralize 100 units of heparin.
  - **Low molecular weight heparin (LMWH) overdosage:** If most recent LMWH dose has been administered within the last 4 hours, use 1 mg protamine per 1 mg (100 units) LMWH; a second dose of 0.5 mg protamine per 1 mg (100 units) LMWH may be given if activated partial thromboplastin time (APTT) remains prolonged 2–4 hours after the first dose.

ADVERSE EFFECTS: May cause hypotension, bradycardia, dyspnea, and anaphylaxis. Excessive administration beyond that needed to reverse a heparin effect may cause bleeding as a paradoxical coagulopathy.

PYRIDOXINE (VITAMIN B$_6$)

INDICATIONS AND USE: For treatment of pyridoxine-dependent seizures; to prevent or treat vitamin B$_6$ deficiency; treatment of drug-induced deficiency (eg, isoniazid or hydralazine); treatment of acute intoxication of isoniazid or hydralazine.

ACTIONS: Vitamin B_6 is essential in the synthesis of gamma-aminobutyric acid (GABA), an inhibitory neurotransmitter in the CNS; GABA increases the seizure threshold. Pyridoxine is also required for heme synthesis and proteins, carbohydrates, and fats metabolism.
SUPPLIED: Injection, oral liquid.
ROUTE: PO, IM, IV.
DOSAGE:

- **Pyridoxine dependent seizures:** 100 mg IV single test dose, followed by a 30-minute observation period. If a response is seen, begin maintenance of 50–100 mg PO daily.
- **Dietary deficiency:** Children, 5–25 mg/day PO for 3 weeks, then 1.5–2.5 mg/day in multivitamin product.

ADVERSE REACTIONS: Sensory neuropathy (after chronic administration of large doses), seizures (following IV administration of very large doses), nausea, decreased serum folic acid concentration, respiratory distress.

PYRIMETHAMINE (DARAPRIM)
ACTION AND SPECTRUM: Folic acid antagonist selective for plasmodial dihydrofolate reductase. Activity highly selective for plasmodia (cidal) and *Toxoplasma gondii*.
SUPPLIED: Tablets (an oral suspension can be prepared by pharmacist).
ROUTE: PO.
DOSAGE:

- **Newborns and infants:**
  - **Toxoplasmosis:** 2 mg/kg/day divided every 12 hours for 2 days, then 1 mg/kg/day daily together with sulfadiazine for 6 months followed by 1 mg/kg/day 3 times weekly with sulfadiazine and leucovorin (oral folinic acid) (5–10 mg 3 times/week) should be administered to prevent hematologic toxicity for the next 6 months.
- **Children ≥1 month of age:**
  - **Prophylaxis for first episode of *Toxoplasma gondii*:** 1 mg/kg/day once daily with dapsone plus oral folinic acid (5 mg every 3 days).
  - **Prophylaxis for recurrence of *Toxoplasma gondii*:** 1 mg/kg/day once daily given with sulfadiazine or clindamycin, plus oral folinic acid (5 mg every 3 days).

PHARMACOKINETICS: Hepatic metabolism.
ADVERSE EFFECTS: Anorexia, vomiting, abdominal cramps, megaloblastic anemia, leukopenia, thrombocytopenia, pancytopenia, atrophic glossitis, rash, seizures, and shock.
COMMENTS: Administer with feedings if vomiting persists. Give sulfadiazine alone in empiric therapy of toxoplasmosis until the diagnosis is ruled out. Dose reduction is necessary in hepatic dysfunction.

RANITIDINE (ZANTAC)
INDICATIONS AND USE: Short-term treatment of duodenal and gastric ulcers, gastroesophageal reflux disease, upper gastrointestinal bleed and hypersecretory conditions.
ACTIONS: Histamine (H_2) receptor antagonist; competitively inhibits the action of histamine on the gastric parietal cells, inhibits gastric acid secretion.
SUPPLIED: Injection, oral syrup.
ROUTE: PO, IV.
DOSAGE:

- **Loading dose:** 1.5 mg/kg/dose IV then 12 hours later maintenance.
- **Maintenance** 1.5–2 mg/kg/day divided every 12 hours IV.
- **Continuous infusion:** 1.5 mg/kg/dose as loading dose followed by 0.04–0.08 mg/kg/hour infusion (or 1–2 mg/kg/day).
- **Oral:** 2–4 mg/kg/day divided every 8–12 hours. Maximum: 6 mg/kg/day.

ADVERSE EFFECTS: Constipation, abdominal discomfort, sedation, malaise, leukopenia, thrombocytopenia, elevated serum creatinine, bradycardia, and tachycardia.
COMMENTS: Dose adjustment needed in renal dysfunction. Injection contains 0.5% phenol. No short-term toxicity is noted. May add the daily dose to the total PN regimen and infuse over 24 hours to avoid the need for intermittent dosing.

RIFAMPIN (RIFADIN, ROFACT)
ACTION AND SPECTRUM: A broad-spectrum antibiotic that exerts its bacteriostatic action by inhibiting DNA-dependent RNA polymerase activity. It is effective against mycobacteria, *Neisseria* spp., and Gram-positive cocci (eg, staphylococci). It is used to eliminate meningococci from asymptomatic carriers; and for prophylaxis in contacts of patients with *Haemophilus influenzae* type B infection. If used as monotherapy, resistance develops rapidly; therefore, rifampin should always be used in combination with other agents for synergistic effect.
SUPPLIED: Capsules (oral suspension can be compounded by the pharmacy), injection.

ROUTE: PO, IV.

DOSAGE:

- **Synergy for *Staphylococcus aureus* infections:**
  - **Neonates:** 5–20 mg/kg/day PO/IV in divided doses every 12 hours with other antibiotics.
- **H. *influenzae* prophylaxis:**
  - **Neonates <1 month:** 10 mg/kg/day every 24 hours for 4 days.
  - **Infants and children:** 20 mg/kg/day every 24 hours for 4 days, not to exceed 600 mg/dose.
- **Nasal carriers of *S. aureus*:**
  - **Children:** 15 mg/kg/day divided every 12 hours for 5–10 days in combination with other antibiotics.
- **Meningococcal prophylaxis:**
  - **<1 month:** 10 mg/kg/day in divided doses every 12 hours for 2 days.
  - **Infants and children:** 20 mg/kg/day in divided doses every 12 hours for 2 days, not to exceed 600 mg/dose.
- **Tuberculosis:**
  - **Infants and children:** 10–20 mg/kg/day in divided doses every 12–24 hours.

PHARMACOKINETICS: Highly lipophilic; crosses the blood-brain barrier and is widely distributed into body tissues and fluids, Hepatic metabolism, undergoes enterohepatic recycling. Half-life is ~3–4 hours.

ADVERSE EFFECTS: Gastrointestinal irritation (anorexia, vomiting, and diarrhea), hypersensitivity (rash, pruritus, and eosinophilia), drowsiness, ataxia, blood dyscrasias (leukopenia, thrombocytopenia, and hemolytic anemia), hepatitis (rare), and elevation of serum urea nitrogen and uric acid levels. Causes pink to red discoloration of urine.

COMMENTS: Rifampin should always be in combination with other agents. Administer by slow IV infusion over 30 minutes to 3 hours at 6mg/mL concentration. Extravasation may cause local irritation and inflammation. *Note:* A potent enzyme inducer of hepatic metabolism. Patients receiving digoxin, phenytoin, phenobarbital, or theophylline may have a substantial decrease in the serum concentration of these drugs after starting rifampin. Careful monitoring of serum drug concentrations is necessary.

SILDENAFIL (VIAGRA, REVATIO)

INDICATIONS AND USE: (Revatio) Treatment of persistent pulmonary hypertension of the newborn (PPHN) refractory to treatment with inhaled nitric oxide; to facilitate weaning from nitric oxide (ie, to attenuate rebound effects after discontinuing inhaled nitric oxide); secondary pulmonary hypertension following cardiac surgery.

ACTIONS AND SPECTRUM: Selective phosphodiesterase-type 5 (PDE-5) inhibitor. PDE-5 is found in the pulmonary vascular smooth muscle, vascular and visceral smooth muscle, corpus cavernosum, and platelets. PDE-5 is responsible for the degradation of cyclic guanosine monophosphate (cGMP). Normally, nitric oxide (NO) activates the enzyme guanylate cyclase, which increases the levels of cGMP; cGMP produces smooth muscle relaxation. Inhibition of PDE-5 by sildenafil increases the cellular levels of cGMP which potentiate vascular smooth muscle relaxation, particularly in the lung where there is high PDE5 concentrations. Sildenafil causes vasodilation in the pulmonary vasculature and, to a lesser extent, in the systemic circulation.

SUPPLIED: Tablets.

ROUTE: PO. An oral suspension may be compounded by pharmacist.

DOSAGE: *Note:* Limited pediatric information exists; most pediatric literature consists of case reports or small studies and a wide range of doses have been used; further studies are needed.

- **Neonates:** 0.3 to 1 mg/kg/dose every 6 to 12 hours. Some studies have used 2 mg/kg/dose.
- **Infants and children:** Initial: 0.25–0.5 mg/kg/dose every 4–8 hours; increase if needed and if tolerated to 1 mg/kg/dose every 4–8 hours; doses as high as 2 mg/kg/dose every 4 hours have been used in several case reports.

PHARMACOKINETICS: Metabolism is via the liver via cytochrome P450 isoenzyme CYP3A4 (major) and CYP2C9 (minor). Major metabolite is formed via N-desmethylation pathway and has 50% of the activity as sildenafil.

ADVERSE EFFECTS: Use in neonatal and pediatric patients should be limited and considered experimental. The safety and efficacy in pediatric patients have not been established. There is short-term concern for worsening oxygenation and systemic hypotension; concern for increased risk of retinopathy of prematurity and platelet dysfunction.

COMMENTS: Significant increases in sildenafil concentrations may occur when used concurrently with CYP3A4 inhibitors (eg, azole antifungal agents, cimetidine and erythromycin) Concurrent use with heparin may have an additive effect on bleeding time. Use of sildenafil with vitamin K antagonists may increase risk of bleeding (primarily epistaxis).

SODIUM ACETATE

INDICATIONS AND USE: Correction of metabolic acidosis through the conversion of acetate to bicarbonate; sodium replacement.

ACTIONS AND SPECTRUM: Sodium acetate is metabolized to bicarbonate on an equimolar basis, which neutralizes hydrogen ion concentration and raises the blood and urine pH. Sodium is the primary extracellular cation.

SUPPLIED: Injection: 2 mEq/mL; 4 mEq/mL.

ROUTE: IV; hypertonic solution must be diluted prior to IV administration- maximum rate of infusion 1 mEq/kg/hour.

DOSAGE: If sodium acetate is desired over sodium bicarbonate (dosing similar to sodium bicarbonate).

- **Metabolic acidosis:** Based on the following formulas if blood gases and pH measurements are available: Neonates, infants, and children:

$$HCO_3^- \text{ (mEq)} = 0.3 \times \text{weight (kg)} \times \text{base deficit (mEq/L)}$$

or

$$HCO_3^- \text{ (mEq)} = 0.5 \times \text{weight (kg)} \times [24-\text{serum } HCO_3^- \text{ (mEq/L)}]$$

ADVERSE EFFECTS: Hypernatremia, hypokalemic metabolic alkalosis, hypocalcemia, edema.

COMMENTS: Use with caution with hepatic failure, congestive heart failure (CHF).

SODIUM BICARBONATE (VARIOUS)

INDICATIONS AND USE: Management of metabolic acidosis; alkalinization of urine; stabilization of acid base status in cardiac arrest and treatment of life-threatening hyperkalemia.

ACTIONS: Alkalinizing agent that dissociates to provide bicarbonate ion, which neutralizes hydrogen ions, and raises the pH of the blood and urine.

SUPPLIED: Injection.

ROUTE: IV.

DOSAGE:

- **Initial dose:** 1–2 mEq/kg IV slowly over 30 minutes.

$$\text{Dose in mEq} = 0.3 \times \text{weight (kg)} \times \text{base deficit (mEq/L)}$$

or

$$\text{Dose in mEq} = 0.5 \times \text{weight (kg)} \times [24-\text{serum } HCO_3^- \text{ (mEq/L)}].$$

ADVERSE EFFECTS: Rapid correction of metabolic acidosis with sodium bicarbonate can lead to intraventricular hemorrhage, hyperosmolality, metabolic alkalosis, hypernatremia, hypokalemia, and hypocalcemia.

COMMENTS: Use with close monitoring of arterial blood pH. Use only when adequate ventilation confirmed. Routine use in cardiac arrest is not recommended. Avoid extravasation; tissue necrosis can occur due to the hypertonicity of $NaHCO_3$. For direct IV administration: in neonates and infants, use the 0.5 mEq/mL solution or dilute the 1 mEq/mL solution 1:1 with sterile water for injection (SWI); administer slowly (maximum rate in neonates and infants: 10 mEq/minute); for infusion, dilute to a maximum concentration of 0.5 mEq/mL in dextrose solution and infuse over 2 hours (maximum rate of administration: 1 mEq/kg/hour).

SODIUM POLYSTYRENE SULFONATE (KAYEXALATE)

INDICATIONS AND USE: Treatment of hyperkalemia.

ACTIONS: Cation exchange resin that removes potassium by exchanging sodium ions for potassium ions in the intestine before the resin is passed from the body.

SUPPLIED: Powder for suspension, suspension (in 33% sorbitol) (1.25 g/5 mL, containing 4.1 mEq of sodium ion/g).

ROUTE: PO, PR.

DOSAGE: 1 g/kg/dose PO every 6 hours or every 2–6 hours PR. 1 g of resin will exchange 1 mEq of sodium for 1 mEq of potassium.

ADVERSE EFFECTS: Large doses may cause fecal impaction. Hypokalemia, hypocalcemia, hypomagnesemia, and sodium retention may occur.

COMMENTS: Small amounts of magnesium and calcium may also be lost in binding. When using the powder for oral administration, dilute in 3–4 mL fluid per g of resin; 10% sorbitol, water, or syrup may be used as diluent. When using powder for rectal administration, dilute in water or 25% sorbitol at a concentration of 0.3–0.5 g/mL; retain enema in colon for at least 30–60 minutes or several hours, if possible.

SPIRONOLACTONE (ALDACTONE)

INDICATIONS AND USE: Primarily used in conjunction with a thiazide diuretic in the treatment of hypertension, congestive heart failure, and edema when prolonged diuresis is desirable.

ACTIONS: Competes with aldosterone for receptor sites in the distal renal tubules; increases sodium chloride and water excretion while conserving potassium and hydrogen ions; it also may block the effect of aldosterone on arteriolar smooth muscle.

SUPPLIED: Tablets (oral suspension can be compounded by the pharmacy).

ROUTE: PO.
DOSAGE: 1–3 mg/kg/day divided every 12–24 hours.
ADVERSE EFFECTS: Hyperkalemia, dehydration, hyponatremia, hyperchloremic metabolic acidosis and gynecomastia (usually reversible).
COMMENTS: Contraindicated in hyperkalemia, anuria, and rapidly deteriorating renal function. Monitor potassium closely when giving potassium supplements.

STREPTOKINASE (KABIKINASE, STREPTASE)

INDICATIONS AND USE: Thrombolytic agent used for the treatment of systemic thrombosis.
ACTIONS: Promotes thrombolysis; activates conversion of plasminogen to plasmin; plasmin degrades fibrin, fibrinogen and other procoagulant proteins into soluble fragments.
SUPPLIED: Powder for injection.
ROUTE: IV.
DOSAGE: Safety and efficacy in children has not been established.
- **Loading dose:** 2000 units/kg IV over 30–60 minutes.
- **Maintenance:** 2000 units/kg/hour as continuous infusion for 6 to 12 hours. Titrate the dose to maintain the thrombin time at 2–5 times the normal control value.

ADVERSE EFFECTS: May cause severe spontaneous bleeding, hypersensitivity and anaphylactic reactions, fever (common), and chills. Contraindicated in patients with streptococcal infection within the last 2 months, any internal bleeding, gastrointestinal bleeding or major surgery within the last 10 days. Antibodies to streptokinase may remain for 3 to 6 months following initial dose. If repeat thrombolytic therapy is indicated use another agent.
COMMENTS: Before starting therapy, obtain a baseline thrombin time, activated partial thromboplastin time, prothrombin time, hematocrit, and platelet count; repeat all tests every 12 hours. It is desired to maintain the thrombin time at 2–5 times normal and the prothrombin time and activated partial thromboplastin time as 1.5–2 times normal. Prepare final infusion solution to a concentration of 1000 units/mL in D₅W. Begin heparin therapy during or immediately upon completion of streptokinase therapy. Failure of thrombolytic agents in newborns/neonates may occur due to low plasminogen levels. Clot lysis may be more effective by the administration of fresh-frozen plasma. **Antidote:** Aminocaproic acid (loading dose 200 mg/kg IV or PO stat, followed by a maintenance dose of 100 mg/kg/dose IV or PO every 6 hours for up to 10 days after the procedure). *Note:* Limited experience in neonates.

SULFACETAMIDE SODIUM (BLEPH-10)

ACTION AND SPECTRUM: Interferes with bacterial growth by inhibiting bacterial folic acid synthesis. Used for the treatment and prophylaxis of conjunctivitis. Spectrum includes *Staphylococcus aureus, Streptococcus pneumoniae, Haemophilus influenzae,* and *Moraxella* spp.
SUPPLIED: Ophthalmic solution and ointment.
ROUTE: Ophthalmic.
DOSAGE: Instill 1–2 drops into each eye every 1–3 hours initially, then increase the time interval as the condition responds; apply ointment to each eye 1–4 times/day and at bedtime. Usual 7–10 days.
ADVERSE EFFECTS: May cause burning and stinging sensation of eyes, increased sensitivity to light, blurred vision and pruritus.
COMMENTS: Contraindicated in infants <2 months of age.

SULFADIAZINE (VARIOUS)

ACTION AND SPECTRUM: Acts via competitive antagonism of *p*-aminobenzoic acid, an essential factor in folic acid synthesis. Spectrum of action includes both Gram-positive and Gram-negative organisms. In neonatology, used primarily as adjunctive treatment for *Toxoplasma gondii* in combination with pyrimethamine.
SUPPLIED: Tablets. Pharmacist can compound oral suspension.
ROUTE: PO.
DOSAGE:
- **Congenital toxoplasmosis: Newborns:** 100 mg/kg/day divided every 12 hours for 12 months in conjunction with pyrimethamine 1 mg/kg/day once daily and supplemental folinic acid (5 mg every 3 days) for first 6 months, then pyrimethamine (1 mg/kg/day 3 times/week) and folinic acid (10 mg 3 times/week) for the next 6 months.
- **Toxoplasmosis: Children:** 120–200 mg/kg/day divided every 6 hours in conjunction with pyrimethamine (2 mg/kg/day divided every 12 hours for 3 days) followed by 1 mg/kg/day once daily (maximum dose: 25 mg/day) with supplemental folinic acid (5–10 mg every 3 days).

ADVERSE EFFECTS: Hypersensitivity (fever, rash, hepatitis, vasculitis, and lupus-like syndrome), neutropenia, agranulocytosis, thrombocytopenia, aplastic anemia, Stevens-Johnson syndrome, and crystalluria (keep urine alkaline, maintain adequate hydration and urine output high). Kernicterus may occur.
COMMENTS: Avoid use in neonates, except for treatment of congenital toxoplasmosis. *Folinic acid* supplementation necessary to prevent folic acid deficiency.

TICARCILLIN DISODIUM (TICAR)

SPECTRUM: Semisynthetic extended-spectrum penicillin that possesses anti–*Pseudomonas* activity and has good coverage against enteric Gram-negative organisms. Inhibits bacterial cell wall synthesis.
SUPPLIED: Injection.
ROUTE: IM, IV (infuse over 30 minutes).
DOSAGE:

- **Neonates:**
  - **Postnatal age ≤7 days:**
    - **≤2000 g:** 150 mg/kg/day IV in divided doses every 12 hours.
    - **>2000 g:** 225 mg/kg/day IV in divided doses every 8 hours.
  - **Postnatal age >7 days:**
    - **<1200 g:** 150 mg/kg/day in divided doses every 12 hours.
    - **1200–2000 g:** 225 mg/kg/day in divided doses every 8 hours.
    - **>2000 g:** 300 mg/kg/day in divided doses every 6–8 hours.
- **Infants and children:**
  - **IM:** 50–100 mg/kg/day IM in divided doses every 6–8 hours.
  - **IV:** 200–300 mg/kg/day IV in divided doses every 4–6 hours; doses as high as 400 mg/kg/day divided every 4–6 hours have been used in acute pulmonary exacerbations of cystic fibrosis. Maximum dose: 24 g/day.

PHARMACOKINETICS: Mostly excreted in urine as unchanged drug.
ADVERSE EFFECTS: Hypersensitivity reactions with eosinophilia; hypernatremia and hypokalemia; inhibition of platelet aggregation; hyperbilirubinemia, elevation of AST, ALT, BUN, and serum creatinine.
COMMENTS: Avoid IM use if possible. Caution with high sodium content (contains 5.2 mEq of sodium/g of ticarcillin disodium).

TICARCILLIN DISODIUM AND CLAVULANATE POTASSIUM (TIMENTIN)

SPECTRUM: Combination antibiotic of ticarcillin (a carboxypenicillin) and clavulanic acid (a β-lactamase inhibitor). Clavulanate expands activity of ticarcillin to include β-lactamase producing strains of *Staphylococcus aureus, Haemophilus influenzae, Moraxella catarrhalis, Bacteroides fragilis, Klebsiella, Prevotella, Pseudomonas aeruginosa, Escherichia coli,* and *Proteus* species.
SUPPLIED: Injection.
ROUTE: IV.
DOSAGE Timentin (ticarcillin/clavulanate) is a combination product; each 3.1 g vial contains 3 g ticarcillin disodium and 0.1 g clavulanic acid. Dosage recommendations are based on ticarcillin component. Maximum dose: 400 mg/kg/day not to exceed 18–24 g/day.

- **Term neonates and infants <3 months:** 200–300 mg ticarcillin component/kg/day divided every 6–8 hours.
- **Infants ≥3 months and children <60 kg:**
  - **Mild to moderate infections:** 200 mg ticarcillin component/kg/day divided every 6 hours.
  - **Severe infections outside the CNS:** 300 mg ticarcillin component/kg/day in divided doses every 4–6 hours.

PHARMACOKINETICS: Ticarcillin, renal (tubular secretion); clavulanic acid, hepatic and renal.
ADVERSE EFFECTS: Eosinophilia, leukopenia, inhibition of platelet aggregation, prolongation of bleeding time, neutropenia, hemolytic anemia, thrombocytopenia, hypernatremia, hypokalemia, elevations in AST, ALT, BUN, and serum creatinine, and thrombophlebitis.
COMMENTS: Use with caution and modify dose in patients with renal impairment, Sodium content of 1 g: 4.51 mEq.

TOBRAMYCIN SULFATE (NEBCIN)

ACTION AND SPECTRUM: Aminoglycoside antibiotic that alters bacterial protein synthesis resulting in alteration in cell membrane permeability that ultimately leads to bacterial cell death. Used for the treatment of documented or suspected infections caused by susceptible Gram-negative bacilli including *Pseudomonas aeruginosa* and non–pseudomonal enteric bacillus infection, which is more sensitive to tobramycin than gentamicin based on susceptibility tests. Usually used in combination with a β-lactam antibiotic.
SUPPLIED: Injection, solution for nebulization, ophthalmic, and ophthalmic ointment.
ROUTE: IM, IV (infuse over 30 min), topical (ophthalmic), inhalation.
DOSAGE:

- **Neonates:**
  - **Preterm <1000 g:** 3.5 mg/kg/dose IM/IV every 24 hours.
  - **0–4 weeks, <1200 g:** 2.5 mg/kg/dose IM/IV every 18 hours.
  - **Postnatal age ≤7 days:**
    - **1200–2000 g:** 2.5 mg/kg/dose IM/IV every 12 hours.
    - **>2000 g:** 2.5 mg/kg/dose IM/IV every 12 hours.
  - **Postnatal age >7 days:**
    - **1200–2000 g:** 2.5 mg/kg/dose IM/IV every 8–12 hours.
    - **>2000 g:** 2.5 mg/kg/dose IM/IV every 8 hours.

- **Infants and children <5 years:** 2.5 mg/kg/dose IM/IV every 8 hours.
- **Ophthalmic:** Instill 1–2 drops into each eye every 4 hours or more often if infection is severe, or apply a small amount of ointment into each eye 2–3 times/day or for severe infections every 3–4 hours.
- **Inhalation:** 150 mg twice daily nebulized has been used for difficult to manage NICU patients. Monitor serum levels after two days of therapy.

ADVERSE EFFECTS: See Gentamicin Sulfate.

COMMENTS: Reserve for cases resistant to gentamicin sulfate. Obtain serum peak and trough concentrations at about the third maintenance dose. Desired serum peak concentration is 4–12 mcg/mL (sample obtained 30 minutes after the infusion is complete); desired serum trough concentration is 0.5–2 mcg/mL (sample obtained 30 minutes to just before the next dose).

TROMETHAMINE (THAM)

INDICATIONS AND USE: Treatment of metabolic acidosis in mechanically ventilated patients with significant hypercarbia or hypernatremia. Not indicated for the treatment of metabolic acidosis due to bicarbonate deficiency.

ACTIONS: Alkalinizing agent that acts as a proton (hydrogen ion) acceptor; combines with hydrogen ions and their associated anions of acids (lactic, pyruvic, carbonic, and other metabolic acids) to form bicarbonate and buffer to correct acidosis. It buffers both metabolic and respiratory acids; limiting carbon dioxide generation. The resulting salts are then renally excreted.

SUPPLIED: Injection, 0.3 molar solution (1 mmol = 120 mg = 3.3 mL = 1 mEq Tham).

ROUTE: IV.

DOSAGE:
- **Method 1:** 3.3–6.6 mL/kg (1–2 mmol/kg) of undiluted solution infused in a large vein over 1 hour.
- **Method 2:** Dose (mL) = weight (kg) × 1.1 × base deficit (mEq/L).
- **Maximum dose** in neonates with normal renal function is ~5 to 7 mmol/kg/24 hours.

ADVERSE EFFECTS: Respiratory depression, apnea, thrombophlebitis, venospasm, alkalosis, hypoglycemia, and hyperkalemia. Avoid infusion via low-lying umbilical venous catheters due to associated risk of hepatocellular necrosis; severe local tissue necrosis and sloughing may occur if solution extravasates; administer via central line or large vein slowly.

COMMENTS: Contraindicated in anuria, uremia, salicylate toxicity and chronic respiratory acidosis. Administration beyond 24 hours is not recommended. Monitor for hyperkalemia and pH especially with renal dysfunction.

UROKINASE

INDICATION AND USE: Thrombolytic agent indicated for the lysis of acute pulmonary emboli. Unlabeled/investigational uses include treatment of deep venous thrombosis, myocardial infarction.

ACTIONS: Promotes thrombolysis; activates conversion of plasminogen to plasmin; plasmin degrades fibrin, fibrinogen and other procoagulant proteins into soluble fragments.

SUPPLIED: Vial, powder for injection.

ROUTE: IV.

DOSAGE: The safety and efficacy in children has not been established. The activated partial thromboplastin time (aPTT) should be <2 times the normal before urokinase therapy is begun and before starting anticoagulants following the urokinase infusion.
- **Arterial thrombosis, loading dose:** 4400 units/kg IV over 10 minutes then 4400 units/kg/hour for 6 to 12 hours. Heparin therapy should be initiated during or immediately following the completion of thrombolytic therapy.

ADVERSE EFFECTS: Major bleeding, anaphylaxis, bronchospasm, allergic reaction, fever, gastrointestinal (GI) hemorrhage.

COMMENTS: Contraindicated in patients with any internal bleeding, GI bleeding, major surgery within the last 10 days.

URSODIOL (ACTIGALL)

INDICATIONS AND USE: (Unlabeled use). To facilitate bile excretion in infants with biliary atresia; treatment of cholestasis secondary to parenteral nutrition (PN); improve the hepatic metabolism of essential fatty acids in patients with cystic fibrosis and gallbladder stone dissolution.

ACTIONS: A hydrophobic bile acid that decreases the cholesterol content of bile and bile stones by reducing the secretion of cholesterol from the liver and decreases the fractional reabsorption of cholesterol by the intestines.

SUPPLIED: Tablet, capsule. An oral suspension can be compounded by the pharmacist.

ROUTE: PO.

DOSAGE:
- **Biliary atresia:**
  - **Infants:** 10–15 mg/kg/day PO once daily.

- **Total parenteral nutrition–induced cholestasis:**
  - **Infants and children:** 30 mg/kg/day PO in 3 divided doses.
- **Improvement in the hepatic metabolism of essential fatty acids in cystic fibrosis:**
  - **Children:** 30 mg/kg/day PO in 2 divided doses.

PHARMACOKINETICS: Absorbed well orally. **Metabolism:** Undergoes extensive enterohepatic recycling; following hepatic conjugation and biliary secretion, the drug is hydrolyzed to active ursodiol, where it is recycled or transformed to lithocholic acid by colonic microbial flora. Half-life: 100 hours.

ADVERSE EFFECTS: Rash, diarrhea, biliary pain, constipation, stomatitis, flatulence, nausea, vomiting, abdominal pain, elevated liver enzymes.

COMMENTS: Dissolution of gallstones may take several months, use with caution in patients with nonvisualizing gallbladder and patients with chronic liver disease.

VANCOMYCIN HYDROCHLORIDE (VANCOCIN)

ACTION AND SPECTRUM: Bactericidal action by interfering with bacterial cell wall synthesis. Active against most Gram-positive cocci and bacilli, including streptococci, staphylococci (including methicillin-resistant staphylococci), clostridia (including *Clostridium difficile*), *Corynebacterium* spp., and *Listeria monocytogenes*. Bacteriostatic against enterococci. No cross-resistance with other antibiotics has been reported. It is the drug of choice against methicillin-resistant staphylococci.

SUPPLIED: Injection, oral solution.

ROUTE: IV, Intrathecal, PO.

DOSAGE:

- **Neonates:**
  - **Postnatal age ≤7 days:**
    - **<1200 g:** 15 mg/kg/day IV every 24 hours.
    - **1200–2000 g:** 10–15 mg/kg/dose IV every 12–18 hours.
    - **>2000 g:** 10–15 mg/kg/dose IV every 8–12 hours.
  - **Postnatal age >7 days:**
    - **<1200 g:** 15 mg/kg/day given IV 24 hours.
    - **1200–2000 g:** 10–15 mg/kg/dose IV every 8–12 hours.
    - **>2000 g:** 15–20 mg/kg/dose IV every 8 hours.
- **Infants >1 month and children:** 40 mg/kg/day IV in divided doses every 6–8 hours.
- **Intrathecal/intraventricular:** Neonates: 5–10 mg/day.
- **Oral (antibiotic-associated pseudomembranous colitis):** *Note:* Metronidazole is the drug of initial choice per 2006 Red Book recommendations). Children: 40 mg/kg/day in divided doses every 6 hours for 7–10 days; not to exceed 2 g/day.

PHARMACOKINETICS: Renally excreted. Half-life is 6–10 hours.

ADVERSE EFFECTS: Allergy (rash and fever), ototoxicity (with prolonged serum peak concentrations >40 mcg/mL), nephrotoxicity (higher incidence with trough concentrations >10 mcg/mL) and thrombophlebitis at the site of injection. Rapid infusion may cause rash, chills, and fever ("red-man" syndrome) mimicking anaphylactic reaction. Apnea and bradycardia without other signs of "red-man" syndrome have also been associated with rapid infusion. Infuse dose over at least 60 minutes.

COMMENTS: Therapeutic range: Serum peak level between 25–40 mcg/mL; 30 to 40 mcg/mL when treating meningitis (sample drawn 60 minutes after the infusion is completed) and serum trough level of 5–15 mcg/mL; experts recommend 15 to 20 mcg/mL when treating MRSA pneumonia, endocarditis or bone/joint infections (sample drawn 30 minutes prior to scheduled dose). In general, draw serum peak and trough levels around the fourth maintenance dose. Monitor serum creatinine, blood urea nitrogen (BUN), and urine output. If staphylococci exhibit tolerance to the drug, combine it with an aminoglycoside, with or without rifampin. Oral doses are poorly absorbed.

VARICELLA-ZOSTER IMMUNE GLOBULIN (VariZIG)

INDICATIONS AND USE: For protection of infants of mothers with varicella-zoster infections (chickenpox) within 5 days before or 48 hours after delivery, of postnatally exposed preterm infants <1000 g or <28 weeks' gestation regardless of maternal history, and of postnatally exposed premature infants ≥28 weeks' gestation whose maternal history is negative for varicella.

ACTIONS: Passive immunity through infusion of immunoglobulin G (IgG) antibodies. Protection lasts 1 month or longer. VariZIG does not reduce the incidence but acts to decrease the risk of complications.

SUPPLIED: Injection.

ROUTE: IM.

DOSAGE: <10 kg: 125 units = 1 × 125 unit vial minimum dose: 125 units; do not give fractional doses. Maximum dose is 625 international units.

ADVERSE EFFECTS: Pain, erythema, swelling, rash at the site of injection, and, rarely, anaphylaxis.

COMMENTS: Best results are achieved if VariZIG is given within 96 hours after exposure. It is obtained through FFF Enterprises (Temecula, California) (1-800-843-7477).

VECURONIUM BROMIDE (NORCURON)

INDICATIONS AND USE: Skeletal muscle relaxation and paralysis in infants requiring mechanical ventilation or surgery, or to facilitate endotracheal intubation.

ACTIONS: Nondepolarizing muscle relaxant that competitively antagonizes autonomic cholinergic receptors. Onset of action is 1–2 minutes with a duration that varies with dose and age.

SUPPLIED: Powder for injection.

ROUTE: IV.

DOSAGE:

- **Neonates:** 0.1 mg/kg/dose then maintenance: 0.03–0.15 mg/kg IV push every 1–2 hours as needed.
- **Infants >7 weeks to 1 year:** 0.1 mg/kg/dose; repeat every hour as needed; may be administered as a continuous infusion at 1–1.5 mcg/kg/minute (0.06–0.09 mg/kg/hour).

ADVERSE EFFECTS: May cause hypoxemia with inadequate mechanical ventilation; bronchospasm, apnea, arrhythmias, tachycardia, hypotension, hypertension.

COMMENTS: Causes less tachycardia than pancuronium bromide. When used with narcotics, decreases in heart rate and blood pressure have been observed.

VITAMIN A

INDICATIONS AND USE: Treatment and prevention of vitamin A deficiency; to reduce the risk of chronic lung disease in high risk premature neonates with Vitamin A deficiency.

ACTIONS: Vitamin A is required for growth and bone development, vision, reproduction, and differentiation and maintenance of epithelial tissue. Retinol is the parent compound of vitamin A, and the form that is transported within the body. Retinol is released from the liver and is bound to serum retinol binding protein (RBP), which facilitates absorption, transport and mediation of the biological activity. The pulmonary histopathologic changes seen in patients with bronchopulmonary dysplasia (BPD) are similar to those seen with Vitamin A deficiency. Retinol metabolites exhibit potent and site-specific effects on gene expression as well as lung growth and development.

SUPPLIED: Injection.

ROUTE: IM, PO (contained in multivitamin preparations).

DOSAGE:

- **Prevention of bronchopulmonary dysplasia in premature infants:** 5000 units IM 3 times a week for 4 weeks.
- **Prophylactic therapy for children at risk for developing deficiency:**
  - **Infants ≤1 year:** 100,000 units PO every 4–6 months.
  - **Children >1 year:** 200,000 units PO every 4–6 months.
- **Recommended daily allowance (RDA):**
  - **<1 year:** 375 mcg PO (1250 units).
  - **1–3 years:** 400 mcg PO (1330 units).
- **Daily dietary supplement:**
  - **Infants up to 6 months:** 1500 units PO.
  - **Children 6 months to 3 years:** 1500–2000 units.

ADVERSE EFFECTS: Concomitant use with glucocorticoids should be avoided, as it significantly raises plasma vitamin A concentrations. Seen only with doses that exceed physiologic replacement. Monitor for signs of toxicity: full fontanel, lethargy, irritability, hepatosplenomegaly, edema, and mucocutaneous lesions.

VITAMIN D₂ (ERGOCALCIFEROL, CALCIFEROL, DRISDOL)

INDICATIONS AND USE: To prevent or treat rickets, to treat hypoparathyroidism and to manage hypocalcemia resulting from vitamin D deficiency.

ACTIONS: Stimulates calcium and phosphate absorption from the small intestine; promotes secretion of calcium from bone to blood; promotes renal tubule phosphate resorption; acts on osteoblasts to stimulate skeletal growth and on the parathyroid glands to suppress parathyroid hormone synthesis and secretion.

SUPPLIED: Oral solution, 8000 units/mL; injection.

ROUTE: PO.

DOSAGE:

- **2008 AAP statement on the Prevention of Rickets and Vitamin D Deficiency in Infants, Children and Adolescents (Wagner et al: Pediatrics 122 (5):1142–52).**
  - **Neonates and children:** Breastfed and partially breastfed infants should be supplemented with 400 international units of vitamin D beginning in the first few days of life and continuing until the daily consumption of vitamin-D fortified formula or milk is 1 liter per day or 1 quart per day; also non-breast-fed infants who are ingesting less than 1000 mL/day of vitamin D-fortified or milk and children and adolescents who do not obtain 400 international units of vitamin D per day through vitamin D-fortified milk and foods should receive a vitamin D supplement of 400 international units per day.
- **Dietary supplementation:**

- **Premature infants:** 400–800 international units, up to 30,000 international units/day.
- **Infants and healthy children:** 400 international units/day.
- **Hypoparathyroidism:** 8000 units/kg daily for 1 to 2 weeks to safely and quickly correct hypocalcemia followed by maintenance dose of 2000 units/kg daily.

COMMENTS: Excessive doses may lead to hypervitaminosis D, manifested by hypercalcemia and its associated complications (1 mcg = 40 USP units).

VITAMIN E (*DL*-α-TOCOPHEROL ACETATE) (AquaSOL E)

INDICATIONS AND USE: Treatment or prevention of vitamin E deficiency.

ACTIONS: Antioxidant that prevents oxidation of vitamin A and C; protects polyunsaturated fatty acids in membranes from attack by free radicals and protects red blood cells against hemolysis by oxidizing agents.

SUPPLIED: Drops, 50 units/mL.

ROUTE: PO.

DOSAGE: **Premature or low birth weight neonates:** 5 to 25 units PO/day diluted with feedings. Do not give simultaneously with iron; will decrease iron absorption.

COMMENTS: Physiologic serum vitamin E levels are 0.8 to 3.5 mg/dL. Serum levels should be monitored when pharmacologic doses of vitamin E are administered. Liquid preparation is very hyperosmolar (3620 mOsm/kg H_2O) and should be diluted (1 mg of *dl*-α-tocopherol acetate = 1 unit).

VITAMIN K$_1$ (PHYTONADIONE) (AQUAMEPHYTON, MEPHYTON)

INDICATIONS AND USE: Prevention and treatment of hemorrhagic disease of the newborn and vitamin K deficiency.

ACTIONS: Required for the synthesis of blood coagulation factors II, VII, IX, and X. Because vitamin K$_1$ may require 3 hours or more to stop active bleeding, fresh-frozen plasma, 10 mL/kg, may be necessary when bleeding is severe. The drug has no antagonistic effects against heparin.

SUPPLIED: Tablets, injection.

ROUTE: PO, IM, IV, subcutaneous. For IV administration, dilute in D$_5$W or normal saline (maximum concentration: 10 mg/mL with infusion rate not to exceed 1 mg/minute; usual rate 15–30 minutes).

DOSAGE:

- **Neonatal hemorrhagic disease:**
  - **Prevention:** 1 mg IM at birth.
    - **Preterm infant <32 weeks' gestation:**
      - **Birthweight >1000 g:** 0.5 mg IM at birth.
      - **Birthweight <1000 g:** 0.3 mg/kg IM at birth.
  - **Treatment:** 1–2 mg IM/day.
- **Vitamin K deficiency due to drugs, malabsorption, or decreased synthesis of vitamin K:**
  - **Infants and children:** 2.5–5 mg/day PO day or 1–2 mg subcutaneous, IM, IV, as a single dose.
- **Oral anticoagulant overdose:** 0.5–2 mg/dose IV every 12 hours as needed. (Monitor the serial prothrombin time and partial thromboplastin time for response.)

ADVERSE EFFECTS: Relatively nontoxic. Hemolytic anemia and kernicterus have been reported in neonates given menadiol sodium diphosphate (vitamin K$_3$ [Synkavite]). Severe hypersensitivity or anaphylactic reactions have been associated with IV administration of vitamin K$_1$. Efficacy of treatment with vitamin K$_1$ is decreased in patients with liver disease.

ZIDOVUDINE (RETROVIR) (AZT, ZDV)

INDICATIONS AND USE: Treatment of HIV infection in combination with other antiretroviral agents; chemoprophylaxis to reduce perinatal HIV transmission; prophylactic treatment of neonates born to HIV-infected mothers.

ACTIONS: Nucleoside reverse transcriptase inhibitor (NRTI) that inhibits HIV viral polymerases and DNA replication.

SUPPLIED: Syrup; injection.

ROUTE: IV, PO.

DOSAGE:

- **Premature Infants <35 weeks' gestational age (GA) at birth:**
  - **Initial dose:** 2 mg/kg/dose PO every 12 hours or 1.5 mg/kg/dose IV every 12 hours.
  - **Increase to every 8 hours as follows:**
    - **GA at birth <30 weeks:** Increase above dose to every 8 hours at 4 weeks of age.
    - **GA at birth ≥30 weeks:** Increase above dose to every 8 hours at 2 weeks of age.
- **Neonates and infants <6 weeks:** 2 mg/kg/dose PO every 6 hours or 1.5 mg/kg/dose IV every 6 hours.
- **Infants ≥6 weeks and children:** 160 mg/m^2/dose PO every 8 hours. Maximum: 200 mg every 8 hours. Twice daily dosing is not FDA approved in children, but some investigators use 180–240 mg/m^2/dose every 12 hours to improve compliance; data on this dose in children is limited.

- **IV continuous infusion:** 20 mg/m^2/hour.
- **IV intermittent infusion:** 120 mg/m^2/dose every 6 hours.

ADVERSE EFFECTS: The most frequent are granulocytopenia and severe anemia. Others include thrombocytopenia, leukopenia, diarrhea, fever, seizures, insomnia, cholestatic hepatitis, and lactic acidosis.

COMMENTS: Use with caution in patients with impaired hepatic function, bone marrow compromise, or folic acid or vitamin B$_{12}$ deficiency.

INTERACTIONS: Concurrent acetaminophen, probenecid, cimetidine, indomethacin, morphine, and benzodiazepines may increase toxicity as a result of decreased glucuronidation or reduced renal excretion of zidovudine. Concomitant acyclovir may cause neurotoxicity; ganciclovir and flucytosine may cause severe hematologic toxicity as a result of synergistic myelosuppression. Ribavirin and zidovudine are antagonistic and should not be used concurrently.

133 Effects of Drugs and Substances in Pregnancy and Breast-Feeding

The chapter provides some summary data on commonly used drugs and substances that may be taken by the mother during pregnancy and breast-feeding. A more comprehensive listing of over 800 medications is available on line at www.neonatologybook.com. Regardless of the designated risk category or presumed safety, no drug or substance should be used during pregnancy or breast-feeding unless it is clearly needed and the potential benefits clearly outweigh the risks.

The table lists the generic medication name and in parentheses the Food and Drug Administration (FDA) fetal risk category as of the fall of 2008 (see later). Reported pregnancy-adverse events and comments are presented based on the available reports in the literature. Next, breast-feeding compatibility is noted. At the present time there is no formally FDA-sanctioned breast-feeding category, and the system used here is discussed later. Lastly, any reported effects on lactation or on infant effects based on breast milk consumption are noted. The editorial board has made an attempt to summarize the data based on the best information available for an individual agent where sources disagree. These data are subject to change as new information becomes available. The reader is advised to consult the FDA and manufacturer's web site for the latest information concerning risks of these medications.

U.S. FDA FETAL RISK CATEGORIES (AS OF FALL 2008)[1]

CATEGORY A

Adequate studies in pregnant women have not demonstrated a risk to the fetus in the first trimester of pregnancy; there is no evidence of risk in the last two trimesters.

---

[1]Note: In late 2008, the FDA proposed changes to their labeling system in *Summary of Proposed Rule on Pregnancy and Lactation Labeling* (http://www.fda.gov/cder/regulatory/pregnancy_labeling/summary.htm; Accessed October 24, 2008). Under FDA's proposed rule, the labeling would contain two subsections: one on pregnancy and one on lactation. Current pregnancy labeling uses five categories: A, B, C, D, and X. The categories do not always distinguish between risks based on human versus animal data findings or between differences in frequency, severity, and type of fetal developmental toxicities. The proposed rule would remove the categories from the labeling of all drug products. Both the pregnancy and lactation subsections would have three principal components: a risk summary, clinical considerations, and a data section. Once implemented, this will affect how medications are labeled in the future. Check www.fda.gov for updates on this pending rule.

CATEGORY B
Animal studies have not demonstrated a risk to the fetus, but there are no adequate studies in pregnant women.

or

Animal studies have shown an adverse effect, but adequate studies in pregnant women have not demonstrated a risk to the fetus during the first trimester of pregnancy, and there is no evidence of risk in the last two trimesters.

CATEGORY C
Animal studies have shown an adverse effect on the fetus, but there are no adequate studies in humans. The benefits from the use of the drug in pregnant women may be acceptable despite its potential risks.

or

There are no animal reproduction studies and no adequate studies in humans.

CATEGORY D
There is evidence of human fetal risk, but the potential benefits from the use of the drug in pregnant women may be acceptable despite its potential risks.

CATEGORY X
Studies in animals or humans or adverse reaction reports, or both, have demonstrated fetal abnormalities. The risk of use in pregnant women clearly outweighs any possible benefit.

BREAST-FEEDING COMPATIBILITY

As noted, no formal system exists for categorizing drugs or substances ant their effect on breast-feeding, lactation, and effects on the infant. The following system is used in this book:

CATEGORY (+) : Generally compatible with breast-feeding.

CATEGORY (–) : Avoid with breast-feeding. Toxicity can be seen.

CATEGORY (CI) : Contraindicated.

Drug (FDA Fetal Risk Category)	Pregnancy-Adverse Events and Comments	Breast-Feeding Compatibility	Effect on Lactation and Adverse Effects on Infant
Acebutolol (B; D if 2nd and 3rd trimester)	IUGR. Bradycardia and hypotension in infant exposed near term. Can cause transient hypoglycemia.	–	Excreted into breast milk. May cause bradycardia and hypotension.
Acetaminophen (B)	Safe for short-term use. In long-term and overdose: fetal and neonatal death with hepatorenal toxicity.	+	Excreted in breast milk. AAP: compatible.
Acetazolamide (C)	Not associated with malformations.	+	Excreted in breast milk. AAP: compatible.
Acetohexamide (C)	Human studies: no increase in congenital malformations. ACOG recommends insulin for gestational diabetes. Causes symptomatic hypoglycemia and seizures in newborn. Monitor infant's glucose after birth.	–	No studies; effects unknown. Risk of hypoglycemia.
Acyclovir (B)	No adverse effects seen.	+	AAP: compatible.
Adenosine (C)	No adverse effects reported. High IV doses: potential fetal toxicity.	+	No studies. Drug unlikely excreted into breast milk.
Albuterol (C)	Fetal tachycardia, hypoglycemia, risk of polydactyly, transient fetal hyperglycemia, and atrial flutter, and decreased incidence of RDS.	+	No studies. Probably compatible.
Alfentanil (C; D if prolonged or high doses near term)	Risk in 3rd trimester. No adverse effects. Respiratory depression.	+	Excreted into breast milk. Significance of amount unknown.
Allopurinol (C)	Few studies.	+	Drug excreted in breast milk. AAP: compatible.
Alprazolam (D)	Neonatal withdrawal may occur.	–	Excreted in breast milk. Risk of withdrawal, lethargy, weight loss, and adverse effects on neurodevelopment. AAP: effect unknown but of concern.
Alteplase (C)	Risk of hemorrhage in mother.	+	Unknown excretion. Risk to infant minimal.
Amikacin (C; D per manufacturer)	No adverse effects in fetus. Test for ototoxicity.	+	Drug excreted in breast milk. Observe infant for changes in bowel flora, allergies, and use caution when interpreting culture results.
Amiloride (B; D if gestational hypertension)	Few human studies. Hypospadias reported.	+	No studies. Drug likely excreted in breast milk. Probably compatible.
Aminocaproic acid (C)	Few human studies.	–	No human lactation studies. Drug likely excreted into breast milk. Best to avoid breast-feeding.
Aminopterin (X)	Malformations not found with 2nd and 3rd trimester use. Need long-term studies.	CI	Antineoplastic agent; contraindicated.
Amiodarone (D)	Risk in human studies. Transient bradycardia, IUGR, prolonged QT, SGA, goiter, hypo/transient hyperthyroidism. Test thyroid function of infant.	–	Excreted into breast milk. Possible hypothyroidism. AAP: effect unknown but of concern.
Amitriptyline (C)	Association with congenital malformations. Neonatal withdrawal and urinary retention seen.	–	Drug and metabolites excreted in breast milk. Use may be of concern.
Ammonium chloride (B)	Three possible malformations reported. Acidoses in mother and fetus when taken near term.	+	No studies. Probably compatible.

(Continued)

Drug (FDA Fetal Risk Category)	Pregnancy-Adverse Events and Comments	Breast-Feeding Compatibility	Effect on Lactation and Adverse Effects on Infant
Amoxapine (C)	Studies too small to access risk.	−	Drug and its metabolites excreted in breast milk. Use may be of concern.
Amoxicillin (B)	No congenital defects, fetal or neonatal risk.	+	Excreted in breast milk. Observe infant for changes in bowel flora, allergies, and use caution in interpreting culture results.
Amphetamine (C)	Not teratogenic. Prematurity, IUGR, intrauterine death, and cerebral injuries seen.	CI	AAP: contraindicated.
Amphotericin B (B)	No adverse effects on fetus reported.	+	No human data; probably compatible.
Ampicillin (B)	Probably not teratogenic.	+	Drug excreted in breast milk. Observe infant for changes in bowel flora, allergies, and use caution in interpreting culture results. Monitor for diarrhea.
Aspartame (B; C if PKU)	Not a risk to fetus.	+	Use cautiously if mother or infant has PKU.
Aspirin (C; D if in 3rd trimester)	Risk in 1st, 3rd trimester. High 1st trimester dose: ↑perinatal mortality, teratogenicity, and IUGR. Risk of IC hemorrhage, DA closure, PPHN, ↓ in clotting. Acetaminophen preferred.	−	Excreted into breast milk. May affect platelet function.
Atenolol (D)	Monitor for symptoms of β-blockade for 48 hours after delivery. May cause IUGR and lower birthweight.	−	Excreted in breast milk. Monitor for signs of β-blockade.
Atracurium (C)	No adverse effects. Safe in the last part of pregnancy; studies have not been done in early pregnancy.	+	No studies. Probably compatible.
Atropine (C)	Parasympatholytics are associated with minor malformations.	+	AAP: compatible.
Azatadine (B)	No association found between the drug and birth defects.	+	No studies. Probably compatible.
Azathioprine (D)	Risk in human studies. Leukopenia and thrombocytopenia, immunosuppression, IUGR, transient chromosomal aberrations, and congenital defects reported.	−	Potential for toxicity with active metabolites.
Azithromycin (B)	Few human studies.	+	Few studies. Drug accumulates in breast milk. Probably compatible.
Aztreonam (B)	No studies. No adverse effects located.	+	Drug excreted into breast milk. AAP: compatible.
Bacampicillin (B)	No studies of fetal risk available.	+	Potential problems are changes in bowel flora and allergies. Use caution in interpreting culture results.
Bacitracin (C)	Not associated with congenital malformations.	+	No studies. Topical use compatible.
Baclofen (C)	Few human studies; No adverse effects located.	+	Few studies. AAP: compatible.

(*Continued*)

Drug (FDA Fetal Risk Category)	Pregnancy-Adverse Events and Comments	Breast-Feeding Compatibility	Effect on Lactation and Adverse Effects on Infant
Belladonna (C)	Risk of hypospadias, eye and ear malformations, and respiratory tract anomalies with 1st trimester use.	+	No studies. Probably compatible. See Atropine.
Benazepril (C 1st trimester; D 2nd, 3rd trimester)	Hypocalvaria, renal defects, IUGR, prematurity, and severe neonatal hypertension. Oligohydramnios causes limb contractures, persistent PDA, craniofacial deformation, pulmonary hypoplasia, and death.	+	No studies. Probably compatible.
Benztropine (C)	Possible association with minor malformations and cardiovascular defects. Paralytic ileus was seen.	+	No studies. Probably compatible.
Betamethasone (C; D if 1st trimester)	1st trimester use associated with orofacial clefts. Hypoglycemia, leukocytosis, adrenal suppression, LBW with decrease in head circumference, transient constriction of ductus arteriosus seen.	+	No studies. Drug likely excreted. Probably compatible.
Bethanechol (C)	No reports of fetal risk; studies limited.	–	Few studies. Drug likely excreted in breast milk. Abdominal pain and diarrhea reported in infant.
Bisacodyl (C)	No human studies. Bulk-forming laxatives preferred.	+	No studies. Drug likely excreted into breast milk.
Bismuth subsalicylate (C)	Use only in first half of pregnancy. See Aspirin.	–	Use with caution or avoid.
Bleomycin (D)	Human studies imply risk. Leukopenia with neutropenia, alopecia, and chromosomal aberrations seen.	–	No studies available. Potential toxicity; avoid.
Bretylium (C)	No studies. May cause maternal hypotension, with risk to fetus.	–	No studies. Avoid breast-feeding.
Bromocriptine (B)	Not a risk to the fetus.	CI	Suppresses lactation. AAP: use with caution.
Brompheniramine (C)	Increased risk of malformations if taken during 1st trimester. Risk of RLF in premature infant exposed to antihistamines last 2 weeks in utero.	+	AAP: compatible.
Buclizine (C)	Risk of fetal malformations. Risk of RLF in premature infant exposed to antihistamines during last 2 weeks in utero.	+	No studies. Probably compatible.
Budesonide (B for inhaled; C for oral)	Inhaled: not significant risk for congenital defects. Small risk between nasal budesonide and cardiac defects.	+	No studies. Drug likely excreted in breast milk. Manufacturer: don't breast-feed if using the Pulmicort Turbuhaler.
Butalbital (C; D if prolonged or high doses at term)	Few studies. No malformations seen. Observe for neonatal withdrawal.	–	No studies available.
Butorphanol (C; D if prolonged or high doses near term)	Risk in 3rd trimester. No fetal malformations reported; respiratory depression and withdrawal syndrome may occur.	+	Few studies. Probably compatible.
Caffeine (B)	Moderate consumption does not pose risk to fetus. Can see in infant: LBW, fine tremors, tachypnea, fetal sleep pattern and behavioral changes, PACs, and tachyarrhythmias.	+	Excreted into breast milk. Monitor for irritability and poor sleeping. No effect with moderate intake (2–3 cups/day).

(Continued)

Drug (FDA Fetal Risk Category)	Pregnancy-Adverse Events and Comments	Breast-Feeding Compatibility	Effect on Lactation and Adverse Effects on Infant
Calcitonin-salmon (C)	No congenital defects reported. Increase in calcitonin concentration in fetal serum.	+	No studies; drug not likely excreted. May inhibit lactation.
Calcitriol (C; D if doses above RDA)	Vitamin D analog. Can see mild transient hypercalcemia in infant.	+	High-dose in mothers lead to elevated levels of Vitamin D_2 in breast milk and hypercalcemia in breast-fed infants. Caution.
Captopril (C 1st trimester; D 2nd, 3rd trimester)	Hypocalvaria, renal defects, IUGR, prematurity, severe neonatal hypotension, limb contractures, pulmonary hypoplasia, intrauterine fetal death, and oligohydramnios can be seen. Monitor renal function and blood pressure in infant.	+	Drug is excreted in low amounts. AAP: compatible.
Carbachol ophthalmic medication (C)	No studies of fetal risk available.	+	No studies. Probably compatible.
Carbamazepine (D)	Associated with increase in malformations: cleft palate, CV defects, urinary tract defects, and NTDs. A fetal carbamazepine syndrome has been discussed. Vitamin K deficiency with hemorrhagic disease and transient cholestatic hepatitis has been seen.	+	Risk of bone marrow suppression if taken chronically.
Carbarsone (D)	Contains arsenic, which has been associated with CNS lesions. Avoid.	CI	Contraindicated. No studies available.
Carbenicillin (B)	No malformations seen.	+	No studies; drug likely excreted in low amounts. Observe infant for allergies, changes in bowel flora, and use caution in interpreting culture results.
Carbimazole (D)	May cause scalp defects and other congenital malformations.	+	New studies: no toxicity. AAP: compatible.
Casanthranol (C)	No reports of fetal anomalies.	+	Few studies. Probably compatible. Observe for diarrhea.
Cascara sagrada (C)	Higher risk for benign tumors but confirmation needed.	+	Few studies. Probably compatible. Observe for diarrhea.
Cefaclor (B)	Risk of congenital defects, but other factors may be involved.	+	Excreted into breast milk in low amounts. Observe infant for changes in bowel flora, allergies, and use caution in interpreting culture results. Compatible.
Cefadroxil (B)	No association with congenital defects.	+	Excreted into breast milk. Observe infant for changes in bowel flora, allergies, and use caution in interpreting culture results.
Cefamandole (B)	No teratogenic risk seen.	+	Excreted into breast milk in low amounts. Observe infant for changes in bowel flora, allergies, and use caution in interpreting culture results.
Cefatrizine (B)	No studies of fetal risk.	+	No reports of use.
Cefazolin (B)	No adverse effects seen.	+	Excreted into breast milk in low amounts. Observe infant for changes in bowel flora, allergies, and use caution in interpreting culture results.

(Continued)

Drug (FDA Fetal Risk Category)	Pregnancy-Adverse Events and Comments	Breast-Feeding Compatibility	Effect on Lactation and Adverse Effects on Infant
Cefonicid (B)	No studies in pregnancy.	+	Excreted into breast milk. Observe infant for changes in bowel flora, allergies, and use caution in interpreting culture results.
Cefoperazone (B)	No adverse newborn effects noted.	+	Excreted into breast milk. Observe infant for changes in bowel flora, allergies, and use caution in interpreting culture results.
Ceforanide (B)	No studies in pregnancy.	+	No studies. Drug likely excreted in breast milk. Observe infant for changes in bowel flora, allergies, and use caution in interpreting culture results.
Cefotaxime (B)	No teratogenic risk seen.	+	Excreted into breast milk. Observe infant for changes in bowel flora, allergies, and use caution in interpreting culture results.
Ceftazidime (B)	No reports of fetal risk.	+	Excreted into breast milk. Observe infant for changes in bowel flora, allergies, and use caution in interpreting culture results.
Ceftizomine (B)	No reports of fetal risk.	+	Excreted into breast milk. Observe infant for changes in bowel flora, allergies, and use caution in interpreting culture results.
Ceftriaxone (B)	Possible association with cardiovascular defects.	+	Excreted into breast milk. Observe infant for changes in bowel flora, allergies, and use caution in interpreting culture results.
Cefuroxime (B)	No adverse newborn effects noted.	+	Excreted into breast milk. Observe infant for changes in bowel flora, allergies, and use caution in interpreting culture results.
Cephalexin (B)	Risk of congenital defects, other factors may be involved.	+	Excreted into breast milk. Observe infant for changes in bowel flora, allergies, and use caution in interpreting culture results.
Cephalothin (B)	No adverse newborn effects noted.	+	Excreted into breast milk. Observe infant for changes in bowel flora, allergies, and use caution in interpreting culture results.
Cephapirin (B)	No studies available. Safe for use in pregnancy.	+	Excreted into breast milk. Observe intant for changes in bowel flora, allergies, and use caution in interpreting culture results.
Cephradine (B)	Risk of congenital defects, other factors may be involved.	+	Excreted into breast milk. Observe infant for changes in bowel flora, allergies, and use caution in interpreting culture results.
Chloral hydrate (C)	No adverse effects reported.	+	Excreted into breast milk. AAP: compatible. Observe infant for drowsiness.
Chlorambucil (D)	Contraindicated in 1st trimester. Unilateral agenesis of kidney and ureter and cardiovascular anomalies. May cause LBW.	CI	No studies. Avoid breast-feeding.

(Continued)

Drug (FDA Fetal Risk Category)	Pregnancy-Adverse Events and Comments	Breast-Feeding Compatibility	Effect on Lactation and Adverse Effects on Infant
Chloramphenicol (C)	Avoid at term because of risk for gray syndrome (cardiovascular collapse).	−	Excreted into breast milk. Risk of bone marrow depression. Observe infant for changes in bowel flora and use caution in interpreting culture results. AAP: effect unknown but of concern. Observe for vomiting after feeding, intestinal gas, refusing to breast-feed, and falling asleep at the breast.
Chlordiazepoxide (D)	At term, neonatal depression with hypotonia up to 1 week reported. Neonatal withdrawal syndrome.	−	No studies. Drug likely excreted into breast milk. Avoid
Chlorhexidine (B)	No adverse effects in the newborn have been reported.	+	Unknown excretion. Rinse nipples if used.
Chloroquine (C)	There may be a small increased risk of birth defects in human studies.	+	Drug excreted into breast milk. AAP: compatible.
Chlorothiazide (C; D if used in gestational hypertension)	1st trimester: risk of congenital defects in mothers with CV disorders. May cause hypoglycemia, hyponatremia, thrombocytopenia, hypokalemia, hemolytic anemia, and death. Monitor infant's electrolytes, platelet count, and serum glucose after birth.	+	Monitor infant electrolytes and platelets.
Chlorpromazine (C)	Avoid use near term. Paralytic ileus, extrapyramidal syndrome, neonatal hypotonia, lethargy, and jaundice seen.	−	Excreted into breast milk. Observe infants for sedation. APP: effect unknown but of concern.
Chlorpheniramine (B)	Possible association with fetal malformations reported. Increased risk of RLF in premature infant exposed to antihistamines during last 2 weeks in utero.	+	No studies available.
Chlorpropamide (C)	Causes symptomatic hypoglycemia. Monitor infant's serum glucose for 5 days after birth. Can see hyperbilirubinemia, polycythemia, and hyperviscosity.	−	Excreted in breast milk; may cause hypoglycemia.
Chlortetracycline (D)	Avoid because they may cause yellow staining of teeth, inhibition of bone growth, maternal liver toxicity, and congenital defects.	+	Excreted in low amounts. Observe infant for changes in bowel flora, allergies, and use caution in interpreting culture results.
Chlorthalidone (B; D if gestational hypertension)	Risk for congenital malformations. May cause hypoglycemia, thrombocytopenia, hyponatremia, hypokalemia, and death. Monitor infant's electrolytes, platelet count, and glucose.	+	May suppress lactation. Adverse effects not reported. Monitor infant's electrolytes and platelets.
Cholecalciferol (C/D if used in doses above RDA)	May be associated with supravalvular aortic stenosis syndrome which is associated with hypercalcemia of infancy.	+	Drug excreted in small amounts. Monitor calcium levels of infant if mother taking pharmacologic doses of vitamin D.
Cholestyramine (B)	Not systemically absorbed but may cause vitamin deficiency in fetus.	+	No studies. Long-term use: vitamin deficiency in the mother and infant.
Ciclopirox (B)	No studies. No adverse effects.	+	No studies. Exposure to infants negligible.

(Continued)

Drug (FDA Fetal Risk Category)	Pregnancy-Adverse Events and Comments	Breast-Feeding Compatibility	Effect on Lactation and Adverse Effects on Infant
Cimetidine (B)	No increased risks of congenital malformations. Has antiandrogenic effects.	+	Use with caution. May suppress gastric acidity and cause CNS stimulation. AAP: compatible.
Ciprofloxacin (C)	Questionable association with congenital anomalies. Use with caution in 1st trimester.	+	Few studies. Drug likely excreted in breast milk. AAP: compatible. Manufacturer: wait 48 hours after last dose before feeding.
Cisplatin (D)	Few studies. Leukopenia with neutropenia seen.	CI	Excreted in breast milk; breast feeding contraindicated.
Clindamycin (B)	No adverse effects.	+	Excreted in breast milk. Observe infant for changes in bowel flora, allergies, and use caution in interpreting culture results. AAP: compatible.
Clofibrate (C)	No human studies. No adverse effects. Avoid near term, especially premie because of limited capacity for glucuronidation of this med.	−	No studies. Drug likely excreted in breast milk. Avoid breast-feeding because of risks.
Clomiphene (X)	May cause neural tube defects and other fetal malformations.	−	No studies. May reduce lactation.
Clonazepam (D)	Risk of fetal and neonatal toxicity. Avoid in 1st trimester. May cause apnea and paralytic ileus of the small bowel.	−	Excreted in breast milk. Test serum levels in infant and monitor for apnea, respiratory and CNS depression.
Clonidine (C)	Few human studies; cannot define risk.	+	Excreted in breast milk. Long term follow-up unknown.
Clorazepate (D)	Congenital malformations associated with in utero exposure to other benzodiazepines.	−	No studies. Drug likely excreted in breast milk. AAP: effects unknown but of concern. Observe for sedation and drowsiness.
Clotrimazole (B)	Questionable association with a decrease in the prevalence of undescended testis.	+	Minimal absorption, unlikely levels of this antifungal agent in breast milk.
Cloxacillin (B)	Possible association with cardiovascular defect.	+	No studies. Drug likely excreted into breast milk. Observe infant for allergies, changes in bowel flora, and use caution in interpreting culture results.
Cocaine (C/X if nonmedicinal use)	Major toxicity: withdrawal, SIDS, neurophysiologic and multisystem abnormalities (see ✿).	CI	Cocaine intoxication in infant from maternal intranasal use (hypertension, tachycardia, mydriasis, and apnea) and topical use on mother's nipples (apnea and seizures).
Codeine (C/D if prolonged or high doses near term)	If addicted or high doses in 2nd or 3rd trimester or at delivery, toxicity can occur. Respiratory depression and withdrawal syndrome can be seen.	−	Short-term therapy ok with close monitoring in healthy full-term. Long-term therapy not compatible with breast-feeding. Observe infant for sedation, lethargy, and poor feeding. AAP: compatible.
Colchicine (D)	Few studies but no malformations. Questionable association of Down syndrome and colchicine. Can cause azoospermia. Use with caution.	+	Excreted into breast milk. No adverse effects. Wait 8 to 12 hours after dose.
Colistimethate (C)	No adverse effects reported.	+	Drug excreted in low amounts. Observe infant for changes in bowel flora, allergies, and use caution in interpreting culture results.

(Continued)

Drug (FDA Fetal Risk Category)	Pregnancy-Adverse Events and Comments	Breast-Feeding Compatibility	Effect on Lactation and Adverse Effects on Infant
Corticotropin (C)	No adverse effects. Corticosteroids may cause congenital malformations.	+	No studies available. Probably compatible.
Cortisone (C/D if 1st trimester)	Human studies: increase in cleft lip with or without palate, decrease in birthweight, and questionable association with cataracts.	+	Unknown excretion.
Cromolyn sodium (B)	No associations between the medication and congenital defects.	+	No studies.
Cyclacillin (B)	No malformations seen.	+	No studies; drug likely excreted in breast milk. Observe infant for allergies, changes in bowel flora, and use caution in interpreting culture results.
Cyclamate (C)	Causes cytogenetic effects in lymphocytes. No association between these effects and congenital malformations.	+	No studies available.
Cyclizine (B)	Risk of RLF in premature infants exposed to antihistamines during last 2 weeks in utero.	+	No studies available.
Cyclophosphamide (D)	Fetal malformations from 1st-trimester exposure: pancytopenia, leukopenia, IUGR, anemia, bone marrow hypoplasia, LBWs, stillbirth, and neonatal death. Use by father before conception: malformations in infant.	CI	Risk relating to immune suppression, growth, and carcinogenesis. May cause neutropenia and thrombocytopenia. AAP: drug may interfere with cellular metabolism.
Cycloserine (C)	Few studies. No adverse fetal effects. Use with caution.	+	Excreted into breast milk. No risks.
Cyclosporine (C)	Few studies. Thrombocytopenia, leukopenia, DIC, hypoglycemia, and IUGR have been seen in infants.	−	Excreted into breast milk. Possible immune suppression; unknown effect on growth or association with carcinogenesis. AAP: a drug that could interfere with cellular metabolism.
Cyproheptadine (B)	Few studies. Questionable association with oral clefts and hypospadias.	+	No studies. Increase in sensitivity of infants to antihistamines. Monitor for agitation, poor sleeping pattern, and feeding problems.
Cytarabine (D)	May cause chromosomal abnormalities and congenital anomalies with maternal or paternal use before conception. Pancytopenia, LBW, chromosomal aberrations, and intrauterine fetal death.	CI	No studies. Contraindicated because of risks.
Dacarbazine (C)	No studies.	−	No studies. Risk of toxicity: hemopoietic depression.
Dactinomycin (C)	Few studies. LBW and stillbirth have been reported.	−	No studies. Risk of toxicity to infants.
Dalteparin (B)	Less risk than from standard unfractionated heparin or no therapy.	+	No studies. Drug not likely excreted in breast milk. Risk negligible.
Danazol (X)	May cause virilization with disorder of sex development of female infants and female pseudohermaphroditism.	CI	No studies. Avoid breast feeding.
Dantrolene (C)	Few studies. No fetal or newborn effects when used before delivery.	−	Excreted into breast milk. Wait 2 days after last dose.
Dapsone (C)	Not a major risk. Hemolytic anemia and hyperbilirubinemia seen in an infant.	−	Excreted in breast milk. May cause hemolytic anemia in G6PD deficiency.

(Continued)

Drug (FDA Fetal Risk Category)	Pregnancy-Adverse Events and Comments	Breast-Feeding Compatibility	Effect on Lactation and Adverse Effects on Infant
Deferoxamine (C)	Few studies: no adverse effects. May cause low iron levels, requiring iron in infants.	+	No studies. Drug likely excreted; effects unknown.
Demeclocycline (D)	Contraindicated in 2nd and 3rd trimester. Avoid because they may cause yellow staining of teeth, inhibition of bone growth, maternal liver toxicity, and congenital defects.	+	Excreted in low amounts. Remote possibility of dental staining and inhibition of bone growth. Observe infant for changes in bowel flora, allergies, and use caution in interpreting culture results.
Desipramine (C)	No malformations. Withdrawal syndrome reported.	−	Drug excreted; effects unknown but of concern.
Desmopressin (B)	No adverse effects reported.	+	Compatible.
Dexamethasone (C/D if 1st trimester)	Association with nonsyndromic orofacial clefts. Benefits: decrease in incidence and severity of RDS, decrease in incidence and mortality from intracranial hemorrhage, and increased survival of premature infants. Given to stimulate fetal lung maturation.	+	No studies. Drug likely excreted in breast milk.
Dextroamphetamine (C)	Risk in human studies. Withdrawal can occur. Illicit use: risk of IUGR, premature birth, increase in morbidity.	−	Amphetamine concentrated in breast milk. No adverse effects seen. AAP: compatible.
Dextromethorphan (C)	Not a major teratogen.	+	No studies. Drug likely excreted. Probably compatible. Use alcohol-free preparation.
Diatrizoate (D)	May suppress fetal thyroid function when given intra-amniotic. Monitor for hypothyroidism.	+	Probably compatible.
Diazepam (D)	Risk low for congenital malformations. May cause floppy infant syndrome and withdrawal. Decreased fetal movements and loss of beat-to-beat variability.	−	May cause infant sedation and weight loss. May accumulate in infants. AAP: effects unknown but of concern. Not recommended.
Diazoxide (C)	Risk in 3rd trimester. Can cause maternal hypotension. May cause transient fetal bradycardia and hyperglycemia. Alopecia, hypertrichosis lanuginosa, and a decrease in ossification of the wrist can be seen if used in the last 19–69 days of pregnancy. Use with caution or not at all.	−	No studies.
Diclofenac (B; D if 3rd trimester or near delivery)	May close ductus arteriosus in utero, cause PPHN, inhibition of labor, and spontaneous abortion. NSAIDs: congenital malformations.	+	No studies. Drug likely excreted in breast milk. AAP: other NSAIDs compatible.
Dicloxacillin (B)	No congenital malformations seen.	+	No studies. Observe infant for allergies, changes in bowel flora, and use caution in interpreting culture results.
Didanosine (B)	Increased risk of congenital malformations seen with 1st-trimester use.	CI	No studies. Drug likely excreted in breast milk. Effects unknown. CDC recommends HIV-infected mothers in developed countries should not breast-feed.

(Continued)

Drug (FDA Fetal Risk Category)	Pregnancy-Adverse Events and Comments	Breast-Feeding Compatibility	Effect on Lactation and Adverse Effects on Infant
Dienestrol (X)	Increase in cardiovascular defects, eye and ear anomalies, and Down syndrome. Contraindicated.	+	No adverse effects. Possible decrease in nitrogen and protein content and milk volume.
Diethylstilbestrol (DES) (X)	Complications of reproductive system of female: carcinoma of cervix and vagina. Complications of the reproductive system and GU abnormalities, including neoplasms, in male. An increase in psychiatric illness (depression and anxiety) was seen in both males and females.	CI	No studies. Possible decreased milk volume and decreased nitrogen and protein content.
Digoxin (C)	No defects reported. Neonatal death from maternal overdose of digitoxin.	+	Excreted in small amounts.
Dihydrotachysterol (A/D if above the RDA)	May be associated with supravalvular aortic stenosis syndrome, which is associated with hypercalcemia of infancy.	+	Monitor for increased calcium levels if mother taking pharmacologic doses.
Diltiazem (C)	Few studies. Questionable association with CV defects. No increase in major congenital malformations.	+	Excreted into breast milk. Probably compatible.
Dimenhydrinate (B)	Questionable association with CV defects and inguinal hernia. No association with fetal malformations. Risk of RLF in infant exposed to antihistamines during last 2 weeks in utero.	+	No studies. Drug likely excreted in breast milk. Caution: infants have increased sensitivity to antihistamines.
Diphenhydramine (B)	May cause cleft palate and withdrawal. Risk of RLF in premature infant exposed to antihistamines during last 2 weeks. Avoid with temazepam.	+	Excreted in breast milk. Manufacturer: contraindicated because of increase in sensitivity of newborns to antihistamines.
Diphenoxylate (C)	No congenital abnormalities. No association between congenital defects and med.	−	Active metabolite likely excreted in breast milk. Potential toxicity. AAP considers atropine as compatible.
Dipyridamole (B)	Few studies. No congenital defects. Decrease in the incidence of stillbirth, IUGR, placental infarction.	+	Excreted into breast milk; effect unknown. Probably compatible.
Disopyramide (C)	Risk in 3rd trimester. No congenital abnormalities.	+	Excreted into breast milk. No adverse effects.
Disulfiram (C)	Not a major teratogen. No alcohol while on this drug.	−	No studies. Drug likely excreted into breast milk. Effects unknown.
Dobutamine (B)	Few studies.	+	No studies available. Probably compatible.
Docusate (calcium, potassium, sodium) (C)	No congenital malformations. Possible hypomagnesemia with use.	+	Probably compatible. Monitor nursing infant for diarrhea.
Dopamine (C)	Few studies: no adverse risks.	+	No studies. Probably compatible.
Doxepin	No congenital malformations. Questionable association with polydactyly. One study showed IQ (significantly) and language was negatively associated with the number of depression episodes after delivery.	−	Drug excreted into breast milk. Adverse effects: drowsiness, shallow respirations, hypotonia, poor suckling and swallowing, vomiting, and hyperbilirubinemia. Avoid breast-feeding. AAP: effect unknown but of concern.

(Continued)

Drug (FDA Fetal Risk Category)	Pregnancy-Adverse Events and Comments	Breast-Feeding Compatibility	Effect on Lactation and Adverse Effects on Infant
Doxorubicin (D)	Contraindicated in 1st trimester. Fetal malformations have been reported.	CI	Concentrated in milk. May cause immune suppression. AAP: drug may interfere with cellular metabolism of the infant.
Doxycycline (D)	Contraindicated in 2nd and 3rd trimester. During pregnancy may cause: yellow staining of teeth, inhibition of bone growth, maternal liver toxicity, and congenital defects.	+	Excreted into breast milk in low concentrations. Theoretical dental staining and inhibition of bone growth is remote. Observe infant for changes in bowel flora, allergies, and use caution in interpreting culture results with sepsis evaluation. AAP: compatible.
Doxylamine (A)	Probably safe. Increase in congenital malformations but not secondary to medication.	+	No studies. Drug likely excreted in breast milk. Effects unknown. Monitor for sedation and other antihistamine actions.
Droperidol (C)	Few human studies: low risk.	−	No studies. Drug likely excreted; effects unknown.
Echinacea (C)	Safety needs to be established.	−	Avoid use.
Edrophonium (C)	No congenital malformations. Transient muscular weakness seen in 20% of newborns whose mothers have myasthenia gravis.	+	No studies. Nonionized drug fraction may be excreted. Effects unknown.
Enalapril (C 1st trimester; D 2nd, 3rd trimester)	Risk in 2nd and 3rd trimester. Teratogenic: renal defects and hypocalvaria. IUGR, fetal hypotension, limb contractures, anuria oligohydramnios, and death. Monitor renal function and blood pressure in the newborn.	+	Drug excreted in small amounts. AAP: compatible.
Encainide (B)	Few human studies. Maternal benefit exceeds fetal risk.	+	Drug excreted in breast milk. Effects unknown. Probably compatible.
Enoxaparin (B)	Because of relatively high molecular weight, not expected to cross placenta.	+	No studies. Drug unlikely excreted in breast milk. Risk insignificant.
Ephedrine (C)	Minor fetal malformations may be associated with use during 1st trimester. Fetal tachycardia and increase in beat-to-beat variability.	−	Few studies. Observe infant for irritability, excessive crying, and disturbed sleeping patterns. Avoid breast-feeding.
Epinephrine (C)	1st trimester use: fetal malformations. Use any time: inguinal hernia. May cause decreased uterine blood flow.	−	No studies available.
Epoetin alfa (C)	No major risk to fetus. Thrombosis is a complication for mother.	+	No studies; excretion unlikely. No risk expected.
Epoprostenol (B)	Few human studies. Benefits outweigh potential risks to fetus.	+	No studies. Amount in breast milk probably insignificant.
Ergotamine (X)	Larger or more frequent doses: fetal toxicity and teratogenicity. Use during 1st trimester: increase in major birth defects. May cause intrauterine fetal death. Can cause fetal distress.	CI	Vomiting, diarrhea, and convulsions. May hinder lactation. AAP: use with caution.
Erythromycin (B)	No reports of malformations. Avoid estolate salt: can induce hepatotoxicity in pregnant patients.	+	Excreted in low amounts. No adverse effects. Observe infant for changes in bowel flora, allergies, and use caution in interpreting culture results.
Esmolol (C)	May decrease uterine blood flow: fetal hypoxia. Bradycardia, hypoglycemia, poor feeding, and hypotonia may occur. β-blockade in infant.	+	No studies. Unlikely breast feeding would occur.

(Continued)

Drug (FDA Fetal Risk Category)	Pregnancy-Adverse Events and Comments	Breast-Feeding Compatibility	Effect on Lactation and Adverse Effects on Infant
Estradiol (X)	Contraindicated. In utero exposure: developmental changes in psychosexual performance of boys, less heterosexual experience, and fewer masculine interests.	+	Less than 10% of vaginal dose (50 or 100 mg) in breast milk. AAP: compatible.
Estrogens, conjugated (X)	Contraindicated. Fetal malformations (increase in Down syndrome, CV defects, and eye and ear abnormalities).	+	No adverse effects. May decrease milk volume, nitrogen, and protein content.
Ethacrynic acid (B; D if used in gestational hypertension)	Decrease in placental perfusion and ototoxicity in mother and newborn. Not recommended.	+	No studies. Manufacturer: do not breast feed.
Ethambutol	No abnormalities. Concern: long-term ocular damage.	+	Excreted into breast milk. AAP: compatible.
Ethosuximide (C)	May cause congenital anomalies.	+	Drug excreted; no effects seen. AAP: compatible.
Famotidine (B)	Few studies. No adverse effects.	+	Drug excreted; effects unknown. Potential risk; however AAP: compatible with breast-feeding.
Felodipine (C)	Limited studies. No increase in congenital malformations in 1st trimester.	+	No studies. Drug likely excreted.
Fenoprofen (B/D if used in 3rd trimester or near delivery)	Risk in 1st and 3rd trimester. NSAIDs: congenital malformations. Constriction of ductus arteriosus in utero, PPHN, and inhibition of labor.	+	Drug excreted in small amounts; effects unknown.
Fentanyl (C; D if used for long term or at high doses near term)	Risk in 3rd trimester. No malformations. Respiratory depression and withdrawal syndrome.	+	Drug excreted in low concentrations. AAP: compatible.
Ferrous sulfate (A)	No adverse effects.	+	Compatible. With supplementation, ~0.25 mg/day excreted into breast milk.
Flecainide (C)	No congenital defects. May cause hyperbilirubinemia. Loss of fetal heart rate variability and accelerations.	+	Drug excreted; effects unknown. AAP: compatible.
Fluconazole (C)	Few studies. Continuous 1st-trimester doses of 400 mg/day or more may be teratogenic. Low doses safe.	+	Excreted into breast milk; no toxicity reported. AAP: compatible.
Flucytosine (C)	Contraindicated in 1st trimester. No defects but fluorouracil may produce fetal malformations.	−	No studies. Avoid, potential risks.
Fluorouracil (D/X according to manufacturer)	Avoid in 1st trimester: fetal malformations. 3rd trimester: cyanosis and jerking and LBW (any time).	CI	No studies. Drug excreted in breast milk. Contraindicated because of risk.
Fluoxetine (C; D if 2nd half of pregnancy)	Human studies show it is not a major teratogen, but minor anomalies were seen. SSRI: LBW, prematurity, withdrawal, respiratory distress, PPHN, neonatal serotonin syndrome, possible abnormal neurobehavior later on.	−	Long-term studies not done. Manufacturer: do not breast-feed. AAP: effects unknown but of concern. Maternal benefits may outweigh risks to nursing infant. Reduced weight gain seen.

(Continued)

Drug (FDA Fetal Risk Category)	Pregnancy-Adverse Events and Comments	Breast-Feeding Compatibility	Effect on Lactation and Adverse Effects on Infant
Fluphenazine (C)	Risk in 3rd trimester. Upper respiratory distress and rhinorrhea, difficulty feeding and vomiting, choreoathetoid movements, and arching of the body.	−	No studies. Drug likely excreted in breast milk. AAP: effects unknown but of concern.
Flurazepam (X)	Sleepiness, drowsiness, and lethargy if given before delivery. No congenital anomalies reported.	−	No studies. Drug likely excreted in breast milk. AAP: effects are unknown but of concern.
Folic acid (A/C if above RDA)	Folate deficiency: fetal anomalies (neural tube defects most common), abortions, placenta previa, LBW, premature delivery, placental abruption.	+	Excreted into breast milk. No adverse effects.
Foscarnet (C)	Observe for fetal renal toxicity by monitoring amniotic fluid volume.	CI	No studies. Drug likely excreted in breast milk. Contraindicated because of risk.
Furazolidone (C)	No congenital defects. Hemolytic anemia in G6PD-deficient infant if given at term.	−	No studies available.
Furosemide (C; D if used in gestational hypertension)	Questionable association with hypospadias.	+	Excreted into breast milk. No adverse effects.
Gabapentin (C)	Few studies. Possible developmental toxicity. Jaundice and intermittent tremors in infant.	+	No studies. Drug likely excreted in breast milk but effect unknown.
Ganciclovir (C)	Potential for fetal toxicity.	−	No studies. Potential risks. Avoid.
Gentamicin (C)	Potentiation of magnesium sulfate–induced neuromuscular weakness. Monitor infant for ototoxicity.	+	Drug is excreted in small amount. Observe for bloody stools and diarrhea. AAP: compatible.
Ginkgo biloba (C)	No studies. Best to avoid.	−	No studies. May contain other compounds. Safest course is to avoid.
Glyburide	Hypoglycemia, hyperbilirubinemia, and polycythemia seen in infants.	+	Nondetectable levels in breast milk. Glucose levels normal. Probably compatible.
Glycopyrrolate (B)	Questionable association with minor fetal malformations.	+	No studies. Probably compatible. See Atropine.
Gold sodium thiomalate (C)	Few studies. Long-term follow-up required.	+	Gold excreted and absorbed into breast milk. Possible risk. Some don't recommend breast-feeding. AAP: compatible.
Griseofulvin (C)	Few studies. Medication is tumorigenic, embryotoxic, and teratogenic in animals. Possible association with conjoined twins.	−	No studies. Potential of tumorigenicity and toxicity. Avoid.
Guaifenesin (C)	Compatible. Questionable increase in inguinal hernias.	+	No studies. Probably compatible.
Haloperidol (C)	Avoid in 1st trimester. Limb defects seen. Tardive dyskinesia if exposure during pregnancy.	−	Excreted into breast milk; effect unknown. Use of concern. Decrease in psychomotor and mental development.
Heparin (C)	Possible association with CV defects and other malformations.	+	Not excreted in breast milk.
Hepatitis A vaccine (C)	Inactivated vaccine, compatible.	+	No studies. Probably compatible.
Hepatitis B vaccine (C)	No adverse effects; use after 1st trimester.	+	No studies. Probably compatible.

(Continued)

Drug (FDA Fetal Risk Category)	Pregnancy-Adverse Events and Comments	Breast-Feeding Compatibility	Effect on Lactation and Adverse Effects on Infant
Heroin (B/D if prolonged therapy or high doses near term)	Risk in 3rd trimester. May cause: congenital malformations, jaundice, RDS, low Apgar scores, withdrawal, LBW, and increased perinatal mortality. Long-term effects: lower height and weight, impaired organizational, perceptual, and behavioral abilities.	CI	Excreated in breast milk and causes addition in infant.
Human papillomavirus vaccine (B)	Limited studies, no toxicity reported. ACOG states to avoid in pregnancy.	+	Infants had more acute respiratory illnesses in the mothers who had the vaccine within 30 days.
Hydralazine (C)	Risk in 3rd trimester. No congenital abnormalities. Bleeding, thrombocytopenia, fetal distress, fetal premature atrial contractions, lupuslike syndrome in newborn.	+	Excreted into breast milk. No adverse effects. AAP: compatible.
Hydrochlorothiazide (B)	Not teratogenic. May cause hypoglycemia, thrombocytopenia, hyponatremia, hypokalemia, and death. Monitor infant's electrolytes, platelet count, and serum glucose.	+	May suppress lactation. Thrombocytopenia may occur. AAP: compatible.
Hydrocodone (C/D if prolonged or high doses near term)	Possible association with congenital malformations seen in 1st trimester. Respiratory depression or withdrawal syndrome.	+	No studies. Drug likely excreted in breast milk. Observe infant for GI problems, sedation, and changes in feeding.
Hydromorphone (B/D if prolonged therapy or high doses near delivery)	No malformations. Withdrawal and respiratory depression can occur.	+	Excreted into breast milk. Effects unknown.
Hydroxychloroquine (C)	Lower doses: not significant fetal risk. Higher doses: unknown fetal risk.	+	Excreted in small amounts. Breast-feeding with caution. Once-weekly doses reduced drug exposure. AAP: compatible.
Hydroxyzine (C)	Studies reveal low risk. Decrease in platelet aggregation and fetal heart rate variability. Near term: withdrawal and seizures can occur.	+	No studies. Drug likely excreted; effects unknown.
Hyperalimentation, parenteral (C)	Try to prevent maternal complications.	+	Compatible.
Ibuprofen (B; D if 3rd trimester or near delivery)	May cause closing of ductus arteriosus in utero, PPHN, oligohydramnios. NSAIDs: oral clefts, gastroschisis, and cardiac defects.	+	Excreted in minimal amounts. AAP: compatible.
Imipramine (C)	Fetal malformations, withdrawal syndrome, and urinary retention.	−	Excreted into breast milk; effects unknown but may be of concern.
Immune globulin (C) (intramuscular or intravenous)	No adverse effects.	+	No studies. Probably compatible.
Indomethacin (B/D if used for greater than 48 hours or after 34 weeks' gestation)	Risk in 1st and 3rd trimester. Delayed labor, premature closure of ductus arteriosus, PPHN, decrease in fetal urine output, unilateral pleural effusion, periventricular leukomalacia, IVH, impaired renal function, renal failure, intestinal perforation, and death. NSAIDs: congenital malformations.	+	Excreted into breast milk. AAP: compatible.

(Continued)

Drug (FDA Fetal Risk Category)	Pregnancy-Adverse Events and Comments	Breast-Feeding Compatibility	Effect on Lactation and Adverse Effects on Infant
Insulin, regular (B)	Poorly controlled diabetes: increased risk of congenital defects and fetal macrosomia.	+	Digested in infant's GI tract.
Interferon-Alfa (all types) (C)	Limited studies. Use with caution.	+	Drug excreted in small amounts. AAP: compatible.
Iodine (D)	Risk in 2nd and 3rd trimester. Transient hypothyroidism, goiter, and cardiomegaly can be seen in infant.	+	AAP: compatible; may affect thyroid activity of infant.
Isoetharine (C)	Use in 1st trimester: possible risk of minor malformations, inguinal hernia, and clubfoot.	+	No studies. Probably compatible.
Isoniazid (C)	Not teratogenic. Hemorrhagic disease of the newborn seen.	+	Drug excreted into breast milk. Observe for peripheral neuritis or hepatitis. AAP: compatible.
Isoproterenol (C)	Use in 1st trimester: possible risk of minor fetal malformations.	+	No studies available.
Isosorbide dinitrate/mononitrate (C)	No studies available.	+	No studies available.
Isotretinoin (X)	With 1st-trimester use: severe birth defects. Use contraception 1 month before, during, and 1 month after.	−	Unknown excretion. Risk of toxicity.
Itraconazole (C)	Studies do not show a significant risk of major anomalies. Safest course is to avoid in 1st trimester.	−	Excreted in breast milk. Potential effects not studied. Can accumulate in tissues. Avoid breast-feeding.
Kanamycin (D)	Eighth cranial nerve damage. Ototoxicity and hearing loss with deafness can occur.	+	Low concentrations in breast milk. Observe infant for changes in bowel flora, allergies, and use caution in interpreting culture results.
Ketoconazole (C)	Questionable risk of limb malformations with oral med. Compatible with topical.	+	Excreted in breast milk; effects unknown. AAP: compatible.
Labetalol (C)	In 1st trimester: association with malformations. If near delivery: hypotension and bradycardia. Monitor infant for 48 hours after birth. IUGR.	+	Monitor for hypotension and bradycardia.
Lactulose (B)	No information available.	+	No studies. Probably compatible.
Lamotrigine (C)	Risk in humans. In 1st trimester, risk of oral clefts. If taken with valproate, increase in major defects.	−	May be of concern. Monitor infant's serum lamotrigine concentration. Observe for adverse effects.
Levofloxacin (C)	Avoid in pregnancy (especially 1st trimester): risk of arthropathy and cartilage damage.	+	Excreted into breast milk. Effects unknown. AAP: other fluoroquinolones compatible.
Levorphanol (C; D if prolonged periods or high doses at term)	No congenital anomalies. Risk in 3rd trimester. Respiratory depression and withdrawal syndrome.	+	No studies. Drug likely excreted in breast milk. Long-term effects need to be studied.
Levothyroxine (A)	1st-trimester use: cardiovascular anomalies, Down syndrome, and polydactyly. Maternal hypothyroidism: LBW and lower neuropsychological development of infants.	+	Compatible; does not interfere with neonatal thyroid screening.
Lidocaine (B)	Tachycardia, bradycardia, low Apgar. Lower scores on tone and muscle strength. In 1st trimester: risk of respiratory tract anomalies, tumors, and inguinal hernias.	+	Drug excreted in small amounts. Low risk to infant. AAP: compatible.

(Continued)

Drug (FDA Fetal Risk Category)	Pregnancy-Adverse Events and Comments	Breast-Feeding Compatibility	Effect on Lactation and Adverse Effects on Infant
Lindane (B)	Limited studies. Neurotoxicity, seizures, and aplastic anemia, possible hypospadias.	+	No studies. Drug likely excreted into breast milk. Abstain for 4 days after discontinuing drug.
Liothyronine (A)	No adverse effects. Maternal hypothyroidism: LBW and lower neuropsychological development.	+	Does not affect thyroid screening programs.
Lisinopril (C 1st trimester; D 2nd, 3rd trimester)	Risk in 2nd or 3rd trimester. Discontinue use. ACE inhibitors: malformations, fetal death. Chronic renal failure, IUGR, fetal distress, hypocalvaria, and renal insufficiency.	+	No studies. Drug likely excreted in breast milk. AAP: compatible.
Lithium (D)	Cardiac defects when used in 1st trimester and toxicity in newborn when used near term.	–	Milk levels average 40% of maternal levels. AAP: use with caution. Monitor for cyanosis, hypotonia, and bradycardia, monitor blood levels in infant.
Liotrix (A)	No adverse effects.	+	Compatible.
Loperamide (B)	Limited studies. Association with cardiovascular defects and lower birth weights.	+	No studies. AAP: compatible.
Loratadine (B)	Not a major teratogen. Loratadine OK if not in the 1st trimester.	+	Drug excreted in breast milk. Risk low. AAP: compatible.
Lorazepam (D)	Risk in 1st and 3rd trimester. Neonatal respiratory depression and hypotonia.	–	Unknown but of concern if exposure prolonged.
Losartan (C 1st trimester; D 2nd, 3rd trimester)	Risk in 2nd and 3rd trimester. Monitor newborn's BP and renal function. Avoid use: IUGR, oligohydramnios, PDA, hypocalvaria, anuria of the newborn, limb contractures, and stillbirth.	+	No studies. Drug likely excreted. Effects unknown. AAP: compatible.
Lovastatin (X)	Malformations seen. Avoid use.	CI	Contraindicated: risk of toxicity.
Magnesium sulfate (B)	Neonatal respiratory depression, loss of reflexes, and muscle weakness, fetal hypocalcemia with congenital rickets, hypotonia, and a decrease in GI motility. Observe infants during the first 24–48 hours.	+	AAP: compatible.
Mannitol (C)	No adverse effects.	+	No studies. Probably compatible.
Maprotiline (B)	May cause oral cleft. Limited studies.	–	Excreted in low amount. Clinical significance unknown.
Measles vaccine (X by manufacturer and ACOG)	Contraindicated. Avoid pregnancy after vaccine (30 days to 3 months).	+	Compatible with breast-feeding.
Mechlorethamine (D)	Contraindicated in 1st-trimester use. Fetal malformations with 1st-trimester use and LBW with use any time.	CI	No studies. Drug likely excreted in breast milk. Risks for toxicity; breast-feeding contraindicated.
Meclizine (B)	Possible fetal malformations. Association with ocular malformations. Risk of RLF in premature infant exposed to antihistamines during last 2 weeks.	+	No human lactation studies. Drug likely excreted into breast milk. Probably compatible. Caution: newborns and premature infants have increased sensitivity to antihistamines.
Meclofenamate (B/D if used in 3rd trimester or near delivery.)	Risk in 1st and 3rd trimester. Delayed labor, premature closure of ductus arteriosus, and PPHN. NSAIDs: congenital malformations.	+	No studies. Drug likely excreted into breast milk; effects unknown. AAP: NSAIDs compatible with breast-feeding.

(Continued)

Drug (FDA Fetal Risk Category)	Pregnancy-Adverse Events and Comments	Breast-Feeding Compatibility	Effect on Lactation and Adverse Effects on Infant
Medroxyprogesterone (X)	Not recommended: risk of fetal malformations. Growth retardation within 4 weeks of conception.	+	AAP: compatible.
Melphalan (D)	May cause IUGR. Contraindicated in 1st trimester.	CI	No studies. Drug likely excreted. Risk of toxicity in infant.
Meperidine (B/D if prolonged treatment or high doses near term)	Respiratory depression and withdrawal. EEG changes in the neonate, transient decrease in oxygenation.	+	Excreted in breast milk. No effects seen. AAP: compatible.
Mephobarbital (D)	May cause withdrawal and hemorrhagic disease of newborn. With 1st-trimester exposure: cardiac defects and cleft lip/palate.	–	Monitor for sedation and withdrawal. Use caution. (See Phenobarbital).
Mercaptopurine (D)	Risk in 3rd trimester. Fetal malformations, pancytopenia, LBW, IUGR, myelosuppression, and hemolytic anemia seen in infants.	–	No studies. Drug likely excreted. Risk for toxicity. Avoid breast-feeding.
Meropenem (B)	Safe for use 28 weeks' gestation or later. Use before 28 weeks unknown.	+	No studies. Drug likely excreted, effects unknown.
Mesalamine (B)	Maternal benefits appear to outweigh risks to fetus.	–	Drug excreted in small amount. Risk of adverse effects (allergic reaction and diarrhea) in nursing infant. AAP: use with caution.
Mesoridazine (C)	Unknown. Questionable association with congenital malformations.	–	Excreted in breast milk. AAP: effect on infant unknown but of concern.
Metaproterenol (C)	Possibly polydactyly. May cause fetal tachycardia and neonatal hypoglycemia.	+	No studies. Probably compatible. Monitor infant for tachycardia, hypoglycemia, and tremor.
Methadone (B/D if prolonged treatment or high doses at term)	Risk in 3rd trimester. May cause withdrawal syndrome, LBW, and death. Thrombocytosis and hyperbilirubinemia seen in newborn.	+	Drug excreted in low concentrations. AAP: compatible.
Methamphetamine (C)	With medical use, risk is low for anomalies. Withdrawal symptoms. With abuse: preterm labor, placental abruption, fetal distress, postpartum hemorrhage, IUGR, feeding difficulty, drowsiness, and lassitude that may last several months.	CI	AAP: contraindicated.
Methaqualone (D)	Not recommended.	–	No studies available.
Methenamine (C)	Probably compatible.	+	Excreted in breast milk. No adverse effects reported.
Methimazole (D)	May cause scalp defects and other malformations.	+	Risk of interfering with thyroid function.
Methotrexate (X)	Methotrexate embryopathy in 1st trimester. In 2nd or 3rd trimester: fetal toxicity and mortality.	CI	May accumulate in tissues; cytotoxic; interferes with cellular metabolism.
Methoxsalen (C)	No congenital malformations. Long-term effects (eg, cancer) need to be studied.	–	No studies; drug acts as photosensitizer. Stop feeding and discard milk for at least 24 hours.
Methyldopa (B)	No congenital malformations. Monitor for hypotension 48 hours after delivery.	+	Limited studies; probably compatible
Methylene blue (C/D if intra-amniotically)	Risk in 2nd and 3rd trimester. Possibly associated with fetal malformations.	+	No studies available.
Methylphenidate (C)	Few human studies.	–	Excreted in breast milk. Observe infant for CNS stimulation, decreased appetite, insomnia, and irritability.

(Continued)

Drug (FDA Fetal Risk Category)	Pregnancy-Adverse Events and Comments	Breast-Feeding Compatibility	Effect on Lactation and Adverse Effects on Infant
Metoclopramide (B)	No adverse effects reported.	–	Increases milk production. Effects unknown but of concern.
Metolazone (B/D if used in gestational hypertension)	May cause risk of congenital defects if taken in 1st trimester. Hypoglycemia, thrombocytopenia, hyponatremia, hypokalemia, and death. Monitor infant's electrolytes, platelet count, and serum glucose.	+	May suppress lactation. Monitor infant's electrolytes and platelets.
Metoprolol (C/D if 2nd or 3rd trimester)	Monitor infant for hypotension and bradycardia 48 hrs after birth. IUGR if early in 2nd trimester; decrease in placenta weight if in 3rd trimester.	–	Monitor for bradycardia and hypotension.
Metronidazole (B)	Possible fetal malformations with 1st-trimester use. Questionable risk of carcinogenic potential.	–	If one dose, hold feeding for 12-24 hours; if multiple, do not breast-feed. Medication is carcinogenic and mutagenic.
Miconazole (C)	No adverse effects.	+	No studies available.
Mineral oil (C)	May inhibit maternal absorption of fat-soluble vitamins (A, D, E, and K) if taken long term.	+	No studies.
Minocycline (D)	Contraindicated in 2nd and 3rd trimester. May cause yellow staining of teeth, inhibition of bone growth, maternal liver toxicity, and congenital defects.	+	Excreted into breast milk. Observe infant for changes in bowel flora, allergies, and use caution interpreting culture results.
Minoxidil (C)	May cause hypertrichosis. Decreases in blood pressure that could affect placental perfusion. Questionable cause of malformations; best to avoid in 1st-trimester.	+	Drug likely excreted; no adverse effects seen.
Misoprostol (X)	Teratogenic and congenital malformations.	–	Significant diarrhea in infant.
Mithramycin (see Plicamycin (X)			
Montelukast (B)	Human studies are lacking.	+	No studies. Probably compatible.
Morphine (C/D if long-term or high dose near delivery)	Risk of inguinal hernia, respiratory depression when used during labor. Monitor for neonatal withdrawal.	+	Excreted in breast milk. AAP: compatible. Long-term effects unknown.
Mumps vaccine (C)	Risk of malformations. Don't use.	+	No studies available; probably compatible.
Nadolol (C; D if 2nd or 3rd trimester)	Bradycardia and hypotension if exposed near term. Monitor blood pressure and heart rate. IUGR, tachypnea, hypothermia, hypoglycemia, and cardiorespiratory depression.	–	Risk for toxicity. Monitor for bradycardia and hypotension.
Nafcillin (B)	No adverse effects.	+	No studies available. (See Penicillin.)
Nalbuphine (B/D if prolonged or high doses near term)	Respiratory depression, fetal distress, and withdrawal syndrome.	+	No studies. Drug likely excreted. Amounts insignificant.
Nalidixic Acid (C)	Limited studies. Pyloric stenosis.	+	Drug excreted, amounts insignificant. AAP: compatible.
Naloxone (B)	No adverse effects.	+	No studies available.
Naltrexone (C)	Few studies. Changing opioid receptors and altering behavior is of concern.	–	No studies. Drug likely excreted. Effects unknown. Adverse effects: alteration of opioid receptors and altered levels of some hormones.

(Continued)

Drug (FDA Fetal Risk Category)	Pregnancy-Adverse Events and Comments	Breast-Feeding Compatibility	Effect on Lactation and Adverse Effects on Infant
Naproxen (C/D if used in 3rd trimester or near delivery)	Risk in 1st trimester of structural anomalies. 3rd trimester: closure of ductus arteriosus with resulting PPAN. Avoid use near term.	+	Drug excreted in breast milk; effects unknown. AAP: compatible.
Neomycin (C)	No malformations. Ototoxicity (risk of deafness low).	+	No studies. Drug excreted. Amount probably insignificant.
Neostigmine (C)	No malformations. Transient muscular weakness seen in 20% of infants whose mothers have myasthenia gravis.	+	No studies. Drug likely excreted; effects unknown.
Niacin (A/C if doses above RDA)	Possible association of pregnancy-induced hypertension.	+	Compatible with breast-feeding.
Niacinamide (A/C if doses above RDA)	Possible association of pregnancy-induced hypertension.	+	Compatible with breast-feeding.
Nicardipine (C)	Limited studies. Hypotension and bradycardia may occur. Monitor infant for 48 hours after birth.	+	Probably compatible. No studies.
Nicotine (transdermal, others) (D)	Prematurity, placenta previa, PROM, placental abruption, growth retardation, LBW, SIDS, abnormal neurobehavioral development, and increase in certain childhood diseases, retinal abnormalities, increase in major birth defects.	−	Unknown. Smoking not recommended. No studies on nicotine replacement.
Nifedipine (C)	Severe effects when combined with magnesium sulfate.	+	Drug excreted. Breast-feed 4 hours after dose. AAP: compatible.
Nitrofurantoin (B)	No adverse effects. Hemolysis if given near term avoid near delivery.	+	Excreted in breast milk. Monitor infants with G6PD deficiency for hemolytic anemia.
Nitroglycerin (B/C per manufacturer)	No adverse effects. Fetal heart changes (loss to beat-to-beat variability, late decelerations, and bradycardia).	+	No studies available.
Nitroprusside (C)	Fetal bradycardia. Risk of cyanide accumulation in fetus.	−	No studies available.
Norethynodrel (X)	Question of cardiac malformations, hypospadias, and masculinization of female infants.	+	↓ Wt gain, ↓ milk production, and content of milk changed. Probably significant only in malnourished mothers. AAP: compatible with breast-feeding.
Norfloxacin (C)	Not a risk of malformations. Use caution during 1st trimester. Best to avoid.	+	No studies. Drug likely excreted.
Nortriptyline (C)	May cause fetal malformations and urinay retention.	−	Excreted in breast milk; no adverse effects. Long-term concern for effects on neurobehavior. AAP: effect unknown but of concern.
Novobiocin (C)	May cause hyperbilirubinemia if used near term.	+	Excreted in breast milk. No adverse effects. Observe infant for changes in bowel flora, allergies, and use caution when interpreting culture results.
Nystatin (C)	No adverse effects.	+	Poorly absorbed. Excretion would not occur.
Octreotide (B)	Data too limited to assess safety.	+	Expect excretion. No studies.
Omeprazole (C)	Teratogenic risk low. Questionable risk of cardiac defects. Avoid in 1st trimester.	−	Few studies. Drug likely excreted; effects unknown. Avoid use.
Ondansetron (B)	No adverse effects.	+	No studies. Drug likely excreted; effects unknown.

(Continued)

Drug (FDA Fetal Risk Category)	Pregnancy-Adverse Events and Comments	Breast-Feeding Compatibility	Effect on Lactation and Adverse Effects on Infant
Oral contraceptives (all classes) (X)	Risk of anomalies (VACTERL) low. May cause masculinization of females and hyperbilirubinemia.	+	Causes dose-dependent suppression of lactation. Decreased weight gain, milk production, and nitrogen and protein content of human milk are associated with this drug. Changes probably only significant in malnourished mothers. Use lowest dose possible. AAP: compatible.
Oxacillin (B)	No adverse effects.	+	Excreted in low amounts. Observe infant for changes in bowel flora, allergies, and use caution when interpreting culture results.
Oxazepam (D)	Teratogenic syndrome. CNS defect, growth retardation, and dysmorphic features.	−	Monitor for lethargy. EEG: sedation-type pattern.
Oxprenolol (C/D if 2nd or 3rd trimester)	Bradycardia and hypotension in infants if near term. Monitor blood pressure and heart rate. May cause IUGR.	−	Monitor for hypotension and brady-cardia.
Oxycodone (B/D if long term or at high doses near delivery)	Withdrawal syndrome and respiratory depression. No congenital malformations.	+	Observe for sedation, feeding difficulties, and GI side effects.
Oxymetazoline (C)	No risk. Higher dose and frequency: persistent late FHR decelerations.	+	No studies.
Oxymorphone (B/D if long term or at high doses near delivery)	Withdrawal syndrome and respiratory depression. No congenital malformations.	+	No studies.
Pancuronium Bromide (C)	No data. Decreased accelerations and beat-to-beat variability. Observe for newborn depression.	+	No studies. Excreted in trace amounts; effects unknown.
Paregoric (B/D if prolonged or high dose near delivery)	Wthdrawal syndrome and respiratory depression. No malformations reported.	+	Probably excreted; limited studies.
Paroxetine (D)	Risk of congenital malformations, cardiac defects, withdrawal, jaundice, hypoglycemia, respiratory distress, LBW, prematurity, neonatal serotonin syndrome, neonatal behavioral syndrome, PPH, and abnormal neurobehavior with SSRI.	−	Effect unknown but of concern.
Penicillamine (D)	Connective tissue abnormalities (cutis laxa).	−	No studies. Some say avoid use.
Penicillin G (all forms) (B)	Adverse effects unlikely.	+	Observe infant for changes in bowel flora, allergies, and use caution in interpreting culture results.
Pentamidine (C)	Aerosolized pentamidine had no adverse effects.	CI	No studies.
Pentobarbital (D)	Withdrawal syndrome and hemorrhagic disease in newborn.	−	Excreted in breast milk; effects unknown.
Permethrin (B)	No adverse effects.	+	No studies. Little drug excreted.
Perphenazine (C)	No adverse effects.	−	Excreted into breast milk. AAP: effect unknown but of concern.
Phenazopyridine (B)	No adverse effects.	+	No data available.

(*Continued*)

Drug (FDA Fetal Risk Category)	Pregnancy-Adverse Events and Comments	Breast-Feeding Compatibility	Effect on Lactation and Adverse Effects on Infant
Phenobarbital (D)	Withdrawal syndrome, hemorrhagic disease in newborn, fetal malformations, and neurodevelopmental problems.	–	Monitor for sedation and withdrawal. AAP: major adverse effects, use caution.
Phenylephrine (C)	Fetal malformations reported. Constriction of uterine vessels.	+	No studies. Drug likely excreted; effects unknown.
Phenytoin (D)	May cause fetal hydantoin syndrome, tumors, and hemorrhagic disease in newborn.	+	Monitor for methemoglobinuria (rare).
Phytonadione (C)	No adverse effects reported.	+	Give vitamin K at birth.
Pindolol (B/D if 2nd or 3rd trimester)	Bradycardia and hypotension in infants exposed near term. Monitor BP and HR. May cause IUGR.	–	Monitor for hypotension and bradycardia.
Piperacillin (B)	No adverse effects.	+	Excreted into breast milk. Observe infant for changes in bowel flora, allergies, and use caution interpreting culture results.
Pneumococcal vaccine (C)	No adverse effects reported.	+	No studies. Probably compatible.
Polymyxin B (B)	No reports of congenital defects.	+	No studies available.
Potassium chloride (A)	Follow potassium levels in mother.	+	Compatible.
Potassium citrate (A, C by manufacturer)	No adverse effects. Follow potassium levels in mother.	+	No studies. Probably compatible. Observe for GI problems in infant.
Potassium gluconate (A)	No adverse effects. See Potassium chloride.	+	Compatible with breast-feeding. No adverse effects.
Pravastatin (X)	Contraindicated; cholesterol and cholesterol products are important in fetal development.	CI	No studies. Excreted into breast milk. Risk of toxicity. Avoid.
Prazosin (C)	Few studies.	–	No studies. Drug excreted; effects unknown.
Prednisone (C/D if 1st trimester)	Immunosuppression and cataracts. Small risk of fetal malformations such as orofacial clefts.	+	AAP: compatible.
Primaquine (C)	No congenital defects. Hemolysis if given near term in patients with G6PD deficiency.	+	No studies available.
Primidone (D)	Possible risk of fetal malformations, tremors, jitteriness, and hemorrhagic disease of newborn. Give vitamin K at birth.	+	Drug excreted in breast milk. AAP: use with caution. Monitor for sedation.
Probenecid (C)	No congenital defects reported.	–	Excreted into breast milk. Observe for diarrhea.
Procainamide (C)	No congenital anomalies or adverse fetal effects.	+	Drug likely excreted. AAP: compatible; effects unknown.
Procarbazine (D)	Fetal malformations and LBW. Contraindicated in 1st trimester.	CI	No studies. Drug likely excreted. Contraindicated because of risk of tumorigenicity.
Prochlorperazine (C)	Rare fetal malformations.	–	Sedation in nursing infant a possible side effect.
Promazine (C)	Rare fetal malformations. May cause hyperbilirubinemia in infant.	–	No studies. Drug likely excreted. Monitor for sedation.

(Continued)

Drug (FDA Fetal Risk Category)	Pregnancy-Adverse Events and Comments	Breast-Feeding Compatibility	Effect on Lactation and Adverse Effects on Infant
Promethazine (C)	Respiratory depression when given at term (*controversial*). Transient behavioral and EEG changes in infant.	+	Drug likely excreted; effects unknown.
Propantheline (C)	Question of minor malformations.	+	No studies available.
Propofol (B)	Can see hypotonia, irritability, somnolence, and low Apgar scores.	+	Drug excreted into breast milk.
Propoxyphene (C/D if long term)	May cause fetal malformations and neonatal withdrawal syndrome.	+	Excreted into breast milk. AAP: compatible.
Propranolol (C/D if 2nd, 3rd trimester)	May cause LBW, IUGR, respiratory depression at birth, neonatal hypoglycemia, polycythemia, hyperbilirubinemia, thrombocytopenia, hypocalcemia with convulsions, fetal bradycardia, and hypotension. Monitor respirations and heart rate for 24–48 hours if exposed near term.	+	AAP: compatible. Monitor for hypotension and bradycardia.
Propylthiouracil (D)	Fetal malformations reported. Reversible hypothyroidism and goiter in infant.	+	AAP: compatible. Monitor thyroid function of infant.
Protamine (C)	No adverse effects reported.	+	No studies available.
Pseudoephedrine (C)	Minor fetal malformations. Avoid in 1st trimester.	+	AAP: compatible. Monitor for agitation.
Pyridostigmine (C)	May cause microcephaly and CNS problems; 20% of infants whose mothers have myasthenia gravis have muscular weakness.	+	Excreted into breast milk. AAP: compatible.
Pyridoxine (A)	Fetal malformations unlikely. Convulsions seen (intrauterine and infant).	+	AAP: compatible.
Pyrimethamine (C)	Probably no birth defects. Give folic acid during 1st trimester.	+	Excreted into breast milk. AAP: compatible.
Quinidine (C)	Safe for fetus. Thrombocytopenia in infants in few cases.	+	Few studies. AAP: compatible.
Quinine (D, X per manufacturer)	Malformations of limbs, CNS, heart, and GI tract and deafness. Hemolysis in G6PD infants. Auditory and optic nerve damage. Avoid.	+	Excreted into breast milk; G6PD should be R/O. APP: compatible.
Ranitidine (B)	Not a major teratogen.	+	Excreted in breast milk; ↓ gastric acidity, effects unkown. AAP: similar drug compatible.
Ribavirin (X)	No abnormalities seen. Avoid.	−	No studies. Drug likely excreted; effects unknown.
Rifampin (C)	May cause hemorrhagic disease of newborn.	+	Excreted into breast milk. AAP: compatible.
Ritonavir (B)	Few human studies. Maternal benefits outweigh fetal risks.	CI	No studies. Drug likely excreted. Effect unknown. CDC: HIV-infected mothers in developed countries should not breast-feed.
Rubella vaccine (C)	Risk of congenital rubella syndrome.	+	Compatible.
Secobarbital (D)	May cause hemorrhagic disease of newborn and withdrawal.	+	Excreted into breast milk. AAP: compatible; effects unknown
Senna (C)	No adverse effects reported.	+	Observe for diarrhea. AAP:compatible.
Silicone implants (C)	Compatible.	+	AAP: ok to breastfeed.

(*Continued*)

Drug (FDA Fetal Risk Category)	Pregnancy-Adverse Events and Comments	Breast-Feeding Compatibility	Effect on Lactation and Adverse Effects on Infant
Spectinomycin (C)	No adverse effects reported.	+	No studies available.
Spironolactone (C/D for gestational hypertension)	No adverse effects. Risk of antiandro-genic effects. Diuretics not recom-mended for GA HT.	+	Unknown excretion; effect unknown AAP: compatible
Streptokinase (C)	No adverse effects reported.	+	No studies. Exposure risk low.
Streptomycin (D)	May cause eighth cranial nerve damage and ototoxicity.	+	Excreted into breast milk. Observe infant for changes in bowel flora, allergies, and use caution in inter-preting culture results.
Succinylcholine (C)	Not teratogenic. Respiratory depression in infant with genetic trait for atypi-cal cholinesterase.	+	Compatible.
Sucralfate (B)	No adverse effects reported.	+	Drug minimally excreted.
Sufentanil (C, D if long term or high amounts near term)	Dose-related respiratory depression and negative effects on neurobehavior may occur in the infant.	+	Drug likely excreted. Effects unknown.
Sulfasalazine (B/D near term)	No congenital anomalies. Risk of jaun-dice and kernicterus when given near term.	–	May cause bloody diarrhea in infants. AAP: give with caution.
Sulindac (B/D if 3rd trimester or near delivery)	Small risk of congenital anomalies, clos-ing of ductus arteriosus in utero, PPHN, and suppression of renal function.	–	No studies. Risk of toxicity.
Tacrolimus (C)	Reversible hyperkalemia, renal toxicity, IUGR, and premature delivery. Questionable association with cardiomyopathy.	+	Excreted into breast milk. Monitor infants levels.
Tamoxifen (D)	Avoid during pregnancy. Possible human teratogenicity.	CI	Inhibits lactation.
Temazepam (X)	Few human studies. Avoid this drug and diphenhydramine: resulted in stillbirth.	–	Excreted into breast milk. AAP: effect unknown but of concern. Observe infant for sedation and changes in feeding.
Terbutaline (B)	Transient fetal tachycardia and neonatal hypoglycemia.	+	AAP: compatible.
Testosterone (X)	Contraindicated. 1st-trimester: mas-culinization and clitoral hypertrophy in female fetuses, fused or partially fused labia, and possibly absent vagina. Clitoral hypertrophy exposure at any gestational age.	CI	Suppresses lactation.
Tetanus/Diphtheria Toxoid (adult) (C)	Unknown fetal risk.	+	No human lactation studies.
Tetanus Toxoid/ Reduced Diph-theria Toxoid and Acellular Pertus-sis Vaccine Adsorbed (TDaP) (C)	No adverse effects.	+	Compatible.
Tetracycline (D)	Avoid: may cause permanent yellow-brown staining of teeth, inhibition of bone growth, maternal liver toxicity, and congenital defects.	+	Drug likely excreted. Observe infant for changes in bowel flora, aller-gies, and use caution in inter-preting culture results .
THC (marijuana) (X)	Contraindicated. LBW, leukemia, risk of VSDs, increased alcohol effect, adverse effects on neurobehavior, mild neonatal withdrawal.	CI	AAP: contraindicated.

(Continued)

Drug (FDA Fetal Risk Category)	Pregnancy-Adverse Events and Comments	Breast-Feeding Compatibility	Effect on Lactation and Adverse Effects on Infant
Theophylline (C)	May cause transient tachycardia, irritability, and vomiting at birth. No congenital effects reported.	CI	AAP: compatible. Monitor for irritability.
Thiabendazole (C)	No adverse effects reported.	+	No studies. Drug likely excreted; effects unknown.
Thioguanine (D)	May cause fetal malformations and chromosomal abnormalities.	CI	No studies. Risk of toxicity (tumors in nursing infants).
Thiotepa (D)	Avoid in 1st trimester. Studies limited in 2nd and 3rd trimester.	CI	No studies. Drug likely excreted. Risk for toxicity (tumors in nursing infants).
Thiothixene (C)	Limited information.	–	No studies. Drug likely excreted; effects unknown.
Ticarcillin (B)	No adverse effects reported.	+	Drug excreted. Observe infant for changes in bowel flora, allergies, and use caution in interpreting culture results.
Timolol (C/D if 2nd or 3rd trimester and used systemically)	May cause IUGR, bradycardia, and hypotension in infants exposed near term. Monitor blood pressure and heart rate.	–	Monitor for β-blockade. AAP: compatible.
Tobramycin (C/D from manufacturer)	No congenital defects. Potentiation of magnesium sulfate–induced neuromuscular weakness. Monitor infant for ototoxicity.	+	Excreted into breast milk. Observe infant for changes in bowel flora, allergies, and use caution when interpreting culture results.
Tolazamide (C)	Near term: prolonged neonatal hypoglycemia.	–	No studies. Drug likely excreted; effects unknown.
Tolbutamide (C)	Near term: prolonged neonatal hypoglycemia. Has caused neonatal thrombocytopenia.	–	Excreted into breast milk. AAP: compatible. Monitor for jaundice and hypoglycemia.
Tolmetin (C, D if 3rd trimester or near delivery)	Congenital anomalies reported. May cause closing of ductus arteriosus in utero and PPHN.	+	Excreted into breast milk. AAP: compatible.
Tretinoin (systemic) (D)	Teratogenic. Retinoic acid embryology: contraindicated.	+	No studies available. Probably compatible.
Tretinoin (topical) (C)	Topically, teratogenic risk minimal.	+	Minimal absorption. Probably compatible.
Triamterene (C; D for gestational hypertension)	May decrease placental perfusion, maternal hypovolemia.	+	No studies. Drug likely excreted into breast milk. Probably compatible.
Trimethoprim/ Sulfamethoxazole (C; D if near term)	Teratogenic defects: cardiovascular, neural tube defects, and possibly oral clefts.	+	Excreted into breast milk. AAP: compatible.
Tripelennamine (B)	No adverse effects reported.	+	No studies. Probably compatible; manufacturer: contraindicated because of increased sensitivity of infants to antihistamines.
Urokinase (B)	Low risk.	+	No studies. Probably compatible.
Valproic acid (D)	Risk of neural tube, head, face, digits, GU tract defects, IUGR, fetal distress, hepatotoxicity, hyperglycemia, and hyperbilirubinemia.	–	AAP: compatible.
Vancomycin (B)	No congenital defects. Transient fetal bradycardia.	+	Excreted into breast milk. Observe infant for changes in bowel flora, allergies, and use caution in interpreting culture results.

(Continued)

Drug (FDA Fetal Risk Category)	Pregnancy-Adverse Events and Comments	Breast-Feeding Compatibility	Effect on Lactation and Adverse Effects on Infant
Vasopressin (B)	No fetal malformations.	+	Compatible with breast-feeding
Verapamil (C)	Decreased uterine blood flow, hypotension, and fetal bradycardia.	+	Excreted into breast milk. Limited studies but probably compatible.
Vidarabine (C)	Few studies.	+	No studies. Unknown if excreted.
Vincristine (D)	Congenital defects. Pancytopenia, transient bone marrow hypoplasia, chromosomal aberrations, and IUGR can occur.	CI	No human lactation studies available. Because of risk of toxicity to nursing infant, women should not breast-feed.
Vitamin A (A/X if over RDA)	Severe maternal vitamin A deficiency is teratogenic. Doses above RDA: teratogenic.	+	Compatible with breast-feeding.
Vitamin B$_{12}$ (A if RDA dose; C if over)	No adverse effects reported.	+	Compatible with breast-feeding.
Vitamin C (A if RDA dose; C if over)	No congenital defects. May cause scurvy in infant if used at high doses.	+	Compatible with breast-feeding.
Vitamin D (A if RDA dose; D if over)	May be associated with supravalvular aortic stenosis syndrome, which is associated with hypercalcemia of infancy.	+	Compatible with breast-feeding. Monitor for increased calcium levels if mother is taking pharmacologic doses.
Vitamin E (A if RDA dose; C if over)	No adverse effects reported.	+	Compatible with breast-feeding.
Vitamins, multi (A)	No adverse effects reported	+	Compatible with breast-feeding.
Warfarin (X, per manufacturer)	Major risk of defects. May cause fetal warfarin syndrome and hemorrhage.	+	Compatible with breast-feeding.
Zidovudine (C)	Neonatal anemia and IUGR may occur.	CI	HIV-1-infected mothers in developed countries should not breast-feed.

Based on data from Briggs GG et al (eds): *Drugs in Pregnancy and Lactation*, 8th ed. Philadelphia, PA: Lippincott Williams & Wilkins, 2008; Gomella (eds): *Clinician's Pocket Reference 2009.* New York, NY: McGraw-Hill, 2009; Koren G: *Medication Safety in Pregnancy and Breast-Feeding.* New York, NY: McGraw-Hill, 2007; and manufacturer's package inserts as of October 2008.

Appendix A. Abbreviations Used in Neonatology

A1AT	Alpha 1 antitrypsin	**BG**	Babygram (radiograph that includes the chest and abdomen)
AaDO2	Alveolar to arterial oxygen gradient		
AAP	American Academy of Pediatrics	**bid**	Twice daily
a/A ratio	Arterial to alveolar oxygen ratio	**BIND**	Bilirubin-induced neurologic dysfunction
AATD	Alpha-1 antitrypsin deficiency	**BIOT**	Biotinidase deficiency
ABR	Auditory brainstem response	**BM**	Breast milk
ACAAI	American College of Allergy, Asthma, and Immunology	**BMC**	Bone mineral content
		BOLD	Blood oxygen level dependent
ACOG	American College of Obstetricians and Gynecologists	**BP**	Blood pressure
		BPD	Biparietal diameter; bronchopulmonary dysplasia
ACT	Activated clotting time		
ADH	Antidiuretic hormone	**bpm**	Beats per minute
AED	Automatic external defibrillator	**BPP**	Biophysical profile
aEEG	Amplitude integrated encephalography	**BSEP**	Bile salt export pump
AEP	Auditory evoked potential	**BUN**	Blood urea nitrogen
AFI	Amniotic fluid index	**BW**	Birthweight; body weight
AGA	Appropriate for gestational age	**BWS**	Beckwith Wiedemann Syndrome
AGS	Adrenogenital syndrome	**C**	Cervical; Centigrade
AHA	American Heart Association	**CA**	Community acquired
AI	Aortic insufficiency	**CAH**	Congenital adrenal hyperplasia
AIDS	Acquired immunodeficiency syndrome	**CAM**	Complementary and alternative medicine; cystic adenomatoid malformation
ALT	Alanine aminotransferase		
ALTE	Apparent life-threatening event	**CANMWG**	Chicago Area Neonatal MRSA Working Group
AM	Morning		
Ao	Aortic	**CBC**	Complete blood count
AoI	Aortic isthmus	**CBF**	Cerebral blood flow
AOI	Apnea of infancy	**CBG**	Capillary blood gases
AOP	Apnea of prematurity	**CBS**	Capillary blood sampling
AP	Anteroposterior	**CBV3**	Coxsackievirus B3
Apgar	Appearance, pulse, grimace, activity, respirations	**CCAM**	Congenital cystic adenomatoid malformation
Apo-A	Apolipoprotein A	**CCHB**	Congenital complete heart block
APR	Acute phase reactants	**CDC**	Centers for Disease Control and Prevention
AP-ROP	Aggressive posterior retinopathy of prematurity		
		CDH	Congenital diaphragmatic hernia
APTT	Activated partial thromboplastin time	**CDG**	Congenital disorders of glycosylation
AR	Autosomal recessive	**CF**	Cystic fibrosis
ARC	AIDS-related complex	**CFM**	Cerebral function monitor
ARD	Antibiotic removal device	**CGH**	Comparative genomic hybridization
AREVD	Absent or reversal of end diastolic flow	**CH**	Congenital hydrocephalus
ARF	Acute renal failure	**CHARGE**	Coloboma, heart anomaly, atresia choanae, retarded growth, genital hypoplasia, and ear anomalies
ART	Artificial reproductive technology		
ARV	Antiretroviral drugs		
AS	Aortic stenosis	**CHD**	Congenital hip dislocation; congenital heart disease
ASAP	As soon as possible		
ASD	Atrial septal defect	**CHF**	Congestive heart failure
AST	Aspartate aminotransferase	**CHIME**	Collaborative Home Infant Monitoring Evaluation
ATN	Acute tubular necrosis		
ATP	Adenosine triphosphate	**CID**	Cytomegalovirus inclusion disease
A-V	Arteriovenous	**CIE**	Counterimmunoelectrophoresis
AV	Atrioventricular	**CLD**	Chronic lung disease
A-VO₂	Arteriovenous oxygen	**Cm**	Centimeter
BAEP	Brainstem auditory evoked potential	**CMA**	Chromosomal microarray analysis
BAER	Brainstem audiometric evoked response	**CMV**	Cytomegalovirus
BASD	Bile acid synthetic defect	**CNS**	Central nervous system; Crigler Najjar syndrome
BEEP	Bile salt export pump		
BD	Base deficit	**cP**	Centipoises
BF	Breast-feeding	**CPAP**	Continuous positive airway pressure

CPD	Citrate phosphate dextrose
CPIP	Chronic pulmonary insufficiency of prematurity
CRP	C-reactive protein
CRT	Capillary refill time
CRS	Congenital rubella syndrome
CRYO-ROP	Cryotherapy for retinopathy of prematurity
CS	Congenital syphilis; cesarean section
CSF	Cerebrospinal fluid
CST	Contraction stress test
CTG	Cardiotocography
CVH	Combined ventricular hypertrophy
CVP	Central venous pressure
CVS	Chorionic villus sampling
CT	Computed tomography
cUS	Cranial ultrasound
CXR	Chest x-ray
D	Day; diarrhea
DAT	Direct antibody test (Coombs test)
D25	25% dextrose solution
DBP	Diastolic blood pressure
DC	Direct current
D/C	Discharge or discontinue
DDH	Developmental dysplasia of hip
DDST	Denver Developmental Screening Test
DDX	Differential diagnosis
DES	Diethylstilbestrol
DFA	Direct fluorescent antibody
DHT	Dihydrotestosterone
DI	Diabetes insipidus
DIC	Disseminated intravascular coagulation
DISIDA	Diisopropyl iminodiacetic acid
dL	Deciliter
DM	Diabetes mellitus
DMSA	Dimercaptosuccinic acid
DNPH	2,4-Dinitrophenylhydrazine
DNR	Do not resuscitate
DOA	Dead on arrival
DOCA	Deoxycorticosterone acetate
DP	Dorsalis pedis
DPT	Diphtheria-pertussis-tetanus
DS	Double strength
DSD	Disorder of sex development
DTO	Deodorized tincture of opium
DTPA	Diethylenetriamine penta-acetic acid
DTR	Deep tendon reflexes
DVT	Deep venous thrombosis
D%W	% Dextrose in water
DWI	Diffusion-weighted (magnetic resonance) imaging
Dx	Diagnosis
DXA	Dual energy x-ray absorptiometry
DXM	Dexamethasone
DZ	Disease
EA	Esophageal atresia
EBL	Estimated blood loss
EBV	Epstein-Barr virus
ECG	Electrocardiogram
ECP	Eosinophil cationic protein
ECMO	Extracorporeal membrane oxygenation
ECW	Extracellular water
EDC	Estimated date of confinement
EDV	End diastolic velocity
EEG	Electroencephalogram
EFA	Essential fatty acid
EFM	Electronic fetal monitoring
EHEC	Enterohemorrhagic *Escherichia coli*

EHR	Electronic health records
EIA	Enzyme immunoassay
ELBW	Extremely low birthweight
ELISA	Enzyme-linked immunosorbent assay
EMG	Electromyelogram
EMLA	Eutectic mixture of lidocaine and prilocaine 5% cream
EMR	Electronic medical records
EN	Enteral nutrition
ENNS	Early Neonatal Neurobehavioral Scale
ENT	Ear nose throat
EOS	Early-onset sepsis
EPO	Erythropoietin
ERCP	Endoscopic retrograde cholangiopancreatography
ESR	Erythrocyte sedimentation rate
ESRD	End-stage renal disease
ET, Et	Endotracheal tube/enterostomal therapist; ejection time; expiratory time
ETCOc	End tidal carbon monoxide (concentration)
ETCO$_2$	End-tidal carbon dioxide (concentration)
ETT	Endotracheal tube
F, Fr	French scale (1/3 mm)
FAO	Fatty acid oxidation
FAS	Fetal alcohol syndrome
FBS	Fasting blood sugar; fetal blood sample
Fe	Iron
FE	Fractional excretion
FeNa	Fractional excretion of sodium
FFP	Fresh-frozen plasma
FHR	Fetal heart rate
FHT	Fetal heart tone
FIO$_2$	Fraction of inspired oxygen
FISH	Fluorescence in situ hybridization
FLM	Fetal lung maturity
FRC	Functional residual capacity
FSH	Follicle-stimulating hormone
FSP	Fibrin split products
FTA-ABS	Fluorescence treponemal antibody absorption
FTT	Failure to thrive
FU, F/U	Follow up
FUO	Fever of unknown origin
FVC	Forced vital capacity
FVZS	Fetal varicella zoster syndrome
Fx	Fracture
Fxn	Function
G	Gram, Gravida
GA	Gestational age; general anesthesia
GABA	Gamma-aminobutyric acid
GALE	Uridine diphosphate-galactose-4-epimerase deficiency
GALK	Galactokinase
GALT deficiency	Galactose-1-phosphate uridyltransferase deficiency (produces galactosemia)
GBS	Group B streptococcus
GBV-C	Hepatitis G virus
G-CSF	Granulocyte colony-stimulating factor
GDM	Gestational diabetes mellitus
GE	Gastroesophageal
GER (GERD)	Gastroesophageal reflux (disease)
GFR	Glomerular filtration rate
GGT	Gamma-glutamyl transferase
GGTP	Gamma-glutamyl transpeptidase
GI	Gastrointestinal
GM-CSF	Granulocyte macrophage colony-stimulating factor

GM/IVH	Germinal matrix/intraventricular hemorrhage	**Hx**	History
G$_x$P$_x$Ab$_x$LC$_x$	Shorthand for gravida/para/abortion/ living children (subscript variables represent numbers of each)	**IAP**	Intrapartum antibiotic prophylaxis
		IAT	Indirect antiglobulin technique
		ICAM-1	Intercellular adhesion molecule-1
		ICH	Intracranial hemorrhage
G$_x$P$_x$0000	First zero, full term; second zero, premature; third zero, abortion; fourth zero, living children	**ICN**	Intensive care nursery
		ICP	Intracranial pressure
		ICPH	Intracerebellar parenchymal hemorrhage
G6PD	Glucose-6-phosphate dehydrogenase	**ICS**	Intercostal space
Gt, gtt	Drop, drops	**ICW**	Intracellular water
GTT	Glucose tolerance test	**I&D**	Incision and drainage
GU	Genitourinary	**ID**	Internal diameter
GVHD	Graft-versus-host disease	**IDAM**	Infant of drug-abusing mother
HAA	Hepatitis-associated antigen	**IDDM**	Insulin-dependent diabetes mellitus
HAART	Highly active antiretroviral therapy	**IDM**	Infant of diabetic mother
HAV	Hepatitis A virus	**I:E**	Inspiratory-to-expiratory ratio
HBcAg	Hepatitis B core antigen	**IEM**	Inborn errors of metabolism
HBeAg	Hepatitis B e antigen	**IFA**	Immunofluorescent antibody assay
HBIG	Hepatitis B immune globulin	**IG**	Immunoglobulin
HBP	High blood pressure	**I/G**	Insulin-to-glucose ratio
HBsAg	Hepatitis B surface antigen	**IGF**	Insulin growth factor
HBV	Hepatitis B virus	**IHPS**	Idiopathic hypertrophic pyloric stenosis
HC	Head circumference	**IL**	Interleukin
hCG	Human chorionic gonadotropin	**IM**	Intramuscular
HCM	Health care maintenance	**IMV**	Intermittent mandatory ventilation
HC-MRSA	Healthcare MRSA	**INF**	Intravenous nutritional feedings
Hct	Hematocrit	**iNO**	Inhaled nitric oxide
HCTZ	Hydrochlorothiazide	**INR**	International normalized ratio
HCV	Hepatitis C virus	**I&O**	Intake and output
HCY	Homocystinuria	**IODAM**	Infant of drug-abusing mother
HD	Hirschsprung disease	**IODM**	Infant of diabetic mother
HDN	Hemolytic disease of the newborn	**IPPB**	Intermittent positive-pressure breathing
HDV	Hepatitis D virus	**IPV**	Inactivated poliovirus vaccine
HEENT	Head, eyes, ears, nose, and throat	**IQ**	Intelligence quotient
HELLP	Preeclampsia with *h*emolysis, *e*levated *l*iver enzymes, and *l*ow *p*latelet (count)	**ISG**	Immune serum globulin
		IT	Intrathecal
		I/T	Ratio of immature to total neutrophils
HEPPV	High-frequency positive-pressure ventilation	**It**	Inspiratory time
		ITP	Idiopathic thrombocytopenic purpura
HEV	Hepatitis E Virus	**IU**	International unit
HFJV	High-frequency jet ventilation	**IUGR**	Intrauterine growth restriction
HFNC	High-flow nasal cannula	**IUT**	Intrauterine transfusion
HFO	High-frequency oscillation	**IV**	Intravenous
HFOV	High-frequency oscillatory ventilation	**IVC**	Inferior vena cava; intravenous cholangiogram
HFV	High-frequency ventilation		
Hgb	Hemoglobin	**IVH**	Intraventricular hemorrhage
HGV	Hepatitis G virus	**IVIG**	Intravenous immunoglobulin
HHV	Human herpes virus	**IVP**	Intravenous pyelogram; IV push
Hib vaccine	*Haemophilus influenzae* type b vaccine	**IWL**	Insensible water loss
HIDA	Hepatobiliary scan	**JEB**	Junctional epidermolysis bullosa
HIE	Hypoxic ischemic encephalopathy	**JODM**	Juvenile-onset diabetes mellitus
HIG	Hyperimmune globulin	**K**	Potassium
HIV	Human immunodeficiency virus	**KC**	Kangaroo care
HLA	Human leukocyte antigen	**Kcal**	Kilocalorie
HLHS	Hypoplastic left heart syndrome	**Kg**	Kilogram
HMD	Hyaline membrane disease	**KU**	Klobusitzky unit
HO	History of	**KUB**	Kidneys, ureter, bladder
H&P	History and physical examination	**L**	Liter
HPA	Platelet-specific antigen	**LA**	Left atrium; lactic acidosis
HPF	High-power field	**LAD**	Left axis deviation; left atrial diameter; left anterior descending
HPI	History of present illness		
HPLC	High performance liquid chromatography		
HR	Heart rate	**LAE**	Left atrial enlargement
HSM	Hepatosplenomegaly	**LANE**	Mnemonic for meds acceptable thru ETT (*l*idocaine, *a*tropine, *n*aloxone, *e*pinephrine)
HSV	Herpes simplex virus		
H/t	Head-to-trunk ratio		
HT	Healing touch	**LBBB**	Left bundle branch block
HTN	Hypertension	**LBC**	Lamellar body count

LBW	Low birthweight
LBWL	Low birthweight "lytes"
LC	Living children
LCAD	Long-chain acyl-CoA dehydrogenase
LCHAD	Long chain 3 hydroxyacyl CoA dehydrogenase
LCPUFAs	Long-chain polyunsaturated fatty acids
LGA	Large for gestational age
LH	Luteinizing hormone
LLL	Left lower lobe
LLQ	Left lower quadrant
LMWH	Low molecular weight heparin
LMP	Last menstrual period
LMX4	Liposomal lidocaine cream
LOS	Late-onset sepsis
LP	Lumbar puncture
LPM	Liters per minute
LR	Lactated Ringer's solution
LV	Left ventricle
LVED	Left ventricular end diastolic
LVES	Left ventricular end systolic
LVH	Left ventricular hypertrophy
LVO	Left ventricular output
L-S ratio	Lecithin-to-sphingomyelin ratio
L3-L4	Third lumbar to fourth lumbar vertebral space
M	Molar
m	Meter
MAC	Minimum alveolar concentration; *Mycobacterium avium* complex
MAP	Mean arterial pressure
MAS	Meconium aspiration syndrome
Max	Maximum
MBC	Minimum bactericidal concentration
MCAD	Medium chain acyl CoA dehydrogenase deficiencies
MCH	Mean cell hemoglobin
MCHC	Mean cell hemoglobin concentration
MCA	Multiple congenital abnormalities
MCAD	Medium chain acyl CoA dehydrogenase deficiency
MCA PSV	Middle cerebral artery peak systolic velocity
MCT	Medium-chain triglyceride
MCV	Mean cell volume
MDT	Metered dose inhaler
mEq or meq	Milliequivalent
Mg	Magnesium
MHTPA	Micro hemoagglutination test for *Treponema pallidum*
MIC	Mean inhibitory concentration
Min	Minute
mL	Milliliter
mm	Millimeter
MMA	Methylmalonic acidemia
MMR	Measles mumps rubella (vaccine)
mOsm	Milliosmolality
MPO-ANCA	Myeloperoxidase-antineutrophil cytoplasmic antibody
MRA	Magnetic resonance arteriography
MRCP	Magnetic resonance cholangiopancreatography
MRI	Magnetic resonance imaging
MRSA	Methicillin-resistant *Staphylococcus aureus*
MRV	Magnetic resonance venography
MS	Mitral stenosis; morphine sulfate; mass spectrometry
MS/MS	Tandem mass spectrometry
MSAF	Meconium stained amniotic fluid
MSAFP	Maternal serum levels of α-fetoprotein
MSUD	Maple syrup urine disease
MTCT	Mother-to-child transmission
MV	Minute volume
MVI	Multiple vitamin infusion
MVP	Maximum vertical pocket; mitral valve prolapse
N/A	Not applicable
Na	Sodium
NAA	Nucleic acid amplification
NANN	National Association of Neonatal Nurses
NAT	Nucleic amplification testing
NAVEL	Mnemonic for groin muscle (*n*erve, *a*rtery, *v*ein, *e*mpty space, *l*ymphatic)
NBS	New Ballard score
NCPAP	Nasal CPAP
NCV	Nerve conduction velocity
NE	Norepinephrine, neonatal encephalopathy
NEC	Necrotizing enterocolitis
NEAL	Mnemonic for ETT administered medications (*n*aloxone, *e*pinephrine, *a*tropine, and *l*idocaine)
NG	Nasogastric
NHLBL	National Heart Lung and Blood Institute
NICHD	National Institute of Child Health and Human Development
NICU	Neonatal intensive care unit
NIDCAP	Newborn Individualized Developmental Care and Assessment Program
NIPPV	Nasal intermittent positive pressure ventilation
NKA	No known allergies
NKDA	No known drug allergy
NKH	Nonketotic hyperglycinemia
nl	Normal
NMR	Nuclear magnetic resonance
NNACS	Neonatal Neurologic and Adaptive Capacity Score
NORD	National Organization for Rare Disorders
NP	Nasopharyngeal
NPCPAP	Nasopharyngeal continuous positive airway pressure
NPO	Nothing by mouth
NRP	Neonatal resuscitation program
NRTI	Nucleoside reverse transcriptase inhibitor
NS	Normal saline
NSAID	Nonsteroidal anti-inflammatory drug
NSR	Normal sinus rhythm
NST	Nonstress test
NT	Nasotracheal; (fetal) nuchal translucency
NTA	Nontreponemal antibody
NTA tests	Nontreponemal antibody tests (VDRL, RPR, ART)
NTB	Necrotizing tracheobronchitis
NTBC	[2-Nitro-4 (trifluoromethyl) benzoyl]-1-3-cyclohexanedione)
NTDS	Neural tube defects
NTE	Neutral thermal environment
NVP	Nevirapine
OA	Organic aciduria/acidemia
OAE	Otoacoustic emissions
OB	Obstetrics
OBSN	Observation
OCP	Oral contraceptive pill
OCT	Oxytocin challenge test
OD	Outer diameter
OFC	Occipital frontal circumference

OG	Orogastric
17-OHP	17-hydroxyprogesterone
OI	Oxygen index
OM	Otitis media
OMIM	Online mendelian inheritance of man
Ophth	Ophthalmic
OR	Operating room
OSA	Obstructive sleep apnea
Osm	Osmolality
OTC	Over the counter (nonprescription drug); ornithine transcarbamylase deficiency
OU	Both eyes (*oculus unitas*)
OWB	Oscillating waterbed
Oz	ounce
P	Para (the number of viable [>20 wks] births)
PA	Pulmonary artery; posteroanterior; pulmonary atresia
PAC	Premature atrial contraction
PaCO$_2$	Partial pressure of carbon dioxide, arterial
PAF	Platelet activating factor
PaO$_2$	Partial pressure of oxygen, arterial
PAO$_2$	Partial pressure of oxygen, alveolar
PAPP-A	Pregnancy-associated plasma protein A
PAT	Paroxysmal atrial tachycardia
Paw	Mean airway pressure
P&PD	Percussion and postural drainage
PB	Periodic breathing
PBF	Pulmonary blood flow
PBLC	Premature birth living child
PCA	Postconceptional age; primary cutaneous aspergillosis
PCG	Pneumocardiogram
PCN	Penicillin
PCP	*Pneumocystis jiroveci* pneumonia; phencyclidine
PCR	Polymerase chain reaction
PCT	Procalcitonin
PCVC	Percutaneous central venous catheter
PDA	Patent ductus arteriosus
PDH	Pyruvate dehydrogenase
PE	Pleural effusion; physical examination; pulmonary embolus
PEA	Pulseless electrical activity
PEEP	Positive end expiratory pressure
PET	End tidal CO$_2$ monitoring; partial exchange transfusion
PetCO$_2$	Partial pressure of end tidal carbon dioxide
PFC	Perfluorocarbons; persistent fetal circulation
PFFD	Proximal focal femoral deficiency
PFIC	Progressive familial intrahepatic cholestasis
PFO	Patent foramen ovale
PFT	Pulmonary function test
PG	Phosphatidylglycerol
PGI$_2$	Prostacyclin (epoprostenol)
PGE1	Prostaglandin E1
PHH	Posthemorrhagic hydrocephalus
PI	Pulsatility index
PICC	Percutaneous inserted central catheter
PID	Pelvic inflammatory disease
PIE	Pulmonary interstitial emphysema
PIH	Post-infections hydrocephalus
PILG	Perfluorocarbon induced lung growth
PIP	Peak inspiratory pressure
PIV	Peripheral intravenous
PKU	Phenylketonuria

PLAST	Percussion, lavage, suction, turn
PLV	Partial liquid ventilation
PM	Afternoon and night
PMH	Past medical history
PMN	Polymorphonuclear neutrophil
PN	Parenteral nutrition
PNA	Postnatal age
PNCV	Peripheral nerve conduction velocity
PO	By mouth
P&PD	Percussion and postural drainage
PPD	Purified protein derivative
PPH	Persistent pulmonary hypertension
PPHN	Persistent pulmonary hypertension of newborn
PPN	Peripheral parenteral nutrition
PPROM	Preterm premature rupture of membranes
PPS	Peripheral pulmonic stenosis
PPV	Positive-pressure ventilation
PR	Per rectum
PRBC	Packed red blood cells
PRN	As needed
PROM	Premature rupture of membranes
PT	Prothrombin time
PTB	Preterm birth
PTH	Parathyroid hormone
PTT	Partial thromboplastin time
PTX	Pneumothorax
PUBS	Percutaneous umbilical blood sampling
PUV	Posterior urethral valves
PVC	Premature ventricular contraction
PVD	Posthemorrhagic ventricular dilation
PVH	Periventricular hemorrhage
PVHI	Periventricular hemorrhagic infarction
PV-IVH, PVH-IVH	Periventricular (hemorrhage) intraventricular hemorrhage
PVL	Periventricular leukomalacia
PVR	Peripheral vascular resistance; pulmonary vascular resistance
PVS	Percussion, vibration, and suctioning
Q	Every
Qd	Everyday
qXh	Every X hours
qid	Four times daily
qod	Every other day
Quad screen	Quadruple screen test (maternal serum α-fetoprotein, total human chorionic gonadotropin, unconjugated estriol, inhibin A)
RA	Right atrium
RAD	Right axis deviation
RAE	Right atrial enlargement
RAH	Right atrial hypertrophy
RAST	Radioallergosorbent test
RBBB	Right bundle branch block
RBC	Red blood cell
RDA	Recommended dietary allowance
RDS	Respiratory distress syndrome
rFVIIa	Recombinant factor VII, activated
RFI	Renal failure index
Rh	Rhesus factor
rhAPC	Recombinant human activated protein C
R-HuEPO	Recombinant human erythropoietin
RIA	Radioimmunoassay
RL	Ringer's lactate
RLF	Retrolental fibroplasia
RLL	Right lower lobe
RLQ	Right lower quadrant
RML	Right middle lobe

R/O	Rule out
ROM	Range of motion; rupture of membranes
ROP	Retinopathy of prematurity
ROS	Review of systems
RPR	Rapid plasma reagin (test)
RSV	Respiratory syncytial virus
RT	Rubella titer; respiratory therapy; radiation therapy
RTA	Renal tubular acidosis
RTPCR	Reverse transcriptase polymerase chain reaction
RUL	Right upper lobe
RUQ	Right upper quadrant
RV	Right ventricle; residual volume
RVH	Right ventricular hypertrophy
RVT	Renal vein thrombosis
Rx	Treatment
Rxn	Reaction
s	Without
SA	Sinoatrial
SAE	Serious adverse event
SAH	Subarachnoid hemorrhage
SaO_2	Oxygen saturation of arterial blood
SBP	Systolic blood pressure
SC	Subcutaneous
SCAD	Short chain acyl-CoA dehydrogenase deficiency
SCM	Sternocleidomastoid muscle
SD	Standard deviation
SDH	Subdural hemorrhage
SEH	Subependymal hemorrhage
SEM	Systolic ejection murmur; skin, eyes, and mouth
SEP	Sensory evoked potential
SSEP	Somatosensory evoked potential
SGA	Small for gestational age
SGOT	Serum glutamic oxaloacetic transaminase
SGPT	Serum glutamic pyruvic transaminase
SIADH	Syndrome of inappropriate antidiuretic hormone
SIDS	Sudden infant death syndrome
SIMV	Synchronized intermittent mandatory ventilation
SIP	Spontaneous intestinal perforation
SK	Streptokinase
SLE	Systemic lupus erythematosus
SMX	Sulfamethoxazole
SNC	Selective neonatal chemoprophylaxis
SNHL	Sensorineural hearing loss
SnMP	Sn (tin)-mesoporphyrin
SOAP	Mnemonic for S (Subjective), O (Objective), A (Assessment), P (Plan)
SOB	Shortness of breath
S/P	Status post
SpO_2	Pulse oximetry measurement of blood oxygenation saturation
SQ	Subcutaneous
SSRI	Selective serotonin reuptake inhibitors
SSSS	Staphylococcal scalded skin syndrome
STA	Specific antitreponemal antibody; specific treponemal tests
stat	Immediately
STD	Sexually transmitted disease
Supp	Supplement; suppository
Susp	Suspension
SVC	Superior vena cava

SVD	Spontaneous vaginal delivery
SvO_2	Venous oxygen saturation
SVT	Supraventricular tachycardia
SWC	Sleep wake cycle
Sx	Symptom
Sz	Seizure
TA	Tricuspid atresia
TA-GVHD	Transfusion-associated graft-versus-host disease
TAPVR	Total anomalous pulmonary venous return
TAR	Thrombocytopenia and absent radius (syndrome)
TB	Tuberculosis
TBG	Thyroid-binding globulin
TBLC	Term birth, living child
TBW	Total body water
TcB	Transcutaneous bilirubin
$TcPCO_2$	Transcutaneous carbon dioxide tension
$TcPO_2$	Transcutaneous oxygen tension
TD	Transdermal
TD_xFLMII	Commercial fetal lung maturity assay
TEF	Tracheoesophageal fistula
TENS	Transcutaneous electric nerve stimulation
TEWL	Transepidermal water loss
TFT	Thyroid function test
TGA	Transposition of the great arteries
TGV	Transposition of the great vessels
T&H	Type and hold
THAM	Tris (hydroxymethyl) aminomethane (tromethamine)
THAN	Transient hyperammonemia of the newborn
Ti	Inspiratory time
tid	Three times daily
TLC	Total lung capacity
TLV	Total liquid ventilation
TM	Tympanic membrane
TNF	Tumor necrosis factor
TOF	Tetralogy of Fallot
TORCH	Toxoplasmosis, other, rubella, cytomegalovirus, herpes simplex
TORCHS	As above plus syphilis
tPA	Tissue plasminogen activator
TPN	Total parenteral nutrition
TRH	Thyrotropin releasing hormone
TRALI	Transfusion-related acute lung injury
TSB	Total serum bilirubin
TSH	Thyroid-stimulating hormone
TT	Thrombin time
TTN	Transient tachypnea of newborn
TTV	Torque teno virus; transfusion-transmitted virus
TV	Tidal volume
Type 2 DM	Type 2 diabetes mellitus
U	Unit(s). (Note: Do not use; dangerous abbreviation)
UA	Umbilical artery
U/A	Urinalysis
UAC	Umbilical artery catheter
UDCA	Ursodeoxycholic acid
UDPGT	Uridine diphosglucuronyl acid
UGI	Upper gastrointestinal
UK	Urokinase
ULN	Upper limits of normal
UPEP	Urine protein electrophoresis
UPI	Uteroplacental insufficiency
UPJ	Ureteropelvic junction

UPJO	Uteropelvic junction obstruction	VLCFA	Very long chain fatty acids
URI	Upper respiratory infection	VP	Ventriculoperitoneal shunt
US	Ultrasound	V/Q	Ventilation-perfusion
UTI	Urinary tract infection	VSD	Ventricular septal defect
UV	Umbilical vein	VSS	Vital signs stable
UVC	Umbilical vein catheter	VT	Ventricular tachycardia
VA	Venoarterial	V_T	Tidal volume
VACTERL	Vertebral, anal, cardiac, tracheal,	VUE	Villitis of unknown etiology
	esophageal, renal, limb (anomalies)	VUR	Vesicoureteral reflux
VBG	Venous blood gas	VZV	Varicella zoster virus
VC	Vital capacity	VZIG	Varicella-zoster immune globulin
VCUG	Voiding cystourethrogram	WBC	White blood cell
VDRL	Venereal disease research laboratory	WF	White female
VEGF	Vascular endothelial growth factor	WM	White male
VEP	Visual evoked potential	WNL, wnl	Within normal limits
VER	Visual evoked response	WNV	West Nile virus
VF	Ventricular fibrillation	WPW	Wolff-Parkinson-White syndrome
VISA	Vancomycin intermediate *Staphylococcus*	XR	Extended release
	aureus	ZDV	Zidovudine
VLBW	Very low birthweight	ZnMP	Zinc metalloporphyrin

Appendix B. Apgar Scoring

Apgar scores are a numerical expression of the condition of a newborn infant on a scale of 0–10. The scores are recorded at 1 and 5 min after delivery and become a permanent part of the health record. If there is a problem an additional score is given at 10 minutes. A score of 7–10 is normal (10 is very unusual), 4–7 usually requires some resuscitative measures, and less than 3 requires immediate resuscitation. They have clinical usefulness not only during the nursery stay but at later child health visits when clinical status at delivery may have a bearing on current diagnostic assessments. The system was originally described by Virginia Apgar, MD, an anesthesiologist, in 1952 and first published in 1953.

	Score		
Sign	**0**	**1**	**2**
Appearance (color)	Blue or pale	Pink body with blue extremities	Completely pink
Pulse (heart rate)	Absent	Slow (<100 beats/min)	>100 beats/min
Grimace (reflex irritability)	No response	Grimace	Cough or sneeze
Activity (muscle tone)	Limp	Some flexion	Active movement
Respirations	Absent	Slow, irregular	Good, crying

Appendix C. Blood Pressure Determinations

Table C–1. REPRESENTATIVE 95TH AND 97TH PERCENTILES FOR SYSTOLIC BLOOD PRESSURE IN INFANTS

Study	Technique	Gestation	Age	Systolic Blood Pressure (mm Hg) 95th Percentile	97th Percentile
American Academy of Pediatrics Second Task Force	First auscultation or Doppler ultrasonogram	Term	Day 1 Day 8–30	96 104	
Brompton	Mean of 3 Doppler ultrasonograms	Term	Day 4 6 wks	95[a] 113[a]	
Northern Neonatal Nursing Initiative	Mean of 3 or more Doppler ultrasonograms	Term	Day 1 Day 10		82 111
		24 wk	Day 1 Day 10		57 71
		28 wk	Day 1 Day 10		62 83
		32 wk	Day 1 Day 10		67 94
		36 wk	Day 1 Day 10		74 104

[a]Awake.
Adapted from Watkinson M: Hypertension in the newborn baby. *Arch Dis Child Fetal Neonatal Ed* 2002;86:F78

Table C -2. BLOOD PRESSURE RANGES IN PREMATURE INFANTS ACCORDING TO BODYWEIGHT

Birthweight (g)	Mean Pressure	Systolic (mm Hg)	Diastolic (mm Hg)
501–750	38–49	50–62	26–36
751–1000	35.5–47.5	48–59	23–36
1001–1250	37.5–48	49–61	26–35
1251–1500	34.5–44.5	46–56	23–33
1501–1750	34.5–45.5	46–58	23–33
1751–2000	36–48	48–61	24–35

Based on data from Hegyi T et al: Blood pressure ranges in premature infants: 1. The first hours of life. *J Pediatr* 1994;124:627.

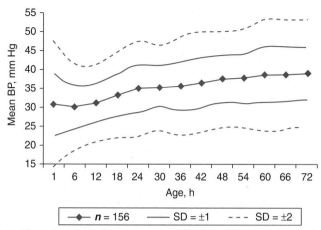

APPENDIX FIGURE C–1. Mean blood pressure of all infants 401–1000 g during the first 72 hours of life. (*Reproduced, with permission, from Faranoff JM et al: Treated hypotension is associated with neonatal morbidity and hearing loss in extremely low birth weight infants.* Pediatrics 2006;117;1131-1135).

Appendix D. Chartwork

ADMISSION HISTORY

Many hospitals are now using EMR (electronic medical records) or EHR (electronic health records). These are often in a preformatted template to be completed electronically. Because there are many different formats, there is no all-inclusive EMR example. The following section provides an overview of the basic history, progress note, admission orders, and discharge summary. Chapter 5 outlines the newborn physical examination.

ADMISSION HISTORY

A. **Identification (ID).** State the name, age, sex, and weight of the infant. Include whether the patient or mother was transported from another facility or whether the infant was born at home or within the hospital.
   Infant James, a 3-h-old 1800-g white male, is an inborn patient from Baltimore, Maryland.
B. **Chief complaint (CC).** The major problems of the patient are usually listed in the order of severity of disease process or occurrence.
   1. *Respiratory distress syndrome.*
   2. *Suspected neonatal sepsis.*
   3. *Premature birth living child (PBLC).*
C. **Referring physician.** Include the name, address, and telephone number of the referring physician.
   Dr. Macaca Mulatta, Benjamin Franklin Medical Center, Chadds Ford, PA;(946) 854-8881
D. **History of present illness (HPI).** The HPI is more helpful if it is divided into four separate paragraphs.
   1. **Initial statement.** This part of the HPI includes the patient's name, gestational age, birthweight, sex, age of the mother, and the number of times she has been pregnant along with the number of her living children.

2. **Prenatal history.** Discuss the maternal prenatal care and record the number of prenatal clinic visits. Include any medications the mother was taking, any pertinent prenatal tests done, and the results.

3. **Labor and delivery.** Include a detailed history of the labor and delivery: type of delivery, type of anesthesia, any medication used, and any fetal monitoring (including results).

4. **Infant history.** Discuss the initial condition of the infant and the need for resuscitation, and write a detailed description of what occurred. Include the Apgar scores and discuss when the infant became symptomatic or when problems were first noted.

> *Infant James is a 1800-g white male delivered to a 19-year-old G_2 now P_2, LC_2 married white female.*

> *The mother had excellent prenatal care. She had her first prenatal visit at approximately 8 weeks' gestation and then saw her obstetrician routinely. She was on no medications nor does she have any history of ethanol or cigarette abuse.*

> *She had rupture of membranes (ROM) at 33 weeks with some mild contractions. At that time, she was seen by her obstetrician, who confirmed the premature rupture of the membranes. She was admitted to the hospital and started on IV ritodrine in an attempt to stop the labor. Vaginal and rectal GBS cultures were obtained. IV penicillin was initiated. Because of a positive GBS culture, penicillin was continued during tocolysis. External fetal monitoring had been normal until 4 h after the Pitocin induction, at which time it showed late decelerations. At this point, an emergency cesarean delivery was performed. General anesthesia was used, and the infant was delivered within 6 min.*

> *The infant was delivered depressed at birth, with 1-min Apgar of 4. He required bagmask ventilation with 100% oxygen. No medications were needed. The 5-min Apgar was 7. The infant appeared poorly perfused and had poor color without oxygen. He was stabilized and transported on 100% oxygen to the NICU.*

E. **Family history (FH).** The family history should include any previous complicated births and their history, miscarriages, neonatal deaths, or premature births. Also include any major family medical problems (eg, hemophilia, sickle cell disease).

> *Mrs. James had 1 prior uncomplicated vaginal delivery that went to term. There is a history of myelodysplasia in infant James's maternal first cousin.*

F. **Social history (SH).** In the social history, include a brief statement discussing the parent's age, marital status, siblings, occupation, and where they are from.

> *The parents live in Chadds Ford. Mother is a 19-year-old mushroom farm worker and cares for their 2-year-old daughter; the father is 24 years and works in the local museum as a custodial worker.*

G. **Physical examination.** See Chapter 5.

H. **Laboratory data.** List the admission laboratory and radiology results.

I. **Assessment.** State your evaluation of the infant's problems. It can include a list of suspected and potential problems as well as a differential diagnosis.

1. *Respiratory distress syndrome: Because the infant is premature, hyaline membrane disease must be considered. Pneumonia is also a likely cause because of the maternal history of suspected chorioamnionitis.*

2. *Suspected neonatal sepsis: Because of the positive GBS culture and the premature onset of labor, there is an increased septic risk in this infant. Certain pathogens need to be ruled out. Group B streptococcus is the most common pathogen in this age group, but Listeria monocytogenes and Gram-negative pathogens should be considered.*

3. *Premature birth living child: The infant is at 33 weeks' gestation by Ballard examination.*

J. **Plan.** Include the therapeutic and diagnostic plans for the infant. (See section on "Admission Orders.")

PROGRESS NOTES

The most commonly used format for daily progress notes is the *SOAP* method. *SOAP* is an acronym; S = subjective, O = objective, A = assessment, and P = plan. Each problem should be discussed in this format. First, state the problems you are to discuss in the order of severity or occurrence and assign a number to them. Then discuss each problem in the *SOAP* format as outlined next.

A. **Subjective (S)**. Include an overall subjective view of the patient by the physician.
B. **Objective (O)**. Include data that can be objectively gathered, usually in three areas:
   1. **Vital signs (temperature, respiratory rate, pulse, blood pressure).**
   2. **Pertinent physical examination.**
   3. **Laboratory data and other test results.**
C. **Assessment (A)**. Include evaluation of the preceding data.
D. **Plan (P)**. Discuss the medication changes, laboratory orders, and any other new orders as well as the treatment plan.
E. **Example.** The following is an example of part of a progress note using the SOAP format.

Problem 1. Respiratory distress syndrome
S: Infant James is now 4 days old and doing much better. He has been able to wean down to 30% oxygen with good arterial gases.
O: Vital signs: temperature 98.7, respirations 52, pulse 140, blood pressure 55/35.
Physical examination: The peripheral perfusion appears good with no obvious cyanosis. There is no grunting or nasal flaring, but the infant has mild substernal and intercostal retractions. The chest sounds slightly wet. Laboratory data and other test results: Arterial blood gases on 30% oxygen—pH 7.32, CO_2 48, O_2 67, 97% saturation. Chest radiograph shows mild haziness in both lung fields.
A: Infant James has resolving mild hyaline membrane disease.
P: The plan is to wean the oxygen as long as his arterial Pao_2 is >55.
Problem 2. Suspected neonatal sepsis—Follow with "SOAP" note.
Problem 3. Premature birth living child (PBLC)—Follow with "SOAP" note.

ADMISSION ORDERS

The following format is useful for writing admission orders. It involves the mnemonic *A.D.C. VAN DISSEL: A*dmit, *D*iagnosis, *C*ondition, *V*ital signs, *A*ctivity, *N*ursing procedures, *D*iet, *I*nput and Output, *S*pecific drugs, *S*ymptomatic drugs, *E*xtras, and *L*aboratory data. Most centers now have online physician ordering templates.

A. **Admit.** Specify the location of the patient (neonatal intensive care unit, newborn nursery) and the attending physician in charge and the house officer along with their paging numbers.
B. **Diagnosis.** List the admitting diagnoses.
   1. *Respiratory distress syndrome.*
   2. *Suspected neonatal sepsis.*
   3. *Premature birth living child.*
C. **Condition.** Note whether the patient is in stable or critical condition.
D. **Vital signs.** State the desired frequency of monitoring of vital signs. Specify rectal or axillary temperature. Rectal temperature is usually done initially to obtain a core temperature and also to rule out imperforate anus. Then, monitor axillary temperature. Other parameters include blood pressure, pulse, and respiratory rate. Weight, length, and head circumference should also be obtained on admission.
E. **Activity.** All are at bed rest but one can specify "minimal stress or hands-off protocol" here. This notation is used for infants who react poorly to stress by dropping their oxygenation, as in patients with persistent pulmonary hypertension. At most centers, it means to handle the infant as little as possible and record all vital signs off the monitor.
F. **Nursing procedure.** Respiratory care (ventilator settings, chest percussion and postural drainage orders, endotracheal suctioning with frequency). Also require that a daily weight and head circumference be recorded. The frequency of Dextrostix (or Chemstrip-bG) testing is included in this section because it is a bedside procedure.

G. **Diet.** All infants admitted to the neonatal intensive care unit are usually made NPO (nothing by mouth) for at least 6–24 h until they are accessed and stabilized. When appropriate, write specific diet orders.

H. **Input and output (I and O).** Request that the nursing staff record accurate input and output of each infant. This record is especially important for infants on intravenous fluids and those just starting oral feedings. Specify how often you want the urine tested for specific gravity and glucose.

I. **Specific drugs.** State drugs to be administered, giving specific dosages and routes of administration. It is useful to also include the milligrams-per-kilogram-per-day dose of the drug to allow cross-checking and verification of the dose ordered. An example is as follows:

 Ampicillin 150 mg IV q12h (300 mg/kg/d divided q12h).

 For all infants, order the following medications at the time of admission.

 1. Vitamin K (see Chapter 132) is given to prevent hemorrhagic disease of the newborn.

 2. Erythromycin eyedrops (see Chapter 132) are given to prevent gonococcal ophthalmia.

J. **Symptomatic drugs.** These drugs are not routinely used in a neonatal intensive care unit and would include such items as pain and sleep medications.

K. **Extras.** Any other orders required but not included above, such as roentgenography, electrocardiography, and ultrasonography.

L. **Laboratory data.** Include laboratory data drawn on admission, plus routine laboratory orders with frequency (eg, arterial blood gases q2h, sodium and potassium bid).

DISCHARGE SUMMARY

The following information is written at the time of discharge and provides a summary of the infant's illness and hospital stay.

A. **Date of admission.**

B. **Date of discharge.**

C. **Admitting diagnosis.**

D. **Discharge diagnosis.** List in order of occurrence or severity.

E. **Attending physician and service caring for the patient.**

F. **Referring physician and address.**

G. **Procedures.** Include all invasive procedures.

H. **Brief history, physical examination, and laboratory data on admission.** Use the admission history, physical examination, and laboratory data as a guide.

I. **Hospital course.** The easiest way to approach this section of the discharge summary is to discuss each problem in paragraph form.

J. **Condition at discharge.** A complete physical examination is done at the time of discharge and included in this section. It is important to include the discharge weight, head circumference, and length so that growth can be assessed at the time of the patient's initial checkup. Also include the type and amount of formula the patient is on and any pertinent discharge laboratory values.

K. **Discharge medications.** Include the name(s) of medication(s), the dosage(s), and length of treatment. If the patient is being sent home on an apnea monitor, it is helpful to include the monitor settings and the planned course of treatment.

L. **Disposition.** Note where the patient is being sent (outside hospital, home, foster home).

M. **Discharge instructions and follow-up.** Include instructions to the parents on medications and when the patient is to return to the clinic (and exact location). It is helpful to indicate tests that need to be done on follow-up and any results that need to be rechecked (eg, bilirubin, repeat phenylketonuria screen).

N. **Problem list.** Same list as the discharge diagnosis list.

Appendix E. Growth Charts

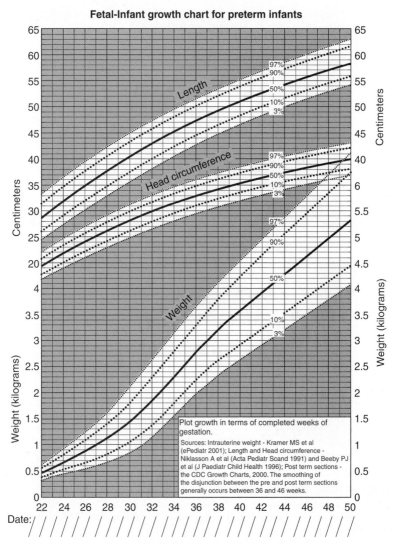

APPENDIX FIGURE E–1. Growth charts for infants. (*From Fenton TR: A new growth chart for preterm babies: Babson and Benda's chart updated with recent data and a new format.* BMC Pediatrics *2003,3:13. Open Access article: http://www.biomedcentral.com/1471-2431/3/13.*)

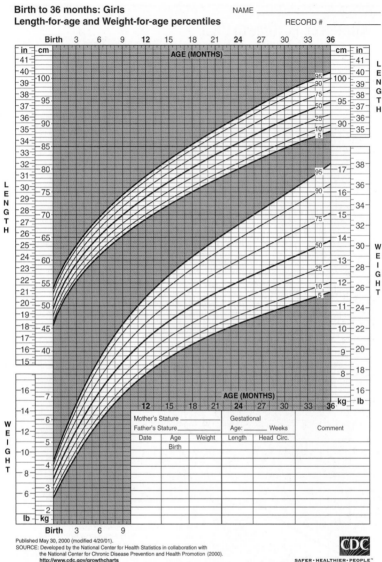

Birth to 36 months: Girls
Length-for-age and Weight-for-age percentiles

NAME _____

RECORD # _____

APPENDIX FIGURE E–2. Growth chart for girls: length and weight, birth to 36 months. (*From NCHS, National Center for Health Statistics. Available at: http://www.cdc.gov/nchs/about/major/nhanes/growthcharts/clinical_charts.htm, Accessed September 23, 2008.*)

Birth to 36 months: Girls
Head circumference-for-age and
Weight-for-length percentiles

NAME _____

RECORD # _____

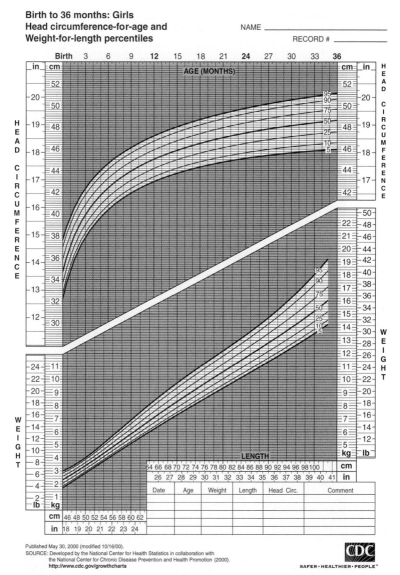

Published May 30, 2000 (modified 10/16/00).
SOURCE: Developed by the National Center for Health Statistics in collaboration with
the National Center for Chronic Disease Prevention and Health Promotion (2000).
http://www.cdc.gov/growthcharts

APPENDIX FIGURE E–3. Growth chart for girls: head circumference and weight, birth to 36 months. (*From NCHS, National Center for Health Statistics. Available at: http://www.cdc.gov/nchs/about/major/nhanes/growthcharts/clinical_charts.htm. Accessed September 23, 2008.*)

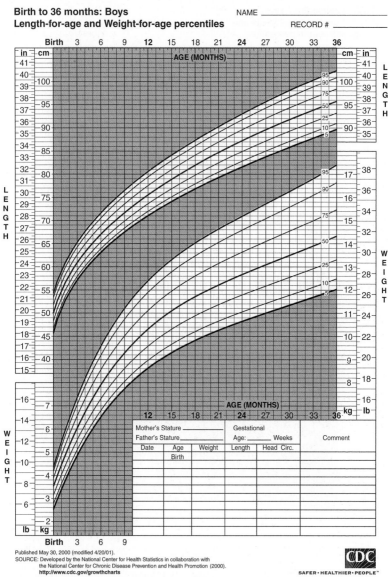

APPENDIX FIGURE E–4. Growth chart for boys: length and weight, birth to 36 months. (*From NCHS, National Center for Health Statistics. Available at: http://www.cdc.gov/nchs/ about/major/nhanes/growthcharts/clinical_charts.htm. Accessed September 23, 2008.*)

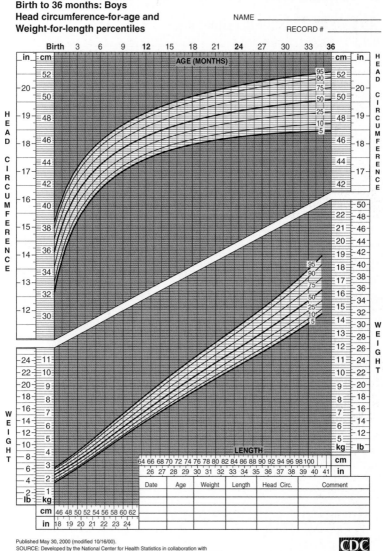

APPENDIX FIGURE E–5. Growth chart for boys: head circumference and weight, birth to 36 months. (*From NCHS, National Center for Health Statistics. Available at: http://www.cdc.gov/nchs/about/major/nhanes/growthcharts/clinical_charts.htm. Accessed September 23, 2008.*)

Appendix F. Isolation Guidelines

The following table, Transmission-Based Precautions for Perinatal/Neonatal Patients in conjunction with Standard Precautions, is based on current knowledge and practices in the fields of epidemiology, pediatrics, and perinatology. Published resource references are listed immediately following the table.

Instructions for using Precautions for Perinatal/Neonatal Patients Table:

- Each disease is considered individually so that only precautions indicated to interrupt transmission for that disease are recommended.
- The column "Maternal Precautions" describes the precautions to be used by staff providing care to the mother.
- The column "Neonatal Precautions" describes the precautions to be used by staff, patients, or visitors in contact with the neonate.
- Staff should assess the mother's ability to wash hands correctly and comply with precautions when determining the appropriateness of permitting rooming in.

Precautions shall be initiated for suspected as well as confirmed infectious diseases/conditions.

TRANSMISSION BASED PRECAUTIONS FOR PERINATAL PATIENTS IN CONJUNCTION WITH STANDARD PRECAUTIONS

Infection/Disease	Maternal Precautions	Neonatal Precautions	Room-in	Mother May Visit in Nursery	Breast-feeding	Additional Considerations
AIDS/HIV Positive	Standard	Standard Bathe baby ASAP when stable	Yes	Yes	No HIV may be transmitted through breast milk.	Recommend tuberculosis testing for mother. Begin treatment for infant with AZT within 6–12 hours of birth and continue treatment for 6 weeks. Refer to AAP Red Book. Report AIDS to Health Department.
Chickenpox (see Varicella)						
Chlamydia Trachomatis	Standard	Standard	Yes	Yes	Yes	Topical prophylaxis is ineffective for *Chlamydia* ophthalmic disease. Treatment for *Chlamydia* conjunctivitis and pneumonia is systemic Erythromycin for 14 days.
Cytomegalovirus (CMV)	Standard	Standard	Yes	Yes	Yes	No additional precautions for pregnant healthcare workers.
Diarrhea	Standard	Standard	Yes	Yes	Yes	
Gonococcal Ophthalmia Neonatorum	Standard	Standard	Yes After 24 hours of maternal treatment with antibiotics.	Yes After 24 hours of maternal treatment with antibiotics.	Yes After 24 hours of maternal treatment with antibiotics.	Prophylactic use of topical 0.5% Erythromycin ophthalmic or 1% tetracycline ointment at birth should be performed to prevent ophthalmic neonatorum.

(Continued)

TRANSMISSION BASED PRECAUTIONS FOR PERINATAL PATIENTS IN CONJUNCTION WITH STANDARD PRECAUTIONS (*CONTINUED*)

Infection/Disease	Maternal Precautions	Neonatal Precautions	Room-in	Mother May Visit in Nursery	Breast-feeding	Additional Considerations
						Newborns born to mothers with active gonorrhea should receive a single dose of ceftriaxone 125 mg IV or IM. For low birthweight neonates, the dose is 25–50 mg/kg of body weight. Cefotaxime (100 mg/kg) in a single does is an alternative. Refer to Perinatal Guidelines 2007, page 333.
Group B Streptococcal Infections	Standard	Standard	Yes	Yes	Yes	Follow Center for Disease Control and Prevention guidelines for laboratory testing and antibiotic treatment recommendations.
Hepatitis A, B, C	Standard	Standard	Yes	Yes	Yes	Early hepatitis B immunization is recommended for all medically stable infants with birth weights > 2 kg, regardless of maternal status. The American Academy of Pediatrics recommend that infants born to HBsAg positive mothers, including preterm and low birthweight infants, receive the initial dose of hepatitis B vaccine within 12 hours of birth. Report to Health Department.

| Herpes Simplex Virus (HSV) Neonatal Infection or Positive Culture in Absence of Disease | Contact Gown and gloves | Yes If baby is at low risk of infection. | Yes | Yes If no vesicular herpetic lesion in the breast area and all active skin lesions are covered. | Cultures obtained from conjunctiva, oral pharynx or skin lesion 24–48 hours or later after birth are more likely to identify neonatal infection. A positive culture obtained ≥ 24 hours after birth needs immediate antiviral treatment, even in the absence of symptoms. Neonates with HSV should be managed in a facility that provides level III subspecialty care and consultation. A mother with HSV infection should be taught to wash her hands carefully and use a clean barrier to ensure that the neonate does not come in contact with the lesions. A mother with herpes labialis (cold sore) should not kiss or nuzzle her newborn until the lesions have cleared. Refer to Perinatal Guidelines, 2007, page 315. |

(Continued)

TRANSMISSION BASED PRECAUTIONS FOR PERINATAL PATIENTS IN CONJUNCTION WITH STANDARD PRECAUTIONS (*CONTINUED*)

Infection/Disease	Maternal Precautions	Neonatal Precautions	Room-in	Mother May Visit in Nursery	Breast-feeding	Additional Considerations
Lice (see Pediculosis)						
Measles (Rubeola)	Airborne Masks for those susceptible. Labor, delivery, and post-partum recovery should take place in a private room with negative pressure, nonrecirculating air with door closed. If mother is transferred to the delivery room for the actual delivery, mother to wear mask during transfer and delivery.	Airborne Masks for those susceptible. Private room with negative pressure, nonrecirculating air with door closed.	No	No	No Until mother is noncontagious.	Contagious during prodrome and for 4 days after onset of rash. Report to Health Department.

Methicillin Resistant *S. aureus* **(MRSA)**	Contact Gown and gloves	Contact Gown and gloves	Yes	Yes Follow contact precautions.	Yes	Apply Contact Precautions for infection or known colonization.
Mumps (Infectious Parotitis)	Droplet Masks within 3 ft of patient. Private room.		No	No	No Until mother is noncontagious.	Contagious for 9 days after onset of swelling. Report to Health Department.
Pediculosis (Lice)	Contact For 24 hours after treatment, gown and gloves.	Contact For 24 hours after treatment, gown and gloves.	Yes	Yes	Yes	Exposed individuals and household contacts should be examined and treated if infected. Instruct mother to clean breasts before feeding, if medication is applied to that area. Stress good hand hygiene with special attention to area under fingernails.
Pertussis (Whooping Cough)	Droplet Masks within 3 ft of patient. Private room.	Droplet Masks within 3 ft of patient. Private room.	No	No	No Until mother is noncontagious.	Contagious for 5 days after start of effective therapy. Report to Health Department.

(Continued)

TRANSMISSION BASED PRECAUTIONS FOR PERINATAL PATIENTS IN CONJUNCTION WITH STANDARD PRECAUTIONS (*CONTINUED*)

Infection/ Disease	Maternal Precautions	Neonatal Precautions	Room-in	Mother May Visit in Nursery	Breast-feeding	Additional Considerations
Respiratory Syncytial Virus (RSV)		Contact and droplet Gown, gloves, mask within 3 ft of the patient.	Yes	Yes May visit private room or cohort.	Yes	Parent education is essential to avoid transmission of the virus. The importance of hand hygiene should be emphasized in all settings. Prophylaxis to prevent RSV in newborns at increased risk for severe disease, particularly those with chronic lung disease receiving medical management on a long-term basis is available. Refer to Perinatal Guidelines, 2007, page 322. Contagious for duration of illness.
Rubella (German Measles) Maternal	Droplet Masks within 3 ft of patient. Private room, masks for those susceptible		Yes	No	No	Contagious for 7 days after onset of rash. Susceptible persons stay out of room, if possible. Report to Health Department.
Rubella (German Measles) Congenital		Contact	Yes	Yes	Yes	Continue contact precautions until 1 year of age unless nasopharyngeal and urine cultures after 3 months of age are negative for rubella virus.

		Gown and gloves				Susceptible persons stay out of room, if possible. Report to Health Department.
Scabies	Contact For 24 hours after treatment, gown and gloves.	Contact For 24 hours after treatment, gown and gloves.	Yes	Yes	Yes	Treatment of exposed individuals and household contacts is recommended. Instruct mother to clean breasts before feeding, if medication is applied to that area. Stress good hand hygiene.
***Staphylococcus aureus* (not MRSA)**	Standard	Standard	Yes	Yes	Yes	Two or more concurrent cases of impetigo related to a nursery or a single case of breast abscess in a nursing mother or infant is presumptive evidence of an epidemic, report immediately to attending physician and Infection Control.
Syphilis	Standard	Standard	Yes	Yes	Yes	Healthcare workers and parents should wear gloves when handling the neonate until 24 hours of treatment with antibiotics. Report to Health Department.

(Continued)

TRANSMISSION BASED PRECAUTIONS FOR PERINATAL PATIENTS IN CONJUNCTION WITH STANDARD PRECAUTIONS

Infection/Disease	Maternal Precautions	Neonatal Precautions	Room-in	Mother May Visit in Nursery	Breast-feeding	Additional Considerations
Tuberculosis (TB) **1. Mother with recent positive purified protein derivative (PPD) and no evidence of active TB.**	Standard	Standard	Yes	Yes	Yes	Infant should be tested: PPD at 4 to 6 weeks of age, at 3 to 4 months of age, and 12 months of age.
2. Mother with minimal disease, or disease has been treated for 2 or more weeks and is determined by Pulmonary or Infectious Disease to be noncontagious at delivery.	Standard	Standard	Yes	Yes	Yes	Infant should have CXR and PPD at 4 to 6 weeks of age; if negative, retest at 3 to 4 and 6 months of age. Report to Health Department.

3. Mother with current pulmonary or laryngeal active TB and suspected of being contagious at time of delivery.	Airborne N95 respirator for healthcare workers. Labor, delivery, and post-partum care in private room with negative pressure, nonrecirculating air with door closed. If mother is transferred to the delivery room for the actual delivery, mother to wear mask during transfer and delivery.	Standard	No Until mother is determined to be noncontagious.	No Until mother is determined to be noncontagious.	No Until mother is determined to be noncontagious.	Infant should be given INH until 6 months of age, then repeat PPD. If PPD is positive, continue INH for a total of 12 months. Report to Health Department.
4. Mother has extra-pulmonary spread of TB (ie, miliary, bone, meningitis, etc.)	Standard	Standard	No Until mother is determined to be noncontagious.	No Until mother is determined to be noncontagious.	No Until mother is determined to be noncontagious.	Infant should be given INH until 6 months of age, then repeat PPD. If PPD is positive, continue INH for a total of 12 months. Report to Health Department.

(Continued)

841

TRANSMISSION BASED PRECAUTIONS FOR PERINATAL PATIENTS IN CONJUNCTION WITH STANDARD PRECAUTIONS (*CONTINUED*)

Infection/Disease	Maternal Precautions	Neonatal Precautions	Room-in	Mother May Visit in Nursery	Breast-feeding	Additional Considerations
Varicella (Chickenpox) or Herpes Zoster in Immunocompromised Mother or if Disseminated Maternal	Airborne Masks for those susceptible Labor, delivery and post-partum care in private room with negative pressure, nonrecirculating air with door closed. If mother is transferred to the delivery room for the actual delivery, mother to wear mask during transfer and delivery.		No Until mother's lesions have crusted.	No Until mother's lesions have crusted.	No Until mother's lesions have crusted.	Continue airborne precautions until all lesions are crusted. May be contagious 1–2 days before the onset of rash. Persons who have had chickenpox do not need to wear a mask. Hospitalized patients should be discharged prior to the 10th day following exposure, if possible. Exposed susceptible patients should be placed on airborne precautions beginning 10 days after exposure and continue until 21 days after last exposure, or until 28 days if varicella-zoster immune globulin. (VZIG) given.

| Varicella-Newborn or Exposure to Varicella | Airborne Masks for those susceptible. Private room with negative pressure, nonrecirculating air with door closed. | Yes | Yes May visit private room or cohort. | Yes Unless mother has lesions. | Hospitalized patients should be discharged prior to the 10th day following exposure, if possible. Begin precautions 10 days after exposure and continue until 21 days after last exposure, or until 28 days if VZIG given. |

Modified from guidelines issued by Kaiser Permanente Hospital, Fontana, CA.

References

American Academy of Pediatrics and The American College of Obstetricians and Gynecologists: *Guidelines for Perinatal Care.* 6th ed. Atlanta, GA: AAP/ACOG, 2007.

Centers for Disease Control: Guidelines for Isolation Precautions in Hospitals. Atlanta, GA: U.S. Department of Health and Human Services, 2007.

Centers for Disease Control: Guidelines for Infection Control in Health Care Personnel. Atlanta, GA: U.S. Department of Health and Human Services, 1998.

Young TE, Magnum B Neofax®: *A Manual of Drugs Used in Neonatal Care.* 20th ed. Montvale, New Jersey: Thomson Healthcare, 2007.

Committee on Infectious Diseases, American Academy of Pediatrics: Red Book: Report of the Committee on Infectious Disease. In Pickering LE (ed). American Academy of Pediatrics, 2006.

Appendix G. Temperature Conversion Table

Celsius	Fahrenheit	Celsius	Fahrenheit
34.0	93.2	37.6	99.6
34.2	93.6	37.8	100.0
34.4	93.9	38.0	100.4
34.6	94.3	38.2	100.7
34.8	94.6	38.4	101.1
35.0	95.0	38.6	101.4
35.2	95.4	38.8	101.8
35.4	95.7	39.0	102.2
35.6	96.1	39.2	102.5
35.8	96.4	39.4	102.9
36.0	96.8	39.6	103.2
36.2	97.1	39.8	103.6
36.4	97.5	40.0	104.0
36.6	97.8	40.2	104.3
36.8	98.2	40.4	104.7
37.0	98.6	40.6	105.1
37.2	98.9	40.8	105.4
37.4	99.3	41.0	105.8

Celsius = (Fahrenheit − 32) × 5/9.
Fahrenheit = (Celsius × 9/5) + 32.

Appendix H. Weight Conversion Table[a]

Ounces	1 lb	2 lb	3 lb	4 lb	5 lb	6 lb	7 lb	8 lb
				Grams				
0	454	907	1361	1814	2268	2722	3175	3629
1	482	936	1389	1843	2296	2750	3204	3657
2	510	964	1418	1871	2325	2778	3232	3686
3	539	992	1446	1899	2353	2807	3260	3714
4	567	1021	1474	1928	2381	2835	3289	3742
5	595	1049	1503	1956	2410	2863	3317	3771
6	624	1077	1531	1985	2438	2892	3345	3799
7	652	1106	1559	2013	2466	2920	3374	3827
8	680	1134	1588	2041	2495	2948	3402	3856
9	709	1162	1616	2070	2523	2977	3430	3884
10	737	1191	1644	2098	2552	3005	3459	3912
11	765	1219	1673	2126	2580	3033	3487	3941
12	794	1247	1701	2155	2608	3062	3515	3969
13	822	1276	1729	2183	2637	3090	3544	3997
14	851	1304	1758	2211	2665	3119	3572	4026
15	879	1332	1786	2240	2693	3147	3600	4054

[a]Values represent weight in grams.
To convert from kilograms to pounds, multiply kilograms by 2.2.
To convert from pounds to grams, multiply pounds by 454.

Index

Entries denoted by an italic *f* or *t* indicate figures, tables, or notes, respectively. Major discussions are in boldface type. When a drug trade name is listed, the reader is referred to the generic name.